VIDEO CON

MW01257522

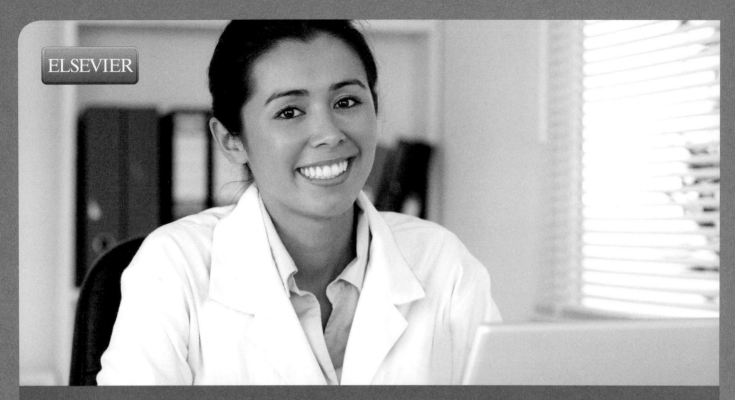

SMALL ANIMAL
DIAGNOSTIC
ULTRASOUND

Third Edition

John S. Mattoon, DVM, DACVR
Consultant
Adjunct and former Professor of Radiology, Department of Veterinary Clinical Sciences
College of Veterinary Medicine
Washington State University
Pullman, Washington

Thomas G. Nyland, DVM, MS, DACVR
Professor Emeritus, Department of Surgical and Radiological Sciences
School of Veterinary Medicine
University of California, Davis
Davis, California

3251 Riverport Lane
St. Louis, Missouri 63043

SMALL ANIMAL DIAGNOSTIC ULTRASOUND, THIRD EDITION   978-1-4160-4867-1

Notice

Veterinary Medicine is an ever-changing field. Standard safety precautions must be followed, but as new research and clinical experience broaden our knowledge, changes in treatment and drug therapy become necessary or appropriate. Readers are advised to check the most current product information provided by the manufacturer of each drug to be administered to verify the recommended dose, the method and duration of administration, and the contraindications. It is the responsibility of the treating veterinarian, relying on experience and knowledge of the animal, to determine dosages and the best treatment for each individual animal. Neither the Publisher nor the editor assumes any liability for any injury and/or damage to animals or property arising from this publication.

The Publisher

Library of Congress Cataloging-in-Publication Data

Small animal diagnostic ultrasound / [edited by] John S. Mattoon, Thomas G. Nyland.—Third edition.
     p. ; cm.
   Includes bibliographical references and index.
   ISBN 978-1-4160-4867-1 (hardcover : alk. paper)
   I. Mattoon, John S., editor of compilation.   II. Nyland, Thomas G., editor of compilation.
   [DNLM: 1. Dog Diseases—ultrasonography.   2. Cat Diseases—ultrasonography.   3. Diagnostic Imaging—veterinary.   SF 991]
   SF772.5
   636.089′60754—dc23
                                                                      2013042514

Content Strategy Director: Penny Rudolph
Content Development Specialist: Brandi Graham
Publishing Services Manager: Jeff Patterson
Senior Project Manager: Tracey Schriefer
Design Direction: Ashley Miner

Printed in Canada

Last digit is the print number: 9 8 7 6 5 4 3 2

Working together to grow libraries in developing countries

www.elsevier.com • www.bookaid.org

First, we'd like to dedicate this edition to all the residents we have mentored over the years. Without your continuous, sometimes incessant inquisitiveness and dedication to learning, academia would be a soulless journey. All of you have helped us become better veterinary radiologists. You have in fact mentored us, and for that we are eternally grateful.

We'd also like to dedicate this text to our radiology colleagues too numerous to mention. You have influenced our careers in so many important ways.

We can never forget the animals. They too have taught us innumerable life lessons and without them we would lead a very dreary existence.

Finally to our wives, Jennifer and Anita, for their enduring patience, understanding, and love during preparation of this edition, and throughout our professional careers.

JSM, TGN

CONTRIBUTORS

Livia Benigni, DVM, MRCVS, CertVDI, DECVDI, PGCertAP
Lecturer in Veterinary Diagnostic Imaging
Department of Clinical Sciences and Services
The Royal Veterinary College
University of London
North Mymms
Hatfield, United Kingdom
Musculoskeletal System

Clifford R. Berry, DVM, DACVR
Professor of Radiology
Department of Small Animal Clinical Science
College of Veterinary Medicine
University of Florida
Gainesville, Florida
Advanced Ultrasound Techniques
Abdominal Ultrasound Scanning Techniques

John D. Bonagura, DVM, MS, DACVIM (Cardiology, Internal Medicine)
Professor and Head of Clinical Cardiology Services
Department of Veterinary Clinical Sciences
College of Veterinary Medicine
The Ohio State University
Columbus, Ohio
Heart

Virginia Luis Fuentes, MA, VetMB, PhD, CertVR, DVC, DACVIM, DECVIM
Professor of Veterinary Cardiology
Department of Clinical Sciences and Services
The Royal Veterinary College
North Mymms
Hatfield, United Kingdom
Heart

Allison M. Heaney, DVM, MS, DACVIM (Cardiology)
Midwest Veterinary Cardiology
Boulder, Colorado

Christopher R. Lamb, MA, VetMB, DACVR, DECVDI, MRCVS, FHEA
Professor of Radiology
Department of Clinical Sciences and Services
The Royal Veterinary College
University of London
North Mymms
Hatfield, United Kingdom
Musculoskeletal System

Martha Moon Larson, DVM, MS, DACVR
Professor of Radiology
Department of Small Animal Clinical Sciences
College of Veterinary Medicine
Virginia-Maryland Regional College of Veterinary Medicine
Blacksburg, Virginia
Liver

Christopher S. MacKay, DVM, MS, DACVR
Assistant Professor
Department of Environmental and Radiological Health Science
College of Veterinary Medicine & Biomedical Sciences
Colorado State University
Fort Collins, Colorado
Eye

Dana A. Neelis, DVM, MS, DACVR
Animal Imaging
Irving, Texas
Neck
Thorax
Gastrointestinal Tract
Adrenal Glands

Rachel Pollard, DVM, PhD, DACVR
Associate Professor
Department of Surgical and Radiological Sciences
School of Veterinary Medicine
University of California, Davis
Davis, California
Ultrasound-Guided Aspiration and Biopsy Procedures
Advanced Ultrasound Techniques

H. Mark Saunders, VMD, DACVR
Lynks Group, PLC
Shelburne, Vermont

William R. Widmer, DVM, DACVR
Professor Emeritus, Veterinary Radiology
Department of Veterinary Clinical Sciences
College of Veterinary Medicine
Purdue University
West Lafayette, Indiana
Peritoneal Fluid, Lymph Nodes, Masses, Peritoneal Cavity, Great Vessel Thrombosis, and Focused Examinations
Urinary Tract

Tamara Wills, DVM, MS, DACVP
Pullman, Washington
Ultrasound-Guided Aspiration and Biopsy Procedures

Allison Zwingenberger, DVM, DACVR, DECVDI
Associate Professor
Department of Surgical and Radiological Sciences
School of Veterinary Medicine
University of California, Davis
Davis, California
Musculoskeletal System

PREFACE

Veterinary ultrasound continues to evolve. Once an imaging modality found primarily in academic institutions and used by specialists, its use is now commonplace in general private practice and across all species. Veterinary ultrasound has attained an almost indispensible place in the daily practice lives of veterinarians all over the world.

Nonetheless, much work remains to be done in proper education in this exciting discipline. The biggest challenge appears to be in helping students and veterinarians realize ultrasound's true potential in day-to-day practice; to make ultrasound an extension of their clinical assessment mind-set, a "test" useful in evaluation of the myriad of presenting clinical signs seen each and every day. Thus the underlying goal of this third edition is to be a part of that process, serving as a practical yet detailed resource for general practice veterinarians, residents and interns, and veterinary students.

The third edition has grown considerably. Thanks to the scientific endeavors of our veterinary colleagues from all parts of the world, hundreds of new scientific references are available, addressing literally every aspect of diagnostic ultrasound. Hundreds of new and updated images have been added, including cytology and gross anatomic specimens. As in past editions, essential physics, instrumentation, and Doppler ultrasound are covered in Chapter 1, to which artifacts has been added for added continuity. Chapter 2 addresses ultrasound-guided fine needle aspirates and tissue core biopsy techniques, with color cytologic images of commonly diagnosed diseases. Chapter 3 is a collection of the most recent trends in diagnostic ultrasound, documenting sure but steady evolution. Beginning with "how-to" Chapter 4, successive chapters are arranged anatomically from "head to toe" (cranial to caudal).

This new edition also includes access to **smallanimal ultrasound.com**. This companion website features more than 100 ultrasound video clips, which correlate to images found in Chapters 5 through 18. An icon is used to indicate when a video is available online, appearing next to the relevant figure. The videos cover a wide range of topics, ranging from calcified thyroid carcinoma to bacterial prostatitis presented with perineal swelling.

We hope our efforts will inspire you. After all, it is you who will move diagnostic ultrasound to levels yet to be seen.

JOHN S. MATTOON, DVM, DACVR

THOMAS G. NYLAND, DVM, MS, DACVR

ACKNOWLEDGMENTS

The third edition of *Small Animal Diagnostic Ultrasound* was long in the making. It was a true labor of love and would not have been possible without the dedicated efforts of many, many people. Some contributed by co-authoring chapters. Many contributed not through the written word but through collegial advice, images, snippets and pearls, and scientific engagement.

To Tomas Baker, Dr. Livia Benigni, Peter Brunelli, Dr. Kip Berry, Dr. David Biller, Dr. John Bonagura, Michele Carbone, Dr. Dongwoo Chang, Dr. Mario Codreanu, Dr. Alexandru Diaconescu, Paul Fisher, Dr. Virginia Fuentes, Dr. Lorrie Gaschen, Dr. Gary Haldorson, Guy Hammond, Dr. Allison Heaney, Dr. Hock Gan Heng, Dr. Vasiliy Kuznetsov, Dr. Chris Lamb, Dr. Marti Larson, Dr. Daniel Lescai, Dr. Gregory Lisciandro, Dr. Maria Lopina, Dr. Fraser McConnell, Dr. Taka Miyabayashi, Dr. Jerzy Gawor, Dr. Dana Neelis, Dr. Chris MacKay, Dr. Bob O'Brien, Dr. Dominique Penninck, Dr. Sandrino Plantos, Dr. Rachel Pollard, Dr. Federica Rossi, Dr. Val Samii, Dr. H. Mark Saunders, Dr. Kathy Spaulding, Dr. Viktor Szatmári, Dr. Rick Widmer, Dr. Robert Williams, Dr. Tamara Wills, Dr. Erik Wisner, Dr. Junghee Yoon, Dr. Ben Young, Dr. Sarah Young, and Dr. Allison Zwingenberger, you have our most sincere thank you. Your efforts will forever be appreciated and never forgotten.

Special thanks go to Drs. Dana Neelis, Chris MacKay, and Carmela Pratt for their help in reviewing chapters for this third edition. Your dedication to reading drafts and leading discussions during your residencies made a big difference in the final product, and made class a little less tedious, too.

A special thank you to Dr. Teresa Luther (WSU Class of 2008), who took the challenge to locate pathology and surgical specimens for this text during her veterinary college years. We only wish we could have used them all!

The Biomedical Communications Unit (BCU) at WSU is truly an outstanding group of professionals. Their expertise and unwavering support were instrumental during manuscript preparation. Thank you Rich Scott, Henry Moore Jr., Bob Mitchell, and Chuck Royce.

We give our heartfelt thanks to WSU radiology colleagues Dr. Greg Roberts, Dr. Russ Tucker, and Dr. Tom Wilkinson. Without their support, the third edition would have never been completed. Also to my (JSM) Department Chair, Dr. Bill Dernell, for his encouragement, year after year of my annual review goal of completing this text.

It is important to us to acknowledge the many people who contributed to the first and second editions of *Small Animal Diagnostic Ultrasound*. Your efforts provided the foundation, without which a third edition would not have been possible or so widely anticipated.

And of course, *Small Animal Diagnostic Ultrasound*, third edition, would have never been possible without the absolutely mind-boggling patience and support from the great people at Elsevier. We would like to give special thanks to Brandi Graham, who prodded us along with tactful and timely emails. And to Penny Rudolph, whose golden voice of calm helped soothe us through some rough times. Thank you Jeanne Robertson for your fantastic, superb new illustrations and updates of prior material. Thank you to Tracey Schriefer for her invaluable proofreading and editing expertise. And we would be remiss if we did not thank Tony Winkle, our first editor for this project.

Although this may seem strange, we'd also like to recognize each other! Three editions of this textbook would not have been possible without the sheer joy and enthusiasm we experienced working together. The summation of our efforts could never have been achieved by either of us alone. Our enduring friendship made all of this possible. This was a career-long opportunity for both of us to be part of the evolution and maturation of veterinary ultrasound, and we hope that some of our boundless enthusiasm has been conveyed to you!

JOHN S. MATTOON, DVM, DACVR

THOMAS G. NYLAND, DVM, MS, DACVR

CONTENTS

CHAPTER 1

Fundamentals of Diagnostic Ultrasound

John S. Mattoon • Thomas G. Nyland

Diagnostic ultrasound uses very high frequency sound waves that are pulsed into the body, and the returning echoes are then analyzed by computer to yield high-resolution cross-sectional images of organs, tissues, and blood flow. The displayed information is a result of ultrasound interaction with tissues, termed acoustic impedance, and does not necessarily represent specific microscopic or macroscopic anatomy. Indeed, organs may appear perfectly normal on an ultrasound image in the presence of dysfunction or failure. Conversely, organs may appear abnormal on ultrasound examination but be functioning properly. This basic tenet must be understood and respected for diagnostic ultrasound to be used properly.

High-quality ultrasound studies require a firm understanding of the important physical principles of diagnostic ultrasound. In this introductory chapter, we strive to present the necessary fundamental physical principles of ultrasound without excessive detail. In-depth sources on the subject are recommended to interested readers.[1-5] These textbooks uniformly stress that image quality depends on knowledge of the interaction of sound with tissue and the skillful use of the scanner's controls. Ultrasound examinations are highly interactive; a great deal of flexibility is often required for good images to be obtained. Accurate interpretation depends directly on the differentiation of normal and abnormal anatomy. Unlike with other imaging modalities, interpretation is best made at the time of the study. It is very difficult to render a meaningful interpretation from another sonographer's static images or video clips.

BASIC ACOUSTIC PRINCIPLES

Wavelength and Frequency

Sound results from mechanical energy propagating through matter as a pressure wave, producing alternating compression and rarefaction bands of molecules within the conducting medium (Figure 1-1). The distance between each band of compression or rarefaction is the sound's *wavelength* (λ), the distance traveled during one cycle. *Frequency* is the number of times a wavelength is repeated (cycles) per second and is expressed in hertz (Hz). One cycle per second is 1 Hz; 1000 and 1 million cycles per second are 1 kilohertz (kHz) and 1 megahertz (MHz), respectively. The range of human hearing is approximately 20 to 20,000 Hz. Diagnostic ultrasound is characterized by sound waves with a frequency up to 1000 times higher than this range. Sound frequencies in the range of 2 to 15 MHz and higher are commonly used in diagnostic ultrasound examinations. Even higher frequencies (20 to 100 MHz) are used in special ocular, dermatologic, and micro-imaging applications.

Frequencies in the millions of cycles per second have short wavelengths (submillimeter) that are essential for high-resolution imaging. The shorter the wavelength (or higher the frequency), the better the resolution. Frequency and wavelength are inversely related if the sound velocity within the medium remains constant. Because sound velocity is independent of frequency and nearly constant (1540 m/sec) in the body's soft tissues[1,5] (Table 1-1), selecting a higher frequency transducer will result in decreased wavelength of the emitted sound, providing better axial resolution (see Figure 1-1, *A*, and Figure 1-2). The relationship between velocity, frequency, and wavelength can be summarized in the following equation:

$$\text{Velocity (m/sec)} = \text{frequency (cycles/sec)} \times \text{wavelength (m)}$$

The wavelengths for commonly used ultrasound frequencies can be determined by rearranging this equation (Table 1-2).

Propagation of Sound

Diagnostic ultrasound uses a "pulse echo" principle in which short pulses of sound are transmitted into the body (see Figure 1-1, *C*). Propagation of sound occurs in longitudinal pressure waves, along the direction of particle movement as shown in Figure 1-1. The speed of sound (propagation velocity) is affected by the physical properties of tissue, primarily the tissue's resistance to compression, which depends on tissue density and elasticity (stiffness). Propagation velocity is increased in stiff tissues, decreased in tissues of high density. Fortunately the propagation velocities in the soft tissues of the body are very similar, and it is therefore assumed that the average velocity of diagnostic ultrasound is 1540 m/sec.

The assumption of a constant propagation velocity (1540 m/sec) is fundamental to how the ultrasound machine calculates the distance (or depth) of a reflecting surface. Suppose it takes 0.126 ms from the time of pulse until the return of the echo. The depth of the reflective surface would be calculated as follows:

$$1540 \text{ m/sec} \times 0.126 \text{ ms} \times 1 \text{ sec}/1000 \text{ ms} = 0.194 \text{ m or } 19.4 \text{ cm}$$

This value must be divided by 2 to account for the trip to and from the reflector, so the depth of the reflective surface equals 9.70 cm.

It should be intuitive then that if the sound travels through fatty tissue at 1450 m/sec, the reflector depth will be erroneously calculated as greater (or deeper) than it actually is. This is termed *speed propagation error*, discussed and illustrated further in later sections that focus on artifacts.

Further, when the ultrasound beam encounters gas (331 m/sec) or bone (4080 m/sec), marked velocity differences in

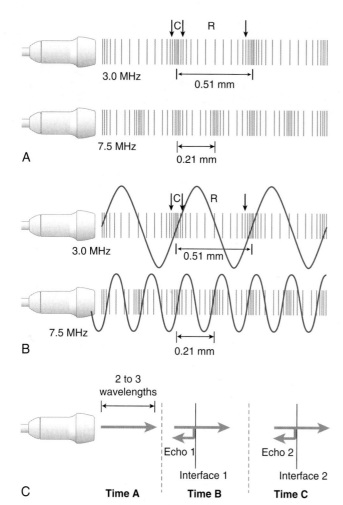

Figure 1-1 Ultrasound waves and echoes. A, Ultrasound emitted from the transducer is produced in longitudinal waves consisting of areas of compression (C) and rarefaction (R). **B,** The wavelength, depicted overlying the longitudinal wave, is the distance traveled during one cycle. Frequency is the number of times a wave is repeated (cycles) per second. The wavelength decreases as frequency increases. Switching from a lower frequency to a higher frequency transducer (e.g., from 3.0 to 7.5 MHz) shortens the wavelength and provides better resolution. **C,** In pulsed ultrasound systems, sound is emitted in pulses of two or three wavelengths rather than continuously as seen in A and B. A portion of the sound is reflected, whereas the remainder is transmitted as it passes through interfaces in tissues.

these media result in high reflection and improper echo interpretation with characteristic reverberation and shadowing artifacts (see later sections on artifacts) (Figure 1-3). This strong reflection is due to a combination of an abrupt change in sound velocity and the density of the media (acoustic impedance) at a soft tissue–bone or soft tissue–air interface. Acoustic impedance is discussed later in this chapter.

The *depth* to which sound penetrates into soft tissues is directly related (but inversely proportional) to the frequency employed. Higher frequency sound waves are attenuated more than lower frequency waves, so attempts to improve resolution by increasing frequency result in decreased penetration. By recognizing this important inverse relationship, the ultrasonographer selects the highest frequency transducer that will penetrate to the desired depth.

TABLE 1-1

Velocity of Sound in Body Tissues

Tissue or Substance	Velocity (m/sec)
Air	331
Fat	1450
Water (50° C)	1540
Average soft tissue	1540
Brain	1541
Liver	1549
Kidney	1561
Blood	1570
Muscle	1585
Lens of eye	1620
Bone	4080

Data from Curry TS III, Dowdey JE, Murry RC Jr. *Christensen's Physics of Diagnostic Radiology.* 4th ed. Philadelphia: Lea & Febiger; 1990.

Reflection and Acoustic Impedance

The echoes reflected from soft tissue interfaces toward the transducer form the basis of the ultrasound image. Interfaces that are large relative to beam size are known as *specular reflectors.* Interfaces that are not at a 90-degree angle to the ultrasound beam reflect sound away from the transducer and do not contribute to image formation. Therefore scanning from different angles may improve image quality as different interfaces become perpendicular to the beam. An example illustrating the importance of a 90-degree incidence angle is shown in Figure 1-4.

The velocity of sound within each tissue and the tissue's density determine the percentage of the beam reflected or transmitted as it passes from one tissue to another. The product of the tissue's density and the sound velocity within the tissue is known as the tissue's *acoustic impedance,* which refers to the reflection or transmission characteristics of a tissue. For simplification, the density differences between tissues can be used to estimate acoustic impedance in soft tissue because sound velocity is assumed to be nearly constant. Acoustic impedance can be defined by the following equation:

$$\text{Acoustic impedance } (Z) = \text{velocity } (v) \times \text{tissue density } (p)$$

It is the impedance difference between tissues that counts. The amplitude of the returning echo is proportional to the difference in acoustic impedance between two tissues as the sound beam passes through their interface. There are only small differences in acoustic impedance among the body's soft tissues (Table 1-3).[6] This is ideal for imaging purposes because only a small percentage of the sound beam is reflected at such interfaces, whereas the majority is transmitted and available for imaging deeper structures.

Bone and gas have high and low acoustic impedances, respectively. Air is less dense and more compressible than soft tissue and transmits sound at a lower velocity. Bone is more dense and less compressible than soft tissue and transmits sound at a higher velocity. This means that when the sound beam encounters a soft tissue–bone or soft tissue–gas interface, nearly all sound is reflected and little is available for imaging deeper structures (Table 1-4; see Figure 1-3). This effect represents a high acoustic impedance mismatch. Distal acoustic shadowing is produced deep to the bone or gas

Axial Resolution

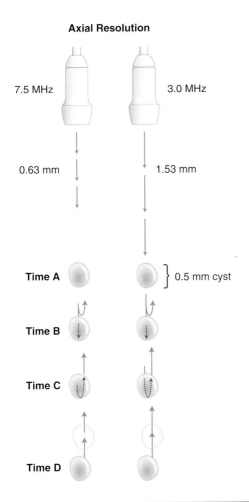

Transducer	Wavelength	Spatial pulse length*	Maximum axial resolution
3.0 MHz	0.51 mm	1.53 mm	0.765 mm
7.5 MHz	0.21 mm	0.63 mm	0.315

*Assumes 3 wavelengths/pulse

Figure 1-2 **Axial resolution.** Higher frequency transducers produce shorter pulses than lower frequency transducers because the wavelength of the emitted sound is shorter. Pulse length actually determines axial resolution but is directly dependent on the wavelength from the beam. In this example, the near and far walls of a cyst can be resolved if the echoes returning to the transducer from each wall remain distinct. The echo from the near wall must clear the wall before the echo from the far wall returns to merge with it. The ability to resolve the cyst is dependent on the pulse length and distance between walls. Axial resolution cannot be better than half the pulse length. In this example, a 0.5-mm cyst could theoretically be resolved with a 7.5-MHz but not a 3.0-MHz transducer because of the superior axial resolution of the higher frequency. However, resolution of this degree is never achieved because of the inherent limitations of current ultrasound scanners.

because little sound penetrates. Increasing output intensity or increasing gain will not improve penetration but merely increases artifacts, such as reverberation echoes. The sonographer must find an "acoustic window" that avoids bone and gas when imaging the abdomen. For the same reason, an acoustic coupling gel is used between the transducer and skin for all ultrasound examinations to eliminate interposed air.

TABLE 1-2

*Commonly Used Ultrasound Frequencies**

Frequency (MHz)	Wavelength (mm)
2.0	0.77
3.0	0.51
5.0	0.31
7.5	0.21
10.0	0.15

*Assume velocity = 1.54 mm/μsec (1540 m/sec).

TABLE 1-3

Acoustic Impendence

Tissue or Substance	Acoustic Impedance*
Air	0.0004
Fat	1.38
Water (50° C)	1.54
Brain	1.58
Blood	1.61
Kidney	1.62
Liver	1.65
Muscle	1.70
Lens	1.84
Bone	7.8

Data from Curry TS III, Dowdey JE, Murry RC Jr. *Christensen's Physics of Diagnostic Radiology.* 4th ed. Philadelphia: Lea & Febiger; 1990.
*Acoustic impedance (Z) = ×10⁶ kg/m²-sec.

TABLE 1-4

Sound Reflection at Various Interfaces

Interface	Reflection (%)
Blood-brain	0.3
Kidney-liver	0.6
Blood-kidney	0.7
Liver-muscle	1.8
Blood-fat	7.9
Liver-fat	10.0
Muscle-fat	10.0
Muscle-bone	64.6
Brain-bone	66.1
Water-bone	68.4
Soft tissue–gas	99.0

Data from Hagen-Ansert SL. *Textbook of Diagnostic Ultrasonography.* 3rd ed. St Louis: Mosby; 1989.

Scattering and Speckle
Most echoes displayed on the ultrasound image do not arise from large specular reflectors, such as the surface of organs, but from within the organs. When the ultrasound beam encounters small uneven interfaces less than the incident wavelength (submillimeter) in the parenchyma of organs, *scattering* occurs. This is also termed *diffuse* reflection or *nonspecular* reflection and is independent of beam angle. Acoustic

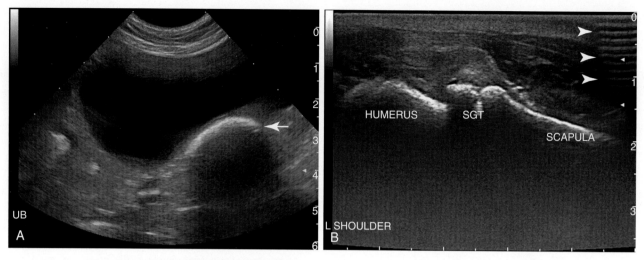

Figure 1-3 Strong reflectors of ultrasound. A, Gas within the descending colon (*arrow*) creates a very echogenic, curved interface deep to the anechoic urinary bladder. Secondary lobe artifacts are present creating false echoes within the normally anechoic urine. Acoustic shadowing is present deep to the colon. It is not as complete (clean) a shadow as that created by mineral. **B,** The body surface of the proximal humerus, supraglenoid tubercle (*SGT*), and scapula are highly reflective, creating a vividly hyperechoic outline of the left shoulder of this puppy with septic arthritis. There is a reverberation artifact in the upper right corner of the image created by poor transducer-skin contact (*arrowheads*). Acoustic shadowing is present deep to the bone surfaces.

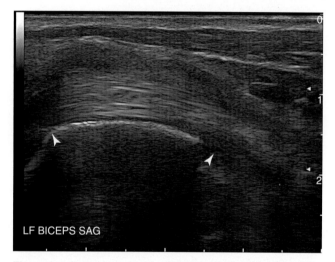

Figure 1-4 Importance of angle of incidence of the ultrasound beam. Multiple, parallel, echogenic fibers of the biceps tendon are well visualized across the center of the image because the ultrasound beam is perpendicular (90 degrees) to them. As the tendon bends away to the right and left, the echogenicity of the tendon is lost (*arrowheads*). The ultrasound beam is now off-incidence (no longer perpendicular) to the tendon, refracted away. This artifact could be mistaken for tendon pathology.

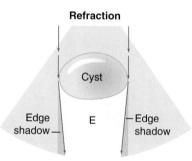

Figure 1-5 Refraction of ultrasound. Refraction of the ultrasound beam produces a shadow distal to curved structures. The structure must propagate sound at a velocity different from that of the surrounding medium. This phenomenon is often referred to as critical-angle shadowing or edge shadowing. Outward refraction of the beam is seen when the sound velocity is higher in the structure than in the surrounding medium. This occurs when sound passes from retroperitoneal fat through the curved surface of the kidney. In the case of a liver or kidney cyst, sound refraction is inward (focused) because velocity within the cyst is lower than in liver or kidney tissue. Distal enhancement (*E*) is also seen deep to cysts because of a decreased attenuation compared with surrounding tissue.

impedance mismatches are small compared with those of specular reflectors, and the returned weak echoes can be imaged only because they are abundant and tend to reinforce one another, producing ultrasound *speckle*. These echoes contribute to the parenchymal "texture" seen in abdominal organs but *may not represent actual anatomy, gross or microscopic.* This type of scattering increases with higher frequency transducers so that texture is appreciably enhanced.

Refraction

The velocity change occurring as a sound wave passes from one medium to another causes the beam to bend if the interface between the media is struck at an oblique angle. This can produce an artifact of improper location for an imaged structure. Altering the beam's direction is called refraction. Refraction along with reflection also contributes to a thin, echo-poor area that is lateral and distal to curved structures, such as the gallbladder or a cyst (Figure 1-5). This effect is termed an *edge shadow*.

Attenuation

The ultrasound beam is transmitted into the body as acoustic energy, quantified as acoustic power (*P*) expressed in watts (W) or milliwatts (mW) per unit time, or intensity (*I*), which accounts for the cross-sectional area of the ultrasound beam ($I = W/cm^2$). *Attenuation* is the collective term that describes the loss of acoustic energy as sound passes through tissues. Echoes reflected back toward the transducer are also attenuated in an identical manner. Sound attenuation (volume loss) is generally measured in decibels (dB) rather than intensity or power.

Factors that contribute to attenuation are absorption (heat loss), reflection, and scattering of the sound beam. Absorption refers to conversion of a sound pulse's acoustic (mechanical) energy to heat. This is primarily due to frictional forces as the molecules of the transmitting medium move back and forth longitudinally in response to the passage of a sound wave. Heat production within tissues is important when the biological effects and safety of ultrasound are considered.

Of great importance is that the amount of attenuation is directly proportional to the frequency of the ultrasound beam; higher frequencies are attenuated much more than lower frequencies in a given medium. This means that any attempt to improve resolution by increasing the frequency invariably decreases penetration. The attenuation is substantial and is equal to approximately 0.5 dB/cm/MHz in soft tissues over the round-trip distance. This is an essential concept because it dictates transducer selection, overall and depth (time) dependent gain (TGC) settings, and system power.

Dark areas (shadowing) are noted distal to highly attenuating structures (mineral, air), whereas lighter areas (enhancement) are seen distal to tissues with low sound attenuation (fluid). Some disease processes, such as severe hepatic lipidosis, cause abnormal attenuation of ultrasound in soft tissues.

INSTRUMENTATION

All diagnostic ultrasound machines, regardless of cost or features, consist of several basic components. A pulser energizes piezoelectric crystals within the transducer, emitting pulses of ultrasound into the body. Returning echoes are received by the transducer and processed (by the receiver) to form an image that is viewed on a monitor.

Pulser
Ultrasound imaging is based on the pulse-echo principle. This means that sound is produced by the transducer in pulses rather than continuously (see Figures 1-1 and 1-2). The pulser (or transmitter) applies precisely timed high-voltage pulses to the piezoelectric crystals within the transducer, which then emits short bursts of ultrasound into the body. The image is formed from the echoes returning to the transducer from the tissues after each pulse. Therefore adequate time must be allowed for all echoes to return before the transducer is pulsed again. Typically, sound is transmitted less than 1% of the time; the transducer is waiting for all echoes to return more than 99% of the time. When the crystal is pulsed, approximately two or three wavelengths are emitted in each pulse before a backing block in the transducer dampens the vibration. Thus the spatial pulse length is commonly two or three wavelengths. A higher frequency transducer emits shorter wavelengths, and therefore correspondingly shorter pulses, than a lower frequency transducer (see Figures 1-1 and 1-2). It is the pulse length, in turn dependent on transducer frequency, that determines the ability to separate points along the axis of the sound beam, termed *axial resolution*. The pulse length is commonly 0.1 to 1.0 mm. Axial resolution cannot be better than half the pulse length because of the overlap of returning echoes reflected off closely spaced interfaces.[1]

There are two points of clinical importance with regard to the pulser. One is that the ultrasonographer can adjust the voltage applied to the transducer by use of the *power* control. Simply stated, the power control is a volume control

adjusting the acoustic energy (or loudness, in decibels) that is transmitted into the body. The louder the pulses going into the body, the louder the returning echoes, which in turn creates an overall brighter image. The power control is the only operator adjustment that affects sound transmitted into the body. All other controls affect the returning echoes at the level of the receiver. Although it would be useful to have unlimited acoustic energy so that image brightness would never be an issue, the U.S. Food and Drug Administration (FDA) regulates the maximum output of ultrasound scanners for patient safety. The permissible acoustic energy in part depends on the type of examination selected. For example, settings used with pediatric subjects have a lower maximum output than those used with adults.

Second, the rate of the pulses can also be controlled; this is termed *pulse repetition frequency* (PRF). It is fundamentally important that the time between ultrasound pulses be long enough to allow returning echoes to reach the transducer before the next pulse of sound is emitted. If a pulse of transmitted sound occurs too soon, overlap with the returning echoes creates erroneous data. This requirement is particularly significant when using Doppler ultrasound, which is explained later in the chapter. For reference, PRFs of less than 1 kHz to 10 kHz or higher are necessary in diagnostic ultrasound.

Transducer
The transducer (commonly referred to as a scan head or probe) plays the dual role of transmitter *and* receiver of ultrasound through use of piezoelectric crystals. As noted, piezoelectric crystals vibrate and emit sound when voltage is applied to them by the pulser. The range of frequencies emitted by a particular transducer depends on the characteristics and thickness of the crystals contained within the scan head.

Modern transducers are capable of multifrequency operation, termed *broad bandwidth*. A range of frequencies are produced, composed of a preferential (central) frequency in addition to higher and lower frequencies. Advances in transducer technology allow simultaneous imaging of the near and far fields with sound waves of different frequencies. This allows the maximal resolution possible for a given depth without having to switch transducers. The use of broad bandwidth technology has several advantages. From a practical standpoint, the transducer may be operated at higher or lower frequencies for increased resolution or increased penetration for deeper structures, respectively (Figure 1-6). It has also allowed manufacturers to achieve better image resolution by capturing the spectrum of frequencies produced by insonated tissues. Speckle artifact can be reduced by *frequency compounding*, a technique that adds together speckle patterns generated at different frequencies, resulting in an increase in image contrast.

Receiver
When the piezoelectric crystals within the transducer encounter acoustic pressure waves from returning echoes, small voltages are produced. These electrical signals are processed by the ultrasound computer (the receiver), ultimately creating a diagnostic image. Manipulating these weak electrical signals by selecting various scanner controls (processing parameters) to create the best possible image is largely operator dependent and constitutes the "art" of diagnostic ultrasound.

Scanner Controls
Scanner controls permit the operator to maximize image quality; less than ideal or improper settings degrade the image. It must be emphasized that adjustments may directly affect image interpretation. Organs can be made hyperechoic or hypoechoic, or their parenchymal texture displayed as course

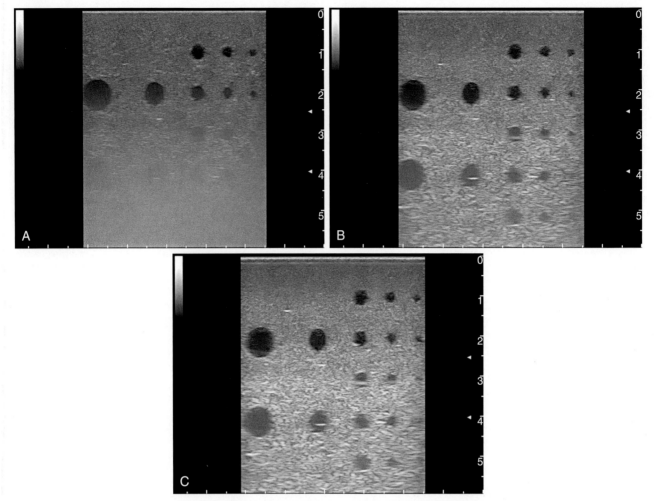

Figure 1-6 Broadband transducer frequency effect on image quality and depth penetration. A linear array broadband (4 to 13 MHz) transducer was used to make these images of an ultrasound phantom. The only parameter difference between images is the portion of the frequency range selected (high, midband, and low). Two focal points are present, at depths of 2.5 and 4 cm. Overall depth of the displayed image is 59 mm. **A,** Operating at 13 MHz, there is good visualization of the first two rows of cysts in the near field, at depths of 1 and 2 cm. Poor depth penetration of the high frequency 13 MHz selection does not allow adequate ultrasound beam penetration for visualization of the deeper rows of cysts, located at 3, 4, and 5 cm. **B,** Operating at midband of the frequency spectrum there is better penetration of the ultrasound beam to 5 cm, allowing recognition of the deeper cysts. Note how the deeper tissue has become brighter. **C,** At the lower frequency range (4 MHz), the cysts at 4 and 5 cm are more clearly seen and the overall image is brighter.

or fine, depending on the selection and adjustment of the many operator controls. Controls are given a variety of names, depending on the manufacturer (Figure 1-7), but their functions are similar despite the inconsistency in names. Understanding and learning to effectively operate ultrasound equipment is one defining difference between experienced and inexperienced sonographers.

There is only one control to alter the intensity of sound output from the transducer (the power control); all other controls are used to adjust amplification of the returning echoes. Gain and TGC controls are the most important operator controls, and these must be mastered to yield the best possible image. Additionally, they must be adjusted throughout an examination, accounting for differences in patient thickness and area examined (e.g., liver versus urinary bladder). There are a plethora of additional controls used to optimize the image. These include dynamic range, gray-scale display

maps, edge filters, persistence, and scan line density. Figure 1-8 illustrates many of the controls as indicated on the image display screen.

Ultrasonography is based on the pulse-echo principle, as discussed previously. A pulse of sound is emitted from the transducer after a special piezoelectric crystal contained within the scan head is vibrated and quickly dampened. The pulse-repetition frequency is the number of pulses occurring in 1 second, typically in the thousands of cycles per second. The frequency of sound emitted depends on a crystal's inherent characteristics. The crystal's vibrations are immediately dampened by a backing block so that only a short pulse length of two or three wavelengths is emitted. The crystal then remains quiet while waiting for returning echoes reflected from tissues within the body. These echoes vibrate the crystal again, producing small voltage signals that are amplified to form the final image.

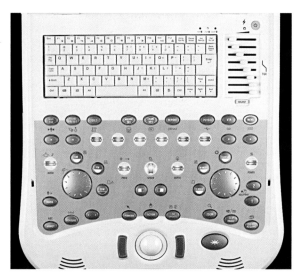

Figure 1-7 Ultrasound operator controls. The sonographer must become familiar with the controls so that image optimization becomes routine. The controls are labeled with text or icons for easy identification of function. An alphanumeric key board is seen in the top of the image. To the right are the TGC controls. The large wheel on the right is the gain control for B- and M-mode, and the power toggle is seen at upper right. Doppler controls are centered around the gain wheel on the left and the lower row of blue toggle switches. Familiarity with personal computers should allow most operators to become comfortable with the controls in a relatively short time despite the rather ominous array of knobs and switches. (MyLab 30, Biosound Esoate, Indianapolis, IN)

A timer is activated at the moment the crystal is pulsed so that the time of each echo's return can be determined separately and placed at the appropriate location on the video monitor. The elapsed time represents the distance (depth) from the transducer where a particular echo originated. An average speed of sound within soft tissues (approximately 1540 m/sec) is assumed by all ultrasound equipment. The elapsed roundtrip time must be halved and multiplied by 1540 m/sec to determine the actual distance of the reflecting interface from the transducer (Figure 1-9). Echoes arising from the deepest tissues return to the transducer later than those from superficial structures. A dot representing each returning echo is placed on the video monitor at the appropriate depth according to the time it took for the echo to return. Ultrasound instruments are calibrated to interpret and display the depth in centimeters (rather than time of return) automatically. A gray scale is also assigned to each dot corresponding to the amplitude or strength of the returning echo. The current convention is to display low-intensity echoes as nearly black, medium-intensity echoes as various shades of gray, and high-intensity echoes as white (white-on-black display). Some scanners may be capable of reversing this display so that high-intensity echoes are displayed as black and low-intensity echoes as nearly white (black-on-white display), although this format is used infrequently today.

The human eye can distinguish only about 10 to 12 shades of gray on a video monitor. Most ultrasound systems are designed to acquire a wider range of levels (32 to 128 levels or more) and fit them into the dynamic range of the monitor using special compression, expansion, or mapping schemes. Images can be postprocessed so that shades of gray can be assigned in various ways from the acquired signals. When gray

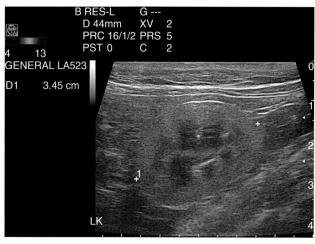

Figure 1-8 Screen information: deciphering displayed ultrasound parameters. An explanation of the letters and numbers depicted on the ultrasound image is offered here to help demystify the plethora of postprocessing controls available. Adjustment allows the image to be fine-tuned. Each manufacturer has its own nomenclature and method of information display, but there is commonality in function. In this sagittal image of the left kidney (*LK*) the transducer indicator is directed cranially; thus the cranial pole of the left kidney is to the left, caudal to the right. All manufacturers have some form of transducer mark that corresponds to a symbol on the edge of the image, usually the company icon. A wide-band high-frequency (4 to 13 MHz) linear-array transducer has been used for these images (designated LA523). The transducer is being operated the higher end of its frequency range, indicated by the small bar graph position (toward 13) in the far upper left icon, and the B RES-L denotation (B-mode, RES = resolution, L = lower part of the highest frequency range) within the upper left header. Just below this is the total depth of field, 44 mm (D 44 mm). Two focal points have been used (*small green arrowheads*) to maximize resolution at the depth of the kidney. The small tick marks along the right y-axis and the x-axis represent 5 mm increments, the larger tick marks indicate 1 cm. PRC 16/1/2: This denotes three different image processing programs and the corresponding machine settings. P = dynamic range, 16. Dynamic range is the difference in loudness between the weakest returning echoes and the strongest. A higher dynamic range yields more shades of gray, whereas a lower dynamic range yields a more black and white image (higher contrast). Abdominal imaging uses a wider dynamic range, whereas in cardiology a narrower range is used to maximize contrast. Tendon and ligament exams are often optimized in between. On this machine, dynamic range is indicated in numerals. On others, the value is given in decibels (dB). A wide dynamic range could be 90 dB, a narrow range, 50 dB. R = enhancement, 1. Enhancement is a setting to increase or decrease edge definition. C = line density, 2. Line density is the number of ultrasound scan lines shown. Increasing the line density increases detail; decreasing line density results in a faster frame rate at the expense of image detail. PST 0: Indicates the gray-scale map selected G —: Indicates the gain setting, not displayed on a captured image XV 2: Denotes "X View," a proprietary image-viewing program PRS 5: Persistence level. Persistence is how long each successive frame is overlapped with the next image frame. A long persistence yields a very smooth image, and excessive persistence results in a blurred image. C 2: Denotes dynamic contrast D1 3.45 cm: The measurement of the left kidney (*LK*) length, between the electronic cursors. (MyLab 30, Biosound Esoate, Indianapolis, IN)

levels are assigned, priority can be given to weaker signals so that subtle changes in parenchymal reflection amplitude are represented by separate shades of gray. Conversely, strong signals can be assigned more gray values when weaker echoes are unimportant. The resultant change in image contrast theoretically displays only the most clinically relevant information. Operator-selectable postprocessing curves using linear or logarithmic functions are preinstalled on many machines. In some cases, the curves can be customized by the sonographer.

The ultrasound beam and the returning echoes are attenuated as they pass through tissues. The farther away a reflecting interface is from the transducer, the weaker the returning echo will be. The ultrasound scanner's controls are designed to either increase the intensity of sound transmitted into tissues (power control) or electronically amplify returning echoes to compensate for this attenuation, termed gain and time-gain compensation (TGC) controls. In most cases, the TGC controls are also used to suppress strong echoes returning from superficial structures in the near field. The prime objective of manipulating the scanner's controls is to produce uniform image brightness throughout the near and far fields.

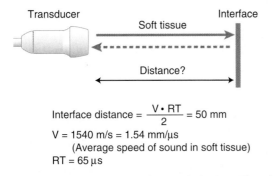

Interface distance = $\dfrac{V \cdot RT}{2}$ = 50 mm

V = 1540 m/s = 1.54 mm/μs
    (Average speed of sound in soft tissue)
RT = 65 μs

Figure 1-9 Distance determination by round-trip time. The ultrasound scanner determines the distance to a reflecting interface by halving the round-trip time (*RT*) from the beginning of a sound pulse until the echo's return and multiplying it by the average speed of sound in soft tissue (*V*). If the RT takes 65 μsec, the distance to the interface is 50 mm.

Power (Intensity, Output) Control

The power control modifies the voltage applied to pulse the piezoelectric crystal, thereby regulating the intensity of the sound output from the transducer. The greater the voltage spike, the larger the vibration amplitude (intensity) transmitted into tissues. Increasing the power also results in a uniform increase in the amplitude of returning echoes. The power should be set as low as possible to obtain the best resolution and prevent artifacts. This is done by choosing an appropriate transducer frequency that will penetrate to the area of interest without requiring excessive power levels. Whenever possible, the gain or TGC controls should be used to maximize the amplification of returning echoes, enabling as low a power setting as possible (Figures 1-10 and 1-11).

Overall Gain (Amplification) Control

The overall gain control affects the amplification of returning echoes, directly responsible for overall image brightness. All ultrasound machines have a *gain control* that causes *uniform amplification* of all returning echoes regardless of their depth of origin (Figures 1-12 and 1-13).

Time-Gain (Depth-Gain) Compensation Controls

The time-gain compensation (TGC) controls are used to produce an image that is *balanced* in brightness, from near field to far field. Echoes returning from deeper structures are weaker than those arising from superficial structures because of increased sound attenuation. The echo return time is directly related to the depth of the reflecting surface, as described previously. To selectively compensate for the weaker echoes arriving at the transducer from deeper structures, the gain is increased as the length of echo return time also increases. This compensation process is graphically represented by a TGC curve displayed on many ultrasound monitors (Figure 1-14). The TGC curve represents the gain setting in effect *at any particular depth*.

Because the near field echoes produce a brighter image while echoes from deeper structures are more attenuated and thus darker, the operator must use the TGC controls to reduce near field brightness while increasing the brightness of the far field. TGC controls are usually a series of slider controls that

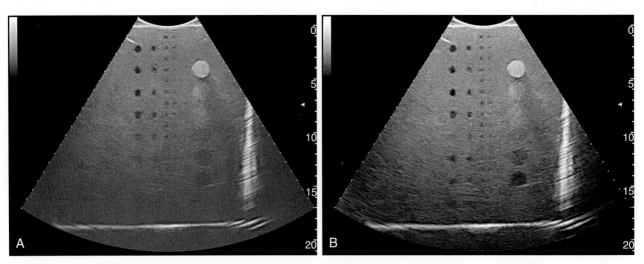

Figure 1-10 The effects of power output on image quality. Overall gain (40%), TGC, and all other parameters are identical for both images; only the power output has been changed. **A,** 10% power output. **B,** 100% power output. The image is slightly brighter because of the increase in power. Note the better visualization of the deeper, far-field structures. Images were made using a broadband (1 to 8 MHz) large curved-array transducer operating in the highest frequency range, using an ultrasound phantom. Power output has less effect on image brightness than overall gain.

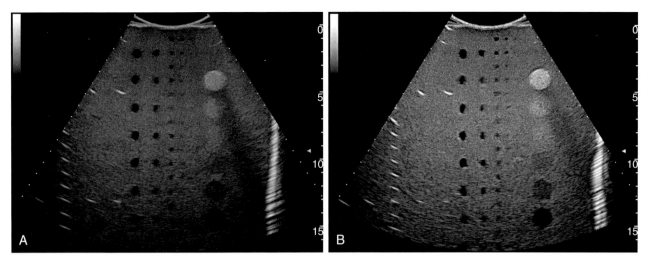

Figure 1-11 The effects of power output on image quality when using harmonic imaging. Overall gain (30%), TGC and all other parameters are identical for both images; only the power output has been changed. **A,** 10% power output. Note the overall brightness of the image and poor visualization of the far-field structures. **B,** 100% power output. Brightness of the image has increased compared to **A.** The deeper cystic structures are now easily identified. These images were made using a broadband (1 to 8 MHz) large curved-array transducer using harmonics and an ultrasound phantom. Power output has a greater effect on image brightness when using harmonic mode compared to standard, nonharmonic mode images.

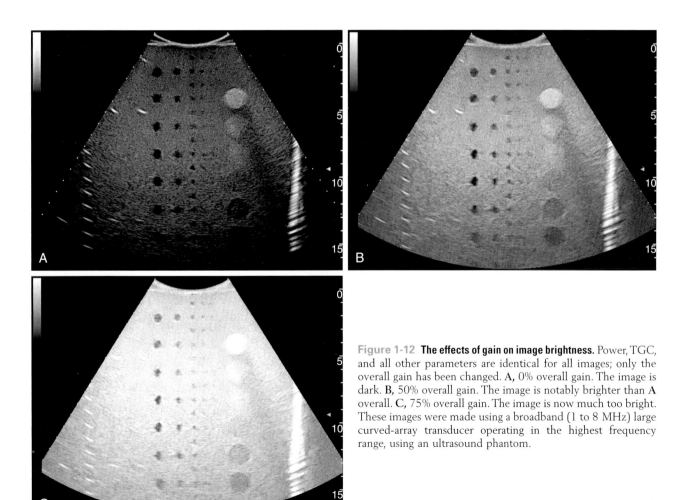

Figure 1-12 The effects of gain on image brightness. Power, TGC, and all other parameters are identical for all images; only the overall gain has been changed. **A,** 0% overall gain. The image is dark. **B,** 50% overall gain. The image is notably brighter than **A** overall. **C,** 75% overall gain. The image is now much too bright. These images were made using a broadband (1 to 8 MHz) large curved-array transducer operating in the highest frequency range, using an ultrasound phantom.

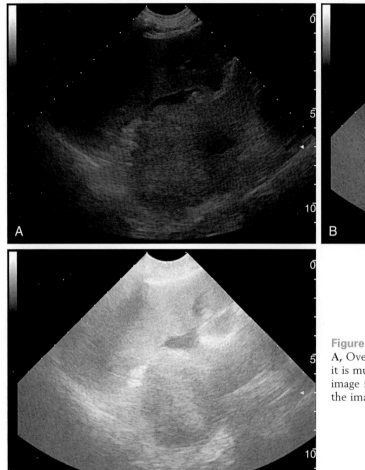
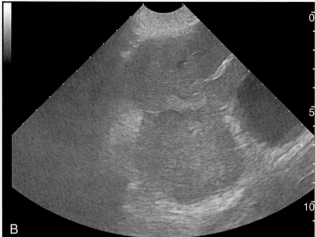
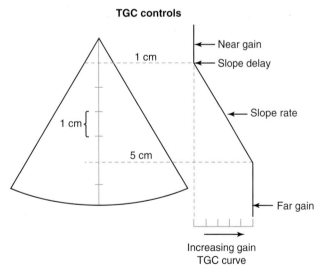

Figure 1-13 **The effects of gain on image quality.** Liver mass. **A,** Overall gain in too low; the image is not diagnostic because it is much too dark. **B,** Overall gain is in the proper range; the image is diagnostic quality. **C,** Overall gain is much too high; the image is too bright, rendering it nondiagnostic.

Figure 1-14 **TGC controls.** The purpose of the time-gain compensation (TGC) controls is to produce uniform image brightness throughout the depth of display by compensating for attenuation of the sound beam in tissue. Control settings are represented graphically by a TGC curve (seen to the right of the real-time image in this example). The curve shows the relative gain applied at any particular depth. Increasing gain (amplification of returning echoes) with increasing depth is represented by displaying the curve farther to the right as one moves downward.

allow you to intuitively adjust the TGC (see Figure 1-7). Moving the top sliders to the left reduces near field brightness, whereas moving the middle and bottom sliders to the right increases image brightness accordingly. The names and appearance of the controls may vary (knobs, slider controls, or touch screen), but they all function similarly to adjust the gain at various depths. This may be represented graphically on screen, or the shape of the TGC curve may be inferred by the position of the sliders. The first part of the TGC curve may consist of a straight portion that represents the first few centimeters of depth in the displayed image under the near gain control. Near gain is applied uniformly throughout this depth. The near gain control is misnamed because it usually functions to *suppress* strong echoes from superficial structures in the near field. The TGC controls on some older ultrasound scanners are less refined, with near and far field controls in addition to an overall gain control.

Proper TGC adjustment is fundamental for proper image display. Once the image is adjusted for uniform brightness from near to far field, the overall gain is then applied to increase (or decrease) the entire image to the sonographer's preference. Proper TGC and overall gain adjustment is such an important function that top-end machines now have automated TGC controls. A simple push of a button adjusts the image based on scanner parameters and the characteristics of the tissues examined. In human medicine, this is a time-saving feature. However, experience has shown that automated TGC may not provide an optimum image in veterinary patients. Figure 1-15 shows the effects of improper and proper TGC adjustment.

Dynamic Range

Another important operator control is dynamic range, which is the amount of compression applied to the wide range of amplitude of the returning echoes; it is often expressed in decibels. Dynamic range in part controls the contrast of the ultrasound image. Relatively narrow dynamic range (e.g., 0 to 45 dB) results in images that have higher contrast (more black and white), whereas larger dynamic range (e.g., 0 to 60 dB) yields images with higher latitude or more shades of gray. In echocardiography, a narrower dynamic range is used, whereas in abdominal imaging a larger range of displayed echo amplitudes is preferred. Dynamic range is preset for a variety of machines but may be adjusted by the operator when needed (Figure 1-16).

Gray-Scale Maps

A variety of gray-scale maps are available on all newer ultrasound machines. These postprocessing curves can dramatically alter image appearance. In general, gray-scale maps that display more shades of gray (higher latitude) are preferred for abdominal imaging, whereas those displaying more contrast are used in echocardiography. Gray-scale maps can often be customized as part of user determined presets. Figure 1-17 shows the effect of different gray-scale settings.

Colorized Gray-Scale Maps

Many ultrasound machines allow colorization of gray-scale images. Although not commonly used, sometimes applying a colorizing map to a gray-scale image increases lesion conspicuity. Figure 1-18 illustrates a variety of colorized gray-scale maps.

Modes of Image Display

There are three modes of ultrasound signal display, two of which are used more frequently in clinical applications in veterinary medicine (Figure 1-19).

A-Mode

The least frequently used mode of image display is A-mode (amplitude mode), but it has special use for ophthalmic examinations and other applications requiring precise length or depth measurements, including back fat determination in production animals. A-mode is the simplest of the three modes. The echo's origin and amplitude are displayed as spikes originating from a vertical baseline (see Figure 1-19A). The transducer is located at the top of the baseline. Depth is represented by a progression from the top to the bottom of the baseline. Therefore the position of the spikes along the baseline represents the depth at which the echoes originated. The height of the spikes above the baseline represents the amplitude of returning echoes. In dedicated A-mode machines (e.g., for ophthalmic applications), the baseline may be displayed horizontally, with the transducer's location represented at the far left of the baseline, with increasing depth along the baseline to the right.

B-Mode

B-mode (brightness mode) displays the returning echoes as dots whose brightness or gray scale is proportional to the amplitude of the returned echo and whose position corresponds to the depth at which the echo originated along a single line (representing the beam's axis) from the transducer (see Figure 1-19, B). B-mode is usually displayed with the transducer positioned at the top of the screen and depth increasing to the bottom of the screen.

M-Mode

M-mode (motion mode) is used for echocardiography along with B-mode to evaluate the heart. M-mode tracings usually record depth on the vertical axis and time on the horizontal axis (see Figure 1-19, C). The image is oriented with the transducer at the top. The single line of B-mode dots described before, with brightness (gray scale) proportional to echo amplitude, is swept across a video monitor or recorded on a strip chart recorder. The motion of the dots (change in distance of reflecting interfaces from the transducer) is recorded with respect to time. The echo tracings produced with M-mode are useful for precise cardiac chamber and wall measurements and quantitative evaluation of valve or wall motion with time.

Real-Time B-Mode

Real-time B-mode scanners display a moving gray-scale image of cross-sectional anatomy. This is accomplished by sweeping a thin, focused ultrasound beam across a triangular, linear, or curvilinear field of view in the patient many times per second. The field is made up of many single B-mode lines, as described before. Sound pulses are sent out and echoes received back sequentially along each B-mode line of the field until a complete sector image is formed. Each line persists on the display monitor until it is renewed by a subsequent sweep of the beam. A malfunctioning transducer can dramatically illustrate how the image is composed of a series of separate lines (Figure 1-20). A narrow beam diameter enables the formation of a tomographic cross-sectional image, which is only a few millimeters thick. The beam may be steered mechanically or electronically through the field, with the frame rate (image renewal time) dependent on the depth displayed. The frame rate must be slower for displaying deeper depths because more time is needed for the echoes to return to the transducer. Sagittal, transverse, dorsal, and oblique planes through the body may be obtained by changing the transducer's orientation on the skin. The two basic types of real-time B-mode scanners are mechanical sector scanners and arrays of various configurations. The most versatile real-time sector scanners are also capable of A-mode and M-mode image production.

Types of Transducers

Essentially all current diagnostic ultrasound machines use transducers composed of multiple piezoelectric elements (up to several hundred), termed *arrays* (Figure 1-21, B-E). Because of the complex electronics used to form the image (beam steering), these transducers are termed *electronic*. The configuration of the array defines the type of electronic transducer, its application, and the appearance of the image on the monitor. Electronic array transducers are in contrast to older mechanical technology in which a single piezoelectric crystal was oscillated to create an image. Figure 1-22 shows the common types of transducers used in small animal diagnostic ultrasound.

The real-time *sector* scanner is named because the screen image produced by the transducer has a sector or triangular field of view (see Figure 1-21, A, B, D, E). The sector image has also been described as pie, wedge, or fan shaped. The sector angle is commonly 90 degrees, but narrower or wider angles may be selected by the user for specific purposes (Figure 1-23). Wide angles increase the field of view width for abdominal scanning at the expense of reduced frame rate. Narrow fields are useful when the desired viewing region is small or when an increase in frame rate is needed, such as during cardiac imaging of patients with high heart rates. The advantage of a sector scanner is that the image produced is divergent and therefore offers a wider field of view at greater image depth. Conversely, the primary disadvantage is that the first few centimeters of the near field is composed of the tiny tip of the sector, rendering near-field imaging difficult at best.

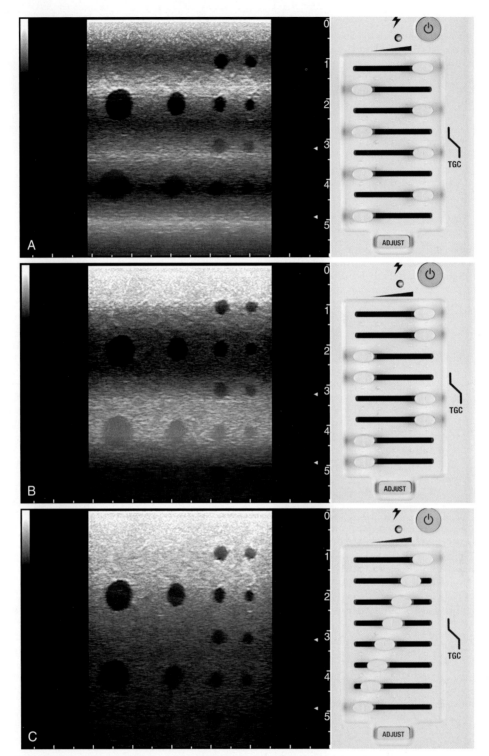

Figure 1-15 Time-gain compensation (TGC) effects. Slide controls with corresponding effects on the ultrasound image set for demonstration purposes. Slides to the right increase gain at the corresponding image depth (increase image brightness), while slides to the left decrease gain (decrease image brightness). **A,** Alternating increases (to right) and decreases (to left) of the TGC slides and resultant ultrasound image (*a*). **B,** Alternating increases and decreases of the TGC slides and resultant ultrasound image (*b*). **C,** TGC slides positioned exactly opposite of normal settings, with increases in near-field gain (upper slides to the right) and decreases in far-field gain (slides to the left), with resultant incorrect ultrasound image that is too bright in the near field and too dark in the far field (*c*).

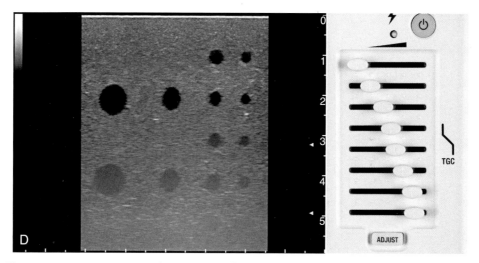

Figure 1-15, cont'd D, Typical TGC setting for proper balance of image brightness. There is a relative near-field reduction in gain (top slides to the left) and far-field increase in gain (bottom slides to the right) to produce an image with equal brightness from near to far (*d*). These images were made using a broadband (4 to 13 MHz) linear array transducer and an ultrasound phantom. All parameters are identical except the position of the TGC controls.

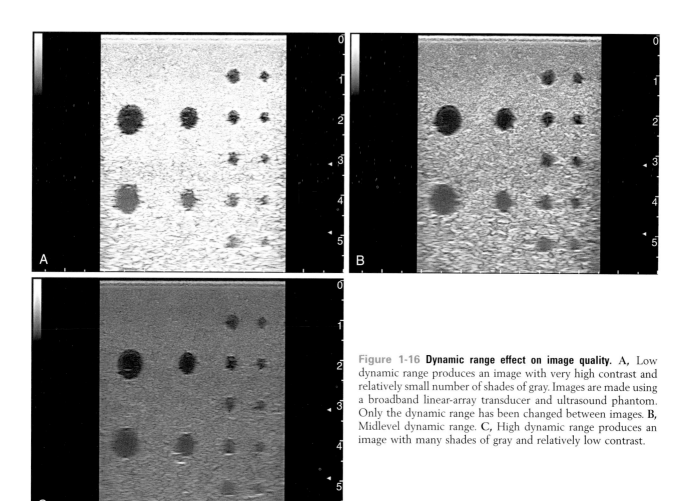

Figure 1-16 **Dynamic range effect on image quality. A,** Low dynamic range produces an image with very high contrast and relatively small number of shades of gray. Images are made using a broadband linear-array transducer and ultrasound phantom. Only the dynamic range has been changed between images. **B,** Midlevel dynamic range. **C,** High dynamic range produces an image with many shades of gray and relatively low contrast.

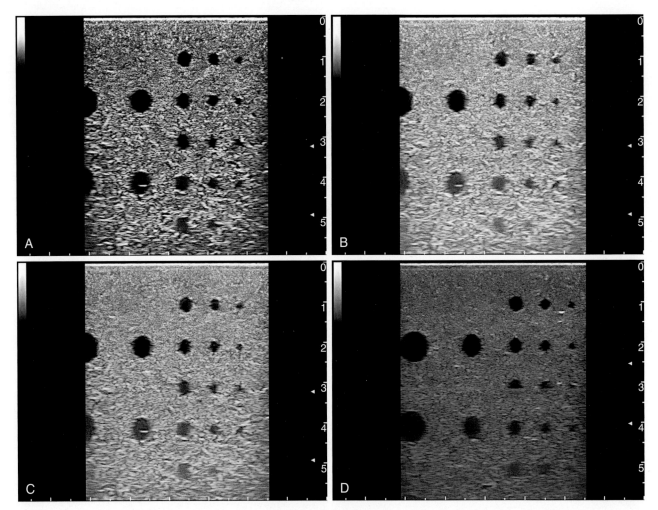

Figure 1-17 **Gray-scale maps.** Representation of the ultrasound image can be altered by choosing various gray-scale maps (postprocessing curves). Generally speaking, maps with more shades of gray are preferred for abdominal imaging, whereas maps that emphasize greater contrast are used for cardiac and musculoskeletal imaging. Gray-scale maps can often be customized as part of user determined presets. **A,** Very high contrast gray-scale map. **B,** High contrast gray-scale map. **C,** Medium contrast gray-scale map. **D,** Low contrast gray-scale map.

Sector scanners may be classified as either mechanical or electronic, depending on the method used to sweep the beam through the sector field.

Sector scanners, whether mechanical or electronic, have the disadvantage of limited near-field visibility compared with linear-array or large curvilinear-array transducers. Sector scanners are particularly useful for evaluation of deeper structures and other structures, such as the heart, to which access is limited by a narrow intercostal window.

Mechanical Sector Scanners

A mechanical sector scanner sweeps the beam through the field of view by to-and-fro oscillation of a solitary piezoelectric crystal to generate a real-time image (see Figure 1-21, *A*). More advanced multifrequency mechanical transducers use three crystals of different frequencies in circular rotation to create a sector image. Mechanical sector scanners do not allow variable focusing, and the moving parts are subject to wear. High image quality relative to cost have made them attractive, and although they are no longer used in the most modern abdominal and cardiac clinical machines, they are still manufactured for use in very high frequency transducers (20 MHz

and higher) for ocular imaging and in research applications using laboratory animals.

Arrays

Piezoelectric arrays may be formed in a variety of configurations: Linear, small and large curvilinear, phased, and annular arrays. Precise timing is used in firing these combinations of elements to change the direction of the beam. This enables the beam to be steered electronically, providing real-time images in a linear or sector format. These types of transducers are reliable because they have no moving parts. The instrumentation associated with ultrasound imaging is continuously evolving, and the interested reader is referred to an excellent in-depth discussion of transducer characteristics and instrumentation for further details.[3]

Linear Array

A linear-array transducer has multiple crystals arranged in a line within a bar-shaped scan head (see Figures 1-21, *C*, and 1-22, *D, E*). The narrow beam is swept through a *rectangular* field by firing the transducer's crystals sequentially. More than one crystal is fired at a time, and focusing at selected depths

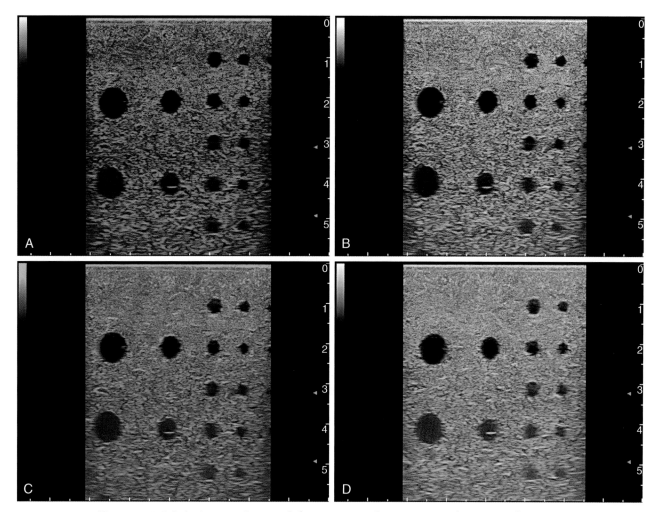

Figure 1-18 Colorized gray-scale maps. Colorizing gray-scale images may enhance normal anatomy or lesion conspicuity. **A**, Orange. **B**, Violet. **C**, Green. **D**, Yellow.

can be achieved by varying the number and sequence of elements fired. Linear-array transducers are available in a variety of sizes and frequency ranges, and their hallmarks are that they offer the highest available scanning frequency (e.g., 7-13 MHz or higher) and provide the largest near-field image (equal to the transducer length) (Figure 1-24). For these reasons, experienced sonographers use a linear array whenever possible. In general, they can be used for abdominal imaging in most small animal patients. Linear-array transducers provide the best possible resolution and are used in near-field examination.

There are limitations of a linear-array transducer. Their configuration requires a relatively large skin contact area compared to small sector scanners, which makes it difficult to position the scan head under the sternum or within intercostal spaces. And although the rectangular field of view is advantageous for superficial structures, far field width of view is limited because of the lack of beam divergence (think of it as tunnel vision) (Figure 1-25, *A*). However, this drawback has been overcome with the latest in linear array technology in which a trapezoidal image is created and effectively increases the width of the far field (see Figure 1-25, *B*). This is accomplished by laterally steering the crystals on each end of the transducer. Figure 1-26 illustrates the practical use of the trapezoidal feature while scanning an enlarged kidney. Finally, because of the higher frequencies used, linear-array transducers have a relatively shallow maximum depth of field (generally 10 cm or less) (see Figure 1-25).

Curvilinear Array

Curvilinear-array transducers are linear arrays shaped into convex curves (see Figures 1-21, *D, E* and 1-22, *B, C*). This arrangement produces a sector image with a wider far field of view than that of linear arrays. These transducers are available in a variety of sizes and frequencies suitable for many applications and they allow focusing. Small radius curved arrays (microconvex) are the best general purpose transducers for abdominal imaging in small animal medicine. They have a very small contact area (footprint) and are available in relatively high frequency ranges (e.g., 3 to 9 MHz) (see Figure 1-22, *B*). These transducers are also used in pediatric human medicine. Curved-array transducers with larger radiuses are generally only available in low to midrange frequencies (e.g., 1 to 8 MHz) and are useful for imaging the abdomen of the largest patients (including humans). Large curved-array transducers have a larger near field of view compared to those obtained with smaller curved arrays but have a much larger footprint (see Figure 1-22, *C*). This, along with lower resolution of the large curved-array transducers, limits their utility for most small animal practitioners in all but the largest patients. Figure 1-27, *A, B*, compares microconvex and large convex-array transducer images.

Phased Array

Phased-array sector transducers align the piezoelectric crystals in a short linear or block configuration, creating a sector field

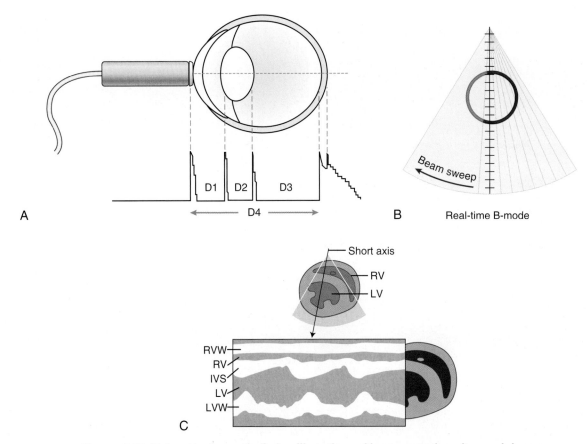

Figure 1-19 **Modes of ultrasound display illustration, with accompanying ultrasound images.** **A,** A-mode. **B,** B-mode. **C,** M-mode.

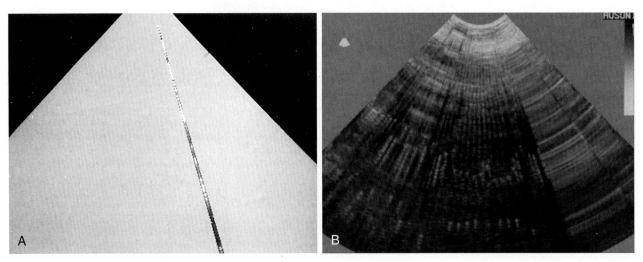

Figure 1-20 **Scan line.** **A,** Only one scan line was recorded during the sweep of the ultrasound beam through the sector arc because of a malfunctioning transducer. This illustrates how multiple scan lines are required to form the complete sector image during each sweep of the beam. **B,** This image of a malfunctioning transducer clearly illustrating how the collection of scan lines combine to form the composite image.

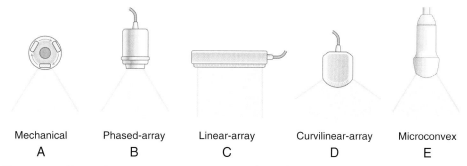

Mechanical   Phased-array   Linear-array   Curvilinear-array   Microconvex
    A   B   C   D   E

Figure 1-21 **Types of real-time transducers.** A, Mechanical sector scanner (rotating head type). B, Phased-array sector scanner. C, Linear-array scanner. D, Large curvilinear-array (convex) sector scanner. E, Microconvex (small curvilinear-array) sector scanner.

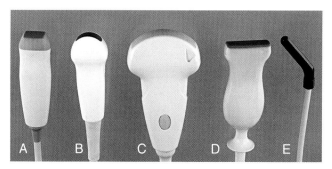

Figure 1-22 **Commonly used transducers in small animal diagnostic ultrasound.** A, Phased array. B, Microconvex. C, Large convex array. D, Linear array. E, Intraoperative linear array.

of view by firing multiple transducer elements in a precise sequence electronically (see Figures 1-21, *B*, and 1-22, *A*). The beam is steered in different directions and can be focused at various levels, which yields a wide field of view at deeper depths even with a small transducer (see Figure 1-27, *C*). Phased-array transducers are generally designed for cardiac applications, offering very high frame rates needed for critical assessment as well as a small footprint necessary for intercostal work. A state-of-the-art cardiac suite might have three phased-array transducers available, ranging in center frequencies of 2 to 3 MHz, 5 to 7 MHz, and 10 MHz or higher for the smallest patients.

Annular Array

Annular-array transducers have multiple transducer elements arranged in rings, hence the name. This arrangement permits precise focusing in both lateral and elevation (azimuth) planes. However, a disadvantage of this type of array is that the beam must be steered mechanically to produce a real-time image. This makes it more susceptible to wear than electronic arrays. Annular arrays are not commonly used today.

Transducer Selection

The basic tenet in transducer selection is to always use the highest frequency that permits adequate penetration to the desired depth. This pertains not only to selecting a specific transducer but also to properly using its broadband capability. For example, the liver of a large dog may require use of the 3-MHz portion of a 3- to 9-MHz broadband transducer, whereas examination of the more superficial kidneys may allow use of the 9-MHz portion of the frequency spectrum for best resolution. Even a linear-array transducer could be used to visualize the kidneys.

In private small animal practice, a microconvex (small curved array) transducer is requisite, offering the most versatility. Its broad frequency range (e.g., 3 to 9 MHz) and small footprint allow its use on most small patients, from cats to dogs up to the size of a Labrador Retriever or German Shepherd, with an effective penetrating depth of 12 to 15 cm. A broadband high-frequency linear-array transducer is preferred for small parts imaging and achieving the best resolution in smaller patients, but it would be difficult to use as the only probe in most practices because of its limited depth capability and larger footprint. A large, lower frequency curved-array transducer is generally required for large patients (rottweilers, Great Danes, mastiffs), but many practices are financially limited to two probes. Specialty practices and universities usually have a multitude of transducers to choose from, including several phased-array transducers for cardiac use in different size patients, a transesophageal transducer, a very high frequency linear array (up to 20 MHz), and perhaps an intraoperative transducer.

IMAGE QUALITY: SPATIAL RESOLUTION

Spatial resolution is the ability to separate two closely spaced objects. We must consider spatial resolution of the ultrasound beam in three image planes: along the axis, lateral to the axis, and perpendicular to the axis. Figure 1-28 illustrates the three-dimensional nature of the ultrasound beam.

We have discussed the first image plane, *axial resolution*, at the beginning of the chapter under Basic Acoustic Principles. To summarize, the higher the transducer frequency and shorter the pulse length, the better the axial resolution (see Figures 1-1 and 1-2). As sonographers, we have control of which frequency transducer we select, but we have no control over pulse length.

The second image plane is termed *lateral resolution* and refers to the ability to resolve adjacent points *perpendicular* (side-by-side) to the ultrasound beam axis along the plane of the scan (Figure 1-29). Lateral resolution is determined by the *width* of each individual ultrasound beam, and the resolution varies with the transducer frequency and the distance from the transducer. The *focal point* is the center of the narrowest part of the beam along the beam axis. Resolution decreases with distance from the focal point, but acceptable lateral resolution is found for several centimeters along the beam axis on either side of the focal point (focal zone). Modern day electronic transducers allow the sonographer to maximize lateral resolution by manually focusing the ultrasound beam at a selected depth (or depths, because multiple focal points can be selected) (Figure 1-30, *C, D*). Figure 1-31 shows the effect of focal point placement and image resolution.

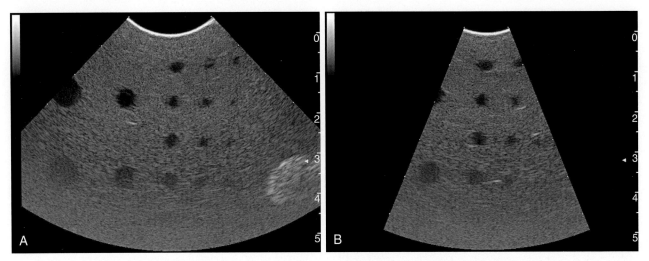

Figure 1-23 Sector angle. A, The sector angle of the microconvex transducer is 90 degrees. Note the wide field of view. The frame rate was 32 frames per second (fps). **B,** The sector angle of this microconvex transducer is now set to 45 degrees. The field width is notably reduced; however, the frame rate increased to 62 fps.

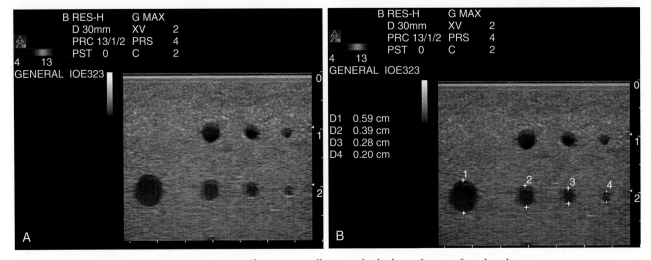

Figure 1-24 Linear array image. These images illustrate the high resolution of modern linear array transducers. **A,** A linear array transducer produces a rectangular image without field-of-view divergence. It yields exquisite near-field detail. This image of an ultrasound phantom was made using an intraoperative broadband linear-array probe operating at 13 MHz and a depth of 3 cm (30 mm). **B,** Electronic cursors were used to obtain axial measurements of the small cysts within the ultrasound phantom, ranging from approximately 6 to 2 mm, left to right (D1-D4). The tick marks along the bottom of the image represent 5 mm (*small tick marks*) and 1 cm (*large tick marks*); the near-field width is approximately 3 cm. The vertical scale is clearly denoted (0, 1, 2 cm). Note the focal points are placed precisely at the level of the two rows of cysts for optimizing image resolution.

Newer ultrasound technology allows automatic variable dynamic focusing. In dynamic scanning, the depth of the focal point is continuously changed along the beam axis during scanning. This technique effectively extends the focal zone length to the entire depth of the display.

Focusing cannot be done with fixed-focus mechanical transducers, but knowledge of the point where the beam is narrowest (focal point) for a given transducer allows placement of the region of interest at the point of maximal lateral resolution.

Standoff pads can be used to place a particular near-field structure deeper into the image and into the focal zone. Alternatively, the operator can change transducers to place the area of interest within the focal zone of a particular mechanical transducer.

A third type of resolution, *elevation* (or *azimuth*) resolution, refers to the ability to resolve adjacent points *perpendicular* to the beam axis and scan plane. Elevation resolution is determined by slice *thickness* in the plane perpendicular to the beam axis and scan plane (see Figures 1-28 and 1-30, *B*). Azimuth is a function of transducer design and cannot be specifically adjusted by the sonographer.

Axial resolution is superior to lateral resolution or elevation resolution. Consequently, all measurements should be taken along the beam axis, if possible (see Figure 1-24, *B*).

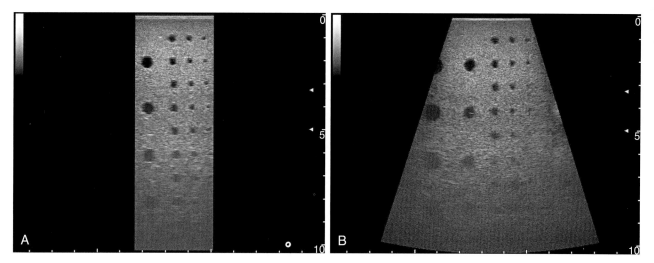

Figure 1-25 **Linear array narrow field of view at depth. A,** Using the same ultrasound phantom and transducer as in Figure 1-24, the image is now made at a depth of 10 cm. Note the very narrow field of view and how small the image has become. Also, even at operating at the lowest part of the frequency spectrum (4 MHz) at maximum gain, the deeper cystic structures and parenchyma are poorly resolved. **B,** Same image as A, but using trapezoidal feature available on some linear array transducers. Note the much wider far field of view.

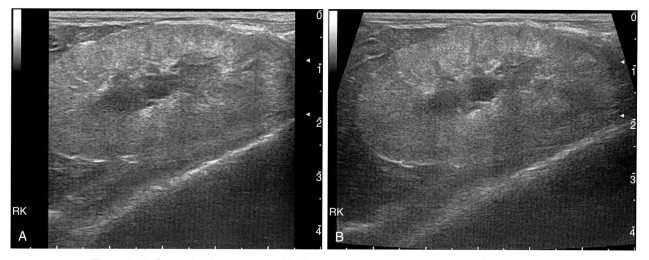

Figure 1-26 **Conventional versus trapezoidal linear transducer array image display.** This image of an abnormal right kidney (*RK*) in a cat illustrates the usefulness of trapezoidal display when using a linear-array transducer. **A,** Sagittal image using conventional linear array display shows that the entire length of the kidney cannot be displayed because it is longer than the transducer. The field of view is not wide enough to encompass the entire kidney. **B,** Sagittal image with trapezoidal feature allows imaging of the entire length of the kidney because of the diverging far field and resultant trapezoidal image.

SPECIAL NEW IMAGING MODES

Tissue Harmonic Imaging

As we have learned, ultrasound travels at different velocities in various soft tissues and within fat, yet the ultrasound computer processes returning echoes at a constant value of 1540 m/sec. This nonlinear propagation of ultrasound through tissues causes phase aberrations, resulting in distortion of the ultrasound image. Harmonic imaging is a technique used to reduce noise and clutter within an ultrasound image by reducing the effects of phase aberrations. It is available on many modern ultrasound machines and at times can be extremely useful.

Harmonic frequencies consist of integral multiples of the lowest fundamental frequency emitted by the transducer. For example, if f represents a fundamental frequency of 4 MHz, $2f$ is the second harmonic frequency, 8 MHz. Simply stated, instead of listening for returning echoes generated by the fundamental frequency, in harmonics mode the transducer listens for harmonic frequencies. Since harmonic ultrasound beams are narrower and the frequencies have lower *amplitude* than the fundamental frequency, images generated contain

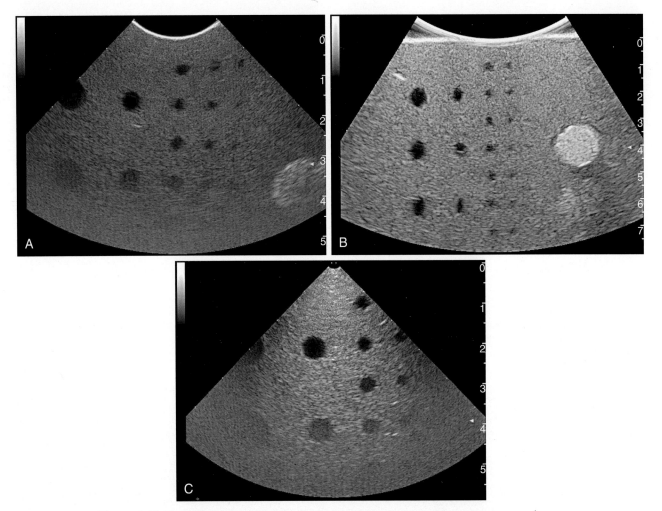

Figure 1-27 Electronic sector array transducer image comparison. A, Microconvex curved-array transducer image. The sector is narrower in the near field when compared to a large curved array transducer, a result of the small size of the transducer tip and compact placement of the piezo-electric crystals. This is the most common and versatile transducer for small animal abdominal imaging. This image was made using a broadband transducer operating in the center of its 3- to 9-MHz range and 54-mm depth. **B,** Large curved-array transducer adjusted for an 8-cm depth of field. Note the sector image with a broad near-field view provided by a large curved array configuration. These transducers are used for large patients because of their lower frequency and better penetration. This image was made using a broadband transducer operating in the high frequency region of its 1 to 8 MHz range. **C,** Phased-array transducer. The sector shape of the image is quite pronounced, with very little useful information in the first few centimeters of depth. Phased-array transducers are used principally for cardiac ultrasound. This image was made using a broadband transducer operating in the central region of its 4- to 11-MHz range, at 58-mm depth.

less side lobe and slice thickness artifact, less reverberation, and less scatter, and they yield higher spatial resolution.

Harmonic imaging is of particular benefit in imaging the urinary bladder, often with less artifact superimposed on the anechoic "canvas" of urine (Figure 1-32). Harmonic imaging is also valuable in larger patients, because formation of harmonic frequencies increases with scanning depth. Conversely, harmonic imaging is of little value in scanning very superficial structures.

In practice, the use of harmonics to improve image quality is variable. In some patients, it has an amazingly positive effect, in others there is apparent image degradation. Image quality also varies within patients. For example, it may effectively improve image quality while scanning the urinary bladder but may not improve the quality of a liver examination. Nonetheless, some sonographers prefer to routinely scan in harmonic mode. Harmonic imaging is frequently used with ultrasound contrast agents and is discussed in detail in Chapter 3.

Spatial Compounding
Spatial compounding is a newer technology developed to increase image quality by reducing the deleterious effect of speckle. Conventional ultrasound beams are directed in a single, fixed angle relative to target tissues. With spatial compounding, multiple scan lines and scan angles are used to scan tissues (Figure 1-33). This increases the effect of primary beam echo generation (because there are more of them) but diminishes the effects of off-incidence scatter. The result is improved image contrast. The sonographer usually has several spatial compounding selections to choose from that vary in application (e.g., near field versus far field), number of scan lines used, and so on.

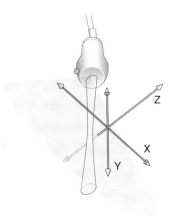

Figure 1-28 Three planes of ultrasound beam resolution. Axial resolution (Y) is along the beam axis and is determined by pulse length. Lateral resolution (X) is perpendicular to the beam axis along the plane of the scan. The diameter (width) of the beam in the X direction determines lateral resolution. Elevation or azimuth resolution (Z) is perpendicular to both the beam axis and scan plane. The diameter (height, or slice thickness) of the beam in the Z direction determines elevation resolution. Both lateral resolution and elevation resolution vary with transducer frequency and distance from the transducer. Axial resolution is always better than lateral or elevation resolution.

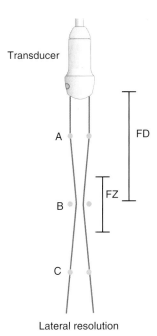

Figure 1-29 Lateral resolution. Lateral resolution is determined by the beam's diameter. In focused ultrasound beams, the diameter of the beam is narrowest at the focal point (B). Higher frequency transducers produce narrower beams. The distance between the transducer and focal point is the focal distance (FD). Acceptable lateral resolution is obtained for a short distance along the beam's axis on either side of the focal point within the focal zone (FZ). Increased beam width at other distances from the transducer (A and C) results in poorer lateral resolution.

A recent publication has described the effects of spatial compounding in veterinary medicine.[7] Multiple ring-down artifacts created by multiple scan lines interacting with a single source are characteristic of spatial compound imaging (see Figure 1-33, B). Imaging of the urinary bladder was

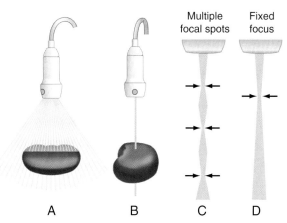

Figure 1-30 Ultrasound beam. A, Real-time ultrasound image is produced by sweeping a thin, focused beam across a sector (shown) or rectangular (not shown) field. **B,** When the ultrasound image (or beam) is viewed 90 degrees to **A,** beam thickness is seen, which is known as azimuth or elevation resolution. This corresponds to the Z-plane in Figure 1-28. **C, D,** Illustrations of the width of a single beam of ultrasound, showing multiple focal points (C) or a single focal point (D). This corresponds to the X-plane (lateral resolution) in Figure 1-28; also see Figure 1-29 Lateral resolution.

improved with reduction or elimination of clutter. Increased width and reduced intensity of acoustic shadowing and reduction or elimination of edge shadowing was observed. No effect on acoustic enhancement was observed, contrary to what has been reported in human sonography.[8] Despite the theoretical advantages of spatial compounding, its overall usefulness in routine clinical veterinary imaging is still debated. As shown in Figure 1-34, image smoothing that occurs with spatial compounding renders a slightly blurry image that is particularly evident when reviewing still images.

Extended Field of View
Extended field of view technology allows the sonographer to build a static, *panoramic* image by moving the transducer along the axis of the transducer face (x-axis). Extended field of view imaging partially compensates for ultrasound's relatively narrow field of view. It is useful in helping establish spatial and anatomic relationships in extensive or multiorgan disease (Figure 1-35).

Three-Dimensional Ultrasound
Three-dimensional (3-D) ultrasound has been available a number of years, but its utility in veterinary medicine has yet to be defined. Surface rendering and volumetric information can be obtained, allowing review of static images from endless perspectives. In human medicine, 3-D ultrasound is routinely used for gynecology, obstetrics, and infertility examinations and in cardiology. Real-time 3-D is termed *4-D ultrasound.* 4-D ultrasound requires very advanced equipment and has found only limited use in the most advanced echocardiology applications.

IMAGE ORIENTATION AND LABELING

Consistent orientation and labeling of the ultrasound image are important for systematic interpretation of scans. The following discussion is limited to abdominal scanning because the procedures for echocardiography and other areas of the body are covered in later chapters. There is no universally accepted standard for abdominal image orientation in

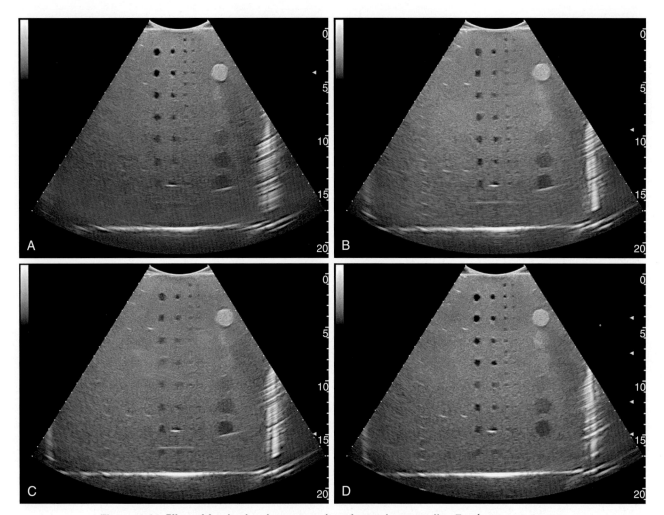

Figure 1-31 Effect of focal point placement and number on image quality. Focal points minimize lateral ultrasound beam width and thus increase lateral resolution at that depth. These images show the effects of a single focus placed in the near field (**A**), midfield (**B**), and far field (**C**). Four focal points are shown (**D**), maximizing the image quality from near to far field. The images were made using a large curved array broadband transducer (1-8 MHz) operating in its mid-band imaging an ultrasound phantom. Only the focal points have been changed between images. Note how this transducer easily images to the 20-cm depth of the phantom. **A,** The single focus is placed at 4 cm, with excellent detail of the near-field cysts and large hyperechoic nodule. The deeper cysts and nodules are poorly visualized. **B,** The single focus is placed at 9-cm depth. There is better visualization of the mid and deeper cysts and nodules compared to **A. C,** The single focus is placed at 15-cm depth. This has increased the conspicuity of the deepest cystic structures and hypoechoic nodules at the expense of the midfield structures. **D,** Four focal points are shown, at 4, 7, 12, and 15 cm, producing the best overall image quality. The trade off is a reduction in frame rate when multiple focal points are used (e.g., 32 Hz to 10 Hz).

veterinary medicine. We use the following basic orientation standards, as do the editors of most veterinary journals. The beginner should remember that the top of the image is where the transducer contacts the patient (usually the skin surface) regardless of how the transducer is oriented. Most machines allow a vertical or horizontal change in the monitor's orientation to correspond to the transducer's orientation.

For abdominal scanning, the animal may be positioned on the table in dorsal recumbency with the head oriented away from the sonographer (or in lateral recumbency; scanning methodology is discussed in detail in Chapter 4). The top of the image on the monitor represents the transducer's position on the skin of the ventral abdomen. In the sagittal and dorsal planes, cranial is at the sonographer's left on the image (Figure 1-36, *A*). In the transverse plane, the right side of the animal is at the sonographer's left on the image (see Figure 1-36, *B*). The orientation of the image on the screen depends on the orientation of the transducer. Nearly every transducer has an indicator mark, such as a light, rib, bump, or dimple (see Figure 1-36, *C*), which corresponds to the edge of the ultrasound image on the screen (see Figure 1-8). For abdominal scanning, the transducer indicator is pointed cranially for sagittal and dorsal scan planes, and toward the operator for transverse scans. The screen indicator mark is positioned to the left edge of the image for abdominal scanning and to the right edge of the image for echocardiography.

If the transducer is placed on the right or left lateral aspect of the abdomen in dorsal or lateral recumbency, the top of the

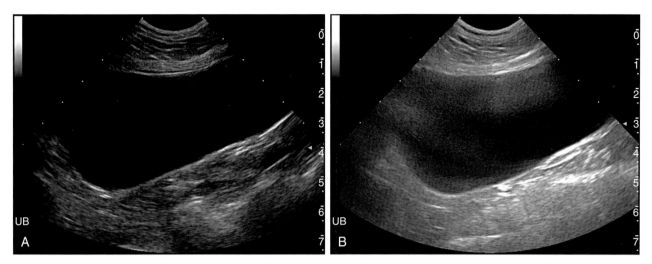

Figure 1-32 **Harmonic imaging. A,** Normal urinary bladder image using harmonic imaging. The bladder wall and surrounding tissues are very well delineated and the urine is anechoic and free of side lobe artifact. **B,** Urinary bladder image without harmonics. Compared to **A,** note the increase in artifact overlying the urinary bladder.

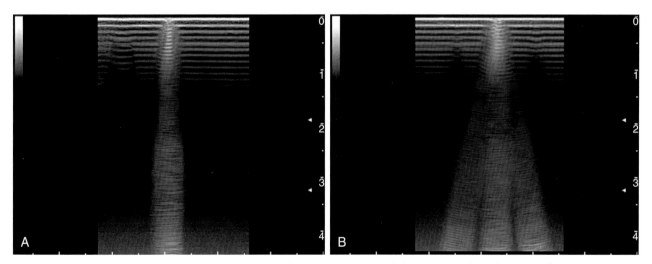

Figure 1-33 **Spatial compound imaging.** These images were made by touching a hypodermic needle transversely across the contact surface of a linear-array transducer. **A,** Nonspatial compound image. A single, strong reverberation ring-down artifact is seen arising from the metallic needle. This comet-tail artifact also illustrates the degradation of lateral resolution as the field of view becomes deeper. **B,** Spatial compound image. The identifying feature of compound imaging is the presence of multiple (three in this example) radiating comet-tail artifacts arising from the needle, a single point source.

viewed image on the monitor corresponds to the animal's right or left side, respectively (see Figure 1-36, *B*). If the image is obtained in a dorsal plane from the right or left lateral abdomen, cranial is at the sonographer's left on the image. When such an image is obtained from the right lateral abdomen in a transverse plane, ventral is at the sonographer's right on the image, and dorsal is to the left. From the left lateral abdomen in a transverse plane, ventral is at the sonographer's left on the image and dorsal to the right. Some sonographers may prefer to orient the displayed image so that the transducer is positioned to the left or right on the screen instead of the top. Not all machines are able to rotate the image, but it does more accurately represent the actual orientation of the sector image as it passes through the body.

Oblique planes are identified as sagittal oblique, transverse oblique, or dorsal oblique, according to whether the section is nearest to the sagittal, transverse, or dorsal plane. The plane used and the animal's right or cranial aspect should be marked on all scans.

Some confusion results when the sections through abdominal organs are named. A *plane* refers to the section through the entire body, whereas an *axis* or a *view* generally refers to the organ itself. For example, a long-axis or longitudinal view of a dog's stomach corresponds to an image in the transverse plane through the body. A short-axis or transverse view of the kidney would be done in nearly a transverse plane through the body, but a long-axis (longitudinal) view of the kidney could consist of an image in either a sagittal or dorsal plane.

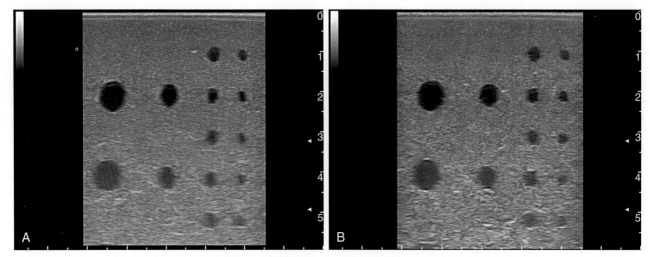

Figure 1-34 **The effect of spatial compounding on image quality.** One noticeable effect of compound imaging (**A**) is a smoother, slightly blurry image when compared with conventional (noncompound) imaging (**B**).

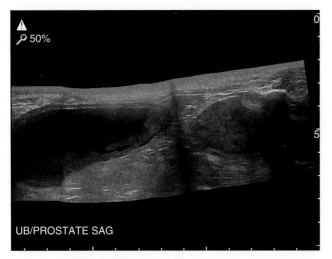

Figure 1-35 **Extended field of view image.** This extended field of view image of a urinary bladder neoplasm and prostatic enables a panoramic view of the extensive nature of the disease process.

Clear, consistent annotation of scan planes, axes, and views on hard copy or video clips is essential for communicating the findings to those not present during the examination.

IMAGE INTERPRETATION AND TERMINOLOGY

Ultrasonography is a technique that images anatomy in any desired tomographic plane. Therefore the sonographer must be familiar with normal three-dimensional anatomy to recognize artifacts, interpret normal variations, and detect pathologic changes. Publications correlating normal sectional anatomy of the dog and cat with ultrasonography, computed tomography, and magnetic resonance images provide excellent references for interpretation.[9-14] Some of the most useful resources for ultrasound imaging, however, are anatomy textbooks. Familiarity with gross anatomy, organ relationships, and vascular landmarks are extremely important, and every seasoned ultrasonographer has a plethora of anatomy texts at his or her disposal.

Box 1-1

Order of Increasing Echogenicity of Body Tissues and Substances

Bile, urine
Renal medulla
Muscle
Renal cortex
Liver
Storage fat
Spleen
Prostate
Renal sinus
Structural fat, vessel walls
Bone, gas, organ boundaries

As we have learned, specular echoes originate from interfaces at right angles to the ultrasound beam. These echoes produce boundaries between structures much as they would appear in a gross anatomic cross-section. For example, specular echoes are seen at arising from the surface of organs or at the walls of vessels. In contrast, nonspecular or scattered echoes summate to produce detectable parenchymal echoes and do not depend on the orientation of the small structures with respect to the beam. A dot on the screen does not necessarily represent a specific structure, and any relationship to the resulting image may be indirect. The parenchymal texture of organs is presumably related to the quantity and distribution of scattered echoes from the connective tissue framework. A mixture of specular and scattered echoes form ultrasound images, but the complex mechanism of echo production within tissues is not yet fully understood.

Blood or fluid that does not contain cells or debris is usually black on ultrasound images because few echoes are returned, although this is not always the case. As fluid gains viscosity from increased protein, cells, or debris, it may become more echogenic. There are exceptions to this and echogenicity is not a reliable indicator of fluid composition.

Normal parenchymal organs and body tissues are visualized as various shades of gray, which is fairly constant from animal to animal (Box 1-1). Diseases that diffusely involve

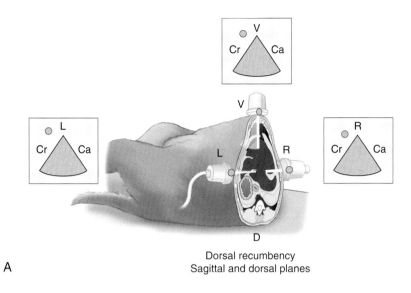

A
Dorsal recumbency
Sagittal and dorsal planes

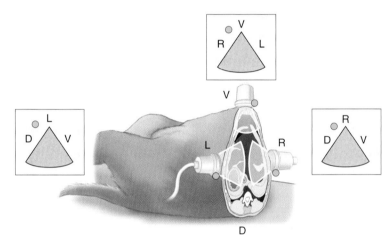

B
Dorsal recumbency
Transverse planes

Figure 1-36 **Transducer orientation and anatomy.** Image orientation and labeling in the sagittal and dorsal (**A**) and transverse (**B**) planes with the animal in dorsal recumbency. The drawings within the squares represent the ultrasound images of various transducer positions on the abdomen. **C,** Various forms of transducer orientation marks. *Ca,* Caudal; *Cr,* cranial; *D,* dorsal; *L,* left; *R,* right; *V,* ventral.

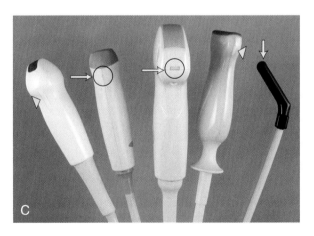

C

abdominal organs or tissues may alter the usual echogenicity relationship. Fat is generally thought to be highly echogenic, but low-level echoes are returned from fat in certain areas of the body, such as subcutaneous tissues of obese animals. Structural fat may be more echogenic than storage fat because of increased connective tissue content. Connective tissue usually appears highly echogenic, but certain uniform areas of fibrosis with few interfaces may actually appear relatively echo-free.

This is presumably because of the presence of relatively few interfaces at right angles to the beam.

Regions distal to highly attenuating structures, such as bone or gas, appear dark on the image because of shadowing. Artifacts such as shadowing must be differentiated from actual echo-poor regions produced by fluid or necrosis. Areas distal to regions of low sound attenuation may appear bright owing to an artifact termed *acoustic enhancement*. This

TABLE 1-5

Image Texture

Dot size	Small (fine), Medium, Large (coarse)	Uniform (regular, homogeneous)
		Nonuniform (irregular, heterogeneous)
Dot spacing	Close, Wide	Uniform (regular, homogeneous)
		Nonuniform (irregular, heterogeneous)

appearance must not be confused with regions of actual increased echogenicity.

Terms that are used to describe the appearance of ultrasound images should relate to a tissue's echo intensity (brightness), attenuation, and image texture (Box 1-2). These terms describe the ultrasound appearance relative to surrounding tissue or other structures. Terms using density, such as high- or low-echo density, are best avoided because a tissue's echogenicity is not always related to its density.

High attenuation and low attenuation are terms properly used to compare the appearance of a tissue or structure with surrounding echogenicity after the TGC controls have been adjusted. Specific terms, such as acoustic shadowing and distal acoustic enhancement, are commonly used to describe high and low sound attenuation by evaluating the echoes deep to a mass.

Terms used to describe image texture are perhaps the most difficult to standardize because interpretation is subjective. However, the size, spacing, and regularity of dots are important (Table 1-5). The dots may be small, medium, or large, and they may be closely or widely spaced. In addition, size and spacing may be uniform (regular, homogeneous) or nonuniform (irregular, heterogeneous).

Fine or coarse parenchymal texture refers to small or large dot size, respectively. A uniform texture suggests similar size and spacing of dots throughout the parenchyma. A heterogeneous texture suggests that the dot size, spacing, or both may vary throughout the parenchyma.

Uniform and nonuniform (homogeneous and heterogeneous) can refer to either echogenicity or texture. Therefore one should specify the echogenicity and texture separately. For example, one should specify heterogeneous parenchymal echogenicity or heterogeneous parenchymal texture, or both. Merely stating that there is a heterogeneous parenchymal appearance is confusing because echogenicity, texture, or both may be nonuniform.

IMAGING PITFALLS AND ARTIFACTS

Ultrasound artifacts are incorrect representations of anatomy or function (e.g., blood flow) and are ubiquitous, encountered to some degree during *every* ultrasound examination.[15-17] There are a variety of ultrasound artifacts that the sonographer must recognize and contend with because they may obscure normal anatomy or disease, or they may be misinterpreted as pathology. These can include equipment artifacts, technique artifacts, patient motion (always an issue in veterinary medicine), and artifacts resulting from the interaction of ultrasound with tissues. To recognize many of the artifacts produced during scanning, the ultrasonographer must be familiar with the interaction of ultrasound with tissues, as we have discussed. You will quickly observe, if you haven't already, that what you see on the ultrasound display may not be the true story. An excellent review of ultrasound artifacts was published in the veterinary literature by Kirberger (1995).[17]

Some artifacts are caused by improper use of equipment, control settings, or scanning procedures and can be avoided. These are discussed in Chapter 4. Other artifacts are beyond operator control and are inherent to basic physical assumptions made by even the most modern ultrasound technology. Assumptions are that ultrasound travels in a straight line and at a constant velocity, that echoes originate only from objects located in the primary beam axis, and that echo strength is related to the reflecting or scattering properties of the tissue or organ. Ultrasound artifacts occur when one or more of these assumptions are violated, displaying anatomic structures that are not real, missing, misplaced, or of incorrect echogenicity, shape, or size. Although many artifacts are deleterious, others are useful and can enhance interpretation (e.g., acoustic enhancement, acoustic shadowing, reverberation). Kremkau (2011) has nicely categorized ultrasound artifacts into those of propagation and attenuation.[1]

PROPAGATION ARTIFACTS

Secondary Lobe Artifact

Secondary lobe artifacts (commonly known as side-lobe and grating lobe) produce "ghost images" of off- axis structures (out of sight) on the displayed image (Figure 1-37, *A*). Secondary lobe artifacts are produced by minor secondary beams of ultrasound traveling off-axis to the primary beam. When secondary lobes of sufficient intensity interact with a highly reflective interface and return to the transducer, the returning echoes are erroneously displayed along the path of the main ultrasound beam even though they did not originate within the main beam. Curved surfaces, such as the diaphragm, bladder, and gallbladder, and a highly reflective interface, such as air, are common conditions in which side-lobe artifacts occur (see Figure 1-37, *B*). Secondary echoes are considerably less intense than those originating within the main beam, and they are best seen within anechoic structures such as the urinary and gallbladder where they create *pseudosludge* (Figure 1-38). Pseudosludge is a term indicating the presence of erroneous echoes within an anechoic structure, such as the urinary and gallbladder, resembling real abnormal bile or urine. Secondary lobes exhibit a threshold effect and will disappear or

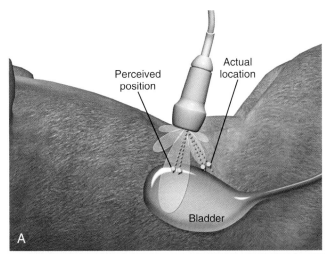

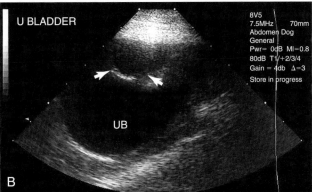

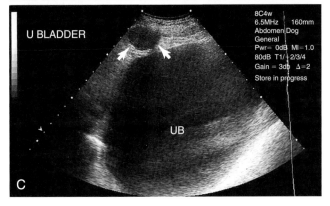

Figure 1-37 **Side lobe (secondary lobe) artifact. A,** Schematic representation of side-lobe artifact. Two strong reflective points (actual position) within one of the side lobes return a significant amount of energy that is erroneously displayed on the axis of the main beam (perceived position). **B,** Side-lobe artifact (*arrows*) within the urinary bladder (*UB*). **C,** The nearly anechoic round artifact in **B** is created by a hematoma (*arrows*) ventral to the urinary bladder (*UB*), easily seen in its true position by repositioning a lower frequency transducer.

be greatly reduced in brightness with lower instrument settings (gain, power), whereas real echoes persist. Secondary lobe artifacts may disappear when the focal point of an electronic transducer is positioned deeper or a different transducer is used (see Figure 1-37, C); these artifacts also vary in shape and intensity with different transducers. It is safe to say that secondary lobe artifacts are ubiquitous.

We have used the term secondary lobe to include side-lobe and grating lobe artifacts because in practice, both create erroneous ghost images overlying the primary image and are essentially indistinguishable. Technically, side-lobe artifacts can occur with any type of transducer, single-element or array; grating lobe artifacts occur only with array transducers, created by the interaction of multiple piezoelectric elements.[1] Side lobes occur just slightly off-axis of the primary beam, whereas grating lobes are produced at larger angles. An in vitro study was performed to reproduce side-lobe and grating lobe artifacts with different transducer types and to recognize these artifacts in vivo.[18] In that article, artifacts produced in vitro were recognized in vivo when a highly reflective object such as urinary bladder wall was imaged adjacent to an anechoic region (urine).

Slice Thickness Artifact

Slice thickness artifact resembles secondary lobe artifact by placing spurious echoes within an image, usually overlaying an anechoic structure. Indeed, the two artifacts may be indistinguishable at first glance. In the bladder and gallbladder, slice thickness artifact can mimic the presence of sediment (pseudosludge) (see Figure 1-38, *A, B*). Slice thickness artifact, as the name implies, occurs when part of the ultrasound beam's thickness (azimuth or Z-plane) is straddling the wall of a cystic structure such that part of the beam is inside and part of it is outside. Echoes originating from this part of the beam are erroneously displayed within the cystic structure on the image. The echoes disappear when the entire width of the beam is placed within the cystic structure. Slice thickness artifact is similar to the partial volume effect described in computed tomography (CT) and magnetic resonance imaging (MRI).

There are ways to differentiate this artifact from the true sediment. True sediment usually has a flat interface, whereas the surface of pseudosediment is curved. True sediment is always within the dependent portion of the bladder or gallbladder so changing the position of the animal will change the location of the sediment. The pseudosediment interface remains perpendicular to the incident beam, whereas the true sediment interface changes with position (see Figure 1-38, C). In addition, slice thickness artifact can be reduced by using higher frequency transducers and imaging within the focal zone. Slice thickness artifact is more prevalent with mechanical transducers because of large far-field beam divergence. Today's arrayed transducers have a much narrower beam width caused by electronic focusing.

Reverberation, Ring-Down, and Comet-Tail Artifacts

Reverberation artifacts (repetition artifacts) occur when the ultrasound beam repeatedly bounces between two highly reflective surfaces (usually gas or metal), or between the transducer and a strong reflector. Ultrasound is entirely reflected back from the gas and then bounces back and forth between the probe and the gas, creating multiple echoes from one ultrasound pulse (Figure 1-39). The number of reverberation images depends on the penetrating power of the beam and the sensitivity of the probe. If the echoes are sufficiently strong, they will be displayed as multiple repeating reflections deep to the real reflector (Figure 1-40) The skin-transducer interface is a common site of reverberation artifact (termed external reverberation), (see Figure 1-3, *B*). Internal reflectors, such as bone, gas, or metal, are also common causes of internal repetition. Reverberation differs according to the size, location, nature, and number of reflectors encountered. Classic examples of this artifact are the internal echoes created by superficial gas-filled bowel segments (see Figure 1-40) and the contact artifact created by the presence of a highly reflective interface (air) between the probe and the patient (see Figure 1-3, *B*).

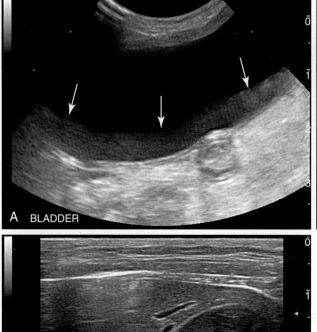

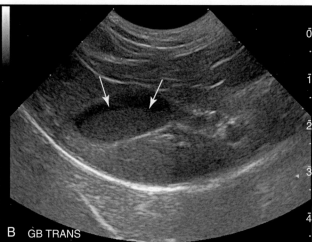

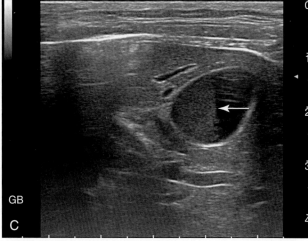

Figure 1-38 **Pseudosludge.** Pseudosludge is another manifestation of side lobe artifact. Both secondary (side) lobe and slice thickness artifacts can create the false impression of sludge within the urinary or gallbladder. **A,** Pseudosludge in urinary bladder, seen as an echogenic band in the far field of the urinary bladder *(arrows)*. **B,** Pseudosludge in the gallbladder, seen as a convex area of echogenicity within the majority of the lumen *(arrows)*. **C,** True sludge in the gallbladder. Note the distinct, flat interface of the echogenic bile with anechoic bile *(arrow)*. This is a transverse image obtained from the right side of the cranial abdomen; right is at the top of the image, ventral is to the right, and dorsal is to the left (see 1-36A for orientation).

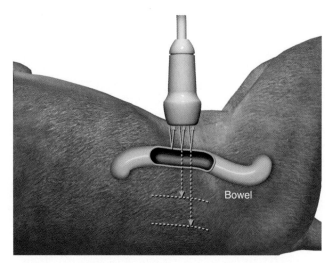

Figure 1-39 **Reverberation artifact.** Illustration showing the principle of the ultrasound reverberation artifact. In this example, the ultrasound beam reflects strongly off gas within the lumen of the bowel, so strongly that a portion of it then echoes off the transducer. This repeats itself, creating regularly spaced echogenic interfaces that are progressively deeper into the image.

The diffuse echoes between each reverberation are called ring-down artifacts, created by a bugle-shaped fluid interface trapped between at least two layers of gas bubbles.[17] Ring-down artifact has been described at the surface of diseased lung[19] and is commonly encountered when imaging the gastrointestinal tract.[17] The streaky nature of ring-down artifact has caused it to be confused with the comet-tail artifact. Although both artifacts contain a series of closely spaced echoes, which may even appear as a solid streak, ring-down and comet-tail artifact have completely different origins. Ring-down artifacts are streaks that are deep to gas pockets, whereas comet-tail artifacts are created by ultrasound interaction with metallic objects.[17]

The comet-tail artifact is easily recognized by a series of closely spaced, discrete, very bright, small echoes.[20] Comet-tail artifacts arise because of the very large acoustic impedance mismatch between metal and surrounding tissue. Comet-tail artifact is frequently encountered with metallic objects such as foreign bodies (e.g., gunshot pellets) or a biopsy needle. Figure 1-33 shows the striking appearance of comet-tail artifacts created by a metallic object (hypodermic needle).

Reverberation, ring-down and comet-tail artifacts are usually an annoyance, obscuring deeper structures. However, they can be a useful artifact if detected in unexpected locations, such as the peritoneal cavity (bowel rupture) or within external soft tissues where an abscess or metallic pellet is present.

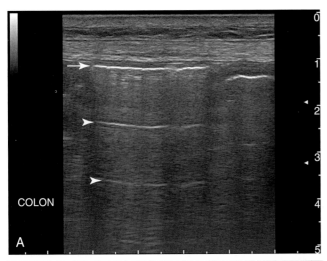

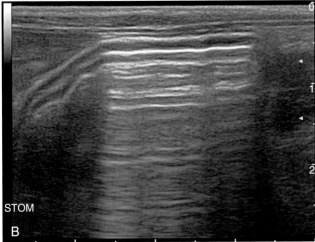

Figure 1-40 **Reverberation artifacts. A,** Reverberation artifact is seen in this image of the colon. The most superficial echogenic line is the true gas interface within the colon (*arrow*). Two repeating echogenic linear artifacts are seen in the deeper tissues, equally spaced (*arrowheads*). Note that the brightness of the repeating echoes diminishes with depth, due to attenuation. In between the reverberation artifacts there are echoes termed ring-down artifact. **B,** Reverberation and ring-down artifact created by gas within the stomach. The repeating lines of reverberation are not as distinct as in **A,** and the ring-down artifact is more pronounced.

Mirror Image Artifact (Multipath)

Errors in interpreting the location of an organ or structure can occur when a large reflector such as the diaphragm-lung interface is encountered. In these conditions, the most common artifact is the mirror image (Figure 1-41).

Mirror image artifacts are produced by curved, strongly reflective interfaces such as the diaphragm-lung interface. Part of the insonating beam is reflected back into the liver at an off-incident angle. The echoes from the liver return to the transducer along the same path through the diaphragm-lung interface. The ultrasound machine assumes that the sound pulse and the reflected echoes travel to and from the transducer in a straight line. If the echo return time is delayed because of multiple reflections (multipath), the machine places echoes of more superficial structures at deeper locations (cranial to the diaphragm) along the beam axis. A mirror image is produced in this erroneous position because of the increased round-trip time (Figure 1-42).

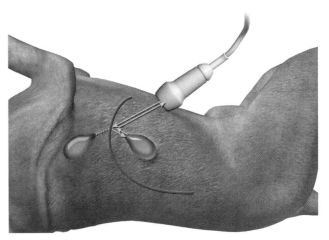

Figure 1-41 **Mirror image artifact.** In this illustration, the ultrasound has reflected off the curved surface of the lung-diaphragm interface and is now on course to interact with the gallbladder. Returning echoes follow the same course, eventually reaching the transducer. Because of the prolonged time it took for the reflected echoes to return, the gallbladder is now erroneously positioned deeper into the field of view, as is the surrounding liver. The true liver and gallbladder will also be seen in their proper positions.

The mirror image of the liver mimics this organ in the thoracic cavity immediately cranial to the diaphragm. This artifact may simulate a diaphragmatic hernia or lung consolidation. This artifact can occasionally occur wherever a highly reflective, curved interface exists. Mirror image artifacts may be seen when scanning the pelvic inlet (colon) or neck (trachea) and may occur in very unexpected locations.

Refraction

As discussed earlier, refraction is part of the normal interaction of ultrasound with tissue. But, refraction also produces misleading artifacts. Refraction of the ultrasound beam occurs when the incident sound wave traverses tissues of different acoustic impedances. The sound wave transmitted to the second medium changes direction (Figure 1-43). This may cause a reflector (e.g., an organ) to be improperly displayed. Numerous in vivo refraction artifacts, such as ghost artifact and organ duplication, have been described in humans. Ghost artifact, also called double-image artifact and split-image artifact, is a common artifact in pelvic examinations in women.[21,22] The rectus muscle and its associated variable prism of fat act as a lens to refract the ultrasound beam.[23,24] The refraction error appears as a double image. This artifact may lead to misdiagnosis and errors in measurement.

Organ duplication or even triplication artifact has similar physical characteristics. Kidneys in obese human patients are a common site for this artifact.[25] Refraction occurs between the spleen or liver and the adjacent fat and creates a duplication of the kidney. The artifacts of shadowing and enhancement, also partially due to refraction, are discussed separately.

Propagation Speed Error

Propagation speed error occurs when two tissues in the near field to an organ have different propagation velocities. This artifact can cause the borders of organs to be erroneously mildly displaced and appear irregular. It can also affect precise measurement of structures or lesions. A common example of this is the spleen and fat overlying the left kidney (Figure 1-44). Because the speed of ultrasound is about 1540 m/sec

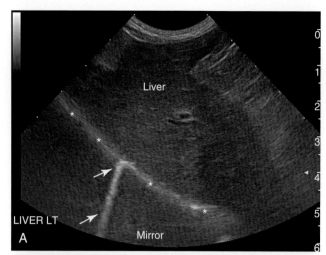

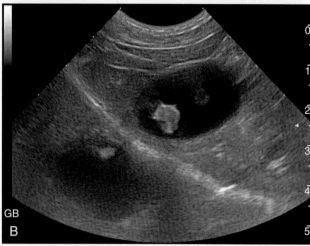

Figure 1-42 **Mirror image artifact.** **A,** An anomalous image of the liver (*Mirror*) has been placed into the thorax, to the left of the echogenic lung surface (******). A solitary ring-down artifact is seen, indicating an irregularity to the lung surface (*arrows*). **B,** In this example, the liver, gallbladder, and gallstones are seen as mirror images to the left of the lung/diaphragm interface.

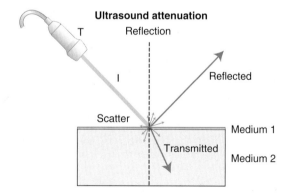

Figure 1-43 **Attenuation.** Illustration of reflection, refraction (transmitted beam), and scattering of the incident ultrasound beam as it crosses media of different acoustic impedances (Medium 1, Medium 2). *I,* Incident beam; *T,* Transducer.

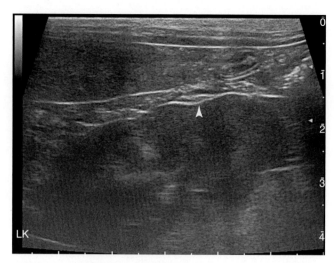

Figure 1-44 **Speed propagation error.** The surface of the left kidney (*LK*) is artifactually depressed (*arrowhead*) because the ultrasound is traveling slower through fat directly adjacent to it in the near field. The spleen is adjacent to the kidney in the near field to the left, and a loop of small intestine is to the right.

in the spleen but a bit slower in fat (1450 m/sec), the portion of the kidney deep to the fat is erroneously displayed as slightly deeper than it really is, yielding an uneven margin. This is because the ultrasound computer assumes a velocity of all ultrasound to be 1540 m/sec.

In people, fatty hyperechoic masses in the liver are associated with artifactual posterior displacement of the diaphragm. This erroneous displacement is explained by the lower speed of sound in fat, which lengthens the return time of echoes and hence increases the distance.[26] Other examples of erroneous diaphragmatic displacement are seen with abdominal or pleural effusion. The diaphragmatic discontinuity is due to sound beam refraction at the interface between the liver and the fluid.[27]

ATTENUATION

Shadowing

Acoustic shadowing appears as an area of low-amplitude echoes (hypoechoic to anechoic area) deep to structures of high attenuation. Acoustic shadowing results from nearly complete reflection or absorption of the sound.[28,29] The greater the amount of the beam's cross-section attenuated, the greater is the shadowing.[1] This artifact can be produced by gas or bone (see Figure 1-3). In the case of a soft tissue–gas interface, 99% of the sound is reflected, and the resulting shadow appears "dirty" (inhomogeneous) owing to multiple reflections or reverberations, or both (see Figure 1-3*A*). In the case of a soft tissue–bone interface, a significant portion of the ultrasound beam is absorbed; therefore reverberations are absent, and a "clean" (uniformly black) shadow is created (Figure 1-45). Urinary calculi and gallstones tend to behave like bone and create a strong, clean acoustic shadow (Figure 1-46). Barium in high concentration in a segment of bowel can also produce acoustic shadowing. It should be noted that small amounts of diluted barium may not shadow at all or be differentiated from intraluminal gas.

However, the concept of dirty and clean shadowing is far from absolute. On occasion, gas produces a sharp, clean shadow, and conversely, calcified structures can create dirty shadows. Size, location relative to the focal zone, transducer frequency, and composition of a calculus are critical to identification of distal shadowing. The calculus must be near the focal zone of the transducer and be at least as wide as the incident beam to create an obvious acoustic shadow.[30]

Calculi placed in a phantom do not necessarily produce an acoustic shadow. If calculi are placed in a wide part of a focused beam, there is insufficient attenuation of the beam and there is no apparent shadow.[17,31] Shadow characteristics appear to be independent of the internal composition of the structure; instead, they depend on the reflecting surface properties.[31,32]

Edge Shadowing

An acoustic shadow is occasionally seen distal to the lateral margins of rounded or cystic structures. This has been explained by the lower acoustic velocity through a fluid-filled structure, which refracts the ultrasonic beam at the fluid-tissue interface (see Figure 1-5).[30] This refraction at the margins of rounded structures is also called edge shadowing. It is regularly seen at the edges of a rounded structure, such as the bladder, gallbladder, adrenal gland, kidney, and even at the medulla-diverticulum junction of the kidney (Figure 1-47).

In vivo and in vitro studies have been performed to better understand the apparently confusing behavior of an incident beam on a circular region of higher or lower velocity. In a higher velocity region, the reflected beam is diverging because of the shape of the reflecting interface, and the refracted beam is also diverging (defocusing) because of variation in refracted angles across the beam. In a lower velocity circular region, the reflected beam is again diverging, whereas the refracted beam is now converging (focusing) because of the lens action of the region. In addition to this behavior, changes in the echo's size (caused by the focusing action and differential attenuation between the liquid within the cyst and the surrounding tissue) also induce edge shadowing.[29]

Scanning the caudal abdomen of a patient with peritoneal effusion, one can see a central, poorly echogenic portion of the bladder wall mimicking a wall defect[33] (Figure 1-48). The artifactual bladder wall defect is a result of acoustic shadowing caused by beam refraction.

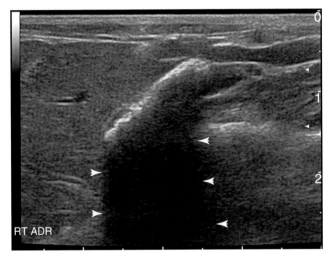

Figure 1-45 Acoustic shadowing. A mineralized right adrenal gland in a cat shows a complete ("clean") acoustic shadow (*arrowheads*), seen as an anechoic void deep to the echogenic surface of the adrenal gland.

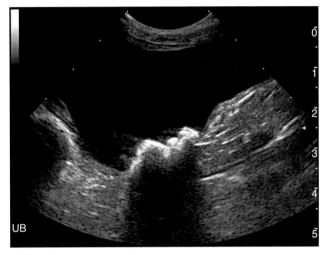

Figure 1-46 Acoustic shadowing. Multiple cystic calculi are creating a complete acoustic shadow.

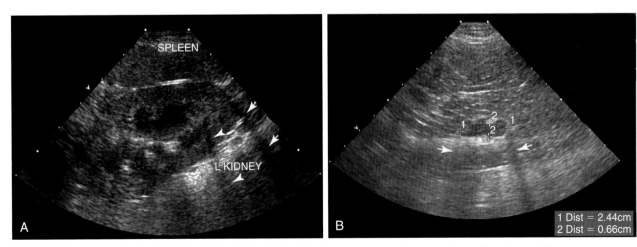

Figure 1-47 Edge shadowing. A, Dark edge shadows can be seen arising from the edges of the kidney (*arrows*) and the corticomedullary interface within the kidney (*arrowheads*). Additional edge artifacts are present but not annotated. **B,** Edge shadowing (*arrows*) can occur even from very small structures such as this adrenal gland, located between electronic cursors.

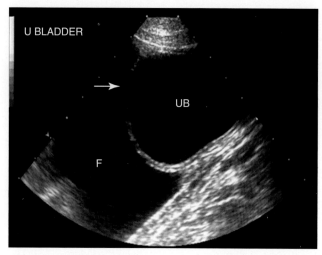

Figure 1-48 Edge shadowing. An edge shadowing is creating the false impression of a defect within the urinary bladder wall (*arrow*). Anechoic peritoneal fluid is present (*F*).

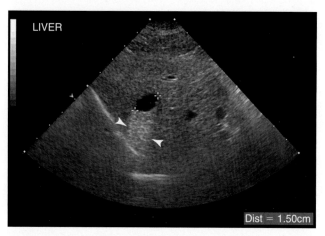

Figure 1-49 Acoustic enhancement. The liver parenchyma deep to the small anechoic liver cyst (between electronic cursors) is brighter than surrounding liver tissue at the same depth (*arrowheads*). This is because the ultrasound beam is not attenuated as it travels through the cyst and therefore has higher energy than adjacent ultrasound that has traveled through liver parenchyma. This is termed acoustic enhancement.

Enhancement

Acoustic enhancement (also called enhancement, through-transmission) represents a localized increase of echo amplitude occurring distal to a structure of low attenuation (Figure 1-49). On an ultrasound scan, enhancement appears as an area of increased brightness; this is commonly seen distal to both the gallbladder and the urinary bladder. This artifact is helpful in differentiating cystic structures from solid, hypoechoic masses. Cysts often have smooth, discrete borders; abscesses, granulomas, and tumors usually have irregular, ill-defined borders, whose forms also assist in differentiating different types of masses.

Enhancement and shadowing can also occur where they are unexpected. Hyperechoic masses with distal enhancement and anechoic masses with distal shadowing are occasionally seen. To understand these apparently contrary statements, we must return to some basic ultrasound physics. Attenuation of the sound beam is a result of absorption, reflection, and scattering; absorption is the principal contributor in a soft tissue

(see Figure 1-43). Therefore echogenicity (scattering level) and attenuation may not be correlated, and high and low echogenicity with either high or low attenuation are possible. Indeed, an echoic mass associated with distal enhancement indicates low attenuation through the lesion, despite the high echogenicity that probably occurs from scattering.

DOPPLER ULTRASONOGRAPHY

Doppler ultrasonography is the physical interaction of ultrasound with flowing blood; the Doppler effect occurs when ultrasound is reflected from moving blood cells. The reflected sound has a different frequency than the insonating frequency, the *Doppler shift*, which can be displayed in several ways to study blood flow. It can also be heard, because the Doppler shift is in the range of human hearing.

Doppler ultrasonography is used to detect the presence of blood flow, as well as direction, speed, and character of flow within vessels. It can differentiate blood vessels from nonvascular tubular structures (e.g., dilated bile ducts or renal diverticula). Doppler ultrasonography is also used to determine the presence of flow when thrombosis is suspected, and it has become essential in the detection of portosystemic shunts. In cardiology, Doppler is invaluable in detection of valvular insufficiencies, valvular and outflow stenoses, and septal defects. It is an accurate, noninvasive method of determining velocity, allowing calculation of blood flow and blood pressure.

Doppler ultrasonography can be simply classified as spectral or color (or a combination), based on how blood flow information is displayed. More correctly, perhaps, is to recognize that there are really four types of Doppler ultrasound based on physical principles of image formation: pulsed wave, continuous wave, color Doppler, and power color Doppler. Pulsed wave and continuous wave Doppler are termed *spectral* Doppler, displaying quantitative information as a time-velocity waveform along *x* and *y* axes (Figure 1-50, *A*). Color and power Doppler use color map overlays of blood flow on real-time, two-dimensional gray-scale images to display information (Figure 1-50, *B*, *C*). *Duplex* Doppler ultrasonography refers to simultaneous display of pulsed or continuous wave spectral Doppler tracings and B-mode images (Figure 1-51, *A*). *Triplex* Doppler is the combination of B-mode and color and spectral Doppler display information (Figure 1-51, *B*).

In veterinary practice, color and power Doppler are used more extensively than pulsed wave (PW) or continuous wave (CW), because interpretation of color maps is easier and more intuitive than assessing spectral maps. Spectral Doppler is used daily in veterinary cardiology practice where precise measurement of blood flow is necessary. In abdominal imaging, one of the principle uses of spectral Doppler is differentiating arterial from venous blood flow and assessing waveforms of the portal vein and caudal vena cava. Clinical use of Doppler is presented in organ-specific chapters.

An in-depth review of the physical principles of Doppler ultrasonography is encouraged for the interested reader, because it is well beyond the scope of this textbook.[1]

PRINCIPLES OF DOPPLER

The Doppler effect, as it pertains to ultrasonography, results from an apparent shift in sound frequency as sound waves are reflected from moving targets, usually blood cells. If motion is toward the transducer, the frequency of the returning echoes is higher than that of the transmitted sound (a positive shift). If the motion is away from the transducer, the echoes have a lower frequency than the transmitted sound (a negative shift)

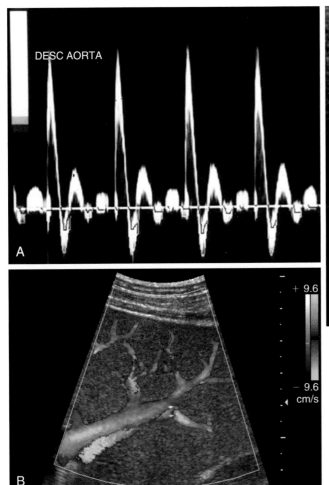

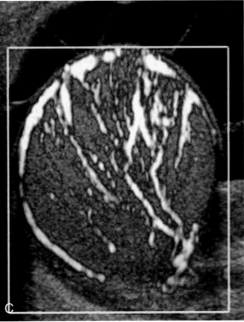

Figure 1-50 **Spectral, color, and power Doppler.** A, Spectral Doppler displays blood flow information in the form of a graph, with the *y*-axis representing blood velocity, the *x*-axis representing time. B, Color Doppler displays blood flow information as a color map overlay on a real-time B-mode image. C, Power Doppler also displays blood flow information as a color map overlay on a real-time B-mode image, although the type of information differs from color Doppler.

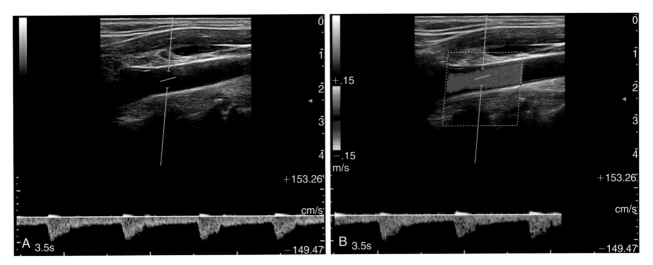

Figure 1-51 **Duplex and triplex Doppler.** A, Duplex Doppler displays spectral Doppler and real-time B-mode together on the ultrasound screen. B, Triplex Doppler displays spectral Doppler and color or power Doppler together with a B-mode image.

(Figure 1-52). The difference between the transmitted and received frequencies is known as the Doppler shift. The greater the Doppler shift, the greater the velocity. However, the Doppler shift will not be as great if the transmitted beam is not parallel to blood flow. A correction factor must be applied that takes into account the incident angle of the transmitted beam. The Doppler equation describes this relationship:

$$f = 2Fv\cos(a)/c$$

where f (Hz) is the Doppler shift frequency (frequency difference between the transmitted and reflected sound), F (Hz) is the original transmitted sound frequency, v (m/sec) is the velocity of the moving target, a is the angle between the incident beam and the target's direction of motion, and c is the speed of sound in the body (1540 m/sec for soft tissue). The equation is usually rearranged to solve for the velocity of the target as follows:

$$v = fc/2F\cos(a)$$

Figure 1-53 shows the relationship of the Doppler beam and angle of incidence to the blood vessel. As the incident beam becomes parallel to the direction of blood flow [angle of

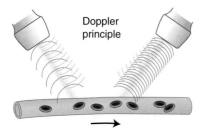

Figure 1-52 The Doppler principle. This illustration depicts the most fundamental principle of Doppler ultrasonography. Blood flow is from left to right. Blue waves represent the insonating Doppler ultrasound frequency for each transducer. The transducer on the left is positioned so that blood flow is moving away from the ultrasound beam. The returning reflected ultrasound waves (red) are further apart depicting a lower returning frequency, known as a negative Doppler shift. The transducer on the right is directing its ultrasound beam toward the oncoming blood flow. The resultant returning ultrasound frequency is higher (more closely spaced red waves), a positive Doppler shift.

incidence approaches zero and cos(a) approaches 1], a maximal frequency shift is produced and the angle has minimal effect on the resulting calculations. The objective of Doppler evaluation is to orient the incident beam as parallel to flow as possible to prevent calculation errors associated with large incident angles. This is possible on evaluation of flow in the heart and great vessels but difficult on evaluation of flow in peripheral vessels traveling nearly parallel to the skin's surface. An angle of incidence of less than 60 degrees is desired but often difficult to obtain. Small changes in incident angle above 60 degrees result in significant changes in calculated velocity.

The most important concept with Doppler is that the frequency of the returned echoes is compared with the original frequency of the transmitted sound. The difference is usually in the kilohertz range and audible when sent to the loudspeaker of the Doppler unit. Information is also visually presented on the video monitor as a Doppler spectral display consisting of frequency shift (kHz) or velocity (cm/sec) on the vertical axis versus time on the horizontal axis. It may also be viewed as a color map.

PULSED WAVE DOPPLER ULTRASONOGRAPHY

With pulsed wave (PW) Doppler ultrasonography, sound is transmitted in pulses as in real-time B- and M-mode imaging. The site of the echo's origin can be determined precisely by the time delay for return. Echoes arising from moving blood will arrive at the transducer during a discrete interval corresponding to the vessel's *depth*. If the echoes during this interval are the only ones accepted and processed, the frequency difference between the transmitted and reflected sound from that particular blood vessel can be determined. This process is known as *range gating*, in which the gate is opened and closed to accept echoes only from a particular depth. Superimposition of the gate's location (depth) and the size of the gate *(sample volume)* on the two-dimensional display, in the form of a movable rectangular cursor, enables precise placement within the region of interest (see Figure 1-53). The gate cursor can be moved along a line drawn parallel to the incident beam on the screen. Superimposed on the gate is a longer linear cursor that can be rotated so that it is aligned parallel to the direction of blood flow. This cursor permits determination of the transmitted beam's incident angle to the direction of flow (see Figure 1-53).

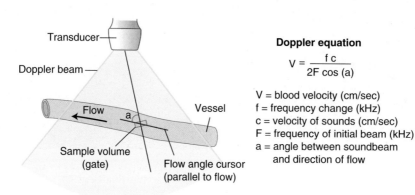

Doppler equation

$$V = \frac{fc}{2F\cos(a)}$$

V = blood velocity (cm/sec)
f = frequency change (kHz)
c = velocity of sounds (cm/sec)
F = frequency of initial beam (kHz)
a = angle between soundbeam and direction of flow

Figure 1-53 Duplex Doppler ultrasonography. Duplex Doppler ultrasonography superimposes a Doppler beam indicator and sample volume (gate) on a real-time B-mode image display. The Doppler beam indicator represents the angle of the incident beam. The sample volume shows the location and size of the area sampled. A manually rotated cursor can be aligned parallel to a blood vessel to determine the beam's incident angle to the vessel.

The transducer used for pulsed Doppler ultrasonography is the same as that used for real-time B- and M-mode imaging. For modern electronic transducers, when the PW Doppler is in use, a real-time B-mode image may be simultaneously displayed on the screen, allowing proper placement of the Doppler cursor (duplex, triplex Doppler). Older mechanical transducers dictate that either a Doppler image or a B-mode image are displayed at one time. In this case, the operator can toggle between real-time Doppler or B-mode images, or the machine can be set to update images periodically (e.g., every 2 seconds).

Pulsed wave is the most commonly used type of spectral Doppler because it is readily available on nearly all modern transducers and it possesses depth discrimination. Its major limitation is that it cannot accurately assess very high blood flow (e.g., as seen with aortic or pulmonary stenosis), becoming "overloaded" by higher velocities (aliasing).

CONTINUOUS WAVE DOPPLER ULTRASONOGRAPHY

Continuous wave (CW) Doppler ultrasonography is also used to determine blood flow and direction, but it uses a special transducer with two crystals that is not by itself capable of two-dimensional imaging. Sound is transmitted and received *continuously* by use of the separate transmitting and receiving crystals. *Continuous wave Doppler ultrasonography does not possess depth discrimination.* Therefore anything moving within the path of the beam is sampled, including multiple vessels or heart chambers (this concept is important because we later discuss the difference between a CW spectral waveform and PW Doppler). However, continuous wave Doppler ultrasonography can measure much higher flow velocities than pulsed Doppler ultrasonography can, because sampling is continuous with no waiting for echoes to return. Continuous wave Doppler ultrasonography is essential for recording high velocities distal to stenotic lesions. This is the major advantage of CW Doppler and it is used extensively in echocardiology.

In the days before multielement transducers, the exact path of the CW beam needed to be determined blindly, by the characteristics of the Doppler spectral and/or audible Doppler shift. Phased array transducers now allow CW Doppler spectral display with periodically updated real-time B-mode images. Though essential for echocardiography, CW Doppler is not generally necessary for abdominal ultrasonography.

INTERPRETATION OF THE DOPPLER SPECTRAL DISPLAY

As noted, spectral Doppler is either pulsed wave or continuous wave . Both display a *spectrum* of Doppler frequencies. The Doppler spectral display presents flow information as a function of time. Time is plotted on the horizontal axis, and velocity is plotted on the vertical axis (Figure 1-54). The horizontal baseline in the Doppler spectral tracing indicates the point of zero frequency shift (no flow) in the returning echoes. By convention, the spectral tracing is *above* the zero baseline when the returned echo frequency is higher than the transmitted frequency, with flow directed *toward* the transducer. A tracing *below* the baseline indicates that flow is directed *away* from the transducer, and the returned frequency is lower than the insonating frequency (see Figure 1-52).

The width (vertical thickness) of the spectral trace at any point in time indicates the range of blood cell velocities (frequency shifts) present. A large range of flow velocities at a

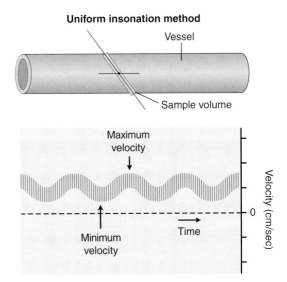

Uniform insonation method

Figure 1-54 Spectral Doppler display: uniform insonation method. The Doppler spectral display shows velocity or frequency shift on the vertical axis and time on the horizontal axis. Flow is directed toward the transducer if the tracing is above the baseline and away from the transducer if the tracing is below the baseline. The width of the tracing represents the range of blood cell velocities (frequency shifts) encountered; the gray scale within the tracing represents the number of blood cells traveling at a particular velocity. The uniform insonation method can be used to determine the average flow velocity within a vessel. The sample volume encompasses the entire vessel with the uniform insonation method. Therefore the spectral display reflects the range of all velocities within the vessel.

particular point in the pulse cycle is called *spectral broadening,* seen as increased width of the waveform. This is usually seen with significant vessel narrowing and turbulence. Excessive gain or changes in the gray-scale dynamic range, large sample volumes, or placement of the sample volume too close to the vessel wall may falsely suggest spectral broadening and lead to diagnostic error.

The gray-scale brightness (echogenicity) of the tracing represents the *number* of red blood cells traveling at a particular velocity. The brightness (gray scale) of the waveform is also used to represent the amplitude of each frequency component. As for B-mode imaging, brightness is affected by Doppler gain settings, discussed later in the section, Doppler Controls.

There is one important difference between a PW and CW spectral tracing. Because CW data is not depth specific but includes blood flow at all depths along the cursor, the area under the spectral waveform is nearly always filled in with echoes of varying brightness. By contrast, a PW tracing showing plug flow will have an anechoic area under the waveform, because all the blood cells are moving at essentially the same velocity (no spectral broadening) (Figure 1-55). In other words, a typical CW waveform will show the ultimate expression of spectral broadening.

As noted, ultrasound scanners have the ability to automatically calculate average frequency shift, or velocity. Average blood flow may then be calculated by multiplying the average velocity by the cross-sectional area of the vessel. The vessel's diameter and blood velocity may change during the cardiac cycle or with respiration, which is displayed on the spectral tracing. Average vessel diameter and velocity must be used to obtain reliable measurements of average blood flow.

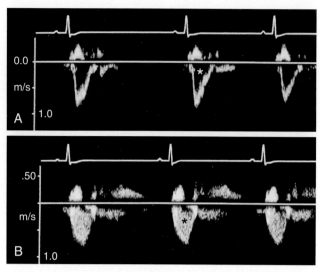

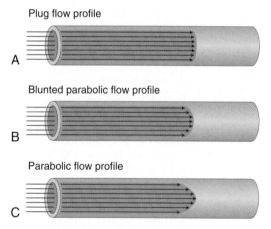

Figure 1-55 Comparison of Pulse Wave and Continuous Wave Doppler Spectral Waveforms. These waveforms are of the right ventricular outflow tract of a normal dog. **A,** Pulse wave Doppler showing very uniform blood velocity, with a large anechoic area under the spectral tracing (*white* *). **B,** Continuous wave Doppler shows an echogenic area under the spectral tracing filled with echoes (*black* *), termed spectral broadening.

Figure 1-56 Blood flow velocity profiles. Blood flow velocity profiles are different in arteries and veins and vary with the vessel's size. Plug profiles are found in larger arteries (**A**), whereas blunted parabolic (**B**) and parabolic (**C**) profiles are characteristic of smaller vessels.

Blood normally flows faster near the center of a vessel's lumen and slower near its walls. The flow profile is different in arteries and veins and varies with the vessel's size and location. Large arteries may have a plug flow profile (Figure 1-56, *A*), whereas smaller vessels have a blunted parabolic (see Figure 1-56, *B*) or parabolic (see Figure 1-56, *C*) flow. A spectrum of shift frequencies is returned if the entire lumen is sampled.

If the sample volume is adjusted to sample the entire lumen of the vessel, a spectrum of returned frequencies representing all velocities present within the lumen is displayed (see Figure 1-54). As noted, the width of the tracing indicates the range of velocities present within the sample volume. The gray scale (brightness) in any portion of the tracing represents the relative number of blood cells traveling at that particular velocity. The tracing is usually displayed as white on black so

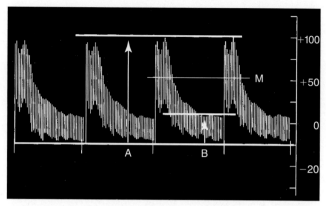

Figure 1-57 Resistive flow indices. Doppler flow indices are used to characterize resistance to flow in peripheral vascular beds. These indices are based on the peak systolic velocity or frequency (*A*), the end-diastolic velocity or frequency (*B*), and the mean velocity or frequency (*M*). The most commonly used indices are the systolic-to-diastolic ratio [S/D = A/B], the resistive index [RI = (A − B)/A], and the pulsatility index [PI = (A − B)/M]. These indices have been advocated over absolute velocity measurements because they are independent of the angle of insonation and less subject to error. Changes in these indices may help identify alterations in vascular resistance associated with transplant rejection, parenchymal dysfunction, or malignant disease.

that the whitest areas of the tracing represent the greatest number of red blood cells. The average velocity depends on the percentage of cells traveling at a particular velocity throughout the cardiac or respiratory cycle. It is not sufficient to use the middle of the Doppler spectral tracing as the average velocity because the number of cells at a particular velocity (gray scale) is not taken into account. The average velocity or frequency shift is calculated automatically on most Doppler ultrasound units. Broadening (increased width) of the spectral tracing is seen in such diseases as valvular stenosis, regurgitation, and intracardiac shunting because turbulence causes an increased range of velocities.

Arteries are easily identified with spectral Doppler by their pulsatile waveform. By comparison, most veins have relatively nonpulsatile waveforms, with lower average velocities than arteries. The venae cavae and hepatic veins are exceptions and are discussed in Chapter 5.

Stenosis of vessels is associated with large frequency shifts in both systole and diastole at the point of maximal narrowing. Turbulent flow is noted in the poststenotic regions. Analysis of these changes allows prediction of the degree of vessel narrowing. Resistance to flow in the vascular bed distal to the point of measurement can also be estimated. Increased resistance reduces diastolic flow. Doppler indices such as the systolic-to-diastolic ratio (S/D), resistive index (RI), and pulsatility index (PI) allow comparison of flow in systole and diastole (Figure 1-57). These indices are used to evaluate stenosis, thrombosis, or more commonly, increased resistance to flow in peripheral vessels.

COLOR DOPPLER

Most modern Doppler units will color-code blood velocity measurements over a wide area of the field of view and superimpose this information on the two-dimensional B-mode gray-scale image (Figure 1-58). Using pulsed wave Doppler technology, signals from moving red blood cells are displayed in color as a function of their motion toward or away from the transducer. The amount of color saturation also indicates the relative velocity of the cells. For example, yellows, oranges, and reds may represent flow directed toward the transducer, with yellow-white representing the highest measured velocities. Flow away from the transducer may be represented as shades of blue and green, with the highest velocities displayed as green-white. Figure 1-59 depicts the relationship and differences of color and spectral Doppler.

Color Doppler obtains *mean* flow velocity information over a large area rather than specific velocities at a localized site within tissue (Figure 1-60). This is accomplished by obtaining frequency shift information from many sample volumes (gates) along a single line instead of from the single sample volume used with conventional pulsed wave Doppler. Color flow displays are easier to interpret, and there is less risk of missing important flow information because a wide area is evaluated simultaneously. In addition, small vessels are

easier to visualize than with conventional imaging. Vessels identified with color Doppler (or power Doppler) can then be critically assessed using pulsed wave Doppler if necessary.

The color Doppler bar displayed on the screen represents mean velocity of the sampled area, the color map (Figure 1-61). The bar is divided by a thin black line representing no blood flow (0 velocity). Above and below center are the color maps. Usually red-yellow hues are above and blue hues below center. In this example, blood flow towards the transducer is depicted as red, and blood flow away from the transducer is blue. The deep shades of color represent low velocities, and the lighter shades or change in color represent higher velocities. There are velocity scale indicators at each end of the bar that represent the maximum mean velocity that can be displayed without aliasing. The smaller the number, the more sensitive the system is in detecting low flow. Conversely, higher numbers indicate the ability to map higher velocity blood flow without aliasing. These numbers are directly related to the pulse repetition frequency (PRF), discussed momentarily. All color Doppler machines have a variety of

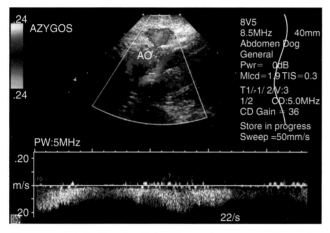

Figure 1-58 **Color Doppler.** Color flow and conventional Doppler imaging (parallel cursors represent the sample volume) can be obtained simultaneously with higher end ultrasound units. Color flow Doppler information is superimposed on the two-dimensional display and is useful to identify a variety of vascular abnormalities. One can simultaneously determine arterial versus venous flow, flow velocity, and direction of flow and obtain a Doppler spectral display.

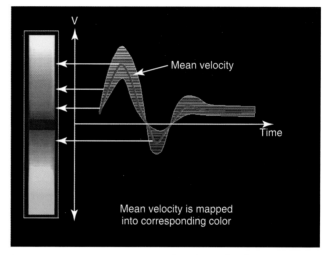

Figure 1-60 **Mean velocity map.** The relationship between pulsed wave Doppler and mean velocity information is displayed with color Doppler.

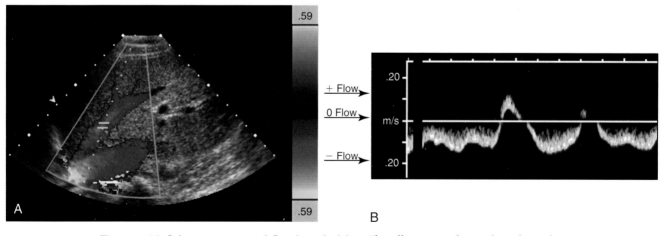

Figure 1-59 **Color versus spectral Doppler principles.** This illustration shows the relationship between color Doppler (A) pulsed wave (PW) (B). Within the large sector window on the color display (A), PW technology is used to sample frequency shifts and create a color map overlay of blood flow on a B-mode image. The thin black band between the red and blue color map represents 0 flow. Color Doppler displays mean velocity, not peak velocity, as does PW Doppler.

color maps to choose from, represented by color bars (Figure 1-62). It is important to note that the color bar can be reversed (Figure 1-63). This is routinely done in human vascular ultrasound studies so that arteries appear as red and veins, as blue.

Velocity-variance (VV) is another type of color Doppler map (bar), depicting the amount of blood flow variance in addition to velocity (Figure 1-64). Laminar blood flow has little or no variance, whereas high variance is seen in areas of stenosis. Velocity-variance bars depict mean velocity on the vertical axis (identical to the color Doppler bar just described), and the horizontal axis of the bar represents variance; the lowest variance is along the left side of the bar, the highest variance along the right. VV maps are used primarily in echocardiology. As for conventional color Doppler maps, a variety of VV maps are available, depending on user preference and application.

Two disadvantages of color flow Doppler imaging are that (1) only *mean* velocity in a particular area is displayed, and (2) the maximal velocity that can be detected is limited. Color Doppler is also relatively insensitive to low flow volumes. Additionally, color Doppler imaging is angle dependent, similar to spectral Doppler imaging; it is subject to aliasing

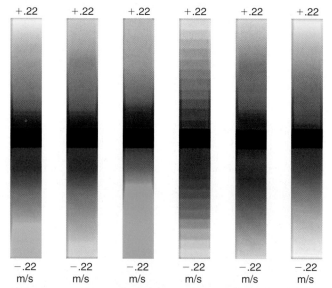

Figure 1-62 **Color Doppler color bars.** A variety of color Doppler maps are available, represented by color bars. The color bars indicate mean velocity and direction. The number at the top and bottom of each bar represents the maximum mean velocity displayed before aliasing occurs. Increasing the pulse repetition frequency (PRF) creates a larger number and thus the ability to sample higher velocities. Conversely, lowering the PRF reduces the scale and increases Doppler sensitivity to lower velocity blood flow.

Figure 1-61 **The color Doppler bar.** Color represents mean velocity at sample area. Velocity scale indicators appear at each end. Toward the transducer is one color (i.e., red), away from the transducer is another (i.e., blue). Shade indicates the velocity of blood flow. Deep shades indicate low velocities, lighter shades or a change in color indicates higher velocities. Baseline or 0 velocity is depicted as black, between the blue and red hues.

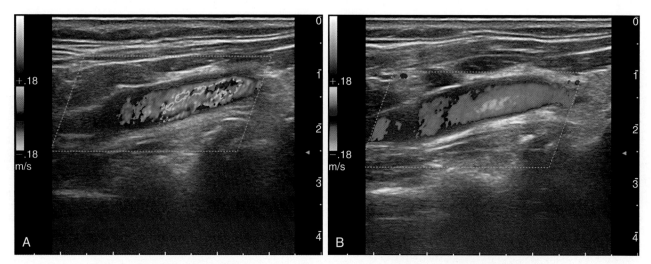

Figure 1-63 **Color bar reversal.** **A,** The color Doppler bar is displayed with red above baseline, blue below. In this example, blood flow is blue and from right to left, away from the transducer (below baseline, blue). **B,** The color bar has been reversed so that blue is now above baseline and red is below. The blood vessel is now seen as red. Blood flow is still from right to left, away from the transducer, since red is below baseline. This figure illustrates that color flow maps do not necessarily indicate arterial versus venous blood.

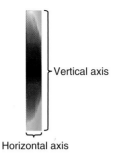

Figure 1-64 **Velocity variance color bar.** Another way to map color Doppler blood flow is the velocity-variance (VV) map. Mean velocity is depicted on the vertical axis (as with standard color Doppler bar), and in addition, variance of blood flow is depicted horizontally across the color bar.

and noise artifacts, and it may not represent the entire Doppler spectrum. Therefore the precision is not as high as what is obtainable with a full spectral analysis using conventional pulsed or continuous wave Doppler ultrasonography. Color flow Doppler examination is presently best used to detect flow abnormalities that may be missed with the discrete, small-volume sampling techniques of conventional Doppler ultrasonography. Fortunately, all color flow Doppler units are also capable of conventional, range-gated Doppler spectral analysis. Therefore more precise data can be obtained and quantitated from these areas with use of standard Doppler techniques.

POWER DOPPLER

Power Doppler displays a color map overlay on real-time B-mode images, just as with color Doppler. However, the blood flow information presented is much different. Power Doppler ultrasonography displays the *integrated power, energy,* or *strength* of the Doppler signal instead of the mean frequency shift used with color Doppler imaging (Figure 1-65).[34] It is the *concentration* of the red blood cells that determines the power of the Doppler. There is no aliasing with power Doppler ultrasonography because frequency shift is not displayed and power Doppler is essentially independent of angle of insonation (see Figure 1-68, *D*). This makes power Doppler very sensitive to slow flow and detection of small and deep blood vessels. The trade-off is that information regarding flow velocity, turbulence, and direction is unavailable, although some manufactures now offer directional power Doppler, combining pulsed wave technology with power Doppler (see Figure 1-67, *C*).

Unlike color Doppler ultrasonography, in which noise may appear as any color in the image, power Doppler ultrasonography allows assignment of a homogeneous background color to noise. This permits higher gain settings and lower pulse repetition frequencies, with increased sensitivity for flow detection in small vessels and those with slow flow. The amplitude of noise signals is much lower than the blood echo amplitude, resulting in an excellent signal-to-noise ratio; the noise amplitude does not corrupt blood echo amplitude. This allows power Doppler to display blood flow to virtually the noise floor. The main disadvantage of power Doppler is that it is more sensitive to artifactual *motion* (patient or transducer), and the frame rate tends to be slower than with color Doppler imaging.

The power Doppler color bar differs from the color Doppler bar. First, the power Doppler bar is read *horizontally.* The energy signal is coded to a color map where different hues

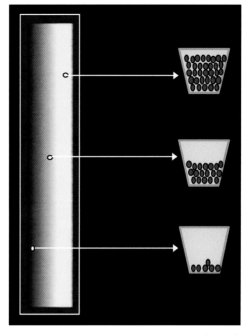

Figure 1-65 **Power Doppler.** Energy is proportional to echo amplitude. Each energy signal is assigned a unique hue. Hue is related to the number of blood cells in a sample volume. Hue is not related to velocity of blood.

TABLE 1-6

Comparison of Power versus Color Doppler: Advantages and Disadvantages

ADVANTAGES (+) AND DISADVANTAGES (−)	
Power Doppler	**Color Doppler**
− No velocity	+ Velocity
− No direction	+ Direction
+ Sensitivity	− Sensitivity
+ No aliasing	− Aliasing artifact
+ Angle to flow independence	− Angle to flow dependence

correspond to different energy levels; each hue represents a different number of moving blood cells. Color brightness is related to the *number* of moving blood cells, not the mean velocity as with color Doppler. Darker hues to the left represent lesser numbers of blood cells, whereas to the right the lighter hues represent higher numbers of blood cells (Figure 1-66). The user can select a number of different color maps from a menu; color maps differ by manufacturer.

Figure 1-67 shows the differences in color and power Doppler image displays. Table 1-6 compares and summarizes the advantages and disadvantages of power Doppler and color Doppler.

INSTRUMENTATION

Doppler instruments are available on mechanical sector and various array scanners. Mechanical scanners must stop movement of the crystals to perform Doppler evaluations, and the two-dimensional image is frozen while the Doppler sample is

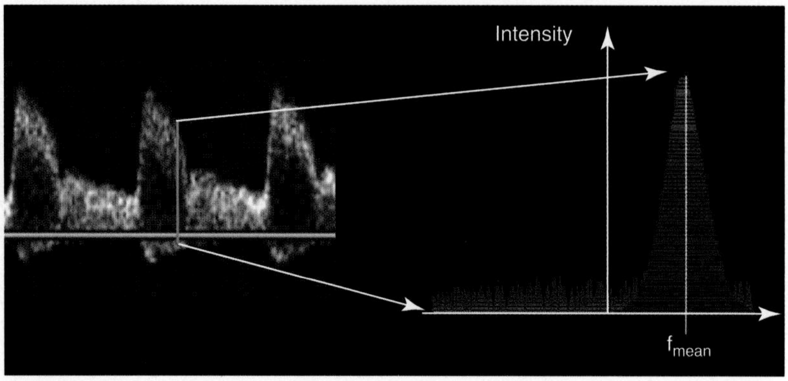

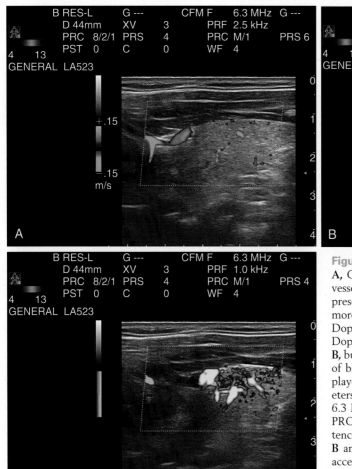

Figure 1-66 Power Doppler color bar. Energy is the summation of all echo intensities present in a power density spectrum. It is the area under the power density spectrum curve.

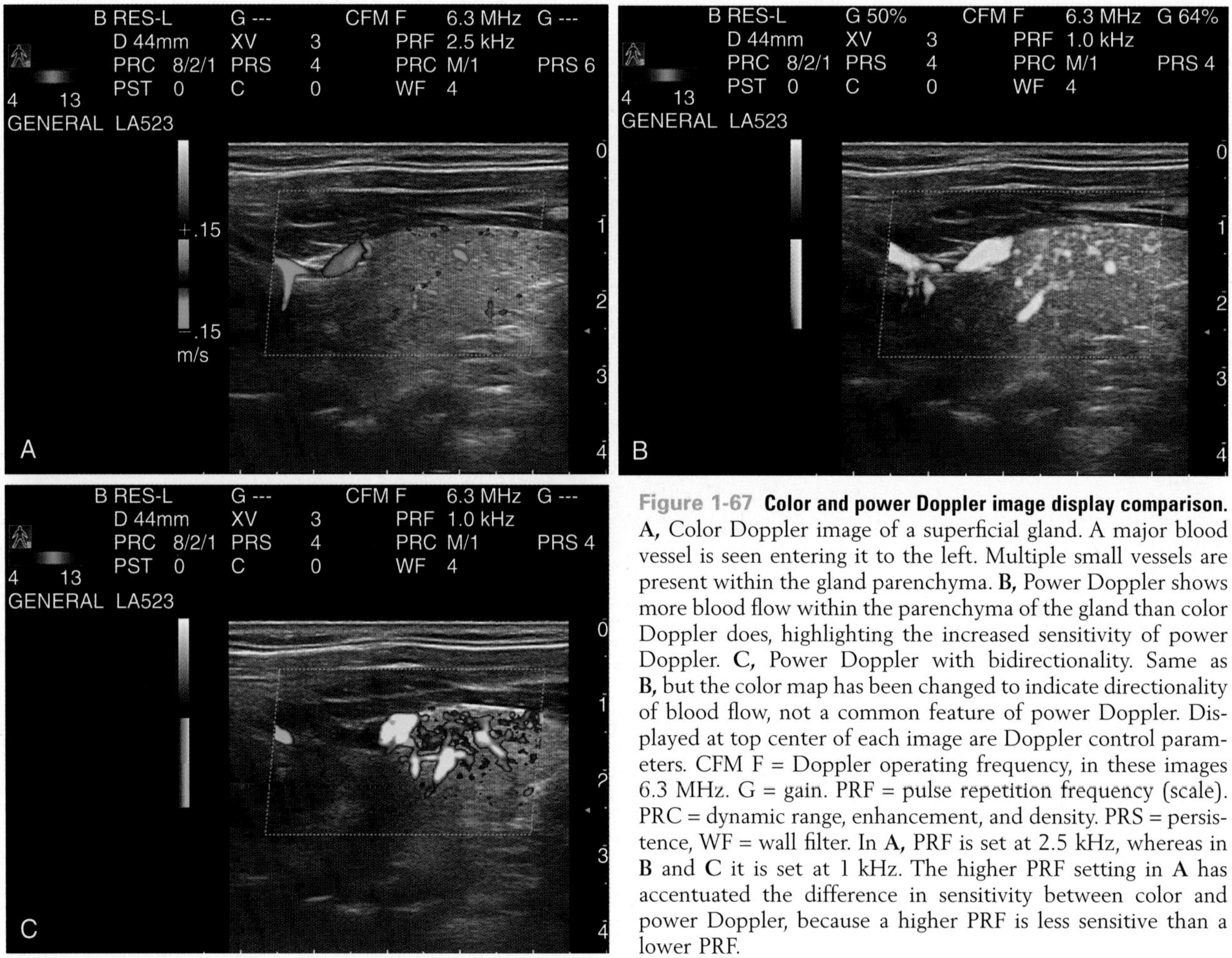

Figure 1-67 Color and power Doppler image display comparison. A, Color Doppler image of a superficial gland. A major blood vessel is seen entering it to the left. Multiple small vessels are present within the gland parenchyma. **B,** Power Doppler shows more blood flow within the parenchyma of the gland than color Doppler does, highlighting the increased sensitivity of power Doppler. **C,** Power Doppler with bidirectionality. Same as **B,** but the color map has been changed to indicate directionality of blood flow, not a common feature of power Doppler. Displayed at top center of each image are Doppler control parameters. CFM F = Doppler operating frequency, in these images 6.3 MHz. G = gain. PRF = pulse repetition frequency (scale). PRC = dynamic range, enhancement, and density. PRS = persistence, WF = wall filter. In **A,** PRF is set at 2.5 kHz, whereas in **B** and **C** it is set at 1 kHz. The higher PRF setting in **A** has accentuated the difference in sensitivity between color and power Doppler, because a higher PRF is less sensitive than a lower PRF.

taken. The image may be updated at frequent intervals selected by the operator, but simultaneous imaging and Doppler sampling are not possible. Therefore movement of the transducer or animal during acquisition of Doppler data requires repositioning of the Doppler gate in the desired location with use of two-dimensional imaging.

Array scanners are capable of acquiring nearly simultaneous image and flow information by special phasing of pulses because there are no moving parts. The Doppler pulse is interspersed between imaging pulses. It is much easier to maintain the sample volume in the desired location with array scanners while acquiring Doppler data.

DOPPLER CONTROLS

The Doppler controls are usually grouped logically into one section of the ultrasound machine, separate from B-mode imaging and other controls. Basic controls include buttons or switches to select the type of Doppler desired (pulsed wave, continuous wave, color Doppler, or power Doppler), Doppler cursor, sample volume or gate, angle correction, gain, Doppler transducer frequency, pulse repetition frequency (scale), color maps, baseline adjustment, priority, wall filter, persistence, and various postprocessing maps similar to those available for B-mode imaging (see Figure 1-7).

To begin a spectral Doppler exam, the Doppler beam indicator is aligned, usually with a track ball, with the target vessel. For pulsed wave Doppler, the sample volume (gate) is then placed within the vessel lumen, its size adjusted appropriately. The flow angle cursor is then adjusted to be perfectly parallel to the vessel (see Figures 1-53 and 1-54). The machine will default to a preset pulse repetition frequency (PRF). Once the Doppler is activated, a spectral waveform should appear and an audible signal should be heard. If no signal is registered, the PRF is lowered until a spectral tracing is seen. Or, if the signal is overloaded (aliasing), the PRF is increased to reduce sensitivity. With continuous wave Doppler, only the Doppler beam indicator is placed because there is no gate (no depth discrimination).

For color Doppler, the sample area is placed over the region of interest (see Figure 1-58 or any of the color Doppler figures). Once activated, a color map should appear indicating blood flow. If it does not, the PRF is reduced (increasing sensitivity) until flow is seen.

One of the more difficult aspects of Doppler ultrasonography is proper alignment of the Doppler cursor with blood vessels. Recall that the best and most accurate signal is achieved when the vessel is parallel to the Doppler signal (parallel to the Doppler beam cursor). In many instances, blood vessels are more perpendicular than parallel, rendering a weak or nonexistent signal. Figure 1-68 shows the effect of insonation angle on Doppler signal and image.

Patient motion is another common hindrance in obtaining high quality Doppler images. Patient restlessness, respiratory and cardiac motion, and even gastrointestinal peristalsis create "flash" artifacts in both spectral and color Doppler (Figure 1-69). Proper use of Doppler takes practice and a thorough understanding of both the physical principles and the plethora of Doppler controls. This cannot be overemphasized; Doppler

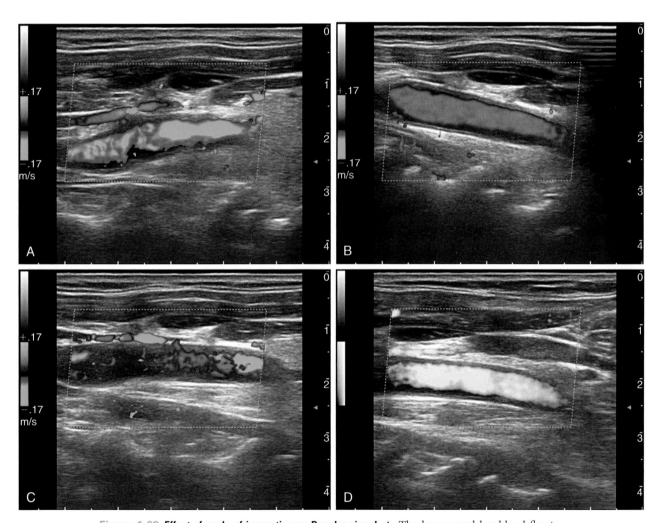

Figure 1-68 Effect of angle of insonation on Doppler signal. A, The large vessel has blood flowing away from the transducer and is displayed in blue. The smaller, more superficial vessel is coded in red, indicating blood flow is toward the transducer. **B,** By simply altering transducer angle, blood in the large vessel in A is now coursing toward the transducer; blood flow is mapped as red. The smaller vessel in A is not seen. **C,** The transducer face is now parallel with the blood vessels, the Doppler insonation angle at essentially 90 degrees. In this instance, the signal is very poor signal, which is indicated by poor filling of the lumen. Also of note is the mixture of red and blue within the vessel; directionality cannot be determined in this circumstance. **D,** Power Doppler image showing good filling of blood vessel lumens. This shows the independence of angle of insonation when using power Doppler.

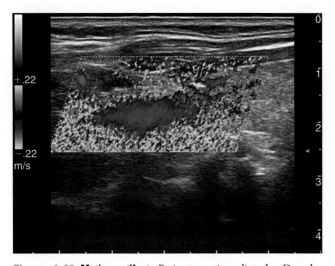

Figure 1-69 Motion artifact. Patient motion disturbs Doppler image acquisition and is recognized by flashes of color that are unrelated to blood flow. Motion can be from patient restlessness or discomfort, but also from respiration, cardiac motion, rapid movement of the transducer, and even gastrointestinal tract peristalsis.

misdiagnoses are common. Figure 1-67 explains displayed Doppler control parameters.

Gain

Doppler ultrasonography has its own dedicated gain control, independent from B-mode gain (see Figure 1-7). The principles and function of the gain control discussed for B-mode imaging similarly apply to Doppler ultrasound. TGC controls are not used for color Doppler, however. If gain is insufficient, the image will be too dark (no spectral signal or no color); too much gain creates an image that is too bright and laden with artifact (Figures 1-70 and 1-71). The rule of thumb for setting Doppler gain is to increase it until artifactual speckle occurs and then reduce just to the point where the speckle disappears. Spectral and color Doppler gain are independent of each other and independent of the B-mode gain.

Pulse Repetition Frequency

Pulse repetition frequency (PRF) is the number of ultrasound pulses emitted per unit time. It is one of the most useful and critical controls for both spectral and color Doppler. On some machines the PRF is referred to as *velocity scale* or *scale*. Increasing or decreasing the PRF increases or decreases the

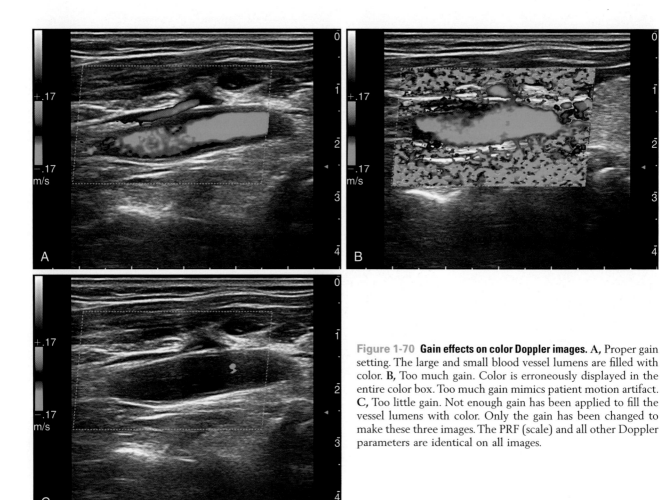

Figure 1-70 Gain effects on color Doppler images. A, Proper gain setting. The large and small blood vessel lumens are filled with color. **B,** Too much gain. Color is erroneously displayed in the entire color box. Too much gain mimics patient motion artifact. **C,** Too little gain. Not enough gain has been applied to fill the vessel lumens with color. Only the gain has been changed to make these three images. The PRF (scale) and all other Doppler parameters are identical on all images.

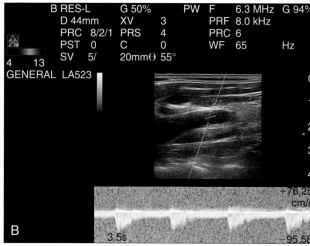

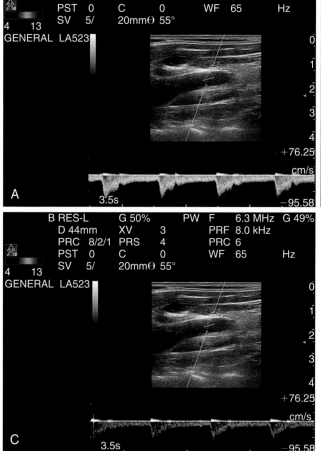

Figure 1-71 Effects of gain on pulsed wave (spectral) Doppler images. A, Proper spectral gain setting (G = 66%). The background is essentially anechoic with only a hint of faint background speckle. **B,** Gain is much too high (G = 94%). The background is now artifactually echoic (white) and the spectral tracing is difficult to identify. **C,** Gain is too low (G = 49%). These images were made using the same Doppler parameters; only the gain setting has been changed. Pulsed wave (PW) Doppler information is displayed in the upper right corner of the image, similar to that explained for color Doppler in Figure 1-67. In addition, the bottom line of text in the upper left corner indicates a sample volume (gate) of 5 mm, a depth of PW sampling of 20 mm, and a Doppler angle of insonation of 55 degrees. The sample volume indicator marks and the flow angle cursor can be seen overlying the center of the vessel.

velocity scale. In Doppler imaging, a high PRF (e.g., 6 or 8 kHz) is required for accurate assessment of high flow vessels, such as the aorta and renal, carotid, and other arteries. A low PRF (e.g., 250 to 2000 Hz) is used for visualizing organ parenchymal vasculature and detecting small vessels. However, using a low PRF makes the ultrasound very sensitive to motion artifact.

Recall that ultrasound pulses must be spaced far enough apart to allow returning echoes to reach the transducer before the next pulse of sound is emitted. If a pulse of transmitted sound occurs too soon, overlap with the returning echoes creates erroneous data. Using a PRF that is too low causes the Nyquist limit to be exceeded and allows aliasing to occur (discussed shortly under Artifacts). Using a PRF that is too high renders the Doppler insensitive to anything but the highest of blood flow. In this case, low flow within organs or smaller vessels may be erroneously overlooked, or an avascular misdiagnosis may be made. Therefore using the lowest possible PRF allows detection of the smallest flow, whereas higher flows require upward adjustment for proper display (Figure 1-72).

Doppler Transducer Frequency
Similar to available B-mode transducer frequencies, the sonographer can select the most appropriate Doppler frequency. This is independent of the B-mode frequency employed. Doppler sensitivity improves with higher frequencies, but increased sound attenuation limits the depth of penetration. Therefore the highest frequency that will penetrate to the

required depth should be used, as in conventional ultrasound imaging. Higher frequencies are used for small structures and for tissues and organs whenever possible. Lower frequency Doppler is used for penetrating deeper structures, such as the liver, and in very large patients who are difficult to scan. Using a lower frequency may be necessary to improve the quality of a Doppler signal obtained at higher frequency.

Baseline Control
The Doppler baseline can be adjusted up or down, in both spectral and color Doppler. This control can be adjusted to eliminate aliasing in many instances without resorting to changes in PRF or transducer frequency (see Figure 1-75, A, B).

Persistence
As with B-mode, Doppler persistence is frame averaging, adding "history" to the current image. It affects temporal resolution, smoothes the image, and fills the vessel, and some level of persistence is usually indicated. However, at high levels it may reduce hemodynamic information (Figure 1-73).

Color Write Priority
Some ultrasound machines allow the sonographer to prioritize the percentage of the ultrasound beam dedicated to B-mode gray scale versus Doppler image. This can be useful in optimizing the Doppler image or the simultaneous B-mode image, depending on need. Altering the B-mode gain has the same effect.

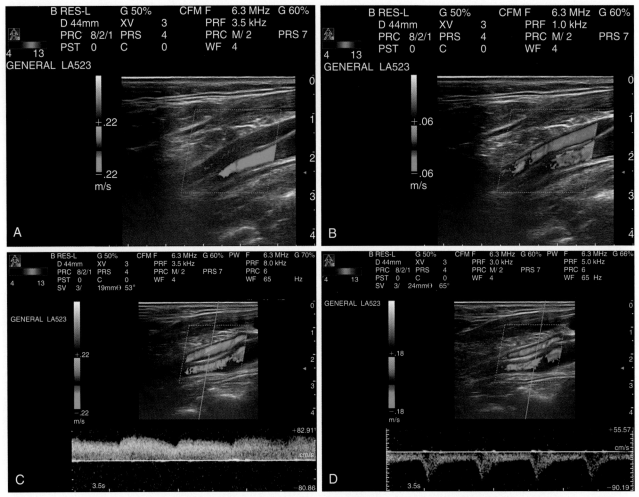

Figure 1-72 Effects of pulse repetition frequency (PRF) on Doppler display. Two blood vessels of different flow velocities are seen adjacent to each other. To accurately display the blood flow within these two vessels, two different PRF settings must be used. This example illustrates that, although Doppler settings may be correct for one vessel, they may not be correct for an adjacent one. Their Doppler appearance is directly affected by PRF setting. **A,** Within the color Doppler sample area (*dotted green lines*), the near blood vessel is only faintly color-coded (red), whereas the deeper blood vessel is well filled with color (blue). The PRF is 3.5 kHz, with a scale of ±0.22 meters/second (m/sec) mean velocity displayed. In this example, the PRF is too high to accurately display the slow flow in the near blood vessel (i.e., not sensitive enough), but it is properly adjusted to accurately display the faster flow within the deeper blood vessel. **B,** In this image, the PRF has been decreased to 1 kHz, resulting in a color bar scale of ±0.06 m/sec. The slow blood flow in the near vessel is now accurately displayed. However, the deeper vessel color map is incorrect (it should be blue, away from the transducer as seen in **A**). The PRF is too low for an accurate color map display. The mean velocity has exceeded 0.06 m/sec and wrapped around to the upper portion of the color, displayed as red. This is an example of color Doppler aliasing. **C,** In this triplex Doppler image, both blood vessels are color mapped properly, reliably determining blood flow direction. Pulsed wave Doppler has been applied to the near vessel. The spectral tracing shows a relatively nonpulsatile wave form (venous) above the baseline, indicating blood flow is toward the transducer (consistent with the color Doppler information). The PW PRF is 8 kHz and the true blood velocity is approximately 60 cm/sec (the PW scale is about ±80 cm/sec). **D,** The PW sampling gate has been shifted to the deeper vessel, showing an arterial wave form below the baseline on the spectral tracing. Note the baseline has shifted, with +55 cm/sec above and −90 cm/sec below. The full complement of user information is available along the header of triplex images **C** and **D**. B-mode information is on the far left (plus PW sample size, depth, and Doppler angle), color Doppler information is in the center, and PW information is to the right.

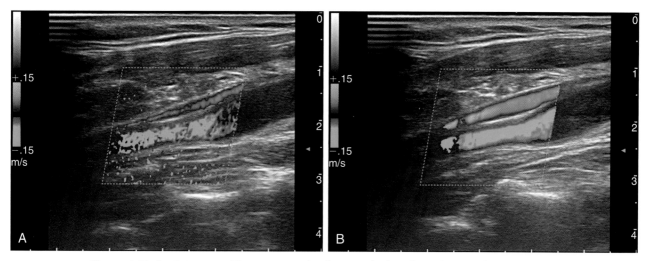

Figure 1-73 **Persistence. A,** No persistence has been applied to this color Doppler image. Note the poor color mapping of both vessels and the sharp, grainy appearance. **B,** High persistence allows good color mapping of the blood vessels. Note the smoother appearance of the image compared to **A.**

Wall Filters

The wall filter in a Doppler system eliminates high-amplitude, low-frequency echoes originating from slow-moving reflectors such as the vessel wall. Ideally, this cleans up the spectral display and prevents masking of low-amplitude, high-frequency echoes arising from slow blood flow. However, improper use of the wall filter may also remove signals from low-velocity blood flow and result in interpretation errors. Therefore the setting should be kept as low as possible, usually in the range of 50 to 100 Hz.

IMPORTANT DOPPLER ARTIFACTS

Aliasing and Range Ambiguity Artifact

Pulsed wave and color Doppler imaging reconstruct Doppler shift signals from regularly timed pulsed samples of information. Outgoing and incoming pulses must be timed to prevent overlap, or aliasing occurs. High velocity blood flow induces aliasing. It also occurs when sampling deeper vessels, because the PRF is reduced to allow time for echoes from a pulse to return before the next series of pulses is transmitted.

In more detail, pulsed wave Doppler (including color Doppler) has a maximal frequency shift that can be interpreted unambiguously; this frequency is known as the Nyquist limit. The sampling rate of the ultrasound must be twice the highest frequency shift present in the returning echoes for blood flow information to be interpreted correctly. When the Nyquist limit is exceeded, aliasing occurs. Portions of the spectral display representing the highest shifted frequencies produce false signals by wrapping around to the opposite side of the baseline. The derived frequency is much lower than the actual Doppler shift. Signals may be displayed as a negative shift and appear or "alias" as lower frequencies on the Doppler spectral display (Figures 1-74 and 1-75, *A*). If the next pulse is transmitted before all echoes are returned, range ambiguity could result. For color Doppler, aliasing is seen as "wraparound" of one color spectrum to the other (Figure 1-76; also see Figure 1-72, *B*).

Aliasing can be reduced or eliminated in several ways. As discussed, the baseline can be shifted to allow the entire

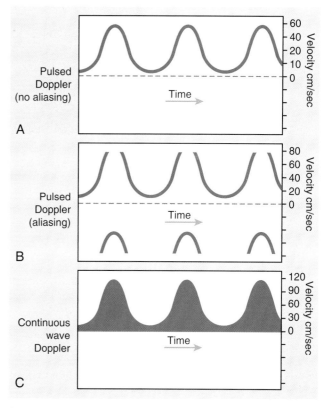

Figure 1-74 **Aliasing illustration.** Aliasing occurs when the pulsed Doppler sampling rate is too slow to correctly record the frequency shift produced by high blood flow. The highest frequency shift that can be interpreted correctly is known as the Nyquist limit. **A,** The pulsed Doppler spectral display properly records flow without aliasing if the Nyquist limit has not been exceeded. **B,** Aliasing is recognized with high blood flow when the Nyquist limit has been exceeded by wrapping around of the pulsed Doppler spectral tracing to the opposite side of the baseline. **C,** High-velocity flow is properly displayed when continuous wave Doppler imaging is employed.

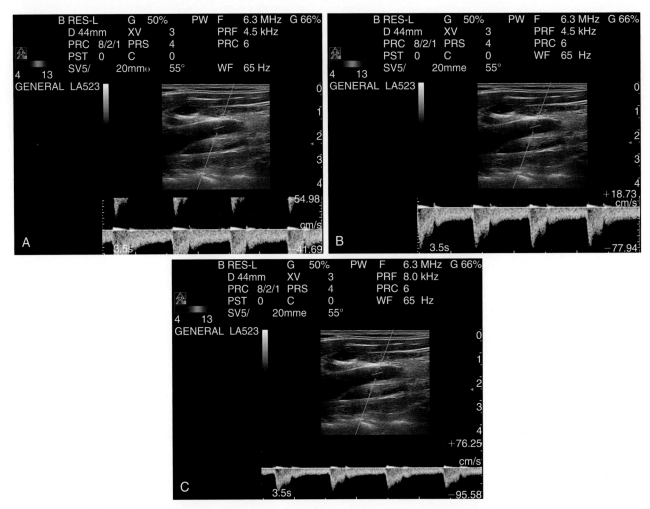

Figure 1-75 **Pulsed wave Doppler aliasing, pulse repetition frequency (PRF), and baseline position.** **A,** Aliasing of a pulsed wave (PW) spectral tracing made using a pulse repetition frequency (PRF) of 4.5 kHz. The PRF is too low to accurately display the velocity of the blood flow, creating the wraparound aliasing artifact. **B,** Moving the baseline up or down, depending on direction of blood flow, is one method that may eliminate aliasing. In this example, raising the baseline to accommodate the entire height of the spectral tracing was possible. Now, 18 cm/sec is displayed above baseline, whereas approximately 78 cm/sec is displayed below. This is enough to display the waveform velocity of approximately 70 cm/sec. The PRF of 4.5 kHz is unchanged. **C,** Another method to eliminate aliasing is to increase the PRF. By increasing the PRF from 4.5 kHz to 8 kHz, the spectral waveform is easily accommodated. Note the size of the wave form has diminished as the scale has increased to 95.58 cm/sec below and 76.25 cm/sec above the relatively centered baseline. As for **B,** the maximum velocity of this artery is approximately 70 cm/sec.

height (velocity or Doppler shift) to be displayed (see Figure 1-75, *B*). The pulse-repetition rate (velocity scale) can be increased (e.g., from 1 kHz to 3 kHz) (see Figures 1-75, *C,* and 1-76, *B*). Lastly, a lower frequency Doppler pulse can be selected (e.g., 7 MHz to 4 MHz).

High pulse-repetition rates are possible at shallow depths because echoes return quickly. Therefore high flow velocities can be measured at shallow depths with pulsed Doppler ultrasonography. At deeper depths, the pulse rate must be slower to accommodate echo return before the next pulse is transmitted. The maximal velocities that can be measured are also correspondingly less. An unwanted side effect of a high pulse-repetition rate is possible range ambiguity and the creation of ghost sample volumes, as discussed next. Aliasing will occur with pulsed Doppler ultrasonography if high flow velocities are present in deeper vessels, because the sampling rate will be inadequate to measure the true velocity.

High pulse-repetition rates increase the Nyquist limit but may produce range ambiguity if all the echoes from a previous pulse have not returned by the time of the next pulse.[35] Depth discrimination is partially lost because flow velocity information will be sampled from multiple sites. This can create artifacts in B-mode as well as Doppler ultrasound imaging. In spectral Doppler, this effect causes supplemental ghost sample volumes to appear on the display in addition to the primary sample volume, informing the operator that range ambiguity is present (Figure 1-77). This is acceptable if the supplemental sampling sites can be positioned outside of any other vessels so that flow information is limited to the primary sample volume. If aliasing occurs, switching to a lower frequency transducer or increasing the incident angle of the beam closer to 90 degrees may reduce the magnitude of the frequency shift and eliminate aliasing.[6] However, small changes in incident angle above 60 degrees result in significant changes in

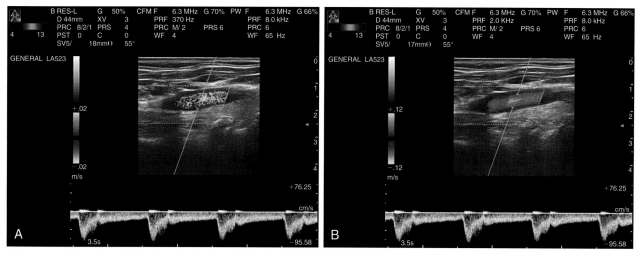

Figure 1-76 **Color Doppler aliasing and pulse repetition frequency (PRF). A,** The PRF is nearly as low as it can be at 370 Hz, a setting that is very sensitive to low blood flow. However, when used to evaluate this relatively high velocity blood vessel, a mosaic color map of blues and reds develops within its lumen, an example of color Doppler aliasing. Note that the spectral tracing is not showing aliasing because the PW PRF is set correctly at 8 kHz. This emphasizes the independence of color Doppler and PW Doppler controls. **B,** One method to correct aliasing is to increase the PRF, making the Doppler less sensitive. In this example, the PRF has been raised form 370 Hz to 2 kHz. The color map now properly displays vessel blood flow. Aliasing can be confused with turbulence from stenosis, so recognition of it is important in certain circumstances.

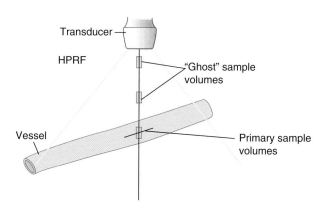

Figure 1-77 **Range ambiguity.** Range ambiguity occurs with pulsed Doppler ultrasonography when the sampling frequency is too high to allow the return of all echoes before the next pulse is transmitted. High pulse-repetition frequency (HPRF) helps prevent aliasing with pulsed Doppler ultrasonography when high blood flow is present. Depth discrimination is partially lost. The appearance of supplemental (ghost) sample volumes on the display indicates that range ambiguity is present, and sampling will also occur from these areas. This is acceptable if the secondary sample volumes are positioned outside of blood vessels and flow is recorded from the primary sample volume only.

calculated velocity. Therefore any errors in the incident angle calculation will result in large errors in the velocity determination. High blood flow velocities and deep vessels require the use of continuous wave Doppler ultrasonography, but depth discrimination is lost. The region of interest must be the only site of blood flow within the beam with continuous wave Doppler ultrasonography.

Twinkling Artifact

The twinkling artifact produces a color flow Doppler signal from a strongly reflective, hyperechoic structures such as cystic calculi. It was first described in human medical literature in 1996[36] and has since been studied in veterinary medicine.[37] The twinkling artifact does not always occur, but does so more commonly when the surface of a calculus is rough or irregular. It occurs regardless of the calculus composition. Interestingly, urinary bladder crystalluria was more commonly detected by the presence of the twinkling artifact than by urinalysis.[37] We have seen the twinkling artifact in a variety of species and locations (Figure 1-78).

SAFETY OF DIAGNOSTIC ULTRASOUND

Longer pulse durations and higher pulse repetition frequencies are used with Doppler ultrasonography than with other ultrasound operating modes. The higher energy transmitted with Doppler ultrasonography has the potential of causing adverse biological effects because of tissue heating. In some commercially available instruments, there is preliminary evidence to suggest that temperatures may increase on the order of 1° C at soft tissue–bone interfaces if the focal zone of the transducer is held stationary. This may have significance in fetal examinations. Nonthermal effects have also been described, but there is disagreement about the relevance with current diagnostic practices. Acoustic cavitation, defined as the formation or activity of bubbles in an ultrasound field, is the nonthermal phenomenon of most concern.

The principle of ALARA (as low as reasonably achievable) for ultrasound exposure should always be practiced. However, there have been no confirmed adverse biological effects reported in patients or instrument operators by exposure to ultrasound intensities and conditions typical of today's examination practices and equipment. Nevertheless, it remains prudent to minimize exposure to the patient and operator. It is especially important to limit exposure with pulsed or continuous wave Doppler instruments, in which the beam is on for a higher percentage of the time, sometimes at greater intensity levels, than with conventional ultrasound imaging.

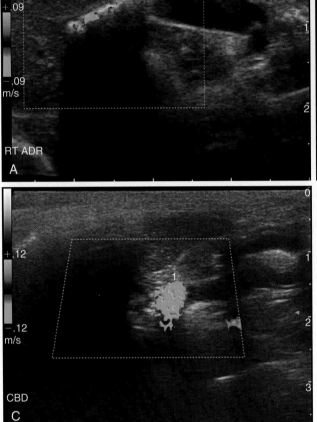
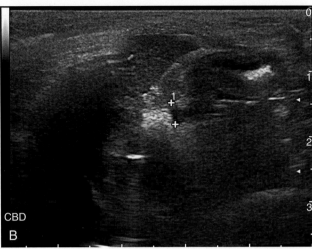

Figure 1-78 **Twinkling artifact. A,** Twinkling artifact arising from mineralization of a feline adrenal gland. Just deep to the irregular mineralized surface of the adrenal gland, color Doppler signal is observed, a twinkling artifact. Strong acoustic shadowing is also present. **B,** A large calculus is present within a dilated common bile duct (*CBD*), showing acoustic shadowing. **C,** Same image as **B,** with color Doppler showing a vivid color Doppler twinkling artifact.

Present knowledge indicates that the benefits of ultrasound clearly outweigh any potential risks, but maintaining power levels as low as possible and keeping the exposure time to a minimum make sense until more information becomes available. Kremkau[1] has written an excellent, comprehensive chapter on the safety of ultrasound. The authoritative source for information on the subject has been produced and published by the Bioeffects Committee of the American Institute of Ultrasound in Medicine (AIUM).[38,39]

REFERENCES

1. Kremkau FW. *Sonography Principles and Instruments.* 8th ed. Philadelphia: Elsevier Saunders; 2011.
2. Hagen-Ansert SL. Foundations of Sonography. In: Hagen-Ansert SL, editor. *Textbook of Diagnostic Ultrasonography.* 6th ed. St Louis: Mosby-Elsevier; 2006. p. 3–32.
3. Merritt CRB. Physics of Ultrasound. In: Rumack CM, Wilson SR, Charboneau JW, editors. *Diagnostic Ultrasound.* 3rd ed. St Louis: Elsevier-Mosby; 2005. p. 3–34.
4. Middleton WD, Kurtz AB, Hertzberg BS. *Ultrasound: The Requisites.* 2nd ed. St Louis: Elsevier-Mosby; 2004. p. 3–27.
5. Bushberg JT, Seibert JA, Leidholdt EM, et al. Ultrasound. In: *The Essential Physics of Medical Imaging.* 2nd ed. Philadelphia: Lippincott Williams & Wilkins; 2002. p. 469–553.
6. Curry TS III, Dowdey JE, Murry RC. Ultrasound. In: *Christensen's Physics of Diagnostic Radiology.* 4th ed. Philadelphia: Lea & Febiger; 1990. p. 323–71.
7. Heng HG, Widmer WR. Appearance of common ultrasound artifacts in conventional vs. spatial imaging. *Vet Radiol Ultrasound* 2010;**51**:621–7.
8. Merritt CR. Technology Update. *Radiol Clin North Am* 2001;**39**:385–97.
9. Feeney DA, Fletcher TF, Hardy RM. *Atlas of Correlative Imaging Anatomy of the Normal Dog: Ultrasound and Computed Tomography.* Philadelphia: WB Saunders; 1991.
10. Smallwood JE, George TF II. Anatomic atlas for computed tomography in the mesaticephalic dog: Thorax and cranial abdomen. *Vet Radiol Ultrasound* 1993;**34**:65–83.
11. Smallwood JE, George TF II. Anatomic atlas for computed tomography in the mesaticephalic dog: Caudal abdomen and pelvis. *Vet Radiol Ultrasound* 1993;**34**:143–67.
12. Assheuer J, Sager M. *MRI and CT Atlas of the Dog.* Oxford: Blackwell Science; 1997.
13. Samii VF, Biller DS, Koblik PD. Normal cross-sectional anatomy of the feline thorax and abdomen: Comparison of computed tomography and cadaver anatomy. *Vet Radiol Ultrasound* 1998;**39**:504–11.
14. Samii VF, Biller DS, Koblik PD. Magnetic resonance imaging of the normal feline abdomen: An anatomic reference. *Vet Radiol Ultrasound* 1999;**40**:486–90.

15. Park RD, Nyland TG, Lattimer JC, et al. B-mode gray-scale ultrasound: Imaging artifacts and interpretation principles. *Vet Radiol* 1981;**22**:204–10.

16. Herring DS, Bjornton G. Physics, facts and artifacts of diagnostic ultrasound. *Vet Clin North Am Small Anim Pract* 1985;**15**:1107–22.

17. Kirberger RM. Imaging artifacts in diagnostic ultrasound: A review. *Vet Radiol Ultrasound* 1995;**36**:297–306.

18. Barthez PY, Leveille R, Scrivani PV. Side lobes and grating lobes artifacts in ultrasound imaging. *Vet Radiol Ultrasound* 1997;**38**:387–93.

19. Louvet A, Bourgeois JM. Lung ring-down artifact as a sign of pulmonary alveolar-interstitial disease. *Vet Radiol Ultrasound* 2008;**49**:374–7.

20. Ziskin MC, Thickman DI, Goldenberg NJ, et al. The comet tail artifact. *J Ultrasound Med* 1982;**1**:1–7.

21. Sauerbrei EE. The split image artifact in pelvic ultrasonography. *J Ultrasound Med* 1985;**4**:29–34.

22. Buttery B, Davison G. The ghost artifact. *J Ultrasound Med* 1984;**3**:49–52.

23. Muller N, Cooperberg PL, Rowley VA, et al. Ultrasonic refraction by the rectus abdominis muscles: The double image artifact. *J Ultrasound Med* 1984;**3**:515–19.

24. Vendeman FN, Meilstrup JW, Nealey PA. Acoustic prism causing sonographic duplication artifact in the upper abdomen. *Invest Radiol* 1990;**25**:658–63.

25. Middleton WD, Melson GL. Renal duplication artifact in ultrasound imaging. *Radiology* 1989;**173**:427–9.

26. Taylor KJW. *Atlas of Ultrasonography.* 2nd ed. New York: Churchill Livingstone; 1985.

27. Middleton WD, Melson GL. Diaphragmatic discontinuity associated with perihepatic ascites: A sonographic refractive artifact. *AJR Am J Roentgenol* 1988;**151**:709–11.

28. Sommer FG, Filly RA, Minton JM. Acoustic shadowing due to refractive and reflective effects. *AJR Am J Roentgenol* 1979;**132**:973–9.

29. Robinson DE, Wilson LS, Kossoff G. Shadowing and enhancement in ultrasonic echograms by reflection and refraction. *J Clin Ultrasound* 1981;**9**:181–8.

30. Sommer FG, Taylor KJW. Differentiation of acoustic shadowing due to calculi and gas collections. *Radiology* 1980;**140**:399–403.

31. Rubin JM, Adler RS, Bude RO, et al. Clean and dirty shadowing at US: A reappraisal. *Radiology* 1991;**181**:231–6.

32. Weichselbaum RC, Feeney DA, Jessen CR, et al. Relevance of sonographic artifacts observed during in vitro characterization of urocystolith mineral composition. *Vet Radiol Ultrasound* 2000;**41**:438–46.

33. Douglass JP, Kremkau FW. Ultrasound corner: The urinary bladder wall hypoechoic pseudolesion. *Vet Radiol Ultrasound* 1993;**34**:45–6.

34. Rubin JM, Bude RO, Carson PL, et al. Power Doppler US: A potentially useful alternative to mean frequency-based color Doppler US. *Radiology* 1994;**190**:853–6.

35. O'Brien RT, Zagzebski JA, Delaney FA. Ultrasound corner: range ambiguity artifact. *Vet Radiol Ultrasound* 2001;**42**:542–5.

36. Rahmouni A, Bargoin R, Herment A, et al. Color Doppler twinkling artifact in hyperechoic regions. *Radiology* 1996;**199**:269–71.

37. Louvet A. Twinkling artifact in small animal color-Doppler sonography. *Vet Radiol Ultrasound* 2006;**47**:384–90.

38. AIUM Bioeffects Consensus Report. *J Ultrasound Med* 2008;**27**:499–644.

39. *American Institute of Ultrasound in Medicine: Medical ultrasound safety.* 2nd ed. Laurel, MD: American Institute of Ultrasound in Medicine; 2009.

CHAPTER 2
Ultrasound-Guided Aspiration and Biopsy Procedures

John S. Mattoon • Rachel Pollard • Tamara Wills • Thomas G. Nyland

Percutaneous ultrasound-guided aspiration and biopsy procedures have become routine in small animals because precise needle placement is possible with continuous real-time monitoring, even for deep-seated lesions.[1-10] The percentage of positive diagnostic samples is increased, and there is improved speed and safety compared with other biopsy methods. Ultrasound equipment is portable, general anesthesia may be unnecessary, and exposure to ionizing radiation is eliminated. However, ultrasound-guided biopsy is not possible when gas or bone prevents visualization of the biopsy region. In this case, computed tomography or fluoroscopy becomes the imaging modality of choice. The size, type, and location of the lesion ultimately determine the biopsy method chosen.

Special sonoendoscopic transducers developed for use in humans allow transesophageal, transgastric, transduodenal, transvaginal, and transrectal imaging and biopsy procedures.[11-14] These transducers may have applications in animals as they become affordable and more widely available to veterinary clinicians.

EQUIPMENT

A sector, curvilinear, or linear-array transducer can be used for ultrasound-guided biopsies. The linear-array transducer is preferred for superficial structures because of superior visibility of the near field. The near field is poorly seen with a sector scanner unless an offset is used to position the area of interest farther from the transducer within the wider portion of the beam. If an offset is used, an indirect or freehand biopsy technique is preferred, as discussed later, because sterility is otherwise difficult to maintain. With either type of transducer, the biopsy site should be placed within the focal zone of the transducer for best resolution.

A dedicated linear-array biopsy transducer may have a groove, a slot, or a central hole for guidance of the needle but these are rarely used in veterinary medicine. External needle guides may also be attached to conventional linear-array and sector scan heads (Figure 2-1). The guide may be composed of plastic or metal, depending on the manufacturer. Some devices allow release of the needle from the guide after it has been placed into the lesion. All guides accommodate needles of various sizes and functions to hold the needle within the plane of the ultrasound beam. The dedicated linear-array biopsy transducer must be gas or chemically sterilized before each procedure. With an external guide, only the guide itself needs to be sterilized because the transducer is covered with a sterile sleeve before the guide is attached (see Figure 2-1, *A*, and *B*).

Alternatively and more commonly, a sterilized guide is attached to a *sanitized* transducer (see Figure 2-1, C). External guides are inexpensive compared with dedicated biopsy transducers, and multiple guides can be purchased and sterilized in advance. Biopsy guides may be disposable, or they can be reused after autoclave, gas, or chemical sterilization. Some inexpensive plastic guides or inserts that adjust for various needle sizes come presterilized and may be economically discarded after use.

Ultrasound scanners with biopsy guide capability indicate the needle's path by means of lines or other markers superimposed on the video display (Figure 2-2). The lesion is placed along the line or marker while the needle is advanced to the required depth under continuous monitoring. The distance to the lesion from the skin surface may be estimated by the screen's centimeter scale or with electronic cursors.

During the procedure, supplies for ultrasound-guided biopsy should be easily accessible from a well-stocked room, supply cart, or supply bag, depending on whether ultrasound procedures are performed away from the ultrasound area with portable equipment. Specialized types of biopsies, such as intracranial and intra-operative procedures, may require dedicated transducers, holders, and most definitely sterile coverings.

PREPARATION OF THE PATIENT

When there is a significant risk of bleeding or when highly vascular lesions are being sampled, the patient should be examined for hemostatic disorders before *tissue-core biopsies*. This assessment is made from the history, physical examination, laboratory work, and other diagnostic procedures. In a study of a large number of dogs and cats undergoing ultrasound-guided biopsies, minor complications were seen in over 20% of the cases and major complications were seen in 6% of the cases.[15] Significant bleeding was seen with thrombocytopenia. Dogs with prolonged one-stage prothrombin time (OSPT) and cats with prolonged activated partial thromboplastic time (aPTT) were more likely to have complications than patients with normal values. Therefore screening tests such as platelet count, prothrombin time, partial thromboplastin time, and bleeding time are generally indicated. However, routine *fine needle aspiration using small gauge needles (e.g., 22- to 25-gauge) for cytologic diagnosis* usually require no special preparation unless there is a high risk of bleeding. Fine-needle aspiration (FNA), also known as fine-needle aspiration cytology (FNAC), fine-needle aspiration biopsy (FNAB), and needle aspiration biopsy (NAB), should not be confused with tissue-core biopsy, because the latter

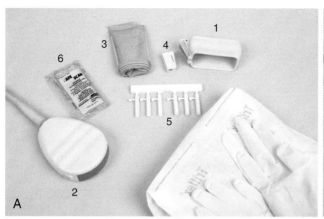
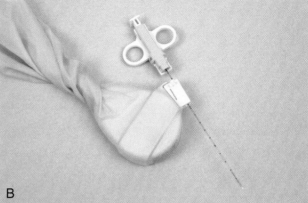
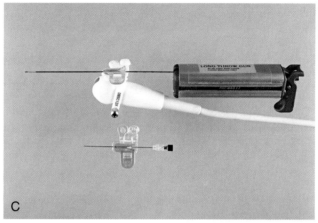

Figure 2-1 **Biopsy guide. A,** The ATL external biopsy guide system (Advanced Technology Laboratories, Bothell, WA) consists of a collar (*1*) that fits around the transducer (*2*), which can be covered with a sterile sleeve (*3*). A disposable external needle guide (*4*) containing an appropriate insert (*5*) for the size of needle used is then snapped onto the collar's protrusion. The biopsy needle is thereby fixed within the plane of the ultrasound beam during insertion. Sterile ultrasound gel (*6*) is also used to maintain aseptic technique. **B,** The assembled ATL biopsy system is shown with an automated biopsy needle (E-Z Core, 18-gauge Single Action Biopsy Needle, Products Group International, Lyons, CO). **C,** The Esaote external biopsy guide system (Esaote, Genoa, Italy) consists of a plastic collar secured with a thumb screw to the transducer to which a biopsy guide attaches. In this photograph, the color-coded 18-gauge biopsy guide is attached to the collar, and an 18-gauge biopsy needle and automatic biopsy gun are in place (Manan PRO-MAG 2.2, Manan Medical Products, Inc., Wheeling, IL). Pictured below is an unattached 22-gauge biopsy guide with a spinal needle in place. This device allows the needle to be removed from the guide if desired once the target is reached.

uses larger gauge needles to harvest tissue and is therefore considered to be a more risky procedure.

The skin over the biopsy site should be clipped and prepared aseptically. In many cases, FNA can be performed without chemical restraint or local anesthesia. Multiple injections of local anesthetic may be more painful than a single needle pass for aspiration biopsy, and the anesthetic itself be painful. Sometimes it is difficult to localize exactly where the needle will pass through the skin, or the entrance site changes because of patient motion. Local anesthesia may be required in some instances, depending on the type of biopsy performed and the animal's temperament, and some sonographers routinely use it.

Placement of an intravenous catheter for tissue-core biopsies facilitates the administration of chemical sedation and permits access for resuscitative procedures, if necessary. Some aspiration and all tissue-core biopsies are facilitated by the use of intravenous short-acting anesthesia, such as a combination of intravenous ketamine hydrochloride and diazepam, dexmedetomidine (Dexdomitor) and butorphanol (Torbugesic), or

intravenous propofol (Diprivan) for sedation, unless contraindicated by the animal's condition. In many cases, a half-dose provides sufficient restraint, with the remainder given as needed. No local anesthesia is required. Agents that promote panting or splenic enlargement should be avoided when possible. Panting causes excessive movement and gas ingestion, whereas splenic enlargement sometimes interferes with biopsies of abdominal masses or the left kidney. General inhalation anesthesia is rarely required except to prevent movement during the biopsy of small masses adjacent to vital structures (breath hold), but for some practitioners the added safety margin of inhalation anesthetics and intubation is preferred.

GENERAL TECHNIQUES

The shortest distance and safest path between the skin surface and the lesion or region to be sampled should be chosen. The needle should not pass through more than one body cavity (pleural, peritoneal, retroperitoneal) or abdominal organ, if

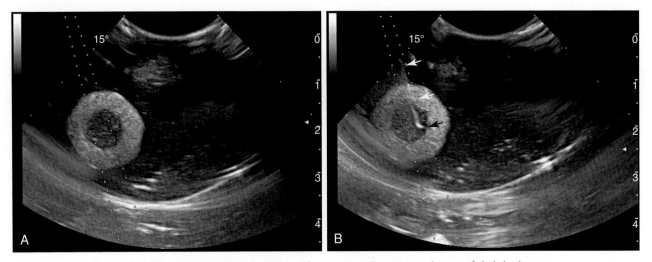

Figure 2-2 **Biopsy guide monitor display. A,** Electronic markers (two columns of slightly diverging *small white dots*) indicate the path the needle will travel when using the biopsy guide, which is 15 degrees (*15°*) relative to the axis of the ultrasound beam. The lesion or area to be sampled is placed along the path before the needle is inserted. **B,** The position of the needle (*arrows*) can be monitored continuously during insertion and at the actual time of biopsy. The tip of the needle is indicated by the black arrow. These images were made using a gelatin biopsy phantom and a microconvex sector transducer. The model for the target lesion is a green olive with a pimento center (see Figure 2-8).

possible. A separate needle should be used for each location if multiple biopsy samples are taken. These procedures prevent the spread of infection or neoplasia to other locations. The biopsy site should be selected with ultrasound and the skin prepared aseptically over a wide area. Sterile acoustic coupling gel can be used but is generally not necessary if the skin is kept moist with alcohol. Samples are best obtained without the presence of gel fragments. Draping is not necessary unless there is a potential for the aspiration or biopsy site to become contaminated during the procedure. The three methods for biopsy guidance are the indirect technique, the freehand technique, and the needle guidance system.[13,14]

Indirect Guidance

Indirect needle guidance refers to removal of the transducer after the angle and depth of needle insertion have been determined from the ultrasound image. Applying firm skin pressure with the hub of a needle can temporarily mark the site if necessary. The needle is then inserted blindly after sterile skin preparation. A needle stop may be used to mark the correct depth of needle placement. The needle should be placed shortly after the transducer is removed to avoid changes in alignment or depth caused by the patient's movement. The indirect technique is mostly used in animals during therapeutic thoracocentesis, abdominocentesis, and cystocentesis when large quantities of fluid are present.

Freehand Guidance

Freehand puncture is accomplished by holding the transducer in one hand and inserting the biopsy needle with the other (Figure 2-3).[4] This technique is the most versatile and most common, and it is used for both aspiration and tissue-core biopsy acquisition. The needle is continuously visualized if it is kept within the plane of the beam. Practice is required to maintain the entire needle's length within the beam so that the tip can be accurately localized. It is recommended that the sonographer use their dominant hand to guide the needle, and use their nondominant hand to hold the transducer. This may seem foreign at first, because most of us scan with our

dominant hand. However, the important aspect of using ultrasound guidance for needle techniques is precise placement of the needle, and this can be best accomplished when the dominant hand guides the needle. Your ability to throw a ball with your dominant arm compared with your nondominant arm provides a good analogy. Which arm has more control?

The area of needle entry is prepared aseptically. The transducer is cleansed using an approved aseptic solution, usually dilute alcohol (please see manufacture recommendations for approved cleaning agents; some may harm the transducer). This is easily accomplished by placing an alcohol-soaked surgical sponge or cotton ball over the tip of the transducer during skin preparation to prevent later contamination from an unclean transducer. We have used this technique for many years and have found it to be satisfactory and without complications.

There may be circumstances where absolute sterility is essential (e.g., immunocompromised patients, intraoperative ultrasound, more involved interventional techniques). In these cases, the surgically gloved operator covers the transducer with a sterile surgical glove or sterile-fitted sleeve supplied by the manufacturer. This is accomplished by rolling the glove or sleeve inside out, adding gel to the inside, and stretching it over the transducer without contaminating the outer surface of the covering. If a surgical glove is used with a sector transducer, the head is usually placed within the thumbhole to minimize trapped air. If the needle is to be inserted immediately adjacent to the transducer, caution must be used to prevent touching the transducer with the needle. Using the free-hand guidance method, the needle can often be inserted in a direction more perpendicular to the ultrasound beam than with an attached needle guide, resulting in maximal visibility (see Figure 2-3, *E-G*).

Needle Guidance Systems

The needle guidance system, which uses a biopsy guide attached to the transducer, is the easiest biopsy method (see Figures 2-1 and 2-2). However, it can be physically limiting. Bony structures may interfere with placement of the

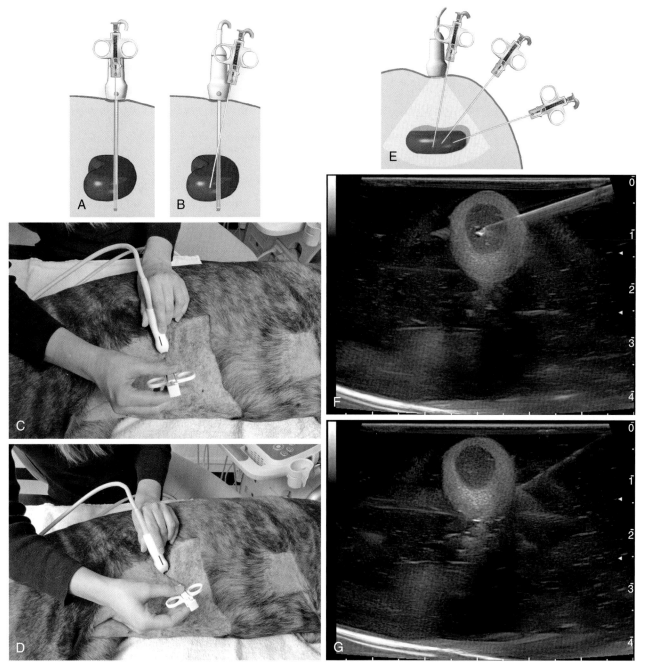

Figure 2-3 **Freehand technique.** This method of biopsy is accomplished by holding the transducer in one hand while the needle is inserted with the other. It takes practice to maintain the needle within the beam plane, but the technique allows the needle to be inserted nearly perpendicular to the beam, which maximizes visibility. This method also allows guided aspiration or biopsy of structures closer to the skin surface than when an external biopsy guide is used. **A,** Proper needle alignment. It is important to keep the entire length of the needle within the plane of the ultrasound beam so that it can be properly visualized. This is done automatically with a biopsy guide but is the responsibility of the operator with freehand biopsy. **B,** Improper needle alignment. If the needle is inserted oblique to the plane of the beam as shown here, only a portion of the needle will be visualized. This results in incorrect needle placement and the operator is unaware of true needle placement, which can have disastrous, deadly results. **C** and **D,** Examples of freehand aspiration with the needle properly (**C**) and improperly (**D**) aligned with the transducer and plane of the ultrasound beam. Note the position of the needle relative to the center of x-axis of the transducer, indicated by the red vertical ridge on the transducer. **E,** Needle visibility relative to the angle with the ultrasound beam. Maximal needle visibility is obtained when the needle is placed at right angles to the beam. However, it is also important to place the needle close to the transducer so that the entire path can be visualized during insertion from the skin surface. In practice, ideal needle placement depends on the transducer type, shape of the beam, and depth to the target. This illustration depicts a microconvex sector transducer. **F** and **G,** Examples of needle visibility relative to the angle with the ultrasound beam (a linear array transducer was used). Ideal visualization of the needle occurs when it is nearly perpendicular to the axis of the ultrasound beam (**F**). Needle becomes poorly visualized as it becomes less perpendicular to beam axis (**G**). These images were made using a biopsy phantom with 25-gauge needles.

transducer or insertion of the needle, and because of the fixed angle of needle insertion, this system may not permit biopsy of structures, especially those that are superficial. We have found the biopsy guide to be most beneficial for targeting very deep, small lesions that can be quite challenging using the freehand method.

The biopsy guide is attached with or without a sterile transducer sleeve, as noted for freehand guidance. The lesion or biopsy site is localized, and the position of the guide on the skin surface is noted. It is important that the animal remain still to prevent a change in the lesion's position relative to the skin surface. A stab incision of the skin with a No. 11 blade usually facilitates passage of the tissue core biopsy needle because larger gauge needles are used (typically 14 to 18 gauge). It also helps alleviate deviation of the needle from the plane of the ultrasound plane. This is not usually required with a thin, rigid needle (e.g., hypodermic or small gauge spinal needle). Though most of our FNA procedures are done without local or general anesthesia, ketamine plus diazepam, propofol sedation, or light anesthesia is usually used for tissue-core biopsies.

PRINCIPLES OF NEEDLE SELECTION AND BIOPSY

Needle Selection

Ultrasound-guided aspiration and tissue-core biopsies are routinely performed in veterinary medicine. Aspiration procedures are used to obtain material for culture or biochemical or cytologic analysis. A tissue-core biopsy is used primarily to obtain material for histologic analysis, although samples can also be cultured, specially stained, or otherwise analyzed. Figure 2-4 shows commonly used aspiration and biopsy needles.

Aspirations are generally preferred with small solid masses (<1 cm diameter), cystic lesions, and highly vascularized lesions, or when diffuse cellular infiltration with lymphoma or mast cell tumor is suspected. If the aspiration sample is nondiagnostic, it may be followed by a tissue-core biopsy. Tissue-core biopsies are preferred with large masses and other types of diffuse organ disease or when histologic evaluation is needed. The decision to perform an aspiration or tissue-core biopsy and the type of needle selected are determined by the lesion to be sampled, the suspected abnormality, and the risk to the patient. Regardless, it must be recognized that aspiration samples are smaller than those acquired from tissue-core biopsy, and results of their analysis may not match the final histologic diagnosis. For example, results of fine-needle aspiration of the liver agreed with histologic outcome in 30.3% of dogs and 51.2% of cats in one study.[16] A different study looking at splenic aspiration biopsies found agreement with histology in 61.3% of dogs and cats.[17]

Cyst aspiration can be done with a thin needle (21 to 25 gauge), whereas an abscess containing thick, purulent contents often requires a larger bore needle. Aspiration of tumor masses for cytologic analysis can usually be done with a 21- or 22-gauge needle, or even smaller, but tissue-core biopsies require 14- to 18-gauge needles for an adequate sample. Larger bore needles are easier to visualize and provide superior samples but have been associated with higher complication rates, particularly hemorrhage (see Figure 2-4, C).[18,19] Smaller biopsy needles may result in tissue crushing or fragmentation yielding a less diagnostic sample.[20] Therefore the smallest needle that yields an adequate specimen should be chosen. As a general rule, we prefer 25-gauge needles for all aspirates, and if samples do not yield a good specimen smear, a larger needle is used. For biopsies, a 16-gauge needle seems

a good compromise of commonly available 14-to 18-gauge needles. For cats, smaller dogs, and other small patients, an 18-gauge needle is preferred for safety, whereas 14-gauge needles are used in larger patients.

The shape of the needle tip also influences the yield from aspiration procedures. A needle with a beveled tip produces a higher positive yield than do needles with circumferential or other types of sharpened tips.[21] Thin-walled needles yield larger specimens for tissue-core biopsies, but they tend to be flexible and deviate from the beam plane unless a special metal alloy is used to increase stiffness.[22]

Needle visibility can be a significant issue when trying to ensure accurate placement, particularly when sampling focal lesions. A larger bore needle is easier to visualize and can be used if it does not increase complication risks. Ensuring that the needle is placed within the focal zone of the transducer also increases visibility. Electronically focused transducers are able to vary the focal depth to match the needle's path, and multiple focal points can be used to maximize needle visualization. Injection of a small amount of sterile saline or air through the needle may also help localize the needle's tip during scanning. Wiggling the needle, moving the stylet in and out,[22] and rocking the transducer to better position the needle within the beam plane are additional techniques commonly used to assist with needle visualization. Care must be exercised when moving the needle; to minimize tissue laceration, it is always best to rock the transducer to localize the needle rather than move the needle.

A 21- to 25-gauge injection needle that is 1.0 to 1.5 inch or longer is commonly used for freehand fine needle aspiration. It may be used alone (Figure 2-5, A) with a pincushion technique described later or be attached to a syringe (usually preloaded with air) (see Figure 2-5, B). Alternatively, an extension set can be attached to the needle and syringe (see Figure 2-5, C), a technique we generally use to drain large quantities of fluid, because more flexibility is offered when changing full syringes.

Our preferred method for FNA sample collection is actually a *nonaspiration technique*, termed the *pincushion technique*. The needle is placed into the lesion and rapidly moved in and out within the lesion several times (not wiggled side-to-side). The goal is to fill the needle with diagnostic cells without undue blood contamination. We adopted this technique many years ago after recognizing that applying negative pressure (aspiration) when sampling vascular organs such as the spleen often led to blood cell contamination and a nondiagnostic sample. A recent article supports the validity of nonaspiration technique for obtaining high quality cytologic samples of the dog and cat spleen.[23] A syringe preloaded with air facilitates injection of the sample onto a slide. If the smear is deemed inadequate, negative pressure is then used to acquire a more substantial sample.

For guided aspiration samples or for very deep lesions, the most commonly used needle is a 20- or 22-gauge disposable spinal needle that is 3.5 inches (9 cm) or longer and has a stylet and beveled tip (see Figure 2-4). Spinal needles are relatively inexpensive, and the length is adequate to pass through the biopsy guide and still reach most lesions. Ordinarily the stylet is removed and a syringe is attached *after* the needle is placed within the lesion. This keeps the needle free of other cell types as the needle passes through more superficial tissues before reaching the target. However, some investigators recommend removing the stylet and attaching the extension tubing before placing the needle, a technique that will be described later.[4] The stiffness of a spinal needle allows it to penetrate skin without a stab incision and minimizes its deviation from the beam plane. However, the diamond tip can be painful when passing through the skin, and local anesthesia or

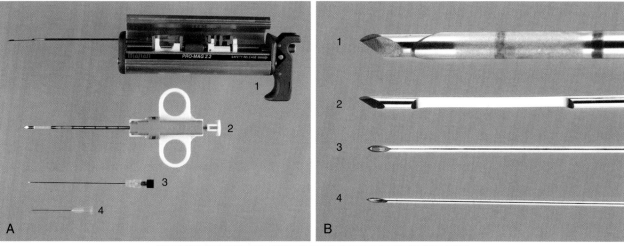

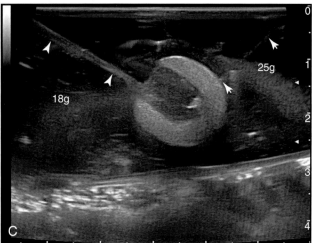

Figure 2-4 **Aspiration and biopsy needles.** **A,** Examples of needles for aspiration or tissue-core biopsy: (*1*) the Manan biopsy gun is a nondisposable spring-loaded automatic device that uses disposable needles (shown in place) for tissue-core biopsy, and (*2*) the spring-loaded semiautomatic E-Z Core biopsy needle (Products Group International, Lyons, CO) are examples of needles used for tissue-core biopsy. The spinal needle (*3*) and injection needles (*4*) are the most frequent types for FNA and fluid aspiration. Biopsy and aspiration needles are available in a variety of gauges and lengths. **B,** Examples of needle tips: (*1*) closed 14-gauge E-Z Core biopsy needle for tissue-core sample (needle *2* in **A**), (*2*) 18-gauge tissue core biopsy needle showing the sample notch (needle *1* in **A**), and typical beveled tips (*3*, spinal needle; *4*, injection needle) for aspiration biopsy or fluid aspiration (needles *3* and *4* in **A**). Note that the biopsy needles have a coated surface (light gray near the tip to increase needle visualization) and dark bands on the needle shaft representing 1-cm depth marks. **C,** Effect of needle gauge (diameter) on needle visualization. The larger 18-gauge needle on the left (*arrowheads*) is better visualized than the smaller 25-gauge needle on the right (*arrows*), although in this example the tip of the 25-gauge needle is brighter than the 18-gauge tip.

moderate sedation may be necessary when using a spinal needle.

Tissue-core biopsies are most easily performed with spring-loaded semiautomatic biopsy needles or a fully automatic, spring operated biopsy "gun," using 14- to 18-gauge needles, although other types of needles may be satisfactory (see Figure 2-4).[24,25] In most instances, spring-loaded biopsy devices provide better samples than hand-deployed needles, although a recent publication has shown satisfactory results using a manual biopsy device on canine cadaver organs and clinical patients.[26] The biopsy samples from spring-loaded biopsy needles or guns are usually free of tearing or crush artifacts that sometimes accompany manual methods. These needles typically have a 17-mm notch in the tip of the inner trocar to hold the biopsy sample. Semiautomatic biopsy needles and some biopsy guns are available to accommodate shorter needle throws with smaller sample notches for biopsy of smaller lesions and smaller patients.

There is a safety advantage in using a spring-loaded disposable *semiautomatic biopsy needle*, because the operator *manually* advances the inner trocar, which can be observed sonographically. The outer cutting needle is spring-loaded and is activated once the inner trocar is properly placed. Disposable semiautomatic biopsy needles cost the same as the disposable needles used for the biopsy guns and are available in a variety of gauges and lengths. The disposable semiautomatic needles have become the preferred biopsy instrument for many practitioners.

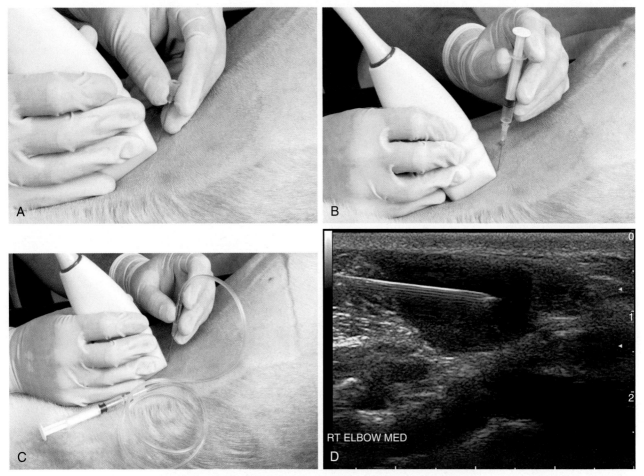

Figure 2-5 Fine-needle aspiration techniques. A, Needle only. **B,** Needle attached to air preloaded syringe. **C,** Needle attached to extension tube with preloaded syringe. **D,** Spinal needle (often used for deeper lesions). The needle is seen as highly echogenic line across the screen. Reverberation artifact is present. The needle is very visible because it is at a 90-degree angle to the ultrasound beam of this linear array transducer. The needle is embedded in a hypoechoic nodule of the elbow. The diagnosis was a histiocytic sarcoma.

A biopsy gun is considered fully automatic. It is a precision piece of medical equipment, has a powerful spring system, will last a lifetime, and is priced accordingly. A biopsy gun uses disposable needles, available in a variety of gauges and lengths. After placing the needle into the gun, the gun is cocked, readying it for sample collection. The operator pushes a button and the inner trocar is spring advanced, and the outer cutting needle is then immediately advanced by a second spring mechanism. The operator must know *the exact travel path and advancement length* of the biopsy gun "throw" and account for this distance so that deeper tissue is not unexpectedly sampled, potentially with disastrous results (Figure 2-6). As an example, the biopsy gun shown in Figures 2-1, *C,* and 2-4, *A,* has 2.2 cm of needle advancement, which is typical of longer throw biopsy guns using needles with a 1.7-cm tissue sample notch. Shorter throw biopsy guns are available, and some are adjustable. It is important to use the correct needle for the throw of the gun. We do not advocate resterilization and reuse of these needles; they become dull and quality of the tissue sample may suffer.

Aspiration and Biopsy Technique

Aspiration of moderate to large amounts of fluid can be done blindly or with indirect or freehand guidance. A three-way valve and extension tubing can be used to remove large amounts of fluid. Over-the-needle plastic catheters can also be inserted to help decrease the risk of injury during drainage.

Solid lesions are aspirated by guiding the needle to the lesion under direct visualization. The needle tip is moved up and down in 1- to 2-cm excursions while maintaining several milliliters of negative suction (see Figure 2-5). The needle can also be rotated to help increase cytologic yield.[21] Suction should be released before the needle is removed; this prevents sampling outside the lesion and retains the contents primarily within the needle. Aspiration of blood should be prevented because it will dilute the sample. If processing will be delayed, the syringe should be preloaded with 2 mL of sterile saline to flush the needle's contents into a test tube.[27] Immediate cytologic examination after each aspiration is preferred to reduce the number of passes required for a positive sample.

As mentioned previously, a nonaspiration technique has also been advocated to obtain cytologic samples.[23,28] The reported accuracy of this technique varies in the literature, but it seems to provide better samples with less blood dilution. The needle is moved up and down several centimeters within the lesion or until a small amount of fluid is seen within the hub of the needle.

Tissue-core biopsies are performed by advancing the needle to the desired depth, while taking into account the additional

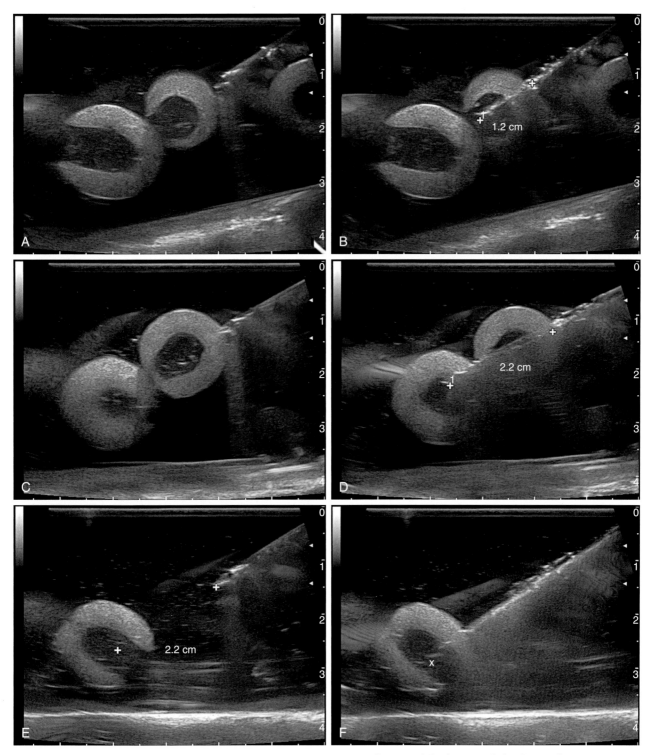

Figure 2-6 Needle advancement (biopsy throw). Knowing the size of the lesion and the throw of the biopsy needle is critical to prevent overshooting the target. A biopsy phantom using olives as target lesions has been used to create these images. **A,** A short-throw (1.2 cm) automatic biopsy gun is used with an 18-gauge needle. The tip of the needle is placed on the edge of the target, which measures approximately 15 mm in diameter. **B,** Deployment of the biopsy gun in **A** advances the needle 1.2 cm (between electronic cursors), provided the gun is held perfectly stationary. The tip of the needle is within the central portion of the target, safely harvesting a core sample (having advanced 1.2 cm). **C,** A long-throw (2.2 cm) automatic biopsy gun is used with an 18-gauge needle. The tip of the needle is placed on the edge of the target, which measure approximately 15 mm in diameter. **D,** Deployment of the biopsy gun in **C** advances the needle 2.2 cm (between electronic cursors), provided the gun is held perfectly stationary. The needle has passed through the target lesion with the tip now in the second, deeper positioned olive. This is an example of improper needle advancement and can have serious consequences (e.g., if the unintended sample is a major blood vessel). **E,** In this example, the distance of the biopsy needle throw is calculated for a lesion that is smaller than the throw length. The tip of the needle of this 2.2 cm throw automatic biopsy gun is positioned 2.2 cm from the center of the target (between electronic cursors). **F,** Deployment of the biopsy gun in **E** advances the needle precisely into the calculated center (x) of the target (while holding the gun perfectly stationary).

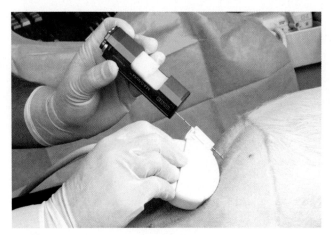

Figure 2-7 **Tissue-core biopsy of the liver.** One operator can obtain a tissue-core biopsy specimen with an automated biopsy gun. The needle can be placed by the freehand technique or with an external biopsy guide (as shown here). A spring-loaded single use needle with or without a guide may also be used. The Bard Magnum biopsy gun (Bard Biopsy Systems, Tempe, AZ) shown here is a nondisposable device that takes disposable needles for tissue-core biopsy. The length of the tissue core sampled may be adjusted with this device, which may also be sterilized, if desired.

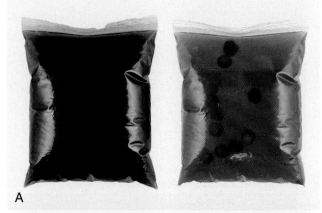

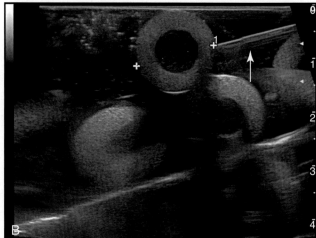

Figure 2-8 **Biopsy phantom. A,** To practice fine needle aspirations and biopsy technique, a gelatin phantom is recommended. Green olives have been suspended in gelatin within a zip-lock bag. The phantom on the left was made using dark purple food coloring so that the target lesions (olives) are not visible to the naked eye. The sonographer must rely solely on the ultrasound image for needle guidance. The phantom on the right is translucent, showing olive targets suspended within the gelatin. A translucent phantom may be best for those just learning needle placement technique. **B,** Ultrasound images of green olives with pimento make an excellent target for practicing hand-eye coordination of ultrasound-guided aspiration and biopsy technique. Olives appear as a target lesions, with a thick hyperechoic rim surrounding a hypoechoic center. The olive in the near field measures 1.5 cm in diameter (between electronic cursors). An aspiration needle (*arrow*) is present with the tip slightly indenting the olive.

distance that the needle might travel when deployed. The sterile needle is loaded into the gun with nonsterile technique, using the hub for handling. The needle shaft remains sterile because sterile plastic tubing covers its length. The tubing is removed immediately before the biopsy. The needle shaft does not touch the gun during operation. Regardless of whether a biopsy gun or spring-loaded single-use device is used, an assistant uses a sterile injection needle to remove the biopsy sample from the specimen notch. The sample can be placed in formalin or a sterile container for culture or impression smears. Because the needle shaft remains sterile, the needle can be reloaded into the biopsy gun for multiple biopsies of the same organ or site. If more than one organ is to be sampled, use of a new needle is recommended to prevent spread of infection or neoplasia. Figure 2-7 shows a biopsy gun being used with a guide to obtain a liver sample.

A biopsy phantom made out of a gelatin-filled plastic ziplock bag (or an empty intravenous fluid bag or barium enema bag) is useful to practice hand-eye coordination for freehand or guided biopsy techniques (Figure 2-8). Olives (green, with pimento) or other suitable items for imaging are suspended within the phantom while the gelatin solidifies. The operator can practice keeping the needle within the plane of the beam and inserting needles at various angles with the freehand technique.

Potential Complications

The potential complications of ultrasound-guided biopsy vary with the experience of the operator, type of biopsy, size of the needle, and nature of the lesion. Complications are much less common than with blind techniques. Aspiration procedures should initially be performed with 25- to 27-gauge needles if there is a high potential for bleeding, such as in patients with thrombocytopenia.[15] This can be followed by a larger bore needle or tissue-core biopsy if required. Hemorrhage, as discussed previously, is usually minor and self-limited if there are no coagulation abnormalities and a small-gauge needle is used. If it is available, color Doppler imaging to help avoid vascular structures before biopsy will reduce complications. In one report in small animals, significant hemorrhage was found in

less than 5% and death in less than 1% of all procedures.[3] In another study of 195 dogs and 51 cats that underwent 233 ultrasound-guided biopsies or fine-needle aspirations, 1.2% had major complications and 5.6% had minor localized hemorrhage.[29]

A recent report on cats undergoing liver biopsy describes a high fatality rate (19%) when a fully automatic biopsy gun was used. No deaths occurred when a semiautomatic biopsy needle was used.[30] The deaths were explained by intense vagotonia and shock resulting from the pressure wave generated by the strong spring mechanism of the automated biopsy gun. Although we have not experienced this horrible complication in our practices, we have heard similar tales from practitioners worldwide. Biopsy guns must be used with caution, if at all, in cats and other small patients.

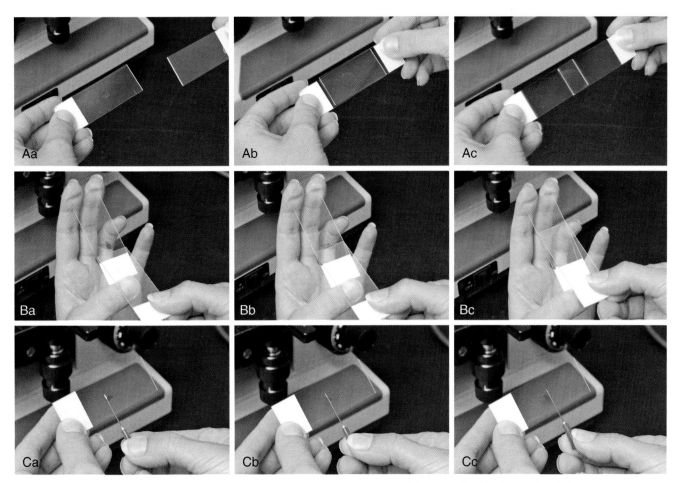

Figure 2-9 Slide techniques. A, Squash (a, b, c). One clean slide is gently placed over the slide containing fresh (not dried) sample material and the slides are gently pulled apart using no downward pressure. This will help spread the cells into a monolayer to allow for accurate cytologic evaluation. **B,** Smear (a, b, c). This technique is similar to a blood smear and pushes the sample across the slide gently to spread out the cells for cytologic evaluation. This is often used on fluid samples. **C,** Needle (a, b, c). This technique is performed by rolling an unused needle parallel to the slide to gently spread out the sample. There will likely be thick areas of the slide that may not be of good cytologic quality, but a monolayer can be seen along the edges to help with cell evaluation. This technique is often recommended for densely cellular samples that contain predominantly broken cells using other methods.

Complications can vary with the type of biopsy (fine-needle aspiration versus tissue-core biopsy), the organ examined, and the nature of the lesion sampled. Sepsis or peritonitis is possible, although rare, when an abscess or infected lesion is sampled. Appropriate broad-spectrum antibiotics should be administered prophylactically until results of bacterial culture and sensitivity studies are obtained. A thick lesion wall usually prevents leakage after aspiration. The diagnostic benefit clearly outweighs the risk in most cases. Penetration of adjacent structures, particularly bowel, during aspiration does not seem to increase the risk of complications.[29] Seeding of tumor along the needle track has been infrequently reported in veterinary patients and appears to be associated with transitional cell carcinoma of the bladder in dogs[31,32] and pulmonary adenocarcinoma in cats.[32]

Slide Preparation Techniques for Fine Needle Aspirates

In our practices, fine-needle aspirations are the mainstay of ultrasound-guided diagnostics procedures, performed multiple times every day. Proper preparation of microscope slides

from needle aspirations is just as important as obtaining a proper sample. Nothing is more frustrating than submitting a slide that is determined to be nondiagnostic because of poor slide preparation technique. First, the slides should be carefully wiped clean with a tissue or clean shirtsleeve. This removes any film and debris (tiny glass particles) that are often present even in a newly opened box of slides. A clean slide allows a smooth smear to be made. The squash technique is popular and easy to master (Figure 2-9, *A*). Another is the smear technique (see Figure 2-9, *B*), similar to making a blood smear. Last is the needle technique (see Figure 2-9, *C*), in which a clean needle is used to spread the sample on the slide.

FINE NEEDLE ASPIRATION AND BIOPSY OF SPECIFIC ORGANS AND LOCATIONS

Brain and Spinal Cord

Intraoperative procedures of the brain and spinal cord have been used sparingly in animals but have the potential to provide the same benefit as comparable neurosurgical

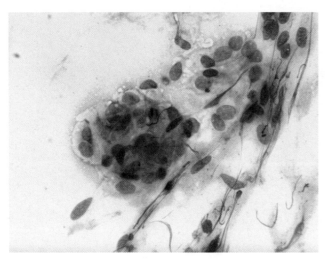

Figure 2-10 Meningioma. An aspirate of an extradural mass in the cervical region of a dog contains cohesive clusters of cells that range from elongate to oval with mild pleomorphism admixed with strewn nuclei. (Wright-Giemsa; ×50.)

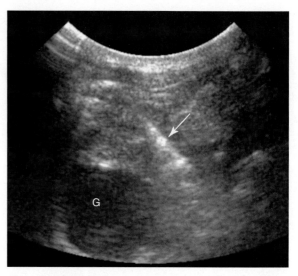

Figure 2-11 Biopsy of a retrobulbar mass in a cat. A freehand tissue-core biopsy of the retrobulbar mass is performed while taking care to avoid the globe (G) and optic nerve. Needle positioning is often difficult because of interference by the bony orbit. The biopsy needle is seen in the mass (*arrow*).

procedures in humans.[33] Although brain biopsy is commonly done with computed tomographic guidance, intraoperative sonography has also been used in humans and animals to guide needle placement for brain biopsies and to assist with localization and resection of brain lesions.[33-42] A craniotomy or burr hole permits transducer placement on the dura or cortical surface. The biopsy is done freehand, using a biopsy guide, or the transducer may be held with specialized devices to minimize movement. In some cases, the transducer is removed from a locked probe guide and replaced with a needle guidance system that is fixed at the same angle. The biopsy can then be done without direct ultrasound visualization.

Ultrasound guidance has also been used to place ventricular shunt catheters in infants, to evaluate arteriovenous malformations at surgery, and to assist in cerebral artery bypass operations.[38] Potential future applications include guidance for transdural laser ablation of specific areas of the brain.

Intraoperative spinal sonography has been helpful to accurately demarcate the borders of masses within the cord or spinal canal in humans and dogs (Figure 2-10).[33,38,43,44] In addition, the best site for biopsy of solid portions of complex masses can be determined. Ultrasonography can also provide immediate feedback regarding the adequacy of mass resection. Other uses of intraoperative ultrasound in dogs include assistance with surgical management of cervical spondylomyelopathy,[45] removal of herniated disks, assessment of the adequacy of decompression during laminectomy, and discospondylitis.[44]

A recent report describes the use of ultrasound-guided fine-needle aspiration to diagnose malignant peripheral nerve sheath tumors in the brachial plexus in dogs.[46]

Periorbital tissues

Although only one report of ultrasound guided intervention into the periorbital soft tissues is present in the veterinary literature,[47] we have used this technique at our institutions for many years. Typically an aspiration biopsy is attempted first, using a 20- to 22-gauge injection needle, with tissue-core biopsy to follow if the sample is nondiagnostic (Figure 2-11). A biopsy guide is difficult to use for these lesions because the approach is often limited by surrounding bony structures. Thus a free-hand technique is frequently used. The globe, optic nerve, and orbital vasculature must all be avoided during these procedures.

Soft Tissues of the Cervical Region

High-frequency ultrasonography has been used to evaluate the thyroid gland, parathyroid gland, and other surrounding structures in the cervical region of the dog and cat.[48-54] Fine-needle aspiration biopsy guided by direct palpation has been done successfully, but ultrasound may detect and enable aspiration of smaller lesions or structures not readily palpated. A 10- to 13-MHz or higher linear-array transducer is preferred to obtain the best near-field visualization. In many cases, there is clinical or laboratory evidence of thyroid or parathyroid disease and aspiration is not needed. For those that may require aspiration, a 21- to 25-gauge needle may be introduced freehand, adjacent to the transducer in the same plane as the beam. Doppler ultrasound is useful in preaspiration or prebiopsy assessment of cervical masses, because thyroid carcinomas are common in dogs and very well vascularized; thus they often hemorrhage after aspiration or biopsy. Figure 2-12 shows characteristic cytology of a dog thyroid carcinoma and a feline thyroid adenoma. As for many lesions, tissue-core biopsy specimens are sometimes necessary if aspiration biopsies are inconclusive or unsuccessful.

Bone

Traditionally, ultrasonography has not been used to evaluate bone lesions owing to the inability of ultrasound to penetrate the cortex. However, evaluation becomes possible when there are breaks in the cortex (Figure 2-13). Fine-needle aspirates of bony lesions have proven useful in distinguishing osteosarcoma from other types of bone tumors and usually can differentiate neoplasia and infectious bony lesions. Bone aspirates are now commonly performed in our practices. The feasibility of ultrasound-guided fine-needle aspiration biopsy of suspected neoplastic lesions of bone has been reported in a preliminary study of 22 dogs and 1 cat.[55] Radiographic evidence of a destructive or destructive-productive bone lesion was identified in the appendicular skeleton of 20 animals and in the axial skeleton of 3. It was concluded that ultrasound-guided aspiration biopsy, if diagnostic, may help prevent the need for anesthesia and a tissue-core biopsy in some cases (see Figure 2-13, C). However, if the aspiration biopsy finding is negative or inconclusive, a tissue-core biopsy and histologic

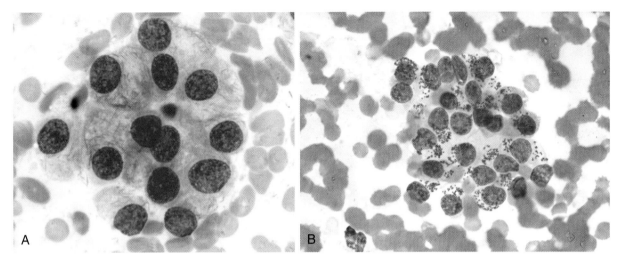

Figure 2-12 **A,** Thyroid carcinoma. Aspirates from a cervical mass in a dog reveal cohesive clusters of round to polygonal cells exhibiting mild to moderate pleomorphism. Canine thyroid carcinomas often appear uniform cytologically, and histopathologic evaluation is often recommended for complete characterization. (Wright-Giemsa; ×100.) **B,** Thyroid adenoma. A fine-needle aspirate from a feline mass in the thyroid region reveals a cohesive cluster of round to slightly cuboidal cells exhibiting mild pleomorphism and containing few to several dark blue to black granules (tyrosine granules). (Wright-Giemsa; ×100.)

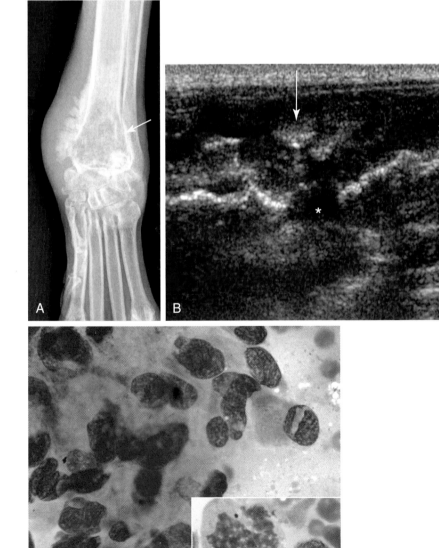

Figure 2-13 **Aspiration of bone. A,** Radiograph of the distal radius of a dog with a primary osteosarcoma (*arrow*) showing regions of production and destruction. Ultrasound guided aspiration is possible because breaks in the cortex are present. **B,** The normally smooth periosteal surface is irregular with mineralization elevated from the cortex (*arrow*). A break in the cortex is seen (*) and is the best location into which to place the biopsy needle. **C,** Aspirates reveal numerous pleomorphic spindle cells associated with eosinophilic material (osteoid). The inset contains a mitotic figure, commonly observed cytologically. (Wright-Giemsa; ×100.)

evaluation should be performed in all cases. In this series, 18 lesions were sarcomas, 3 were carcinomas, 1 was a bone cyst, and 1 was inconclusive. Ultrasound-guided aspiration biopsy was of diagnostic value in 11 of 23 cases (47.8%). A more recent study showed diagnostic bone aspiration samples were obtained in 32 of 36 canine osteosarcomas with high sensitivity and specificity.[56]

Thorax

Ultrasound-guided techniques facilitate sampling of pleural fluid, and pulmonary, mediastinal, and thoracic wall lesions, provided that there is adequate contact between the lesion and the chest wall (Figure 2-14) or pleural fluid is present.[9,57-77] Recent thoracic radiographs should be compared with the ultrasound findings before interventional procedures, and spectral or color Doppler techniques are used to exclude masses of vascular origin and to avoid normal vascular structures.

Linear-array transducers may provide the best visualization of pleural nodules because of a wide near-field view but are encumbered by a large transducer face that dictates positioning within the intercostal space. A small sector scanner such as a microconvex probe works well within an intercostal space because of its small footprint, but does not offer the best near field image. A biopsy guide, if it can be used, facilitates placement of the needle in small lesions. It is unnecessary for large lesions. A guide may be difficult to use in small patients or when ribs interfere with proper placement. The freehand technique is recommended in these cases and is the preferred and most commonly used technique.

We routinely aspirate thoracic masses with regular injection needles of 22- to 27-gauge or spinal needles of 21- to 22-gauge by the freehand technique. Extension tubing may be attached to the needle before the biopsy. This provides a closed system and decreases the risk of lung laceration during movement of the patient.

Cytologic evaluation of thoracic fluid is nearly always indicated and often diagnostic. Ultrasound is a very effective modality to safely obtain pleural fluid samples. There is minimal risk of hemorrhage if the heart and great vessels within the mediastinum are carefully avoided, and pneumothorax risk is minimal as well. Figure 2-15 shows examples of commonly encountered and cytologically diagnosed pleural effusions and cranial mediastinal mass lesions.

Biopsy of larger masses (>2.5 cm) has been successfully done with spring-loaded biopsy devices, although the risk of complications is greater than with aspiration.[25] Should a pulmonary mass be sampled, core biopsy specimens should be taken from the nonaerated portions of the mass to reduce the risk of pneumothorax, avoiding blood vessels and the periphery of the lesion. It is important that needle travel not extend outside the mass during the biopsy. Biopsy-induced pneumothorax, if it occurs, is usually minor and self-limited with no treatment required. No significant complications have been

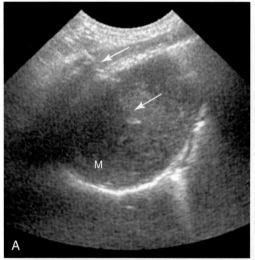
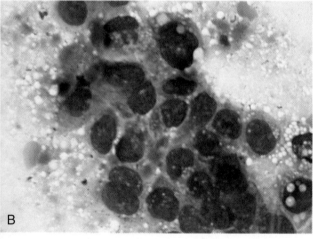
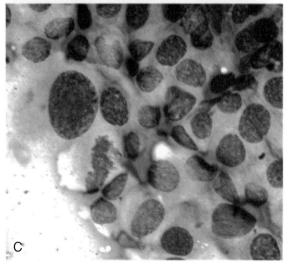

Figure 2-14 Fine needle aspiration of a pulmonary mass and commonly encountered lung neoplasms. A, The mass is easily visible because contact with the pleural surface is present. The needle (*arrows*) has been guided between the ribs and is visible within the mass (*M*). Note that the needle is placed distant to the aerated lung surrounding and deep to the mass. **B,** Carcinoma. Aspirates of a lung mass from a dog contain several cohesive clusters of epithelial cells exhibiting multiple criteria of malignancy including moderate anisocytosis and anisokaryosis, nuclear molding, and an increased mitotic rate. (Wright-Giemsa; ×100.) **C,** Histiocytic sarcoma. Lung aspirate from a dog with predominantly round to occasionally spindle shaped cells exhibiting marked pleomorphism. (Wright-Giemsa; ×100.)

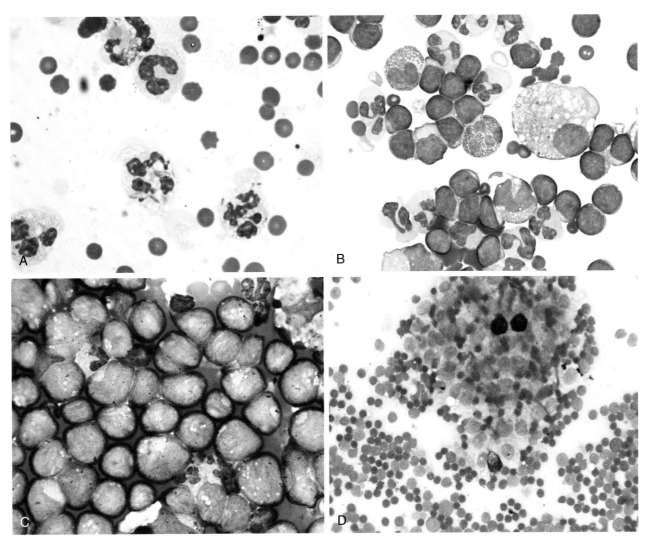

Figure 2-15 **Cytology of commonly encountered pleural effusions. A,** Pyothorax. Thoracic fluid from a cat reveals numerous degenerate neutrophils admixed within a proteinaceous background containing red blood cells. Bacteria are observed intracellularly (center of image) and also extracellularly (not shown). (Wright-Giemsa; ×100.) **B,** Chylous effusion. A cytospin preparation of thoracic fluid from a cat reveals several small lymphocytes (smaller than a neutrophil) with few eosinophils and a macrophage containing punctuate vacuoles. (Wright-Giemsa; ×100.) **C,** Lymphosarcoma from effusion, cranial mediastinal mass, or both. A cytospin preparation of thoracic fluid from a dog reveals numerous large lymphocytes containing few microvacuoles. (Wright-Giemsa; ×100.) **D,** Canine thymoma. Aspirates of a canine cranial mediastinal mass reveal a mixed population of cells including epithelial cells admixed with numerous, predominantly small lymphocytes and few scattered mast cells. (Wright-Giemsa; ×50.)

encountered with use of these techniques during more than 25-years at our institutions. When feasible, ultrasound-guided thoracic aspirations and biopsies are preferred over computed tomography or fluoroscopic techniques because they are simple, safe, and low cost.

Abdomen

In small animals, abdominal ultrasound-guided fine needle aspirations and biopsies are generally performed with the animal in lateral or dorsal recumbency on a V-shaped, padded trough or surgery table. Sedation and local anesthesia are administered as needed, depending on the type of aspiration or biopsy and temperament of the animal. The shortest distance to the biopsy site should be noted during the initial ultrasound examination.

Because of the safety and ease of fine-needle aspirates, nearly all abnormalities seen are aspirated instead of biopsied, with biopsy to follow if cytology is inconclusive or nondiagnostic. This procedure works well in our hospitals because we have in-house clinical pathology laboratory service. Results are available quickly after sampling, which allows resampling or biopsy the same day if needed. Sending cytology samples out for next day service is problematic if the results are inconclusive, so many practitioners prefer to perform a more definitive tissue core biopsy instead of fine-needle aspirations. Also remember that there is not always good agreement between cytologic and histologic findings. Additionally, findings from small tissue cores obtained with a biopsy needle do not always agree with results from larger samples obtained with laparoscopy or laparotomy. One of the most important lessons

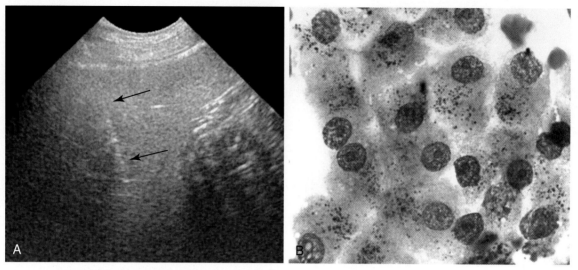

Figure 2-16 **Fine needle aspirate of the liver. A,** A freehand fine-needle aspiration of the liver is performed in a region devoid of vessels and biliary structures. For diffuse liver disease, the left liver lobes are typically chosen for biopsy. The needle (*arrows*) is visualized within the liver. **B,** Feline liver: Fine-needle aspirate from a normal liver. (Wright-Giemsa; ×100.)

learned over the years is to develop a good, synergistic working relationship with your clinical pathologist.

Liver
In our practices, nearly all liver alterations seen on ultrasound or found on serum biochemistries are aspirated, with possible biopsy to follow if cytology is inconclusive or not diagnostic. The techniques for liver fine-needle aspirates and biopsy with various blind and guided methods have been reviewed.[8] With use of ultrasonography, the transducer must be positioned under the sternum by applying sufficient pressure to displace overlying gas-filled stomach (see Figure 2-6). This is not necessary if the liver is markedly enlarged. The specimen can be taken while the liver is viewed in a sagittal, transverse, or dorsal plane as long as the thickness of the liver parenchyma is adequate to fully accommodate needle travel during the procedure (Figure 2-16). Penetration of the pleural cavity should be avoided if an intercostal approach is used.

Biopsy or aspiration of the liver is routinely done in the left medial or left lateral lobe away from the diaphragm, central hilar vessels, gallbladder, and apex of the heart. This may not be possible when solitary focal lesions are present or if the liver is small, requiring the sonographer to be very certain of needle direction and depth. As noted, aspiration is usually the first-line procedure of choice for liver disease, with or without sonographic abnormalities. Aspirates of solid, cystic, complex, or highly vascular lesions, or diffuse disease are routinely performed. This may be followed with a tissue-core biopsy if the aspirate is nondiagnostic and biopsy of the solid portion of the lesion can be done safely. To reduce the chance of bleeding and possible peritoneal dissemination of tumor or infection, the capsular surface of the liver is avoided during sampling. With focal lesions, it is helpful to include more normal-appearing liver at the margin of a lesion. When diffuse liver disease is present, two or three samples in different locations are taken to ensure an adequate, representative specimen. Lesions that appear highly vascular may be avoided in favor of surgical biopsy unless a suitable nonvascular region can be identified. Assessment of vascularity is facilitated with Doppler ultrasonography before the biopsy. In cases of very small livers, acoustic windows may be difficult or impossible to obtain, rendering ultrasound-guided biopsy (or even aspirates) unsafe, with deference to surgical methods. In some cases, breath-hold technique under general anesthesia displaces a small liver caudally enough for a safe transcostal window to be obtained.

As we know, there are limitations in cytologic findings obtained from fine-needle aspirates, with discordant results when compared to tissue biopsy.[78] An interesting recent study compared ultrasound findings with cytology in dogs with suspected liver disease.[79] It was found that liver masses 3 cm or larger, ascites, hepatic lymph node abnormalities, and an abnormal spleen were most predictive of hepatic neoplasia on cytology, whereas liver nodules smaller than 3 cm were most predictive of a cytologic diagnosis of vacuolar hepatopathy. Realizing some limitations of cytology for definitive diagnoses, there are a number of common diseases that can be fairly reliably diagnosed via high quality fine needle aspirates. These include diffuse diseases such as lymphoma, mast cell disease, vacuolar hepatopathy (usually steroid hepatopathy in dogs, lipidosis in cats), cholestasis, hepatitis, and cholangiohepatitis. Hepatic cancers are often diagnosed with cytology but are more apt to require tissue-core biopsies for a more specific diagnosis. Figure 2-17 shows examples of liver disease diagnosed from cytology.

Gallbladder and Biliary Tract
Several ultrasound-guided techniques involving the biliary system have been developed for use in humans and may have applications in veterinary medicine. These include diagnostic gallbladder aspiration, gallbladder aspiration biopsy, diagnostic cholecystography, percutaneous cholecystostomy, and treatment of cholelithiasis.

Gallbladder aspiration with a small needle (20 to 22 gauge) to obtain bile for culture has been investigated as a method for diagnosis of acute cholecystitis in humans.[80,81] A positive Gram stain (1+ bacteria or white blood cells) or culture having 1+ bacterial growth was found to indicate acute cholecystitis in 87% of patients.[81] However, the researchers also reported that a negative Gram stain or culture did not necessarily exclude the disease in their series of patients.[81] High levels of antibiotics had been administered to many of their patients, which may have influenced the culture results. Therefore further investigation was recommended. It is now currently

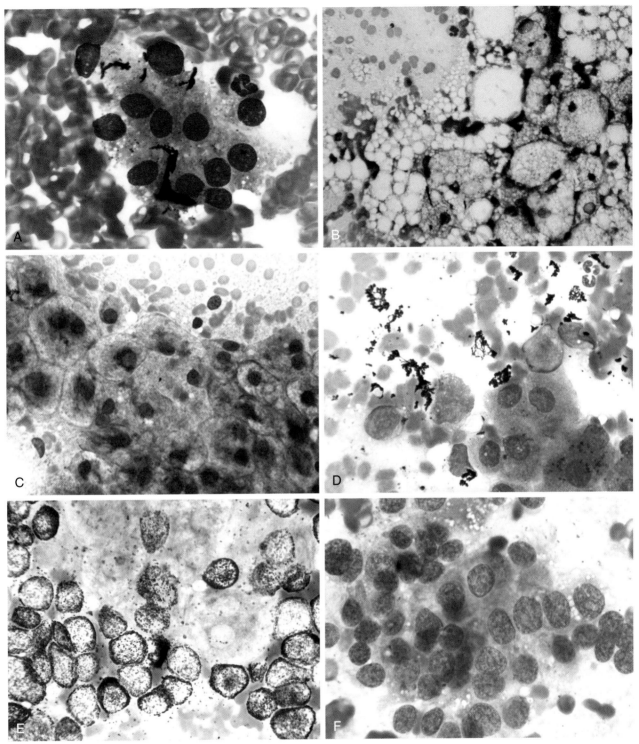

Figure 2-17 **Cytologic examples of commonly diagnosed liver disease. A,** Cholestasis. Liver aspirate from a dog with cholestasis. Note the dark green to black thick bile casts situated between hepatocytes. (Wright-Giemsa; ×100.) **B,** Lipidosis. Liver aspirate from a cat with hepatic lipidosis. The hepatocytes are distended by coalescing, variably sized, clear vacuoles. (Wright-Giemsa; ×100.) **C,** Vacuolar hepatopathy. Liver aspirate from a dog with vacuolar change compatible with glycogen deposition. The majority of hepatocytes contain wispy to slightly vacuolated cytoplasm. (Wright-Giemsa; ×100.) **D,** Lymphoma. Aspirate of canine liver contains large lymphocytes admixed with well-differentiated hepatocytes; scattered lymphoglandular bodies and purple granular material (ultrasound gel) are also present. (Wright-Giemsa; ×100.) **E,** Mast cell disease. Canine liver aspirates reveal numerous granulated mast cells admixed with a cluster of well-differentiated hepatocytes. (Wright-Giemsa; ×100.) **F,** Hepatic carcinoma. Liver aspirate from a dog with histopathologically diagnosed hepatic carcinoma. The cohesively clustered cells are disorganized and exhibit moderate pleomorphism with loss of normal hepatocyte morphology. (Wright-Giemsa; ×100.)

Continued

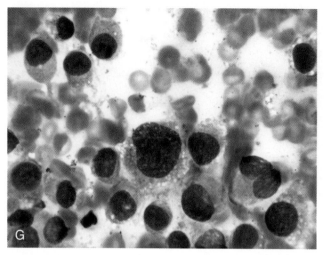

Figure 2-17, cont'd **G,** Histiocytic sarcoma. Liver aspirate from a dog with no normal hepatocytes present. The predominant cells are round to occasionally spindle-shaped, exhibiting marked pleomorphism. Few mitotic figures are noted. Additional features including multinucleated cells, nuclear atypia, and cytoplasmic vacuolation were noted in other areas of the cytology slide. (Wright-Giemsa; ×100.)

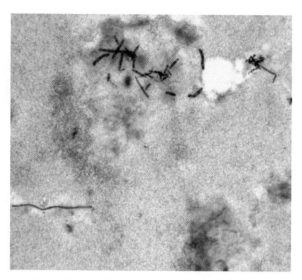

Figure 2-18 **Cholecystitis.** Direct preparation of bile fluid contains numerous large bacterial rods over an eosinophilic background with clumps of pale basophilic material and scattered golden bile pigment. (Wright-Giemsa; ×100.)

thought that percutaneous aspiration of the gallbladder is safe in humans but may lack utility for diagnosis of acute cholecystitis. Complications from gallbladder aspiration with use of small-bore needles are rare in human patients without obstructions. Aspiration of masses associated with the gallbladder wall in humans, with use of a small needle, have likewise been reported to carry minimal risk of complications.[82] Primary or undifferentiated carcinomas of the gallbladder wall have been diagnosed by this method.

Ultrasound-guided cholecystocentesis has been reported in healthy dogs[83] and cats[84] with no apparent side effects. A ventral abdominal approach is used to guide a 22-gauge needle into the fundus of the gallbladder, and bile is aspirated for culture and cytology. A report of three dogs with extrahepatic biliary obstruction secondary to pancreatitis indicated that ultrasound-guided therapeutic drainage of the gall bladder was successful for managing cholestasis until blockage of the common bile duct had resolved.[85] However, one of four cats with cholecystitis or acute neutrophilic cholangitis suffered gallbladder rupture following ultrasound-guided cholecystocentesis.[86]

Ultrasound-guided cholecystocentesis has become a moderately common procedure in our hospitals; it is straightforward and without complications. It may be indicated when hepatobiliary biochemical alterations are present (or absent) and there is abnormal bile on the ultrasound examination. Clinical signs of gallbladder disease may be mild and nondescript, and there has been historical reluctance to sample bile, especially if blood work is normal or not entirely suggestive of hepatobiliary disease. In our opinion, gallbladder sludge and debris should be assessed carefully, especially in cats, and not automatically discarded as incidental (Figure 2-18). We typically do not aspirate bile that has characteristics of a mucocele, especially if the wall is very thin or difficult to discern, for fear of rupture.

A small gauge needle is used (22- to 25-gauge injection or spinal needle) and bile is submitted for cytology and culture. As much bile as possible is drained from a single puncture, but unless asked to do so, repeated attempts to completely drain the gallbladder are not made. Needle passage through

the liver has been recommended, because the surrounding liver parenchyma will likely seal the puncture in the gallbladder wall. If a small gauge needle does not yield a sample, a larger size may be used, but in our experience, infected bile is usually thin and watery. Mucus is usually difficult to aspirate even with an 18-gauge needle, a clue that you are dealing with a mucocele.

Percutaneous cholecystography has been used in humans to opacify the biliary system before surgery when transhepatic cholangiography under fluoroscopic guidance has failed.[87-89] The risk of leakage was reported to be greatest with biliary obstruction or the use of larger bore needles. Gallbladder leakage was less likely if the needle passed through the hepatic parenchyma before entering the gallbladder, possibly because of tamponade of the puncture by the liver.[90]

Percutaneous cholecystostomy has been used to treat acute cholecystitis or temporarily relieve biliary obstruction in extremely ill patients, allowing their clinical condition to improve before surgical cholecystectomy,[87,91] and we have occasionally been asked to do this. A variety of specialized catheter systems have been developed that allow percutaneous placement of the catheter into the gallbladder under ultrasound guidance. Catheter dislodgment is prevented by the formation of a loop or accordion configuration in the distal intraluminal portion of the catheter. Techniques for percutaneous gallbladder ablation with ultrasound guidance are also under investigation. These methods may help treat patients that are too ill for surgical cholecystectomy. Cholelithiasis in humans has previously been treated with percutaneous techniques such as basket removal, fragmentation, and contact stone dissolution. However, these methods are less frequently used today.

Spleen

The spleen may be aspirated to sample focal lesions or to help determine the cause of diffuse splenomegaly. Aspiration of sonographically normal spleen is also common in our practices if clinically indicated, as a normal appearing spleen may not be normal at all (mast cell disease, lymphoma). Aspiration procedures are most useful in detecting lymphosarcoma or mast cell involvement of the spleen, as well as extramedullary hematopoiesis, hyperplasia, and even metastatic disease. Two

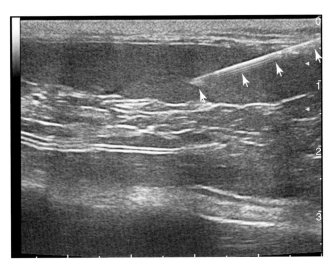

Figure 2-19 **Aspiration biopsy of the spleen in a cat.** Routine splenic aspiration biopsy is nearly always performed by the free-hand method and does not require a biopsy guide. The 25-gauge needle (*arrows*) can be identified within the spleen. Note the characteristic metal comet-tail reverberation artifact from the needle. Although the 25-gauge needle is very small, it is well visualized because it is nearly at a right angle to the incident ultrasound beam of this linear array transducer, the focal points are properly positioned, and a high frequency (13 MHz) was used. Aspiration and biopsy needles are generally not seen with this degree of clarity (see Figure 2-23, *A*).

recent publications have stressed the importance of aspiration cytology of the spleen (and liver) for staging mast cell disease in dogs.[92,93] Unfortunately, splenic hemangiosarcoma, which is common in dogs, is more difficult to definitively diagnose cytologically. A 22- or 25-gauge injection needle is used with a freehand method in most cases (Figure 2-19). A pincushion aspiration technique is advocated and should be stopped as soon as blood is seen in the needle hub. This prevents dilution of the sample with blood, which makes interpretation difficult. The aspirate should be evaluated immediately and the aspiration repeated if necessary. No complications have been encountered with splenic aspirates or tissue core biopsies if coagulation parameters are normal. The sonographer should avoid exiting the opposite side of the spleen with the needle; two puncture sites bleed more than a single entry puncture. Figure 2-20 illustrates cytologically diagnosed diffuse and nodular splenic diseases.

Tissue-core biopsies of the spleen have historically been avoided by many because of a perceived high potential for hemorrhage. However, in a preliminary investigation, 22 anesthetized dogs underwent splenic biopsy with an 18-gauge needle and the automated Biopty gun[94]; 3 dogs were found to have a 60-mL blood loss and 7 dogs had an average 30-mL loss, whereas 12 dogs had no detectable hemorrhage. The specimens were of high quality in 70% of the cases. Lower quality samples were attributed to red pulp congestion caused by anesthesia. In a follow-up clinical study of seven cases, the investigators reported that high-quality splenic biopsy specimens were obtained with no complications. They also concluded that tissue-core biopsies of the spleen might be of poor quality or nondiagnostic if the spleen is engorged. Others have since described similar findings.[10] A more recent investigation concluded that splenic biopsies were indeed safe to perform and provided information that complements analysis of fine-needle aspirates.[95]

In our experience, tissue-core biopsies of solid splenic masses are useful and can be performed safely if an aspirate

is nondiagnostic. However, both aspirates and biopsies of complex splenic masses containing fluid-filled cystic structures (e.g., many hemangiosarcoma lesions) are less useful and often nondiagnostic because of blood dilution or sampling of nonneoplastic portions of hemorrhagic tumor. As a general rule, most complex splenic masses are surgically removed without prior FNA or biopsy. Thoracic radiographs and ultrasound of the heart are commonly performed additional diagnostic procedures in these cases.

Pancreas

Pancreatic biopsy is performed to differentiate pancreatitis or pancreatic abscess from pancreatic neoplasia. Differentiation of pancreatic diseases is difficult because clinical signs, laboratory values, and appearance on imaging studies are often similar. Pancreatic carcinoma and pancreatitis also commonly coexist in the same patient. Overall, we perform comparatively few aspirations and even fewer biopsies on the pancreas compared to the liver, spleen, and kidney. However, we have not experienced any deleterious effects from the aspirations and biopsies we have performed during the past 25 years.

In humans, the yield from aspiration biopsies of the pancreas has been less rewarding than for liver. This is because tumor and pancreatitis are commonly found together, yielding a high percentage of inconclusive aspirates. Sampling of the inflammatory or necrotic portions of a mass may also lead to a false-negative diagnosis. However, a fluid aspirate may help determine whether there is associated infection. Nevertheless, the sensitivity for diagnosis of pancreatic carcinoma ranges from 64% to 100% with no false-positive results.[96]

The 9-cm, 20- to 22-gauge spinal needle has been shown to provide excellent samples of pancreatic masses in humans. Aspiration biopsies may be done by back-and-forth needle movements as described previously or by using rotary drilling motions with continuous suction during advancement of the needle. Figure 2-21 is an example of fine needle aspiration cytology of canine pancreatitis.

Complications associated with aspiration biopsy of the pancreas in humans are unusual. However, severe acute pancreatitis sometimes develops for unexplained reasons. Acute pancreatitis was the main complication observed, especially when normal pancreatic tissue was penetrated in sampling small lesions.[97,98] In one review of 184 pancreatic biopsies, 5 patients (3%) developed acute pancreatitis, and all of them had lesions smaller than 3 cm.[99] Seeding of tumor along the needle track has been reported infrequently and is not presently considered a contraindication to biopsy in humans.[97,100]

In humans, tissue-core biopsy specimens of the pancreas obtained by an automated biopsy gun and an 18-gauge needle have also been used successfully for diagnosis of malignant pancreatic disease.[101] However, we recommend aspiration of pancreatic lesions unless the mass is large. This is to avoid traversing normal pancreatic tissue or possibly penetrating adjacent vital structures in the pancreatic region. A recent article has compared the effect of pancreatic tissue sampling on serum pancreatic enzyme levels in normal dogs.[102] Ultrasound-guided aspiration did not cause an elevation in pancreatic lipase values or serum trypsin-like immunoreactivity. Intraoperative aspiration and clamshell tissue biopsy, however, were associated with increased serum trypsin-like immunoreactivity and mild peracute necrosis, inflammation, hemorrhage, and fibrin deposition. An elevation in canine-specific pancreatic lipase was not seen during the time frame of the study.

Pancreatic pseudocysts are easily aspirated, but subsequent leakage may cause peritoneal irritation. Therefore a 22-gauge or smaller needle should be used for diagnostic aspiration. The recurrence rate is high in humans after treatment by aspiration drainage alone.[103] Surgical treatment or external catheter drainage is still the preferred therapeutic procedure.[104] In dogs, pancreatic pseudocysts usually resolve without treatment provided that they are not infected.

Gastrointestinal Tract

Surgical intervention is usually required to relieve bowel obstruction or to treat hemorrhage associated with gastrointestinal masses. Therefore biopsy specimens are often obtained at surgery. However, focal masses associated with the gastrointestinal tract may be aspirated without risk with a small gauge needle to obtain material for cytologic diagnosis.[6,105-107]

A tissue-core biopsy sample can be safely taken of large solid masses if clinically indicated. The bowel lumen should be avoided to reduce the chance of subsequent fistula formation or peritonitis. The risk of bleeding, leakage, or dissemination of tumor or infection can be diminished by taking the sample entirely within the mass rather than cutting through the outer serosal surface.

Aspiration (or tissue core biopsy with a 20-gauge needle) of segmental or diffusely thickened bowel is routinely performed and can be diagnostic (Figure 2-22). However, there are very real limitations with this method, especially with normal appearing or mildly thickened bowel. Diagnostic samples can be difficult to obtain, and inflammatory bowel disease may be difficult to differentiate from lymphoma, two of the most common causes of bowel thickening. Aspiration of regional lymph nodes is commonly done with intestinal aspirates, but even so, misdiagnoses can occur.[108] For these reasons, the most reliable diagnostic test is full thickness biopsy of intestine and lymph node samples obtained at surgery or by laparoscopy.

Kidney

Aspiration and tissue-core biopsies of diffuse kidney disease or masses are performed with procedures similar to those used for other abdominal organs. It is very important to direct the needle away from the renal hilus; laceration of a renal artery or vein will be lethal. Typically, the caudal pole of the left

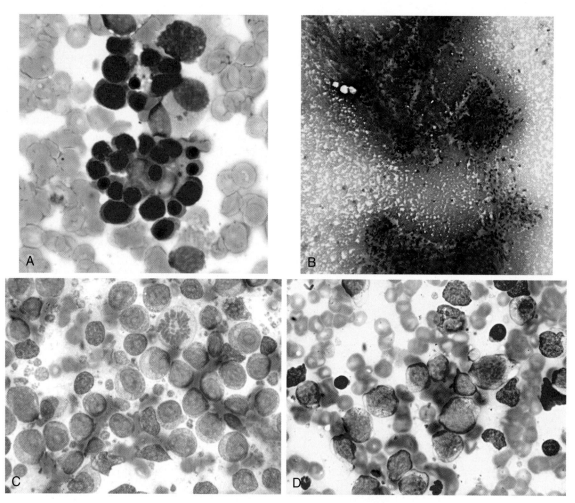

Figure 2-20 Cytologically diagnosed diffuse and nodule splenic disease. A, Canine extramedullary hematopoiesis (EMH). Fine needle aspirates of canine spleen containing numerous erythroid precursors. Large megakaryocytes and myeloid precursors can also be seen. (Wright-Giemsa; ×100.) **B,** Splenic hyperplasia. Splenic aspirate from a dog containing numerous clumps of splenic reticular stromal cells with increased numbers of lymphocytes. There may also be a mild increase in plasma cells. (Wright-Giemsa; ×10.) **C,** Lymphosarcoma. Canine splenic aspirate diffusely containing numerous large lymphocytes, each with a prominent nucleolus surrounded by lymphoglandular bodies (basophilic bits of cytoplasm); mitotic rate is increased. (Wright-Giemsa; ×100.) **D,** Granular lymphoma. Aspirate of a canine spleen containing a predominance of large lymphocytes with perinuclear clusters of few eosinophilic granules. (Wright-Giemsa; ×100.)

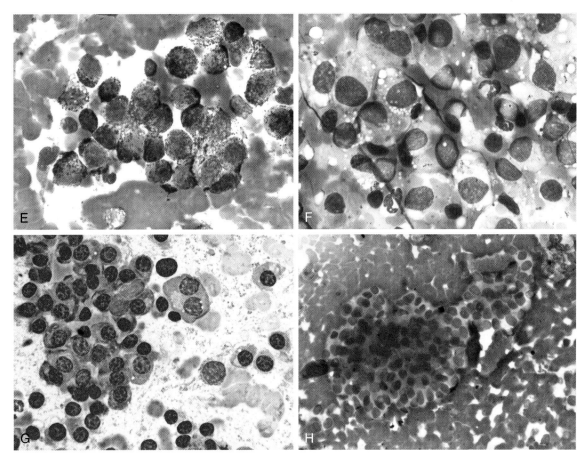

Figure 2-20, cont'd **E,** Mast cell tumor (MCT). Canine splenic aspirates reveal numerous round cells containing variable quantities of purple granules (mast cells) present in loose clusters and individually. (Wright-Giemsa; ×100.) **F,** Histiocytic sarcoma. Canine splenic aspirates reveal high numbers of spindle-shaped to round cells containing few cytoplasmic vacuoles and exhibiting moderate pleomorphism. Erythrophagocytosis is noted in several of the cells. (Wright-Giemsa; ×100.) **G,** Multiple myeloma. Aspirates from a canine spleen reveal sheets of plasma cells, which are occasionally binucleated and exhibit mild to moderate pleomorphism. (Wright-Giemsa; ×100.) **H,** Adenocarcinoma metastasis. Aspirate from a canine spleen containing cohesively clustered round to cuboidal cells, occasionally in acinar-like formations. (Wright-Giemsa; ×100.)

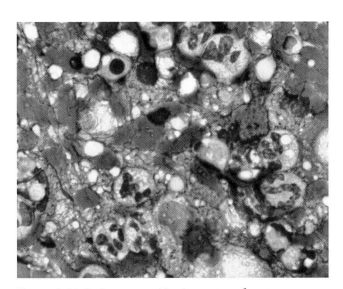

Figure 2-21 **Canine pancreatitis.** Aspiration of canine pancreas reveals numerous neutrophils, including a few pyknotic cells (upper left), admixed between amorphous eosinophilic strands of strewn nuclear debris or fibrin. (Wright-Giemsa; ×100.)

kidney is sampled because it is often easiest to access (Figure 2-23). The cranial pole of the left kidney or caudal pole of the right kidney is also usually accessible. A 22- or 25-gauge injection needle is preferred for aspiration. Aspiration of the kidney is routinely performed when lymphosarcoma is a primary differential diagnosis, and in nearly all cases, cytologic analysis leads to a definitive diagnosis (Figure 2-24). Mast cell tumor, amyloidosis, and some cases of pyelonephritis (Figure 2-25) are amenable to cytologic diagnosis. Cysts are not usually aspirated if they meet all of the ultrasound criteria for a simple renal cyst and are not associated with clinical signs. However, aspiration may be indicated if the cyst has a thick or irregular wall, internal echoes, or septations, or if a solid mass is seen arising from the wall of the cyst.

In many cases of renal insufficiency or failure, especially with normal appearance on sonography, structural alterations of glomeruli and renal tubules must be determined with histopathology, and tissue-core biopsies become necessary. This is also true in cases for which a previous fine-needle aspiration was nondiagnostic. However, because of high renal blood flow and potential complications from hemorrhage, renal biopsies are performed on a relatively limited and very selective basis. A commonly heard comment from around the world is that renal insufficiency or failure is treated the same regardless of

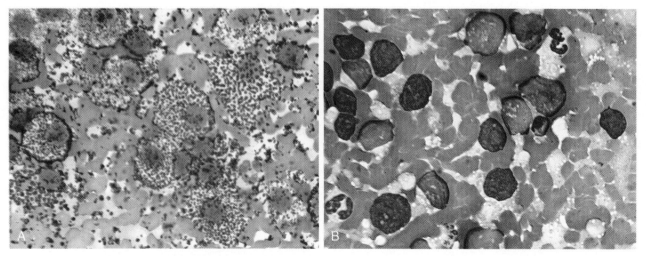

Figure 2-22 Aspiration cytology of gastrointestinal disease. A, Mast cell tumor. Aspirate of a feline small intestine contains numerous well-granulated mast cells are observed within a blood contaminated background. (Wright-Giemsa; ×100.) **B,** Lymphoma. Aspirates from a thickened feline stomach wall are highly cellular, containing a predominance of large lymphocytes admixed with lymphoglandular bodies and numerous red blood cells. (Wright-Giemsa; ×100.)

etiology, and the high risk versus treatment benefit of biopsy is often respected. A 16- or 18-gauge spring-loaded biopsy needle is usually preferred because it leaves a smaller puncture and perceived reduced risk of hemorrhage; 14-gauge needles are used in very large patients. However, it has been shown that renal biopsy tissue obtained with an 18-gauge needle is often deficient in glomeruli and crushed or fragmented, whereas 14-gauge needle samples were all of excellent quality.[20] This same study also showed that laparoscopic renal biopsies were of higher quality and obtained with less hemorrhage than ultrasound-guided biopsies. From communication with many practitioners in the United States and abroad, laparoscopic renal biopsies are preferred by those trained in this technique. The primary reasons cited are better quality of samples and ability to control hemorrhage.

Kidney biopsies in cats are usually done by immobilizing the kidney with transducer pressure, bringing it close to the ventral abdominal skin surface, and performing a biopsy of the lateral kidney cortex percutaneously with freehand ultrasound guidance. Biopsy with a guidance system is more difficult to perform on feline kidneys than on canine kidneys because of their small size and mobility. Biopsy of canine kidneys is usually done under ultrasound guidance either by the freehand technique or with use of external biopsy guides.

The caudal pole of the left kidney is the preferred tissue-core biopsy site when diffuse kidney disease is suspected. In most cases, two or three specimens are taken to ensure an adequate sample. The lateral cortex of the cranial or caudal pole of either kidney can be sampled from the ventral abdomen, but the hilar region should be avoided because of proximity to the pelvis and larger blood vessels. The position of the biopsy needle relative to the hilum is best determined by viewing the kidney in the sagittal plane. Also, the biopsy plane should not be directed medially, where the aorta or caudal vena cava may be accidentally punctured (a good motto to follow regardless of organ sampled!). Firm transducer pressure helps displace overlying bowel while the biopsy needle is inserted to the surface of the caudal pole. It is important to position the needle in this location so that cortical tissue and glomeruli are included in the sample. Deep penetration of the medulla and opposite kidney surface should be avoided, if possible. If the spleen is large, biopsy of

the left kidney may be difficult. However, the spleen and bowel can usually be avoided by judicious use of transducer pressure. Biopsy of the right kidney is slightly less desirable because of its cranial location and proximity to the pancreas. However, with proper technique, biopsy of the right kidney can also be successfully performed when diffuse disease is suspected.

Inadvertent penetration of the bowel or spleen with a small needle during aspiration biopsy is of no clinical consequence. Penetration of these organs with larger cutting needles should be prevented by using firm transducer pressure. We are not aware of any bowel- or spleen-related complications after hundreds of kidney biopsies at our institution. Drugs that cause splenic enlargement should be avoided to minimize potential interference from the spleen.

Complications of percutaneous renal biopsies in humans include renal, subcapsular, perirenal, and collecting system hemorrhage; urinary leaks and fistulas; arteriovenous malformations; and arteriocalyceal fistulas.[109-111] Complications such as perirenal hemorrhage and hematuria have been reported in small animals, but these have generally been limited to the immediate postbiopsy period.[1,20,112-114] Complications other than mild hemorrhage are rare, although persistent hemorrhage has been noted occasionally. Cats and miniature breed dogs seem more prone to hemorrhage in our experience. Hematuria is rare and usually resolves without treatment. However, hematuria was noted in one case for 10 days after a renal biopsy. This complication usually resolves without treatment and should be treated conservatively unless the hemorrhage is severe, blood clots obstruct the ureter, or the duration is longer than 2 weeks.

The patient must be monitored closely after kidney biopsy because the potential for hemorrhage is greater than with other organs. Monitoring should consist of an immediate postbiopsy scan of the kidney and bladder for signs of hemorrhage, serial packed cell volume determinations at 30-minute intervals if indicated, and close observation of vital signs for at least 4 to 6 hours.

The effect of ultrasound-guided renal biopsies on renal function has been investigated in cats and dogs.[115,116] It was found that unilateral renal biopsies in cats had minimal effect on renal function. Serial renal biopsies in dogs showed no

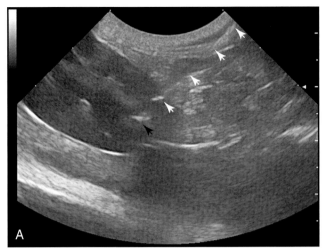

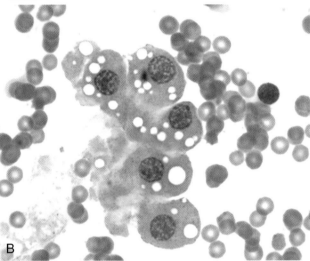

Figure 2-23 **Kidney fine needle aspirate. A,** Fine needle aspiration (25 gauge) of a normal cat kidney is usually performed in the cranial or caudal pole (shown) when diffuse disease is suspected. The needle (*arrows*) is only partially visible because a small needle and microconvex sector transducer were used. The black arrow denotes the tip of the needle. **B,** Fine needle aspirate from the normal cat kidney in **A.** Renal tubule epithelial cells are often vacuolated in cats. (Wright-Giemsa; ×100.)

differences in GFR between biopsied and control kidneys and only minimal changes that might be mistaken for progressive renal disease. A recent report has described the use of contrast harmonic ultrasound to evaluate postbiopsy renal parenchyma, both short and long term.[117] The authors found contrast harmonic imaging to be better for detecting postbiopsy lesions (22 out of 22 dogs) compared to conventional ultrasound (14 out of 22 dogs).

Adrenal Masses

In humans, adrenal masses of 2 to 3 cm or larger have been aspirated with ultrasound guidance. The most common indication is to confirm metastatic disease from a known primary malignant neoplasm elsewhere.[118] Human radiologists must be familiar with management of a hypotensive crisis should a pheochromocytoma be inadvertently sampled.[119,120] Adrenal masses may also be highly vascular, and assessment of vascularity with Doppler ultrasonography before biopsy is strongly recommended.

In the early years of veterinary ultrasound, adrenal aspirates and even biopsies were commonly performed by specialists. Today the trend has reversed because of improved biochemical tests and advancement of computed tomography and magnetic resonance imaging in assessment of adrenal disease, as well as personal observation of serious side effects from catecholamine release in a small number of patients. Little has been written on the subject in the veterinary literature. Ultrasound-guided biopsy of two dogs with adrenal hyperplasia[121] and one dog with an adrenal neuroblastoma[122] has been reported; no complications were described. Although an adrenal biopsy may be uneventful, there is the potential for a hypertensive or paradoxical hypotensive crisis if a pheochromocytoma is inadvertently sampled.[123] Close proximity to the aorta and caudal vena cava also increase risk. As in humans, intraoperative excision biopsies of pheochromocytomas are preferred because appropriate support staff and drugs are available to handle adverse reactions.

Urinary Bladder

Ultrasound is routinely used to atraumatically obtain urine samples. Bladder masses, which are nearly always neoplastic, are easily aspirated with a 22- to 25-gauge injection or spinal needle. However, implantation of tumor cells along the needle track has been reported, although the true frequency remains unknown.[31,32] We routinely employ ultrasound-guided aspiration of bladder masses via urethral catheter.[124] Ultrasonography is used to determine the position of the catheter adjacent to the bladder or urethral mass while "traumatic catheterization" and aspiration is performed to harvest cells (Figure 2-26). An end-port or side-port catheter may be used.

Prostate

As noted for urinary bladder masses, percutaneous aspirations or tissue biopsies have been associated with needle tract seeding, and therefore some practitioners use ultrasound to guide intraluminal traumatic catheterization to safely obtain samples (Figure 2-27, *A*) Percutaneous prostatic aspiration or tissue-core biopsies are still performed; however, they are usually obtained from the caudoventral abdomen lateral to the prepuce. A transrectal approach has also been reported and compared with the prepubic approach.[125] The parenchyma of the prostate in the intact male is slightly more echogenic than that of other abdominal organs, which may make needle visualization more difficult.[1] In the case of aspiration biopsies, a spinal needle is often necessary to reach the prostate, and jiggling the needle or moving the needle stylet may be necessary to improve visualization of the needle. Rocking the transducer may also help to position the needle better within the plane of the beam. Tissue-core biopsies are done in either a sagittal or transverse plane, ideally with use of an automated device and a 16- or 18-gauge needle. The pubis sometimes interferes with biopsy if the prostate is small or situated deep within the pelvic canal. As for essentially all ultrasound-guided samples, we perform many more aspirations than biopsies because of the ease of the procedure and comfortably reliable results.

Aspiration of intraparenchymal cysts or cavitary lesions for culture is recommended when prostatitis is suspected. A case series of 13 dogs undergoing ultrasound guided prostatic abscess and cyst drainage indicated that culture and sensitivity testing of the aspirated fluid was useful for diagnostic and therapeutic purposes.[126] Tissue-core biopsies are done when solid mass lesions or diffuse disease is present. However, cystic lesions and infection may also be present with prostatic neoplasia. Therefore a tissue biopsy should be performed in addition to aspiration when neoplasia is suspected. If possible, multiple areas within the prostate should be sampled, because

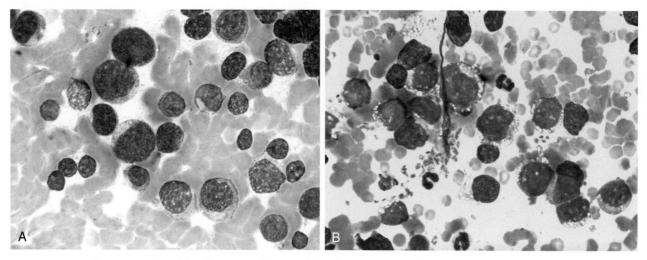

Figure 2-24 **Renal Lymphoma. A,** Feline renal lymphoma. Aspirates from an enlarged cat kidney contain numerous large lymphocytes and fewer small lymphocytes with scattered lymphoglandular bodies. (Wright-Giemsa; ×100.) **B,** Canine renal lymphoma. Aspirates from an enlarged, multi-nodular dog kidney contain numerous large lymphocytes (2 to 4 times the size of a neutrophil) with scant basophilic cytoplasm, often containing microvacuoles. The large lymphocytes often contain indistinct nucleoli. Lymphoglandular bodies, few neutrophils, and red blood cells are also observed. (Wright-Giemsa; ×100.)

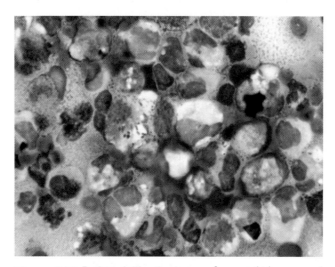

Figure 2-25 **Pyelonephritis.** Aspirates of a cat kidney reveal numerous markedly degenerate neutrophils with clusters of cocci and rod-shaped bacteria observed intracellularly (center of image). (Wright-Giemsa; ×100.)

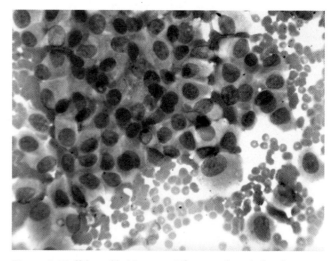

Figure 2-26 **Urinary bladder mass.** Ultrasound-guided catheterization from a mass in the trigone of the bladder from a dog reveal numerous large cohesive clusters of round to polygonal epithelial cells exhibiting moderate pleomorphism, diagnostic for transitional cell carcinoma. (Wright-Giemsa; ×100.)

prostatic diseases can be segmental or isolated within the gland. This results in fewer false-negative diagnoses. One study in a small number of dogs (25) concluded strong agreement between cytologic and histopathologic diagnosis for prostatic disease.[127] Figures 2-27, *B-D,* show examples of cytologic diagnoses of prostatic disease.

In our experience, the incidence of complications from prostatic biopsies is low. Potential complications include hemorrhage, leakage of contents from infected cavitary lesions, and persistent hematuria. The prostatic urethra should be avoided, as inadvertent puncture is not ideal.

During the procedure, be careful to avoid the aorta, vena cava, and iliac vessels that lie close to the prostate. Consider the distance of needle travel during the biopsy so that the dorsal prostate, adjacent vessels, and colon are not penetrated.

It is best to palpate the femoral artery in planning the biopsy route.

Local spread of infection or the development of septicemia after aspiration of intraprostatic abscesses is theoretically possible but has not been encountered with the use of small 21- to 22-gauge spinal needles for aspiration. Many animals are receiving concurrent treatment or will be treated with appropriate antibiotics. We usually do not aspirate paraprostatic cysts because bacteriologic culture is easily obtained at the time of surgical ablation or marsupialization.

Abdominal Lymph Nodes and Masses
Percutaneous aspiration or biopsy of enlarged lymph nodes or a mass of unknown origin is done in a standard manner, usually using a freehand method (Figure 2-28). The

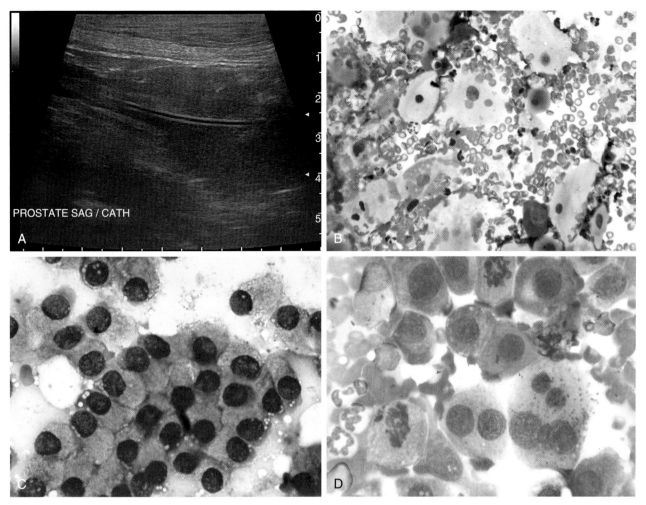

Figure 2-27 Prostate Gland. A, Sagittal ultrasound image of an abnormal prostate gland and urethra with a catheter in place, used to obtain cytologic samples. **B,** Squamous metaplasia and prostatitis. Aspirates of a canine prostate contain numerous squamous epithelial cells with minimal atypia and numerous neutrophils. The squamous metaplasia (confirmed histopathologically) was secondary to a testicular tumor. (Wright-Giemsa; ×100.) **C,** Benign prostatic hyperplasia. Aspiration of a symmetrically enlarged, intact male dog prostate reveals a cohesive cluster of uniform cuboidal cells aligned in rows and containing moderate amounts of basophilic cytoplasm with few microvacuoles. (Wright-Giemsa; ×100.) **D,** Prostatic carcinoma. Aspirates from an asymmetrically enlarged canine prostate gland show exfoliated round to polygonal nucleated cells, present individually and in loose clusters, exhibiting multiple criteria of malignancy (moderate anisokaryosis and anisocytosis, two mitotic figures, and multinucleation) with minimal associated inflammation. (Wright-Giemsa; ×100.)

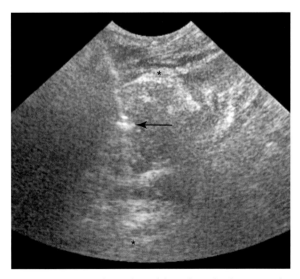

Figure 2-28 Biopsy of a lymph node. This enlarged lymph node (between electronic cursors) was biopsied using a single-use semiautomated biopsy device. The tip of the biopsy needle is in the parenchyma of the lymph node (*arrow*).

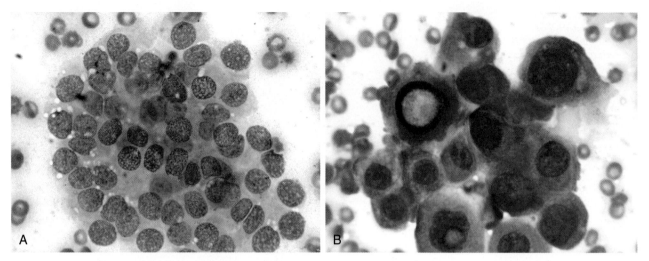

Figure 2-29 **Abdominal lymph node cytology. A,** Apocrine gland adenocarcinoma metastasis. Aspirates of a dog medial iliac lymph node contain no evidence of lymphoid tissue, which has been replaced by cohesive clusters of round to cuboidal cells exhibiting mild to occasionally moderate pleomorphism. This patient had a history of an apocrine gland adenocarcinoma. (Wright-Giemsa; ×100.) **B,** Prostatic carcinoma: Aspirates from a medial iliac lymph node lymph node from a dog with a history of prostatic carcinoma contain numerous cohesive clusters of large polygonal to round nucleated cells exhibiting moderate to marked pleomorphism. Very few lymphoid elements were seen in other areas of the slide to help confirm lymph node origin. (Wright-Giemsa; ×100.)

procedure chosen depends on the size of the lymph node or mass, its distance from the skin surface, and its proximity to vital structures. As for many aspiration or biopsy procedures, the distance between skin surface and lymph node can be reduced by applying firm pressure with the hand, the transducer, or both, before the needle is inserted. This also displaces overlying bowel loops. The sublumbar lymph nodes (medial iliac or others) may be aspirated if they are sufficiently enlarged and the major blood vessels, bladder, and colon can be avoided. Figure 2-29 shows diagnostic cytology of medial iliac lymph node metastasis.

REFERENCES

1. Hager DA, Nyland TG, Fisher P. Ultrasound-guided biopsy of the canine liver, kidney, and prostate. *Vet Radiol* 1985;**26**:82–8.
2. Hoppe FE, Hager DA, Poulos PW, et al. A comparison of manual and automatic ultrasound-guided biopsy techniques. *Vet Radiol* 1986;**27**:99–101.
3. Kerr LY. Ultrasound-guided biopsy. *Calif Vet* 1988; 9–10.
4. Papageorges M, Gavin PR, Sande RD, et al. Ultrasound-guided fine-needle aspiration: An inexpensive modification of the technique. *Vet Radiol* 1988;**29**: 269–71.
5. Smith S. Ultrasound-guided biopsy. *Semin Vet Med Surg (Small Anim)* 1989;**4**:95–104.
6. Penninck DG, Crystal MA, Matz ME, et al. The technique of percutaneous ultrasound guided fine-needle aspiration biopsy and automated microcore biopsy in small animal gastrointestinal diseases. *Vet Radiol Ultrasound* 1993;**34**:433–6.
7. Barr F. Percutaneous biopsy of abdominal organs under ultrasound guidance. *J Small Anim Pract* 1995;**36**: 105–13.
8. Kerwin SC. Hepatic aspiration and biopsy techniques. *Vet Clin North Am Small Anim Pract* 1995;**25**:275–91.
9. Wood EF, O'Brien RT, Young KM. Ultrasound-guided fine-needle aspiration of focal parenchymal lesions of the lung in dogs and cats. *J Vet Intern Med* 1998;**12**: 338–42.
10. de Rycke LM, van Bree HJ, Simoens PJ. Ultrasound-guided tissue-core biopsy of liver, spleen and kidney in normal dogs. *Vet Radiol Ultrasound* 1999;**40**:294–9.
11. Torp-Pedersen S, Lee F, Littrup PJ, et al. Transrectal biopsy of the prostate guided with transrectal US: longitudinal and multiplanar scanning. *Radiology* 1989;**170**: 23–7.
12. Zanetta G, Brenna A, Pittelli M, et al. Transvaginal ultrasound-guided fine needle sampling of deep cancer recurrences in the pelvis: usefulness and limitations. *Gynecol Oncol* 1994;**54**:59–63.
13. Caspers JM, Reading CC, McGahan JP, et al. Ultrasound-guided biopsy and drainage of the abdomen and pelvis. In: Rumack CM, Wilson SR, Charboneau JW, editors. *Diagnostic Ultrasound.* 2nd ed. St. Louis: Mosby–Year Book; 1998. p. 599–627.
14. McGahan JP. Invasive ultrasound principles (biopsy, aspiration, and drainage). In: McGahan JP, Goldberg BB, editors. *Diagnostic Ultrasound: A Logical Approach.* Philadelphia: Lippincott-Raven; 1998. p. 39–75.
15. Bigge LA, Brown DJ, Penninck DG. Correlation between coagulation profile findings and bleeding complications after ultrasound-guided biopsies: 434 cases (1993-1996). *J Am Anim Hosp Assoc* 2001;**37**:228–33.
16. Wang KY, Panciera DL, Al-Rukibat RK, et al. Accuracy of ultrasound-guided fine-needle aspiration of the liver and cytologic findings in dogs and cats: 97 cases (1990-2000). *J Am Vet Med Assoc* 2004;**224**:75–8.
17. Ballegeer EA, Forrest LJ, Dickinson RM, et al. Correlation of ultrasonographic appearance of lesions and cytologic and histologic diagnoses in splenic aspirates from

dogs and cats: 32 cases (2002-2005). *J Am Vet Med Assoc* 2007;**230**:690–6.

18. Andriole JG, Haaga JR, Adams RB, et al. Biopsy needle characteristics assessed in the laboratory. *Radiology* 1983;**148**:659–62.

19. Haaga JR, LiPuma JP, Bryan PJ, et al. Clinical comparison of small-and large-caliber cutting needles for biopsy. *Radiology* 1983;**146**:665–7.

20. Rawlings CA, Diamond H, Howerth EW, et al. Diagnostic quality of percutaneous kidney biopsy specimens obtained with laparoscopy versus ultrasound guidance in dogs. *J Am Vet Med Assoc* 2003;**223**:317–21.

21. Ferrucci JT Jr, Wittenberg J, Mueller PR, et al. Diagnosis of abdominal malignancy by radiologic fine-needle aspiration biopsy. *AJR Am J Roentgenol* 1980;**134**:323–30.

22. Bisceglia M, Matalon TA, Silver B. The pump maneuver: an atraumatic adjunct to enhance US needle tip localization. *Radiology* 1990;**176**:867–8.

23. Leblanc CJ, Head LL, Fry MM. Comparison of aspiration and nonaspiration techniques for obtaining cytologic samples from the canine and feline spleen. *Vet Clin Pathol* 2009;**38**:242–6.

24. Bernardino ME. Automated biopsy devices: significance and safety. *Radiology* 1990;**176**:615–16.

25. Parker SH, Hopper KD, Yakes WF, et al. Image-directed percutaneous biopsies with a biopsy gun. *Radiology* 1989;**171**:663–9.

26. Vignoli M, Barberet V, Chiers K, et al. Evaluation of a manual biopsy device, the "Spirotome", on fresh canine organs: liver, spleen, and kidneys, and first clinical experiences in animals. *Eur J Cancer Prev* 2011;**20**:140–5.

27. Wittenberg J, Mueller PR, Simeone JF. Performing the biopsy. In: Ferrucci JT, Wittenberg J, Mueller PR, editors. *Interventional Radiology of the Abdomen*. Baltimore: Williams & Wilkins; 1985. p. 50–85.

28. Fagelman D, Chess Q. Nonaspiration fine-needle cytology of the liver: a new technique for obtaining diagnostic samples. *AJR Am J Roentgenol* 1990;**155**:1217–19.

29. Leveille R, Partington BP, Biller DS, et al. Complications after ultrasound-guided biopsy of abdominal structures in dogs and cats: 246 cases (1984-1991). *J Am Vet Med Assoc* 1993;**203**:413–15.

30. Proot SJ, Rothuizen J. High complication rate of an automatic Tru-Cut biopsy gun device for liver biopsy in cats. *J Vet Intern Med* 2006;**20**:1327–33.

31. Nyland TG, Wallack ST, Wisner ER. Needle-tract implantation following US-guided fine-needle aspiration biopsy of transitional cell carcinoma of the bladder, urethra, and prostate. *Vet Radiol Ultrasound* 2002;**43**:50–3.

32. Vignoli M, Rossi F, Chierici C, et al. Needle tract implantation after fine needle aspiration biopsy (FNAB) of transitional cell carcinoma of the urinary bladder and adenocarcinoma of the lung. *Schweiz Arch Tierheilkd* 2007;**149**:314–18.

33. Zegel HG, Heller LE. Angeid-Backman E. Intraoperative ultrasound principles. In: McGahan JP, Goldberg BB, editors. *Diagnostic Ultrasound: A Logical Approach*. Philadelphia: Lippincott-Raven; 1998. p. 107–26.

34. Tsutsumi Y, Andoh Y, Inoue N. Ultrasound-guided biopsy for deep-seated brain tumors. *J Neurosurg* 1982;**57**:164–7.

35. Tsutsumi Y, Andoh Y, Sakaguchi J. A new ultrasound-guided brain biopsy technique through a burr hole. Technical note. *Acta Neurochir (Wien)* 1989;**96**:72–5.

36. Enzmann DR, Irwin KM, Marshall WH, et al. Intraoperative sonography through a burr hole: guide for brain biopsy. *AJNR Am J Neuroradiol* 1984;**5**:243–6.

37. Enzmann DR, Irwin KM, Fine M, et al. Intraoperative and outpatient echoencephalography through a burr hole. *Neuroradiology* 1984;**26**:57–9.

38. McGahan JP, Montalvo BM, Quencer RM, et al. Intraoperative cranial and spinal sonography. In: McGahan JP, editor. *Interventional Ultrasound*. Baltimore: Williams & Wilkins; 1990. p. 43–57.

39. Sutcliffe JC, Battersby RD. Intraoperative ultrasound-guided biopsy of intracranial lesions: comparison with freehand biopsy. *Br J Neurosurg* 1991;**5**:163–8.

40. Thomas WB, Sorjonen DC, Hudson JA, et al. Ultrasound-guided brain biopsy in dogs. *Am J Vet Res* 1993;**54**:1942–7.

41. Rubin JM, Chandler WF. Intraoperative sonography of the brain. In: Rumack CM, Wilson SR, Charboneau JW, editors. *Diagnostic Ultrasound*. 2nd ed. St Louis: Mosby–Year Book; 1998. p. 631–52.

42. Fujita K, Yanaka K, Meguro K, et al. Image-guided procedures in brain biopsy. *Neurol Med Chir (Tokyo)* 1999;**39**:502–8, discussion 508–9.

43. Montalvo BM, Falcone S. Intraoperative sonography of the spine. In: Rumack CM, Wilson SR, Charboneau JW, editors. *Diagnostic Ultrasound*. 2nd ed. St. Louis: Mosby–Year Book; 1998. p. 653–69.

44. Nanai B, Lyman R, Bichsel PS. Use of intraoperative ultrasonography in canine spinal cord lesions. *Vet Radiol Ultrasound* 2007;**48**:254–61.

45. Nanai B, Lyman R, Bichsel P. Intraoperative use of ultrasonography during continuous dorsal laminectomy in two dogs with caudal cervical vertebral instability and malformation ("Wobbler syndrome"). *Vet Surg* 2006;**35**:465–9.

46. da Costa RC, Parent JM, Dobson H, et al. Ultrasound-guided fine needle aspiration in the diagnosis of peripheral nerve sheath tumors in 4 dogs. *Can Vet J* 2008;**49**:77–81.

47. Hartley C, McConnell JF, Doust R. Wooden orbital foreign body in a Weimaraner. *Vet Ophthalmol* 2007;**10**:390–3.

48. Wisner ER, Mattoon JS, Nyland TG, et al. Normal ultrasonographic anatomy of the canine neck. *Vet Radiol* 1991;**32**:185–90.

49. Wisner ER, Nyland TG, Feldman EC, et al. Ultrasonographic evaluation of the parathyroid glands in hypercalcemic dogs. *Vet Radiol Ultrasound* 1993;**34**:108–11.

50. Wisner ER, Nyland TG, Mattoon JS. Ultrasonographic examination of cervical masses in the dog and cat. *Vet Radiol Ultrasound* 1994;**35**:310–15.

51. Wisner ER, Theon AP, Nyland TG, et al. Ultrasonographic examination of the thyroid gland of hyperthyroid cats: Comparison to (TcO$_4$-)-Tc-99m scintigraphy. *Vet Radiol Ultrasound* 1994;**35**:53–8.

52. Wisner ER, Nyland TG. Clinical vignette. Localization of a parathyroid carcinoma using high-resolution ultrasonography in a dog. *J Vet Intern Med* 1994;**8**:244–5.

53. Wisner ER, Penninck D, Biller DS, et al. High-resolution parathyroid sonography. *Vet Radiol Ultrasound* 1997;**38**:462–6.

54. Wisner ER, Nyland TG. Ultrasonography of the thyroid and parathyroid glands. *Vet Clin North Am Small Anim Pract* 1998;**28**:973–91.

55. Samii VF, Nyland TG, Werner LL, et al. Ultrasound-guided fine-needle aspiration biopsy of bone lesions: a preliminary report. *Vet Radiol Ultrasound* 1999;**40**:82–6.

56. Britt T, Clifford C, Barger A, et al. Diagnosing appendicular osteosarcoma with ultrasound-guided fine-needle aspiration: 36 cases. *J Small Anim Pract* 2007;**48**:145–50.

57. Ikezoe J, Sone S, Higashihara T, et al. Sonographically guided needle biopsy for diagnosis of thoracic lesions. *AJR Am J Roentgenol* 1984;**143**:229–34.

58. Cinti D, Hawkins HB. Aspiration biopsy of peripheral pulmonary masses using real-time sonographic guidance. *AJR Am J Roentgenol* 1984;**142**:1115–16.

59. O'Moore PV, Mueller PR, Simeone JF, et al. Sonographic guidance in diagnostic and therapeutic interventions in the pleural space. *AJR Am J Roentgenol* 1987;**149**:1–5.

60. Stowater JL, Lamb CR. Ultrasonography of noncardiac thoracic diseases in small animals. *J Am Vet Med Assoc* 1989;**195**:514–20.

61. Ikezoe J, Morimoto S, Arisawa J, et al. Percutaneous biopsy of thoracic lesions: value of sonography for needle guidance. *AJR Am J Roentgenol* 1990;**154**:1181–5.

62. Konde LJ, Spaulding K. Sonographic evaluation of the cranial mediastinum in small animals. *Vet Radiol* 1991;**32**:178–84.

63. Raptopoulos V, Davis LM, Lee G, et al. Factors affecting the development of pneumothorax associated with thoracentesis. *AJR Am J Roentgenol* 1991;**156**:917–20.

64. Tikkakoski T, Lohela P, Leppanen M, et al. Ultrasound-guided aspiration biopsy of anterior mediastinal masses. *J Clin Ultrasound* 1991;**19**:209–14.

65. Wernecke K. Percutaneous biopsy of mediastinal tumours under sonographic guidance. *Thorax* 1991;**46**:157–9.

66. Chang DB, Yang PC, Luh KT, et al. Ultrasound-guided pleural biopsy with Tru-Cut needle. *Chest* 1991;**100**:1328–33.

67. Weingardt JP, Guico RR, Nemcek AA Jr, et al. Ultrasound findings following failed, clinically directed thoracenteses. *J Clin Ultrasound* 1994;**22**:419–26.

68. Yang PC, Chang DB, Yu CJ, et al. Ultrasound-guided core biopsy of thoracic tumors. *Am Rev Respir Dis* 1992;**146**:763–7.

69. Yang PC, Chang DB, Yu CJ, et al. Ultrasound guided percutaneous cutting biopsy for the diagnosis of pulmonary consolidations of unknown aetiology. *Thorax* 1992;**47**:457–60.

70. Yang PC, Lee YC, Yu CJ, et al. Ultrasonographically guided biopsy of thoracic tumors. A comparison of large-bore cutting biopsy with fine-needle aspiration. *Cancer* 1992;**69**:2553–60.

71. Yuan A, Yang PC, Chang DB, et al. Ultrasound-guided aspiration biopsy of small peripheral pulmonary nodules. *Chest* 1992;**101**:926–30.

72. Andersson T, Lindgren PG, Elvin A. Ultrasound guided tumour biopsy in the anterior mediastinum. An alternative to thoracotomy and mediastinoscopy. *Acta Radiol* 1992;**33**:423–6.

73. Tidwell AS. Diagnostic pulmonary imaging. *Probl Vet Med* 1992;**4**:239–64.

74. Malik R, Gabor L, Hunt GB, et al. Benign cranial mediastinal lesions in three cats. *Aust Vet J* 1997;**75**:183–7.

75. Brandt WE. Chest. In: McGahan JP, Goldberg BB, editors. *Diagnostic Ultrasound: A Logical Approach*. Philadelphia: Lippincott-Raven; 1998. p. 1063–86.

76. Brandt WE. The thorax. In: Rumack CM, Wilson SR, Charboneau JW, editors. *Diagnostic Ultrasound*. 2nd ed. St Louis: Mosby–Year Book; 1998. p. 575–97.

77. Tidwell AS. Ultrasonography of the thorax (excluding the heart). *Vet Clin North Am Small Anim Pract* 1998;**28**:993–1015.

78. Willard MD, Weeks BR, Johnson M. Fine-needle aspirate cytology suggesting hepatic lipidosis in four cats with infiltrative hepatic disease. *J Feline Med Surg* 1999;**1**:215–20.

79. Guillot M, Danjou MA, Alexander K, et al. Can sonographic findings predict the results of liver aspirates in dogs with suspected liver disease? *Vet Radiol Ultrasound* 2009;**50**:513–18.

80. McGahan JP, Walter JP. Diagnostic percutaneous aspiration of the gallbladder. *Radiology* 1985;**155**:619–22.

81. McGahan JP, Lindfors KK. Acute cholecystitis: diagnostic accuracy of percutaneous aspiration of the gallbladder. *Radiology* 1988;**167**:669–71.

82. vanSonnenberg E, Wittich GR, Casola G, et al. Diagnostic and therapeutic percutaneous gallbladder procedures. *Radiology* 1986;**160**:23–6.

83. Voros K, Sterczer A, Manczur F, et al. Percutaneous ultrasound-guided cholecystocentesis in dogs. *Acta Vet Hung* 2002;**50**:385–93.

84. Savary-Bataille KC, Bunch SE, Spaulding KA, et al. Percutaneous ultrasound-guided cholecystocentesis in healthy cats. *J Vet Intern Med* 2003;**17**:298–303.

85. Herman BA, Brawer RS, Murtaugh RJ, et al. Therapeutic percutaneous ultrasound-guided cholecystocentesis in three dogs with extrahepatic biliary obstruction and pancreatitis. *J Am Vet Med Assoc* 2005;**227**:1782–6, 1753.

86. Brain PH, Barrs VR, Martin P, et al. Feline cholecystitis and acute neutrophilic cholangitis: clinical findings, bacterial isolates and response to treatment in six cases. *J Feline Med Surg* 2006;**8**:91–103.

87. McGahan JP, Lindfors KK. Percutaneous cholecystostomy: an alternative to surgical cholecystostomy for acute cholecystitis? *Radiology* 1989;**173**:481–5.

88. McGahan JP, Raduns K. Biliary drainage using combined ultrasound fluoroscopic guidance. *J Intervent Radiol* 1990;**1990**:33–7.

89. Creasy TS, Gronvall S, Stage JG. Assessment of the biliary tract by antegrade cholecystography after percutaneous cholecystostomy in patients with acute cholecystitis. *Br J Radiol* 1993;**66**:662–6.

90. Warren LP, Kadir S, Dunnick NR. Percutaneous cholecystostomy: anatomic considerations. *Radiology* 1988;**168**:615–16.

91. McGahan JP. Gallbladder. In: McGahan JP, editor. *Interventional Ultrasound*. Baltimore: Williams & Wilkins; 1990. p. 159–70.

92. Stefanello D, Valenti P, Faverzani S, et al. Ultrasound-guided cytology of the spleen and liver: a prognostic tool in canine cutaneous mast cell tumor. *J Vet Intern Med* 2009;**23**:1051–7.

93. Book AP, Fidel J, Tripp C, et al. Correlation of ultrasound findings, liver and spleen cytology, and prognosis in the clinical staging of high metastatic risk canine mast cell tumors. *Vet Radiol Ultrasound* 2011;**52**(5):548–54.

94. Partington BP, Leveille R, Bradley GA. Ultrasound guided biopsy of the canine spleen. American College of Veterinary Radiology Annual Scientific Meeting 1990.

95. Watson AT, Penninck D, Knoll JS, et al. Safety and correlation of test results of combined ultrasound-guided fine-needle aspiration and needle core biopsy of the canine spleen. *Vet Radiol Ultrasound* 2011;**52**(3):317–22.

96. Fekete PS, Nunez C, Pitlik DA. Fine-needle aspiration biopsy of the pancreas: a study of 61 cases. *Diagn Cytopathol* 1986;**2**:301–6.

97. Smith EH. Complications of percutaneous abdominal fine-needle biopsy. Review. *Radiology* 1991;**178**:253–8.

98. Brandt KR, Charboneau JW, Stephens DH, et al. CT- and US-guided biopsy of the pancreas. *Radiology* 1993;**187**:99–104.

99. Mueller PR, Miketic LM, Simeone JF, et al. Severe acute pancreatitis after percutaneous biopsy of the pancreas. *AJR Am J Roentgenol* 1988;**151**:493–4.

100. Bergenfeldt M, Genell S, Lindholm K, et al. Needle-tract seeding after percutaneous fine-needle biopsy of pancreatic carcinoma. Case report. *Acta Chir Scand* 1988;**154**:77–9.

101. Elvin A, Andersson T, Scheibenpflug L, et al. Biopsy of the pancreas with a biopsy gun. *Radiology* 1990;**176**:677–9.

102. Cordner AP, Armstrong PJ, Newman SJ, et al. Effect of pancreatic tissue sampling on serum pancreatic enzyme levels in clinically healthy dogs. *J Vet Diagn Invest* 2010;**22**:702–7.

103. Gandini G, Grosso M, Bonardi L, et al. Results of percutaneous treatment of sixty-three pancreatic pseudocysts. *Ann Radiol (Paris)* 1988;**31**:117–22.

104. vanSonnenberg E, Wittich GR, Casola G, et al. Percutaneous drainage of infected and noninfected pancreatic pseudocysts: experience in 101 cases. *Radiology* 1989;**170**:757–61.

105. Grooters AM, Biller DS, Ward H, et al. Ultrasonographic appearance of feline alimentary lymphoma. *Vet Radiol Ultrasound* 1994;**35**:468–72.

106. Rivers BJ, Walter PA, Johnston GR, et al. Canine gastric neoplasia: utility of ultrasonography in diagnosis. *J Am Anim Hosp Assoc* 1997;**33**:144–55.

107. Penninck DG, Moore AS, Gliatto J. Ultrasonography of canine gastric epithelial neoplasia. *Vet Radiol Ultrasound* 1998;**39**:342–8.

108. Lingard AE, Briscoe K, Beatty JA, et al. Low-grade alimentary lymphoma: clinicopathological findings and response to treatment in 17 cases. *J Feline Med Surg* 2009;**11**:692–700.

109. Nadel L, Baumgartner BR, Bernardino ME. Percutaneous renal biopsies: accuracy, safety, and indications. *Urol Radiol* 1986;**8**:67–71.

110. Wickre CG, Golper TA. Complications of percutaneous needle biopsy of the kidney. *Am J Nephrol* 1982;**2**:173–8.

111. Gainza FJ, Minguela I, Lopez-Vidaur I, et al. Evaluation of complications due to percutaneous renal biopsy in allografts and native kidneys with color-coded Doppler sonography. *Clin Nephrol* 1995;**43**:303–8.

112. Zatelli A, Bonfanti U, Santilli R, et al. Echo-assisted percutaneous renal biopsy in dogs. A retrospective study of 229 cases. *Vet J* 2003;**166**:257–64.

113. Jeraj K, Osborne CA, Stevens JB. Evaluation of renal biopsy in 197 dogs and cats. *J Am Vet Med Assoc* 1982;**181**:367–9.

114. Osborne CA, Bartges JW, Polzin DJ, et al. Percutaneous needle biopsy of the kidney. Indications, applications, technique, and complications. *Vet Clin North Am Small Anim Pract* 1996;**26**:1461–504.

115. Drost WT, Henry GA, Meinkoth JH, et al. The effects of a unilateral ultrasound -guided renal biopsy on renal function in healthy sedated cats. *Vet Radiol Ultrasound* 2000;**41**:57–62.

116. Groman RP, Bahr A, Berridge BR, et al. Effects of serial ultrasound-guided renal biopsies on kidneys of healthy adolescent dogs. *Vet Radiol Ultrasound* 2004;**45**:62–9.

117. Haers H, Smets P, Pey P, et al. Contrast harmonic ultrasound appearance of consecutive percutaneous renal biopsies in dogs. *Vet Radiol Ultrasound* 2011;**52**(6):640–7.

118. Welch TJ, Sheedy PF 2nd, Stephens DH, et al. Percutaneous adrenal biopsy: review of a 10-year experience. *Radiology* 1994;**193**:341–4.

119. McCorkell SJ, Niles NL. Fine-needle aspiration of catecholamine-producing adrenal masses: a possibly fatal mistake. *AJR Am J Roentgenol* 1985;**145**:113–14.

120. Casola G, Nicolet V, vanSonnenberg E, et al. Unsuspected pheochromocytoma: risk of blood-pressure alterations during percutaneous adrenal biopsy. *Radiology* 1986;**159**:733–5.

121. Besso JG, Penninck DG, Gliatto JM. Retrospective ultrasonographic evaluation of adrenal lesions in 26 dogs. *Vet Radiol Ultrasound* 1997;**38**:448–55.

122. Marcotte L, McConkey SE, Hanna P, et al. Malignant adrenal neuroblastoma in a young dog. *Can Vet J* 2004;**45**:773–6.

123. Gilson SD, Withrow SJ, Wheeler SL, et al. Pheochromocytoma in 50 dogs. *J Vet Intern Med* 1994;**8**:228–32.

124. Lamb CR, Trower ND, Gregory SP. Ultrasound-guided catheter biopsy of the lower urinary tract: technique and results in 12 dogs. *J Small Anim Pract* 1996;**37**:413–16.

125. Zohil AM, Castellano MC. Prepubic and transrectal ultrasonography of the canine prostate: A comparative study. *Vet Radiol Ultrasound* 1995;**36**:393–6.

126. Boland LE, Hardie RJ, Gregory SP, et al. Ultrasound-guided percutaneous drainage as the primary treatment for prostatic abscesses and cysts in dogs. *J Am Anim Hosp Assoc* 2003;**39**:151–9.

127. Powe JR, Canfield PJ, Martin PA. Evaluation of the cytologic diagnosis of canine prostatic disorders. *Vet Clin Pathol* 2004;**33**:150–4.

ULTRASOUND GUIDED THERAPEUTICS

In humans, ultrasound is used as a method to guide a variety of therapeutic interventions. For example, ultrasound has been used to guide needle placement for intralesional chemical ablation procedures, radiofrequency heat ablation, and cryoablation of tumors.[1-8] In addition, ultrasound-guided injection of medications, particularly into joints has been described.[9,10] The potential applications for these less invasive interventional procedures are rapidly expanding in veterinary medicine.

Chemical Ablation
Cervical Lesions
The injection of ethanol into functional thyroid tissue in cats and parathyroid tissue in dogs has been reported.[11-13] In a study involving four hyperthyroid cats with unilateral thyroid nodules, ethanol injections resulted in remission in all cases, with only mild, transient dysphonia as a side effect in one cat.[11] However, a larger study involving seven hyperthyroid cats with bilateral thyroid nodules indicated that ethanol injection resulted in only a transient response to treatment, with all cats eventually becoming hyperthyroid again.[13] Horner syndrome, dysphonia, and laryngeal paralysis, presumably associated with leakage of ethanol into the surrounding soft tissues were all side effects in this case series.

Percutaneous ultrasound guided ethanol ablation of functional parathyroid tumors in dogs has had mixed outcomes.[5,12] In one study, remission was achieved in seven of eight dogs with primary hyperparathyroidism.[12] Six of the seven successfully treated dogs required only one treatment, whereas the seventh dog required two treatments. Laryngeal paralysis secondary to damage to the recurrent laryngeal nerve was suspected in several of the dogs in this report. The paralysis was likely secondary to leakage of ethanol from the injection site into the regional fascial planes. A more recent study describing the outcome of five hyperparathyroid dogs treated with ethanol ablation concluded that all dogs sustained elevated serum calcium levels and were considered treatment failures.[14]

When performing ultrasound-guided ethanol ablation of cervical tumors, the target tissue is isolated with ultrasound and the volume of the lesion to be treated is calculated from the product of the height, length, and width. The volume of 96% ethanol to be injected is estimated as approximately equal to the volume of the target tissue. However, the exact volume to be injected is determined in part by ultrasonographic observation of ethanol dissection through the target tissue during injection (Figure 3-1). An ethanol primed 1.5-inch, 25-gauge injection needle attached to an extension set and 3-mL syringe is placed into the lesion under ultrasound guidance. Ethanol injection is performed slowly, resulting in coagulation necrosis and vascular thrombosis within the treated tissue.[15] Injection should be aborted and the needle redirected should accumulation of ethanol be seen outside of the target tissue. The animal should be fully anesthetized, because this procedure is painful and many important structures such as the carotid artery are located close to the thyroid and parathyroid glands.

Abdominal Lesions
Ethanol ablation of hepatic and renal cysts and hepatic abscesses has recently been described in dogs and cats.[16-19] In the case of renal and hepatic cysts, these lesions are only ablated if the cyst is causing clinical signs of ureteral or biliary obstruction, or if stretching of the organ capsule causes abdominal pain, anorexia, or both. In a series of 22 cases of hepatic and renal cysts, 19 animals treated by ultrasound-guided drainage and alcoholization had resolution of clinical signs 3 to 4 weeks following the procedure.[18] The procedure was aborted in the remaining 3 animals because of hemorrhage. Six animals (5 dogs and 1 cat) underwent ultrasound-guided drainage and alcoholization of hepatic abscesses, with excellent outcome in all cases and no need for surgery.[17]

With the animal under anesthesia, ultrasound is used to locate the lesion and a 22- or 23-gauge spinal needle is introduced percutaneously into the cyst or abscess. The stylet is removed and the lesion is drained slowly; a sample of fluid retained for culture and cytology. Care should be taken to use a syringe that is no greater the two times the volume of fluid to be removed. This will prevent excessive suction and damage to the walls of the lesion. Once the lesion is drained, a volume of 95% ethanol equivalent to one half the amount of removed fluid is injected into the lesion. After 3 minutes, the alcohol is removed and a second alcoholization procedure is performed using a mixture of 95% ethanol and 2% lidocaine. All fluid is removed after 3 minutes and the animal is recovered from anesthesia.[17,18]

Radiofrequency Heat Ablation
As an alternative to ethanol ablation, radiofrequency (RF) heat ablation has been used to treat hyperthyroidism in cats and hyperparathyroidism in dogs.[5,20,21] With the animal under anesthesia, a ground pad is placed onto the abdomen in a shaved region and an RF needle is placed into the lesion using ultrasound guidance. RF-specific needles are available and are typically used in humans. We have adapted a 20- to 22-gauge indwelling catheter, using the stylet to deliver the RF energy and the catheter to shield the surrounding tissue.[21] Applied RF energy results in thermal necrosis at the needle tip. As the

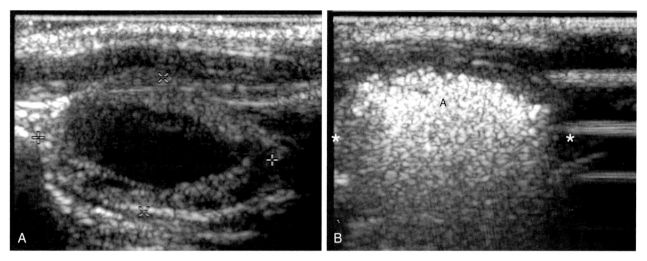

Figure 3-1 **Ethanol ablation of the thyroid gland in a hyperthyroid cat. A,** A sagittal image of a cystic, enlarged thyroid gland (between electronic cursors) is shown. Before ablation, the volume of the gland was calculated. **B,** After 2 mL cystic fluid was removed, 96% ethanol was injected into the cystic part of the thyroid gland (between electronic cursors). Increased echogenicity is caused by small air bubbles in the ethanol (*A*).

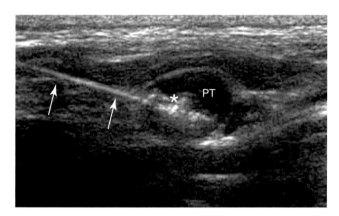

Figure 3-2 **Parathyroid radiofrequency heat ablation in a dog with primary hyperparathyroidism.** The needle (*arrows*) is placed into the enlarged parathyroid gland (*PT*) and radiofrequency energy is applied. As the tissue is heated, gas bubbles are liberated into the tissue around the needle tip (*asterisk*).

tissue heats, gas bubbles transiently develop within the treated area, indicating successful ablation (Figure 3-2). Should gas bubbles develop in the surrounding tissues, the procedure should be stopped and the needle redirected. In humans, a tissue temperature of 60° C causes cell death, so treatment time and RF energy is tailored to this goal. Some custom RF needles provide tissue temperature options. Alternatively, computed tomography (CT) or magnetic resonance imaging (MRI) might be used to ascertain if an entire lesion has been treated.[22,23] We have found that treatment of small lesions (<1.0 cm diameter) for 1.5 minutes at 9 to 16 W appears to be successful, although the needle may need to be re-directed several times to achieve complete thermal necrosis.

This procedure offers several advantages over ethanol ablation. First, RF ablation destroys a discrete volume of tissue at the noninsulated needle tip with no potential for dissection along fascial planes. Moreover, RF ablation does not damage regional vasculature. Blood flow in regional vasculature conveys heat away, thereby sparing the vessel walls. In humans, RF ablation has a higher success rate in comparison to ethanol

ablation, with fewer treatments necessary to achieve remission.[24] The drawback to RF ablation is equipment cost.

In a study of 9 hyperthyroid cats with unilateral or bilateral thyroid nodules, 14 separate ablation procedures were performed.[20] As with ethanol ablation, all cats had a transient resolution of thyrotoxicosis, but hyperthyroidism recurred in all cases. Side effects included Horner syndrome (2 cats) and asymptomatic laryngeal paralysis (1 cat). Results of an early study using RF ablation to threat primary hyperparathyroidism in dogs indicated that 8 of 11 dogs were successfully treated, and 1 dog developed laryngeal paralysis. Needle placement within the lesion was not achieved in the 3 dogs that did not remit, presumably because the lesions were small and the chosen needles were too large.[21] A more recent paper comparing the outcome of parathyroidectomy to ethanol and heat ablation indicated that hypercalcemia was controlled in 44 of 49 (90%) hyperparathyroid dogs treated with RF ablation.[5] Statistically, the outcome was equal to parathyroidectomy and superior to ethanol ablation. The improved success rate implied increasing skill with RF ablation associated with experience.

Joint Injections

Ultrasound is used to guide injection of medications into specific areas, particularly joints. The primary application is for the injection of corticosteroids into the biceps bursa of dogs diagnosed with biceps tenosynovitis. A 25-gauge needle is placed into the biceps bursa under ultrasound guidance, and joint fluid is removed for culture and cytology. Corticosteroids are injected under ultrasound guidance. The injection should not be made directly into the biceps tendon, as this may weaken the tendon fibers.

ADVANCED DIAGNOSTICS

In recent years, ultrasound has been used in combination with other imaging techniques to provide superior diagnostic information. Most frequently, ultrasound is used to guide needle placement for the injection of a contrast agent or radiopharmaceutical to improve the safety and quality of a study acquired with radiography, CT, or nuclear imaging.

Antegrade Pyelography and Pyelocentesis

Antegrade pyelography is a technique that has been described in both dogs and cats for identifying ureteral obstruction.[25-27] It is particularly useful in animals whose renal function is impaired to the point that intravenous pyelography does not result in adequate pelvic and ureteral opacification. Moreover, the risk of contrast medium nephrotoxicity is eliminated because systemic contrast is not administered. When a diagnostic study can be obtained, antegrade pyelography has 100% sensitivity and specificity for identifying ureteral obstruction in cats, which far surpasses results from ultrasound or radiography alone.[26]

To perform the procedure, the animal is placed under general anesthesia and the ventral abdomen is shaved and aseptically cleansed. A 25-gauge, 2.5-inch spinal needle is directed into the dilated renal pelvis from a ventrolateral approach under ultrasound guidance, taking care to avoid the arcuate arteries at the corticomedullary junction. A moderate degree of pelvic dilation should be present to minimize the likelihood of lacerating the collecting system. Typically 1 to 2 mL of urine is removed for culture, and then iodinated contrast media is injected into the pelvis. The volume of contrast media administered is arbitrarily determined based on the degree of resistance to injection but should be roughly equal to the quantity of urine removed. Serial radiography or fluoroscopy is subsequently used to determine if ureteral obstruction is present (Figure 3-3).

Adin and colleagues (2003) reported that complications arose in 8 of 18 studies performed in 7 of 11 cats.[26] The most common complication was leakage of contrast material through the needle tract, which occurred in 8 of 18 studies and rendered 5 studies nondiagnostic. One cat required surgical repair of an iatrogenically lacerated renal pelvis.

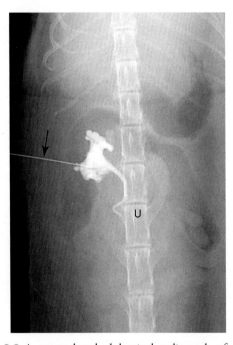

Figure 3-3 A ventrodorsal abdominal radiograph of a cat is shown after a nephropyelogram has been performed. Using ultrasound guidance, the needle (*arrow*) was inserted through the body wall and into the dilated right renal pelvis. Iodinated contrast media was injected after removal of several milliliters of urine. Contrast filling of the obstructed right ureter shows that it terminates abruptly at the level of the cranial aspect of the 4th lumbar vertebra (*U*).

Subcapsular hemorrhage was seen in 6 of 18 kidneys, and intrapelvic hemorrhage occurred in 1 cat. Hemorrhage was not life threatening in any case.

Ultrasound-guided aspiration of urine from the renal pelvis (pyelocentesis) for culture and cytology has been reported[28,29] and is occasionally used when urine samples from the bladder are not diagnostic. The technique has been used not only for urine collection but also for drainage treatment of pyonephrosis.[29]

Splenoportography

Although abdominal ultrasound can be useful for identifying portosystemic shunts, some shunt vessels are difficult to find. Identifying the presence and exact location of the shunt vessel is an important part of presurgical planning. One method for addressing these issues involves direct injection of agitated saline or radiopharmaceuticals into the splenic parenchyma under ultrasound guidance.[30-32] The animal is sedated and a region on the left ventral abdomen is shaved and aseptically prepared. The spleen is isolated ultrasonographically, and agitated saline radiopharmaceutical is injected directly into the splenic parenchyma using a 22-gauge, 1.5-inch needle. Either $^{99m}TcO_4^-$ or ^{99m}Tc-mebrofenin can be used because both radiopharmaceuticals provide superior count density and vessel visualization. Additionally, the radiation dose to the patient and technical staff is less than what is acquired during transrectal scintigraphy.[32-35] ^{99m}Tc-mebrofenin has the added advantage of quantifying liver function.[34] Regardless of the radiopharmaceutical, this technique allows differentiation of single from multiple shunts and can define portoazygous or internal thoracic vein shunts. But it cannot distinguish solitary intrahepatic from extrahepatic shunts. In 10% of cases, leakage of radiopharmaceutical from the spleen into the peritoneal cavity resulted in a nondiagnostic study.[32]

An alternative method for imaging the portal circulation involves ultrasound-guided catheterization of the splenic vein.[36] Because the splenic vein empties directly into the portal vein, this procedure provides direct access to the portal circulation. The animal is anesthetized and the ventral and left lateral abdomen is shaved and aseptically prepared. A target splenic vein is chosen and the ultrasound transducer oriented so that the vascular walls are parallel to the direction of catheter placement. A 17- or 19-gauge spinal needle is introduced into the splenic vein and advanced 0.5 cm into the lumen. A 19- or 22-gauge heparinized catheter is threaded through the needle into the splenic vein and then the portal vein. The catheter is periodically flushed to ensure patency as it is advanced. Once the catheter is sonographically visualized in the splenic or portal vein, the needle is removed and the catheter is secured to the body wall using bandage tape. Iodinated contrast media (8 to 10 mL) is injected into the catheter under fluoroscopic visualization to identify vascular anomalies (Figure 3-4). Although hemorrhage is a potential complication, none occurred in 15 catheterization attempts on 3 experimental dogs; 12 catheter placements were successful.[36]

Ultrasound-Guided Computed Tomography and Radiographic Lymphography

Surgical ligation of the thoracic duct is the definitive treatment for intractable chylothorax. However, the thoracic duct commonly has multiple tributaries, so that identifying the location of a common duct before branching is useful for presurgical planning. Ultrasound-guided lymph node injection of radiographic contrast medium is a recent technique to obtain radiographic or CT thoracic duct lymphangiograms in dogs and cats.[37-41] Two basic approaches have been described: popliteal lymph node injection and mesenteric lymph node injection. Both have proven fairly reliable. A recent study compared the two techniques and concluded that popliteal injection was faster and less painful than mesenteric injections for CT thoracic duct lymphangiography.[41] A common theme from these investigations is the variation in number of thoracic duct branches, and their size and location, which is essential information for presurgical planning and identification of complete ductal ligation following surgery.

With the dog under general anesthesia, the ventral abdomen is shaved and aseptically prepared for mesenteric lymph node

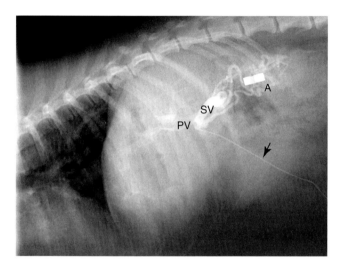

Figure 3-4 A right lateral abdominal radiograph of a dog is shown during injection of iodinated contrast media into a splenic vein catheter. The catheter (arrow) was placed under ultrasound guidance. Contrast media is seen in the splenic vein (SV) and portal vein (PV). In addition, a large plexus of extrahepatic shunting vessels are seen caudal to the splenic vein in the region of previous ligation of a single extrahepatic shunt. A, Ameroid constrictor.

injection.[39-41] Ultrasound is used to identify a mesenteric lymph node. A 25-gauge, 1.5-inch injection needle is guided into the lymph node, and 1 to 2 mL of nonionic, iodinated contrast medium is injected. Contrast medium and small air bubbles can often be seen filling the parenchyma of the lymph node but should not be seen leaking into the peritoneal cavity. Injection should stop if contrast leakage is seen or when the lymph node capsule appears completely filled. CT images are then acquired. (Figure 3-5).

Ultrasound-guided popliteal lymph node injection lymphangiography is a viable and less invasive procedure for assessment of thoracic duct integrity.[38,41] The popliteal lymph node is isolated and held in place by an assistant while the lymph node is injected. Contrast can be seen as echogenic material within the lymph node. Once a pressure threshold has been reached, the contrast material enters the lymphatic ducts to the medial iliac lymph nodes, then proceeds to the cisterna chyli and thoracic duct. Radiographs or CT images can then be made.

Ultrasound-Guided Peritoneography

Animals with suspected diaphragmatic hernia that cannot be confirmed with survey radiographs or ultrasound may undergo ultrasound-guided peritoneography. The animal is placed in right lateral or dorsal recumbency. Sedation is only necessary if the animal is noncompliant. The ventral abdomen is shaved and aseptically prepared near the umbilicus. A 22- to 25-gauge needle is introduced into the peritoneal space under ultrasound guidance, ensuring that a visceral organ is not penetrated. Nonionic iodinated contrast material is injected at a dose of 1.1 mL/kg (2.2 mL/kg if there is copious ascites) and should be seen dissipating into the peritoneal space.[42] The back end of the animal is elevated for 5 minutes; then radiographs of the caudal thoracic and cranial abdominal region are obtained in right and left lateral, dorsoventral, and/or ventrodorsal positions (Figure 3-6).[42]

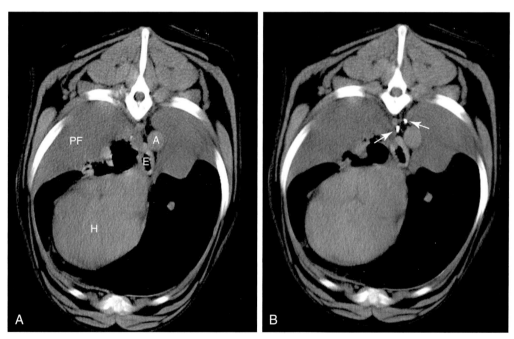

Figure 3-5 **An ultrasound-guided computed tomography lymphangiogram. A,** Before lymphography, the thoracic duct is not visible on this CT image. A, aorta; E, esophagus; H, heart; PF, pleural fluid. **B,** After injecting iodinated contrast into the mesenteric lymph nodes, the thoracic duct can be seen. Two branches are identified at this level (arrows). (Images courtesy Eric Johnson DVM, DACVR School of Veterinary Medicine, University of California, Davis).

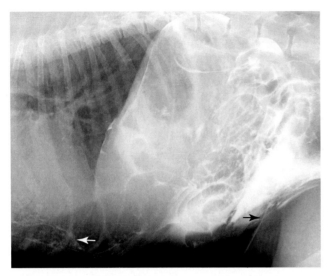

Figure 3-6 An ultrasound-guided peritoneogram has been performed. Nonionic, iodinated contrast material was injected into the abdominal cavity after placing a catheter into the peritoneal space (*black arrow*) under ultrasound guidance. This ensures that a parenchymal organ is not infused with contrast. Contrast media is seen leaking into the thoracic cavity, indicating the presence of a diaphragmatic hernia (*white arrow*).

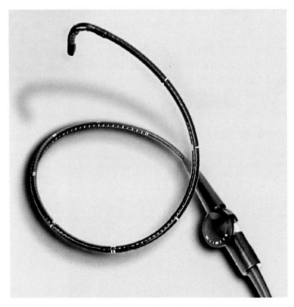

Figure 3-7 An endoscopic, esophageal transducer. (Courtesy of Esaote North America)

Endosonography

Endoscopic ultrasonography refers to the use of small high-frequency transducers incorporated into the tip of an endoscope, providing excellent near-field resolution[43-45] (Figure 3-7). The ultrasonographic endoscope is introduced into a body cavity perorally, transrectally, or transvaginally. Orientation of the probe and topographic recognition are initially difficult but can be facilitated by the use of standard endoscope positions. Endoscopic ultrasonography has been used in human medicine to evaluate the esophagus, stomach, colon, prostate, vagina, uterus, heart, and great vessels. Structures adjacent to the digestive lumen, such as the hilum of the liver,

common bile duct, pancreas, spleen, kidneys, urethra, lymph nodes, and abdominal vessels, can also be optimally imaged. With some instruments, direct endoscopic visualization and biopsy can be combined. Miniature endoscopic Doppler probes have been designed to study the location and flow characteristics of gastrointestinal vessels for identification of suspected bleeding sites.[46,47]

Transesophageal ultrasound has been used for echocardiography since the early 1990s,[48-54] and the sonographic appearance of the dog mediastinum was described in 1998.[54] In 2003, endoscopic ultrasonography was described for the diagnosis of intrathoracic lesions in two dogs[55] and was followed by publication of a review article describing its use for imaging the mediastinum, bronchial lymph nodes, esophagus, and pulmonary lesions. Fine-needle aspiration was also described.[56] Abdominal applications included pancreatic and liver imaging (including portosystemic shunts), and examination of the gastrointestinal tract and lymph nodes. Since then, endoscopic ultrasound has been used to study alimentary lymphoma,[57] and it is a new tool in the diagnosis of feline pancreatitis.[58] Specialized, high-cost equipment and anesthesia requirements will still limit its use in veterinary medicine to university and specialty practices.

Elastography

Recent advances in ultrasound imaging techniques have also included evaluation of sonographic characteristics of the elastic properties of a given tissue in humans, such as breast, pancreas, thyroid, prostate, and hepatic and other abdominal organs.[59-66] Although a relatively new clinical advancement, ultrasound elastography was originally described by Ophir and colleagues[59] in 1991. An external compressive force (usually pressure with the ultrasound transducer) is temporarily applied during the exam, which displaces or strains the tissue being evaluated.

The primary principle of elastography is based on the relative hardness or incompressibility of a tissue as it becomes diseased. Specific mechanical properties of tissues after the application of compression can then be calculated using the precontact and postcontact differences in returning ultrasound frequencies that are displayed as color or gray-scale coded "elastogram" (Figure 3-8). Superimposed over the gray-scale two-dimensional image is the color scaled elastogram. The color scale is based on the degree of tissue hardness (typically displayed in yellow to red) or softness (compressibility; typically displayed in blue to green). In theory, differences in tissue stiffness caused by a variety of pathologies can be determined noninvasively. The stiffness of a given tissue generally tends to increase with disease (sensitive, but nonspecific change). The differences in relative stiffness recorded in the elastogram are based on the change in longitudinal strain that occurs with precompression and postcompression ultrasound recorded by the reflected ultrasound frequencies at depth.

CONTRAST SPECIFIC IMAGING TECHNIQUES

Ultrasound Contrast Agents

The original ultrasound contrast agent consisted of agitated saline and was used to identify right-to-left cardiac shunts. Bubbles liberated in the agitated saline acted as reflectors and appeared as bright swirling echoes on the ultrasound image. Free gas bubbles were too large to pass through the pulmonary circulation, so if they were injected into the venous return to the right heart, the presence of bubbles in the left ventricle indicated a shunt. First generation manufactured ultrasound contrast agents consisted of a synthetic outer shell surrounding

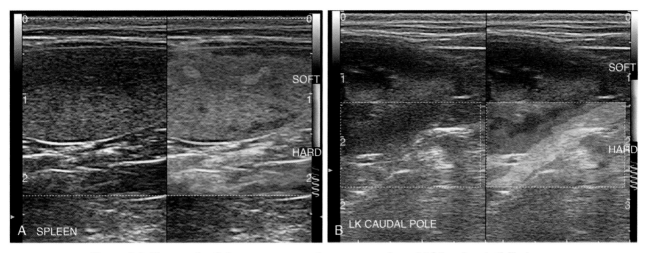

Figure 3-8 **Elastography.** Split screen sonographic images without (*right*) and with (*left*) elastography overlay of a normal (**A**) spleen and (**B**) kidney from an adult dog. **A,** The spleen is predominantly blue (soft or compressible) with a yellow/red (hard) outer fibrous connective tissue capsule and superficial body wall. **B,** The renal medulla is blue (soft or compressible), whereas the outer cortex is red (harder or decreased compressibility). The fatty tissue directly adjacent to the kidney is very soft (green).

air (Levovist, Schering AG). Although an improvement over agitated saline, these agents do not yield a high signal-to-noise ratio.[67]

Second generation ultrasound contrast agents contain high molecular weight gas bubbles stabilized by a lipid, polymer, or albumin shell. Examples of second generation contrast agents include Definity (Bristol-Myers Squibb), Optison (Amersham Health Inc.), and SonoVue (Bracco). Optison is the only commercially available agent with a human albumin shell, and for immunogenic reasons, it is contraindicated in veterinary patients.[68,69] First and second generation agents are small enough to pass through the pulmonary circulation (typically 3 to 10 μm in diameter) and consequently have a longer circulatory half-life than agitated saline. For example, the elimination half-life of SonoVue is 6 minutes.[70] Some agents persist in circulation and are eventually eliminated by the reticuloendothelial system, whereas others are designed to be taken up rapidly by the reticuloendothelial system for organ-specific imaging.

Ultrasound contrast agents have several interesting characteristics. First, they are strictly intravascular and do not leak out into the interstitium. In addition, when insonified, these agents will expand and contract, resulting in the reflection of sound signals at the frequency that the signal was sent (fundamental frequency). However, with lower frequency, higher pressure insonation, ultrasound contrast agents will expand more than they contract, thereby producing reflected echoes that are no longer at the fundamental frequency (Figure 3-9). Finally, if the incident beam is of sufficiently low frequency, high pressure, or both, the contrast microbubble will be destroyed, resulting in a brief but intense signal.[71-73]

Nonlinear Imaging Techniques

B-mode ultrasound has the advantage of producing images in real time with excellent spatial and temporal resolution. However, the task of mapping small blood vessels with ultrasound has previously been difficult, because the acoustic signal from blood may be 34 to 40 dB below that of the surrounding vessel walls. Moreover, for tumor imaging, the flow rate is significantly lower than in normal tissue because of the highly tortuous vessel structure and increased flow resistance.[74] Doppler shifts are overwhelmed by tissue motion when the

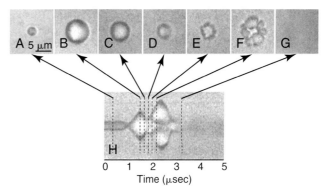

Figure 3-9 This series of photographs shows a single ultrasound contrast microbubble during insonification with an ultrasound pulse. **A,** The bubble before ultrasound. **B,** With ultrasound, the bubble expands. **C,** The bubble then starts to contract. **D,** As the bubble contracts, it starts to fragment. **E,** The fragmented bubble starts to expand again in its oscillatory cycle. **F,** The bubble has broken apart with expansion. **G,** The fragments have dispersed. **H,** This streak image shows the bubble's activity over time. (Images courtesy Katherine Ferrara, PhD, Department of Biomedical Engineering, University of California, Davis)

shift from the vasculature is below 1 cm/sec, which prevents detection of slow flowing capillary blood.[75]

With the addition of microbubble contrast agents, ultrasound becomes sensitive to much smaller vessels and very low flow rates, but still maintains the ability to detect morphologic information from traditional B-mode imaging. Combining power Doppler with ultrasound contrast agents results in improved detection of small vessels, although imaging of capillary sized vessels remains impossible because of limited contrast resolution (Figure 3-10). Contrast enhanced power Doppler has proven useful in humans for evaluating masses in the prostate, breast, and pancreas, among other organs.[76-78] Contrast enhanced power Doppler has not been explored extensively for the assessment of parenchymal organs in veterinary patients. However, it has been used to identify sentinel lymph nodes in dogs with head and neck tumors

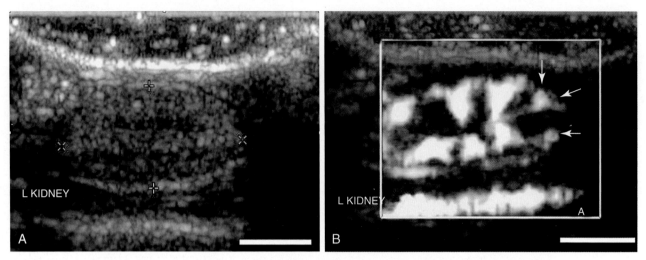

Figure 3-10 **Contrast enhanced power Doppler imaging of a mouse kidney. A,** B-mode image of the left kidney of a mouse is shown in the sagittal imaging plane (between electronic cursors). **B,** Following bolus injection of ultrasound contrast material, power Doppler is applied. Contrast allows visualization of the interlobular arteries of the renal cortex (*arrows*). Enhancement of the aorta (*A*) is also seen. The white bar indicates 0.5 cm. (From Ferrara K, Polard R, Borden M: Ultrasound microbubble contrast agents: Fundamentals and application to gene and drug delivery, *Annu Rev Biomed Eng* 9:415-447, 2007.)

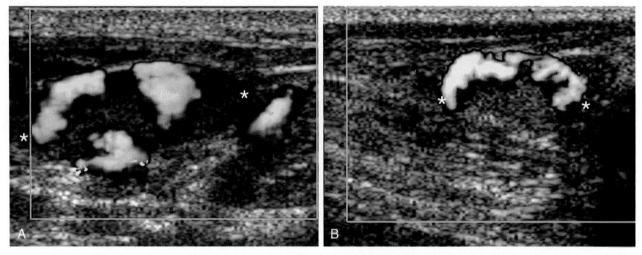

Figure 3-11 Ultrasound contrast medium was injected into the interstitial tissue downstream and allowed to traverse the lymphatics to reach the lymph node. This allowed detection of the sentinel nodes. **A,** Contrast medium was injected into the head, and the cervical lymph node is identified as the sentinel node. Power Doppler imaging allows delineation of the contrast as it fills in this normal node from the periphery to the hilus. **B,** Contrast medium was injected into the metatarsal region and the popliteal lymph node (cursors) is identified as the sentinel node. Power Doppler imaging allows delineation of the contrast as it fills in this normal node from the periphery to the hilus. (Images courtesy Erik Wisner DVM, DACVR School of Veterinary Medicine, University of California, Davis.)

(Figure 3-11),[79,80] assess medial iliac lymph nodes,[81] improve definition of lymph nodes for biopsy,[82] and evaluate normal intestinal vascularity via intraoperative contrast sonography.[83] The technique has also been used to define the contrast enhancement patterns of nodes affected by lymphoma.[84] Lymph nodes infiltrated by lymphoma have a strikingly different vascular pattern than normal lymph nodes.[84] In that study, direct comparison indicated that 2.13 times more vessels were seen with contrast harmonic imaging than power Doppler imaging of the same lymph nodes.

Harmonic Imaging

In an attempt to better visualize the microvasculature, various other ultrasound-based approaches have been described to accentuate the nonlinear contrast agent echoes and repress the echoes generated from surrounding tissue. *Harmonic imaging* is a broad category of techniques that share the common feature of sending an incident beam at one frequency and listening for returned echoes at a harmonic (an integer multiple) of the incident beam (Figure 3-12).[85] For example, a transducer might have a fundamental frequency of 4 MHz but be capable of detecting the second harmonic (8 MHz) or a subharmonic (2 MHz) frequency. Because the harmonic frequency returned to the transducer is of lower amplitude, the fundamental frequency is typically filtered to favor detection of the desired harmonic.

Although harmonic imaging was developed to better visualize nonlinear reflectors such as contrast agents, there are several advantages to using noncontrast imaging. As sound travels through tissue, the tissue is compressed and then expanded. During tissue compression, the ultrasound wave travels at a slightly different speed with the end result being

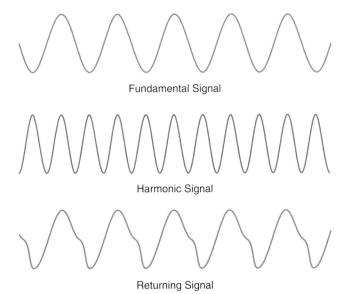

Figure 3-12 In harmonic imaging, an ultrasound pulse of a specific frequency (fundamental signal) is emitted by the transducer. The transducer listens for the emitted frequency as well as the harmonic. What returns to the transducer and is recorded is a combination of the fundamental frequency and the harmonic. (From Ferrara K, Polard R, Borden M: Ultrasound microbubble contrast agents: Fundamentals and application to gene and drug delivery, *Annu Rev Biomed Eng* 9:415-447, 2007.)

a distortion of the wave shape. Depending on the fundamental frequency, this can result in the generation of harmonics at various tissue depths. Tissue harmonic imaging offers the following advantages to B-mode imaging. First, several artifacts are reduced or eliminated. Reverberation, ring-down, and scattering artifacts produced by the interaction of sound with the skin, subcutaneous fat, and body wall are eradicated, because harmonics are not generated until sound penetrates deeper in the tissue. Moreover, acoustic pressure from side lobe artifacts is not high enough to return to the transducer. Finally, the narrower beam results in less volume averaging and improved lateral resolution. The end result is improved image quality (Figure 3-13). Note that settings for tissue harmonic imaging are not the same as those for contrast harmonic imaging, and the two cannot be used interchangeably.

Contrast harmonic imaging relies on the generation of harmonic frequencies from the nonlinear oscillation of ultrasound contrast agents. Most contrast agents produce harmonic signals when insonified at a specific frequency, typically in the 2 to 3 MHz range. In humans, contrast harmonic imaging has been used to improve the visualization and characterization of a variety of neoplastic lesions, including breast, prostate, liver, and kidney. In veterinary medicine, contrast harmonic imaging has been used to evaluate the normal liver,[86] kidney,[87] spleen,[88] and lymph nodes[81] in dogs to establish baseline values for quantitative variables, such as peak intensity, time to peak, and area under the curve. Contrast agent dosage in veterinary patients depends upon the type of agent used and whether a bolus injection or constant rate infusion is used.[68,88-92] Bolus injections are typically useful for qualitative or wash-in and wash-out quantitative assessment of parenchymal organs, whereas constant rate infusions are preferred for destruction-replenishment techniques (see later). The animal is typically not sedated unless compliance is an issue.

In a study by O'Brien and colleagues (2004), contrast harmonic ultrasound for the assessment of malignant liver nodules had very high sensitivity, specificity, positive predictive value, and negative predictive value with an accuracy value of 96.9%.[89] Results of that study indicated that benign nodules would appear isoechoic to surrounding liver parenchyma at the time of peak enhancement, whereas malignant lesions were hypoechoic in comparison to surrounding liver parenchyma. Moreover, most malignant lesions had an early wash-in

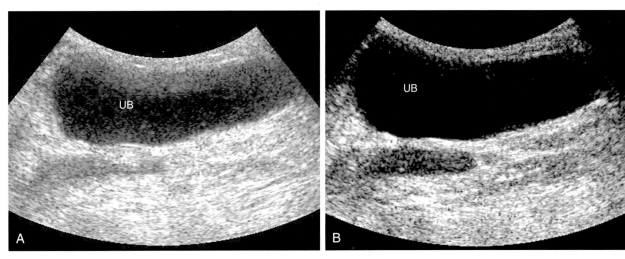

Figure 3-13 The difference between standard B-mode imaging and tissue harmonic imaging is shown. **A,** The urinary bladder (*UB*) is imaged using a 5-MHz transducer. **B,** Harmonic image of the urinary bladder in **A** using the same transducer. Note that the anechoic urine, free of artifactual echoes within the bladder, and the increased conspicuity of the far-field aorta.

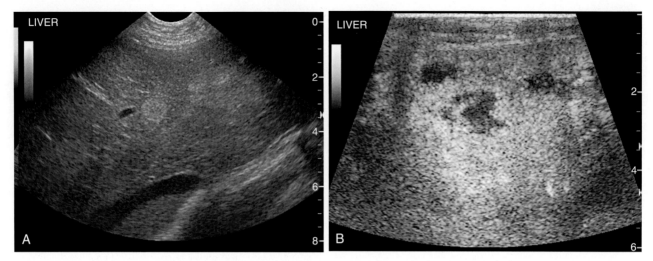

Figure 3-14 Contrast enhanced harmonic ultrasound of metastatic hemangiosarcoma in the liver. **A,** B-mode image of the liver shows subtle hyperechoic liver lesions. **B,** After intravenous contrast media is administered, metastatic nodules appear hypoechoic compared to surrounding normal liver at peak enhancement. (Images courtesy Robert O'Brien, DVM, DACVR, Veterinary Teaching Hospital, University of Illinois.)

phase or poor perfusion in addition to an early wash-out stage. Contrast harmonic imaging can also detect metastatic hemangiosarcoma lesions in the liver that were not identified with B-mode imaging[93] (Figure 3-14). The metastatic lesions appear hypoechoic compared to the contrast-enhanced normal liver surrounding them. In the cat, contrast-enhanced power Doppler imaging has proven useful for assessing vascularity and perfusion of the pancreas, with significantly higher values in animals with symptoms of pancreatic disease.[94]

Contrast-enhanced harmonic imaging has also been used to assess dogs with portosystemic shunts. A cephalic catheter is placed and small (0.1 to 0.2 mL) boluses are administered as needed for diagnosis. Hepatic arterial tortuosity (Figure 3-15) and significantly shorter time to peak (7 ± 2 seconds; reference range 23 ± 7 or 46 ± 20 seconds)[86,92] are seen in dogs with increased arterial blood flow caused by portacaval shunting.[95]

Although a useful technique, contrast harmonic imaging has limitations. Most importantly, because of the inherent properties of the technique, a compromise must be made between image contrast and spatial resolution.[96] The signal-to-noise ratio is low, as is the fundamental frequency used during imaging.

To overcome some of the limitations for contrast harmonic imaging, phase inversion imaging was introduced (Figure 3-16).[97] Phase inversion, also known as pulse inversion, uses two ultrasound pulses that are emitted down each line of sight. The second pulse is inverted in relation to the first. Linear reflectors will send the transmitted pulses back unchanged, such that the sum of the paired waves will cancel and give no signal. However, nonlinear pulse pair responses will alter the pulses so that they no longer cancel when summed. Contrast-enhanced phase inversion imaging is often combined with harmonic imaging; it has been used in experimental animal models[98,99] and in humans to evaluate lesion vascularity.[100-102]

Because ultrasound contrast agents can be destroyed with high pressure, low frequency insonation, destruction-replenishment techniques are under development. A destructive pulse of ultrasound can be used to fragment the contrast agent within the region being imaged (Figure 3-17). Lower pressure, higher frequency, nondestructive pulses can be used to visualize the replenishment of intravascular contrast agent

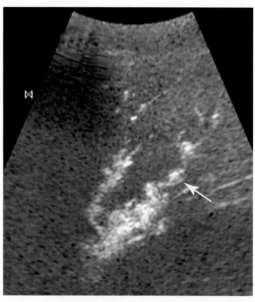

Figure 3-15 Contrast-enhanced harmonic ultrasound image of several branches of the hepatic artery in a dog with a portosystemic shunt. Note the tortuosity of the arterial branches (*arrow*) caused by increased arterial flow to the liver. (Image courtesy Robert O'Brien, DVM, DACVR, Veterinary Teaching Hospital, University of Illinois.)

into the imaging region. This method of evaluation is often called flash-echo imaging. For quantitation purposes, the echo amplitude can be measured as the contrast agent refills the region and the rate of return can be estimated. Such a quantitative destruction-replenishment method was described as early as 1998, where Wei and co-workers[103] proposed the method to assess blood flow velocity in the myocardium. Although still experimental, destruction-replenishment techniques show promise for quantifying tumor response to chemotherapies such as antiangiogenic agents.[104]

Siemens Medical Systems has recently introduced a contrast-specific imaging technique called Cadence contrast pulse sequencing (CPS). This technique allows for contrast

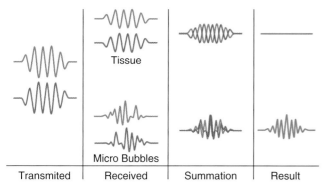

| Transmited | Received | Summation | Result |

Figure 3-16 In a phase inversion scheme, two pulses are transmitted almost simultaneously. The transducer then listens for the return echoes. If the pulses are reflected by a linear reflector such as tissue, they will come back exactly as they were transmitted (*top*). The ultrasound machine sums the returned echoes, which negate each other and yield no signal. If the reflector of the phase inverted pulses is nonlinear, such as with a microbubble (*bottom*), the inverted pulses will be altered upon their return. Therefore their sum will not negate and a signal is detected. (From Ferrara K, Polard R, Borden M: Ultrasound microbubble contrast agents: Fundamentals and application to gene and drug delivery, *Annu Rev Biomed Eng* 9:415-447, 2007.)

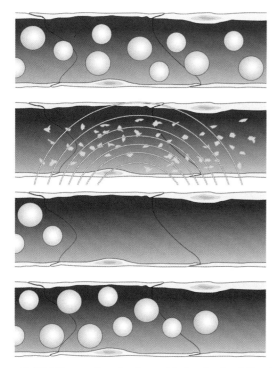

Figure 3-17 Ultrasound contrast agent is freely circulating in the vasculature. In a destruction-replenishment scheme, a strong ultrasound pulse destroys the agent in the imaging plane. Low pressure pulses are then used to observe the contrast agent flowing with the blood back in to the imaging plane. (From Ferrara K, Polard R, Borden M: Ultrasound microbubble contrast agents: Fundamentals and application to gene and drug delivery, *Annu Rev Biomed Eng* 9:415-447, 2007.)

imaging at higher frequencies, thereby improving spatial resolution. Moreover, nonlinear and linear (tissue) echoes can be displayed simultaneously, so that both contrast and anatomic information can be seen.[105] CPS uses a combination of changes in pulse phase and amplitude to selectively minimize tissue echoes and enhance contrast agent echoes. With selective scaling of each received echo and addition of all echoes, linear fundamental tissue signals are rejected and nonlinear microbubble echoes are retained.[105,106] This technique can be used to assess a variety of organ systems and often allows for occult lesion identification (Figures 3-18 to 3-21). An image registration feature is available with CPS, which minimizes motion and improves the accuracy of region-of-interest (ROI) measurements. This system is capable of combining contrast-specific imaging with destruction-replenishment sequencing for the quantitative assessment of regional blood flow (Figure 3-22).

Contrast Agent Bioeffects

The bioeffects associated with ultrasound contrast agents are not fully understood. It has been shown that ultrasound contrast agents, when insonified, are capable of rupturing small vessels.[107] Petechiation and increased vascular permeability of the myocardium have been found in experimental dog models using ultrasound contrast agents imaged with high pressure and low frequency.[108] The greatest concern is that the endothelial damage caused by these agents could liberate tumor cells into the bloodstream or result in damage to and thrombosis of regional capillaries. These theories have neither been proven nor disproven.

More recently, the U.S. Food and Drug Administration (FDA) has issued a warning regarding the use of ultrasound contrast agents in humans because of several cases of anaphylaxis associated with their use. The warning was issued in October 2007 after the FDA had received reports of 11 deaths that occurred between 2001 and 2007 that may have been related to ultrasound contrast administration. An additional 199 serious, nonfatal reactions were also reported, many of which occurred either during or within minutes of administration of the ultrasound contrast agent.

In the warning, the FDA stated that the contrast agents should not be given to patients with acute myocardial infarction, clinically unstable or worsening congestive heart failure, respiratory failure, serious ventricular arrhythmias, emphysema, pulmonary emboli, and certain types of cardiac shunts. Patients receiving the contrast agents must be monitored during the infusion and for 30 minutes following the completion of administration. The implications for veterinary use of ultrasound contrast agents and their potential side effects remain to be seen.

Drug Delivery

Combining drug delivery with contrast-specific imaging techniques is currently a major clinical interest, because this approach offers multiple potential advantages. First, an imaging agent targeted to a specific receptor would allow assessment of whether a given lesion could be treated with a targeted drug-laden microbubble. Additionally, the use of targeted therapeutic agents with imaging properties would allow simultaneous imaging and treatment. Targeted therapies that allow simultaneous imaging directed at dissolution of thrombi, gene and drug delivery for the treatment of tumors, and localized treatment of inflammation have all been described.

Nonspecific methods for ultrasound-guided drug delivery rely on depositing large quantities of a chemotherapeutic agent close to the lesion. The goal is to reduce the overall dose of chemotoxic drugs and thereby to decrease systemic effects. One approach is to systemically inject the pharmaceutical simultaneously with an ultrasound contrast agent and then apply high intensity ultrasound to the target region. In smaller blood vessels, the oscillations of the contrast agent will damage the capillary walls allowing for extravasation of the pharmaceutical (Figure 3-23, *A*).[109,110] Alternatively, drug may be incorporated into the microbubble and increased local

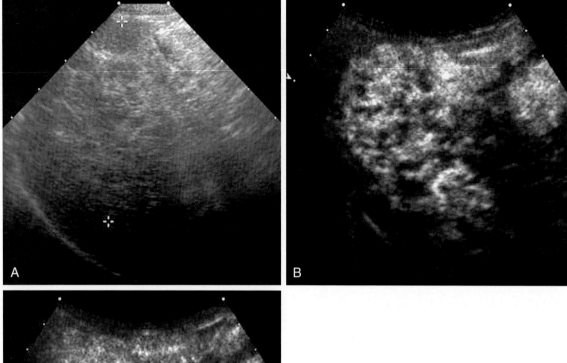

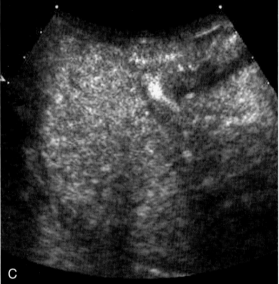

Figure 3-18 Contrast Cadence pulse sequencing (CPS) of a hepatoma. A, B-mode imaging shows a poorly defined mass (cursors) in the liver. **B,** The early phase contrast CPS image shows large vessels within the parenchyma of the mass with more profound enhancement than surrounding normal liver. **C,** Late phase contrast CPS shows equilibration of enhancement between the mass and the surrounding normal liver as is typical in benign lesions. (Images courtesy Robert O'Brien, DVM, DACVR, Veterinary Teaching Hospital, University of Illinois.)

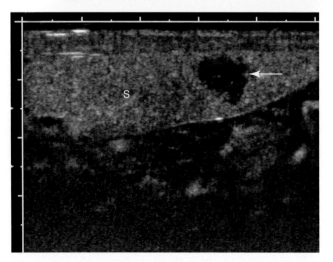

Figure 3-19 Contrast Cadence pulse sequencing (CPS) of a splenic hematoma in a dog. The splenic parenchyma is enhanced (*S*) but the focal hematoma (*arrow*) is not. (Images courtesy Robert O'Brien, DVM, DACVR, Veterinary Teaching Hospital, University of Illinois.)

delivery achieved by rupturing the microbubbles selectively in the feeder vessels of the lesion (see Figure 3-23, *B*).[111,112] However, these methods do not account for the washout of released drug by flowing blood. One proposed method for dealing with this issue is to use optimized radiation pulses of ultrasound to push the microbubbles toward the vascular wall before destroying them. Microbubbles close to the vascular wall will effectively paint the drug onto the endothelium when they are ruptured. Using a fluorescent dye to mark the distribution of the inner oil, combining the radiation force with destructive ultrasound pulses resulted a tenfold increase in oil deposition to cells in vitro when compared to ultrasound alone.[113]

More specific drug delivery may be achieved by attaching a ligand to the outside of the drug-laden microbubble that is directed at a particular surface marker. Endothelial surface markers are particularly attractive targets because certain markers are overexpressed in areas of angiogenesis. If the surface marker is expressed only in the target region, microbubbles will selectively accumulate at the target site. High-intensity ultrasound can be applied locally so that the drug payload is delivered only in the areas where the surface marker is expressed[107,114] (see Figure 3-23, *C*).

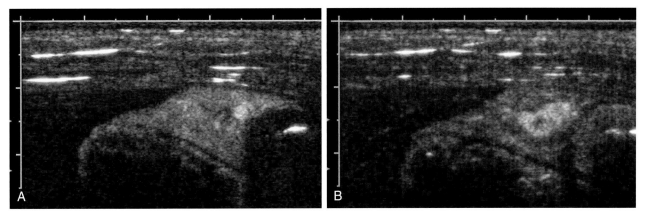

Figure 3-20 **Contrast Cadence pulse sequencing (CPS) of the normal pancreas in a dog. A,** Pancreatic enhancement is uniformly intense at 12 seconds following contrast injection. **B,** Contrast agent has begun to wash out of the pancreatic parenchyma but remains in the vasculature centrally. (Images courtesy Robert O'Brien, DVM, DACVR, Veterinary Teaching Hospital, University of Illinois.)

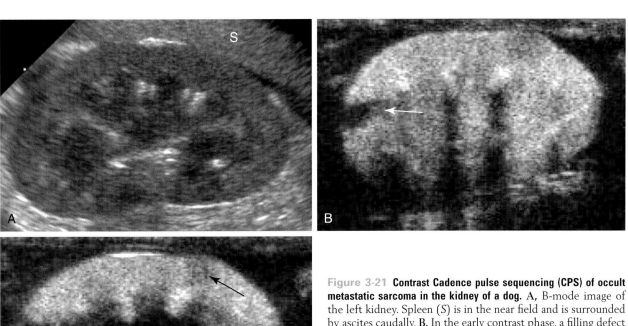

Figure 3-21 **Contrast Cadence pulse sequencing (CPS) of occult metastatic sarcoma in the kidney of a dog. A,** B-mode image of the left kidney. Spleen (*S*) is in the near field and is surrounded by ascites caudally. **B,** In the early contrast phase, a filling defect is seen at the cranial pole (*white arrow*), representing a cortical infarct. **C,** As contrast begins to wash out, the original lesion in the cranial pole remains with a second lesion indentified in the near-field cortex (*black arrow*), representing a metastatic sarcoma lesion. (Images courtesy Robert O'Brien, DVM, DACVR, Veterinary Teaching Hospital, University of Illinois.)

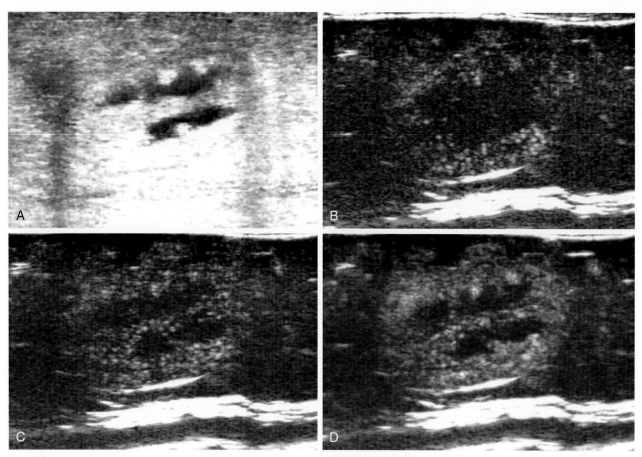

Figure 3-22 **Contrast Cadence pulse sequencing (CPS) of a rat kidney. A,** A destructive pulse destroys all contrast agent in the kidney. **B,** CPS visualizes contrast replenishment into the kidney at 2 seconds while negating most signals from regional tissue. **C,** More contrast is refilling the kidney vasculature at 12 seconds. **D,** 30 seconds after the destructive pulse. (From Ferrara K, Polard R, Borden M: Ultrasound microbubble contrast agents: Fundamentals and application to gene and drug delivery, *Annu Rev Biomed Eng 9:415-447, 2007.*)

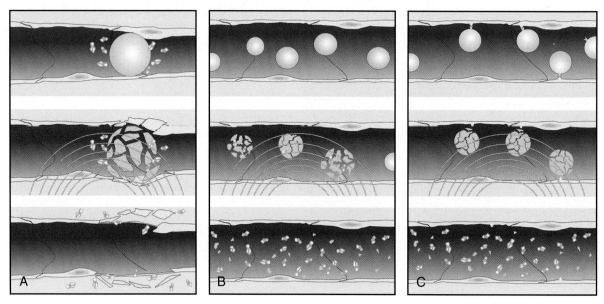

Figure 3-23 **A schematic of drug delivery techniques is shown. A,** Ultrasound contrast agents are freely circulating in small vessels along with drug (*blue particles*). Once a sufficiently strong ultrasound pulse is applied to the area, the contrast agent expands, rupturing the endothelial lining. The drug is then able to extravasate. **B,** Drug-laden ultrasound contrast agents are freely circulating throughout the vasculature. A pulse of ultrasound is applied and ruptures the contrast agent, thereby liberating the drug payload. Because ultrasound is only applied in the region of interest, drug is preferentially delivered locally. **C,** Drug-laden ultrasound contrast agents bearing surface ligands targeted at specific endothelial receptors are freely circulating. The ligand preferentially binds the ultrasound contrast agent in the target region, increasing local agent accumulation. An ultrasound pulse is then applied and liberates the drug payload. (From Ferrara K, Polard R, Borden M: Ultrasound microbubble contrast agents: Fundamentals and application to gene and drug delivery, *Annu Rev Biomed Eng 9:415-447, 2007.*)

REFERENCES

1. Buscarini E, Savoia A, Brambilla G, et al. Radiofrequency thermal ablation of liver tumors. *Eur Radiol* 2005; **15**:884–94.
2. Huppert BJ, Reading CC. Parathyroid sonography: imaging and intervention. *J Clin Ultrasound* 2007;**35**: 144–55.
3. Monchik JM, Donatini G, Iannuccilli J, et al. Radiofrequency ablation and percutaneous ethanol injection treatment for recurrent local and distant well-differentiated thyroid carcinoma. *Ann Surg* 2006;**244**: 296–304.
4. Peng ZW, Liang HH, Chen MS, et al. Percutaneous radio-frequency ablation for the treatment of hepatocellular carcinoma in the caudate lobe. *Eur J Surg Oncol* 2008; **34**:166–72.
5. Rasor L, Pollard R, Feldman EC. Retrospective evaluation of three treatment methods for primary hyperparathyroidism in dogs. *J Am Anim Hosp Assoc* 2007; **43**:70–7.
6. Seror O, N'Kontchou G, Tin Tin Htar M, et al. Ethanol versus radiofrequency ablation for the treatment of small hepatocellular carcinoma in patients with cirrhosis: a retrospective study of efficacy and cost. *Gastroenterol Clin Biol* 2006;**30**:1265–73.
7. Mala T. Cryoablation of liver tumours—a review of mechanisms, techniques and clinical outcome. *Minim Invasive Ther Allied Technol* 2006;**15**:9–17.
8. Schwartz BF, Rewcastle JC, Powell T, et al. Cryoablation of small peripheral renal masses: a retrospective analysis. *Urology* 2006;**68**:14–18.
9. Carson BW, Wong A. Ultrasonographic guidance for injections of local steroids in the native hip. *J Ultrasound Med* 1999;**18**:159–60.
10. Sofka CM, Adler RS. Ultrasound-guided interventions in the foot and ankle. *Semin Musculoskelet Radiol* 2002;**6**: 163–8.
11. Goldstein RE, Long C, Swift NC, et al. Percutaneous ethanol injection for treatment of unilateral hyperplastic thyroid nodules in cats. *J Am Vet Med Assoc* 2001; **218**:1298–302.
12. Long CD, Goldstein RE, Hornof WJ, et al. Percutaneous ultrasound-guided chemical parathyroid ablation for treatment of primary hyperparathyroidism in dogs. *J Am Vet Med Assoc* 1999;**215**:217–21.
13. Wells AL, Long CD, Hornof WJ, et al. Use of percutaneous ethanol injection for treatment of bilateral hyperplastic thyroid nodules in cats. *J Am Vet Med Assoc* 2001;**218**:1293–7.
14. Gear RN, Neiger R, Skelly BJ, et al. Primary hyperparathyroidism in 29 dogs: diagnosis, treatment, outcome and associated renal failure. *J Small Anim Pract* 2005; **46**:10–16.
15. Chow LT, Metreweli C, King WW, et al. Histological changes of parathyroid adenoma after percutaneous injection of ethanol. *Histopathology* 1997;**30**:87–9.
16. Zatelli A, Bonfanti U, D'Ippolito P. Obstructive renal cyst in a dog: ultrasonography-guided treatment using puncture aspiration and injection with 95% ethanol. *J Vet Intern Med* 2005;**19**:252–4.
17. Zatelli A, Bonfanti U, Zini E, et al. Percutaneous drainage and alcoholization of hepatic abscesses in five dogs and a cat. *J Am Anim Hosp Assoc* 2005;**41**:34–8.
18. Zatelli A, D'Ippolito P, Bonfanti U, et al. Ultrasound-assisted drainage and alcoholization of hepatic and renal cysts: 22 cases. *J Am Anim Hosp Assoc* 2007;**43**: 112–16.
19. Agut A, Soler M, Laredo FG, et al. Imaging diagnosis–Ultrasound-guided ethanol sclerotherapy for a simple renal cyst. *Vet Radiol Ultrasound* 2008;**49**:65–7.
20. Mallery KF, Pollard RE, Nelson RW, et al. Percutaneous ultrasound-guided radiofrequency heat ablation for treatment of hyperthyroidism in cats. *J Am Vet Med Assoc* 2003;**223**:1602–7.
21. Pollard RE, Long CD, Nelson RW, et al. Percutaneous ultrasonographically guided radiofrequency heat ablation for treatment of primary hyperparathyroidism in dogs. *J Am Vet Med Assoc* 2001;**218**:1106–10.
22. Clasen S, Pereira PL. Magnetic resonance guidance for radiofrequency ablation of liver tumors. *J Magn Reson Imaging* 2008;**27**:421–33.
23. Schraml C, Clasen S, Schwenzer NF, et al. Diagnostic performance of contrast-enhanced computed tomography in the immediate assessment of radiofrequency ablation success in colorectal liver metastases. *Abdom Imaging* 2008.
24. Livraghi T, Goldberg SN, Lazzaroni S, et al. Small hepatocellular carcinoma: treatment with radio-frequency ablation versus ethanol injection. *Radiology* 1999;**210**: 655–61.
25. Ackerman N, Ling GV, Ruby AL. Percutaneous nephropyelocentesis and antegrade urography: a fluoroscopically assisted diagnostic technique in canine urology. *Vet Radiol* 1980;**21**:117–22.
26. Adin CA, Herrgesell EJ, Nyland TG, et al. Antegrade pyelography for suspected ureteral obstruction in cats: 11 cases (1995–2001). *J Am Vet Med Assoc* 2003;**222**: 1576–81.
27. Rivers BJ, Walter PA, Polzin DJ. Ultrasonographic-guided, percutaneous antegrade pyelography: technique and clinical application in the dog and cat. *J Am Anim Hosp Assoc* 1997;**33**:61–8.
28. Szatmári V, Osi Z, Mancur F. Ultrasound-guided percutaneous drainage for treatment of pyonephrosis in two dogs. *J Am Vet Med Assoc* 2001;**218**:1796–9, 1778–9.
29. Thoresen SI, Bredal WP, Sande RD. Diagnosis, treatment, and long-term follow-up of bilateral, upper urinary tract infection (UTI) in a cat. *J Feline Med Surg* 2002; **4**:213–20.
30. Gómez-Ochoa P, Llabrés-Diaz F, Ruiz S, et al. Ultrasonographic appearance of the intravascular transit of agitated saline in normal dogs following ultrasound guided percutaneous splenic injection. *Vet Radiol Ultrasound* 2010;**51**:523–6.
31. Gómez-Ochoa P, Llabrés-Diaz F, Ruiz S, et al. Use of transsplenic injection of agitated saline and heparinized blood for the ultrasonographic diagnosis of macroscopic portosystemic shunts in dogs. *Vet Radiol Ultrasound* 2011;**52**:103–6.
32. Morandi F, Cole RC, Tobias KM, et al. Use of $^{99m}TCO_4(-)$ trans-splenic portal scintigraphy for diagnosis of portosystemic shunts in 28 dogs. *Vet Radiol Ultrasound* 2005; **46**:153–61.
33. Cole RC, Morandi F, Avenell J, et al. Trans-splenic portal scintigraphy in normal dogs. *Vet Radiol Ultrasound* 2005; **46**:146–52.
34. Morandi F, Cole RC, Echandi RL, et al. Transsplenic portal scintigraphy using 99mTc-mebrofenin in normal dogs. *Vet Radiol Ultrasound* 2007;**48**:286–91.
35. Sura PA, Tobias KM, Morandi F, et al. Comparison of 99mTcO4(-) trans-splenic portal scintigraphy with perrectal portal scintigraphy for diagnosis of portosystemic shunts in dogs. *Vet Surg* 2007;**36**:654–60.
36. Herrgesell EJ, Hornof WJ, Koblik PD. Percutaneous ultrasound-guided trans-splenic catheterization of the

portal vein in the dog. *Vet Radiol Ultrasound* 1999; **40**:509–12.

37. Johnson EG, Wisner ER, Marks SL, et al. Contrast enhanced CT thoracic duct lymphography. *ACVR Proceedings in Veterinary Radiology and Ultrasound* 2006.

38. Naganobu K, Ohigashi Y, Akiyoshi T, et al. Lymphography of the thoracic duct by percutaneous injection of iohexol into the popliteal lymph node of dogs: experimental study and clinical application. *Vet Surg* 2006; **35**:377–81.

39. Johnson EG, Wisner ER, Kyles A, et al. Computed tomographic lymphography of the thoracic duct by mesenteric lymph node injection. *Vet Surg* 2009;**38**:361–7.

40. Kim M, Lee H, Lee N, et al. Ultrasound-guided mesenteric lymph node iohexol injection for thoracic duct computed tomographic lymphography in cats. *Vet Radiol Ultrasound* 2011;**52**:302–5.

41. Millward IR, Kirberger RM, Thompson PN. Comparative popliteal and mesenteric computed tomography lymphangiography of the canine thoracic duct. *Vet Radiol Ultrasound* 2011;**52**:295–301.

42. Wallack ST. *The Handbook of Veterinary Conrast Radiography.* San Diego, CA: 2003.

43. Chak A. Endoscopic ultrasonography. *Endoscopy* 2000; **32**:146–52.

44. Nakata N, Miyamoto Y, Tsujimoto F, et al. Ultrasound virtual endoscopic imaging. *Semin Ultrasound CT MR* 2001;**22**:78–84.

45. Devereaux CE, Binmoeller KF. Endoscopic retrograde cholangio-pancreatography in the next millennium. *Gastrointest Endosc Clin North Am* 2000;**10**:117–33.

46. Martin RW, Gilbert DA, Silverstein FE, et al. An endoscopic Doppler probe for assessing intestinal vasculature. *Ultrasound Med Biol* 1985;**11**:61–9.

47. Wong RC, Chak A, Kobayashi K, et al. Role of Doppler US in acute peptic ulcer hemorrhage: Can it predict failure of endoscopic therapy? *Gastrointest Endosc* 2000; **52**:315–21.

48. Fisher EA, Stahl JA, Budd JH, et al. Transesophageal echocardiography: Procedures and clinical application. *J Am Coll Cardiol* 1991;**18**:1333–48.

49. Kienle RD, Thomas WP, Rishniw M. Biplane transesophageal echocardiography in the normal cat. *J Vet Radiol Ultrasound* 1997;**38**:288–98.

50. Thomas WP. *Clinical applications of transesophageal echocardiography. Proceedings of the Twelfth Annual Veterinary Medical Forum.* Lakewood, Colo: American College of Veterinary Internal Medicine; 1994. p. 312–14.

51. Kramer GA. *Transesophageal echocardiography. Proceedings of the Tenth Annual Veterinary Medical Forum.* Blacksburg, Va: American College of Veterinary Internal Medicine; 1992. p. 618–20.

52. Loyer C, Thomas WP. *Transesophageal echocardiography. Proceedings of the Tenth Annual Veterinary Medical Forum.* Blacksburg, Va: American College of Veterinary Internal Medicine; 1992. p. 621–2.

53. Loyer C, Thomas WP. Biplane transesophageal echocardiography in the dog: Technique, anatomy and imaging planes. *Vet Radiol Ultrasound* 1994;**35**:1–15.

54. St-Vincent RS, Pharr JW. Transesophageal ultrasonography of the normal canine mediastinum. *Vet Radiol Ultrasound* 1998;**39**:197–205.

55. Gaschen L, Kircher P, Hoffmann G, et al. Endoscopic ultrasonography for the diagnosis of intrathoracic lesions in two dogs. *Vet Radiol Ultrasound* 2003;**44**:292–9.

56. Gaschen L, Kircher P, Lang J. Endoscopic ultrasound instrumentation, applications in humans, and potential veterinary applications. *Vet Radiol Ultrasound* 2003;**44**: 665–80.

57. Miura T, Maruyama H, Sakai M, et al. Endoscopic findings on alimentary lymphoma in 7 dogs. *J Vet Med Sci* 2004;**66**:577–80.

58. Schweighauser A, Gaschen F, Steiner J, et al. Evaluation of endosonography as a new diagnostic tool for feline pancreatitis.. *J Fel Med Surg* 2009;**11**:492–8.

59. Ophir J, Cespedes I, Ponnekanti H, et al. Elastography: a quantitative method for imaging the elasticity of biological tissues. *Ultrason Imaging* 1991;**13**:111–34.

60. Tan R, Xiao Y, He Q. Ultrasound elastography: its potential role in assessment of cervical lymphadenopathy. *Acad Radiol* 2010;**17**:849–55.

61. Harvey CJ, Pilcher JM, Eckersley RJ, et al. Advances in Ultrasound. *Clin Radiol* 2002;**57**:157–77.

62. Ophir J, Garra B, Kallell F, et al. Elastographic imaging. *Ultrasound Med Biol* 2000;**26**:S23–9.

63. Yoneda M Suzuki K, Kato S, et al. Nonalcoholic fatty liver disease: US-based acoustic radiation force impulse elastography. *Radiology* 2010;**256**:640–7.

64. Fahey BJ, Nightingale KR, Nelson RC, et al. Acoustic radiation force impulse imaging of the abdomen: demonstration of feasibility and utility. *Ultrasound Med Biol* 2005;**31**:1185–98.

65. Pallwein L, Aigner F, Faschingbauer R, et al. Prostate cancer diagnosis: value of real-time ultrasonography. *Abdom Imaging* 2008;**33**:729–35.

66. Itoh A, Ueno E, Tohno E, et al. Breast disease: clinical application of US elastography for diagnosis. *Radiology* 2006;**239**:341–50.

67. Goldberg BB, Liu JB, Forsberg F. Ultrasound contrast agents: a review. *Ultrasound Med Biol* 1994;**20**: 319–33.

68. Rademacher N, Ohlerth S, Doherr MG, et al. Doppler sonography of the medial arterial blood supply to the coxofemoral joints of 36 medium to large breed dogs and its relationship with radiographic signs of joint disease. *Vet Rec* 2005;**156**:305–9.

69. Yamaya Y, Niizeki K, Kim J, et al. Anaphylactoid response to Optison® and its effects on pulmonary function in two dogs. *J Vet Med Sci* 2004;**66**:1429–32.

70. Schneider M. Characteristics of SonoVue™. *Echocardiography* 1999;**16**:743–6.

71. Chomas JE, Dayton P, Allen J, et al. Mechanisms of contrast agent destruction. *IEEE Trans Ultrason Ferroelectr Freq Control* 2001;**48**:232–48.

72. Sboros V, Moran CM, Pye SD, et al. Contrast agent stability: a continuous B mode imaging approach. *Ultrasound Med Biol* 2001;**27**:1367–77.

73. Tiemann K, Veltmann C, Ghanem A, et al. The impact of emission power on the destruction of echo contrast agents and on the origin of tissue harmonic signals using power pulse- inversion imaging. *Ultrasound Med Biol* 2001;**27**:1525–33.

74. Netti PA, Roberge S, Boucher Y, et al. Effect of transvascular fluid exchange on pressure-flow relationship in tumors: a proposed mechanism for tumor blood flow heterogeneity. *Microvasc Res* 1996;**52**:27–46.

75. el-Fallah AI, Plantec MB, Ferrara KW. Ultrasonic measurement of breast tissue motion and the implications for velocity estimation. *Ultrasound Med Biol* 1997;**23**: 1047–57.

76. Kettenbach J, Helbich TH, Huber S, et al. Computer-assisted quantitative assessment of power Doppler US: effects of microbubble contrast agent in the differentiation of breast tumors. *Eur J Radiol* 2005;**53**: 238–44.

77. Ragde H, Kenny GM, Murphy GP, et al. Transrectal ultrasound microbubble contrast angiography of the prostate. *Prostate* 1997;**32**:279–83.

78. Scialpi M, Midiri M, Bartolotta TV, et al. Pancreatic carcinoma versus chronic focal pancreatitis: contrast-enhanced power Doppler ultrasonography findings. *Abdom Imaging* 2005;**30**:222–7.

79. Lurie DM, Seguin B, Schneider PD, et al. Contrast-assisted ultrasound for sentinel lymph node detection in spontaneously arising canine head and neck tumors. *Invest Radiol* 2006;**41**:415–21.

80. Wisner ER, Ferrara KW, Short RE, et al. Sentinel node detection using contrast-enhanced power Doppler ultrasound lymphography. *Invest Radiol* 2003;**38**:358–65.

81. Gaschen L, Angelette N, Stout R. Contrast-enhanced harmonic ultrasonography of medial iliac lymph nodes in healthy dogs. *Vet Radiol Ultrasound* 2011;**51**:634–7.

82. Gelb HR, Freeman LJ, Rohleder JJ, et al. Feasibility of contrast-enhanced ultrasound-guided biopsy of sentinel lymph nodes in dogs. *Vet Radiol Ultrasound* 2010;**51**:628–33.

83. Jiménez DA, O'Brien RT, Wallace JD, et al. Intraopeartive contrast-enhanced ultrasonography of normal canine jejunum. *Vet Radiol Ultrasound* 2011;**52**:196–200.

84. Salwei RM, O'Brien RT, Matheson JS. Characterization of lymphomatous lymph nodes in dogs using contrast harmonic and Power Doppler ultrasound. *Vet Radiol Ultrasound* 2005;**46**:411–16.

85. Choudhry S, Gorman B, Charboneau JW, et al. Comparison of tissue harmonic imaging with conventional US in abdominal disease. *Radiographics* 2000;**20**:1127–35.

86. Ziegler LE, O'Brien RT, Waller KR, et al. Quantitative contrast harmonic ultrasound imaging of normal canine liver. *Vet Radiol Ultrasound* 2003;**44**:451–4.

87. Waller KR, O'Brien RT, Zagzebski JA. Quantitative contrast ultrasound analysis of renal perfusion in normal dogs. *Vet Radiol Ultrasound* 2007;**48**:373–7.

88. Ohlerth S, Ruefli E, Poirier V, et al. Contrast harmonic imaging of the normal canine spleen. *Vet Radiol Ultrasound* 2007;**48**:451–6.

89. O'Brien RT, Iani M, Matheson J, et al. Contrast harmonic ultrasound of spontaneous liver nodules in 32 dogs. *Vet Radiol Ultrasound* 2004;**45**:547–53.

90. Scharz M, Ohlerth S, Achermann R, et al. Evaluation of quantified contrast-enhanced color and power Doppler ultrasonography for the assessment of vascularity and perfusion of naturally occurring tumors in dogs. *Am J Vet Res* 2005;**66**:21–9.

91. Yamaya Y, Niizeki K, Kim J, et al. Effects of Optison on pulmonary gas exchange and hemodynamics. *Ultrasound Med Biol* 2002;**28**:1005–13.

92. Nyman HT, Kristensen AT, Kjelgaard-Hansen M, et al. Contrast-enhanced ultrasonography in normal canine liver. Evaluation of imaging and safety parameters. *Vet Radiol Ultrasound* 2005;**46**:243–50.

93. O'Brien RT. Improved detection of metastatic hepatic hemangiosarcoma nodules with contrast ultrasound in three dogs. *Vet Radiol Ultrasound* 2007;**48**:146–8.

94. Rademacher N, Ohlerth S, Scharf G, et al. Ultrasonographic Changes of Feline Pancreatic Architecture, Vascularity and Perfusion. *2005 Annual Proceedings American College of Veterinary Radiology* 2007:35.

95. Salwei RM, O'Brien RT, Matheson JS. Use of contrast harmonic ultrasound for the diagnosis of congenital portosystemic shunts in three dogs. *Vet Radiol Ultrasound* 2003;**44**:301–5.

96. Burns PN, Hope Simpson D, Averkiou MA. Nonlinear imaging. *Ultrasound Med Biol* 2000;**26**(Suppl. 1):S19–22.

97. Burns PN, Wilson SR, Simpson DH. Pulse inversion imaging of liver blood flow: improved method for characterizing focal masses with microbubble contrast. *Invest Radiol* 2000;**35**:58–71.

98. Forsberg F, Dicker AP, Thakur ML, et al. Comparing contrast-enhanced ultrasound to immunohistochemical markers of angiogenesis in a human melanoma xenograft model: preliminary results. *Ultrasound Med Biol* 2002;**28**:445–51.

99. Lucidarme O, Nguyen T, Kono Y, et al. Angiogenesis model for ultrasound contrast research: exploratory study. *Acad Radiol* 2004;**11**:4–12.

100. Dietrich CF, Schuessler G, Trojan J, et al. Differentiation of focal nodular hyperplasia and hepatocellular adenoma by contrast-enhanced ultrasound. *Br J Radiol* 2005;**78**:704–7.

101. Hohl C, Schmidt T, Haage P, et al. Phase-inversion tissue harmonic imaging compared with conventional B-mode ultrasound in the evaluation of pancreatic lesions. *Eur Radiol* 2004;**14**:1109–17.

102. Schmidt T, Hohl C, Haage P, et al. Phase-inversion tissue harmonic imaging compared to fundamental B-mode ultrasound in the evaluation of the pathology of large and small bowel. *Eur Radiol* 2005;**15**:2021–30.

103. Wei K, Jayaweera AR, Firoozan S, et al. Quantification of myocardial blood flow with ultrasound-induced destruction of microbubbles administered as a constant venous infusion. *Circulation* 1998;**97**:473–83.

104. Pollard RE, Broumas AR, Wisner ER, et al. Quantitative contrast enhanced ultrasound and CT assessment of tumor response to antiangiogenic therapy in rats. *Ultrasound Med Biol* 2007;**33**:235–45.

105. Phillips P, Gardner E. Contrast-agent detection and quantification. *Eur Radiol* 2004;**14**(Suppl. 8):P4–10.

106. Phillips P. Contrast pulse sequences (CPS): imaging non-linear microbubbles. *IEEE 2001 Ultrasonics Symposium* 2001;**2**:1739–45.

107. Tartis MS, McCallan J, Lum AF, et al. Therapeutic effects of paclitaxel-containing ultrasound contrast agents. *Ultrasound Med Biol* 2006;**32**:1771–80.

108. Miller DL, Driscoll EM, Dou C, et al. Microvascular permeabilization and cardiomyocyte injury provoked by myocardial contrast echocardiography in a canine model. *J Am Coll Cardiol* 2006;**47**:1464–8.

109. Miller DL, Quddus J. Diagnostic ultrasound activation of contrast agent gas bodies induces capillary rupture in mice. *Proc Natl Acad Sci U S A* 2000;**97**:10179–84.

110. Price RJ, Skyba DM, Kaul S, et al. Delivery of colloidal particles and red blood cells to tissue through microvessel ruptures created by targeted microbubble destruction with ultrasound. *Circulation* 1998;**98**:1264–7.

111. Christiansen JP, French BA, Klibanov AL, et al. Targeted tissue transfection with ultrasound destruction of plasmid-bearing cationic microbubbles. *Ultrasound Med Biol* 2003;**29**:1759–67.

112. Hauff P, Seemann S, Reszka R, et al. Evaluation of gas-filled microparticles and sonoporation as gene delivery system: feasibility study in rodent tumor models. *Radiology* 2005;**236**:572–8.

113. Shortencarier MJ, Dayton PA, Bloch SH, et al. A method for radiation-force localized drug delivery using gas-filled liposomes. *IEEE Trans Ultrason Ferroelectr Freq Control* 2004;**51**:822–31.

114. Ellegala DB, Leong-Poi H, Carpenter JE, et al. Imaging tumor angiogenesis with contrast ultrasound and microbubbles targeted to alpha(v)beta3. *Circulation* 2003;**108**:336–41.

CHAPTER 4
Abdominal Ultrasound Scanning Techniques

John S. Mattoon • Clifford R. Berry • Thomas G. Nyland

Expertise in abdominal scanning requires a high level of manual dexterity and eye-hand coordination as well as a thorough understanding of anatomy, physiology, pathophysiology, effects of different body types, and the capabilities and limitations of ultrasound equipment. Of importance to the beginning sonographer is development of a thorough, systematic method for scanning the abdomen. This ensures consistent identification of all organs and structures and more efficient scanning. General applications of abdominal scanning are presented in this chapter with the understanding that it is challenging to appreciate actual scanning technique by reading a textbook. This chapter is intended for those just beginning their abdominal sonography experience. Detailed, specific scanning techniques and anatomic information for each organ system are available in the appropriate dedicated chapters. Because ultrasound is so heavily dependent on anatomic knowledge, novice and experienced sonographers will benefit from the use of reference anatomy texts. It is also noted that there are some sonographic differences between dogs and cats. These are noted throughout this chapter and are compiled in Table 4-1.

POSITIONING OF SONOGRAPHER, PATIENT, AND EQUIPMENT

Proper positioning of the patient and ultrasound machine relative to the sonographer is an important but frequently overlooked consideration for consistency in scanning, ease of equipment adjustment, and comfort of the sonographer (Figure 4-1). For right-handed individuals, the patient should be placed to the sonographer's right, facing ahead. The ultrasound machine is positioned in front of the sonographer, to the left of the patient and within easy reach. Scanning is performed with the sonographer sitting or standing and facing the ultrasound machine. The transducer is held in the right hand, freeing the left hand for adjustment of the controls. Maintaining a forward, frontal view of the ultrasound monitor is essential for short-term and long-term comfort. Scanning while facing the patient and viewing the screen by turning your neck sideways will lead to muscle fatigue and spasms in the neck and shoulder and even cervical nerve injury.

Many sonographers prefer to place the patient in dorsal recumbency (Figure 4-2). Scanning in lateral recumbency, for both the dependent and nondependent surfaces, is another common position (Figure 4-3). Abdominal scanning with the patient standing is useful if the patient is very large, when severe abdominal effusion is present, and for assessment of various organs in certain circumstances (Figure 4-4). Patient positioning is not nearly as important as a thorough, working knowledge of anatomic relationships of abdominal organs and major vascular structures. Indeed, it is not uncommon for experienced sonographers to reposition a patient during an examination in to maximize visualization of a particular structure.

PREPARATION OF THE PATIENT

An ultrasound examination usually requires clipping of the ventral abdominal hair coat. A fine clipper blade, such as No. 40, works well. The cranioventral abdomen should be clipped, from the costal arch cranially to the inguinal region caudally and laterally along the body wall. Patients with short or thin hair coats may not require clipping as long as the hair can be sufficiently moistened. Acoustic gel is applied to the skin to provide the essential acoustic coupling of the transducer to the patient. Acoustic gel is applied liberally over the entire abdomen, either by hand or with the transducer. The patient should be fasted, if possible, so that a distended stomach does not interfere with imaging of the liver (or evaluation of the stomach itself) by the presence of gas, food, and its sheer size. If the urinary system is of prime importance, the patient should not be allowed to urinate immediately before the examination because proper sonographic assessment of the urinary bladder wall thickness requires that it not be empty.

The patient is placed in dorsal recumbency (or other positions as just described) and gently restrained by assistants holding the thoracic and pelvic limbs. A foam pad, foam V-trough pad, or padded V-trough table aids greatly in positioning and restraint. However, deep V-troughs can restrict transducer placement laterally. Use of a deep foam V-trough upside down can be useful in smaller patients. Sedation is usually not necessary. If sedation is required, avoid morphine and its derivatives (panting and aerophagia cause the gastrointestinal tract to become air filled) and xylazine (gastric atony and rapid gas accumulation). General anesthesia may be necessary in rare instances. The basic scanning techniques described refer to the patient in dorsal recumbency unless noted otherwise.

GETTING STARTED

As described in Chapter 1, image orientation should follow standard protocol. Sagittal and dorsal scan planes of the abdomen are oriented so that the cranial part of the patient (or organ) is to the left side of the video monitor. This is achieved by directing the orientation mark on the transducer toward the thorax, assuming that the location of the indicator mark is on the left edge of the image display. If the indicator mark is on the right, the screen may be electronically

TABLE 4-1

Cat versus Dog

Organ	Cat	Dog
Liver	More angular in sagittal plane Concave caudal margin Echogenic fat midline to right Stomach indents on left Less prominent hepatic vasculature	More rounded caudal margin with indentation of stomach across entire caudal surface More visible hepatic and portal veins
Gallbladder	Bi-lobed gallbladder not uncommon Echogenic bile uncommon in healthy cats Commonly follow bile duct to duodenal papilla	Bi-lobed gallbladder rare Echogenic bile more commonly seen in normal patients Rarely follow bile duct beyond neck of gallbladder
Falciform Fat	Thick in most cats Echogenicity and texture very similar to normal liver	Usually thin Echogenicity varies from hypoechoic, isoechoic, hyperechoic to normal liver
Spleen	Thin ≤10 mm Size less affected by sedation or anesthesia Consistent position along left body wall Less apparent splenic veins Finer texture	Size varies greatly (blood reservoir) Position varies; only the head of the spleen is consistently located Splenic veins routinely seen Coarser texture
Stomach	Gastric axis more parallel to spine Pylorus more toward midline Wider pyloroduodenal angle Thick echogenic submucosal fat layer gives "spoked" appearance to empty stomach	Gastric axis perpendicular to spine Pylorus to right of midline Narrow pyloroduodenal angle Thin submucosal layer similar to small intestine
Small Intestine	Thinner duodenal mucosal layer than dogs Ileum often the thickest portion of small intestine Duodenum and jejunum similar thickness	Thick mucosal duodenal layer Duodenum is thickest portion of small intestine
Ileocecocolic junction	Easily, routinely identified Ileocecocolic junction common opening Small cecum Ileocecocolic lymph nodes routinely identified in normal cats	More difficult to identify Ileum enters colon (ileocolic junction) Cecocolic junction is separate Large cecum, usually gas filled, not identifiable Ileocecocolic lymph nodes rarely seen unless enlarged
Pancreas	Left lobe easiest to routinely identify Central pancreatic duct routinely identified, used as landmark Most cats lack an accessory pancreatic duct (minor duodenal papilla)	Right lobe easiest to identify Central pancreatic duct rarely identified in normal dogs Accessory pancreatic duct and minor duodenal papilla normally present in dogs
Kidneys	More oval shape; similar shape on sagittal and dorsal image axes More consistent size More hilar fat deposition Renal cortical fat deposition creates more echogenic cortices in normal cats Right kidney often displaced from renal fossa of caudate liver lobe	Less oval shape, especially on sagittal axis Size varies greatly among various size dogs Less prominent, less common hilar fat deposition Right kidney nearly always in intimate contact with renal fossa of caudate liver lobe
Adrenal glands	Oval (jelly bean) shape No difference in shape between right and left Smaller, more consistent size Mineralization often seen as incidental finding Rarely see layering of adrenal gland	Various shapes: peanut shape, thin elongate, V-shape Right and left shapes often vary Inconsistent size Difficult to thoroughly assess right adrenal gland shape Mineralization often associated with adrenal neoplasia Often see layering of adrenal gland
Urinary bladder	Elongated bladder neck, transition into urethra Smaller, more consistent size Suspended echogenic fat droplets in urine common in normal cats	More abrupt transition of trigone into urethra Inconsistent size Fat droplets rarely seen in normal dog urine
Prostate gland	While present in cats, extremely uncommon to visualize Prostatic disease very rare	Routinely visualized in all male dogs, neutered or intact Prostatic disease common

flipped to the left side. For transverse (short-axis or cross-sectional) scan planes, the right side of the body is placed on the left side of the screen by pointing the transducer's orientation mark to the patient's right (toward the sonographer). These orientations are similar to how most clinicians view abdominal radiographs (ventrodorsal radiographs are viewed with the patient's right side to the left, and lateral radiographs are usually viewed with the cranial abdomen to the left).

If transducer options are available, select the highest frequency available (to maximize resolution) that adequately penetrates the depth of the liver of that particular patient. In large dogs, 5 MHz may be necessary; in most medium and smaller dogs and cats, 7.5 MHz or higher allows an optimal image. The commonly available multifrequency transducers allow lower frequencies to be used in the deeper cranial abdomen in large dogs; higher frequencies are selected, when appropriate, for evaluation of the remaining superficial portions of the liver and other superficial abdominal structures. One should have an idea as to the maximum depth obtainable by the highest frequency of the small curved-array or linear-array transducer that is being used. An 8 or 10 MHz curved-array transducer can easily provide high-quality images up to approximately 8 cm so that all cat and small dog abdomens can be scanned using this high-frequency setting.

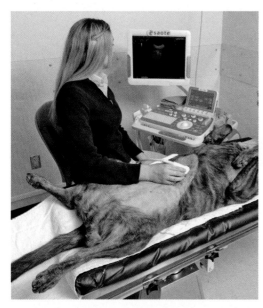

Figure 4-1 **Proper positioning of sonographer, patient, and ultrasound equipment.** The sonographer is sitting facing the machine, scanning the patient with her right hand, her left hand free for manipulating the controls. The patient is placed on a padded table to her right.

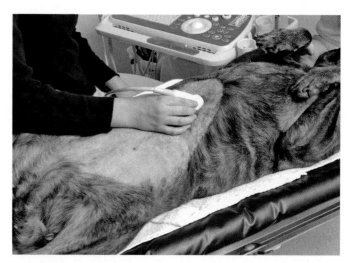

Figure 4-2 The patient has been placed in dorsal recumbency on a padded V-trough table. Most sonographers prefer to image patients in this position. Use of a shallow V-trough table and thin pad allows more lateral accessibility than a deep V-trough foam pad. This patient needed only minimal physical restraint.

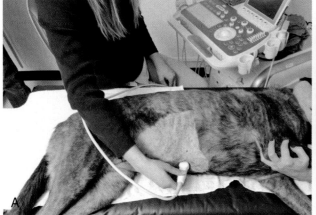
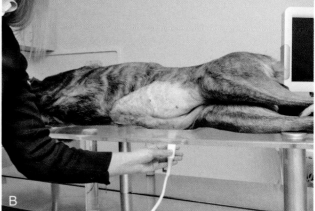

Figure 4-3 **Lateral recumbency for scanning the dependent and nondependent abdomen. A,** The patient is in left lateral recumbency and is being scanned from the nondependent right side. Some sonographers prefer this position for general scanning. Gas accumulation within the nondependent portion of the stomach and intestinal tract can compromise image quality. **B,** The patient is in right lateral recumbency and is being scanned from the dependent right side by use of a port hole table (used primarily for cardiac examinations). This position uses gravity-dependent fluid within the gastrointestinal tract or free within the abdominal cavity as an acoustic window.

User-selectable focal points are set to optimize the image. For general scanning, these may be set at the deepest level to maximize overall image quality, or multiple focal points may be used simultaneously. The disadvantage of using multiple focal points is that a slower frame rate (image acquisition) is necessary. This is deleterious in viewing rapidly moving structures such as the heart. In viewing a specific area of interest, the focal point is set at that specific level to optimize resolution of the area of interest at that depth. The focal point(s) are indicated on the edge of the image by a small arrowhead.

The depth of field is adjusted to allow visualization of the entire depth of the organ or area of interest (Figure 4-5). However, the field coverage should not be so great that the area of interest becomes a small portion of the overall image in the near field (see Figure 4-5, C). Power and gain are set to a visually pleasing gray-scale image that appears uniform throughout the near and far fields (Figure 4-6). This generally requires a reduction in the near-field gain while the far-field gain is preserved with the time-gain compensation (TGC) controls. The TGC curve is usually displayed on the right of the screen. A shift of the curve to the left indicates a reduction in gain at that particular level, whereas a shift to the right indicates increased gain. Once the image is balanced, overall image brightness can be increased or decreased by adjusting the overall gain setting (a separate control) or moving all of the TGC controls in unison. Most equipment also allows the user to adjust the power (output) of the ultrasound beam. A balance between power and overall gain should be reached, using the least amount of power necessary. Gain is the amount of overall amplification applied to the returning ultrasound echoes. This is called postprocessing in that the amplification occurs after the image has already been formed. Power is basically the "volume" or intensity of the ultrasound beam entering the patient. Keeping the power setting to the necessary minimal level reduces the patient's exposure to the biohazards of ultrasound (primarily heat) and reduces image distortion. Images are usually of higher quality when neither power nor gain is at the maximal setting.

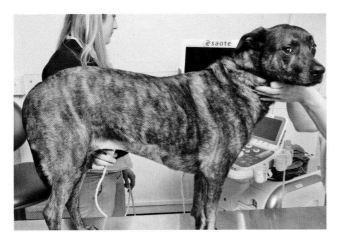

Figure 4-4 Standing position for abdominal scanning. This technique is particularly useful for patients with large peritoneal effusions and for giant-breed dogs that may be difficult to place or maintain in dorsal recumbency. It is also used to reassess a particular area with use of gravity-dependent fluid as an acoustic window. This position is helpful in assessing the gallbladder or urinary bladder in some cases when sediment or calculi are suspected. It is also useful in evaluation of the gastrointestinal tract, particularly the stomach.

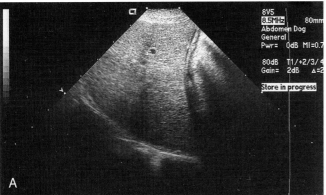

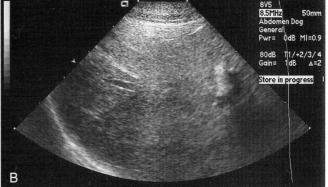

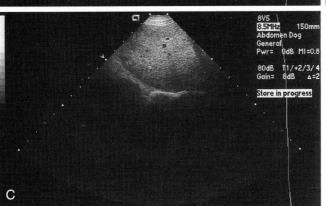

Figure 4-5 Depth of field considerations in a 40-pound shepherd mix. **A,** Correct depth of field. The entire liver is in the field of view. A depth of 8 cm (80 mm) was required. **B,** Depth of field that is too shallow. The dorsal portion of the liver is not in the far field of view. The depth of field was 5 cm (50 mm). **C,** Depth of field that is much too deep. The liver occupies only the upper third of the field of view. Depth was 15 cm (150 mm).

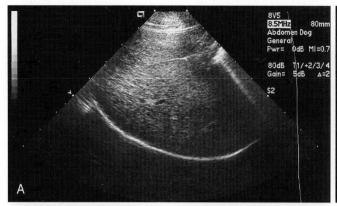
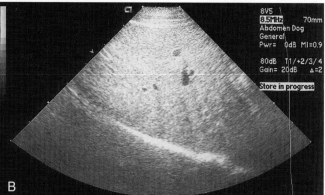
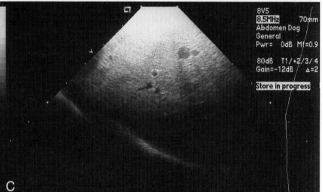

Figure 4-6 **Time-gain compensation (TGC) settings. A,** Correct TGC setting allows a uniform gray-scale image from the near field to the far field. Note that the overall gain setting is 5 dB and the slope of the TGC curve is shifted to the left in the near field, reducing near-field gain (brightness), and to the right in the far field, boosting the deeper tissue echogenicity by increasing gain. **B,** Too much overall gain. The gain has been increased to 20 dB from the image in **A,** resulting in an image that is much too echoic (bright). Note that the TGC curve has not been changed, and the overall brightness is uniform from near field to far field. **C,** Incorrect TGC settings. The upper half of the curve is radically shifted to the right, resulting in increased gain and therefore increased echogenicity in the upper third of the image. The central portion of the image is properly adjusted while the far field is nearly anechoic. Note that the overall gain is only −12 dB.

Most if not all current ultrasound machines allow the user to preset a variety of settings, such as depth, power, gain, and time-gain, and various image-processing parameters, including depth. These may be tailored for abdominal and thoracic imaging and to the size of the patient. For example, with selection of the "cat abdomen" setting, the machine defaults to appropriate predetermined settings for abdominal imaging of a cat or similarly sized small dog.

Many sonographers scan in the order of liver, spleen, stomach, duodenum, pancreas, kidneys, adrenal glands, bladder, prostate, and medial iliac lymph nodes followed by a sweep of the remaining intestinal tract and additional abdominal lymph nodes. The liver, the largest abdominal organ, is located within the deepest portion of the cranial abdomen. Imaging the liver usually requires the most depth of field, power, and gain and in some large patients will require a lower frequency transducer than the remaining abdominal structures. As the rest of the abdomen is scanned, appropriate reduction in power, gain, and depth of field should be made as needed to optimize the image.

For imaging of superficial structures or small patients, a standoff pad may be used.[1] Typical applications include ultrasound examination of the ventral urinary bladder wall, feline spleen, eye, thyroid and parathyroid glands, tendons, and ligaments. A standoff pad is an acoustically inert spacer placed between the transducer and the skin surface of the patient. It allows the most superficial structures of the patient to be visualized. When used with sector-type transducers, the standoff pad places superficial structures deeper into the field of view and out of the near field for optimal visualization. It also places the structure of interest in the focal zone of the transducer. Liberal acoustic coupling gel must be applied between the transducer and the standoff pad as well as between the standoff pad and the patient. With the advent of higher

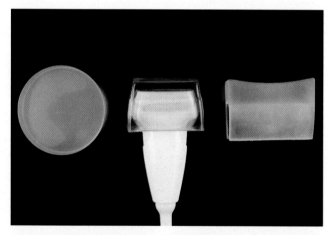

Figure 4-7 **Three types of ultrasound standoff pads.** A popular disk type of standoff is shown in on the left. In the middle is a slip-on type of standoff, which is slipped in place on the transducer. On the right is a universal standoff pad that can be used on most linear-array transducers.

frequency electronic linear- and curved-array transducers, the standoff pad has become less necessary owing to the excellent near-field imaging properties of these transducers. Various examples of the use of standoff pads are present in figures throughout the textbook.

Several types of standoff pads are commercially available (Figure 4-7). The simplest is a silicone disk. Another common type is a molded, hollow standoff that slips onto the end of the transducer. Standoff pads can be made by filling a surgical or examination glove with water. The downside to this is the presence of microbubbles that interfere with image quality. Additionally, when appropriate, a liberal layer (1 cm) of acoustic gel (sterile if required for surgical procedures) could be applied as a spacer; then the transducer is carefully positioned at the very top of the gel.

Although standoff pads can be effectively used in many situations to obtain an image that might otherwise be impossible to acquire, annoying reverberation artifacts can limit their usefulness (see Chapter 1).

TRANSDUCER MOTIONS

There are three principle transducer motions. To increase proficiency in scanning small animal patients, each of these motions should be mastered by the sonographer. The first motion is a distance motion, where the ultrasound transducer is slid along the abdominal wall in a cranial-caudal, lateral, or dorsal-ventral direction. The second motion is a nondistance, angular motion. In this case the transducer remains at the same contact point, but its angle is changed. An example would be in scanning the liver in a deep-chested dog. The

transducer is positioned in longitudinal axis (cranial to the left as seen on the ultrasound screen) and then angled cranially to obtain the cranial-most margin of the liver and lung-diaphragm interface. The third transducer motion is a nondistance, rotational motion. For example, when imaging small parts, the transducer must be rotated ever so slightly (typically millimeters) to get the small part into a long-axis imaging plane for appropriate measurements. Practice and more practice is required to obtain an adequate level of skill when using the transducer.

LIVER

Begin by placing the transducer on the ventral midline directly caudal to the xiphoid process of the sternum, the indicator mark pointing cranially (Figure 4-8). This orients the ultrasound beam in a sagittal plane, positions the image so that cranial is to the left and caudal is to the right, and creates a midline sagittal view of the liver.

In most instances, the liver is readily visualized from this location because the caudal liver margin is in close approximation to the costal arch. Normal exceptions are deep-chested

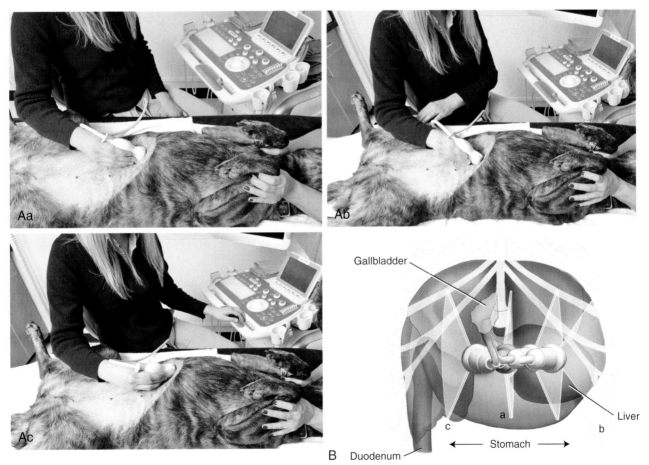

Figure 4-8 **Ultrasound evaluation of the liver in larger patients, sliding the transducer from left to right in sagittal scan planes. A,** Transducer placement for sagittal liver scanning. **a,** The transducer is placed on the ventral abdominal midline at the level of the xiphoid process. The indicator mark on the transducer is directed cranially. **b,** With a sliding motion, the transducer has been moved to the patient's left to image the left side of the liver. **c,** The transducer is now positioned to the patient's right. **B,** Illustration of a ventral view of the cranial abdomen. Sagittal scan planes are used to image the liver. The transducer is moved to the right and left from midline.

Continued

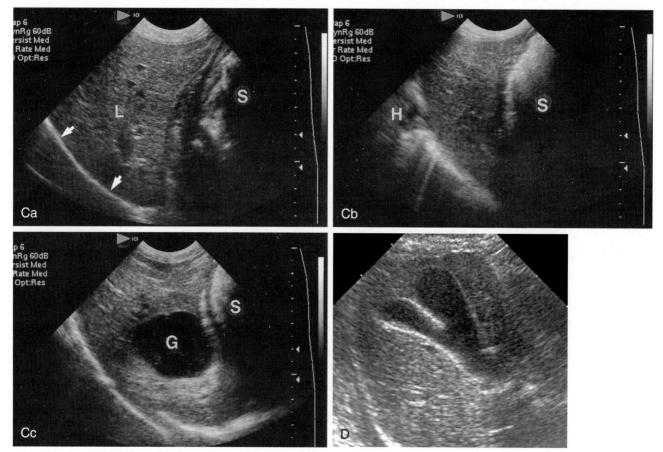

Figure 4-8, cont'd C, Ultrasound images corresponding to **A** and **B**. Note that the indicator mark (*arrowhead*) is to the left of the image, corresponding to the transducer's indicator mark, which is pointing cranially in **B** (the cranial part of the dog is to the left, caudal to the right). The ventral liver margins are noted in the near field adjacent to echogenic falciform fat and body wall. The caudal liver margin is adjacent to the gas-filled stomach. The cranial margin is defined by the diaphragm-lung interface. Note that the cranioventral margin of the liver is not within the sector in any of the three images. **a,** Sagittal midline image of the liver (*L*). The hepatic parenchyma is echogenic with a medium echo texture. The several anechoic round structures are hepatic vessels in cross section. The diaphragm-lung interface is seen as an echogenic curvilinear structure (*arrows*) to the left and in the far field. The air-filled stomach (*S*) is seen in cross section to the right. **b,** Left sagittal image of the liver. The apex of the heart (*H*) is adjacent to the diaphragm-lung interface, and the fundus of the air-filled stomach (*S*) is noted. Note the stomach wall layers and the highly echogenic reverberation artifact created by stomach gas. **c,** Right sagittal image of the liver. The round, anechoic, fluid-filled, thin-walled gallbladder (*G*) is creating distal acoustic enhancement, seen as liver parenchyma, which is more echogenic than surrounding liver tissue. The stomach (*S*) is seen in cross section. **D,** Bi-lobed gallbladder in a cat, a normal finding.

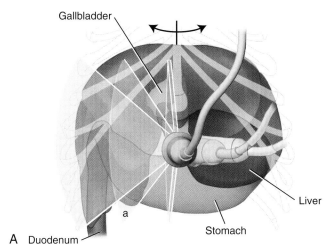

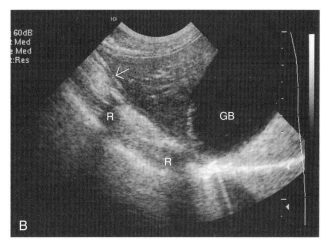

Figure 4-9 **Ultrasound evaluation of the liver in small patients, pivoting the ultrasound beam and fanning from left to right in sagittal scan planes. A,** Illustration of a ventral view of the cranial abdomen. Sagittal scan planes are used to image the liver by fanning the transducer to the left and right from midline. In small patients, the transducer may not need to be slid along the costal arch to view the entire liver, but it may instead be pointed to the right and left, in effect fanning the ultrasound beam to create sagittal images. **B,** Ultrasound image corresponding to position *a* in **A.** The transducer has been directed to the right from a midline position. The small triangle of liver parenchyma is bounded ventrally in the near field by echogenic falciform fat and body wall, caudally by the gallbladder (*GB*), and cranially by the diaphragm (*arrow*) and right lateral body wall. Note the acoustic shadowing created by the ribs (*R*). although depicted in the illustration, the stomach is not seen in this particular ultrasound image.

dogs, in which the liver is more upright and contained farther within the rib cage, and patients with a gas-distended stomach, which effectively closes the acoustic window to the liver. These circumstances necessitate cranial angulation of the ultrasound beam, use of a right- and left-sided intercostal window to visualize the liver, or scanning the patient while standing.

During initial imaging of the liver, machine settings must be adjusted to maximize image quality. The depth of field should be adequate to image the dorsal-most aspect of the liver parenchyma within the far field. Because of the size and solid nature of the liver, gain settings will be high relative to those required for other abdominal structures. Additionally, after a obtaining a global perspective of the hepatic parenchyma, one can divide the liver into thirds (near, mid, and far field) and optimize the image for the hepatic parenchyma in that particular section. This will allow evaluation of more subtle changes using the highest frequency transducer and resolution possible. Always adjust the focal zone to the area of interest (near, mid, or far field).

The liver parenchyma is echogenic, homogeneous, and of medium texture. Anechoic round and tubular vascular structures will be noted, representing hepatic and portal veins. Portal veins have more echogenic walls than the hepatic veins because they have thicker, less organized connective tissue in the vessel walls. This makes the portal vein walls more echogenic off-incidence than hepatic vein walls. Both hepatic and portal vein walls are echogenic when the ultrasound beam in perpendicular to them. In this case, the portal vein walls will be thicker than corresponding hepatic veins. In the dog, the portal veins will dominate the background hepatic architecture when compared to the hepatic veins. Although hepatic and portal veins are not as prominent in the normal cat liver when compared to the dog, the portal veins are still expected to be more prominent when compared to the hepatic veins. The cranial margin of the liver is bounded by an intensely

echogenic curvilinear structure that represents the diaphragm-lung interface. The diaphragm-lung interface (commonly referred to as the diaphragm) serves as a useful landmark for proper orientation and examination of the liver. The only time the sonographer will visualize the true diaphragm and its thickness is when there is a combination of pleural and peritoneal effusions. The caudal margin of the liver is bounded in large part by the stomach. On the left, the stomach or spleen may be adjacent to the liver. On the right, the right kidney is intimately associated with the renal fossa of the caudate liver lobe in the dog. In the cat, typically there is fat separating the cranial pole of the right kidney from the caudate lobe of the liver. During examination of the liver, the sonographer should study not only the appearance of the parenchyma but also the margins of the liver, the porta hepatis, and the contour and appearance of the diaphragm-lung interface. Liver margin evaluation allows detection of protruding nodules and surface irregularities and assessment of rounded margins that occur when the liver enlarges.

Sliding (distance) along the costal arch or pivoting (non-distance, angular motion) the transducer to the left allows imaging of the left side of the liver in the sagittal or sagittal oblique imaging plane. In large dogs, the transducer needs to be moved a relatively large distance along the costal arch. In small patients, little transducer movement is necessary. Simply pivoting or fanning the ultrasound beam may be adequate to image the entire liver (Figure 4-9). The left lateral liver lobe margin can be recognized along the body wall. From here, the transducer is slowly moved back to midline, scanning the entire left half of the liver in the process. In large patients, gently rocking the transducer cranially and caudally is necessary to view the entire cranial-to-caudal dimension of the liver because the entire liver may not fit within the image display (field of view) (Figure 4-10). As the transducer crosses right of midline, the gallbladder is identified as a round or oval anechoic structure with a thin, echogenic wall surrounded by

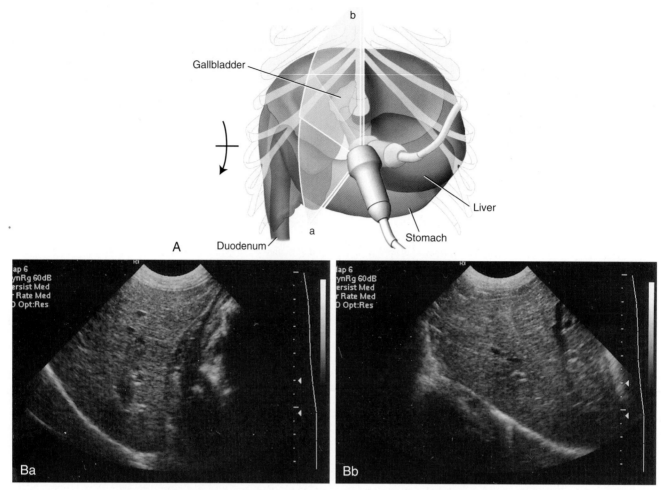

Figure 4-10 **Sagittal images of larger patients showing cranial and caudal direction of the ultrasound beam necessary to image the entire liver.** Because the liver is larger than the field of view of the ultrasound beam, the transducer must be directed cranially and swept left to right to image the cranioventral portion of the liver. **A,** Illustration of a ventral view of the cranial abdomen showing the ultrasound beam in caudal (*a*) and cranial (*b*) sagittal positions. Position *a* shows a midline sagittal scan plane in which the cranioventral portion of the liver is not in the field of view. In position *b*, cranial angulation of the ultrasound beam includes the cranioventral portion of the liver; the caudoventral liver tissue is no longer in the field of view. **B,** Ultrasound images corresponding to positions *a* and *b* in **A**. In **a**, the cranioventral portion of the liver is out of the field of view to the left. In **b**, the cranioventral portion of the liver is in the field of view to the left, but now the caudoventral liver is out of the field of view to the right.

liver parenchyma; it displays distal acoustic enhancement. The gallbladder is located between the right medial lobe laterally and the quadrate lobe medially. The position and volume of the gallbladder varies from patient to patient. It may be positioned near midline or be farther to the right and may contact the diaphragm cranially. In cats, a bi-lobed gallbladder is occasionally present, a normal finding not seen in dogs (see Figure 4-8, *D*). It is important to identify the gallbladder on every examination. In some instances, the neck of the gallbladder can be followed into the cystic duct, which accepts the hepatic ducts from the liver. Extrahepatic and intrahepatic ducts are not normally seen with ultrasound examination, although state-of-the-art equipment is allowing visualization of structures that have previously been hidden from sonographic view. The cystic duct continues as the bile duct, which terminates at the duodenum at the major duodenal papilla, shared with the pancreatic duct. It is relatively uncommon to be able to

follow the bile duct to the duodenal papilla in most dogs unless it is distended. This contrasts to the cat in which the bile duct can often be followed its entire length. The bile duct is ventral (closer in the near field) to the portal vein (Figure 4-11). The portal vein is a large vessel that delivers blood to the liver from the stomach, intestines, pancreas, and spleen. It is located near midline and enters the hilum of the liver (porta hepatis) just dorsal (deeper in the far field) to the bile duct. The caudal vena cava is dorsal and to the right of the portal vein. The right and left hepatic veins can usually be seen entering the caudal vena cava. Transverse abdominal images of this region allow a cross-sectional view of the portal vein to the left and ventral to the caudal vena cava. Although not difficult, imaging of the bile duct, portal vein, and caudal vena cava does require some experience. These structures can at times be difficult to image in some patients because of size, presence of intraabdominal fat, and interference

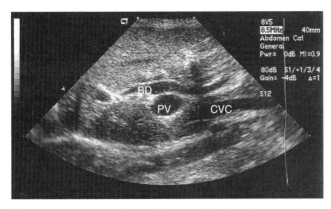

Figure 4-11 Sagittal ultrasound image of the liver in a normal cat. The bile duct (*BD*) is ventral to the portal vein (*PV*), which is ventral to the caudal vena cava (*CVC*).

by duodenal, gastric, or colonic gas. Routine evaluation is encouraged because biliary disease, portosystemic shunts, thrombosis, and other diseases are amenable to ultrasound examination. (See Figure 9-2 for detailed vascular anatomy of the liver.)

After sagittal imaging, the liver should be examined in orthogonal views. This entails transverse, dorsal, and oblique image planes (Figure 4-12). Because of the bony boundaries imposed by the sternum and costal arch, it is technically difficult to completely image the liver in a truly transverse axis. The transducer is placed on midline adjacent to the xiphoid process of the sternum (the transducer's indicator mark facing the right side of the patient, toward the sonographer, so that the right side of the liver is on the left side of the screen). After as much of the liver as possible is examined in a transverse view, the ultrasound beam is directed cranially by tilting

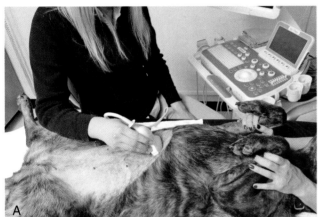
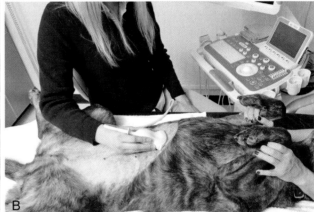

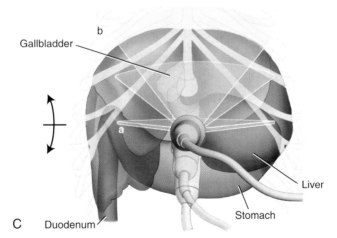

Figure 4-12 **Ultrasound evaluation of the liver, transverse to dorsal plane.** This is a particularly valuable view to examine the right and left portions of the liver. In smaller patients, the right and left portions of the liver may be viewed simultaneously because the ultrasound beam angle is large enough to include the entire liver. **A,** Transducer placement for transverse imaging of the liver. The transducer is placed on midline just caudal to the xiphoid process. The indicator mark on the transducer is positioned to the patient's right, toward the sonographer (not seen). This places the right side of the patient to the left side of the image when the indicator mark on the screen is to the left. **B,** Transducer is now directed into a dorsal plane by directing the ultrasound beam cranially. **C,** Illustration of a ventral view of the cranial abdomen showing transverse to dorsal imaging planes of the liver. A true transverse image is made by placing the transducer on midline at the level of the xiphoid process with the transducer's indicator mark facing to the patient's right (position *a*). By directing the ultrasound beam cranially, oblique and true dorsal images (position *b*) of the liver are seen. *Continued*

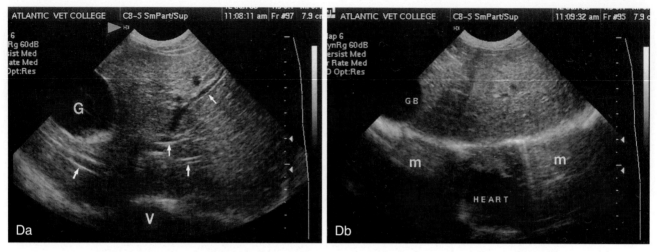

Figure 4-12, cont'd D, Ultrasound images corresponding to positions *a* and *b* in **C. a,** True transverse image of the liver corresponding to position *a* in **C.** The right-sided gallbladder (*G*) is to the left because the indicator mark on the screen is to the left (arrowhead) and the indicator mark on the transducer is pointed to the right (not seen). Portal veins are seen as anechoic tubular structures with echogenic walls (*arrows*). The dorsal liver margin is bounded by the dorsal surface of the peritoneal cavity laterally and centrally by the vertebral column (*V*). Note that the left and right lateral portions of the liver are not displayed because the liver is too wide to be seen in one field of view. **b,** Dorsal image of the liver corresponding to position *b* in **C.** The liver is now thinner because the craniocaudal dimension of the liver is less than the ventrodorsal dimension. The heart is seen in the far field beyond the echogenic line margin of diaphragm-lung interface. Note the mirror image artifact (*m*) of the liver to the left and right of the heart. *GB,* Gallbladder.

the transducer caudally (nondistance, angular motion). The view changes the transverse image to an oblique transverse image and finally a dorsal image as the image plane parallels the sternum. The ultrasound beam plane should then be directed to the right and to the left, again sweeping the beam from a transverse to a dorsal view (Figure 4-13). This imaging plane allows a detailed view of the lateral margins of the liver and the diaphragmatic attachment along the body wall. Transverse to dorsal image views of the liver are informative because the right and left portions of the liver can often be viewed simultaneously and in their entirety in one image display in small patients. Important landmarks visualized during scanning in the transverse to dorsal plane include the left and right hepatic veins converging to the caudal vena cava, the portal vein and its branches, and the gallbladder.

Mirror image artifact is common on scanning of the liver (Figure 4-14; see also Figures 4-12, *Cb,* and 4-13, *D;* see Chapter 1, Figures 1-41 and 1-42). It is important to recognize this artifact because its appearance could be mistaken for a diaphragmatic hernia (see Chapter 17).

FALCIFORM FAT

Falciform fat is located in the near field between the peritoneal surface of the abdomen and the ventral margin of the liver. The falciform fat can be quite thick in normal cats (both thin and obese), but it is a less common finding in dogs, even obese dogs. Recognition of falciform fat is important because its appearance can strongly resemble liver tissue in patients, especially cats. Falciform fat usually has a coarser texture than liver tissue. It is usually hypoechoic or isoechoic to the liver, but can be hyperechoic relative to liver parenchyma (Figure 4-15). Echogenicity of the falciform fat is highly dependent on overall and near-field gain settings. The thin echogenic

margin (capsule) of the liver, separating it from falciform fat, is an important sonographic landmark; however, it can be subtle and not as apparent in cats (see Figure 4-15, *C*). Recognition of falciform fat will help the sonographer avoid an erroneous diagnosis of hepatic enlargement and mistakenly aspirating or biopsying fat instead of liver!

SPLEEN

The size and position of the canine spleen varies greatly, which can complicate a thorough sonographic assessment. A superficial location and potentially large size dictate that multiple sweeps (distance motion) of the ultrasound beam are necessary to image the entire dog spleen. It is essential that the beginning sonographer learn to examine the entire spleen, regardless of size, shape, or position. Failure to do so will sooner or later result in missed splenic disease.

The parenchyma of the spleen is homogeneous and finely textured. It is usually hyperechoic with a finer parenchymal texture relative to the liver. In the hilum of the spleen, the splenic portal vasculature can be readily identified. Branches of the splenic portal veins are often encountered; however, these vessels bifurcate in the splenic parenchyma and taper quickly so that the vasculature is not apparent in the outer half (near field) of the splenic parenchyma. There are fewer large parenchymal vessels seen in the spleen than in the liver. The fibrous capsule of the spleen creates an echogenic margin when the incident ultrasound beam is perpendicular to it. As with the liver, the splenic margins must also be evaluated; they should be smooth and regular.

Scanning the spleen may be thought of in two parts: imaging the head of the spleen and imaging the body-tail (Figure 4-16). The head of the spleen is along the left lateral body wall, caudal and lateral to the stomach, and may be

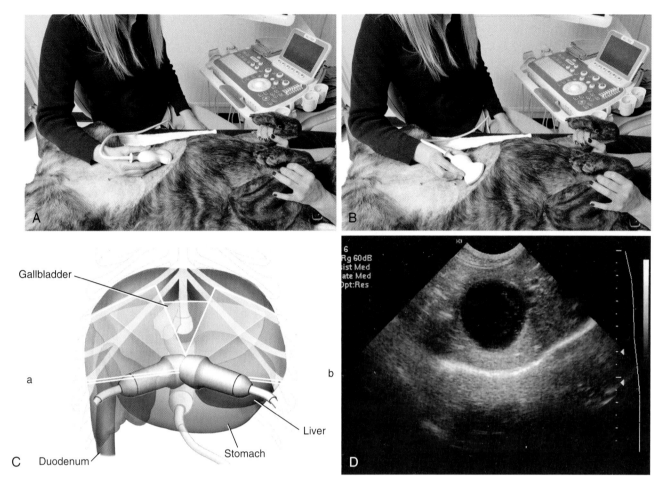

Figure 4-13 **Transverse to dorsal image planes of the liver showing how the transducer must be directed laterally to image the lateral margins of the liver in larger patients. A,** Transducer placement for transverse to dorsal imaging of the right lateral liver. The transducer is directed laterally to the right. The indicator mark on the transducer is positioned to the patient's right, toward the sonographer (not seen). **B,** Transducer placement for transverse to dorsal imaging of the left lateral liver. The transducer is directed laterally to the left. **C,** Illustration of a ventral view of the cranial abdomen showing the ultrasound plane directed toward the right (position *a*) lateral body wall to image the right side of the liver and left (position *b*) lateral body wall. In this illustration, the plane of the ultrasound beams are midway between transverse and dorsal planes. **D,** Ultrasound image corresponding to position A, and *c* in **C.** The right lateral liver is seen with the gallbladder located centrally. Note the thin wall of the gallbladder. Tiny echogenic foci are present within the otherwise anechoic bile. Acoustic enhancement is present distal to the gallbladder. Mirror image artifact of the liver is present in the far field beyond the echogenic diaphragm-lung interface.

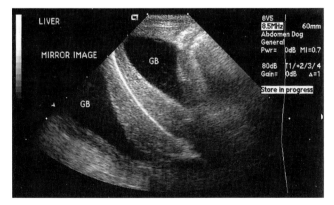

Figure 4-14 **Mirror image artifact of the liver and gallbladder.** The real liver and gallbladder (*GB*) are to the right, the mirror image to the left, separated by the echogenic diaphragm-lung interface.

partially contained within the rib cage. To image the head of the spleen, the transducer is placed in a sagittal location along the left cranial ventral abdomen. The ultrasound beam is directed parallel and adjacent to the left lateral body wall. From this window, the spleen will occupy nearly the entire field of view as the beam is directed through the length of the head of the spleen. Depth of field may be variable and considerable if a large portion of the spleen is present in the perihepatic space. The ultrasound beam is then slowly fanned (nondistance, angular motion) to view the entire thickness of the head of the spleen. The transducer may need to be gently rocked cranially and caudally (nondistance, angular motion) to image the cranial and caudal margins of the head of the spleen.

Orthogonal views of the head of the spleen are obtained by directing the ultrasound beam perpendicular to the left lateral body wall and at right angles to the surface of the spleen. The transducer is moved along the costal arch or

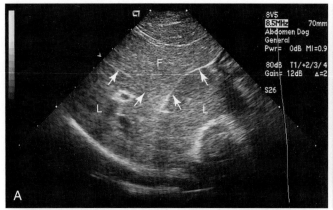

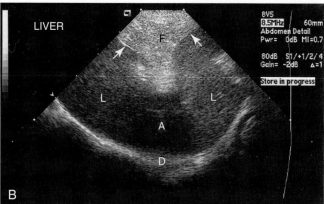

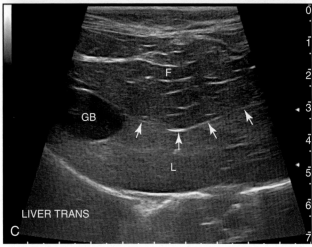

Figure 4-15 Falciform fat. A, Falciform fat (*F*) is similar to the liver parenchyma (*L*) in echogenicity and echo texture in this transverse image of an obese dog. The falciform fat is quite thick. Arrows demarcate the liver margin. **B,** Falciform fat (*F*) is markedly more echogenic than the liver (*L*) in this transverse image of a normal dog. *A,* Acoustic shadow artifact; *D,* diaphragm. **C,** Thick falciform fat (*F*) in a cat, slightly hypoechoic to the deeper liver (*L*) parenchyma. Arrows depict the falciform fat/liver interface. *GB,* Gallbladder.

within the left intercostal spaces laterally. This window may require additional clipping of the hair coat.

Once the head of the spleen has been assessed, the body and tail of the spleen are examined. The depth of field is reduced (e.g., 4 to 5 cm in dogs, 2 to 3 cm in cats) because the normal spleen is not a thick organ. The spleen is superficial and directly adjacent to the ventral abdominal wall, so near-field gain settings must be reduced in most instances. Because the sector width (field of view) is often narrower than the cranial-to-caudal dimension (width) of the canine spleen, dividing the spleen into two or three longitudinal strips during the scanning procedure may be necessary for complete examination.

The transducer is placed along the left side of the cranial abdomen oriented in an approximately sagittal body plane. This allows imaging of the spleen in a transverse axis (cross section). The cranial margin of the spleen is positioned to the left side of the monitor, whereas a portion of the caudal splenic parenchyma is to the right side of the monitor and not visualized in this field of view. Keeping the cranial margin of the spleen in view at all times, the splenic parenchyma is evaluated as the transducer is slowly moved from left to right until the tail end of the spleen is reached. The actual technique of scanning is easiest if the sonographer simply "follows" the spleen on the screen without watching the transducer's path on the patient. Keep in mind that the mid to caudal portion of the spleen is not in the field of view and thus not evaluated during this sweep. The caudal portion of the splenic parenchyma is now evaluated by scanning back toward the head of the spleen. The caudal margin of the spleen is

positioned to the right within the field of view (the previously scanned cranial half of the spleen is now off the screen to the left). The caudal portion of the splenic tail and body are now scanned by slowly sweeping the transducer cranially, from right to left until the head of the spleen is reached. In very large spleens, the central portion of the splenic parenchyma may still need to be scanned to complete the evaluation. This portion may be examined by positioning the spleen within the field of view such that neither the cranial nor caudal splenic margin is seen (thus viewing only the central splenic parenchyma), sweeping the transducer from the left cranial abdomen to the right. In smaller dogs, in all normal cats, and sometimes in larger dogs, the entire body and tail may be imaged in transverse section with one pass of the transducer. In this case, both the cranial and caudal margins of the spleen are seen within the field of view during the sweep of the transducer.

The feline spleen is finely textured and echogenic, similar to the canine spleen but often of seemingly finer texture and perhaps more echogenic. The normal feline spleen is small in width, thickness, and length (Figure 4-17). It tends to be positioned parallel to the left lateral body wall, occasionally resting along the ventral abdominal wall. It is superficial and requires a light transducer touch, marked reduction in near-field gain, and shallow field of view. In many cases, a linear-array transducer (or standoff pad) is necessary to fully assess the spleen, especially if only lower frequency transducers are available. If the machine settings are not correct and too much transducer pressure is applied, it can be easy to overlook the normal feline spleen.

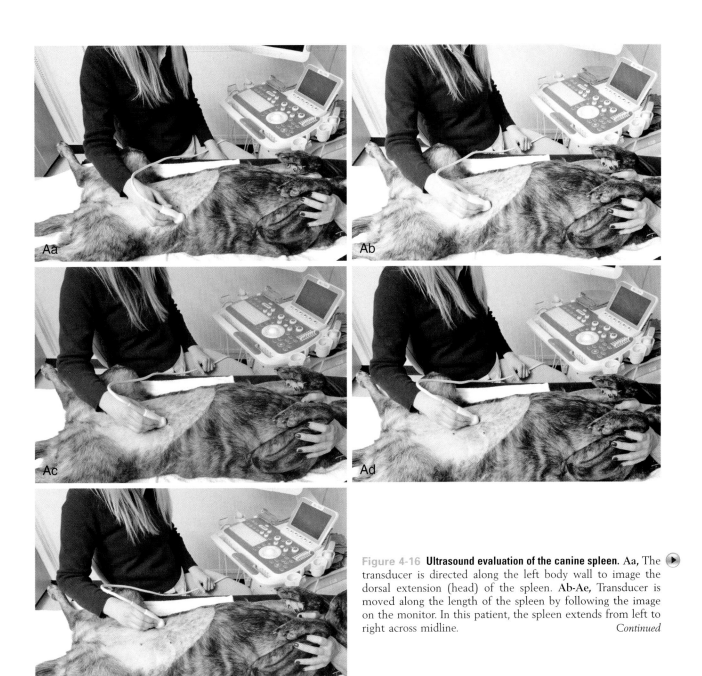

Figure 4-16 Ultrasound evaluation of the canine spleen. Aa, The transducer is directed along the left body wall to image the dorsal extension (head) of the spleen. **Ab-Ae,** Transducer is moved along the length of the spleen by following the image on the monitor. In this patient, the spleen extends from left to right across midline.   *Continued*

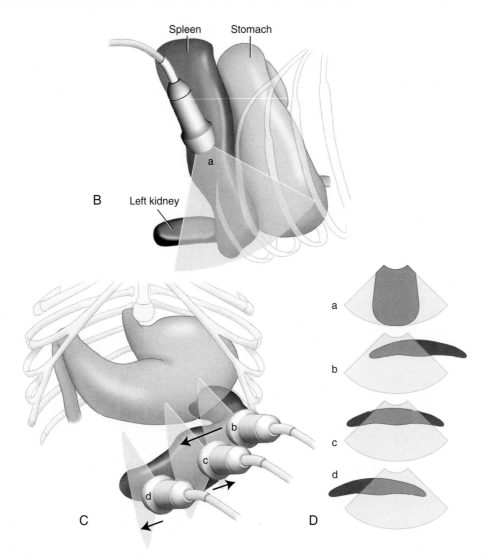

Figure 4-16, cont'd B, Illustration of the left lateral cranial abdomen of a dog in dorsal recumbency. The ultrasound beam is directed along the length of the head of the spleen as it lies along the left lateral body wall (position *a*), as shown in **Aa**. C, Illustration of the ventral view of the canine abdomen showing transducer movement along the long axis of the spleen. The width of the body and tail of the canine spleen may be greater than the field of view of the transducer. Two (*b*, *d*) or three (*b*, *c*, *d*) sweeps may be required to completely image the body and tail of the spleen, depending on size and pathologic changes. D, Illustrations of ultrasound images corresponding to position *a* in **B** and positions *b* to *d* in **C**. **a**, The head of the spleen is seen to occupy the entire field of view. **b**, The cranial half of the spleen is imaged as the transducer is moved from the head of the spleen to the tail, keeping the cranial splenic margin in view to the left of the screen at all times (dotted lines represent the portion of the spleen not imaged during this sweep of the transducer). **c**, The midportion of the spleen is scanned. Cranial and caudal splenic margins are not seen during this central sweep (denoted by dotted lines). **d**, The caudal half of the spleen is imaged while the caudal splenic margin is kept in view at all times. During this sweep of the transducer, the cranial half of the spleen is not seen (*dotted lines*).

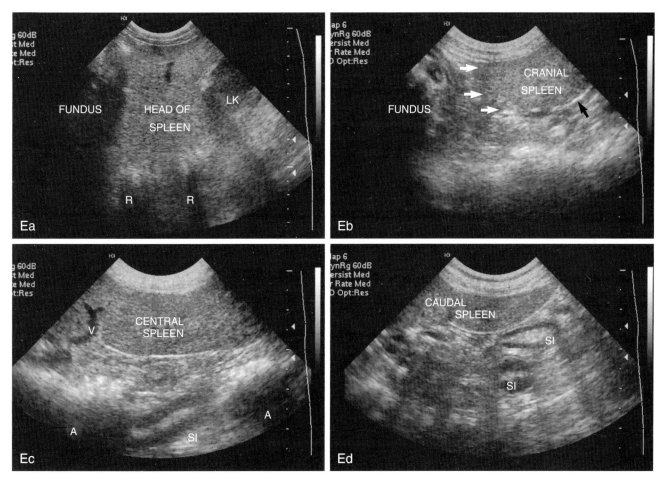

Figure 4-16, cont'd E, Ultrasound images corresponding to positions *a* to *d* in D. **a,** The head of the spleen is a finely textured echogenic structure. A small splenic vessel is seen centrally in the near field as a vertically positioned anechoic tubular structure. Note the thickness of the splenic head when the ultrasound beam is in this plane. The fundus of the stomach is to the left, a portion of the cranial pole of the left kidney (*LK*) is to the right, and ribs (*R*) are creating acoustic shadows dorsally in the far field. **b,** The cranial portion of the body of the spleen is seen. The cranial splenic margin is not clearly delineated because the ultrasound beam is not interacting at right angles to this edge (*white arrows*). Conversely, the dorsal splenic margin is more echogenic because the incident ultrasound beam strikes the capsule at nearly right angles, maximizing reflection and echo formation (*black arrow*). The fundus of the stomach is seen to the left. **c,** The central portion of the spleen is seen, with a branching anechoic splenic vein (*V*). Dorsal to the spleen in the far field are acoustic shadow artifacts (*A*) created by bowel gas and a short segment of small intestine (*SI*). **d,** The caudal margin of the tail of the spleen is present in the near field and fairly well defined. The tail is noticeably thinner than the body of the spleen seen in **b** and **c**. Small intestinal loops (*SI*) are seen dorsal to the spleen.

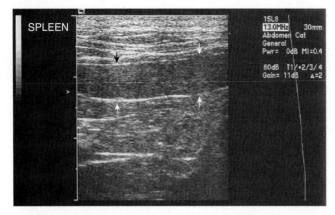

Figure 4-17 Ultrasound image of a normal cat spleen with a linear-array 13-MHz transducer. The gain and time-gain compensation have been adjusted to produce relatively hypoechoic splenic parenchyma. The splenic capsule (*arrows*) is easily seen as a thin linear echogenicity across the entire image because the ultrasound beam from a linear-array transducer is perpendicular to it across the width of the image. The thickness of this normal cat spleen was 5 mm.

STOMACH AND DUODENUM

After the liver and spleen have been thoroughly examined, a logical next step is to image the stomach, gastric outflow tract, duodenum, and region of the pancreas. The anatomic relationship of these organs is illustrated in Figure 4-18. Note that there is a difference of position between the canine and feline stomachs (Figure 4-19). The canine stomach is centrally placed, and the long axis is essentially perpendicular to the vertebral column; the feline stomach is to the left of midline and nearly parallel to the spine.

Attenuation of near-field gain and reduction in overall gain and power settings are usually necessary to optimize image quality of the stomach. The sonographic appearance of the stomach is extremely variable, depending on size and luminal contents (Figure 4-20). In the near field, the stomach wall is seen as a thin, layered, curvilinear structure. Invaginations of the wall into the lumen represent rugal folds. Because stomach gas is routinely present, it rises to the ventral portion of the stomach (near field) and creates acoustic shadowing and reverberation artifact that obscure deeper portions of the stomach from view. If the stomach is fluid-filled or contains sonolucent ingesta, it is possible to examine a larger portion

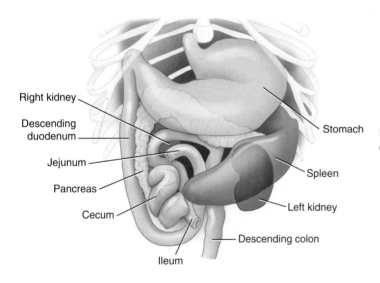

Right kidney

Descending duodenum

Jejunum

Pancreas

Cecum

Ileum

Stomach

Spleen

Left kidney

Descending colon

Figure 4-18 Illustration of the relationship of major abdominal organs in the dog.

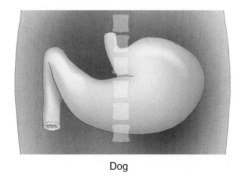

Dog

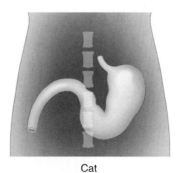

Cat

Figure 4-19 Illustration comparing the difference in position of the canine and feline stomachs. The canine stomach is centered in the cranial abdomen, its long axis essentially perpendicular to the spine. The feline stomach is mostly positioned to the left of midline, and its long axis is nearly parallel to the spine. Note the difference in the relationship between the pylorus and the duodenum between the dog and cat. The cat typically has a much larger pyloroduodenal angle than the dog.

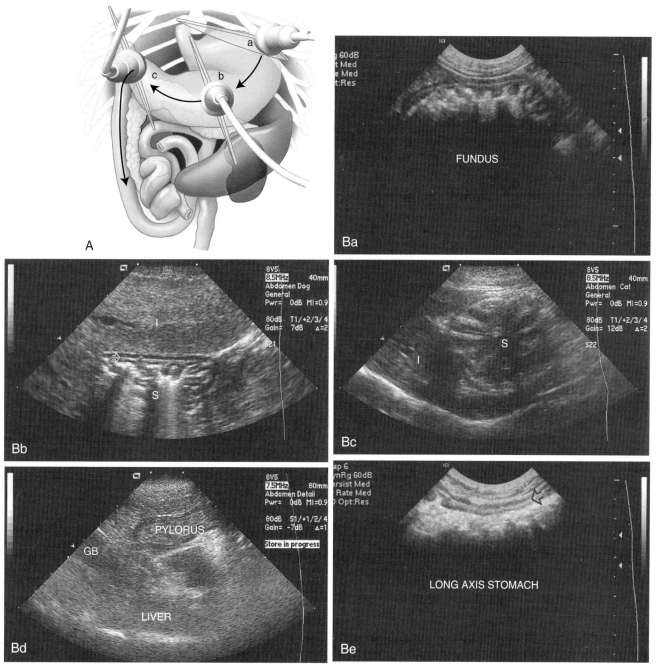

Figure 4-20 **Ultrasound evaluation of the stomach. A,** Illustration of a ventral view of the canine abdomen showing transducer movement in scanning of the stomach (*a, b, c*). **B,** Ultrasound images corresponding to positions *a, b,* and *c* in **A. a,** Sagittal scan plane corresponding to position *a* in **A,** creating a transverse image of the fundus of the stomach. Discrete layers of the stomach wall are easily identified in the near field. Rugal folds are seen as hypoechoic tissue invaginations into the lumen of the stomach. Echogenic gas is present at the gastric-mucosal interface, which is creating acoustic shadows and reverberation artifact, obscuring the contents and lateral and dorsal stomach wall. **b,** Sagittal scan plane corresponding to position *b* in A. In this dog, the stomach (*S*) is nearly empty, and the caudal stomach wall (greater curvature) can be seen to the right. There is enough luminal gas present to obscure the dorsal stomach wall. The layered appearance of the stomach wall is seen (*arrow*). The liver (*I*) is enlarged in this patient and is being used as an acoustic window in the near field. **c,** Sagittal scan plane corresponding to position *b* in A. In this normal cat, the stomach (*S*) is completely empty, allowing visualization of the entire stomach. Note the "spoke wheel" appearance of this empty stomach created by the thick hyperechoic submucosal layer of fat, commonly seen in cats. *l,* Liver. **d,** Sagittal scan plane corresponding to position *c* in **A.** The pylorus is seen in a sagittal axis. *GB,* gallbladder. **e,** Long-axis image of the body of the stomach. Only the ventral, near-field gastric wall (*arrow*) can be seen because of gas reverberation artifact and acoustic shadowing. If the stomach was the organ of interest in this case, it would need to be emptied of air and filled with water or scanned later in the day. Unwanted gastric distention with air occurs because of panting (aerophagia) and with some sedatives (e.g., xylazine, oxymorphone).

of the stomach and perhaps to evaluate gastric contents. If the stomach is empty, the rugal folds and crypts produce a striated pattern or "spoke wheel" pattern, especially in cats, accentuated by the presence of submucosal fat deposition (see Figure 4-20, *Bc*).[2,3]

With the transducer at the level of the xiphoid process and directed in a sagittal body plane, the stomach is seen directly caudal to the liver. In a sagittal body plane, the canine stomach is viewed in a transverse (cross-sectional) axis because it is positioned roughly perpendicular to the long axis of the patient. As noted, this differs from the feline stomach, which is oriented with its long axis more nearly parallel to the spine.

From midline, the transducer is moved to the left, roughly following the costal arch, but moving slightly caudal to include the entire cross section of the stomach within the field of view. To the far left is the fundus of the stomach. From here, the transducer may be slowly moved back toward midline, viewing the body of the stomach in the process. The stomach extends well to the right in dogs; in cats it extends only to near midline. As the transducer is moved to the right, the pyloric antral region of the stomach is identified by location and a reduction in lumen size. The stomach gently curves cranially in transition from the body to the pyloric antrum. Maintaining a transverse section of the stomach at this level requires that the transducer be rotated to some extent clockwise and moved cranially. The wall of the pylorus is thicker owing to increased muscle thickness of its sphincter. The lumen is small and narrow. The pyloric outflow tract leading into the duodenum is visualized as a transition from the muscular portion of the pylorus to the duodenum, which has the typical layered appearance of small intestine (see Chapter 12, Figure 12-8). The transducer must be manipulated to maintain a cross-sectional view of the pyloric outflow tract and duodenum. In dogs, the pyloroduodenal angle is usually quite acute, such that the descending duodenum and pyloric antrum are essentially parallel to each other. In contrast, the cat typically has a more open pyloroduodenal angle (see Figure 4-29). At some point, the transducer must be rotated counterclockwise to image the proximal descending duodenum in cross section, maintaining the lateral aspect of the duodenum to the left on the screen. The duodenum is usually the most lateral small intestinal segment on the right and is typically a millimeter or so thicker than adjacent loops of jejunum. The duodenum can be followed for some distance caudally in most patients, often to the caudal duodenal flexure. Once the duodenum is studied in cross section, the transducer may be rotated 90 degrees for evaluation in a longitudinal axis. Complete visualization of the gastric outflow tract is primarily dependent on the amount of luminal gas present and is somewhat breed dependent. Deep-chested dogs tend to be more difficult to examine because the stomach is partially enclosed within the rib cage, and brachycephalic dogs are usually more aerophagic. Imaging via a right intercostal approach is often beneficial or necessary.[4] The right intercostal approach is valuable for imaging the right side of the liver, the pyloroduodenal angle, the proximal duodenum, and the porta hepatis, including important identification of the aorta, caudal vena cava, and portal vein when in search of portosystemic shunts.

Once the stomach has been viewed in cross section, it is examined along its long axis. Rotating the transducer counterclockwise approximately 90 degrees from a sagittal to a transverse body plane accomplishes this. The transducer may be fanned cranially to produce dorsal oblique images of the stomach. In long-axis orientation, the rugal folds are viewed more longitudinally.

The stomach is assessed for evidence of peristalsis (five or six contractions per minute), the wall is evaluated for thickness (approximately 5 mm) and continuity of layers, and the gastric contents are noted.

PANCREAS

The pancreas is a small, thin, elongate V-shaped hypoechoic organ consisting of right and left lobes connected by the pancreatic body. The left lobe lies between the greater curvature of the stomach and the transverse colon, its lateral extent adjacent to the medial surface of the spleen and cranial pole of the left kidney (Figure 4-21; see also Figure 4-18). The right lobe is located within the mesoduodenum between the dorsomedial surface of the duodenum and the lateral surface of the ascending colon; it extends caudally to the level of the cecum and the caudal duodenal flexure. The right kidney is medial and dorsal to the right lobe of the pancreas. The body of the pancreas connects the two lobes in the angle of the pylorus and duodenum. The portal vein is dorsal and directly adjacent to the body of the pancreas, an excellent vascular landmark for locating the pancreas. The splenic portal vein is another important vascular landmark and is dorsal to the left limb of the pancreas; the splenic vein receives venous drainage from the left pancreatic lobe. These anatomic landmarks are important because their identification allows the sonographer to carefully study the *region* of the pancreas. Often, the pancreas cannot be completely visualized because of the lack in acoustic impedance differences between the pancreas and the surrounding mesentery and fat.

The pancreatic region is examined by scanning the area just caudal to the stomach and gastric outflow tract and medial to the duodenum, similar to the technique described for gastroduodenal imaging. In the now familiar sagittal body plane, the stomach and colon are identified in cross section as two curved echogenic structures (if both contain gas with a characteristic reverberation artifact) in the near field. A cross-sectional image of the left lobe of the pancreas is located between these two structures (see Figure 4-21). The length of the left pancreatic lobe may be studied in cross section by moving the transducer from left to right along the axes of the stomach and transverse colon. The pancreas is usually seen as a poorly marginated, hypoechoic organ. It may be flat and thin, somewhat triangular or lobulated in appearance on this cross-sectional view. A long-axis view of the region of the left lobe of the pancreas is achieved by rotating the transducer 90 degrees counterclockwise into a transverse body plane, just caudal to the stomach and cranial to the transverse colon. Small degrees of nondistance angle motions of the ultrasound beam cranially and caudally allow recognition of the left pancreatic lobe in the area between these two structures (provided the stomach and colon are not touching each other, obscuring the left lobe). Curiously, the left lobe of the pancreas in the cat is usually easier to image than the right, which is opposite of what is typically found in dogs.

The right lobe of the pancreas is located along the mesenteric (dorsomedial) surface of the descending duodenum within the mesoduodenum. Identification of the descending duodenum allows easy assessment of the *region* of the right lobe of the pancreas by directing the plane of the ultrasound beam medial from the descending duodenum. Once the descending duodenum and right pancreatic lobe region have been identified in long axis, the transducer may be rotated counterclockwise approximately 90 degrees to a transverse body plane. In this plane, the descending duodenum is seen in cross section to the left of the screen (lateral), the cross-sectional image of the right kidney medially positioned in the right field of view. The right lobe of the pancreas is within

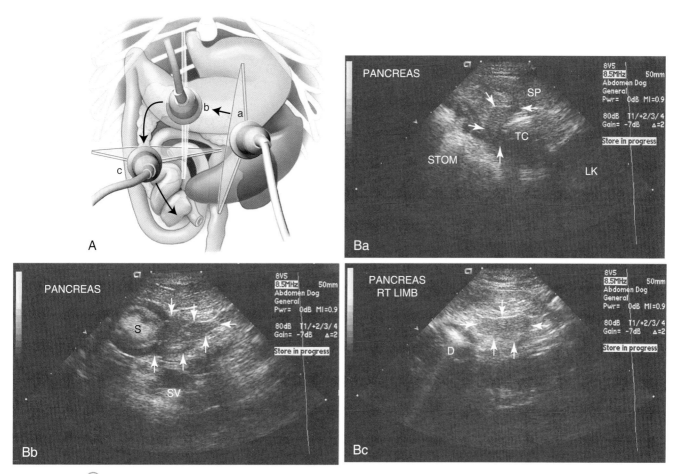

Figure 4-21 **Ultrasound evaluation of the pancreas in transverse section. A,** Illustration of a ventral view of the canine abdomen showing transducer movement in scanning of the pancreas (*a, b, c*). **B,** Ultrasound images corresponding to positions *a, b,* and *c* in **A. a,** Sagittal body plane creating a transverse image of the left lobe of the pancreas. The pancreas (*arrows*) is a small, flat, hypoechoic, homogeneous organ. Landmarks include the stomach (*STOM*), which contains echogenic gas, and the transverse colon (*TC*). In this image, a small portion of the spleen (*SP*) is noted in the near field. *LK,* left kidney. **b,** Left lobe of the pancreas (*arrows*) seen in transverse section as a hypoechoic, homogeneous, triangular structure. The anechoic round structure dorsal to the pancreas is a cross-sectional image of the splenic vein (*sv*). *S,* Stomach. **c,** Right lobe of the pancreas (*arrows*) seen in transverse section. The descending duodenum (*D*) is present in transverse section lateral to the right pancreatic lobe. In this particular instance, the right kidney is not in view.

the mesoduodenum, between the descending duodenum and the right kidney (see Figures 4-21, *A* and *Bc*).

In many cats and dogs, the pancreas is unfortunately not recognized as a discrete structure because it has the same acoustic impedance as the surrounding mesentery and mesenteric fat. It may blend in with the adjacent mesenteric fat; in other patients, it may be identified as a small hypoechoic organ and be seen well. Centrally within each lobe is the longitudinally oriented pancreatic duct, which may be seen as a small anechoic tubular structure, particularly in cats. Its identification in dogs usually indicates pathologic enlargement. It can be differentiated from the right pancreaticoduodenal portal vein based on size or by color, power or pulsed wave Doppler analysis. Nonvisualization of the pancreas rules out the presence of obvious mass lesions, but does not rule out pancreatitis even though specific sonographic abnormalities have not been identified. Conversely, visualization of the pancreas does not imply pathology. The right and left limbs of the pancreas are the most difficult abdominal organs to image routinely; therefore it is difficult to correlate sonographic appearance with the presence or absence of disease.

KIDNEYS

The depth, gain, and focal zone settings necessary to image the kidneys are generally less than those required for imaging the entire liver. Machine settings are similar to those used for imaging of the stomach, duodenum, and pancreas. The relationship of the kidneys relative to adjacent organs is illustrated in Figure 4-22. Figure 4-23, *A* and *B,* shows transducer placement for renal imaging, and Figure 4-23, *C,* illustrates standard renal scan planes. Notice the difference between the true dorsal plane imaging of the kidney (normal renal pelvis seen along the medial renal border in long axis) and a sagittal plane image (central renal pelvis is not visible).

Renal cortical and medullary tissues are evaluated for relative echogenicity and ability to sonographically distinguish the

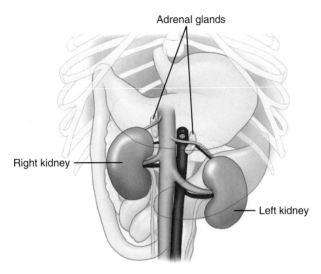

Figure 4-22 Illustration of a ventral view of the canine cranial abdomen showing the anatomic relationship of the kidneys (*RK* and *LK*) with the adjacent stomach, duodenum, pancreas, spleen, and adrenal glands.

cortex from the medulla at a sharp zone or line of transition. The cortical tissue is hyperechoic relative to the medulla, and a distinct, curvilinear demarcation between them should be present. An echogenic rim (corticomedullary rim sign) often separates cortical from medullary tissue. This can be seen in normal and abnormal kidneys. The medullary rim sign is a nonspecific ultrasonographic finding; it is possibly a sentinel sign of subclinical renal disease.[5] The medullary tissue is hypoechoic, sometimes to the degree that inexperienced sonographers may mistake it for hydronephrosis. The kidneys should have a smooth contour with a thin echogenic capsule. The sonographic appearance of the kidneys depends on the image plane and the particular location of the slice of the ultrasound beam.

The standard appearance of the central portion of the kidney when it is viewed in a sagittal plane is of echogenic peripheral cortical tissue surrounding hypoechoic medullary tissue (Figure 4-23, *Ea*, *Eb*, *Ec*, *Ed*). If the sagittal image is oriented medially, close to the hilum, an echogenic "disk" of tissue is often present centrally, representing hilar fat (see Figure 4-23, *Ec*). At this location, cross-sectional views of the renal artery and vein may be seen, whereas the ureter is generally too small to be resolved. The detail of this area depends to a large extent on the quality of the ultrasound equipment used, transducer frequency, and factors relating to the patient (such as obesity). Scanning farther medially, the kidney appears bi-lobed because of the indentation of the renal hilum and renal vessels (see Figure 4-23, *Ed*). If the kidney is imaged far laterally, medullary tissue will not be present, and the resulting image is one of a uniformly echogenic and smaller kidney (see Figure 4-23, *Ea*). The appearance of the kidney in this lateral image must not be mistaken for a pathologically small and echogenic kidney with loss of corticomedullary definition.

The left kidney is caudal to the stomach, dorsal and medial to the spleen along the left side of the abdomen. In dogs, the left kidney is usually imaged with use of the overlying spleen as an acoustic window. With the transducer positioned in a sagittal body plane to the left of midline, the spleen will usually be visualized in the near field as an echogenic, finely textured organ. The left kidney is deep (dorsal) to this and is generally readily found. Once it is visualized, the depth of field

should be adjusted so that the entire kidney is within the image display. The entire kidney is evaluated by gently rocking the transducer medial to lateral in a nondistance, angular motion, keeping the cranial and caudal poles within the field of view. On scanning of the left kidney, splenic tissue is often noted laterally and superficial to the kidney (see Figure 4-23, *Ee*). This occurs because the head of the spleen may curve toward midline dorsally.

Once the kidney is evaluated along its sagittal axis, the transducer is rotated 90 degrees counterclockwise to obtain transverse (cross-sectional) views. The hilum (medial) of the left kidney will be positioned to the left of the image display. Transverse images of the kidney are made from the cranial to caudal poles by sliding the transducer along the length of the kidney (see Figure 4-23, *De*, *Df*, *Ee*, and *Ef*). Mild renal pyelectasia is often best appreciated in this transverse imaging plane of the central hilum.

Some sonographers initially locate the left kidney by positioning the transducer in a transverse body plane on the left side of the abdomen and slowly moving from the stomach caudally until a transverse (cross-sectional or short-axis) image of the kidney is obtained.

Because of its more craniodorsal location and the presence of the pyloric outflow tract and descending duodenum ventrally (within the near field), the right kidney may be more difficult to image than the left. It is generally more dorsal and cranial than the left kidney, and therefore an increase in depth of field and gain may be necessary relative to that required for the left. The right kidney is bounded cranially by the renal fossa of the caudate liver lobe in the dog. Often there is fat separating the cranial pole of the right kidney from the caudate lobe in the cat. The transducer is positioned along the right side of the cranial abdomen just caudal to the costal arch in a sagittal body plane (indicator mark cranial). By slowly sweeping the ultrasound beam laterally and medially (nondistance, angle motion), the right kidney is generally found. It may be necessary in some cases to direct the ultrasound beam cranially, underneath the costal arch. In this case, the right kidney is positioned obliquely or vertically on the screen with the cranial pole in the deeper portion of the field and the caudal pole in the near field (see Figures 4-23, *F* and *G*). This appearance is simply due to angulation of the insonating ultrasound beam and does not indicate the true orientation of the right kidney. Once the right kidney is scanned along its sagittal (long) axis by slowly tilting the transducer toward and away from the sonographer (medial to lateral sweeps), the transducer is rotated counterclockwise approximately 90 degrees to obtain transverse images. The hilum of the right kidney is positioned to the right of the screen. The probe is then moved cranially and caudally for a thorough examination of the right kidney in cross section. One might need to approach from a dorsal 12th or 11th intercostal space to visualize the entire right kidney in deep-chested dogs, with the probe placed along the *lateral* aspect of the abdominal wall between the 12th and 13th ribs or the 11th and 12th ribs, respectively.

A third scan plane by which to image the kidney is a dorsal plane (Figure 4-23, *Dg* and *Eg*). This is achieved by approaching the kidneys from the right or left *lateral* abdominal wall. It is simple to obtain this view from the standard sagittal plane by simply sliding the transducer laterally and rotating your wrist and forearm approximately 90 degrees. The lateral renal cortex is positioned in the near field, and the medial portion of the kidney is in the far field. The kidney has a slightly different sonographic appearance when it is sectioned in this plane. Compared with a sagittal view, the medullary tissue is larger, and the kidney is larger in a lateral to medial dimension. The renal arteries and veins (rarely the ureter) are also viewed in long axis in this plane. The dorsal

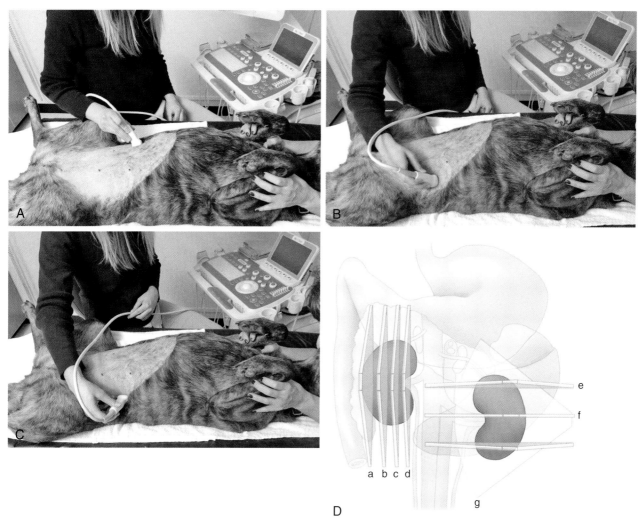

Figure 4-23 **Ultrasound evaluation of the kidneys.** A, Transducer placement for scanning the right kidney (sagittal plane). B, Transducer placement for scanning the left kidney (transverse plane). C, Transducer placement for scanning the left kidney (dorsal plane). Both kidneys are scanned in sagittal, transverse, and dorsal planes from these positions. D, Illustration showing sagittal (*a* to *d*), transverse (*e* and *f*), and dorsal (*g*) image planes through the kidneys. E, Ultrasound images corresponding to planes *a* to *g* in D. **a,** Sagittal image of the lateral cortex of the right kidney in this older dog. Note the lack of medullary tissue this far laterally. The entire kidney is not within the field of view; portions of the cranial and caudal poles are excluded. The kidney is smaller than in images *b* to *d* because the maximal length of the kidney is not present this far laterally. **b,** Sagittal image near the midportion of the right kidney. The renal cortex (*c*) is hyperechoic. A thin band of echogenic tissue (*arrow*) separates the renal cortical tissue (*c*) from the hypoechoic medullary tissue (*m*). **c,** Sagittal image of the right kidney at the level of the renal hilum (*h*). The central, highly echogenic oval area is composed of renal hilar fat and fibrous tissue. This is not quite a true sagittal plane image because the caudal pole of the kidney to the right is smaller than the cranial pole, indicating the off-sagittal nature of the ultrasound beam. This positional artifact must not be interpreted as renal disease. **d,** Sagittal image of the right kidney that is medial to c. This far medial, the kidney is nearly divided into two, with distinct cranial (*cr*) and caudal (*cd*) poles. Anechoic central structures are renal vessels and ureter (*arrows*) surrounded by echogenic fat. **e,** Transverse image of the cranial pole of a canine left kidney (*LK*). The spleen is in the near field and wraps lateral and dorsal to the kidney as well. Two anechoic splenic veins are noted. **f,** Transverse image of the hilum of the left kidney (*LK*). Medial is to the left of the image. Anechoic tubular structures are renal vessels. The spleen is in the near field. **g,** Dorsal image of the left kidney (*LK*). The kidney is larger in a lateral to medial dimension, and there is more medullary tissue than on a sagittal image. A small section of the aorta (*AO*) is noted. The wedge-shaped hypoechoic area adjacent to the lateral renal cortex is an edge shadow artifact. **F,** In some cases the right kidney can be best imaged by positioning the transducer horizontally along the right body wall while directing it cranially under the costal arch and into the caudal pole. This results in positioning the right kidney obliquely or vertically in the image as seen in **G. G,** Vertical orientation of right kidney created by horizontal position of transducer.   *Continued*

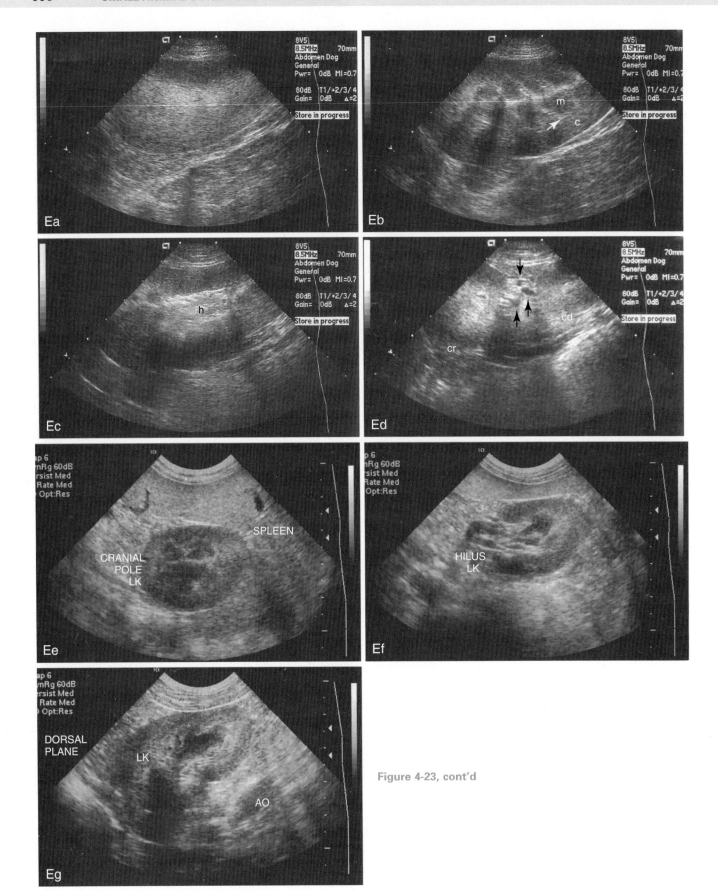

Figure 4-23, cont'd

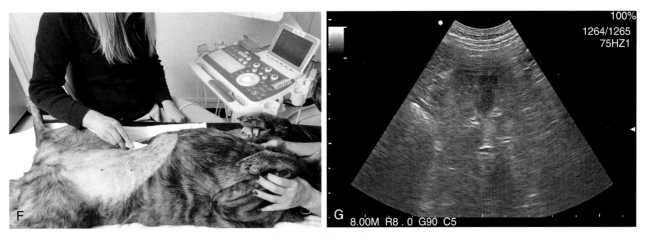

Figure 4-23, cont'd

plane is useful for imaging the adjacent adrenal glands, caudal vena cava, aorta, and portal vein.

ADRENAL GLANDS

The adrenal glands may routinely be identified with experience and equipment of reasonable quality. Anatomically, they are medial to the cranial pole of their respective kidneys. The left adrenal gland lies adjacent to the lateral surface of the aorta, bounded cranially by the cranial mesenteric and celiac arteries, caudally by the left renal artery and vein. The right adrenal gland is in intimate contact with the lateral surface of the caudal vena cava, bounded ventrally by the caudate lobe of the liver and dorsally by sublumbar musculature and the right diaphragmatic crus. The right renal artery and vein form the caudal boundary. The phrenicoabdominal arteries course dorsal to each adrenal gland; the phrenicoabdominal veins cross the ventral surface, often within a small depression.

The adrenal glands can be located in sagittal, transverse, and dorsal image planes. The technique that most consistently identifies the adrenal glands is the dorsal image plane (Figure 4-24). This technique is similar to that described for the kidneys. With location of the left kidney in a dorsal plane, the transducer is positioned to image the cranial renal pole centrally within the image. The typical peanut-shaped hypoechoic left adrenal gland in dogs is found just lateral to the deeper anechoic abdominal aorta seen in long axis. On the right, the hypoechoic adrenal gland is found adjacent to the deeper anechoic long-axis view of the caudal vena cava. The kidneys are usually not present within the scan plane that optimizes visualization of the adrenal gland. Although the size and shape of dog adrenal glands varies considerably, in cats, both glands are typically symmetrical, bean shaped, and smaller than seen in dogs.

The adrenal glands are found less consistently in a sagittal plane by first identifying the cranial pole of either kidney and directing the ultrasound beam medially to locate the aorta or caudal vena cava. The adrenal glands are just lateral to the great vessels and medial to the cranial poles of each kidney. Rarely, all three structures are identified in one image plane. Because of interference from bowel gas and its cranial location within the rib cage, the right adrenal gland is usually more difficult to identify than the left, especially from a sagittal plane. However, a distended stomach or descending colon often create an acoustic barrier to the left adrenal gland. Once the adrenal glands are located in either the dorsal or sagittal plane, they may be imaged in transverse section by simply rotating the transducer counterclockwise approximately 90 degrees. Some sonographers prefer to first find the adrenal glands in transverse section. It is important to remember the regional anatomy of the adrenal glands and use whatever scan position yields the best acoustic window to visualize them.

In addition to the small size, location, and potentially obstructing surrounding structures, the hypoechoic nature of the adrenal glands often makes it very difficult to distinguish them from adjacent vascular structures. With high-resolution equipment, an adrenal cortex and medulla may be seen. Careful attention to the surrounding great vessels is important in cases of adrenal disease; neoplastic invasion and thrombosis of the phrenicoabdominal vein and caudal vena cava can occur.

SMALL INTESTINES AND COLON

The small intestines are assessed by systematically scanning the abdominal cavity in sagittal and transverse scan planes. The depth of field is set to visualize the dorsal-most intestinal tract and then may be decreased to better visualize more superficial bowel segments. The transducer is positioned in a sagittal plane and is moved from left to right and right to left, moving from cranial to caudal to image the entire small intestinal tract. The transducer is rotated 90 degrees, scanning the left, central, and right quadrant in a cranial to caudal manner.

The intestinal tract consists of concentric tissue layers that are seen sonographically as alternating hyperechoic and hypoechoic layers (Figure 4-25; see also Chapter 12, Figure 12-8). The lumen of the small intestine may have anechoic fluid within it, or an echogenic appearance may be due to an admixture of gas and fluid. Gas-filled small intestinal loops create reverberation artifacts and sometimes acoustic shadowing. The inner mucosal-luminal interface is hyperechoic, the mucosal layer is thick and hypoechoic, the thin submucosal layer is hyperechoic, the thin muscle layer is hypoechoic, and the thin outer serosal surface is hyperechoic. These layers are routinely seen with use of newer high-resolution equipment.

Sections of small intestine are viewed sagittally, transversely, and in various oblique images, depending on the transducer and intestinal tract position (see Figure 4-25). The intestinal tract is assessed for uniformity in diameter, wall thickness (3 to 5 mm), discrete wall layers, luminal contents, and peristalsis.

Although the colonic wall has a layered appearance like the small intestine, it is thinner with less obvious layering. It

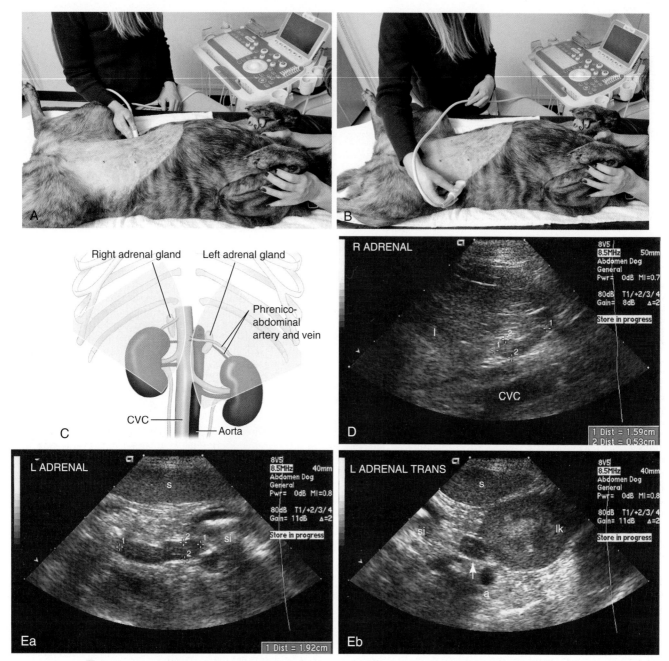

Figure 4-24 **Ultrasound evaluation of the adrenal glands. A,** A dorsal image plane is used to scan the right adrenal gland. **B,** A dorsal image plane is used to scan the left adrenal gland. The transducer position is similar to that used for imaging the kidneys in a dorsal plane. **C,** Illustration showing the dorsal image plane preferred for imaging of the adrenal glands. Note the relationship of the adrenal glands with the caudal vena cava (*CVC*), aorta, and phrenicoabdominal arteries and veins. **D,** Dorsal image of a right canine adrenal gland (between electronic cursors). The adrenal measured 1.59 × 0.53 cm. *CVC,* Caudal vena cava; *l,* liver. **E,** Dorsal (**a**) and transverse (**b**) images of a canine left adrenal gland (*arrow*). Electronic cursors define the dorsal image of the adrenal, measuring 1.92 × 0.41 cm. a, Aorta; *lk,* left kidney; *s,* spleen; *si,* small intestine.

can routinely be identified because of its consistent location (see Figure 4-18) and striking acoustic shadow and reverberation artifacts (Figure 4-26). The colon may be scanned in its entirety, including the junction of small intestine with colon (cat; see Chapter 12, Figure 12-6) or cecum (dog). The ascending colon is adjacent (medial and ventral) to the right kidney and right lobe of the pancreas. The transverse colon is just caudal to the stomach and left lobe of the pancreas, and the descending colon is along the left side of the abdomen. Distally, the descending colon may be seen along the left lateral wall of the urinary bladder (this can vary because the colon is mobile); it becomes dorsal to the urinary bladder as it enters the pelvic inlet. Normal colonic peristalsis is not observed, unlike that in the small intestine.

On a sagittal plane, the colon is seen as an echogenic linear structure (regular or irregular, depending on colonic contents) with acoustic shadowing or strong reverberation artifacts (see Figure 4-26). On transverse sections, the colon is seen as an echogenic curvilinear or crescent-shaped structure with strong artifacts. Familiarity with the appearance of the descending colon is important. Because of its proximity to the urinary bladder, the colon can mimic cystic calculi or lesions within the urinary bladder wall.

URINARY BLADDER

Both sagittal and transverse scans of the bladder should routinely be performed (Figure 4-27). The sagittal scan plane is

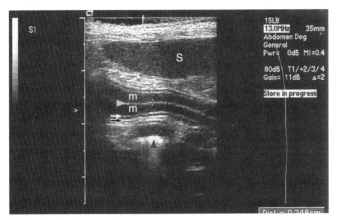

Figure 4-25 Ultrasound evaluation of the small intestine. Sagittal image of a segment of small intestine. Layers of the intestinal wall are clearly seen. Bowel wall thickness is 2.5 mm, measured between the electronic cursors. The outermost linear echogenic layer is serosa (*small black arrow*). The thin hypoechoic to anechoic muscle layer is between the serosa and thin echogenic submucosal layer (*small white arrow*). The mucosa (*m*) is the thickest hypoechoic to anechoic layer, separated by a thin, echogenic, empty lumen (*white arrowhead*). In the far field is a transverse section of small intestine that contains abundant luminal gas (*black arrowhead*), creating strong reverberation artifact and nonvisualization of the opposite intestinal wall. Note how a small amount of subcutaneous fluid (*f*) creates acoustic enhancement of the left side of the image. *S,* Spleen. (13-MHz linear-array transducer.)

achieved by placing the transducer in the caudal abdominal area cranial to the pubis with the indicator mark pointing cranially. The urinary bladder is identified as an anechoic round or oblong structure with a thin, echogenic wall (Figure 4-28). The transducer should be swept slowly back and forth, left to right, to image the entire width of the bladder. If it is greatly distended, the transducer must be positioned cranially and caudally to image the entire length of the bladder. Rotating the transducer 90 degrees counterclockwise produces a transverse image. The transducer is then moved cranially and caudally to image the entire length of the bladder in cross section.

Gain is set at minimum levels, and near-field gain and often far-field gain must be attenuated to prevent artifacts that may obscure pathology (see Figure 4-28, *D*). The bladder is filled with nonattenuating anechoic urine that causes strong distal acoustic enhancement and can obscure the dorsal bladder wall and adjacent structures. The ventral (near-field) bladder wall is superficial and will be obscured by failure to reduce near-field gain. The urinary bladder should be at least moderately full when it is examined. The wall of a nondistended urinary bladder will be artifactually thickened, which can mimic or mask various pathologic conditions.

The sonographer carefully assesses the walls of the urinary bladder and luminal contents. Particular areas of interest are the cranioventral bladder wall (e.g., cystitis, urachal diverticulum), the dorsal bladder wall (e.g., gravity-dependent calculi and sediment), and the trigone region and proximal urethra (e.g., neoplasia). The near-field position of the ventral urinary bladder wall makes it difficult to adequately assess unless technical considerations are optimized. In addition to reducing near-field gain, the use of a standoff pad or a linear-array transducer may be required. This is particularly true for thin or small patients. The cranial-most portion of the urinary bladder wall, which is essentially parallel to the direction of the incident ultrasound beam, will also be difficult to image because of "dropout" caused by refraction or edge artifact (see Chapter 1, Figure 1-48). Reorientation of the incident ultrasound beam relative to the cranial bladder wall may be necessary by angulation of the ultrasound beam caudally from a more cranially positioned transducer. Ultrasound examination with the patient standing is effective in documenting or discounting gravity-dependent echogenic sediment or calculi, adherent blood clots, and mass lesions (see Figure 4-27, *B*).

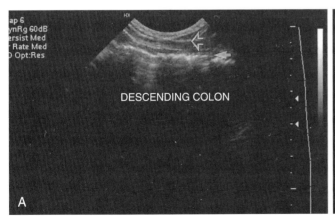
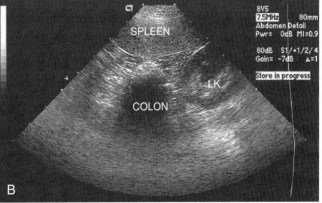

Figure 4-26 Ultrasound evaluation of the colon. A, Sagittal image of the descending colon. The colonic wall is thin (*arrow*), directly adjacent to the body wall (*open arrow*). Irregular, echogenic luminal gas is creating an acoustic shadow. **B,** Sagittal plane through the left cranial abdomen shows the transverse colon in cross section. The spleen and left kidney (*LK*) are noted.

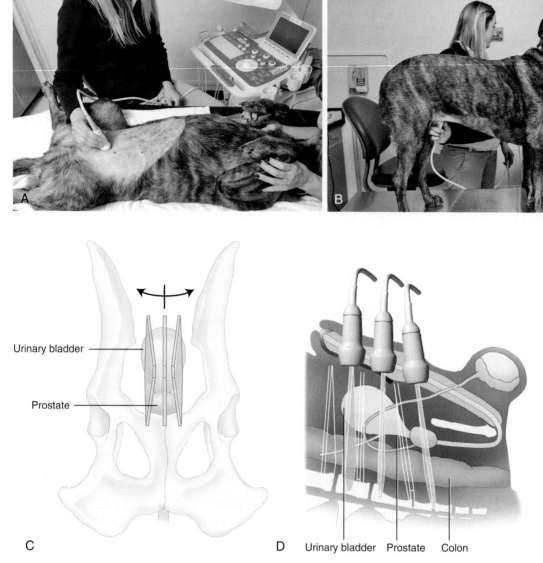

Figure 4-27 Transducer placement and positioning of the patient for ultrasound evaluation of the urinary bladder, prostate, and uterus. A, The transducer is positioned over the caudal abdomen to image the urinary bladder. **B,** Scanning of the urinary bladder with the patient standing is helpful in differentiating movable, gravity-dependent calculi and hematomas from adherent mass lesions. **C,** Illustration of a ventral view of a canine caudal abdomen showing sagittal image planes of the urinary bladder and prostate. **D,** Illustration of a right lateral view of a canine caudal abdomen with the patient in dorsal recumbency showing transverse image planes through the urinary bladder and prostate.

PROSTATE

In male dogs, evaluation of the prostate is simply a caudal extension of the urinary bladder examination (Figure 4-29; see also Figure 4-27). The gain may need to be increased to penetrate the prostatic parenchyma. The transducer is rocked or moved caudally to gain access to the prostate gland, which may be partially within the pelvic inlet. In the sagittal plane, the prostate is seen adjacent to the neck of the bladder as a hyperechoic, homogeneous, finely textured organ (Figure 4-29, A). The long funnel-shaped anechoic region of the trigone of the urinary bladder and proximal urethra can often be followed into the prostate. The prostatic urethra may occasionally be seen. The transverse image of the prostate is obtained by rotating the transducer 90 degrees counterclockwise and sweeping or fanning it cranially and caudally over its entire length

(Figure 4-29, *B*). The margins of the prostate gland are typically well defined by a thin echogenic capsule. The margin should be smooth, and the bi-lobed nature of the prostate is usually appreciated on transverse images. The feline prostate is not evaluated sonographically because of its small size.

UTERUS AND OVARIES

The uterus of a nongravid canine or feline may be imaged under optimal circumstances. The uterus is small, usually less than 1 cm in diameter in dogs and even smaller in cats. It is seen as a long hypoechoic structure directly adjacent to the dorsal surface of the urinary bladder in the appropriate sagittal scan plane (Figure 4-30, *A*). The cervix may be seen as a small, linear echogenic structure directed obliquely within

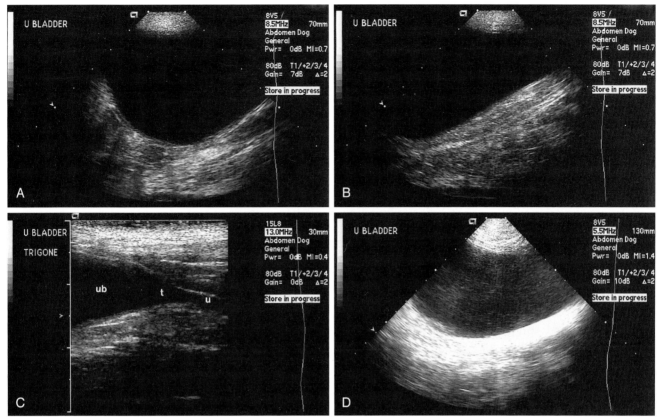

Figure 4-28 **Sagittal ultrasound images of the canine urinary bladder.** A, Cranial urinary bladder, moderately distended with anechoic urine. B, Midportion of the urinary bladder. C, High-detail image of the caudal urinary bladder (*ub*), neck/trigone (*t*), and urethra (*u*). (13-MHz linear-array transducer.) D, Improperly adjusted image of the urinary bladder. Overall gain is too high, resulting in loss of bladder wall visualization and artifactually echogenic urine.

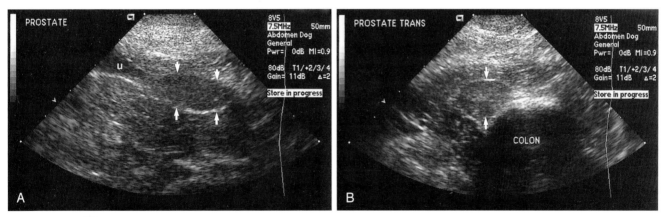

Figure 4-29 **Ultrasound evaluation of the prostate in a neutered 10-year-old canine.** A, Sagittal image of the prostate (*arrows*). The trigone and proximal urethra (*u*) are noted. B, Transverse image of the prostate (*arrows*). As expected, the prostate is very small in this neutered patient, only about 10 mm in thickness. The adjacent colon is a hyperechoic curvilinear structure with strong, clean acoustic shadowing.

the distal portion of the uterine body in a sagittal plane. Rotating the transducer 90 degrees shows the uterus as a small round or oval structure in cross section (see Figure 4-30, *B*). Rarely are the uterine horns imaged in normal, nongravid patients owing to their small size. Normal ovaries in a noncycling patient may be identified with careful study of the area caudal and lateral to each kidney. They are hypoechoic structures when seen, but they often blend with

the adjacent mesentery, making identification difficult (see Figure 4-30, C and D).

ABDOMINAL LYMPH NODES

The abdomen contains a plethora of lymph nodes, divided into parietal and visceral groups[6] (Figure 4-31). The parietal group

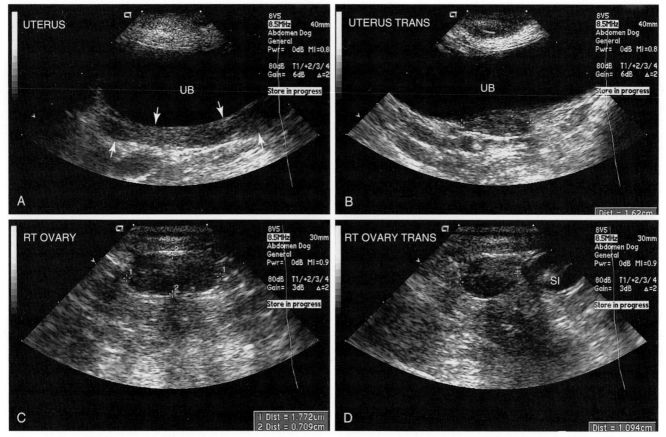

Figure 4-30 **Ultrasound evaluation of the uterus and ovaries in an 11-month-old anestrous canine.** A, Sagittal image of the uterine body (*arrows*). *UB*, Urinary bladder. B, Transverse image of the uterine body (between electronic cursors). The body is flattened and measures 1.62 cm. *UB*, Urinary bladder. C, Sagittal image of the right ovary (between electronic cursors). It measured 1.77 × 0.71 cm. D, Transverse image of the right ovary (between electronic cursors). It measured 1.09 cm. *SI*, Small intestine.

consists of lumbar, aortic, renal, medial iliac, hypogastric, sacral, and deep inguinal (iliofemoral) lymph nodes. Included in the visceral group are hepatic, splenic, gastric, pancreatico-duodenal, jejunal, and colic lymph nodes. Knowledge of afferent and efferent drainage of these nodes can be useful in assessing specific organ abnormalities, including neoplasia, metastatic disease, and in some cases inflammation. Typically, normal lymph nodes are not easily imaged during abdominal ultrasound examinations. Many of the lymph nodes are small and surrounded by mesenteric fat, which makes them difficult to image. However, with newer high-resolution equipment and experience and attention to detail, normal intraabdominal lymph nodes can frequently be visualized.[7] When seen, they are relatively hypoechoic, homogeneous structures and vary in thickness (several millimeters to centimeters) and shape from round or oval to more elongate and fusiform (up to several centimeters or more in length). They may appear nearly anechoic at times, and Doppler examination may be needed to differentiate them from blood vessels. Specific lymph nodes are identified through recognition of specific organ and vascular landmarks. Recognition of generalized or specific lymph node enlargement is important in assessing various disease states.

The lumbar, aortic, and renal lymph nodes are referred to as the lumbar lymph center. They are inconsistently present (or identifiable), small nodes adjacent to the aorta and caudal vena cava. They run from the diaphragm to the level of

the deep circumflex iliac arteries. Afferent lymphatics are from lumbar vertebrae, caudal ribs, lumbar muscles, intercostal muscles, abdominal muscles, aorta, nervous system, diaphragm and peritoneum, kidneys, adrenal glands, abdominal portions of the urogenital system, and mediastinum and pleura. Efferent drainage is to lumbar lymphatic trunks and cisterna chyli.

The medial iliac, hypogastric, and sacral lymph nodes compose the iliosacral lymph center. The medial iliac lymph nodes are the most consistently identified nodes during an ultrasound examination because of their size and consistent location (see Figure 4-31, *D*). They are located in the tissues between the aorta and caudal vena cava, dorsal to the wall of the urinary bladder, which is used as an acoustic window to image this region. The medial iliac lymph nodes are large (up to 4 cm long, 2 cm wide, and 0.5 cm thick in the dog) paired nodes, adjacent to the lateral and ventral surfaces of the caudal vena cava on the right and the aorta on the left. They are positioned at the level of the fifth and sixth lumbar vertebrae, between the deep circumflex vessels and the external iliac artery. They typically are identified by using a dorsal image plane to visualize the shallow angle of the aortic trifurcation, lateral to the aorta and right and left external iliac arteries (see Figure 4-31, *F*). Usually single on each side, they may be double on one or both sides. These nodes receive afferent vessels from the majority of the caudal abdominal structures and organs and portions of the hind limb as well as efferent

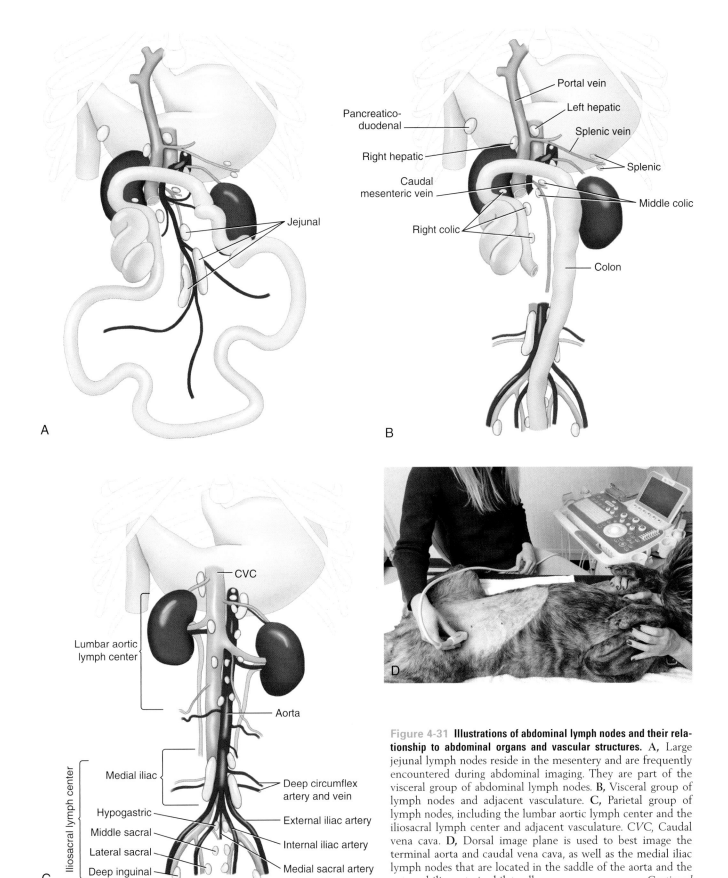

A

B

— Portal vein

— Left hepatic

— Splenic vein

Pancreatico-
duodenal —

Right hepatic —

— Splenic

Caudal
mesenteric vein —

— Middle colic

Right colic —

— Colon

Jejunal

C

— CVC

Lumbar aortic
lymph center

— Aorta

Iliosacral lymph center

Medial iliac

— Deep circumflex
artery and vein

Hypogastric —

— External iliac artery

Middle sacral —

— Internal iliac artery

Lateral sacral —

Deep inguinal —

— Medial sacral artery

D

Figure 4-31 **Illustrations of abdominal lymph nodes and their relationship to abdominal organs and vascular structures. A,** Large jejunal lymph nodes reside in the mesentery and are frequently encountered during abdominal imaging. They are part of the visceral group of abdominal lymph nodes. **B,** Visceral group of lymph nodes and adjacent vasculature. **C,** Parietal group of lymph nodes, including the lumbar aortic lymph center and the iliosacral lymph center and adjacent vasculature. *CVC,* Caudal vena cava. **D,** Dorsal image plane is used to best image the terminal aorta and caudal vena cava, as well as the medial iliac lymph nodes that are located in the saddle of the aorta and the external iliac arteries bilaterally. *Continued*

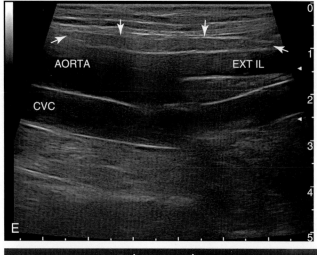

Figure 4-31, cont'd E, The terminal aorta, the branching external iliac artery (*EXT IL*), and the caudal vena cava (*CVC*) are easily visualized as parallel anechoic tubular structures, using a dorsal imaging plane of the caudal abdomen. In the near field a thin, fusiform shaped medial iliac lymph node can be seen (*arrows*). **F,** Two medial iliac lymph nodes in a normal dog (defined by electronic cursors). They are elongate and hypoechoic, measuring 1.80×0.54 cm and 1.21 cm, respectively. A small, anechoic urinary bladder is present in the near field. **G,** Two splenic lymph nodes in a normal dog (defined by electronic cursors). They measured 1.01 and 1.06 cm in length. *LK,* Left kidney; *SPL,* spleen. **H,** A small pancreaticoduodenal lymph node in a normal dog (between electronic cursors, 0.45 cm). This node is hypoechoic and surrounded by echogenic mesentery. *STO,* Stomach. **I,** Jejunal lymph node (*arrows*) in a normal dog. *I,* Intestine; *S,* spleen. **J,** Jejunal lymph node (*LN*) in a dog. The node was nearly anechoic, and color Doppler analysis was used to define its boundaries and adjacent blood vessels. **K,** Middle colic lymph node in a normal dog (between electronic cursors, 0.71 cm). C, Transverse colon.

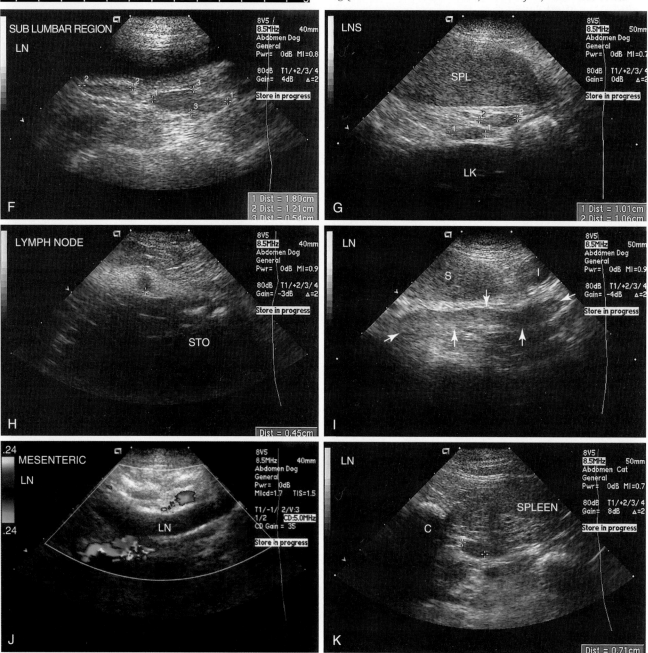

vessels from surrounding lymph nodes. Drainage from the medial iliac lymph nodes is to the lumbar lymph trunk or lumbar aortic lymph nodes. Sonographic identification of the medial iliac lymph nodes has become routine for experienced examiners.

The hypogastric lymph nodes are small, paired nodes caudal to the medial iliac nodes, located between the internal iliac and median sacral arteries. They may be single or multiple. Drainage to these nodes is similar to drainage to the medial iliac lymph nodes. The sacral and deep inguinal lymph nodes are inconsistently present, caudal to the hypogastric nodes.

Hepatic lymph nodes are relatively small nodes that lie on either side of the portal vein near the hilum of the liver. They vary in number. The left is larger (approximately 3 cm long in the dog) and more irregularly shaped than the right, located dorsal to the common bile duct within the lesser omentum. These nodes drain the liver, pancreas, duodenum, and stomach. Efferent vessels form the intestinal lymphatic trunk or plexus.

Three to five small splenic lymph nodes lie along the splenic vein and artery (see Figure 4-31, G). They are usually small but may be up to 4 cm in length. The splenic lymph nodes drain the spleen, liver, pancreas, stomach, esophagus, diaphragm, and omentum. As for the hepatic nodes, efferent splenic node vessels form the intestinal lymphatic trunk.

Gastric lymph nodes, if present, lie in the lesser omentum, close to the lesser curvature and pylorus. They receive afferent vessels from the stomach, esophagus, diaphragm, liver mesentery, and peritoneum. Efferent drainage is to the left hepatic or splenic lymph nodes. A small, consistent pancreaticoduodenal lymph node lies between the pylorus and the right lobe of the pancreas (see Figure 4-31, H); a second node is sometimes found. Lymphatic drainage is from the pancreas, duodenum, and omentum. The pancreaticoduodenal node sends efferent vessels to the right hepatic and right colic lymph nodes.

The jejunal (mesenteric) lymph nodes are the largest lymph nodes in the abdomen (6 cm long, 2 cm wide, and 0.5 cm thick), located within the jejunal mesentery (see Figures 4-31, I and J). They are irregular, even lobulated, and may be triangular in cross section. Multiple nodes are commonly present. The jejunal lymph nodes drain the jejunum, ileum, and pancreas. Efferent vessels form the intestinal trunk or plexus.

The colic lymph nodes consist of right, middle, and left nodes (see Figure 4-31, K). They are within the mesocolon close to the colon and are often multiple. The right colic node is disk shaped and lies medial to the ascending colon near the ileocolic junction. The middle colic node is oval and is caudal to the transverse colon, associated with the caudal mesenteric vein; the cranial portion of the left jejunal lymph node may be in proximity to it. The left colic lymph nodes are within the caudal part of the left mesocolon. They are the smallest of the colic nodes, only several millimeters in length. The colic nodes drain the ileum, cecum, and colon.

ABDOMINAL VESSELS

Major abdominal vessels serve as landmarks to aid identification of major organs and lymph node; consider them a road map of the abdomen. Disease of these vessels also occurs, principally thrombosis and invasion from adjacent neoplastic processes. The sonographer should become familiar with the location and appearance of the abdominal aorta, caudal vena cava, and portal vein as well as important major vessels, such as the celiac and cranial mesenteric arteries, splenic vein, phrenicoabdominal and renal artery and vein, and terminal branches of the aorta and caudal vena cava (see Figures 4-24, C, D, Eb, and 4-31, B, C, E). Particular vessel considerations as they pertain to individual organs and related pathologic processes are discussed in specific chapters.

The aorta and caudal vena cava are the largest and easiest abdominal vessels to image. They are best visualized in the caudal abdomen, with use of the urinary bladder as an acoustic window. In a transverse scan, the aorta is visualized just off midline to the left, the vena cava lying adjacent to it on the right (Figure 4-32). As the scan plane is moved caudally, these vessels bifurcate into the iliac arteries and veins. The external iliac arteries are the first to bifurcate from the aorta, followed by the internal iliac arteries. The common external iliac veins branch off the caudal vena cava in this region; the internal iliac veins arise from the external iliac veins. At this level, multiple, round anechoic cross sections of vessels are identified. The aorta and caudal vena cava can also be longitudinally imaged either in a sagittal plane or in a plane midway between sagittal and dorsal (Figures 4-33, A and B). The aorta is less compressible than the caudal vena cava and has a thicker

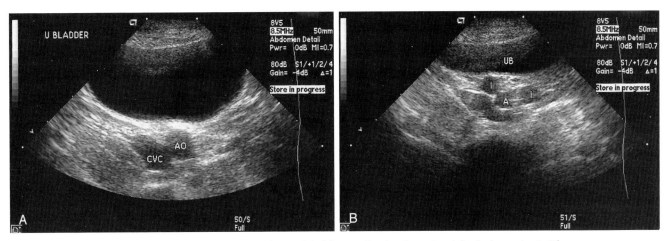

Figure 4-32 **Transverse images of the caudal abdomen showing the major abdominal vessels.** **A,** The caudal vena cava (*CVC*) and aorta (*AO*) are viewed in cross section. The urinary bladder is used as an acoustic window. **B,** Caudally, these vessels have bifurcated. *A,* Aorta; *I,* external iliac arteries; *UB,* urinary bladder.

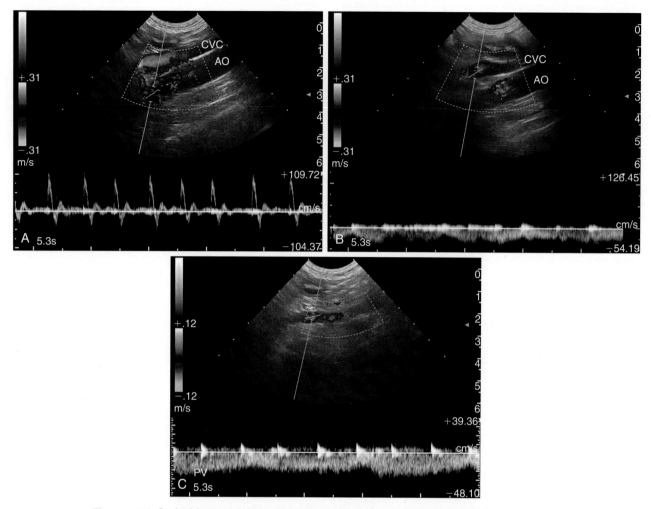

Figure 4-33 Sagittal images of the caudal abdomen showing the major abdominal vessels. A, The caudal vena cava (*CVC*) and aorta (*AO*) are seen as parallel anechoic structures in the right side of the image. Color flow Doppler analysis shows blood flow in the CVC (blue, toward the heart and away from the transducer) and the aorta (red). A pulsed wave Doppler cursor has been placed within the aorta, resulting in a pulsatile arterial spectral Doppler tracing seen below. Aortic blood velocity is approximately 1 m/sec in this example. **B,** Same image as **A** but with the pulsed wave Doppler cursor now placed in the CVC. Note the relatively nonpulsatile nature of the blood flow in the terminal caudal vena cava. This differs from CVC blood flow closer to the heart, which normally has a waveform that mimics right atrial pressure fluctuations. A transverse image of a small intestinal loop is noted in the near field. **C,** Blood flow near the origin of the portal vein. Note the nonpulsatile nature of normal portal blood flow and its relatively low velocity. An adjacent artery (out of the field of view) is creating the positive pulsatile waveforms. Small intestine is noted in the near field.

wall.[8] In addition, aortic pulses can usually be observed. However, one should be aware that the caudal vena cava can appear pulsatile owing to referred motion by the adjacent aorta. In many instances, the sonographer can follow both the aorta and the caudal vena cava cranially to the diaphragm.

The Doppler signal of the normal aorta is characterized by an arterial pulsatile waveform including a peak at systole, small early diastolic reverse flow peak, and low velocity late diastolic flow (see Figure 4-33, *A*). By comparison, the terminal caudal vena cava has a smooth, nonpulsatile Doppler flow signal that occurs during diastole (see Figure 4-33 *B*). The interested reader is referred to two articles addressing abdominal vasculature in exquisite detail.[9,10]

The celiac, cranial mesenteric, and renal arteries can routinely be visualized. The celiac artery arises from the ventral

wall of the aorta caudal to the stomach and branches shortly into the splenic artery to the left and the hepatic artery to the right. The cranial mesenteric artery is the largest branch of the abdominal aorta, arising from its ventral surface just caudal to the celiac artery (Figure 4-34). Figure 4-35 shows the celiac and cranial mesenteric arteries in transverse section as seen using a dorsal image plane. The right renal artery branches off the right lateral surface of the aorta several centimeters caudal to the cranial mesenteric artery, coursing dorsal to the adjacent caudal vena cava. The left renal artery arises from the left lateral surface of the aorta, several centimeters caudal to the right renal artery. The renal arteries may be duplicated, especially on the left side. Assessment of the renal arteries is often best performed in a dorsal (frontal) plane. The patient can be positioned in either right or left lateral recumbency to

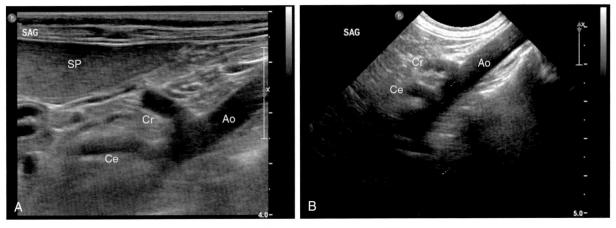

Figure 4-34 Sagittal plane of the celiac (*Ce*) and cranial mesenteric (*Cr*) arteries arising from the ventral surface of the aorta (*Ao*). A, Linear array transducer. SP, spleen. B, Microconvex sector array transducer.

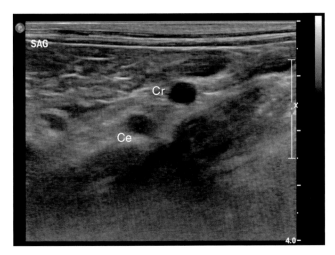

Figure 4-35 Dorsal plane of the aorta just ventral to the abdominal aorta shows the celiac (Ce) and cranial mesenteric artery (Cr) in transverse section. In slang, this view has been referred to as "snake eyes."

facilitate scanning of the contralateral renal artery. In this plane, the renal artery is seen arising from the aorta with a "shepherd's hook" appearance.

The caudal vena cava can be followed cranially and may be seen penetrating the diaphragm and entering the right atrium, especially if ascites or pleural fluid is present. The phrenicoabdominal veins (along with the renal arteries) serve as landmarks for identification of the adrenal glands because they course across the ventral surface of each gland, draining into the caudal vena cava just cranial to the renal veins. The renal veins are ventral to the renal arteries.

The portal vein accumulates blood from the gastrointestinal tract, the pancreas, and the spleen and is formed by the confluence of the mesenteric and splenic veins. It is ventral

to the caudal vena cava. The aorta lies dorsal to these two structures. In a transverse view of the cranial abdomen, the caudal vena cava is situated dorsal and slightly to the right of the portal vein. The aorta is on the midline or slightly to the left. The large splenic vein can be traced from the spleen, caudal to the stomach into the portal vein.

REFERENCES

1. Biller DS, Myer W. Ultrasound scanning of superficial structures using an ultrasound standoff pad. *Vet Radiol* 1988;**29**:138–42.
2. Heng HG, Wrigley RH, Kraft SL, et al. Fat is responsible for an intramural radiolucent band in the feline stomach wall. *Vet Radiol Ultrasound* 2005;**46**(1):54–6.
3. Heng HG, Teoh WT, Sheikh Omar AR. Gastric submucosal fat in cats. *Anat Histol Embryol* 2008;**37**(5):362–5.
4. Brinkman-Ferguson EL, Biller DS. Ultrasound of the right lateral intercostal space. *Vet Clin North Am Small Anim Pract* 2009;**39**(4):761–81.
5. Mantis P, Lamb CR. Most dogs with medullary rim sign on ultrasonography have no demonstrable renal dysfunction. *Vet Radiol Ultrasound* 2000;**41**(2):164166.
6. Bezuidenhout AJ. The lymphatic system. In: Evans HE, editor. *Miller's Anatomy of the dog*. 3rd ed. Philadelphia: WB Saunders; 1993. p. 717–57.
7. Pugh CR. Ultrasonographic examination of abdominal lymph nodes in the dog. *Vet Radiol Ultrasound* 1994;**35**:110–15.
8. Spaulding KA. Helpful hints in identifying the caudal abdominal aorta and caudal vena cava. *Vet Radiol* 1992;**33**:90–2.
9. Spaulding KA. A review of sonographic identification of abdominal blood vessels and juxtavascular organs. *Vet Radiol Ultrasound* 1997;**38**:4–23.
10. Finn-Bodner ST, Hudson JA. Abdominal vascular sonography. *Vet Clin North Am Small Anim Pract* 1998;**28**:887–942.

CHAPTER 5
Eye

Christopher S. MacKay • John S. Mattoon

Ultrasonography has been used since 1956 for the diagnosis of ocular diseases in humans.[1] Veterinary ocular ultrasonography was first described in 1968.[2] Early reports described time-amplitude ultrasonography (A-mode). The use of real-time two-dimensional B-mode ultrasonography in the diagnosis of veterinary ocular disease was reported in 1980.[3] Since then, multiple reports on the normal B-mode ultrasonographic appearance of the canine and equine eye have been published.[4-11]

Ocular ultrasonography is a valuable diagnostic tool because it allows evaluation of the interior of the eye, which may be obscured from direct visualization by any disease that causes ocular opacity. In addition, the retrobulbar soft tissues may be imaged. Although ultrasonography is an excellent ocular imaging modality, the importance of a careful and thorough visual examination of the eye cannot be overemphasized. Advanced imaging techniques such as color Doppler ultrasound, contrast enhanced ultrasound, ultrahigh-frequency (50 to 100 MHz) and high-frequency (20 to 50 MHz) ultrasound of the eye and orbit, once limited to human ocular ultrasonography,[12-25] have been reported in the recent veterinary literature.[26-41] Radiography, computed tomography (CT), and magnetic resonance imaging (MRI) are other diagnostic imaging modalities capable of providing detailed information about the eye, orbit, and periorbital tissues.[42,43]

NORMAL ANATOMY

The canine and feline eye is nearly spherical, measuring between 20 and 25 mm in diameter.[44-46] The vertex of the cornea is called the anterior pole, and the point directly opposite it is the posterior pole. The optic axis is a line connecting the anterior and posterior poles. Meridians are lines on the surface of the eye that connect the poles; the equator is the maximal circumference of the globe midway between the anterior and posterior poles (Figure 5-1).

The eyeball consists of three layers, the external fibrous tunic, the middle vascular tunic (uvea), and the inner nervous tunic (retina). The outer fibrous layer of the eye is composed of the sclera and cornea. The junction of the sclera and cornea is the limbus. This protective layer coupled with intraocular pressure is responsible for the semirigid shape of the eye. The uvea provides nutrition to the eye. It is divided into the iris, the ciliary body (ciliary muscle and ciliary processes), and the choroid (a pigmented vascular structure). The inner nervous layer of the eye is the retina. The intraocular myelinated portion of the optic nerve forms the optic disc. The optic disc is often depressed centrally (physiologic cup),[44,45,47] although it is flush with the surface of the retina in some dogs and

slightly elevated in others.[22] It measures between 1 and 2 mm in diameter in the dog[45,47] and lies slightly ventrolateral to the posterior pole of the eye[45] (Figure 5-2).

The lens of the eye lies in contact with the posterior surface of the iris. It is circular in a transverse plane and elliptic in a sagittal plane. It measures approximately 10 mm in diameter and 7 mm along the optic axis.[44,46,48] The lens is covered by the lens capsule. It is an avascular structure that receives nourishment from the aqueous and vitreous humors (see Figure 5-2).

The eyeball is divided into three chambers, the anterior, posterior, and vitreous chambers. The anterior chamber is bounded by the cornea and the anterior surface of the iris. It communicates with the posterior chamber through the pupil. At the periphery of the anterior chamber is the iridocorneal angle. The small posterior chamber is bounded by the posterior portion of the iris anteriorly and by the anterior lens capsule posteriorly; peripherally it is bounded by the lens zonules, in contact with the vitreous humor. The aqueous humor is present in both the anterior and posterior chambers. It is a clear, colorless fluid that closely resembles cerebrospinal fluid in constitution. The vitreous chamber is bounded by the lens zonules and the posterior lens capsule anteriorly and the retina posteriorly. It is the largest of the three chambers. The vitreous humor (body) occupies the vitreous chamber. It is gelatinous, composed of water (98%), mucopolysaccharides, and hyaluronic acid. Additionally, the vitreous body is reinforced by a fine network of collagen-like fibers (vitrein)[45] (see Figure 5-2).

The orbit is bounded by six bones, the frontal, sphenoid, palatine, zygomatic, maxillary, and lacrimal bones. The bony orbit is incomplete in the dog and cat; the dorsolateral margin is completed by the orbital ligament, which spans the distance from the zygomatic process of the frontal bone to the frontal process of the zygomatic bone. The lacrimal gland is between the dorsolateral aspect of the globe and the orbital ligament. The frontal bone forms the dorsomedial portion of the orbit; the zygomatic bone forms the ventrolateral part. The dorsal surface of the zygomatic salivary gland makes up most of the floor of the orbit. The temporalis muscle surrounds the dorsolateral aspect of the orbit[45] (Figure 5-3).

There are seven extraocular muscles: the dorsal, ventral, medial, and lateral rectus muscles; the dorsal and ventral oblique muscles; and the retractor bulbi muscle. The intraorbital fat pad is found at the posterior pole of the eye, surrounding the optic nerve and lying between it and the extraocular muscles. The internal maxillary artery, a continuation of the external carotid artery, supplies the majority of the globe. The internal maxillary artery branches into the external ophthalmic artery, which in turn gives rise to the

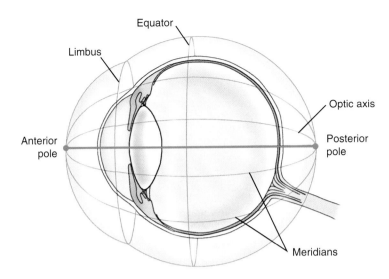

Figure 5-1 Ocular directional terminology.

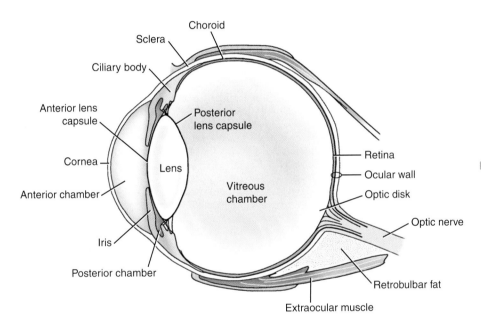

Figure 5-2 Ocular anatomy.

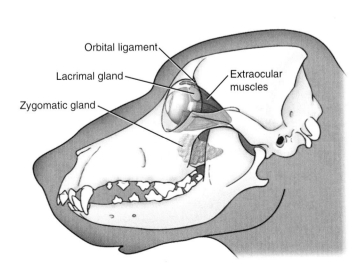

Figure 5-3 Sagittal illustration of the canine orbit demonstrating the extraocular muscles, lacrimal gland, zygomatic salivary gland, and orbital ligament.

short and long posterior ciliary arteries and the anterior ciliary arteries. Venous drainage is through the ophthalmic vein.[45]

EXAMINATION TECHNIQUE

Two main types of ocular ultrasonography have historically been used in human medicine: B-mode and A-mode. Real-time two-dimensional B-mode ultrasonography is the most accessible and commonly used mode in veterinary medicine. The past and current veterinary literature is primarily focused on the B-mode description of the normal and diseased eye. Although A-mode technique is described, and mention of A-mode findings in certain diseases can be found throughout this text, B-mode examination is heavily emphasized. Because B-mode allows a two-dimensional image to be viewed, anatomy is easily discerned. This is in contrast to A-mode ultrasonography, in which the returning echoes are displayed as spikes on a graph with a horizontal and vertical axis (see Chapter 1). A-mode echo patterns indicate the internal composition of lesions, and anterior and posterior echoes allow measurement and characterization. In human medicine, three-dimensional imaging, ultrahigh-frequency ultrasonography, and tissue characterization techniques appear to be superseding A-mode ultrasonography in human ophthalmology. A similar trend is seen in veterinary medicine.

Most small animals can be scanned without the use of sedation, unless the animal is restless because of pain or temperament. Examinations are conducted while the animal sits, stands, or lies in sternal recumbency with the head held steady by an assistant. General anesthesia can also be administered and the animal placed in sternal or dorsal recumbency. However, relaxation of the extraocular muscles during deep anesthesia can cause enophthalmos, third eyelid protrusion and ventral rotation of the globe, which may hinder the examination. Small retractors may be used to keep the eyelids open.

REAL-TIME B-MODE EXAMINATION

Medium-frequency (7.5- to 15-MHz) transducers are well suited for ocular examination because of high resolution capabilities and inherent shallow focal zones (1 to 4 cm). Lower frequency transducers may be best suited for the retrobulbar structures, particularly in larger patients. High-resolution ultrasound (HRUS) transducers with frequencies of approximately 20 MHz, and ultrasound biomicroscopy (UBM) transducers with frequencies between 50 to 100 MHz can be used for detailed imaging of the anterior chamber.[26,32] Transducer placement on the eye is crucial for a successful, high-quality examination.[9] There are two basic techniques. With the corneal technique, the transducer is placed directly on the cornea. The eyelid technique places the transducer directly on the eyelid, coupled with acoustic gel. A standoff pad may be used with either technique to image the anterior portion of the eye.

Corneal Technique
The preferred method is direct placement of the transducer on the cornea after topical ocular anesthesia and appropriate cleaning of the transducer head (e.g., alcohol followed by a saline rinse). This method is necessary for accurate ocular mensuration. The eyelids are spread manually, and the transducer is applied gently to the cornea. Ocular ointment may be used as an acoustic coupling agent, although it is usually not needed because the fluid provided by the topical anesthetic and tear film provides adequate coupling. The direct corneal contact technique allows the best visualization of the vitreoretinal and retrobulbar structures. Imaging of the cornea, anterior ocular structures, and lens requires the use of a standoff pad. It must be emphasized that extreme care is necessary when using the direct corneal technique so that the cornea is not damaged. For this reason, some sonographers prefer to image exclusively through the eyelid.

Eyelid Technique
Placing the transducer directly on the eyelid requires liberal application of a coupling gel. Clipping of the eyelid hair improves image quality by reducing trapped air between the transducer and skin. This technique allows adequate evaluation of the vitreous chamber, the retina, and the deeper orbital structures. The lens may or may not be adequately evaluated. The anterior chamber generally cannot be satisfactorily evaluated with the eyelid placement technique even when a standoff pad is used.[9] Although it is easier to perform, image quality is definitely inferior compared with direct corneal placement of the transducer.

A standoff pad is generally used to image the most superficial structures of the eye, such as the cornea, anterior chamber, ciliary body, and anterior lens capsule; it places these superficial structures within the focal zone of the transducer. The standoff pad can be used with the corneal or eyelid technique. A commercially available standoff pad or a small water-filled balloon (e.g., an examination glove) may be used. The fingers of an examination glove can also be filled with acoustic gel. The commercial pad may be cut to a smaller, more manageable size. Water-filled balloons are less desirable because small air bubbles within the water produce artifacts and reverberation echoes that degrade the image. Some manufacturers produce a transducer with a built-in offset, which is ideal. Molded standoff pads that slip over the tip of the transducer are also available for certain transducers. Standoff pads can be somewhat of a problem because of potential artifacts. With the newer high-frequency transducers designed for small-parts imaging, liberal application of acoustic gel to the eye can provide enough of a standoff to visualize the near-field structures. The eye should be thoroughly rinsed with sterile saline after completion of the examination.

In human ocular ultrasound examination, the transducer is placed on either the cornea or the eyelid. Instead of a flexible standoff pad, a saline immersion technique is preferred.[49,50] It allows the best overall detail of the entire eye. A thin plastic drape with a hole in it is glued around the eye with adhesive and is supported along its periphery by a hoop on a ring stand. Topical anesthesia is applied to the cornea, and the eyelids are held open with small retractors. The drape is then filled with saline warmed to body temperature, and the transducer is placed in the water bath. This technique has also been used in veterinary ocular ultrasound examination.[31] General anesthesia is required. This tedious setup precludes its use for routine screening examinations.

Sagittal, dorsal, and transverse scan plane images of the eye should be obtained during each examination. The ultrasound beam should be placed on the optic axis to produce the standard image. The anterior portion of the image is at the top of the screen; caudal is at the bottom. Whether nasal (medial) and temporal (lateral) structures are placed to the right or left on the screen has not been standardized. What is important is that the ultrasonographer be aware of image orientation so that pathologic changes can be accurately localized. The eye can then be scanned in a sweeping manner to allow visualization of the entire globe and retrobulbar structures (Figure 5-4). The retrobulbar tissues can be imaged through the eye or by placing the transducer caudal to the globe and orbital ligament[51] (see Figure 5-4, C).

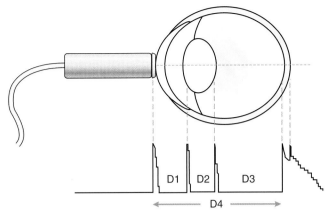

D1 | D2 | D3

D4

Figure 5-5 **A-mode ultrasound scan, optic axis transducer position.** Four echo spikes correspond to the cornea, anterior lens capsule, posterior lens capsule, and posterior ocular wall. The distance between each spike is denoted by D1, D2, and D3; D4 is the total length of the eye.

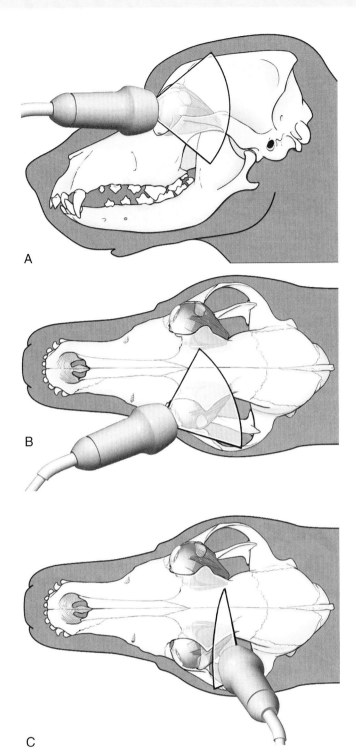

A

B

C

Figure 5-4 Illustration of sagittal (**A**) and dorsal (**B**) image planes of the eye and orbit. The retrobulbar tissues may also be imaged by placing the transducer caudal to the globe (**C**).

A-MODE EXAMINATION

A-mode ultrasonography uses a small ("ice-pick") beam of sound that produces spikes of varying size proportional to returning echo strength at the interfaces of intraocular and retrobulbar structures. Relatively high frequency transducers ranging between 8 and 20 MHz are used. The returning echoes are displayed as spikes on a graph with a horizontal and vertical axis. The vertical (y) axis represents the signal amplitude; the horizontal (x) axis represents elapsed time in microseconds (distance). Measurements of ocular structures (biometry) can be made by multiplying elapsed time (x-axis) by the speed of the ultrasound beam. These calculations are performed automatically by the ultrasound equipment, assuming a constant velocity of ultrasound through the entire eye (velocity of the ultrasound varies, depending on the portion of the eye through which the sound beam is traveling).[52] Calibration can be manually adjusted on some units. In addition to identification and mensuration of normal structures, abnormal intraocular structures producing aberrant echo spikes can be detected.

The corneal contact method after application of local anesthesia is the preferred technique in humans. It is also the reported method in veterinary ocular ultrasonography.[2,53] Coupling gel is not generally needed. Dedicated A-mode ultrasound units have an integral standoff pad or water bath attached to the probe. The scan is generally started along the optic axis, which is recognized by the appearance of the scan (Figure 5-5). The human patient is instructed to look directly at a small light emitted from the center of the transducer, which helps orient the A-mode beam along the optic axis. This technique is obviously not possible in veterinary patients. Once the optic axis is scanned, the transducer is placed at the limbus and redirected to visualize the entire eye. The probe is placed at clock positions corresponding to 6:00, 7:30, 9:00, 10:30, 12:00, 1:30, 3:00, and 4:30. The ultrasound beam is oriented perpendicular to the retina, keeping in mind that the images obtained originate from the opposite chorioretinal layers (e.g., the 6-o'clock probe position corresponds to the retina at the 12-o'clock position)[54] (Figure 5-6).

The owner's manual for a particular dedicated A-mode unit details the various setup procedures and adjustments needed to accurately use the unit.

NORMAL ULTRASOUND ANATOMY

Real-Time B-Mode Examination

The eyelids may be seen using very high quality equipment optimized for near-field imaging, but are usually best imaged with a standoff pad placed on the lid. The eyelids will appear as echoic homogeneous tissue in the near field. With lower frequency transducers, especially sector scanners, the eyelids cannot be well visualized when the transducer is placed directly on them; they become lost or indistinguishable in near-field reverberation artifact. The third eyelid is seen as an echoic structure just deep to the ventral eyelid. Imaging of the eyelids is generally unnecessary because direct visualization is adequate.

A standoff pad may be required to visualize the cornea, which appears as a curvilinear echo in the near field.[4,7,9] Ideally, the standoff pad is placed directly on the cornea because scanning through the eyelid, with or without an offset, often produces reverberation echoes at the transducer-cornea interface that obscure the anatomy. Under optimal conditions, the cornea appears as two parallel echoic lines instead of one, separated by an anechoic corneal stroma[55] (Figure 5-7). An anechoic area deep to the cornea represents the anterior chamber. The iris is difficult to image but can be seen under ideal conditions in contact with the anterior lens

capsule by use of a standoff and a high-frequency transducer.[50,55] The anterior lens capsule appears as an echoic, convex curvilinear structure. It is difficult to image the entire lens capsule because its curvilinear surface leads to peripheral echo dropout due to refraction and reflection of the sound beam. Orienting the ultrasound beam perpendicular to the peripheral portions of the lens surface allows complete visualization of the capsule through multiple images. The interior of the lens is normally anechoic. The posterior lens capsule is identified as a concave curvilinear echo (see Figure 5-7). The equatorial lens capsule and the ciliary body are best seen in animals as echoic structures when the transducer is oriented perpendicular to them with use of a corneal standoff pad.

The vitreous chamber is the anechoic region posterior to the lens. The posterior wall of the eye is seen as a bright curvilinear echo. The three wall layers cannot be individually resolved in the normal state. The optic disc is usually more echoic than the surrounding posterior wall, exhibits shadowing, and usually appears as a slight depression in this surface. Less commonly, the optic disc may be elevated or flush with the retinal surface in the normal animal. The optic nerve is usually seen as a hypoechoic to anechoic, slightly funnel-shaped structure surrounded by hyperechoic retrobulbar fat immediately posterior to the optic disc echo (Figure 5-8). Ultrasonographic mensuration of the optic nerve sheath diameter has been described in dogs.[56] In that study, no significant difference of optic nerve sheath diameter was found between the left and right eyes, and differences in sex, body weight, and age did not significantly affect optic nerve sheath diameter measurements. Significant differences were found between Maltese (1.63 ± 0.23 mm; mean, SD) and Yorkshire Terrier dogs (2.10 ± 0.22 mm), suggesting that breed differences do exist.[56]

The retrobulbar fat is triangular with the base bounded anteriorly by the posterior wall of the globe and bordered laterally by the extrinsic ocular muscles, which converge toward the apex of the orbit at the optic canal. The extrinsic

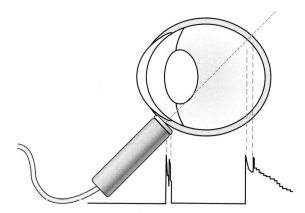

Figure 5-6 A-mode ultrasound scan, limbal transducer position. Note that the lens capsule echo spikes are no longer present. This scan plane is used to fully assess the ocular wall, optic nerve, and extraocular muscles.

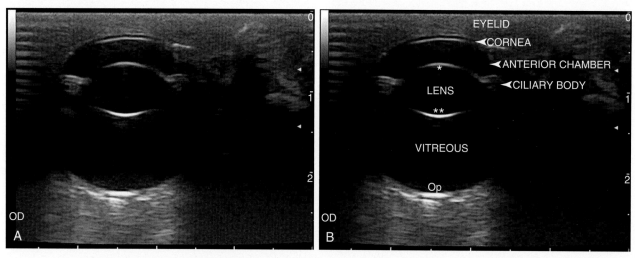

Figure 5-7 B-mode image (**A**) and with annotation (**B**) of a normal dog right eye (*OD*), using the eyelid contact technique. The cornea is seen as a double curvilinear echoic structure deep to the adjacent echoic eyelid. The anterior chamber, between the cornea and the anterior lens capsule, is anechoic. The body of the lens, bounded by the echoic anterior (*) and posterior (**) lens capsule, is anechoic. The ciliary body is seen at the periphery of the lens. The vitreous chamber is anechoic and makes up the greater part of the eye. The optic disc (*Op*) can be seen as a central hyperechoic linear structure when the scan plane is on its axis. The retina makes up the posterior boundary of the vitreous chamber to each side of the optic disc, but cannot be resolved as a discrete structure unless it is detached. The depth of field of this image is too shallow to view the entire retrobulbar space.

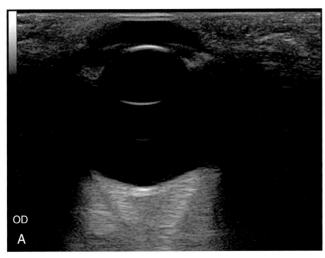
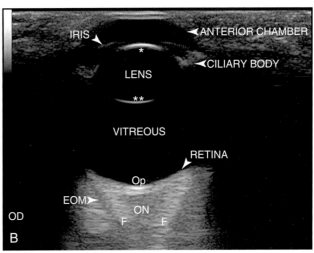

Figure 5-8 B-mode image (**A**) and with annotation (**B**) of a normal dog right eye (*OD*), using a direct corneal technique. This technique usually allows better visualization of the retrobulbar tissues. The anechoic anterior chamber is in the near field. The ciliary body can be seen as an echogenic area of tissue on the periphery of the lens. The body of the lens is bounded by the echoic anterior (*) and posterior (**). In this example, a faint linear echo of the iris can be seen to the right and left of the anterior lens capsule. The optic disc (*Op*) is a focal hyperechoic area at the posterior-most portion of the eye. The hypoechoic optic nerve (*ON*) is bounded by echoic retrobulbar fat (*F*) and hypoechoic extraocular muscle (*EOM*). Note the W appearance of the retrobulbar tissues created by the hypoechoic optic nerve and extraocular muscles surrounded by echogenic retrobulbar fat. The cornea is not well visualized in the very near field because of direct transducer contact.

muscles of the eye are homogeneous, hypoechoic structures with a coarse texture seen deep to the posterior ocular wall just off-axis to the optic nerve, running tangentially to the back of the eye. Fascial planes within the muscles appear as bright linear echoes when they are oriented perpendicular to the ultrasound beam. The overall appearance of the retrobulbar area is that of a W, representing the hypoechoic optic nerve centrally and the extraocular muscles, surrounded by the echogenic fat, peripherally.[57] A V-shaped area is seen if the scan plane is off the optic axis in the vertical plane because the optic nerve is no longer in the image plane. The retrobulbar area is bounded by the bony orbit.

The zygomatic salivary gland can occasionally be imaged ventrally as a hypoechoic structure adjacent to the extraocular muscles on a sagittal scan plane. The temporalis muscle is seen dorsally. The frontal scan plane reveals the region of the frontal sinus nasally and the temporalis muscle laterally. Ultrasound imaging of the lacrimal gland has not been described in the veterinary literature, but it lies dorsolateral to the globe beneath the orbital ligament. The ultrasonographic appearance of the human lacrimal system has been reported.[58] Not all structures can be seen in one scan plane or in every patient. Evaluation of the contralateral eye is recommended for comparison purposes, although the possibility of a bilateral ocular disorder should be kept in mind.

B-mode ultrasonography has been used to measure the axial length of the eye and its internal structures (Figure 5-9).[7,59] A-mode appears to be the standard in human ophthalmology, but a report has shown B-mode to be more accurate than A-mode in determining axial ocular length in the dog.[59] Intraobserver and interobserver repeatability of ocular biometric measurements using standard high resolution B-mode ultrasound in dogs has been reported.[60] In general, acceptable to high repeatability of measurements were found for most structures. Corneal thickness measurements showed the greatest variability, and the authors of that study

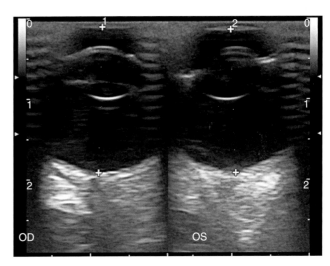

Figure 5-9 Axial ocular length measurements using B-mode ultrasound of the right eye (*OD*) and left eye (*OS*) in a 6-year-old neutered male Pekingese dog. The measurements are nearly identical, 1.81 cm for the right (D1) and 1.78 cm for the left (D2).

concluded that standard B-mode ultrasound is not an accurate method of measuring corneal thickness.[60] Improvement in accuracy and repeatability of measures for smaller structures in the anterior chamber, such as corneal thickness, has been demonstrated with the use of high frequency ultrasound, making this a more appropriate method for measuring corneal thickness and other anterior chamber structures.[27]

The B-mode appearance of the developing prenatal and postnatal canine eye has been described.[61] Quantitative (biometric) and qualitative descriptions are provided, with the eyes becoming visible on ultrasound exam from day 37 of pregnancy onward. A separate study proposes the use of regression analysis to predict the axial globe length in the developing eye, as measured by B-mode ultrasound, in mesocephalic dogs between the ages to 2 weeks to 1 year.[62] The postnatal development of corneal thickness in cats measured by ultrasound biomicroscopy has also been reported.[63]

A number of recent reports in the veterinary literature describe the use of high and ultrahigh frequency ultrasound for imaging of the canine and feline anterior chamber.[26-34] Recent advancements in biomicroscopy transducer design allows for imaging without the use of cumbersome water baths and general anesthesia as described in initial veterinary reports.[64] Improved spatial resolution of HRUS and UBM (20 to 80 μm compared to 300 to 400 μm for a 10-MHz transducer)[26] allows for improved visualization of the cornea, sclera, iris, and lens. Additionally, the iridocorneal angle, ciliary cleft, and posterior chamber can be imaged, making HRUS and UBM valuable diagnostic tools for investigation of glaucoma.[29-31,33,34]

A-Mode Ultrasonography

When a standoff pad or water bath offset is used directly on the cornea and with the ultrasound beam oriented along the optic axis, four major reflecting interfaces can be identified[2,3,50-54,59] (see Figure 5-5). These correspond to the cornea-transducer interface, the anterior lens capsule, the posterior capsule, and the posterior ocular wall (retina, choroid, sclera, retrobulbar structures). The anechoic areas between the spikes correspond to the anterior chamber, the lens, and the vitreous body. Reverberations beyond the retinal spike represent a summation of choroid, sclera, and orbital structures. These structures can be separated from one another by decreasing the system's sensitivity.[54] When the ultrasound beam is directed off the optic axis, or from a limbal position, echoes from the anterior and posterior lens capsule will be diminished or lost because these interfaces are off-incident to the beam. The globe is scanned in a systematic, meridian fashion (see Figure 5-6).

Evaluation of the retrobulbar structures also requires a limbal probe position. The retro-orbital spikes are a continuation of the posterior ocular wall echoes. They are high-amplitude spikes that rapidly decrease in amplitude owing to rapid absorption of sound by the retrobulbar tissues (principally fat). The optic nerve and the extraocular muscles are normal structures that can be identified and measured. The normal appearance of the optic nerve on A-mode evaluation consists of a double-peaked sharp-bordered spike separated by an area of uniform, medium internal reflectivity (Figure 5-10).

Extraocular muscles also have sharply defined borders but appear more echogenic and irregular than the optic nerve because of the presence of fiber bundles (Figure 5-11). Tables of normal values are available and are used to diagnose hyperthyroid-induced ocular myositis and conditions involving the optic nerve in humans.[54]

In A-mode measurements, the sound velocity within different ocular tissues must be used to convert time (horizontal axis) to distance. These values are readily available for the human eye and various species of animals, although the animal data are limited and there is some discrepancy in reported values, especially for the lens.[52,59] Measurements include cornea to anterior lens capsule distance (Dl), anterior to posterior lens capsule (D2), posterior lens capsule to retina (D3), and total length of the eye measured from the cornea to the retina (D4) (see Figure 5-5). One report compared the results of B-mode, A-mode, and direct measurements in normal dogs.[59] Whereas the axial length of the eye (D4) as measured by B-mode correlated well with direct measurements, Dl, D2, and D3 values obtained by B-mode or A-mode were significantly lower than actual measurements. These differences were thought to be related to technical factors such as indentation of the cornea by the transducer or processing techniques (freezing) that would alter the measurements.

Axial ocular length is significantly longer in the human male than in the female.[65,66] This was also found in the dog,[52] but a later independent study reported no significant difference.[59] The lengths of the right and left eyes are equal in all species studied.[52,59,65,66] Dolichocephalic breeds have a longer globe than do mesocephalic breeds.[59]

In veterinary medicine, ocular biometry can be used in establishing lens implant size, calculating lens power, and estimating prosthetic globe size after enucleation.

INTRAOCULAR MASSES

Mass lesions of the globe are produced by neoplasia, infectious and inflammatory disease, and organized hemorrhage. Ocular neoplasia may be primary or metastatic. The majority of non-neoplastic intraocular masses are fungal or hemorrhagic in origin.

General Considerations
B-Mode Examination
Certain basic parameters, such as location, size, shape, and sound attenuation, should be evaluated when the globe is examined for the presence of mass lesions. Concurrent ocular

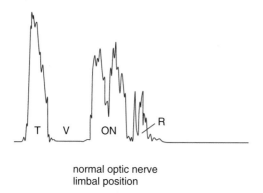

normal optic nerve
limbal position

Figure 5-10 A-mode scan of a normal optic nerve, limbal transducer position. The two tall peaks represent the optic nerve (*ON*). The lower amplitude echoes are retrobulbar tissues (*R*). The anterior echoes are transducer and limbal near-field echoes (*T*). The vitreous (*V*) is anechoic.

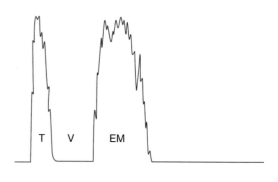

extraocular muscle
limbal position

Figure 5-11 A-mode scan of extraocular muscle (*EM*), limbal transducer position. *T,* Transducer and limbal echoes; *V,* vitreous.

abnormalities may be present, such as vitreal hemorrhage or a detached retina. Because B-mode ultrasonography cannot reliably determine the histologic features of mass lesions, knowledge of certain features of tumors and inflammatory conditions will help the veterinarian develop a sound differential diagnosis. An abundant literature is available for human ocular ultrasound evaluation of intraocular masses, but there are relatively fewer reports in animals.[67-77]

Intraocular masses may be located in the anterior pole, in the ciliary body, anterior to the equator, at the equator, or in the posterior pole. The location of the mass will aid in the differential diagnosis. The mass must be 1 mm or larger to be detected and elevated 2 mm or more for acoustic differentiation.[47,78] Reports in humans indicate that masses can be accurately measured to within 0.5 mm.[78] This is useful for monitoring growth or regression after therapy. Shape may also help differentiate intraocular tumors. Shape has proved useful in the diagnosis of melanomas in humans.[49,50,78] Sound attenuation is also used to differentiate tumor types. An *acoustic quiet zone* and *choroidal excavation* are characteristic of human melanomas.[78] An acoustic quiet zone represents sound attenuation within a mass lesion caused by dense cellularity. The deeper portion shows a relatively hypoechoic parenchyma compared with the more hyperechoic anterior portion of the mass. Choroidal excavation is a concave depression (excavation) of the choroid due to tumor invasion posteriorly only. Acoustic shadowing of normal orbital fat can also occur from sound attenuation distal to highly attenuating tumor masses. The energy of the attenuated sound beam is insufficient to produce echoes in the deeper retro-orbital structures. Therefore these deeper tissues are not visualized. Mineralization within a tumor mass leads to even stronger acoustic shadowing. Retinoblastoma is the tumor that most frequently shows mineralization in humans but has not been reported in small animals.[79,80]

Intraocular Neoplasms

Melanotic tumors are the most common intraocular tumors of animals and humans.[67,69-71,74,76,79-81] They include malignant uveal melanomas as well as melanomas of the eyelid, bulbar conjunctiva, and iris. Uveal melanomas usually arise from the stroma of the ciliary body. From there, they can spread to the iris, filtration angle, posterior portion of the eye, or sclera. Animals may present with uveitis and glaucoma in addition to a darkly pigmented mass originating from the posterior chamber of the eye. Direct visualization of the mass may not be possible when the tumor is small or when the ocular medium is opaque. Ultrasound is valuable in detecting and defining the extent of the mass.

Feline malignant melanomas have a higher rate of metastasis.[79] Anterior uveal melanomas are more common in dogs and cats, whereas posterior uveal (choroidal) malignant melanomas are more prevalent in humans.[79,80,82] The B-mode ultrasonographic appearance of canine anterior uveal (ciliary body) melanomas has been reported.[8,10] These tumors were hyperechoic, displaced the lens, and extended into the vitreous body. An acoustic quiet zone (internal shadowing) was not seen. Distal acoustic shadowing was identified in one case. Interestingly, anterior melanomas in humans do not show an acoustic quiet zone, whereas the more common posteriorly located melanomas do.[78] There do not appear to be any distinguishing B-mode characteristics of canine anterior uveal melanomas at this time, other than location and frequency of occurrence (Figure 5-12). Therefore differential diagnoses for tumors in the anterior uvea or ciliary body region include melanomas, ciliary body adenomas and adenocarcinomas, and metastatic lesions. Ultrasound has been used as an adjunct in the diagnosis of choroidal melanoma,[67,71] and in one cat the

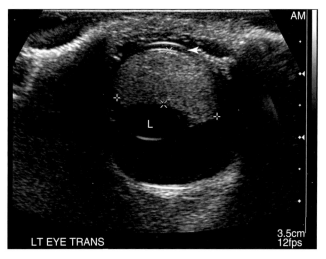

Figure 5-12 Anterior uveal melanoma. The hyperechoic, homogeneous, smoothly marginated mass (between electronic cursors) has obliterated the anterior chamber, is touching the cornea (*arrow*), and has displaced the lens (*L*) posteriorly.

mass was described as a hyperechoic cone-shaped mass bulging toward the vitreous cavity subretinally.[71] Retinal detachment was also identified. We have seen a choroidal melanoma that appeared as a well-defined spherical mass within the posterior most aspect of the posterior chamber, adjacent to the optic disc. The mass was hypoechoic and mildly heterogeneous, with an incomplete hyperechoic rim. (Figure 5-13, *A*) The ultrasound findings corresponded well with magnetic resonance imaging (MRI), where the mass appeared as a well-defined, heterogeneous, T_1 hyperintense/T_2 hypointense spherical mass within the posterior segment (Figure 5-13, *B*).

Two distinct shapes of ocular melanomas have been described in humans. The first is a dome-shaped choroidal melanoma, which is hyperechoic and homogeneous; it may demonstrate an acoustic quiet zone. The overlying retina may be separately visualized as a hyperechoic anterior border of the mass, or it may become detached. The second shape arises when the tumor ruptures Bruch membrane (the choroidal hyaline layer adjacent to the pigmented layer of the retina[83]); its anterior margin loses its dome shape, and the tumor appears mushroom-shaped and heterogeneous. This sign indicates tumor extension and a poorer prognosis. Tumor size has been shown to be the single most important prognosticator of ocular melanomas in humans, with a significantly better prognosis if the tumor is 10 mm or less.[82] Rupture of Bruch membrane was correlated with larger tumors. Choroidal excavation is reported to be present in 42% of all ocular melanomas and has not been described in melanomas originating anterior to the equator.[78] Choroidal excavation was considered to be of high diagnostic significance because it was thought to be unique to melanomas.[78] However, a later report described choroidal excavation with choroidal hemangioma, benign choroidal nevi, and adenocarcinoma.[84]

Ciliary body adenomas and adenocarcinomas are the second most common intraocular tumors in the dog and cat,[81] with adenomas more frequent than carcinomas.[78] Medulloepitheliomas have been reported in animals; some may show teratoid features, such as the presence of cartilage, brain tissue, or skeletal muscle.[79,80] Ciliary adenomas and adenocarcinomas originate from the same general region as most canine and feline melanotic neoplasms (i.e., anterior uvea). The ultrasonographic appearance of these tumors has not been reported.

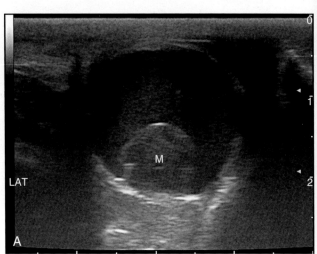
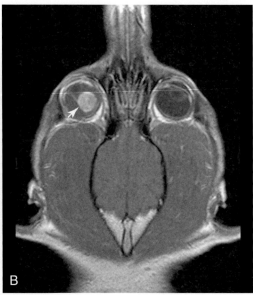

Figure 5-13 Ultrasound (**A**) and MRI (**B**) images of a posterior (caudal) melanoma in an 11-year-old dog presented for blood in the anterior chamber and an absent direct pupillary reflex. **A,** Ultrasound image shows a well marginated mass (*M*) projecting into the vitreous chamber. The vitreous chamber contains diffuse pointlike echoes, proven to be hemorrhage postenucleation. **B,** Dorsal T$_1$-weighted MRI image shows the melanoma as a hyperintense mass within the right vitreous chamber (*arrow*). This image illustrates the exquisite detail offered by MRI.

However, differentiation between adenomas or adenocarcinomas and melanomas may be theoretically possible owing to the multicystic nature of these tumors compared with solid melanomas.[85] Anechoic areas representing cysts may be identified within the tumor mass. In addition, distal acoustic enhancement may be present, which is not apparent with melanomas. Multiple, tiny cystic lesions can also yield a hyperechoic appearance, as has been shown in multicystic disease of other organs (ovaries, kidneys, liver).

The ultrasound appearances of an ocular myxosarcoma and a primary corneal hemangiosarcoma have been described.[72,77] The myxosarcoma was described as a spherical, well-defined mass on the posterior wall of the globe that had moderate homogeneity. The mass protruded from the optic disc and could be followed into the retrobulbar space.[77] The hemangiosarcoma, imaged with biomicroscopy, was described as a large, vascularized, tubular mass extending from the central cornea, and it had small superficial corneal vessels extending to the mass from the limbus.[72]

Ciliary body and iridociliary cysts have been identified in humans and animals. Ciliary body cysts were thin-walled with an anechoic center on ultrasound exam.[73,86] They may be singular or multiple, unilateral or bilateral, and pigmented or nonpigmented; they are either free floating within the aqueous humor or attached to surrounding tissues. Cysts most commonly occur in the Golden Retriever, Labrador Retriever, and Boston Terrier, but have also been described in other breeds including Great Danes.[86,87] Cysts may predispose affected animals to development of glaucoma. Small cysts may not be identified with standard B-mode ultrasound, requiring the use of high- and ultrahigh-frequency ultrasound for detection.[86] Ultrahigh-frequency ultrasound is also useful for differentiation between cysts, solid masses, and cystic masses, such as adenocarcinomas. Treatment for cysts is often conservative, and correct diagnosis is paramount for proper patient management and avoidance of unnecessary surgery or radiation therapy.

Lymphosarcoma is the most common metastatic ocular tumor in the dog and cat.[88,89] It is often bilateral and often associated with disseminated disease. The anterior uvea is frequently involved, sometimes with concurrent intraocular hemorrhage. Squamous cell carcinomas arising from the ear, conjunctiva, and corneal-scleral junction occur. Metastatic carcinomas arising from the mammary glands, thyroid, pancreas, kidney, and nasal cavity have also been described. Meningiomas, canine transmissible venereal tumors, hemangiosarcomas, rhabdomyosarcomas, neurofibrosarcomas, and metastatic melanomas are other potential metastatic neoplasms of the eye, although they are rare.[90]

The ultrasonographic appearance of metastatic ocular tumors has not been previously reported. We have seen a metastatic myosarcoma that appeared as a hyperechoic, heterogeneous, well-marginated mass lesion within the vitreous chamber, centered near the equator. The primary site of origin could not be determined, but the tumor was also found in the liver, pancreas, kidneys, lungs, and heart. Hypertrophic osteopathy of the right femur and tibia was also present. We have also seen a metastatic carcinoma that filled a large portion of the vitreous chamber. It was heterogeneous and well marginated.

Intraocular Hemorrhage and Inflammatory Masses

Infectious and inflammatory disease and hemorrhage of the vitreous chamber can present as intraocular mass lesions. Because they may also present with pointed or membranous echo patterns, they are discussed in the following section.

Endophthalmitis of bacterial or mycotic origin is probably the most common inflammatory conditions producing ultrasonographically identifiable lesions. Blastomycosis is reported to be the most common oculomycosis in the dog.[79] Generalized systemic signs, such as respiratory distress, cough, anorexia, weight loss, and persistent fever, are usually present. The condition is usually bilateral, producing a granulomatous panuveitis. Blindness is common secondary to retinal detachment.

Coccidioidomycosis, cryptococcosis, histoplasmosis, feline infectious peritonitis, and toxoplasmosis also occur and have been associated with infectious uveitis. Oculomycoses are typically choroidal in origin (versus ciliary body). Therefore intraocular fungal disease may be more posteriad than the majority of intraocular tumors. Conversely, hematogenous bacterial ocular infection is reported to more commonly begin in the ciliary body.[79]

An intraocular fungal granuloma in a dog with disseminated disease has been described as a large, irregular, echoic structure within the vitreous chamber.[8,10] We have seen similar vitreal lesions that arise from the choroid, displacing the retina anteriorly and potentially causing detachment. Concurrent retrobulbar involvement can occur (Figure 5-14).

Vitreal hemorrhage can appear as a hyperechoic mass lesion[6,49,54,91] (Figure 5-15). Clot formation can mimic mass lesions of other origin, especially early in the course of disease. Blood clots may be large and have an irregular shape; they may or may not show aftermovement. Concurrent disease may be present, such as retinal detachment. Intraocular hemorrhage is not necessarily evenly distributed. Hemorrhage can also be diffuse and fill the entire vitreous chamber. Lack of blood flow on Doppler interrogation of blood clots potentially allows differentiation from other vascular masses.

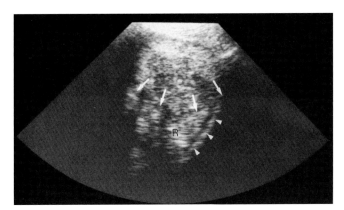

Figure 5-14 **Canine ocular blastomycosis.** This granuloma occupied the entire globe and extended into the retrobulbar tissues (R). Arrows indicate the posterior boundary of the globe; arrowheads depict the margins of the bony orbit. A mechanical transducer was used. (Courtesy Dr. James Hoskinson, Manhattan, Kan.)

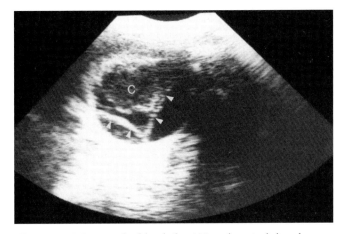

Figure 5-15 Intraocular blood clot (C) with retinal detachment (*arrowheads*). A mechanical transducer was used.

INTRAOCULAR POINTLIKE AND MEMBRANOUS LESIONS

General Considerations
B-Mode Examination
Vitreal lesions can be conveniently classified into one of three groups according to shape. *Pointlike echoes* are small focal echoes that are likely to represent cells within the vitreous body. Multiple pointlike echoes may be an indication of hemorrhage (see Figure 5-13. *A*), white blood cells, or vitreal degeneration. These pointlike echoes can organize into larger, solitary echoic *masses*. In the vitreous chamber, *membranous lesions* are linear echoes that may have a variety of shapes and patterns. Several differential diagnoses exist for membranous lesions. Careful attention to the shape, pattern, and attachment of these membranous lesions will greatly assist the ultrasonographer in making the correct diagnosis. The membrane's relationship to the optic nerve is important. If the membrane attaches to the optic disc, retinal detachment is present. If not, other differential diagnoses must be considered, as discussed in the following.

The distribution and location of vitreal lesions are also important. Vitreal lesions should be separated according to whether they are focal or diffuse and by their location within the chamber (anterior or posterior). Mobility or aftermovements of abnormal structures within the vitreous should be noted during the patient's eyeball movement, as described in humans.

Vitreous Chamber
Diseases of the vitreous chamber include hemorrhage, endophthalmitis, vitreous floaters, vitreal syneresis, asteroid hyalosis, synchysis scintillans, vitreous membrane formation, posterior vitreal detachment, and persistent hyperplastic primary vitreous. The ultrasound appearance of fungal endophthalmitis, hemorrhage, and blood clot formation has been described in animals.[4,6,8,10] A detailed description of the ultrasonographic appearance of the different forms of vitreal degeneration in dogs has also been published.[92]

Hemorrhage
There are multiple causes of vitreal hemorrhage, including trauma, neoplasia, coagulation abnormalities, blood dyscrasias, hypertension, vitreoretinal disease, neovascularization, persistent hyaloid artery, diabetes mellitus, and chronic glaucoma.[90] The role of ultrasonography is to assess the globe for a cause of the hemorrhage and to establish important prognosticators, such as retinal detachment or lens dislocation.

Smaller clots or red blood cells appear as pointlike echoes within the vitreous chamber[4,54,91,93] (Figure 5-16; see also Figure 5-13, *A*). Early vitreal hemorrhage identified on direct examination may not be seen on B-mode scans immediately. Several days may be required until clot formation occurs. In humans, vitreal hemorrhage is seen as diffuse pointlike multiple echoes, not necessarily distributed evenly. Penetrating foreign bodies may leave a linear path of hemorrhage. High mobility of pointlike echoes is a characteristic of vitreal hemorrhage.

Small amounts of hemorrhage will often resolve without treatment after several weeks, although opacities (vitreous floaters) may persist for long periods.[47,90] Fibrous strands called vitreous membranes sometimes develop secondary to clot formation[49,54,91,93] (Figure 5-17; also see Figure 5-16, *B*). They may be innocuous or cause a tractional retinal detachment as they contract. These membranes are often near the optic disc[47] and must be differentiated from retinal detachment. Differentiation between the image of a vitreous membrane and a detached retina can be difficult. The echo produced

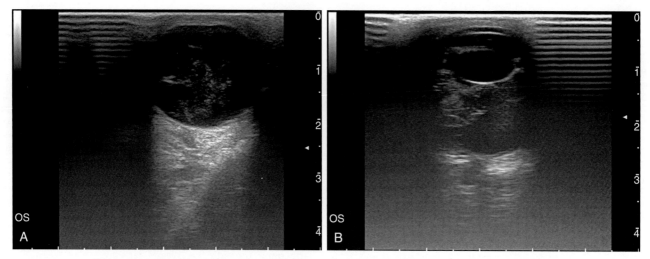

Figure 5-16 **Vitreal hemorrhage. A,** Multiple, pointlike echogenic foci are seen unevenly distributed in the vitreous chamber of this dog who sustained head trauma. **B,** Pointlike hemorrhage and thick, membranous vitreal echoes in a dog with long-standing vitreal hemorrhage.

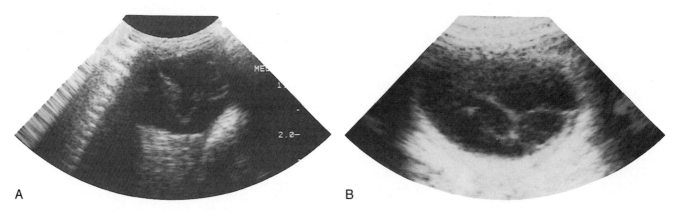

Figure 5-17 **Two examples of vitreal membrane formation secondary to intraocular hemorrhage. A,** The V-shaped appearance of the vitreal membranes could be mistaken for a detached retina. **B,** A more bizarre configuration of vitreal membranes. A mechanical transducer was used.

by the vitreal membranes is of a lower intensity than that of the retina.[49,93] By decreasing the gain, the vitreal membrane echo will disappear sooner than the echo of retinal detachment. Careful evaluation of the relationship of the membranous echoes to the optic disc is also important. Attachments at or near the optic disc are more indicative of a detached retina. Recently, the use of contrast enhanced ultrasound as an aid to differentiate retinal detachment from vitreal membranes has been described. Persistent vascularization of the retina was demonstrated with contrast enhanced ultrasound in all cases of retinal detachment and was 100% accurate in differentiating between retinal detachment and vitreal membranes.[35] Vitreous membranes and retinal detachment may also be present concurrently.

Endophthalmitis
Inflammatory cells in the vitreous may appear identical to diffuse vitreal hemorrhage, with small pointlike lesions demonstrating aftermovement. These infiltrates organize more rapidly than hemorrhage and may produce vitreal membranes. Contraction of these membranes may lead to retinal detachment as described in a Münsterländer dog with endophthalmitis induced by *Candida albicans*,[94] and a cat with panuveitis induced by *Toxoplasma gondii*.[95]

Vitreal Degeneration
Vitreal degeneration encompasses a spectrum of degenerative changes referred to as vitreal syneresis, vitreal floaters, asteroid hyalosis, and synchysis scintillans. Vitreal syneresis a liquefactive degeneration of the vitreous that is seen with aging as a result of depolymerization of hyaluronic acid within the vitreous. Condensation of collagen within the vitreous can also occur with aging and leads to development of vitreal floaters. The ultrasonographic of syneresis and vitreal floaters in dogs is that of poorly reflective, pointlike echoes lying mainly within the ventral aspect of the vitreal chamber in the still eye. The echoes are generally sparse and motile with eye movement. Asteroid hyalosis is a degenerative condition of middle-aged and older dogs in which small foci of calcium-lipid complex (0.03 to 0.1 mm) become diffusely suspended within the vitreous body (Figure 5-18).[78] Asteroid hyalosis has been associated with chronic inflammatory and degenerative ocular disorders but can also be observed spontaneously in older humans and animals. This may be a unilateral or bilateral condition. In humans, these pointlike lesions are seen as multiple, hyperechoic structures and can be extensive, filling the vitreous chamber.[54] They are separated from the retina by a thin anechoic zone and show marked aftermovement. Acoustic shadowing is not a feature of asteroid hyalosis. In dogs, the

ultrasonographic appearance of asteroid hyalosis is that of multiple highly reflective echoes evenly distributed throughout the vitreous that return to their original location after eye movement (see Figure 5-18).[92] Asteroid hyalosis may be associated with posterior vitreal detachment. Ultrasound may be more sensitive than ophthalmoscopic exam for the detection of vitreal degeneration.[92] Synchysis scintillans is the most severe form of vitreal degeneration and results from accumulation of multiple cholesterol crystals within a liquefied vitreous.[92] It is rare in humans and animals, and to the authors' knowledge, the ultrasonographic appearance in animals has not been described.

Posterior Vitreal Detachment

Posterior vitreal detachment appears as a linear or curvilinear convex echo in the posterior portion of the vitreous chamber.[54,96] At first glance, it may appear as a detached retina. It

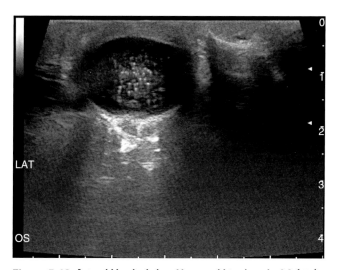

Figure 5-18 Asteroid hyalosis in n 11-year-old terrier mix. Multiple, tiny echogenic foci are present within the vitreous chamber. The image was made in a transverse plane caudal to the lens.

can be differentiated by the fact that the curvilinear echo is attached only anteriorly, not to the optic disc Hemorrhage into the potential space between the vitreous body and the retina can occur.[54,96] Small pointlike echoes may be seen within this region representing red blood cells. Distinct aftermovements will be noted.

Persistent Hyperplastic Primary Vitreous

Persistent hyperplastic primary vitreous is a congenital condition characterized by retrolenticular fibrovascular tissue formation and potential retention of the hyaloid vasculature.[90] The ultrasonographic appearance of persistent hyperplastic primary vitreous in the dog and cat has been described in several publications.[97-102] On B-mode ultrasound evaluation, a funnel-shaped retrolenticular mass is seen with a thin echogenic stalk (persistent hyaloid vasculature) emerging from the lens, coursing along the optic axis to the optic disc (Figure 5-19). Blood flow within the stalk and posterior aspect of the lens may be visible on color or power Doppler interrogation (see Figure 5-19, B). Axial length (D4) is shorter compared with the normal contralateral eye in humans.[54] Cataract formation is often present in the lens of affected eyes.

Retina

Retinal detachment is easily imaged by ultrasound and has been frequently described.[2,4,5,8,10,53]

Detachment of the retina may be partial or complete and result from congenital conditions, trauma, mass lesions, or a multitude of additional disease processes. Intraocular hemorrhage and inflammation can lead to fibrous membrane formation, which contracts and pulls on the retina, detaching it anteriorly. The retina is loosely attached to the choroid, primarily held in place by pressure of the vitreous body. Therefore a perforating injury to the globe may lead to retinal detachment.

Retinal detachment appears as a membranous, linear type of echo on a B-mode scan. Total detachment results in attachment only at the optic disc and the ora serrata, just caudal to the ciliary apparatus. A V or Y shape may be seen on ultrasound evaluation, with the arms representing ora serrata attachment and the base attachment at the optic disc

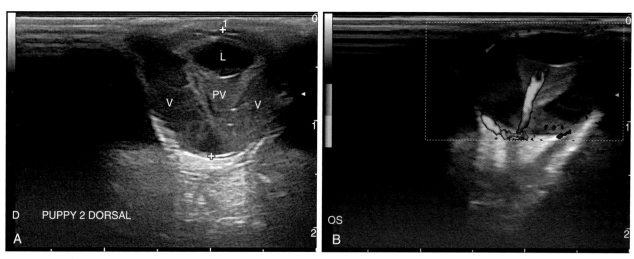

Figure 5-19 Persistent hyperplastic primary vitreous in a 3-week-old puppy. A, An irregular, echogenic funnel-shaped structure (*PV*) is seen posterior to the lens, extending to the posterior ocular wall. There are abnormal echoes within the vitreous chamber (*v*). The lens (*L*) is seen as an anechoic structure in the near field. The electronic cursors are measuring the length of the eye (1.18 cm). **B,** Power Doppler examination shows the persistent hyaloid blood vessel. Note the very vascular nature of the retina.

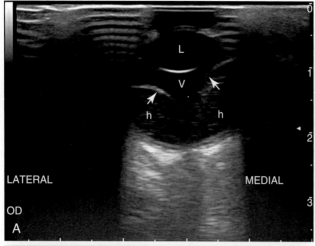

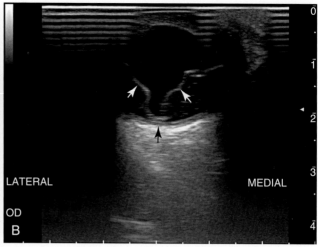

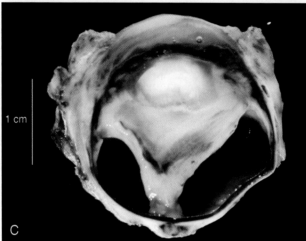

Figure 5-20 **Total retinal detachment. A,** The V-shaped echo in the vitreous chamber is the detached retina (*arrows*). The lens (*L*) is seen in the near field, and the anechoic vitreous is seen just posterior to it. There is subretinal hemorrhage, seen as faint pointlike echoes (*h*). **B,** This example shows a more wavy appearance to the detached retina (*white arrows*). Its attachment to the optic disc is seen (*black arrow*). The anterior-most attachment to the ora serrata is incompletely seen on these images because of edge artifacts created by poor peripheral transducer contact. **C,** Gross specimen of a detached retina, showing the V-shaped, funnel appearance with attachments at the optic disc and peripherally along the ora serrata. (C, courtesy of Washington State University College of Veterinary Medicine, Washington Animal Disease Diagnostic Laboratory, Pullman, WA.)

(Figure 5-20). There may be pointlike echoes in the vitreous chamber representing hemorrhage or exudate, additional membranous echoes depicting vitreal membrane formation, or a mass lesion responsible for the detachment. Careful evaluation is required to make the proper diagnosis because attachment to the optic disc must be demonstrated to differentiate detached retina from posterior vitreal detachment and other vitreal membranous lesions (Figure 5-21; also see Figure 5-20, *B*).

Partial retinal detachment is recognized ultrasonographically as a convex echogenic structure separated from the posterior ocular wall by a zone of sonolucency (Figure 5-22). This retinal elevation may or may not be associated with the optic disc. Differential diagnoses include posterior vitreal detachment and local choroid detachment. Some mobility of the retina is to be expected from either total or partial retinal detachments. Contrast-enhanced ultrasound can be used to aid in the differentiation of partial retinal detachment and vitreal membranes.[35]

Tractional retinal detachment shows a tentlike elevation of the retina that may involve the entire retina or only small portions of it. As mentioned, vitreal membrane formation is responsible for this type of retinal detachment (Figure 5-23).

FOREIGN BODIES

Radiography and ultrasonography are commonly used to search for ocular foreign bodies. Radiography can be used to detect metallic foreign bodies and to assess the bony orbit and

Figure 5-21 Total retinal detachment in a dog with clinical intraocular hemorrhage of several weeks duration. The retina is very thick (*arrows*). Its attachment at the optic disc is shown (*) and the optic nerve (*ON*) is clearly visualized. L, lens.

skull for fractures. Metallic or nonmetallic foreign bodies within or around the eye can be imaged with ultrasound. These include gunshot pellets, metallic fragments, BBs, wood splinters, glass, bone, tooth fragments, and perhaps plant material.

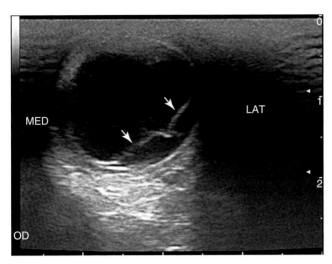

Figure 5-22 Partial retinal detachment in a dog (*arrows*).

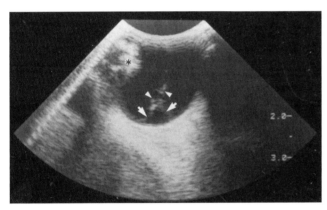

Figure 5-23 Tractional retinal detachment (*arrows*) caused by vitreal membrane formation (*arrowheads*). Intraocular hemorrhage secondary to an anterior uveal neoplasm (*asterisk*) was the inciting cause. A mechanical transducer was used.

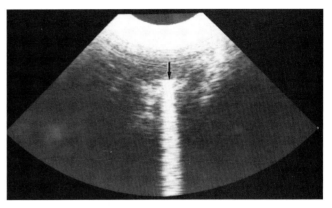

Figure 5-24 **Intraocular metallic foreign body (pellet) (*arrow*).** The eye is unrecognizable because of severe trauma. The comet-tail reverberation artifact is characteristic of metallic foreign bodies. A mechanical transducer was used. (Courtesy Dr. James Hoskinson.)

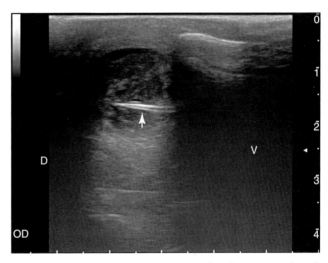

Figure 5-25 **Intraocular porcupine quill.** This dog presented with a mature cataract and a history of a porcupine encounter. Prephacoemulsification ultrasound revealed the presence of an intraocular foreign body, a porcupine quill (*arrow*). The vitreous chamber contains echogenic material consistent with hemorrhage and inflammatory cells.

Metallic foreign bodies, such as a BB, appear as a bright echogenic focus that has a characteristic comet-tail reverberation artifact on B-mode ultrasound evaluation (Figure 5-24). Small metallic or wooden foreign bodies also appear as a bright focal echo. Porcupine quills (Figure 5-25) and wooden foreign bodies may appear as double, linear echogenic bands with distal shadowing.[103] Hypoechoic or echogenic fluid as a result of cellulitis may surround foreign material in the retrobulbar tissues.[104]

Small metallic foreign bodies may not shadow. Small foreign bodies that are in contact with the retina or lie adjacent to any ocular structure may be difficult to differentiate from the surrounding tissue.[105] A metallic foreign body will produce a bright echo regardless of the incident angle of the beam, unlike the bright retinal echo that is produced only when the ultrasound beam is perpendicular to it. Metallic foreign bodies may also be imaged at reduced power or gain settings.

The magnetic versus nonmagnetic qualities of a metallic foreign body can be assessed by applying a pulsed magnetic force while viewing the foreign body ultrasonographically.[91] Displacement confirms a ferromagnetic foreign body.[106] Magnetic extraction of the metallic fragment is occasionally possible. Magnetic fields cannot be applied to BBs because they tend to move away from the applied field, causing further trauma.[107]

The ocular wall may be disrupted in the case of a penetrating missile foreign body, resulting in a ruptured globe. Scleral rupture may be detected on B-mode ultrasound; the most common findings are ill-defined scleral margins and echogenic debris within the anterior and vitreal chambers.[108] Vitreal or uveal herniation commonly occurs through the defect. Vitreal hemorrhage or a detached retina may also be detected. This type of injury can lead to phthisis bulbi, an end-stage eye that is small and distorted and has a diminished axial length. The chorioretinal layers become thickened. Hyperechoic material in the vitreous chamber is representative of old inflammation or infection, fibrosis, or mineralization.

Ultrasound guidance may be used to aid in extraction of retrobulbar foreign bodies.[109]

CORNEA AND IRIS

As noted, the cornea and iris can be difficult to study using conventional ultrasound. Figure 5-26 shows an example of

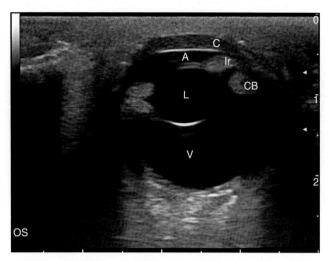

Figure 5-26 Ciliary body edema. Corneal (C), iris (*Ir*) and ciliary body (*CB*) edema. *L*, Lens; *V*, vitreous.

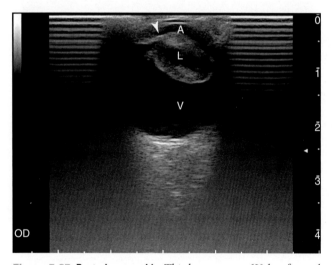

Figure 5-27 Posterior synechia. This lens cataract (*L*) has formed an adhesion (*arrowhead*) between the iris and the anterior lens capsule. *A*, Anterior chamber; *V*, vitreous chamber.

corneal, iris, and ciliary body edema. Figure 5-27 illustrates a small corneal nodule with corneal edema. Posterior synechia is shown in Figure 5-28.

LENS

Normal and pathologic conditions affecting the lens have been studied with ultrasonography in veterinary medicine[2,4,7-10,52,53,57,110-114] (see Figures 5-7 through 5-9). The lens is approximately 7 mm in the anteroposterior dimension (D2) and 10 mm in the transverse or dorsoventral dimension by direct mensuration. The use of ultrasound to measure the axial length has been described in multiple reports.[2,7,52,53,57,114,115] Lens thickness has been shown to increase with age in dogs.[114] Significant differences have been found between A-mode and B-mode measurements versus direct measurements.[53,57] This has been explained by ultrasonographic variables and technique and by differences in the method of obtaining direct measurements.

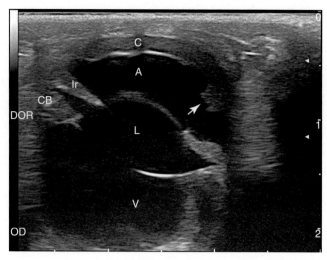

Figure 5-28 Corneal edema in the right eye of a cat of unknown etiology. The cornea (C) is thick and echogenic. A small nodule (*arrow*) is seen protruding into the anterior chamber (*A*). *Ir*, iris; *CB*, ciliary body; *L*, lens; *V*, vitreous chamber. Dorsal is to the left.

Dislocation

Dislocation of the lens may occur secondary to trauma, space-occupying masses, glaucoma, or hereditary predisposition. It is defined as any abnormal location of the lens, with subluxation and complete luxation as subcategories. Subluxation of the lens occurs when the lens tilts away from its normal position. Complete luxation occurs when the peripheral ligamentous attachments of the lens (zonules) are completely ruptured. Figure 5-29 illustrates posterior and anterior lens luxations.

In humans and animals, a lens dislocation posteriorly into the vitreous chamber is seen as a spherical mass that is freely movable on a B-mode scan. We have also observed anterior displacement of the lens with concurrent lens degeneration, which made the lens echoic and easy to image.

Sometimes the lens will not be imaged. Its absence is a sign of abnormal position or perhaps nonexistence (aphakia). Aphakia is a rare condition in humans and animals that is often associated with ocular disorders such as microphthalmia, retinal dysplasia, optic nerve hypoplasia, and dysplastic globe.

Cataracts

Cataracts can be caused by trauma, hereditary predisposition, systemic diseases (e.g., diabetes mellitus), toxins, inflammation, intraocular tumors, and radiation exposure.[6,116] A cataract may develop secondary to reduced nutrition in a luxated lens. A cataract produces abnormal echoes in the normally anechoic lens on B-mode ultrasound evaluation[10,54,55] (Figure 5-30). The anterior and posterior cortices, the nucleus, or all of these become echogenic[111] and may progress to include the entire lens. Ultrasound can differentiate immature, mature, and hypermature cataracts.[110] Immature cataracts show a trend toward reduced thickness, whereas mature cataracts show a trend toward increased thickness on B-mode ultrasound.[114] The lenses of dogs with diabetic cataracts are significantly increased in axial thickness on B-mode ultrasound compared to normal and nondiabetic cataractous lenses (Figure 5-31).[113,114] Diabetic cataractous lenses are predisposed to spontaneous lens rupture as a result of rapid lens intumescence (swelling).[113] Figures 5-32 and 5-33 are examples of lens ruptures. Concurrent retinal detachment is more common

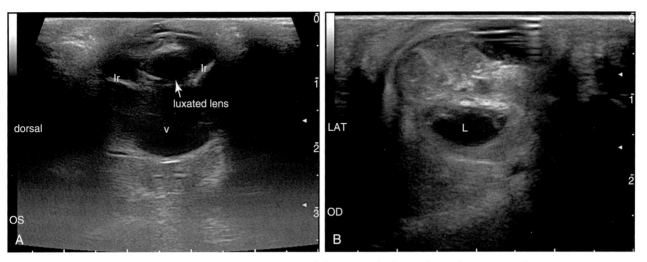

Figure 5-29 Luxation of the lens. A, Anterior dislocation. The lens is located anterior to the iris (*Ir*), within the anterior chamber. *V,* Vitreous chamber. **B,** Posterior lens dislocation (*L*) in a traumatized eye. The eye is nearly unrecognizable; the entire vitreous contains possibly solid echogenic material presumed to be hemorrhage and inflammation.

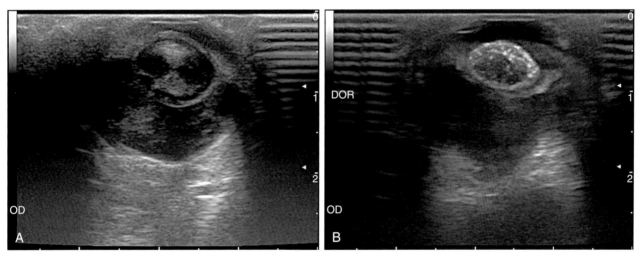

Figure 5-30 Cataracts. A, Abnormal echogenic central portion of the lens is seen. The lens appears swollen. There is vitreal debris present, seen as echogenic substance within the vitreous chamber. **B,** Hypermature cataract, characterized by extremely echogenic lens parenchyma. Dorsal is to the left. *OD,* Right eye.

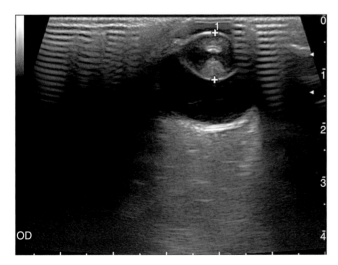

Figure 5-31 Diabetic cataract in the right eye of an 8-year-old female Samoyed. The lens (between electronic cursors, 0.87 cm) is abnormally echogenic and slightly thicker than normal. The left eye was identical.

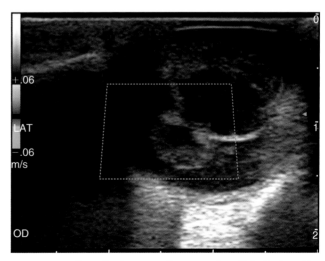

Figure 5-32 Posterior lens capsule rupture in a diabetic dog. The shape of the cataract that has extruded into the vitreous chamber can be recognized in this case. Color Doppler was used to verify a lack of blood flow.

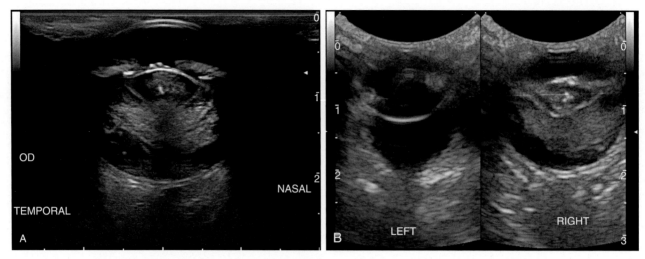

Figure 5-33 **Unilateral posterior lens capsule rupture. A,** High resolution image of the right eye made using an 18-MHz linear-array transducer. The cataract is seen very clearly as abnormal echogenicity in the lens. The defect in the central portion of the posterior lens capsule can be seen, extruding lens parenchyma into the vitreous chamber. **B,** Comparison of right and left eyes. The mature cataract is present within the right lens with posterior rupture into the vitreous chamber. The left eye is normal by comparison. These images are made with a microconvex transducer.

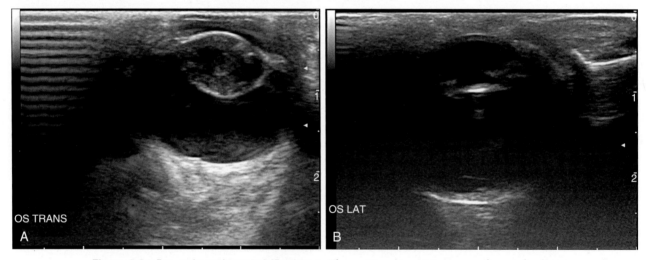

Figure 5-34 **Pre- and postphacoemulsification. A,** The mature cataract is seen as abnormal echogenic lens parenchyma. **B,** Postphacoemulsification, the echogenic lens material has been removed.

with hypermature cataracts and uncommon in eyes with immature cataracts.[110] Nuclear sclerosis does not appear to cause sonographically detectable lesions.[111] Figure 5-34 shows a cataract lens before and after phacoemulsification.

GLAUCOMA

Standard B-mode ultrasonography is useful to measure axial length or to establish the cause of glaucoma or an associated abnormality, such as a luxated lens. Optic disc cupping may also be detected, but it must be differentiated from recession of the optic disc, which can occur normally in some patients.

In human medicine, ultrasound biomicroscopy has become an established and valuable tool for imaging patients with glaucoma and as a research tool for investigating the pathophysiology of the disease.[23,25] Ultrasound biomicroscopy

allows for visualization of the corneal epithelium, corneal endothelium, limbus, iris, ciliary process, and anterior lens capsule (Figure 5-35). Both qualitative and quantitative assessment of the iridocorneal angle and its structures is possible. Standards for quantitative assessment of the anterior chamber and drainage angle structures have been proposed in literature on ultrasonography in humans.[117] Poor interobserver repeatability of measurements have been reported in numerous studies, and software that allows for semiquantitative analysis of the iridocorneal angle structures has been developed, improving both intraobserver and interobserver repeatability of measures.[25] Identification of the scleral spur, a structure not present in the dog or cat eye, is necessary for semiquantitative measurement.

Results of a number of studies investigating the use of ultrasound biomicroscopy for the study of the anterior segment and drainage angle in dogs and cats have been recently reported.[26-34] Since a scleral spur is not present in the dog or

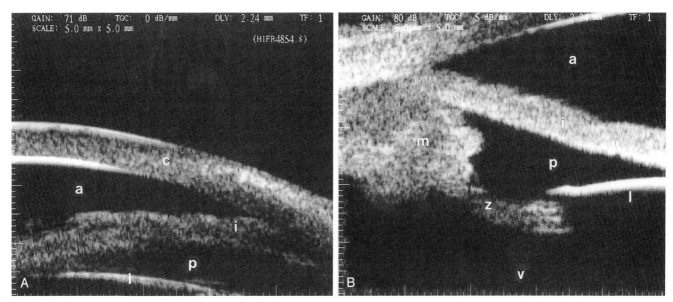

Figure 5-35 **Ocular ultrasound biomicroscopy. A,** Normal eye with use of a 20-MHz ultrasound biomicroscopy unit. **B,** A 20-MHz ocular ultrasound image of the iridocorneal angle in a patient with ciliary body melanoma (*m*). *a,* Anterior chamber; *c,* cornea; *i,* iris; *I,* anterior lens capsule; *p,* posterior chamber; *v,* vitreous chamber; *z,* lens zonules. Large divisions = 1 mm, small divisions = 0.1 mm. (Courtesy Dr. Fred Davidorf and Cynthia Taylor, Columbus, Ohio.)

cat, the use of other landmarks as a basis for quantitative analysis is necessary in dogs and cats. Landmarks used for measurements have varied between species and between studies, and at this time, established and agreed upon guidelines for quantitative measurement of the feline and canine anterior chamber are lacking. Additionally, measurements of certain anterior segment structures may vary between breeds, and recently a regression model to account for breed differences of several measures has been proposed.[31] Intraobserver and interobserver repeatability of measures have been variable across studies but are considered reliable when discrete and easy to recognize landmarks are used.[27] As in human medicine, interobserver variability is greater than intraobserver variability.

Anterior chamber morphology as imaged with biomicroscopy is significantly different between normal cats and those with primary congenital glaucoma.[30] Cats with glaucoma have a significantly smaller angle recess area, diminished ciliary cleft and decreased iris-lens contact. Differences within the anterior segment between female and male dogs have been reported, with females having a significantly smaller angle opening distance.[33] Angle opening distance describes the iridocorneal angle depth, and in that study it was defined as the distance between the end of Descemet membrane and the iris. This finding may partially explain the 2:1 female/male predisposition to primary angle closure glaucoma.[33] Administration of 0.5% tropicamide can alter morphology of the anterior chamber in both cats and dogs.[30,34] Ultrasound biomicroscopy has also been used to investigate the association between anterior segment morphology and risk of postoperative intraocular hypertension in eyes undergoing phacoemulsification.[28]

Although researchers in veterinary medicine are recognizing the benefits of using ultrasound biomicroscopy as a research tool, the clinical practicality and utility of ultrasound biomicroscopy remains to be seen.

Doppler imaging of the orbital and ocular vasculature (see section on Doppler later in this chapter) may also provide insight into the pathophysiology of glaucoma.

RETROBULBAR PATHOLOGY

Ultrasonographic evaluation of the retrobulbar structures is particularly rewarding because they are never seen by direct visualization. Reports of B-mode application in veterinary medicine are available, describing the more common causes of retrobulbar diseases, inflammatory lesions, lymphoma, and hemorrhage.[4,6,9,51,118-124] A-mode and B-mode ultrasound examinations are used extensively in humans to evaluate the retrobulbar tissues. Survey radiography should be used with ultrasonography to assess bone involvement or the presence of a metallic foreign body. Exophthalmos, enophthalmos, a draining periorbital wound, or other clinical signs indicate abnormalities in this area.

General Considerations
B-Mode Examination
Retrobulbar abnormalities may be localized to one of three areas: within the muscle cone (extraocular muscles), which contains the optic nerve and retrobulbar fat; the muscle cone itself; and outside the muscle cone. Lesions within the muscle cone include optic nerve tumors, such as meningiomas and gliomas, and optic neuritis. Cavernous hemangiomas and lymphomas are reported to occur between the optic nerve and the muscle cone in humans.[54,125,126] Thyroid-induced myositis (Graves disease) or eosinophilic myositis may affect one or all of the extraocular muscles.[54,127] Outside the muscle cone, lymphoma, abscesses, foreign bodies, zygomatic or lacrimal gland lesions, or pathologic processes extending from the surrounding bony orbit may be present.

Retrobulbar Masses
Retrobulbar cellular infiltrates and abscesses may occur by extension of tooth root infections or oral inflammatory processes; by extension of disease from the nasal cavity, the sinuses, or the zygomatic salivary gland (Figure 5-36); after penetrating wounds or foreign bodies; or through hematogenous spread of infection or neoplasia. Internal involvement of the eye is rare, as is extension of endophthalmitis into the

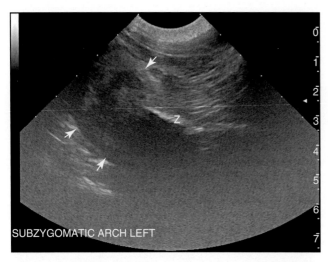

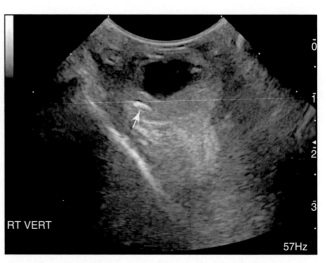

Figure 5-36 Zygomatic salivary gland abscess in a dog with swelling around the left eye. A heterogenous structure was identified in the retrobulbar tissues (*arrows*), an abscessed zygomatic salivary gland. Z, Zygomatic arch.

Figure 5-37 Retrobulbar grass awn (foxtail) cellulitis. A focal hyperechoic structure was identified in the retrobulbar tissues (*arrow*), a grass awn. The periorbital soft tissues are very thickened and the globe is distorted.

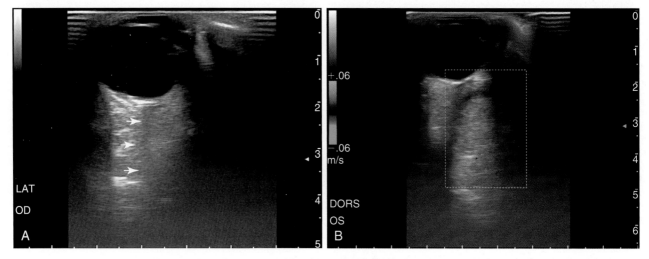

Figure 5-38 Retrobulbar cellulitis. A, A relatively hypoechoic, homogeneous area (*arrows*) distorts the normal adjacent retrobulbar tissues. **B,** Color Doppler image shows no blood flow. In this image plane, the infected tissue has a more defined margin.

retrobulbar space, because the sclera is an excellent barrier. Posterior segment penetration by grass awn foreign bodies have been described in both the dog[128] and cat (Figure 5-37).[104] Most inflammatory lesions are fungal or bacterial in origin, but aberrant migration of *Dirofilaria immitis, Ancylostoma caninum,* and the fly larvae of Diptera has been reported.[79] Cellulitis secondary to retrobulbar infection by *Toxocara canis* in a dog has also been reported.[124]

Retrobulbar cellulitis can be recognized on B-mode evaluation by distortion or obliteration of the normal retrobulbar architecture (Figure 5-38).[118] The hypoechoic appearance of the optic nerve may be lost, with disruption of the retrobulbar fat and disruption or nonvisualization of the extraocular muscles. Diffuse thickening of the retrobulbar tissues with abnormal mixed echogenicity may be present. Cellular infiltrates may cause blunting or indentation of the posterior aspect of the globe (Figure 5-39). It is helpful to compare the affected retrobulbar tissues with those of the contralateral normal eye. The distance between the optic disc echo and the

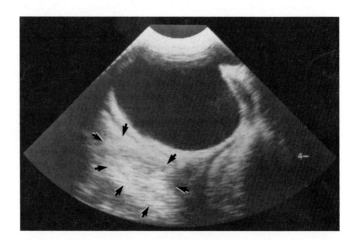

Figure 5-39 Retrobulbar bacterial cellulitis (*arrows*). The cellular infiltrate has distorted the globe and obliterated the adjacent extraocular muscles. A mechanical transducer was used.

posterior bony orbit can help define increased thickness of the retrobulbar tissues.

The ultrasonographic appearance of retrobulbar abscesses has also been reported in animals (Figure 5-40).[6,118] Abscesses are characterized by a well-defined echogenic wall and a hypoechoic to anechoic central area, although this may vary (Figure 5-41). Variations of wall thickness can occur, with smooth or ragged internal margins. An anechoic center indicates homogeneous contents, and distal acoustic enhancement is variable. A well-defined wall may be absent with small abscesses, and the appearance may be that of an anechoic or hypoechoic region. Foreign material may be identified within the hypoechoic regions of abscessation and cellulitis (Figure 5-42; also see Figure 5-37).

A retrobulbar hematoma has been reported in the horse.[119] It appeared as an anechoic, well-circumscribed structure that was not attached to the globe. A hyperechoic structure with acoustic enhancement within the hematoma was thought to be a foreign body or calcification.

Primary tumors of the orbit originate from epithelial and mesenchymal tissues of the globe and orbit. Secondary involvement can occur by extension from the nasal cavity, sinuses, and skull as well as from metastasis from distant sites. Lymphosarcoma, hemangiosarcoma, nasal adenocarcinoma, squamous cell carcinoma (Figure 5-43), osteosarcoma, chondrosarcoma, rhabdomyosarcoma, neurofibrosarcoma, meningiomas, myxosarcoma, anaplastic astrocytoma and lacrimal and zygomatic gland tumors are known to occur. Lymphosarcoma is the most common histologic type of retrobulbar tumor. Concurrent intraocular lymphosarcoma can be present. Bilateral disease is common in both dog and cat. Reports of the B-mode ultrasonographic appearance of lymphosarcoma,

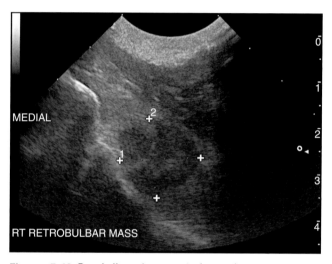

Figure 5-40 **Retrobulbar abscess.** A hypoechoic structure is identified in the retrobulbar space (between electronic cursors, 1.78 × 1.72 cm). This was an abscess, aspirated via ultrasound guidance. Note the globe is not in this image plane.

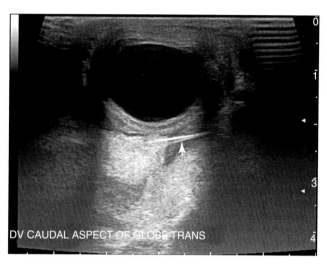

Figure 5-42 **Retrobulbar porcupine quill.** A linear hyperechoic structure (*arrow*) is identified in the retrobulbar tissues, a porcupine quill. Note the highly hyperechoic appearance of the inflamed periorbital and retrobulbar tissues.

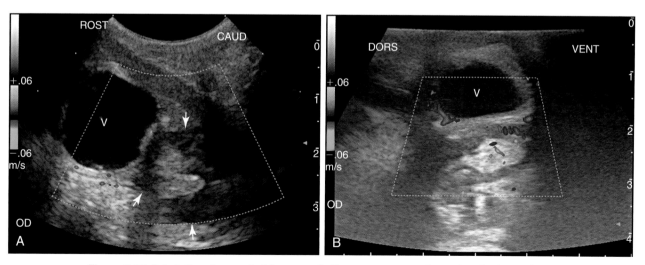

Figure 5-41 **Retrobulbar abscess. A,** A large retrobulbar mass is present (*arrows*) with a hypoechoic, thick, irregular wall and more echogenic center. The mass indents the globe. Color Doppler shows no blood flow within the mass. **B,** A different scan plane of the abscess shows very abnormal architecture of the retrobulbar tissues with distortion of the shape of the globe. Color Doppler shows periorbital blood flow. *Norcardia* was cultured from aspirates obtained under ultrasound guidance. *V,* Vitreous chamber.

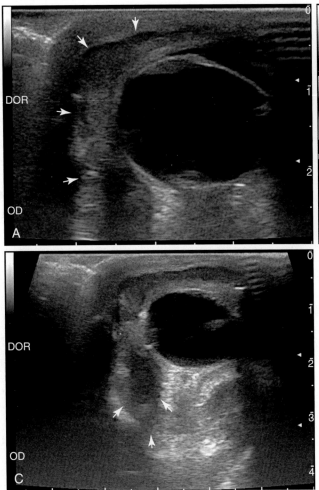

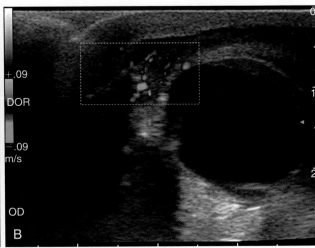

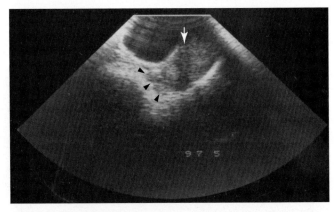

Figure 5-43 Periorbital squamous cell carcinoma in a 12-year-old cat presented for swelling around the right eye. **A,** Close-up view shows soft tissue thickening around the eye (*arrows*). **B,** Color Doppler shows good blood flow to the area. **C,** Deeper field of view shows the soft tissue thickening extends to the retrobulbar space (*arrows*). The histologic diagnosis was squamous cell carcinoma.

chondrosarcoma, osteosarcoma, myxosarcoma, anaplastic astrocytoma and orbital fibrosarcoma in animals are available.[4,118,120,122,129]

Retrobulbar lymphosarcoma has been described as an anechoic, well-defined mass with poor sound transmission that absorbed much of the energy of the sound beam.[4] Irregular borders were noted anteriorly, but no posterior border was present. A focal, hyperechoic retrobulbar lymphoma has been reported in a cat.[118] The same investigator described a lymphoblastic lymphoma in a dog that was initially a diffuse, hyperechoic lesion with irregular margins obliterating the optic nerve; the lesion progressed during a 2-week period to a focal, hypoechoic mass that deformed the posterior aspect of the globe. We have identified retrobulbar lymphosarcomas that appeared as hypoechoic, homogeneous, well-delineated masses. Some lesions had discrete, rounded borders; others had a more irregular outline and shape. These tumors can become large and indent the posterior wall of the globe (Figure 5-44).

The first large ultrasonographic series of retrobulbar lymphomas in humans was reported in 1972.[126] Lymphomas had several characteristic features that included an irregular shape with a lobulated or scalloped tumor margin and good demarcation from the surrounding tissues. Specifically, none of the tumors had a rounded, encapsulated appearance, but they all had a homogeneous, anechoic parenchyma with high acoustic absorption. Sound energy did not penetrate the tumor mass well, with subsequent failure to outline the posterior margin of the tumor. This sound attenuation is due to the solid nature

Figure 5-44 Retrobulbar lymphoma. The hypoechoic mass has a uniform texture, has lobulated borders (*arrowheads*), and indents the globe (*arrow*). A mechanical transducer was used.

of this type of tumor. The anechoic parenchymal pattern is due to the uniform cell populations of lymphomas, which do not possess the acoustic discontinuities needed to cause internal echo formation. Lymphomas occur anywhere within the retrobulbar tissues, can become large, and may indent the posterior wall of the globe.

Osteogenic tumors and chondrosarcoma of the skull can invade the orbital region. These appear as strongly echogenic masses with distal acoustic shadowing that arise from the nasal or dorsal aspect of the orbit.[118] Radiography, CT, or MRI of the skull provide essential diagnostic information regarding these tumors.

The B-mode ultrasonographic appearance of a feline retrobulbar fibrosarcoma has been reported.[129] The tumor was characterized by a hypoechoic to anechoic appearance of the retrobulbar tissues. Normal anatomy was absent, most notably the retrobulbar fat. The posterior wall of the globe was not indented, nor was there any intraocular involvement noted on ultrasound evaluation. This report was unusual in that the cat was presented for enophthalmos. Enophthalmos is a common finding in human patients with metastatic orbital carcinomas originating from the breast and abdomen.[130,131] Enophthalmos is caused by destruction of the retrobulbar fat and by contraction of fibrous tissue.

Zygomatic salivary gland tumors or inflammatory processes may be suggested by the presence of a mass in the ventral aspect of the orbit (see Figure 5-36). Chronic zygomatic salivary gland adenitis has been described secondary to a foreign body; it consisted of an irregular hyperechoic mass that focally indented the posterior ocular wall.[118] The animal was presented for exophthalmos, masseter muscle swelling, and pain on opening its mouth. Survey radiography and sialography may provide additional useful information.

Dogs with myxosarcoma all had pockets of anechoic fluid identified in the retrobulbar space identified on B-mode ultrasound. Pockets varied in size from approximately 1 to 2.5 cm and were single or multiple. A hyperechoic margin to the fluid was present in some dogs. In one case, an irregular hyperechogenic mass lesion was identified within the hypoechoic pocket.[120]

The B-mode ultrasound appearance of an anaplastic astrocytoma in a dog was that of a fusiform, highly echogenic mass measuring approximately 3 cm within the caudoventral region of the orbit. The mass compressed the globe within the region of the optic nerve.[122]

Lacrimal gland tumors or inflammatory processes may be suggested by the finding of a mass in the dorsolateral aspect of the orbit on clinical examination. Primary tumors of the lacrimal gland are reported to be rare in small animals; invasion of the gland by tumors from the surrounding tissues is more common.[132,133] The B-mode and A-mode characteristics of lacrimal gland mixed tumors in humans have been described.[54] Inflammatory or lymphomatous infiltrates are characterized on B-mode evaluation by an enlargement of the lacrimal gland, which is anechoic with well-defined or poorly marginated borders. An epinephrine dacryolith has been reported in an elderly woman being treated for glaucoma with pilocarpine and epinephrine.[134] A hyperechoic, irregular mass was present within a dilated nasolacrimal sac. A-mode and B-mode ultrasonographic appearances of the normal lacrimal system and of a nasolacrimal duct obstruction have also been reported.[58]

The B-mode ultrasound appearance of an orbital lipoma in a dog has been described. The lipoma was well defined and hypoechogenic relative to the surrounding tissues. The lipoma extended from the posterior limit of the orbit to the conjunctival fornix, which was grossly displaced anteriorly.[123]

In a case series describing the ultrasonographic appearance of the retrobulbar space in 50 dogs with confirmed retrobulbar disease, ultrasonographic abnormalities within the retrobulbar space were identified in 43 dogs.[135] Most lesions were unilateral. Neoplasia was identified in 42% of dogs and 30% were diagnosed with retrobulbar abscesses. Roughly half of the neoplastic lesions were primarily orbital, with the remainder originating from the nasal cavity (61% carcinoma, 23% sarcoma, 8% lymphoma, 8% mast cell). Osseous reaction and medial orbital location of a mass were the only features

suggestive of neoplasia. Cavitary lesions were most often associated with salivary mucoceles and retrobulbar abscesses. Significant overlap was otherwise observed between lesions.

A separate study investigated the ability of ultrasound to differentiate between neoplastic and nonneoplastic lesions in cases of unilateral retrobulbar disease in 45 dogs.[43] Out of 45 lesions identified, 29 were neoplastic; 52% of neoplastic lesions were carcinomas, 28% were sarcomas, and 10% were lymphoma. Single cases of hemangiosarcoma, mast cell tumor, and undifferentiated malignancy were also reported. On B-mode ultrasound, neoplastic lesions were more likely to be hypoechoic and homogenous, with well-defined margins and sufficient mass to compress the globe. Neoplastic lesions were also more likely to involve bone, as in the study by Mason et al,[135] and only neoplastic lesions had evidence of mineralization. Fluctuant fluid accumulations were more commonly identified with non-neoplastic lesions. Unlike the study by Mason and colleagues,[135] no preferential location was identified for neoplasms.[43] Aside from ability to demonstrate osseous extension of retrobulbar disease, ultrasound compared favorably with CT findings.

Optic Nerve Pathology

Tumors of the optic nerve include meningioma, glioma, glioblastoma, astrocytoma, neurofibroma, and lymphoma. Reports describing the ultrasonographic appearance of optic nerve tumors in veterinary medicine are sparse. A solitary report describing the B-mode appearance of an anaplastic astrocytoma within the retrobulbar space was identified in the current literature.[122] Meningiomas are rare.[90] In humans, optic nerve tumors, such as gliomas and meningiomas, are located within the muscle cone and enlarge the optic nerve. Echogenic as well as anechoic areas may be present within the mass. The anechoic areas may represent necrosis.[54] The characteristic findings of neurogenic tumors in 17 human patients were reported in 1972.[136] The tumors were round and well demarcated from the surrounding tissues. They had a well-defined anterior margin and high acoustic absorption, leading to dropout and nonvisualization of the posterior extent of the tumor. The tumors were echogenic owing to their heterogeneous cell population. A hypoechoic astrocytoma that was also round and well differentiated from the surrounding retrobulbar tissues has been reported.[137] Meningiomas and gliomas may cause a smooth enlargement of the anterior-most portion of the optic nerve, thus creating a smoothly curved shadow, in contrast to the acute-angled shadow of the normal optic nerve with the retrobulbar tissues.[136] They may indent the posterior ocular wall, and papilledema may be present. These two tumor types are difficult to differentiate by ultrasound evaluation, but meningiomas are reported to have a more irregular appearance and posterior location.[54] We have identified a meningioma in a dog that appeared as a well-defined, fairly homogenous, relatively hypoechoic, bulbous mass in the retrobulbar space immediately caudal to the optic disc (Figure 5-45, A and B). There was no apparent invasion into the globe but the globe was mildly indented by the mass. The ultrasound findings corresponded well with MRI findings, where the mass was visualized as a well-defined T_2 isointense, T_1 hypointense, contrast enhancing, bulbous mass associated with the distal-most aspect of the optic nerve (see Figure 5-45). As with ultrasound, no evidence of invasion into the globe was identified, although invasion into the adjacent aspects of the frontal and olfactory lobes of the brain was identified with MRI.

Toxoplasmosis, cryptococcosis, canine distemper, blastomycosis, feline infectious peritonitis, reticulosis of the central nervous system, and trauma can cause inflammation and enlargement of the optic nerve. Multiple sclerosis is a common

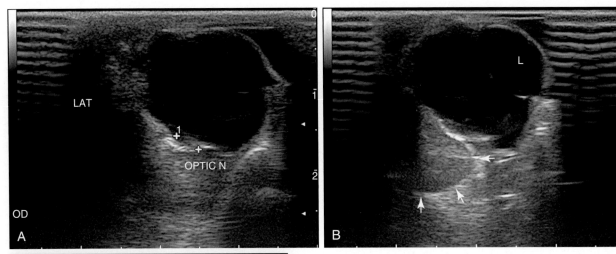

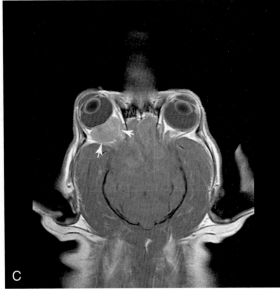

Figure 5-45 Optic nerve sheath tumor (meningioma). A, Homogenous echogenic tissue occupies the retrobulbar space, obliterating the normal W shape created by extraocular muscles, the optic nerve, and retrobulbar fat. Between the electronic cursors (0.32 cm) is a protruding optic disc. The globe is mildly indented by the mass. *L,* Lens. *OD,* right eye. **B,** Similar view as **A,** a lateral boundary of the optic nerve tumor is more readily identified *(arrows).* **C,** Dorsal T₁-weighted MRI image showing superb detail of the optic nerve tumor *(arrows).*

cause of retrobulbar neuritis in humans. Optic neuritis shows diffuse enlargement of the optic nerve.[54] An irregular shape of the anterior portion of the optic nerve, sometimes with a separate echo more proximal in the nerve, may be seen. Possible duplication of the nerve sheath may also occur secondary to perineural enlargement.[138] A protruding optic disc (papilledema) may also be present.

Perineural enlargement may also occur secondary to increased intracranial or cerebrospinal pressure from trauma or neoplasms. Enlargement of the optic nerve with duplication of the optic nerve sheath has been reported in humans.[54] Two echogenic lines are imaged at the periphery of the optic nerve along its axis; the hypoechoic space between these two lines represents a distended subarachnoid space or edematous tissue caused by local capillary leakage. Papilledema may be seen. Differentiation of papilledema from papillitis is difficult, although the disc is reported to be more prominent with edema.[137]

Aplasia, hypoplasia, and optic nerve atrophy may be detected by an absent or small optic nerve on B-mode ultrasonography. The optic nerve may have a narrow, funnel-shaped appearance and is sharply outlined by the retrobulbar fat.[137]

Coloboma is a congenital ocular anomaly resulting from failure of the embryonic ocular cleft to fuse. It often affects the optic disc, appearing as fissures or pits. It is part of the

collie eye syndrome.[53] The B-mode ultrasonographic appearance in humans has been reported.[77] Asymmetrical posterior vitreal herniation surrounding the optic nerve head was seen. Retinal detachment was present, as was subretinal membrane formation.

ORBITAL AND OCULAR VASCULATURE

Color Doppler Evaluation of the Ocular and Orbital Vasculature

The normal ocular and orbital vascular anatomy as imaged with color Doppler ultrasound has been described.[38] The most commonly identified vessels in that study were the external ophthalmic artery, dorsal and ventral external ophthalmic veins, internal ophthalmic artery, anterior ciliary artery and vein, short and long posterior ciliary arteries, primary retinal arteries, and vortex veins. Reference ranges are listed for normal time average velocity (TAV), peak systolic velocity (PSV), end-diastolic velocity (EDV), pulsatility index (PI), and resistive index (RI) for the arteries, and PSV and EDV for the veins. Image reproducibility of the commonly identified vessels was high. RI and PI provide information about the resistance to blood flow within a vessel. In a separate study, the RI and PI measurements of the long posterior ciliary artery in normal unsedated dogs and cats were determined.[36] The suggested upper limit (mean + 2SD) for RI and PI in the long posterior ciliary artery in the cat are 0.72 and 1.02 respectively. The suggested upper limit (mean + 2SD) for the RI of the long posterior ciliary artery in the dog is 0.76, slightly higher than reported in the study by Gelatt-Nicholson and co-workers (0.66).[38] Similarly the suggested upper limit for the PI of the long posterior ciliary artery of 1.68 is higher than the value (1.22) from the same study. Differences in RIs between the two studies may be explained by the sedation used by Gelatt-Nicholson and colleagues (butorphanol tartrate, acepromazine maleate, and atropine sulfate).[38] It is known that healthy dogs sedated with midazolam and butorphanol have significantly higher PI and RI measurements than those from nonsedated dogs.[37] Increases in RI and PI above normal are often associated with decreased vascular perfusion.

Beagle dogs with inherited primary open-angle glaucoma have significantly altered Doppler blood flow velocities and resistive indices in several ocular and orbital vessels as compared to normal Beagle dogs. Specifically, decreased EDVs and increased RIs were found within their short posterior ciliary arteries (main blood supply to the canine optic disc).[39]

Administration of antiglaucoma drugs can also alter blood flow velocities and resistive indices in dogs. The RIs within the short posterior ciliary artery, long posterior artery, and ophthalmic artery are significantly lower in dogs treated systemically with amlodipine (calcium channel blocker) relative to untreated dogs.[40] Topical administration of levobunolol (nonselective beta-adrenergic blocking agent) and dipivefrin (alpha and beta agonist) lead to increased RI, whereas pilocarpine (cholinergic agonist) had no effect on RI in one study.[41]

REFERENCES

1. Mundt GH Jr, Hughes WF Jr. Ultrasonics in ocular diagnosis. *Am J Ophthalmol* 1956;**41**:488–98.
2. Rubin LF, Koch SA. Ocular diagnostic ultrasonography. *J Am Vet Med Assoc* 1968;**153**:1706–16.
3. Johnston GR, Feeney DA. Radiology in ophthalmic diagnosis. *Vet Clin North Am Small Anim Pract* 1980;**10**:317–37.
4. Eisenberg HM. Ultrasonography of the eye and orbit. *Vet Clin North Am Small Anim Pract* 1985;**15**:1263–74.
5. Fourgi L, Ballereau L. L'echographie oculaire chez le chien et le chat. *Prat Med Chir Anim* 1985;**20**:51–5.
6. Miller WM, Cartee RE. B-scan ultrasonography for the detection of space-occupying ocular masses. *J Am Vet Med Assoc* 1985;**187**:66–8.
7. Rogers M, Cartee RE, Miller W, et al. Evaluation of the extirpated equine eye using B-mode ultrasonography. *Vet Radiol* 1986;**27**:24–9.
8. Dziezyc J, Hager DA, Millichamp NJ. Two-dimensional real-time ocular ultrasonography in the diagnosis of ocular lesions in dogs. *J Am Anim Hosp Assoc* 1987;**23**:501–8.
9. Hager DA, Dziezyc J. Millchamp NJ. Two-dimensional real-time ocular ultrasonography in the dog—technique and normal anatomy. *Vet Radiol* 1987;**28**:60–5.
10. Dziezyc J, Hager DA. Ocular ultrasonography in veterinary-medicine. *Semin Vet Med Surg (Small Anim)* 1988;**3**:1–9.
11. Gonzalez EM, Rodriguez A, Garcia I. Review of ocular ultrasonography. *Vet Radiol* 2001;**42**:485–95.
12. Fledelius HC. Ultrasound in ophthalmology. *Ultrasound Med Biol* 1997;**23**:365–75.
13. Coleman DJ, Silverman RH, Daly SM, et al. Advances in ophthalmic ultrasound. *Radiol Clin North Am* 1998;**36**:1073.
14. Williamson TH, Harris A. Color Doppler ultrasound imaging of the eye and orbit. *Surv Ophthalmol* 1996;**40**:255–67.
15. Lieb WE. Color Doppler imaging of the eye and orbit. *Radiol Clin North Am* 1998;**36**:1059.
16. Rosa N, Cennamo G, Breve MA, et al. Power doppler ultrasonography in ocular and orbital diseases. *Ophthalmologica* 1998;**212**(Suppl. 1):99–100.
17. Pavlin CJ, Sherar MD, Foster FS. Subsurface ultrasound microscopic imaging of the intact eye. *Ophthalmology* 1990;**97**:244–50.
18. Pavlin CJ, Harasiewicz K, Sherar MD, et al. Clinical Use of Ultrasound Biomicroscopy. *Ophthalmology* 1991;**98**:287–95.
19. Marchini G, Pagliarusco A, Toscano A, et al. Ultrasound biomicroscopic and conventional ultrasonographic study of ocular dimensions in primary angle-closure glaucoma. *Ophthalmology* 1998;**105**:2091–8.
20. Deramo VA, Shah GK, Baumal CR, et al. Ultrasound biomicroscopy as a tool for detecting and localizing occult foreign bodies after ocular trauma. *Ophthalmology* 1999;**106**:301–5.
21. Downey DB, Nicolle DA, Levin MF, et al. Three-dimensional ultrasound imaging of the eye. *Eye* 1996;**10**:75–81.
22. Cusumano A, Coleman DJ, Silverman RH, et al. Three-dimensional ultrasound imaging—Clinical applications. *Ophthalmology* 1998;**105**:300–6.
23. Nolan W. Anterior segment imaging: ultrasound biomicroscopy and anterior segment optical coherence tomography. *Curr Opin Ophthalmol* 2008;**19**:115–21.
24. Conway RM, Chew T, Golchet P, et al. Ultrasound biomicroscopy: role in diagnosis and management in 130 consecutive patients evaluated for anterior segment tumours. *Br J Ophthalmol* 2005;**89**:950–5.
25. Ishikawa H, Liebmann JM, Ritch R. Quantitative assessment of the anterior segment using ultrasound biomicroscopy. *Curr Opin Ophthalmol* 2000;**11**:133–9.
26. Bentley E, Miller PE, Diehl KA. Use of high-resolution ultrasound as a diagnostic tool in veterinary ophthalmology. *J Am Vet Med Assoc* 2003;**223**:1617–22.
27. Bentley E, Miller PE, Diehl KA. Evaluation of intra- and interobserver reliability and image reproducibility to assess usefulness of high-resolution ultrasonography for measurement of anterior segment structures of canine eyes. *Am J Vet Res* 2005;**66**:1775–9.
28. Rose MD, Mattoon JS, Gemensky-Metzler AJ, et al. Ultrasound biomicroscopy of the iridocorneal angle of the eye before and after phacoemulsification and intraocular lens implantation in dogs. *Am J Vet Res* 2008;**69**:279–88.
29. Crumley W, Gionfriddo JR, Radecki SV. Relationship of the iridocorneal angle, as measured using ultrasound biomicroscopy, with post-operative increases in intraocular pressure post-phacoemulsification in dogs. *Vet Ophthalmol* 2009;**12**:22–7.
30. Gomes FE, Bentley E, Lin TL, et al. Effects of unilateral topical administration of 0.5% tropicamide on anterior segment morphology and intraocular pressure in normal cats and cats with primary congenital glaucoma. *Vet Ophthalmol* 2011;**14**(Suppl. 1):75–83.
31. Kawata M, Tsukizawa H, Nakayama M, et al. Rectification of width and area of the ciliary cleft in dogs. *J Vet Med Sci* 2010;**72**:533–7.

32. Aubin ML, Powell CC, Gionfriddo JR, et al. Ultrasound biomicroscopy of the feline anterior segment. *Vet Ophthalmol* 2003;**6**:15–17.

33. Tsai S, Bentley E, Miller PE, et al. Gender differences in iridocorneal angle morphology: a potential explanation for the female predisposition to primary angle closure glaucoma in dogs. *Vet Ophthalmol* 2012;**15**(Suppl. 1):60–3.

34. Dulaurent T, Goulle F, Dulaurent A, et al. Effect of mydriasis induced by topical instillations of 0.5% tropicamide on the anterior segment in normotensive dogs using ultrasound biomicroscopy. *Vet Ophthalmol* 2012;**15**(Suppl. 1):8–13.

35. Labruyere JJ, Hartley C, Holloway A. Contrast-enhanced ultrasonography in the differentiation of retinal detachment and vitreous membrane in dogs and cats. *J Small Anim Pract* 2011;**52**:522–30.

36. Novellas R, Espada Y, Ruiz de Gopegui R. Doppler ultrasonographic estimation of renal and ocular resistive and pulsatility indices in normal dogs and cats. *Vet Radiol* 2007;**48**:69–73.

37. Novellas R, Ruiz de Gopegui R, Espada Y. Effects of sedation with midazolam and butorphanol on resistive and pulsatility indices in healthy dogs. *Vet Radiol* 2007;**48**:276–80.

38. Gelatt-Nicholson KJ, Gelatt KN, MacKay E, et al. Doppler imaging of the ophthalmic vasculature of the normal dog: blood velocity measurements and reproducibility. *Vet Ophthalmol* 1999;**2**:87–96.

39. Gelatt-Nicholson KJ, Gelatt KN, MacKay EO, et al. Comparative Doppler imaging of the ophthalmic vasculature in normal Beagles and Beagles with inherited primary open-angle glaucoma. *Vet Ophthalmol* 1999;**2**:97–105.

40. Kallberg ME, Brooks DE, Komaromy AM, et al. The effect of an L-type calcium channel blocker on the hemodynamics of orbital arteries in dogs. *Vet Ophthalmol* 2003;**6**:141–6.

41. Choi H, Lee Y, Yeon S, et al. Effects of anti-glaucoma drugs on resistive index of the medial long posterior ciliary artery using color Doppler imaging in Beagle dogs. *J Vet Sci* 2011;**12**:99–101.

42. Penninck D, Daniel GB, Brawer R, et al. Cross-sectional imaging techniques in veterinary ophthalmology. *Clin Tech Small Anim Pract* 2001;**16**:22–39.

43. Boroffka SA, Verbruggen AM, Grinwis GC, et al. Assessment of ultrasonography and computed tomography for the evaluation of unilateral orbital disease in dogs. *J Am Vet Med Assoc* 2007;**230**:671–80.

44. Magrane WG. *Canine Ophthalmology*. 5th ed. Philadelphia: Lea & Fbiger; 1977.

45. Pollock RVH. The eye. In: Evans HE, Christensen CG, editors. *Miller's Anatomy of the Dog*. 2nd ed. Philadelphia: WB Saunders; 1979. p. 1073–127.

46. Martin CL, Anderson BG. Ocular anatomy. In: Gelatt KN, editor. *Veterinary Ophthalmology*. Philadelphia: Lea & Febiger; 1981. p. 12–121.

47. Barrie KP, Lavach JD, Gelatt KN. Diseases of the canine posterior segment. In: Gelatt KN, editor. *Veterinary Ophthalmology*. Philadelphia: Lea & Febiger; 1981. p. 474–517.

48. Prince JH, Diesem CD, Eglitis I, et al. *Anatomy and Histology of the Eye and Orbit in Domestic Animals*. Springfield, Ill: Charles C Thomas; 1960.

49. Coleman DJ. Reliability of ocular and orbital diagnosis with B-scan ultrasound. 1. Ocular diagnosis. *Am J Ophthalmol* 1972;**73**:501–16.

50. Smith ME, Coleman DJ, Haik BG. Ultrasonography of the eye. *Int Ophtlalmol Clin* 1986;**26**:25–50.

51. Stuhr C, Scagliotti R. Retrobulbar ultrasound in the mesaticephalic and dolichocephalic dog using a temporal approach. *Vet Comp Ophthalmol* 1996;**6**:91–9.

52. Schiffer SP, Rantanen NW, Leary GA, et al. Biometric study of the canine eye, using A-mode ultrasonography. *Am J Vet Res* 1982;**43**:826–30.

53. Koch SA, Rubin LF. Diagnostic ultrasonography of the dog eye. *J Small Anim Pract* 1969;**10**:357–61.

54. Shammas JH. *Atlas of Ophthalmic Ultrasonography and Biometry*. St Louis: Mosby; 1984.

55. LeMay M. B-scan ultrasonography of the anterior segment of the eye. *Br J Ophthalmol* 1978;**62**:651–6.

56. Lee HC, Choi HJ, Choi MC, et al. Ultrasonographic measurement of optic nerve sheath diameter in normal dogs. *J Vet Sci* 2003;**4**:265–8.

57. Dallow RL. Ultrasonography of the orbit. *Int Ophtlalmol Clin* 1986;**26**:51–76.

58. Dutton JJ. Standardized echography in the diagnosis of lacrimal drainage dysfunction. *Arch Ophthalmol* 1989;**107**:1010–12.

59. Cottrill NB, Banks WJ, Pechman RD. Ultrasonographic and biometric evaluation of the eye and orbit of dogs. *Am J Vet Res* 1989;**50**:898–903.

60. Boroffka SA, Voorhout G, Verbruggen AM, et al. Intraobserver and interobserver repeatability of ocular biometric measurements obtained by means of B-mode ultrasonography in dogs. *Am J Vet Res* 2006;**67**:1743–9.

61. Boroffka SA. Ultrasonographic evaluation of pre- and postnatal development of the eyes in beagles. *Vet Radiol* 2005;**46**:72–9.

62. Tuntivanich N, Petersen-Jones SM, Steibel JP, et al. Postnatal development of canine axial globe length measured by B-scan ultrasonography. *Vet Ophthalmol* 2007;**10**:2–5.

63. Moodie KL, Hashizume N, Houston DL, et al. Postnatal development of corneal curvature and thickness in the cat. *Vet Ophthalmol* 2001;**4**:267–72.

64. Gibson TE, Roberts SM, Severin GA, et al. Comparison of gonioscopy and ultrasound biomicroscopy for evaluating the iridocorneal angle in dogs. *J Am Vet Med Assoc* 1998;**213**:635–8.

65. Tomlinson A, Phillips CI. Applanation tension and axial length of the eyeball. *Br J Ophthalmol* 1970;**54**:548-53.

66. Larsen JS. Axial length of the emmetropic eye and its relation to the head size. *Acta Ophthalmol* 1979;**57**:76–83.

67. Hyman JA, Koch SA, Wilcock BP. Canine choroidal melanoma with metastases. *Vet Ophthalmol* 2002;**5**:113–17.

68. Blocker T, van der Woerdt A. What is your diagnosis? Cataract, retinal detachment, and a large mass protruding into the vitreous cavity. *J Am Vet Med Assoc* 2000;**217**:23–4.

69. Planellas M, Pastor J, Torres MD, et al. Unusual presentation of a metastatic uveal melanoma in a cat. *Vet Ophthalmol* 2010;**13**:391–4.

70. Miwa Y, Matsunaga S, Kato K, et al. Choroidal melanoma in a dog. *J Vet Med Sci* 2005;**67**:821–3.

71. Semin MO, Serra F, Mahe V, et al. Choroidal melanocytoma in a cat. *Vet Ophthalmol* 2011;**14**:205–8.

72. Haeussler DJ Jr, Rodriguez LM, Wilkie DA, et al. Primary central corneal hemangiosarcoma in a dog. *Vet Ophthalmol* 2011;**14**:133–6.

73. Delgado E, Pissarra H, Sales-Luis J, et al. Amelanotic uveal cyst in a Yorkshire terrier dog. *Vet Ophthalmol* 2010;**13**:343–7.

74. Galan A, Martin-Suarez EM, Molleda JM, et al. Presumed primary uveal melanoma with brain extension in a dog. *J Small Anim Pract* 2009;**50**:306–10.

75. Regnier A, Raymond-Letron I, Peiffer RL. Congenital orbital cysts of neural tissue in two dogs. *Vet Ophthalmol* 2008;**11**:91–8.

76. Yi NY, Park SA, Park SW, et al. Malignant ocular melanoma in a dog. *J Vet Sci* 2006;**7**:89–90.

77. Richter M, Stankeova S, Hauser B, et al. Myxosarcoma in the eye and brain in a dog. *Vet Ophthalmol* 2003;**6**:183–9.

78. Coleman DJ, Abramson DH, Jack RL, et al. Ultrasonic diagnosis of tumors of the choroid. *Arch Ophthalmol* 1974;**91**:344–54.

79. Wilcock BP. The eye and ear. In: Jubb KVF, Kennedy PC, Palmer N, editors. *Pathology of Domestic Animals*. 4th ed. San Diego: Academic Press; 1993. p. 441–528.

80. Cordy DR. Tumors of the nervous system and eye. In: Moulton JF, editor. *Tumors in Domestic Animals*. 3rd ed. Berkeley, Calif: University of California Press; 1990. p. 640–65.

81. Buyukmihci NC. Tumors of the eye. In: Theilen GH, Madewell BR, editors. *Veterinary Cancer Medicine*. 2nd ed. Philadelphia: Lea & Febiger; 1987. p. 635–46.

82. Shammas HF, Blodi FC. Prognostic factors in choroidal and ciliary body melanomas. *Arch Ophthalmol* 1977;**95**:63–9.

83. Bloom W, Fawcett DW. *A Textbook of Histology*. 10th ed. Philadelphia: WB Saunders; 1975.

84. Fuller DG, Snyder WB, Hutton WL, et al. Ultrasonographic features of choroidal malignant melanomas. *Arch Ophthalmol* 1979;**97**:1465–72.

85. Peiffer RL. Ciliary body epithelial tumors. In: Peiffer RL, editor. *Comparative Ophthalmic Pathology*. Springfield, Ill: Charles C Thomas; 1983. p. 183–212.

86. Spiess BM, Bolliger JO, Guscetti F, et al. Multiple ciliary body cysts and secondary glaucoma in the Great Dane: a report of nine cases. *Vet Ophthalmol* 1998;**1**:41–5.

87. Deehr AJ, Dubielzig RR. A histopathological study of iridociliary cysts and glaucoma in Golden Retrievers. *Vet Ophthalmol* 1998;**1**:153–8.

88. Collins BK, Moore CP. Canine anterior uvea. In: Gelatt KN, editor. *Veterinary Ophthalmology*. 2nd ed. Philadelphia: Lea & Febiger; 1991. p. 375–95.

89. Nasisse MP. Feline ophthalmology. In: Gelatt KN, editor. *Veterinary Ophthalmology*. 2nd ed. Philadelphia: Lea & Febiger; 1991. p. 529–75.

90. Curtis R, Barnett KC, Leon A. Diseases of the canine posterior segment. In: Gelatt K, editor. In: Gelatt KN, editor. *Veterinary Ophthalmology*. 2nd ed. Philadelphia: Lea & Febiger; 1991. p. 461–525.

91. McQuown DS. Ocular and orbital echography. *Radiol Clin North Am* 1975;**13**:523–41.

92. Labruyere JJ, Hartley C, Rogers K, et al. Ultrasonographic evaluation of vitreous degeneration in normal dogs. *Vet Radiol* 2008;**49**:165–71.

93. Fielding JA. Ultrasound imaging of the eye through the closed lid using a non-dedicated scanner. *Clin Radiol* 1987;**38**:131–5.

94. Linek J. Mycotic endophthalmitis in a dog caused by *Candida albicans*. *Vet Ophthalmol* 2004;**7**:159–62.

95. Pearce J, Giuliano EA, Galle LE, et al. Management of bilateral uveitis in a *Toxoplasma gondii*–seropositive cat with histopathologic evidence of fungal panuveitis. *Vet Ophthalmol* 2007;**10**:216–21.

96. Innes J, McCreath G, Forrester JV. Ultrasonic patterns in vitreo-retinal disease. *Clin Radiol* 1982;**33**:585–91.

97. Boroffka SA, Verbruggen AM, Boeve MH, et al. Ultrasonographic diagnosis of persistent hyperplastic tunica vasculosa lentis/persistent hyperplastic primary vitreous in two dogs. *Vet Radiol* 1998;**39**:440–4.

98. Allgoewer I, Pfefferkorn B. Persistent hyperplastic tunica vasculosa lentis and persistent hyperplastic primary vitreous (PHTVL/PHPV) in two cats. *Vet Ophthalmol* 2001;**4**:161–4.

99. Gemensky-Metzler AJ, Wilkie DA. Surgical management and histologic and immunohistochemical features of a cataract and retrolental plaque secondary to persistent hyperplastic tunica vasculosa lentis/persistent hyperplastic primary vitreous (PHTVL/PHPV) in a Bloodhound puppy. *Vet Ophthalmol* 2004;**7**:369–75.

100. Bayon A, Tovar MC, Fernandez del Palacio MJ, et al. Ocular complications of persistent hyperplastic primary vitreous in three dogs. *Vet Ophthalmol* 2001;**4**:35–40.

101. Ori J, Yoshikai T, Yoshimura S, et al. Persistent hyperplastic primary vitreous (PHPV) in two Siberian husky dogs. *J Vet Med Sci* 1998;**60**:263–5.

102. Ori JI, Yoshikai T, Yoshimur S, et al. Posterior lenticonus with congenital cataract in a Shih Tzu dog. *J Vet Med Sci* 2000;**62**:1201–3.

103. Hartley C, McConnell JF, Doust R. Wooden orbital foreign body in a Weimaraner. *Vet Ophthalmol* 2007;**10**:390–3.

104. Tovar MC, Huguet E, Gomezi MA. Orbital cellulitis and intraocular abscess caused by migrating grass in a cat. *Vet Ophthalmol* 2005;**8**:353–6.

105. Coleman DJ, Trokel SL. A protocol for B-scan and radiographic foreign body localization. *Am J Ophthalmol* 1971;**71**:84–9.

106. Keeney AH. Indications for ultrasound examination. *Int Ophtlalmol Clin* 1979;**19**:3–7.

107. Ossoinig KC. Standardized echography: basic principles, clinical applications, and results. *Int Ophtlalmol Clin* 1979;**19**:127–210.

108. Rampazzo A, Eule C, Speier S, et al. Scleral rupture in dogs, cats, and horses. *Vet Ophthalmol* 2006;**9**:149–55.

109. Stades FC, Djajadiningrat-Laanen SC, Boroffka SA, et al. Suprascleral removal of a foreign body from the retrobulbar muscle cone in two dogs. *J Small Anim Pract* 2003;**44**:17–20.

110. van der Woerdt A, Wilkie DA, Myer CW. Ultrasonographic abnormalities in the eyes of dogs with cataracts: 147 cases (1986-1992). *J Am Vet Med Assoc* 1993;**203**:838–41.

111. Ori J, Sasa Y, Komiya M, et al. Two-dimensional ultrasonography of the lens in diagnosis of canine cataract and nuclear sclerosis. *J Jpn Vet Med Assoc* 1996;**49**:175–9.

112. Park SA, Yi NY, Jeong MB, et al. Clinical manifestations of cataracts in small breed dogs. *Vet Ophthalmol* 2009;**12**:205–10.

113. Wilkie DA, Gemensky-Metzler AJ, Colitz CM, et al. Canine cataracts, diabetes mellitus and spontaneous lens capsule rupture: a retrospective study of 18 dogs. *Vet Ophthalmol* 2006;**9**:328–34.

114. Williams DL. Lens morphometry determined by B-mode ultrasonography of the normal and cataractous canine lens. *Vet Ophthalmol* 2004;**7**:91–5.

115. Gelatt KN, Samuelson DA, Barrie KP, et al. Biometry and Clinical Characteristics of Congenital Cataracts and Microphthalmia in the Miniature Schnauzer. *J Am Vet Med Assoc* 1983;**183**:99–102.

116. Gelatt KN. The canine lens. In: Gelatt KN, editor. *Veterinary Ophthalmology*. 2nd ed. Philadelphia: Lea & Febiger; 1991. p. 429–60.

117. Pavlin CJ, Foster FS. *Ultrasound biomicroscopy of the eye*. New York: Springer; 1995.
118. Morgan RV. Ultrasonography of retrobulbar diseases of the dog and cat. *J Am Anim Hosp Assoc* 1989;**25**: 393–9.
119. Boroffka SAEB. vandenBelt AJM. CT/ultrasound diagnosis–Retrobulbar hematoma in a horse. *Vet Radiol* 1996;**37**:441–3.
120. Dennis R. Imaging features of orbital myxosarcoma in dogs. *Vet Radiol* 2008;**49**:256–63.
121. Attali-Soussay K, Jegou JP, Clerc B. Retrobulbar tumors in dogs and cats: 25 cases. *Vet Ophthalmol* 2001;**4**: 19–27.
122. Martin E, Perez J, Mozos E, et al. Retrobulbar anaplastic astrocytoma in a dog: clinicopathological and ultrasonographic features. *J Small Anim Pract* 2000;**41**:354–7.
123. Williams DL, Haggett E. Surgical removal of a canine orbital lipoma. *J Small Anim Pract* 2006;**47**:35–7.
124. Laus JL, Canola JC, Mamede FV, et al. Orbital cellulitis associated with Toxocara canis in a dog. *Vet Ophthalmol* 2003;**6**:333–6.
125. Coleman DJ, Jack RL, Franzen LA. High resolution B-scan ultrasonography of the orbit. II. Hemangiomas of the orbit. *Arch Ophthalmol* 1972;**88**:368–74.
126. Coleman DJ, Jack RL, Franzen LA. High resolution B-scan ultrasonography of the orbit. 3. Lymphomas of the orbit. *Arch Ophthalmol* 1972;**88**:375–9.
127. Coleman DJ, Jack RL, Franzen LA, et al. High resolution B-scan ultrasonography of the orbit. V. Eye changes of Graves' disease. *Arch Ophthalmol* 1972;**88**:465–71.
128. Bussanich MN, Rootman J. Intraocular foreign body in a dog. *Can Vet J* 1981;**22**:207–10.
129. Pentlarge VW, Powelljohnson G, Martin CL, et al. Orbital Neoplasia with Enophthalmos in a Cat. *J Am Vet Med Assoc* 1989;**195**:1249–51.
130. Cline RA, Rootman J. Enophthalmos: a clinical review. *Ophthalmology* 1984;**91**:229–37.
131. Reifler D. Orbital metastasis with enophthalmos: A review of the literature. *Henry Ford Hosp Med J* 1985; **33**:171–9.
132. Peiffer RL. Feline ophthalmology. In: Gelatt KN, editor. *Veterinary Ophthalmology*. Philadelphia: Lea & Febiger; 1981. p. 521–68.
133. Gelatt KN. Canine lacrimal and nasolacrimal diseases. In: Gelatt KN, editor. *Veterinary Ophthalmology*. 2nd ed. Philadelphia: Lea & Febiger; 1991. p. 276–89.
134. Bradbury JA, Rennie IG, Parsons MA. Adrenaline dacryolith: detection by ultrasound examination of the nasolacrimal duct. *Br J Ophthalmol* 1988;**72**:935–7.
135. Mason DR, Lamb CR, McLellan GJ. Ultrasonographic findings in 50 dogs with retrobulbar disease. *J Am Anim Hosp Assoc* 2001;**37**:557–62.
136. Coleman DJ, Jack RL, Franzen LA. High resolution B-scan ultrasonography of the orbit. IV. Neurogenic tumors of the orbit. *Arch Ophthalmol* 1972;**88**:380–4.
137. Kerlen CH. B-scan ultrasonography in optic nerve lesions. *Doc Ophthalmol* 1982;**52**:317–25.
138. Coleman DJ, Carroll FD. A new technique for evaluation of optic nerve pathology. *Am J Ophthalmol* 1972;**74**: 915–20.

Dana A. Neelis • John S. Mattoon • Thomas G. Nyland

GENERAL CONSIDERATIONS

Ultrasound examination of the ventral neck poses unique challenges owing to the complexity of the regional anatomy and the relatively small size of the most clinically important anatomic structures and organs. Until recently, high-resolution, small-parts ultrasound capabilities were limited to only a few of the larger veterinary institutions because of the cost of high-end ultrasound machines and special-purpose, high-frequency transducers. With the recent improvements in ultrasound technology and the increased availability of high-resolution transducers, ultrasound imaging of the structures of the ventral neck has become more feasible, indications for ultrasound examination have expanded, and accuracy of diagnosis has improved.

The ultrasound examination of the neck is most often performed in dorsal or lateral recumbency. If scanning in dorsal recumbency, a rolled towel or pad could be used to help straighten the cervical region. Ultrasound examination of this region is best performed with a 10- to 15-MHz linear-array transducer; however, lower frequency (7 to 10 MHz) linear-array or sector-scanning transducers can be used for examination of larger structures. Linear-array transducers have the advantage of eliminating artifact in the near field of the image, but a standoff pad may improve near-field image quality if a sector-scanning transducer is used. Color or pulsed wave Doppler imaging is essential for complete evaluation of blood vessels and vascular tissues such as the thyroid gland. High-resolution ultrasonography of small parts can be used with guided fine-needle aspiration or tissue-core biopsy for definitive diagnosis of lesions of the neck.[1-4]

CAROTID ARTERY AND JUGULAR VEIN

The paired external jugular veins are formed by the convergence of the linguofacial and maxillary veins and lie in the jugular furrows on either side of the ventral neck (Figure 6-1). Paired common carotid arteries run deep to the external jugular veins and course the length of the neck with the vagosympathetic trunk, bifurcating in the cranioventral aspect of the cervical region into external and internal carotid arteries (Figure 6-2). The carotid sinus is located at the origin of the internal carotid artery and appears grossly as a slight, focal dilation of the artery.

The common carotid artery and the carotid bifurcation can be imaged in both the transverse and long axes and serve as excellent anatomic landmarks. They are initially located by placing the transducer in the jugular furrow with the scanning plane directed along the long axis of the neck and at a 45-degree angle between the parasagittal and dorsal planes

(Figure 6-3, imaging plane 1). The common carotid artery and its branches are characterized by an anechoic lumen and a surrounding thick hyperechoic arterial wall (Figures 6-4 and 6-5). Pulsatile blood flow can also be detected on two-dimensional gray-scale images or by Doppler analysis of the vessel lumen (Figure 6-6, *B, C*; also see Figure 6-4, *B*). With the transducer positioned transversely, the carotid arteries appear as small, circular anechoic structures on either side of the trachea (Figure 6-7). The common carotid artery can be traced from the thoracic inlet to the carotid bifurcation in imaging plane 1 and in the transverse plane.

The external and internal carotid arteries are best seen by varying the scanning angle between a dorsal and parasagittal plane. The internal carotid artery is identified in scanning plane 1, arising at an approximately 30-degree angle from the external carotid artery and coursing internally. In some dogs, the carotid sinus can be seen as a focal dilation at the origin of the internal carotid artery and is best imaged in scanning plane 1 at a level ventral to the wing of the atlas[5] (see Figure 6-5). The external carotid artery continues in a straight line rostrally from the common carotid artery. Other anatomic landmarks identified in this plane are the mandibular salivary gland and the digastric muscle viewed obliquely as it crosses the caudoventral aspect of the body of the mandible. The occipital artery can occasionally be identified arising from the external carotid artery immediately cranial to the carotid bifurcation.[5]

The right or left jugular veins are seen in both plane 1 and the transverse plane. Jugular veins are located immediately below the skin surface and have a thin, hyperechoic wall surrounding an anechoic lumen.[5] The jugular veins are seen as anechoic tubular structures during superficial imaging of the cervical region, leading into the thoracic inlet (Figure 6-8). Careful scanning technique may allow identification of additional venous structures, such as the subclavian and internal jugular veins (Figure 6-9). Valves may also be identified within the jugular vein as thin echogenic linear structures with wave-like motion corresponding to movement of the jugular vein (see Figure 6-9).

Because the jugular veins are low-pressure vessels, they easily collapse with transducer pressure. Imaging requires a gentle touch and a high-frequency transducer (preferably linear array). Applying a large volume of coupling gel to the skin overlying the vein and applying minimal transducer pressure can help overcome this. Another method is to image the contralateral jugular vein, using the soft tissues of the neck as a built-in standoff pad. This is accomplished by directing the ultrasound beam in a sagittal oblique plane dorsal to the trachea. The jugular vein on the opposite side of the neck will now be positioned several centimeters deep. Relatively slow jugular vein wall movement is often identified and should not

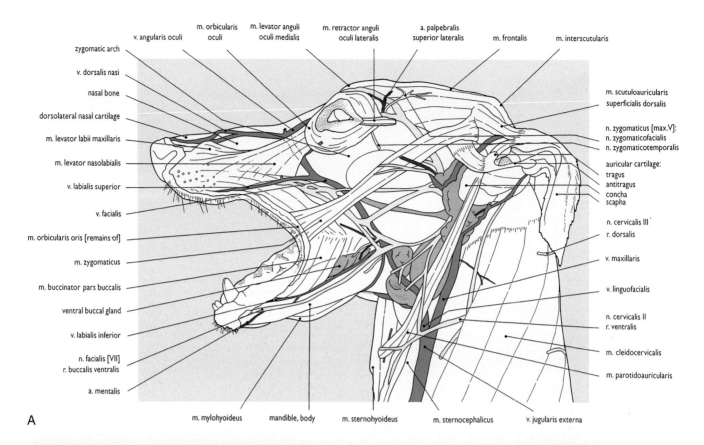

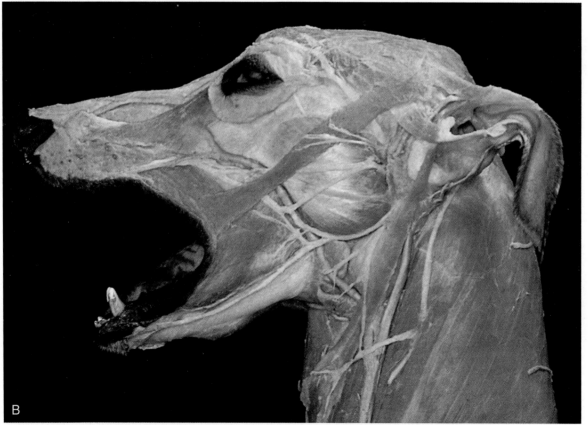

Figure 6-1 Illustration (A) and superficial dissection (B) of the dog head and neck showing jugular vein and branches, mandibular and parotid salivary glands (lateral), and other important anatomic structures that may be studied using ultrasound. (From Done. *Color atlas of veterinary anatomy, vol. 3: The dog and cat.* London: Mosby; 2009.)

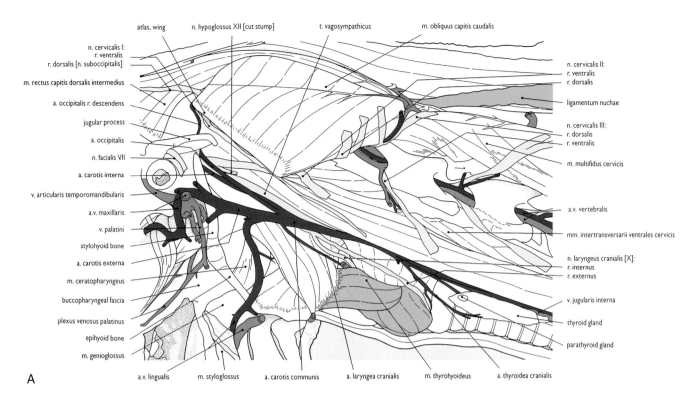

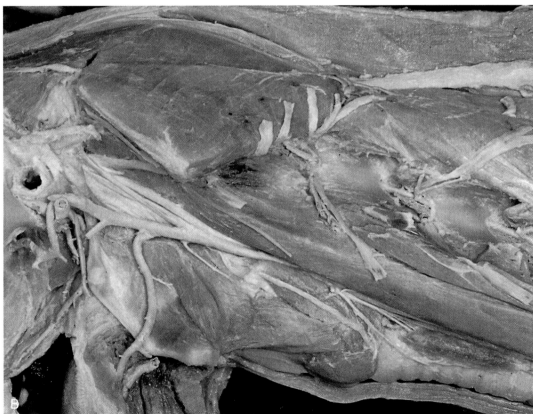

Figure 6-2 Illustration (A) and dissection (B) of the pharyngeal region of a dog. The carotid artery and its branches, and the vagosympathetic trunk are anatomic structures that may be evaluated using ultrasound. (From Done. *Color atlas of veterinary anatomy, vol. 3: The dog and cat.* London: Mosby; 2009.)

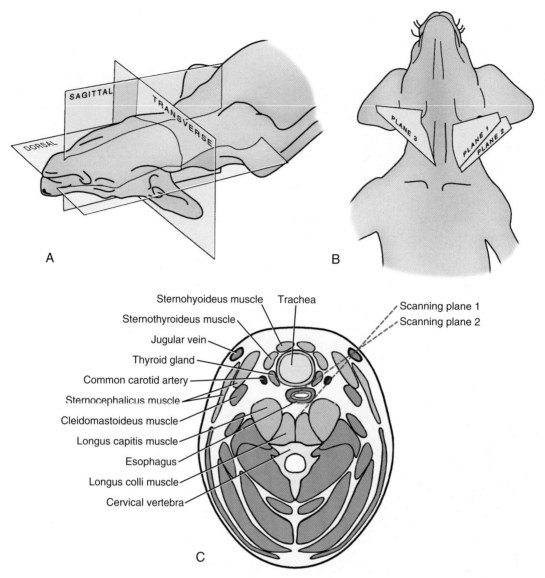

Figure 6-3 **A,** Defined anatomic planes. **B,** Imaging planes used for cervical ultrasound examination. **C,** Transverse section through the neck at the level of the thyroid glands. The approximate angle and anatomic path of imaging planes 1 and 2 are also shown. Structures that can usually be seen on ultrasound examination are labeled.

be confused with arterial pulsatile motion. The jugular veins join the right and left brachiocephalic veins, which in turn drain to the cranial vena cava. The confluence of the brachiocephalic veins into the cranial vena cava forms a Y-shaped anechoic tubular structure that can consistently be imaged (Figure 6-10). This is best imaged in a dorsal plane with the transducer positioned to the right of the trachea and manubrium. Figures 6-6, *A* and *C*, show Doppler evaluation of the jugular vein.

The trachea is readily identifiable because of its characteristic sonographic pattern created by the tracheal rings and acoustic shadowing, reverberation, and mirror image artifact. The long axis of the trachea is seen as a repeating hypoechoic and hyperechoic linear pattern in the near field, representing cartilaginous tracheal rings and fibroelastic annular ligaments of the trachea, respectively (Figure 6-11). A striking mirror image artifact of the trachea may be seen in some instances. In older dogs and in chondrodystrophic breeds, the cartilaginous rings may be mineralized and seen as hyperechoic,

reflective structures instead of hypoechoic cartilage. In cross section, the trachea is a curved, crescent-shaped structure with reverberation or mirror image artifact (Figure 6-12). The esophagus is located to the left of the trachea at the level of the thoracic inlet (see Figure 6-12). It is round, elliptic, or angular in cross section with a well-defined, moderately echogenic muscular wall. Small echogenic foci represent luminal gas centrally. On long axis, a striated pattern is created by echogenic gas within longitudinal folds of esophageal mucosa (Figure 6-13). Swallowing produces peristalsis that can be observed during real-time imaging.

Jugular Vein Thrombosis

Jugular vein thrombosis, a complication of infection, neoplasia, or venous catheter placement, may appear as a solid intraluminal mass of low to moderate echogenicity. Acute thrombi have minimal inherent echogenicity, however, and even total occlusion may appear normal on two-dimensional images. Depending on the cause and age of the thrombus, the lesion

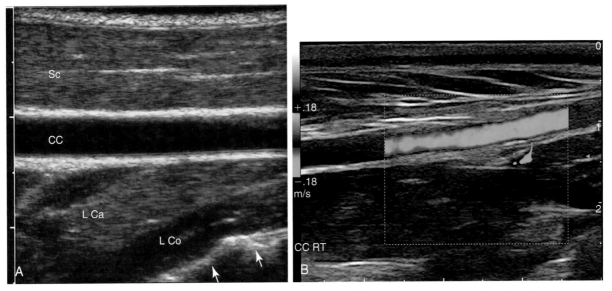

Figure 6-4 **Long-axis view of the common carotid artery (*CC*) of a normal dog in imaging plane 1.** **A,** The arterial lumen is anechoic and the vessel wall is well defined and hyperechoic. The sternocephalic muscle (*Sc*) is seen in the near field and has a characteristic hypoechoic, striated appearance. The longus capitis (*LCa*) and longus colli (*LCo*) are deep to the carotid artery in this imaging plane. The hyperechoic curvilinear structure in the lower right corner of the image represents the ventral margin of the midcervical vertebrae (*arrows*). **B,** Color Doppler longitudinal image of the common carotid artery in a dog. Blood flow is from right to left (the head is to the left).

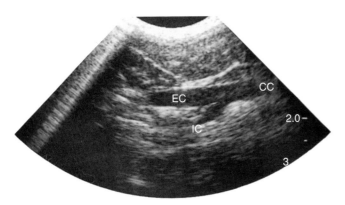

Figure 6-5 **Long-axis view of the carotid bifurcation of a normal dog in imaging plane 1.** The transducer is positioned at the level of the wing of the atlas. The common carotid (*CC*), external carotid (*EC*), and internal carotid (*IC*) arteries can be seen. The slight bulge at the origin of the internal carotid artery is the carotid sinus. A mechanical transducer was used. (From Wisner ER, Mattoon JS, Nyland TG, et al. Normal ultrasonographic anatomy of the canine neck. *Vet Radiol* 1991;32:185–90.)

may have a uniform, heterogeneous or complex appearance (Figure 6-14). The vessel wall may also appear thickened, particularly when thrombosis results from phlebitis, and the lumen is less compressible when transducer pressure is applied. Color or pulsed Doppler evaluation should generally be used to confirm reduced or absent flow (see Figure 6-14, *B*).[6-8]

Thrombi can also form secondary to venous aneurysmal dilations, which have been reported in the head and neck. A saccular dilatation of the left external jugular vein, consistent with a congenital jugular aneurysm, was diagnosed using ultrasound in an 18-month-old dog.[9] Multiple thrombi, which were heterogeneous in echogenicity, were identified within the aneurysm.

Carotid Arterial Thrombosis and Stenosis

Two-dimensional and color Doppler ultrasound examinations are commonly used in people to differentiate carotid artery stenosis from atherosclerotic plaque formation.[10-12] Although atherosclerotic disease is not a major concern in dogs and cats, carotid artery stenosis may occur from other causes, such as trauma, neoplasia, or previous surgery, and ultrasound may be useful in diagnosing the presence and the severity of stenosis. Two-dimensional ultrasound examination will reveal a change in arterial lumen shape or diameter, and color Doppler evaluation may show a change in lumen diameter and flow velocity at the stenosis site.

Arterial thrombi, although uncommon, may occasionally be seen with inflammatory disease or highly vascular invasive malignant neoplasms. The ultrasound findings of arterial thrombi are similar to those described for jugular thrombi.

Arteriovenous Malformations

Arteriovenous malformation may develop as a congenital lesion or as a sequela to trauma, neoplasia, or surgery. In our experience, arteriovenous malformation of the neck is most often associated with thyroid carcinoma. Clinical signs of local venous distention, presence of a bruit or palpable thrill, and evidence of left-sided heart failure from volume overload may be seen. Multiple tortuous, anechoic blood vessels may be seen on ultrasound examination, and most have a variable but distinctly arterial flow pattern on Doppler evaluation. Depending on the cause of the malformation, abnormal vessels may be associated with a mass, and variably echoic thrombi may occur in some vessels[4] (see Figure 6-14, *B* and *C*).

Neoplasia

Cervical ultrasonography can be used to determine the presence and extent of vascular invasion by primary cervical neoplasms and regional metastatic lymph nodes, particularly when surgical management is contemplated. Carotid wall invasion in humans has been described as a loss of discrete

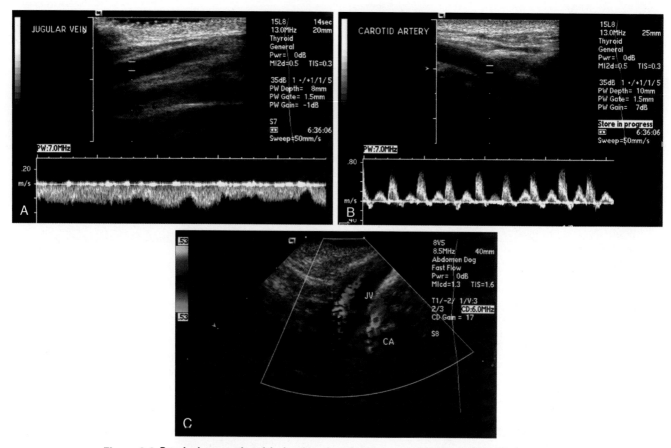

Figure 6-6 Doppler interrogation of the jugular vein and common carotid artery. A 13-MHz linear-array transducer was used for the B-mode images in **A** and **B**; pulsed wave Doppler frequency was 7 MHz. An 8.5-MHz Vector wide view array transducer was used for B-mode images in **C**, with color Doppler operating at 6 MHz. **A,** B-mode long-axis image of the jugular vein with a pulsed wave Doppler gate placed in the vessel lumen (top half of image; the thoracic inlet is to the left). Pulsed wave Doppler tracing shows the characteristic flow profile of the jugular vein. The blood flow is nonpulsatile and is directed below the baseline, indicating flow away from the transducer. Velocity is approximately 0.3 to 0.4 m/sec. **B,** B-mode long-axis image of the common carotid artery with a pulsed wave Doppler gate placed within the arterial lumen (top half of image; the thoracic inlet is to the right). Pulsed wave Doppler tracing shows characteristic pulsatile flow profile of the common carotid artery. Blood flow is directed upward, above the baseline, indicating flow toward the transducer during systole. Doppler signal below the baseline is reverse flow during diastole. Blood flow is approximately 0.6 m/sec. **C,** Color flow Doppler interrogation of the thoracic inlet showing the jugular vein (*JV*) and common carotid artery (*CA*). Blue color mapping within the lumen of the jugular vein indicates flow away from the transducer, toward the thoracic inlet. Red color mapping of the common carotid artery indicates flow toward the transducer, away from the thoracic inlet.

vessel wall echoes that demarcate the lesion from the vessel lumen.[13] In our experience, invasive malignant disease, usually thyroid carcinoma, produces compression and distortion of vessels, incorporation of normal vessels into the invading mass, and marked neovascularity or recruitment of small vessels. Enlarged metastatic or reactive lymph node aggregates may lie adjacent to vessel walls, obscuring both the vessel and node margins.

Carotid body tumors are also occasionally seen in dogs and appear as large, lobulated masses with hypoechoic and complex internal architectural detail and prominent vascularity.[4,14] One report of a presumed carotid body tumor describes its sonographic appearance as a sharply defined mass of uniform echogenicity at the bifurcation of the common carotid artery into the internal and external carotid arteries.[15]

NERVES

With the advanced technology of high frequency transducers and improved image quality, small discrete structures, such as nerves, can be readily identified. Small nerves in the cervical region have been identified in humans using ultrasound.[16] In one study, a linear-array transducer was used to identify the vagosympathetic trunk in 30 clinically normal dogs.[17] The vagosympathetic trunk was consistently located dorsomedial to the common carotid artery. Sonographically, the vagosympathetic trunk appeared as a round hypoechoic structure surrounded by hyperechoic connective tissue; its diameter was approximately 1 mm (mean 1.17 mm). Identification of the vagosympathetic trunk could be helpful in cases where a nerve abnormality is clinically suspected, a mass is identified in the area of the vagosympathetic trunk, or an injection is going to

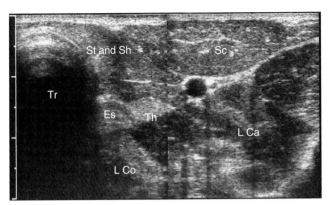

Figure 6-7 Composite transverse image of the left ventral cervical region of a normal dog. The left side of the image is near the ventral midline and the right side is ventrolateral. The transducer was positioned at the level of the left thyroid lobe. The left common carotid artery is the round anechoic structure in the center of the image. The thyroid lobe (*Th*) is positioned slightly medial to the carotid and has a uniform, moderately echoic appearance. Because the trachea (*Tr*) is air filled, only its ventral margin is seen. Reverberation artifact is present, and there is distal shadowing. The esophageal wall (*Es*) is also evident adjacent and slightly medial to the thyroid lobe. The sternocephalic (*Sc*), longus capitis (*LCa*), longus colli (*LCo*), and sternothyroid and sternohyoid (*St and Sh*) muscles all have a characteristic coarse heterogeneous, hypoechoic appearance in cross section. A 13-MHz linear-array transducer was used.

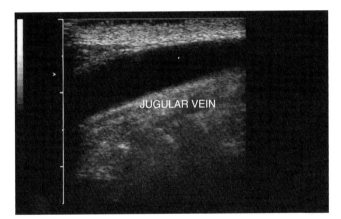

Figure 6-8 Longitudinal axis of a jugular vein. The lumen is anechoic and the wall is thin. Note its superficial location. The jugular vein becomes deeper as it enters the thoracic inlet (to the left).

be made in the same anatomic area. The vagosympathetic trunk in a dog is shown in Figure 6-15, C. A single case report of a neoplastic mass originating from the vagosympathetic trunk has also been described in the dog.[18] This mass was markedly heterogeneous and hypoechoic with multiple hyperechoic shadowing foci of mineral.

THYROID GLAND

The thyroid gland consists of two fusiform lobes, occasionally connected by a thin isthmus, adjacent to the ventral aspect of the tracheal wall and immediately caudal to the larynx. The thyroid gland is imaged on its long axis by first locating the

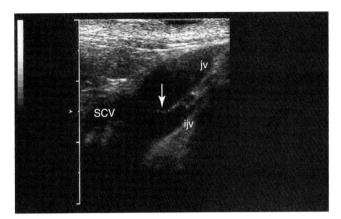

Figure 6-9 Dorsal plane image of the jugular vein (*jv*), subclavian vein (*SCV*), and internal jugular vein (*ijv*) at the level of the thoracic. A valve was present in the jugular vein (*arrow*).

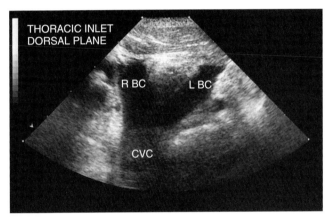

Figure 6-10 Dorsal plane image of the right and left brachiocephalic veins (*R BC, L BC*), entering the cranial vena cava (*CVC*). The brachiocephalic veins are the continuation of the jugular veins.

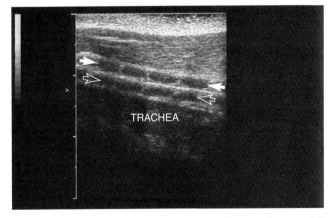

Figure 6-11 Sagittal oblique plane image of the mid to caudal cervical trachea in long axis in a 4-month-old puppy (between solid arrows). The hypoechoic elongate structures are cartilaginous tracheal rings. The smaller echogenic structures between the tracheal rings are the fibroelastic tracheal annular ligaments. A mirror image artifact of the trachea is present deep to the trachea (between open arrows). The sternothyroideus-sternohyoideus muscle is identified in the near field directly adjacent to the trachea as a homogeneous, finely striated structure.

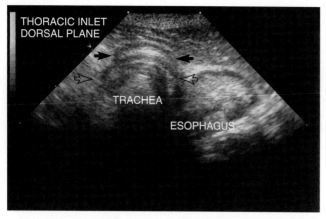

Figure 6-12 The trachea (*solid arrows*) and esophagus in transverse axes near the thoracic inlet. A thin hypoechoic esophageal wall is present with multiple hyperechoic foci centrally representing luminal gas. A mirror image artifact of the trachea is present (*open arrows*).

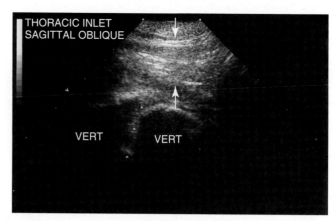

Figure 6-13 Thoracic inlet sagittal plane, left of midline. The esophagus is seen in its long axis (*arrows*). The highly echogenic linear structures represent longitudinal folds of mucosa with small amounts of trapped air. The ventral margins of two caudal cervical vertebrae (*VERT*) are seen as highly echogenic linear structures with complete distal acoustic shadowing. An intervertebral disk space is also seen (*asterisks*).

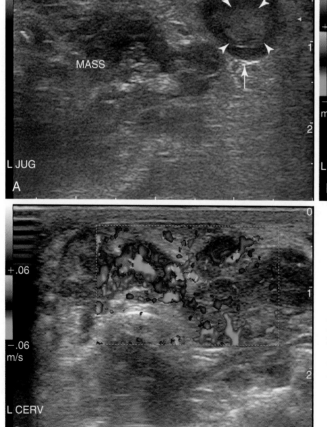

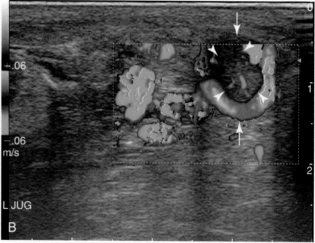

Figure 6-14 Jugular vein thrombosis associated with highly vascular cervical mass in a dog. **A,** An echogenic thrombus (*arrowheads*) is seen in the lumen of the jugular vein (*arrows*). A large, complex mass is present (*MASS*). **B,** Color Doppler shows the filling defect created by the thrombus (*arrowheads*) in the lumen of the jugular vein (*arrows*). Note the large amount of blood flow present within the cervical mass. **C,** Color Doppler of the cervical mass shows its highly vascular nature, not appreciated without the use of Doppler (compare to **A**). The appearance suggests arteriovenous malformation within the tumor.

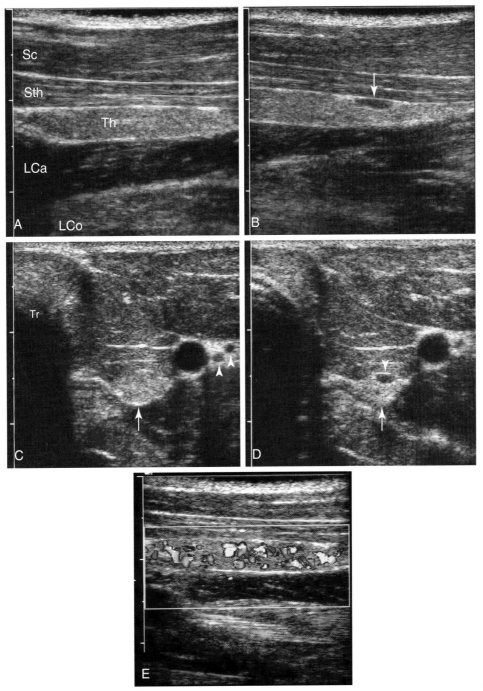

Figure 6-15 A, Long-axis view of a thyroid lobe *(Th)* of a normal dog in imaging plane 2. The thyroid lobe is medial to the carotid artery (not seen) in this imaging plane. Thyroid parenchyma is slightly more echoic and finer textured than adjacent cervical musculature and is surrounded by a thin hyperechoic sheath. The sternocephalic *(Sc)* and sternothyroid *(Sth)* muscles are superficial to the thyroid, and the longus capitis *(LCa)* and longus colli *(LCo)* are seen in the far field. **B,** Same thyroid lobe as in **A** with the transducer positioned slightly more caudally and through a slightly different long-axis plane. A well-defined thyroidal vessel is seen within the thyroid parenchyma *(arrow).* Vascularity was confirmed by verifying blood flow with color Doppler imaging (not shown). **C,** Transverse image of the same thyroid lobe *(arrow).* The common carotid artery serves as a landmark that is lateral and adjacent to the thyroid. Overlying sternocephalic and sternohyoid-sternothyroid muscles are also seen in this image. Shadowing from the trachea *(Tr)* is present on the left. The two smaller circular structures lateral to the common carotid artery are the vagosympathetic trunk and the internal jugular vein *(arrowheads).* **D,** Transverse image of the same thyroid lobe *(large arrow)* with the transducer positioned slightly more caudally. The thyroidal blood vessel seen in long axis in image **B** is now evident *(arrowhead)* and should not be mistaken for a parathyroid gland or thyroid cyst. **E,** Color Doppler image similar to the long-axis image shown in **A** verifies that thyroids are uniformly and highly vascular. This fact should be taken into account before biopsy of thyroid lesions is considered.

common carotid artery in plane 1 in the cranial cervical region. The scanning plane is then rotated ventrally and medially to image the thyroid gland just medial to the common carotid artery (see Figure 6-1, imaging plane 2). If the scan plane is rotated too far, the tracheal wall is seen in its long axis and appears as a prominent hyperechoic continuous line adjacent to which are uniformly spaced, focal hypoechoic regions corresponding to the tracheal cartilage rings[5] (see Figure 6-11). Because the thyroid conforms to the curvature of the tracheal wall, the thyroid lobe may not be seen in its entirety in its long axis without rocking the transducer back and forth slightly.

Thyroid lobes are homogeneous, well marginated, and fusiform (see Figures 6-15 and 6-16). The echogenicity of the thyroid is less than that of the surrounding adventitia but greater than that of the cervical musculature. In medium-sized dogs, each thyroid lobe measures approximately 2.5 to 3 cm and 0.4 to 0.6 cm in the long and short axes, respectively; in cats, the same measurements are 2 cm and 0.2 to 0.3 cm.[5,19,20] In one study of normal beagle dogs, the mean (90% confidence interval) measurements of the thyroid glands were 2.45 cm in length, 0.62 cm in width, 0.53 cm in height, and 0.38 cm^3 in volume, using the equation length × width × height × 0.479. In this study, length had the largest intraobserver and interobserver variability, and height and volume had the lowest variability.[21] Additionally, volume of the thyroid glands has been correlated to body surface area and weight in small, medium, and large dogs.[22] Once the thyroid gland is imaged in plane 2, thyroidal blood vessels can be seen in some dogs by rocking the transducer back and forth (see Figure 6-15, B and D). In the transverse plane, the thyroid gland appears as an oval or roughly triangular structure adjacent and medial to the common carotid artery, deep to the sternohyoid and sternothyroid muscles, and lateral to the trachea[5] (see Figure 6-15, C). A higher frequency transducer (10 to 13 MHz) is necessary to see the normal feline thyroid gland in the transverse plane.[20] Ectopic thyroid tissue may occasionally be found in the caudal cervical region, the thoracic inlet, or the cranial mediastinum and can be missed, either from an inadequate imaging window or from an incomplete examination.

Two-dimensional thyroid ultrasound examination is used to diagnose both diffuse and focal parenchymal disease, to differentiate cystic and solid lesions, and to determine whether lesions are solitary or multiple. Coupled with color Doppler evaluation, it can also be used to differentiate highly vascular from poorly vascular or nonvascular lesions; however, although thyroid lesions can be well characterized anatomically, definitive diagnosis often requires fine-needle or tissue-core biopsy.[4,23,24] In addition, thyroid ultrasound findings may be normal or equivocal despite the presence of abnormal thyroid function.

Thyroid Cysts
Irregularly margined, anechoic cysts, with or without septations, have been found in thyroid lobes of hyperthyroid cats and may also occasionally be seen in dogs as an incidental finding during routine thyroid examination[20] (Figure 6-17). Thyroid cysts can be differentiated from intraparenchymal thyroid blood vessels by verifying a round or oval shape in two imaging planes and by documenting no flow (see Figure 6-17, B). Cystic lesions can be confused with normal parathyroid glands, which are also hypoechoic to anechoic (Figure 6-18). Aspirated fluid from thyroid cysts is usually straw colored, hemorrhagic, or dark brown, often with elevated levels of thyroid hormone.

Hypothyroidism
Ultrasonography of the thyroid glands can also be used to diagnose hypothyroidism. In comparison to euthyroid dogs and dogs with euthyroid sick syndrome, the thyroid glands in dogs with hypothyroidism have been shown to have any or all of the following: a round or oval shape in the transverse plane, a decrease in echogenicity, heterogeneous echogenicity, irregular capsule, abnormal shape, and significant decrease in size.[25-27] In one study, using a cut-off thyroid volume value of 0.05 mL/kg$^{0.75}$ resulted in a sensitivity of 81% and specificity of 96% for hypothyroidism.[25]

Thyroiditis
Thyroiditis associated with production of thyroid hormone antibodies has been found in the dog[28-31] and may be seen in up to one third of dogs with hypothyroidism.[31] Autoimmune thyroiditis, or chronic lymphocytic thyroiditis, is comparable to Hashimoto thyroiditis of humans and is often associated with clinical signs of hypothyroidism. Thyroiditis as a result of extension of cellulitis of the cervical region may also occur; it may be associated with regional lymphadenopathy and abscess formation.

Thyroiditis in humans appears as generalized thyroid enlargement with a nonuniform hypoechoic pattern, with or without a nodular appearance.[3,32-37] The deeper portions of the lobes have a washed-out appearance demonstrating no far wall accentuation, and this appearance is probably due to thyroid inflammation and edema.[35] We have seen a number of dogs with ventral cervical cellulitis or abscesses that have had prominent thyroid lobes with mildly diminished echogenicity and decreased thyroid margin definition. These changes are also likely to be caused by inflammation of the affected thyroid and associated edema formation.

Hyperthyroidism
Ultrasonographic changes in patients, most commonly cats, have been described. When measuring thyroid size on ultrasonography, often the length of the thyroid gland is similar between normal and hyperthyroid cats; however, the overall

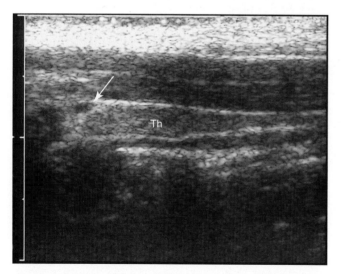

Figure 6-16 Long-axis view of thyroid lobe (*Th*) of a normal cat in imaging plane 2. A thin hyperechoic sheath is seen surrounding the thyroid lobe. Because the thyroid conforms to the curvature of the tracheal wall, the entire thyroid lobe may not be seen without rocking the transducer back and forth slightly. The caudal pole and the middle of the thyroid lobe are well visualized but the cranial pole is obscured in this image. A thyroidal vessel (*arrow*), verified by Doppler analysis (not shown), is seen near the cranial pole.

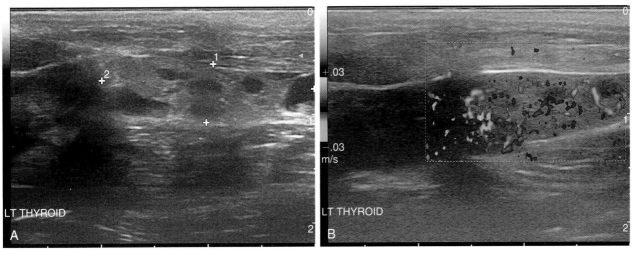

Figure 6-17 **Bilateral thyroid follicular cysts in a 14-year-old Lhasa apso with a 6-month history of elevated calcium. A,** Sagittal image of the left thyroid gland (between electronic cursors; 1.98 cm long, 0.54 cm high). Multiple hypoechoic foci are present within the gland (1 to 2 mm), proven to be thyroid follicular cysts. **B,** Color Doppler examination of the left thyroid gland shows good parenchymal blood flow, with limited signal within the follicular cysts. This dog had bilateral thyroid follicular cystic disease and bilateral parathyroid adenomas (see Figure 6-25).

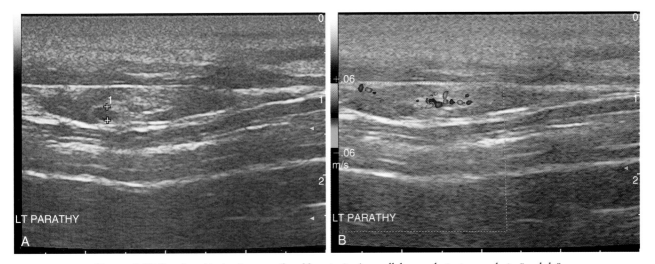

Figure 6-18 **Parathyroid gland versus thyroid cyst. A,** A small hypoechoic to anechoic "nodule" (between electronic cursors, 0.17 cm) in a normal dog's left thyroid gland. **B,** Color Doppler shows good parenchymal blood flow but no flow in the small nodule. This was considered to be an internal parathyroid gland, but lack of blood flow warrants consideration of a small thyroid follicular cyst. This example in a clinically normal dog illustrates the difficulty in differentiating the two. Clinical signs and serum calcium levels must be used to rank probability.

volume is significantly different between the two groups.[20,38] The mean volume for individual lobes in hyperthyroid cats is calculated as maximum length × width × height × π/6. In hyperthyroid cats the volume of the lobes has been reported to be 382 and 572 mm³ on the left and 552 and 782 mm³ on the right.[20,38] In comparison, the mean thyroid lobe volume in normal control cats was determined to be 85 mm.[3,20] Differences between the volumes between the two studies may be due to the method the method used to determine the width of the gland, either an arbitrary value or a measured value. Ultrasound of cat thyroid glands for hyperthyroidism is not universally practiced, given the usefulness of blood work and nuclear medicine in assessing this disease (Figure 6-19).

Neoplasia

Adenomas and carcinomas of the thyroid occur in both the dog[39-44] and cat.[39,44-46] Thyroid ultrasound examination is useful for verifying thyroid origin of a palpable ventral cervical mass. It is also used to characterize known thyroid masses presurgically and to determine the margins of invasive neoplasms. Ultrasound-guided chemoablation or thermal ablation of both benign and malignant thyroid lesions has been used as an alternative to surgery.

Functional thyroid adenomas commonly occur in adult cats and involve both lobes in approximately 70% of affected animals. Ectopic thyroid tissue, either within the caudal cervical region or within the cranial mediastinum, may also

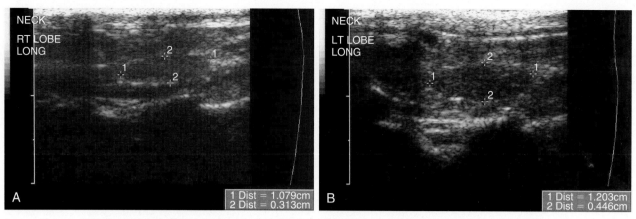

Figure 6-19 **Bilateral, asymmetric feline hyperthyroidism. A,** The right thyroid lobe is essentially normal in size and shape (between electronic cursors). **B,** The left thyroid lobe is larger, more plump, and slightly lobulated compared to the right (between electronic cursors). Nuclear scintigraphy showed this patient had bilateral, asymmetric hyperthyroidism.

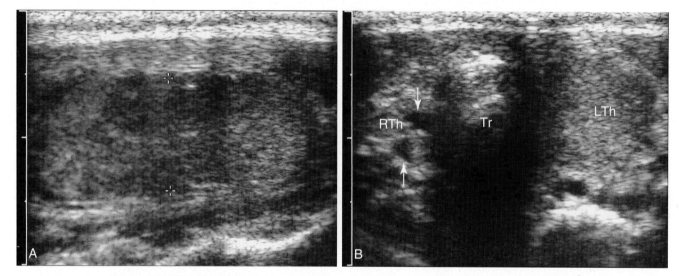

Figure 6-20 **Hyperthyroid cat. A,** Long-axis view of the left thyroid lobe in imaging plane 2. The thyroid lobe measures approximately 9 mm in its short axis and is uniformly hypoechoic. **B,** Short-axis view of the ventral cervical region of the same cat acquired in a transverse imaging plane. In this instance, the transducer was positioned on midline to image both thyroid lobes. The left thyroid lobe (*Th*) is markedly enlarged. Although smaller than the left, the right lobe (*Th*) is also larger than normal, suggesting bilateral hyperthyroidism. Two small, irregularly shaped thyroid cysts (*arrows*) are also present in the right thyroid lobe. Reverberation and shadowing artifacts are owing to air within the trachea (*Tr*).

be present in a small percentage of hyperthyroid cats.[45,47,48] Although thyroid function tests and thyroid scintigraphy are considered the most accurate methods for diagnosis of hyperthyroidism and determination of the anatomic distribution of abnormal thyroid tissue, ultrasound examination can be of value in differentiating morphologically abnormal lobes from normal lobes when scintigraphy is not readily available. Such information may be important for differentiating unilateral from bilateral disease and for determining the affected lobe in patients with unilateral disease when thyroidectomy is contemplated.

Affected thyroid lobes are larger than normal, have well-defined margins, and have a homogeneous to inhomogeneous parenchymal pattern of low echogenicity on ultrasound examination (Figure 6-20; also see Figure 6-19). Some thyroid lobes become tubular and particularly large in the short axis (see Figure 6-20). In some instances, well-defined nodular lesions are surrounded by more normal-looking thyroid parenchyma, whereas the entire thyroid lobe is affected in others. Thyroid lobe margins may become lobulated, and solitary or multicameral cystic lesions often develop within the parenchyma. Ectopic thyroid tissue within the neck can occasionally be identified on ultrasound examination and must be differentiated from lymph nodes and cervical musculature.[20]

Thyroid carcinoma is seen in both the dog[14,39,44,49] and the cat[42,44,46] and may be either nonfunctional or functional.[39,46] In general, carcinomas tend to be unilateral, large, rapidly growing invasive masses that can lead to significant anatomic distortion and upper airway obstruction. Thyroid carcinomas appear ultrasonographically as large, inhomogeneous masses, with variable margination and echogenicity that is usually less than that of normal thyroid tissue (Figures 6-21 to 6-23). Invasion

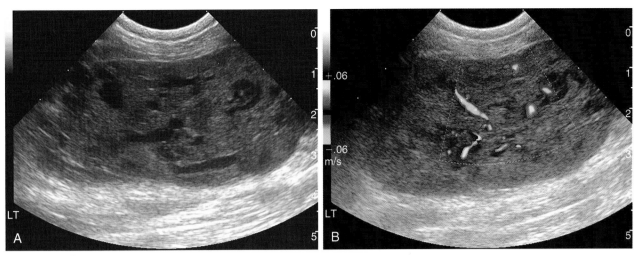

Figure 6-21 **Thyroid carcinoma in a 9-year-old Labrador mix with labored breathing. A,** Sagittal image of a large mass arising from the left thyroid lobe. Multiple anechoic areas are present with in the mass. **B,** Color Doppler shows the anechoic areas are vascular.

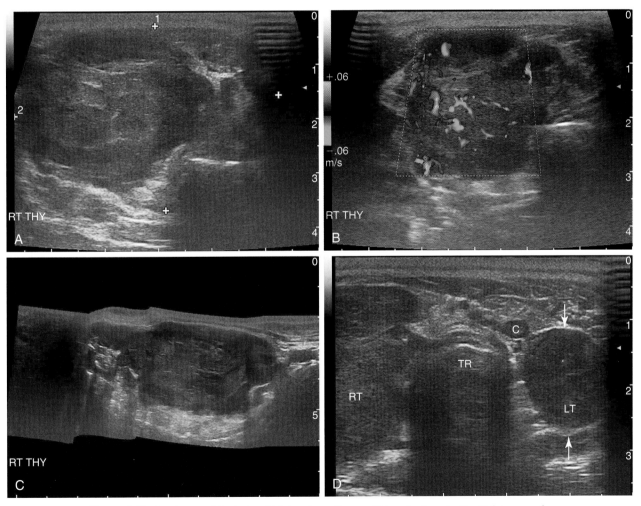

Figure 6-22 **Carcinoma of both thyroid lobes in an 8-year-old beagle dog. A,** Sagittal image of a portion of the right lobe of the thyroid gland showing a complex, solid mass with irregular margins in the deeper tissues (between electronic cursors; 3.40 × 4.95 cm). **B,** Color Doppler shows characteristic high vascularity of thyroid carcinomas. **C,** Extended field of view sagittal image shows the extent of the large right thyroid lobe mass and its irregular margins. **D,** Transverse image shows a portion of the right thyroid lobe mass (*RT*) and the enlarged, abnormal left thyroid lobe (*LT*, *arrows*). C, Common carotid artery; *TR*, trachea.

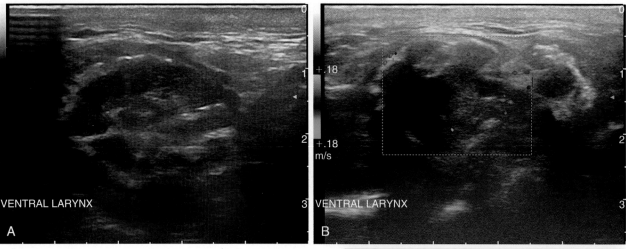

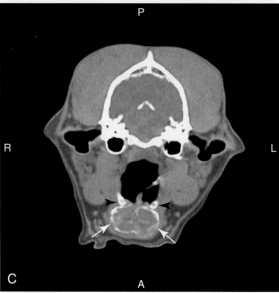

Figure 6-23 **Calcified thyroid carcinoma. A,** A very complex mass is located adjacent to the larynx. It could not be determined sonographically that its origin was the thyroid gland. **B,** The mass is not well vascularized. **C,** A CT examination shows the calcific nature of the mass (*arrows*) and its relationship to the hyoid bones (*black arrowheads*). The CT image is shown in a soft tissue window and level.

of the common carotid arteries, jugular veins, and esophagus may also be detected. Metastasis to regional lymph nodes frequently occurs, and cervical nodes should be evaluated accordingly[4,50] Fine-needle aspiration combined with ultrasound examination is an accurate method for definitive diagnosis and is preferable to tissue-core biopsy because of the rich blood supply and tendency of these lesions to hemorrhage profusely.

Nonsurgical chemoablation of thyroid tissue has been performed in people and dogs with thyroid neoplasia.[50-53] We have performed this technique on a number of dogs with nonresectable invasive thyroid carcinoma as a palliative measure.[50] Absolute ethanol (98% pure medical grade), in a volume adequate to distribute throughout the tumor parenchyma, is injected into the mass by ultrasound guidance. Although precisely calculated injection doses are reported in the human literature, the actual volume depends on the size and tissue characteristics of a particular mass. We use a target volume of at least half the estimated tumor volume initially. Injection is repeated a minimum of four times at 3-week intervals. Initial response varies from significant tumor volume reduction to an arrest of further growth. We currently have inadequate data for intermediate and long-term outcomes. Care must be taken to avoid injecting nearby structures, such as the carotid artery and recurrent laryngeal or vagus nerve. Even with accurate deposition, alcohol diffusion can affect these normal structures. Because these lesions are highly vascularized, systemic alcohol toxicity can also occur when large injection volumes are used.

Ultrasound-guided ethanol ablation of thyroid adenomas in hyperthyroid cats has also been reported with variable results. In the six cats in which the procedure was performed, one died after injection of both lobes, and other cats showed transient signs of Horner syndrome, gagging or laryngeal paralysis, and recurrence of hyperthyroidism. Long-term response of the surviving cats was not reported, although four of five surviving cats were euthyroid at least 2 weeks after injection.[54]

Radiofrequency heat ablation of thyroid nodules using ultrasound guidance has also been performed in cases of feline hyperthyroidism. In one case series of nine cats, the serum total T_4 and thyroxine concentrations decreased following either one or two treatments, and the cats remained euthyroid for an average of 4 months.[55] However, hyperthyroidism eventually recurred in all cats within 0 to 18 months following the procedure. Adverse side effects of the procedure included ipsilateral, transient Horner syndrome in two cases and laryngeal paralysis in one.

Ultrasound is also useful in determining the volume of the thyroid gland for calculation of radiopharmaceutical dose in patients receiving[56] iodine therapy. Ultrasound can also then be used to monitor response to therapy.[57,58] In a population

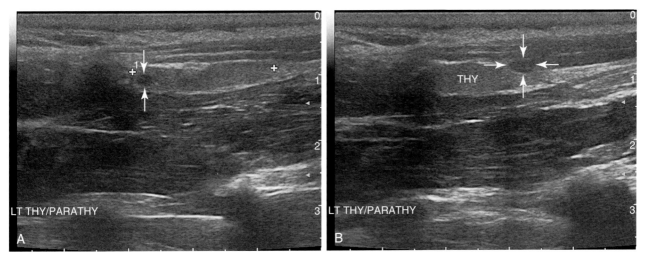

Figure 6-24 **Normal thyroid and parathyroid glands in a dog. A,** Sagittal image of the left thyroid gland (between electronic cursors, 2.20 cm in length) with a cranial, internal parathyroid gland (*arrows*) seen as a small focus of hypoechoic tissue. It measured approximately 1 × 2 mm. **B,** Same thyroid gland (*THY*) with a slightly different sagittal scan plane showing an external, caudally positioned parathyroid gland (*arrows*).

of hyperthyroid cats, sonographically detectable changes in the thyroid glands were detected approximately 6 months following treatment with[56] iodine when compared to the pretreatment examinations. The thyroid glands decreased in volume, became less round and heterogeneous, and had reduced vascularity as assessed with power Doppler imaging.[38]

PARATHYROID GLANDS

There are normally four parathyroid glands in the dog and cat. The two cranially located glands are usually found in the extrathyroidal fascia of the cranial pole of the thyroid gland. The caudal parathyroid glands are more commonly embedded within the parenchyma of the caudal pole of the thyroid. The location and number of parathyroid glands may vary significantly. Abnormalities associated with increased parathyroid function can be divided into primary and secondary hyperparathyroidism. Secondary hyperparathyroidism resulting in parathyroid gland hyperplasia is more common and is usually associated with chronic renal disease or nutritional deficits. Functional parathyroid adenomas are uncommon, and parathyroid carcinomas are rare in the dog and cat.[39] To confuse matters, solitary parathyroid lesions are sometimes characterized histologically as primary hyperplasia or adenomatous hyperplasia. The lines between hyperplasia, adenoma, and adenocarcinoma are blurred, and in all likelihood, these terms represent arbitrary points along a continuum of disease. Fortunately, surgical excision or nonsurgical ablation of a solitary lesion is most often curative, regardless of cell type, which makes the distinction less important.

Parathyroid ultrasound examination is a rapid, low-cost, and noninvasive diagnostic screening test for suspected hyperparathyroidism.[59-64] Preoperative parathyroid localization has been shown to significantly reduce surgical time in humans,[60] and we also find this to be true in dogs and cats.

Normal parathyroid glands are infrequently seen with use of lower frequency transducers (5 to 7 MHz).[5] However, they are often incidental findings when higher frequency transducers (10 to 13 MHz) are used in dogs with normal parathyroid function (Figure 6-24). Normal parathyroid glands appear as well-marginated, round or oval, hypoechoic structures within

or adjacent to the thyroid gland; they typically measure 2 mm or less in diameter, although larger parathyroid glands are occasionally seen in clinically normal dogs. In one recent study of dogs (33 to 78 lb), the average size of the parathyroid glands, as assessed using a high frequency transducer, was 3.3 mm × 2.2 mm × 1.7 mm, which closely matched the gross size of the glands.[65]

The enlarged parathyroid gland is generally round or oval and is anechoic or hypoechoic compared with the surrounding thyroid gland parenchyma.[59,66-70] Larger lesions may also cause far-field enhancement, and they may occasionally be in the midbody of the involved thyroid lobe rather than at either pole. Enlarged parathyroid glands that are isoechoic to thyroid parenchyma have occasionally been seen in humans[67,68] but have not been recognized in dogs or cats.

Accuracy of parathyroid imaging depends on the skill and experience of the sonographer. Errors usually result from small lesion size, poor margination, and ectopia or an inability to differentiate a parathyroid lesion from a blood vessel, thyroid nodule, or cyst.[2,34,64,65,69,71-74] Ultrasound-guided fine-needle aspiration biopsy can be used to differentiate parathyroid lesions from thyroid lesions, but parathyroid hyperplasia, adenoma, and adenocarcinoma cannot be distinguished in this manner.[2,75]

Parathyroid Hyperplasia and Adenoma

Parathyroid hyperplasia, adenomas, and adenocarcinomas appear similar, and differentiation by ultrasonography alone may not be possible.[19,76,77] In a study of 33 dogs with hypercalcemia, dogs with parathyroid lesions measuring 4 mm or larger in diameter had a much greater likelihood of having an adenoma (Figure 6-25) or adenocarcinoma, whereas dogs with lesions less than 4 mm were more likely to have parathyroid hyperplasia.[67] However, in another study of dogs with renal failure, enlargement of the parathyroid glands, which was presumed secondary to hyperplasia of the glands, was greater (size up to 8 mm) in dogs with chronic renal failure when compared to normal dogs and dogs in acute renal failure.[78]

In humans, the presence of multiple enlarged parathyroid glands suggests parathyroid hyperplasia, often from secondary hyperparathyroidism associated with chronic renal insufficiency.[63,79] We have also seen multiple ill-defined, hypoechoic

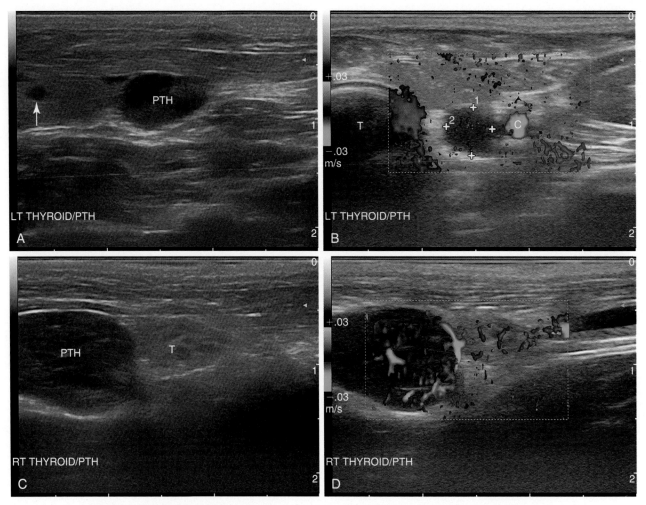

Figure 6-25 **Bilateral parathyroid adenomas and thyroid follicular cysts in a 14-year-old Lhasa apso with a 6-month history of elevated calcium.** **A,** A relatively large hypoechoic nodule (*PTH*) is present associated with the caudal portion of the left thyroid gland (approximately 8 × 4 mm), proven to be a parathyroid adenoma. A small thyroid follicular cyst is seen (*arrow*). **B,** Color Doppler transverse image through the hypoechoic left parathyroid nodule (between electronic cursors, 0.44 × 0.43 cm). Doppler motion artifact is present associated with the trachea (*T*) to the left (red signal); a transverse image of the common carotid artery (*C*) is present to the right, showing blood flow depicted in blue. **C,** Sagittal image of the right thyroid gland (*T*) showing a relatively large hypoechoic parathyroid nodule (*PTH*) associated with the cranial pole. Hypoechoic foci are present within the thyroid tissue as noted for the left. **D,** Color Doppler evaluation of image **C** shows good blood flow within the right parathyroid nodule and the thyroid tissue.

or anechoic nodules, usually measuring 2 mm or less and consistent with parathyroid hyperplasia, in dogs with renal failure.[77]

On the other hand, most patients with solitary lesions have parathyroid adenomas, although solitary primary hyperplastic nodules diagnosed by ultrasonography and confirmed at surgery have been reported in both dogs and humans.[39,76,77,80,81]

In one report of two hypercalcemic cats, ultrasound identified echogenic masses (>1 cm) with anechoic or hypoechoic cavitations in the cervical region; the masses were histologically confirmed as parathyroid adenomas.[82]

Parathyroid adenomas and solitary hyperplastic nodules in people have been treated nonsurgically with moderate success by percutaneous ultrasound-guided ethanol injection.[83-86] In some cases, multiple injections are required, and hypercalcemia can eventually return.[84,86] Despite these drawbacks, nonsurgical treatment has been advocated for those human

patients in whom surgical intervention is unsuitable.[84] Ultrasound-guided chemical ablation of parathyroid adenomas in dogs has also been reported.[70,81] Ethanol (98%) was injected directly into parathyroid glands until there was evidence of ethanol diffusion throughout the mass. In the initial study, a single injection was performed in seven dogs, and two injections were required in one dog.[70] Parathyroid hormone levels were reduced in all dogs soon after injection, and normocalcemia was maintained through 6-month follow-up in all but one dog.

Thermal ablation of parathyroid adenomas has been reported, and initial results suggest that this method may produce a more definitive response than chemoablation.[87] A radiofrequency probe is placed into the lesion with ultrasound guidance, and controlled heat is deposited into the tissue locally until complete ablation occurs. More of these procedures must be performed in dogs to determine their long-term efficacy.

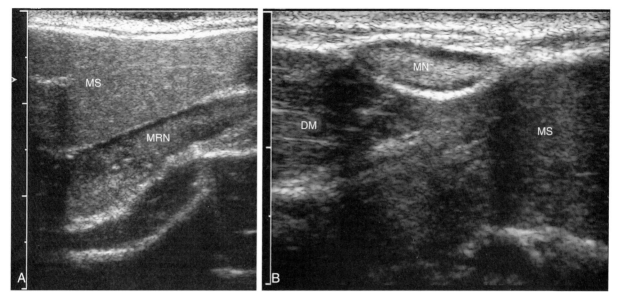

Figure 6-26 **Normal canine retropharyngeal and mandibular lymph nodes. A,** Long-axis view of a medial retropharyngeal lymph node (*MRN*) in imaging plane 3. The node is long and thin with well-defined borders. Node parenchyma is hypoechoic, most noticeably in the peripheral areas corresponding to the subcapsular sinus and cortex. In this example, multiple small target-like structures within the parenchyma could represent lymph node follicles. In most instances, node parenchyma has a more uniform appearance, particularly when lower frequency transducers are used. The uniformly, moderately echoic structure in the near field is the mandibular salivary gland (*MS*). **B,** Superficially located mandibular lymph node (*MN*) in an oblique imaging plane. Characteristics of this node are similar to those described in **A.** The node is superficial and cranial to the mandibular salivary gland (*MS*), and superficial and caudal to the digastric muscle (*DM*). These node groups often consist of two or three closely aggregated nodes.

Parathyroid Carcinoma

Although parathyroid adenocarcinomas may, on average, be slightly larger than adenomas, ultrasound findings are otherwise identical, and differentiation of benign and malignant lesions is not possible.[77,88] In one retrospective review of 19 dogs with carcinoma of the parathyroid glands, a solitary parathyroid nodule was found on ultrasound in 14 of the 17 dogs examined, whereas 3 dogs had additional smaller nodules identified.[89] The size of the nodules ranged from 5 to 25 mm (median, 7 mm) in diameter. Invasion of parathyroid carcinoma into surrounding tissues is described in humans, although no such findings have been reported in dogs and cats.[77,88,90,91]

LYMPH NODES

Major lymph node groups of the head and neck include parotid, mandibular, lateral and medial retropharyngeal, and superficial and deep cervical lymph nodes. Parotid, mandibular, and retropharyngeal lymph nodes are paired; each side consists of a single node or an aggregate node group. The superficial lymphatics consist of a variable number of lymph nodes embedded in fascia on the lateral aspect of the ventral serratus and scalene muscles at the cranial margin of the supraspinous muscle. The deep cervical region has a chain of small lymph nodes near the lateral and ventral wall of the trachea in the cranial, middle, and caudal neck.[92] Most of the lymph nodes of the head and neck are small, measuring 5 mm or less in short-axis diameter and less than 1 cm in length; however, the medial retropharyngeal nodes are typically larger. The medial retropharyngeal lymph nodes have also been measured using ultrasound in presumed normal dogs, with the mean and maximum sizes reported.[93] Regardless of body

weight (1.8 to 59 kg) or age (1 to 15 years) in this population of dogs, the mean (and maximum) measurements were as follows: 2.5 cm (maximum, 5 cm) in length, 1.0 cm (maximum, 2 cm) in width and 0.5 cm (maximum, 1 cm) in height. These measurements are similar to prior references on medial retropharyngeal lymph node size.[92]

Mandibular, retropharyngeal, and larger cervical lymph nodes can be seen in normal dogs and cats when higher frequency transducers are used (Figure 6-26), but because of the variation in size and distribution of normal nodes, each node or node group may not be consistently seen in every patient. When they are seen, normal nodes generally appear as well-defined, hypoechoic oval or elongate structures less than 0.5 cm in short-axis diameter.

Reactive Lymph Nodes and Lymph Node Abscess

Inflammatory lymph nodes are often enlarged to a variable degree and appear homogeneously hypoechoic (Figure 6-27). Loss of definition of the affected lymph node margins is also a common finding and is thought to be caused by edema and cellulitis in those instances in which a regional extranodal inflammatory response is present.[94] Central cavitation of abscessed lymph nodes may also occur and should be differentiated from necrosis and hemorrhage of metastatic nodes. However, differentiation of reactive lymph nodes from metastatic nodes by ultrasound appearance alone can be difficult, and thus ultrasound-guided fine-needle aspirates of the solid components of suspicious nodes are often required for definitive diagnosis.

Neoplasia Metastasis

Because metastatic lymph nodes up to 12 mm in diameter can be missed on physical examination, ultrasonography may

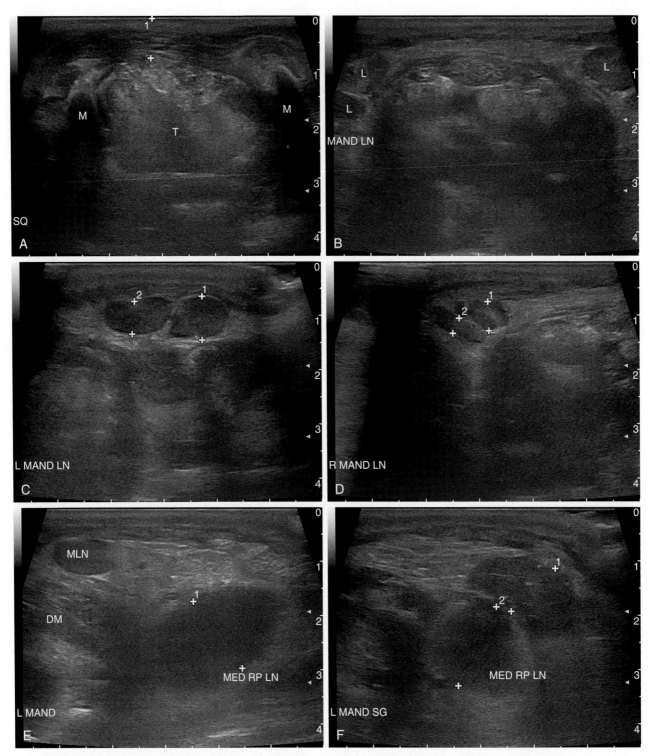

Figure 6-27 Ventral mandibular cellulitis with associated regional lymph node reaction. A, Transverse images through thickened soft tissues ventral to the mandible. *M,* Right and left hemimandibles with acoustic shadowing; *T,* tongue. **B,** Transverse image of the ventral mandible made caudal to *A.* Mandibular lymph node enlargement is present bilaterally (*L*). **C,** Detail image of enlarged left mandibular lymph nodes (between electronic cursors, 0.60 and 0.80 cm). **D,** Detailed image of enlarged right mandibular lymph nodes (between electronic cursors, 0.54 and 0.30 cm). **E,** Enlarged left mandibular lymph node (*MLN*) and retropharyngeal lymph node (1.54 cm between electronic cursors). *DM,* Digastric muscle. **F,** Enlarged left medial retropharyngeal lymph node (*MED RP LN,* D2 1.62 cm between electronic cursors) and its relationship to the left mandibular salivary gland (D1 1.14 cm between electronic cursors).

be used as a rapid adjunctive means to locate metastatic nodes and determine whether muscle, vessel wall, or subcutaneous invasion has occurred.[94-97] Ultrasound examination is particularly useful in conjunction with fine-needle aspiration or biopsy of the lymph node, especially when other criteria for determining node status are equivocal.[98-101]

Researchers have attempted to differentiate benign and malignant lymph nodes based on echogenicity, size, shape, and vascularity; however, metastatic nodes may appear similar to reactive nodes (Figure 6-28). Metastatic lymph nodes are often, but not always, enlarged and are typically hypoechoic compared with surrounding tissue (Figure 6-29). Central necrosis and hemorrhage can also occur with marked enlargement from rapid tumor growth, resulting in nodal parenchyma that appears complex.[94,99,102-104] In humans, criteria for determining malignancy include a short-axis diameter greater than 10 mm, rounding of the normally oval or flattened node shape, and irregular node margins. Short-to-long axis ratios have also been used in people to differentiate malignant from benign nodal disease; a malignant node has a higher ratio, with an average of approximately 0.7. This ratio also appears to apply to superficial lymph nodes in dogs, where malignant nodes have a ratio greater than 0.7[105] (see Figures 6-28 and 6-29). Using the criterion of shape change alone, up to 80% of enlarged lymph nodes are truly metastatic; enlargement of the remainder is caused by benign hyperplasia.[96,106,107]

Doppler assessment of lymph node vascularity has also been used when trying to distinguish between benign and malignant lymphadenopathy using ultrasound. The number of vessels and amount of blood flow in the lymph node was shown to be significantly less in benign lymph nodes when compared to malignant lymph nodes in one study in dogs.[104] Additionally, in an attempt to quantify differences between benign and malignant superficial lymph nodes, assessing the analysis of the spectral Doppler waveforms from intranodal blood flow can be performed. One study determined resistive and pulsatile indices to be higher in cases of malignancy, with metastatic lymph nodes having higher values than lymphomatous, reactive or normal lymph nodes.[105] For the differentiation of neoplasia and inflammation, the cut-off values of resistive index and pulsatile index used in this study were 0.68 and 1.49 respectively. Additionally, in a later study in which

pulsed-wave spectral Doppler analysis was used to distinguish between neoplastic and inflammatory disease in peripheral lymph nodes, the peak systolic velocity–to–end-diastolic velocity ratio using the first spectral tracing was the most accurate diagnostic parameter, with a cut-off value of 3.22.[108] The resistive index value of 0.69 yielded the highest diagnostic accuracy.

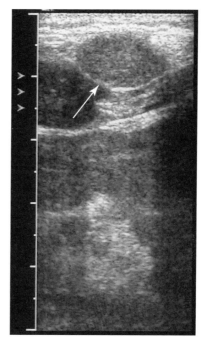

Figure 6-28 Adult dog with regional lymph node metastasis from an invasive thyroid carcinoma; long-axis image of a mandibular lymph node in an oblique imaging plane (*arrow*). Although the node is within normal limits for length, it has a higher than expected short-to-long axis ratio and appears rounded. The heterogeneous structure deep to the node represents a portion of the thyroid carcinoma.

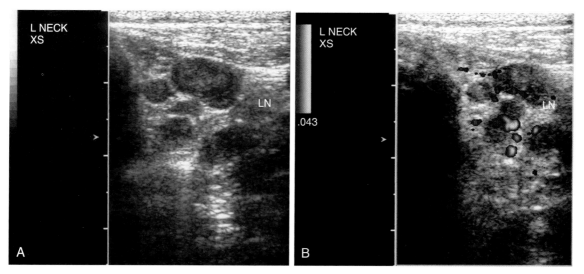

Figure 6-29 **Cervical lymph node metastasis. A,** A collection of small hypoechoic, well-marginated cervical lymph nodes are present. These nodes are normally very small and not visualized. **B,** Power Doppler shows marked peripheral blood flow, whereas the nodes themselves are nearly devoid of flow.

Ultrasound can also be used with microbubble contrast agents to identify sentinel lymph nodes, which are the initial lymph nodes draining a neoplastic mass. In one study, ultrasound contrast identified the sentinel lymph nodes in 8 of 10 dogs, which were all subsequently confirmed with lymphoscintigraphy.[109]

Lymphoma

Multicentric lymphoma with involvement of the regional lymph nodes of the head and neck is common in both the dog and cat. Cervical, retropharyngeal, and mandibular lymph nodes are usually palpable and may become extremely large (Figure 6-30). Lymphomatous nodes have a mildly heterogeneous, hypoechoic appearance and may or may not have distinct margins. In some instances, nodal internal architecture may appear to be preserved (Figure 6-31; also see Figure 6-30, *D*). Because of tissue homogeneity, lymphoma may appear on ultrasound imaging as multiple, distally enhancing, anechoic, cystlike lesions and should not be confused with true cysts. In a human study aimed at differentiating lymphomatous nodes

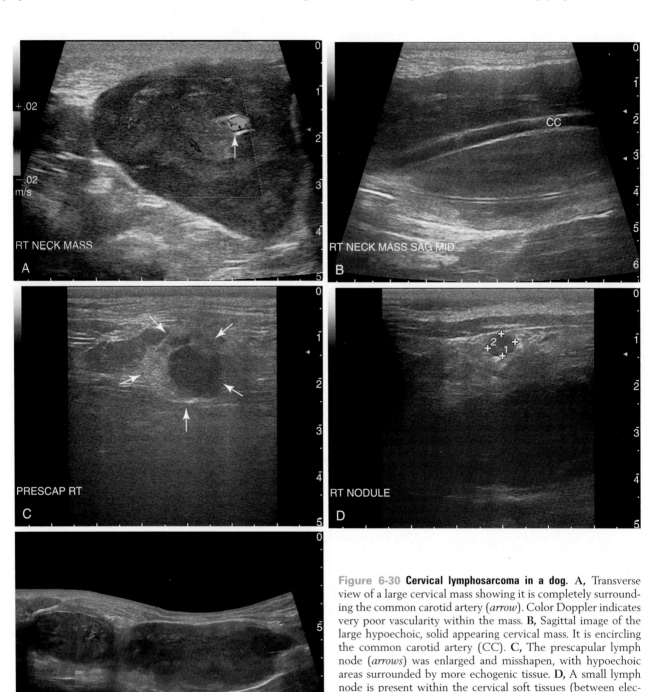

Figure 6-30 Cervical lymphosarcoma in a dog. A, Transverse view of a large cervical mass showing it is completely surrounding the common carotid artery (*arrow*). Color Doppler indicates very poor vascularity within the mass. **B,** Sagittal image of the large hypoechoic, solid appearing cervical mass. It is encircling the common carotid artery (CC). **C,** The prescapular lymph node (*arrows*) was enlarged and misshapen, with hypoechoic areas surrounded by more echogenic tissue. **D,** A small lymph node is present within the cervical soft tissues (between electronic cursors, 0.47 × 0.62 cm). **E,** Extended field of view shows the magnitude of the mass, extending nearly the length of the neck.

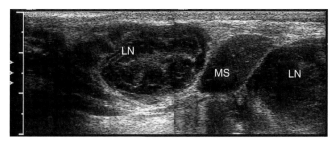

Figure 6-31 Adult dog with massive peripheral lymph node enlargement owing to lymphoma. Large well-defined hypoechoic masses (*LN*) are seen in the region of the mandibular and retropharyngeal lymph nodes in a composite image obtained in an oblique imaging plane. In this example, it appears that some of the normal internal architectural detail of the cranial-most node is preserved. The more hypoechoic periphery may represent infiltrated cortex, and the stellate central region may represent the medullary cords. A diagnosis of lymphoma was confirmed by fine-needle aspiration biopsy. The structure between the two enlarged nodes is the mandibular salivary gland (*MS*).

from metastatic nodes caused by carcinoma, lymphomatous nodes were more homogeneous, were distally enhanced, and did not have evidence of central necrosis.[102] These findings are generally in agreement with our experience in dogs with nodal enlargement from lymphoma. Diagnosis of lymphoma can usually be confirmed with fine-needle aspiration biopsy.[4]

SALIVARY GLANDS

The mandibular salivary gland is caudal to the angle of the mandible in the bifurcation formed by the convergence of the linguofacial and maxillary veins. The mandibular salivary duct courses rostrally and opens onto the sublingual caruncle. The sublingual salivary glands consist of polystomatic glands, located between the first and last cheek teeth, and monostomatic glands, which are further divided into rostral and caudal components. The more compact caudal component is immediately rostral to the mandibular salivary gland and shares a common capsule. The major sublingual duct follows the same path as the mandibular salivary duct. The parotid gland is V shaped and has a lobulated appearance. The gland wraps around the cartilage of the base of the ear dorsally and lies superficial to the dorsal aspect of the mandibular salivary gland ventrally. The parotid duct opens into the buccal vestibule opposite the maxillary carnassial teeth.[110]

The mandibular salivary gland is easily imaged and is a useful reference point in the rostroventral cervical region. In many dogs, the mandibular salivary gland, the medial retropharyngeal lymph node, and the digastric muscle can be seen in the same imaging plane (Figure 6-32, *A* to *C*). The mandibular salivary gland is best seen by first identifying the carotid bifurcation in plane 1, then rotating the transducer approximately 10 to 20 degrees, shifting the rostral aspect of the imaging plane laterally (see Figure 6-32, *A* and *B*, imaging plane 3). The mandibular salivary gland, seen in its long axis in this position, is identified superficial to and slightly rostral to the carotid bifurcation as a well-demarcated oval to triangular structure of moderate echogenicity surrounded by a thin echogenic capsule. Thin, highly echogenic linear streaks are seen within the center of the gland and may represent arborization of the salivary ducts. The gland can also be completely evaluated in its short axis by rotating the transducer 90 degrees from the original imaging position.[5]

On imaging of the mandibular salivary gland, the monostomatic sublingual salivary gland may also be seen in some dogs as a small triangular structure of low echogenicity surrounded by a hyperechoic capsule positioned against the rostral margin of the mandibular salivary gland.[5]

When the ultrasound transducer is swept from ventral to dorsal along the cartilage of the vertical external ear canal, the parotid salivary gland appears as a poorly marginated structure of moderately low echogenicity. It has a more heterogeneous parenchyma than that of the mandibular salivary gland[5] (see Figure 6-32, *D*). The gland is best imaged by placing the transducer in the frontal plane at the base of the ear canal so that the cartilage of the canal is imaged in cross section as a discrete curvilinear structure with distal reverberation echoes. The parotid gland can then be imaged rostral, caudal, and ventral to the canal margin.

Abnormalities of the salivary glands may include neoplasia, sialitis, sialolithiasis, true cysts, and sialoceles caused by previous trauma or inflammation (Figure 6-33).[95] Ultrasound examination is useful in determining whether a mass is intrinsic or extrinsic to the salivary gland but has been relatively nonspecific in delineating the type of abnormality in humans.[111,112]

Salivary Cysts
Cystic lesions are generally of two types: true cysts, which are lined with stratified epithelium; and retention cysts (mucocele), which are lined with granulation tissue. Retention cysts are generally the result of previous inflammation or trauma.[113] Cystic lesions appear as hypoechoic or anechoic regions within the salivary gland. Aspiration may verify the salivary nature of the cystic lesion.

Sialoliths
Clinically significant sialoliths are a rare problem in dogs and cats, and their ultrasonographic appearance has not been reported (see Figure 6-33, *B*). In humans, sialoliths that are 2 mm or larger can be detected and appear as focal echogenic regions associated with far-field shadowing.

Sialitis and Salivary Gland Abscess
Sialitis in humans produces a diffuse enlargement of the gland with sharp margination and a coarser and more inhomogeneous echo pattern than normal.[112] Affected salivary tissue is of variable echogenicity ranging from hypoechoic to hyperechoic compared with normal salivary tissue.[114] This variable echogenicity is also found in dogs with sialadenitis of the zygomatic salivary glands[115] and mandibular salivary glands (see Figure 6-33). Chronic inflammatory lesions are seen as small cystic areas or an inhomogeneous echo pattern owing to inflammation and reactive hyperplasia of intraglandular lymphatic tissue. Intraglandular lymph nodes up to 1 cm in diameter may also be visualized.[114] Abscesses have also been described in humans and appear ultrasonographically as cystic lesions with occasional echoic intracavitary debris present.[111]

Salivary Gland Neoplasia
Salivary neoplasia is uncommon in the dog and rare in the cat, and as such, the ultrasound appearance has not been described.[39,116] In humans, benign adenomas have been characterized as smoothly marginated, slightly inhomogeneous, solid masses that are hypoechoic compared with normal salivary tissue. Carcinomas have been described as hypoechoic and inhomogeneous; they have poorly defined margins, a finding that in combination with enlargement of ipsilateral regional lymph nodes appears to be an important criterion for differentiating benign from malignant disease.[111,114,117]

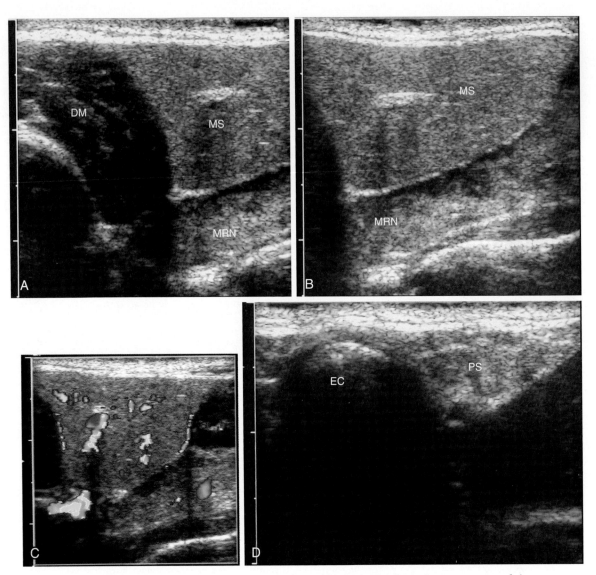

Figure 6-32 Normal adult canine mandibular and parotid salivary glands. A, Long-axis view of the rostral margin of the mandibular salivary gland (*MS*) in imaging plane 3. The parenchyma has a fine, moderately echoic appearance. The digastric muscle (*DM*) is seen as it crosses the angle of the mandible obliquely. The medial retropharyngeal lymph node (*MRN*) is located deep to the mandibular salivary gland. **B,** Same imaging plane as in **A** with the transducer positioned more caudally to include the caudal margin of the mandibular salivary gland. **C,** Color Doppler image of the mandibular salivary gland reveals the rich blood supply of this structure. **D,** Short-axis view of the parotid salivary gland in a transverse imaging plane with the transducer positioned over the external ear canal. Rostral is to the left. The parotid salivary gland (*PS*) appears as a poorly marginated structure of mixed echogenicity adjacent and, in this image, caudal to the shadow cast by the superficial margin of the auricular cartilage and air of the external ear canal (*EC*).

LARYNX AND TRACHEA

Ultrasound appearance of the normal canine and feline larynx has been described. In the dog, anatomic structures that can be detected include the epiglottis, the ventral margins of the cricoid and thyroid cartilages, the cuneiform process of the arytenoid cartilage, and the true and false vocal folds[118,119] (Figure 6-34). Figure 6-35 shows the subtle difference between adduction and abduction of the laryngeal cartilages. In the normal feline patient, the cuneiform process of the arytenoid cartilages and occasionally the vocal cords are visible during ultrasonography of the larynx.[120] Because the normal larynx is air filled, satisfactory imaging planes may be difficult to attain, and only near-field anatomy is seen.

Ultrasonography has been used to diagnose and localize laryngeal masses in cats and dogs. The ultrasound appearances of lymphoma, squamous cell carcinoma, adenocarcinoma, and laryngeal cysts have been described.[120,121] In general, solid masses were heterogeneous and hypoechoic, distorting normal laryngeal lumen margins and sometimes causing luminal compression or partial obstruction. The laryngeal cysts were ovoid or round, well defined and anechoic, and in one report the cyst had marked far-field enhancement. Ultrasonography can also be used to evaluate patients with laryngeal paralysis. In such cases, there is asymmetry or loss of the normal periodic abduction of the arytenoid cartilages, abnormal or paradoxical arytenoid movements, caudal displacement of the larynx, or laryngeal collapse.[120,122] Atrophy of laryngeal

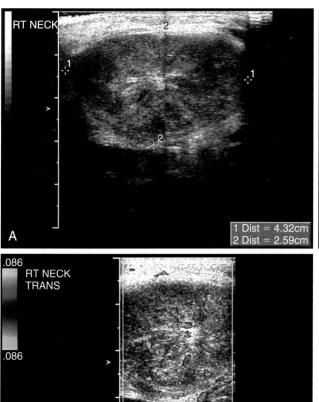

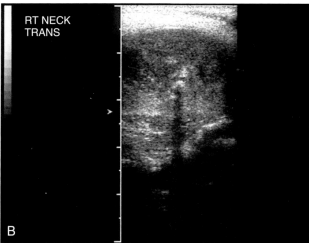

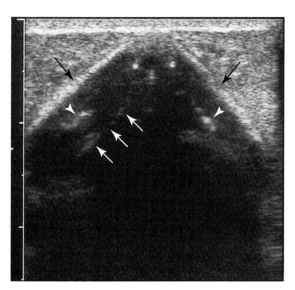

Figure 6-33 **Sialadenitis and sialolith in a dog mandibular salivary gland. A,** Composite image shows an enlarged gland with abnormally heterogenous, striated, radiating parenchyma. **B,** A different image plane shows a focus of intense hyperechogenicity with acoustic shadowing, a sialolith (salivary gland calculus). **C,** Color Doppler examination shows intense blood flow within the gland, consistent with hyperemia and inflammation.

Figure 6-34 Transverse image of a normal canine larynx during inspiration with the transducer positioned on the ventral aspect of the thyroid cartilage (*black arrows*). The ill-defined linear structure on the left represents one of the vocal ligaments (*white arrows*). The highly echoic structures seen bilaterally represent a portion of the arytenoid cartilage (*arrowheads*). Symmetrical movement of these structures is seen during normal respiratory excursions.

musculature may be identified in cases of unilateral paralysis (Figure 6-36).

The trachea can be identified in both transverse and sagittal planes. In the transverse plane, it has a well-demarcated ventral (near-field) margin with reverberation and gas shadowing artifact extending dorsally (see Figures 6-7; 6-12; 6-15, C and D; and 6-25, B). In the sagittal plane, the trachea has a distinct hyperechoic ventral wall with regularly spaced hypoechoic shadows representing cartilage rings and far-field shadowing caused by the presence of intraluminal air[5,123] (Figure 6-37; see also Figure 6-11).

Ultrasonography has been used in humans to diagnose cervical tracheal stenosis[124] and in dogs to diagnose collapse of the cervical trachea by use of simple shape changes in the tracheal margin to characterize the lesion at the time of collapse.[123] It is unlikely, however, that ultrasonography will serve as a satisfactory alternative to radiography or fluoroscopy for diagnosis of tracheal collapse.

TONGUE AND ESOPHAGUS

Muscle support for the base of the tongue consists of the mylohyoid and geniohyoid muscles, which arise from the mandibular rami and extend to the hyoid apparatus. A third muscle, the genioglossus, also arises from the internal margin of the mandibular rami and forms a fan-shaped insertion into the ventral aspect of the tongue. The cervical esophagus originates dorsal to the trachea at the level of the caudal border

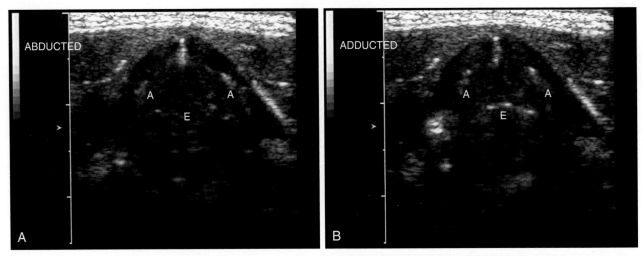

Figure 6-35 **Transverse images of the larynx of a dog during inspiration (A) and expiration (B).** A, During inspiration, there is abduction of the laryngeal cartilages. **B,** During expiration adduction occurs. *A,* Arytenoid cartilage; *E,* epiglottis. Note the subtle differences in arytenoid cartilage location between inspiration and expiration. Though ultrasound can be used to evaluate laryngeal function, direct observation remains the best method to assess laryngeal movement.

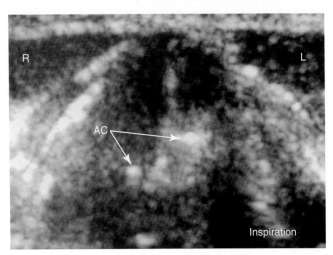

Figure 6-36 **Transverse image of canine laryngeal paralysis obtained during inspiration.** The arytenoid cartilages (*AC*) are asymmetrically positioned; the nonfunctional left cartilage is located on midline, whereas the right is fully abducted. The left arytenoid cartilage is thickened and echogenic. The left laryngeal musculature is atrophied and has a more mottled, echogenic texture than the right.

of the cricoid cartilage in the dog and at the level of the third cervical vertebra in the cat.[110] As it courses caudally, the esophagus shifts position until it lies to the left of the trachea at the thoracic inlet.

The supporting musculature for the tongue can be seen in both the short and long axes by placing the transducer into the intermandibular space (Figure 6-38, *A*). These muscles have a characteristic hypoechoic striated appearance in long axis and a coarse heterogeneous appearance in short axis. The middle and basilar portions of the tongue can also be seen dorsal and adjacent to the genioglossus and have a heterogeneous, hyperechoic appearance.

The esophagus can be imaged from either the left or right of midline, depending on the position of the esophagus in a given patient. In short axis, it appears as a well-defined, roughly circular structure, often with a hyperechoic core

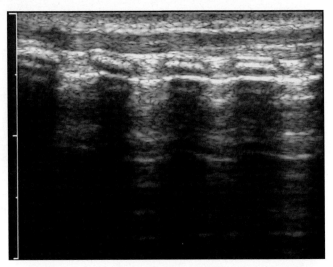

Figure 6-37 Long-axis view of a normal canine trachea obtained by redirecting the transducer slightly medial to the position used for imaging plane 2. The evenly spaced oval structures are the tracheal cartilage rings. In young dogs, cartilage rings often have a more uniformly hypoechoic appearance. The highly echogenic cartilage core and distal shadowing in this dog may be caused by central cartilage mineralization. The hyperechoic undulating line adjacent and internal to the cartilage rings represents the tracheal wall. Reverberation and shadowing are caused by air within the tracheal lumen.

resulting from intraluminal mucus and air. In some instances, distinct adventitial, muscular, and submucosal-mucosal layers can be distinguished (Figure 6-39). The location of the esophagus can be confirmed by identifying esophageal movement after swallowing in the awake patient or by passing an esophageal stethoscope or orogastric tube while imaging the region in the anesthetized animal.[5]

Although only a few reports associated with primary sonographic lesions of the tongue and cervical esophagus have been described in veterinary medicine, ultrasonography is accurate in demonstrating and characterizing such lesions in humans.[125] Neoplastic masses and lesions associated with the

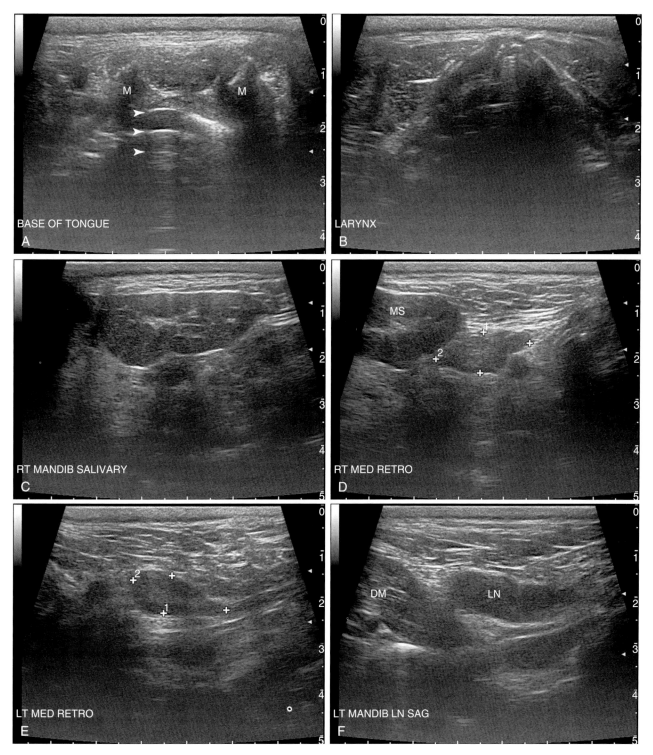

Figure 6-38 Normal anatomy of the base of the tongue and laryngeal region in a dog. A, Transverse image of the ventral mandible. The two rami of the mandible (*M*) create a characteristic and easily identified hyperechoic landmark with acoustic shadowing. Muscular planes are readily identified around and between the rami. Reverberation artifact (*arrowheads*) is present in the far field, created by gas within the oral cavity. **B,** Typical inverted V shape of the larynx. In this image, internal laryngeal anatomy cannot be seen because of interference by air. **C,** Normal long-axis image of the mandibular salivary gland showing its striated appearance. **D,** Right medial retropharyngeal lymph node (between electronic cursors, 0.89 × 2.12 cm) seen in long axis. The right mandibular salivary gland (*MS*) is seen cranial (left) to it. **E,** Long-axis image of the left medial retropharyngeal lymph node (between electronic cursors, 0.83 × 2.15 cm); the left mandibular salivary gland is out of plane. **F,** Left mandibular lymph node (*LN*). The digastric muscle (*DM*) is cranial (to the left) immediately adjacent to the mandibular lymph node.

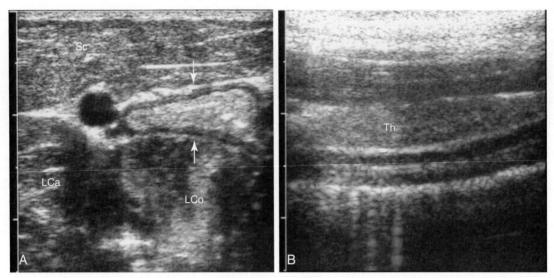

Figure 6-39 Normal adult canine cervical esophagus. A, Short-axis view of the cervical esophagus (*arrows*) and left common carotid artery. Lateral is to the left side of the image. The outer echogenic band is the adventitial layer, the well-defined hypoechoic intermediate region represents the muscular layer, and the moderately echoic internal region represents the submucosal-mucosal layers. The highly echogenic focus in the center of the esophagus is caused by air within the lumen. The sternocephalic (*Sc*), longus capitis (*LCa*), and longus colli (*LCo*) muscles are also seen in this image. **B,** Long-axis view of the cervical esophagus in scanning plane 2. In this image, the esophagus lies adjacent and internal to the thyroid lobe (*Th*) and is completely collapsed. Parallel hypoechoic tissue is separated by echogenic luminal gas.

tongue, including squamous cell carcinoma, rhabdomyoma, and adenocarcinoma, have been identified and described using ultrasound in dogs and cats.[126] Ultrasound can also be used to identify penetrating foreign material within the tongue, although this is more commonly a problem in large animal patients. Additionally, ultrasonography has been used as an adjunct to survey radiography to confirm persistent cervical esophageal dilation in patients with suspected or confirmed megaesophagus. Figure 6-40 shows an example of an esophageal abscess.

CERVICAL MUSCULATURE

Ventral cervical musculature consists of paired sternohyoid, sternothyroid, and sternocephalic muscles that arise from the first sternebra and first costal cartilages and insert on the basihyoid bone, the thyroid cartilage, and the temporal and occipital bones, respectively. Hypaxial muscles consist of paired longus capitis muscles, which arise from the transverse processes of the cervical vertebrae and insert on the ventral surface of the basioccipital bone, and the longus colli muscles, which attach to the ventral aspects of the vertebral bodies and transverse processes of the first through sixth cervical vertebrae. The paired digastric muscles arise from the paracondylar process of the occipital bone, cross over the lateral aspect of the angle of the mandible, and insert on the body of the mandible.[92]

Cervical muscles appear discrete with low echogenicity surrounded by a hyperechoic fascia. Muscle is more mottled and grainy when it is viewed in the transverse or oblique plane.

The digastric muscle is routinely identified by placing the transducer in scanning plane 1 or 3. The digastric muscle can be seen as it crosses the ventral aspect of the angle of the mandible (see Figure 6-32, *A*), and the hyperechoic, curvilinear ventral margin of the mandible can be seen deep and rostral to the digastric muscle.[5]

The sternothyroid, sternohyoid, and sternocephalicus muscles are identified along the length of the ventral neck (see Figures 6-7 and 6-15). Division and separation of the muscles are optimal in the transverse plane in the cranial cervical region (see Figures 6-3 and 6-7). The longus colli and longus capitis muscles are also best recognized in the transverse plane (see Figures 6-7 and 6-39). Muscles can be imaged by sweeping the beam from caudal to cranial along the ventral midline, slightly adjusting the transducer position for optimal visualization of muscle bellies. On transverse scans, the sternohyoid and sternothyroid muscles appear as flat to oval structures of low echogenicity located to the left and right of the trachea (see Figure 6-7). The sternocephalicus muscle is identified lateral to the sternohyoid and sternothyroid muscles (see Figure 6-7). Delineation of discrete muscle bellies is more difficult in the caudal cervical region, presumably because of the convergence of the left and right bellies of the sternocephalicus muscle in this region.[5]

In their long axes, specific muscle groups are more difficult to identify. The long-axis examination is initiated by placing the transducer in the jugular furrow and orienting the beam in plane 1. The sternothyroid, sternohyoid, and sternocephalicus muscles are identified superficial to the common carotid artery and visualized by adjusting the angle of the beam slightly between the dorsal and parasagittal planes (see Figures 6-4 and 6-15). These muscles are also often seen on the side opposite transducer placement. The longus colli and longus capitis are identified deep to the carotid artery (see Figure 6-4). Dorsal to these muscles, the ventral surfaces of the cervical vertebrae are imaged as well-marginated, irregular, noncontinuous hyperechoic lines.[5]

MISCELLANEOUS NECK MASSES

Clinically undifferentiated neck masses not associated with the thyroid, parathyroid, or salivary glands may include

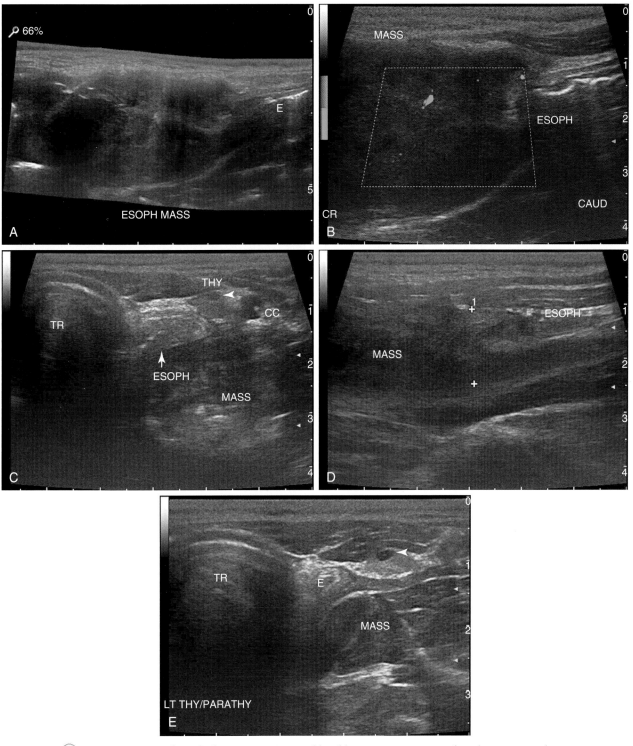

Figure 6-40 Esophageal abscess in a 6-year-old golden retriever presented with gagging and wheezing over a 2-month period (**A-C**). Follow-up ultrasound examination was done after 2 weeks of antibiotic therapy (**D-E**). **A,** Extended field of view image shows a large, complex mass. A portion of normal distal esophagus (*E*) can be seen, identified by normal layering of the esophageal wall and gas within its lumen. **B,** Power Doppler image shows very little blood flow within the mass. The normal distal esophagus can be seen to the right (*ESOPH*). **C,** Transverse images shows a portion of normal esophagus (*ESOPH; arrow*) with a complex mass seen in the deeper cervical tissues. The trachea (*TR*), left thyroid gland (*THY*), parathyroid gland (*arrowhead*) and common carotid artery (CC) are seen. Aspiration was diagnostic for inflammation and abscessation. **D,** Sagittal image of the resolving abscess (*MASS*) now notably smaller in size. **E,** Transverse image similar to **C,** shows a marked reduction in the size of the abscess (*MASS*). *E*, esophagus; *TR*, trachea. The left parathyroid gland (*arrowhead*) can be seen imbedded in the more echogenic thyroid gland.

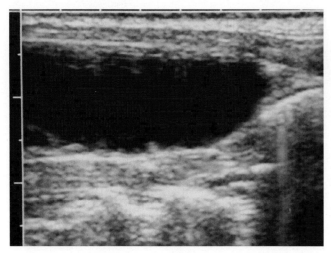

Figure 6-41 **Adult dog with a cystic lesion of undetermined origin.** A thin-walled cyst with anechoic contents and a mildly irregular internal margin is seen in long axis. The mass was located in the ventral cervical region to the left of midline. The origin of the lesion was not determined, but it was thought to be either a branchial or thyroid cyst.

primary neoplasia, metastatic neoplasia, lipomas, cystic lesions, abscess, and hematoma.[4,127,128] Lesions can generally be divided into solid, cystic, and complex categories.[4,127] Complex lesions appear as masses with solid components of varying echogenicity associated with hypoechoic cystic areas sometimes separated by more echogenic septations. Neoplasia often has a solid or complex character; hematoma has a complex or cystic character; and lymphadenitis or a lymph node abscess can appear as any of the three types.[127] Use of a combination of two-dimensional and Doppler ultrasonography is sometimes helpful in determining the vascularity of some neck masses.[129]

Neoplasia
Neoplastic masses can originate from many different structures in the neck. Cervical lipomas have been described as elliptic masses that are hyperechoic to adjacent muscle and contain echogenic striations directed perpendicular to the ultrasound beam.[128] A cervical teratoma in a Boxer dog has also been described near the left mandibular salivary gland.[130]

Cysts
Purely cystic lesions are generally benign and usually of developmental origin. Lesions of this type are rare in the cat and dog.[39] Differentiation of cysts from abscess or hematoma may be made by fine-needle aspiration of fluid contents. The walls of developmental cystic lesions are generally expected to be thinner and to have better defined internal margins (Figure 6-41).

Hematomas
The ultrasound appearance of hematomas varies, depending on stage of development. An acute hematoma may appear as a cystic lesion with a hypoechoic center (Figure 6-42). As the hematoma matures and organizes, it may develop discrete septations, and echogenicity may increase centrally. Well-organized hematomas may also have a thick, well-defined hyperechoic capsule.

Cellulitis, Abscess, and Granuloma
Ultrasonography can be used in cases of inflammatory neck disease to differentiate diffuse cellulitis (Figure 6-43) from

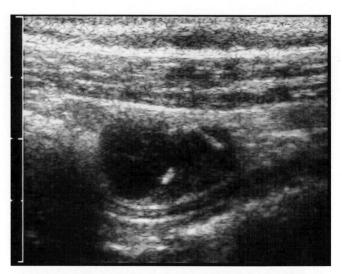

Figure 6-42 **Adult dog with an iatrogenic hematoma.** A moderately well-defined cavitary lesion is seen in long axis. The lesion was located near one of the jugular grooves and arose shortly after jugular phlebotomy was attempted. This image was obtained approximately 24 hours later. Ultrasound findings are typical of an uncomplicated subacute hematoma that has not yet begun to organize significantly.

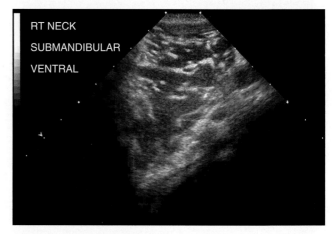

Figure 6-43 **Cellulitis of the ventral mandible.** Hypoechoic strands of tissue separated by hyperechoic strands are typical of cellulitis and seroma formation. Fine-needle aspiration is necessary in many cases to differentiate them.

frank abscess. Margins of anatomic structures are often indistinct, and connective tissue planes are prominent in the presence of diffuse cellulitis, presumably owing to widely distributed edema and inflammation. Abscesses have a cavitary appearance and generally have a thick, irregular wall of high echogenicity. Fluid within the abscess may be of high echogenicity because of the presence of solid material and gas (Figure 6-44). Septations are often present. Cellulitis without abscess formation appears as a diffuse increase in echogenicity associated with a decrease in the definition of normal anatomic structures. Additionally, foreign bodies within the retropharyngeal region, cervical soft tissues, or both, can be identified with ultrasound. Wood foreign bodies within the cervical region have been identified sonographically as hyperechoic linear structures with distal acoustic shadowing (Figure 6-45).[56,131] Figure 6-46 shows the presence of a bony sequestrum, the result of a dog fight.

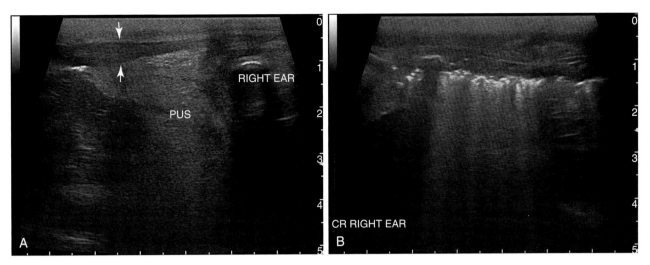

Figure 6-44 Abscess of the right temporal region. A, A thick wall (*arrow*) is seen in the near field of this abscess. The homogeneous echogenic material deep to the thick wall is pus (*PUS*). A transverse image of the horizontal ear canal is seen to the right (*RIGHT EAR*). **B,** A different image plane shows a large amount of highly echogenic gas within the abscess.

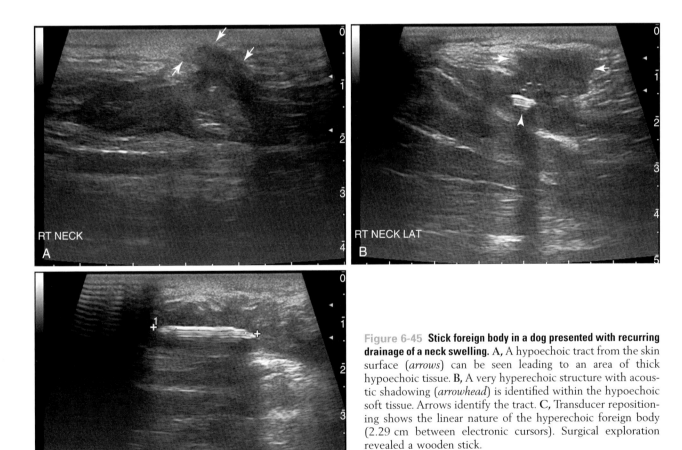

Figure 6-45 Stick foreign body in a dog presented with recurring drainage of a neck swelling. A, A hypoechoic tract from the skin surface (*arrows*) can be seen leading to an area of thick hypoechoic tissue. **B,** A very hyperechoic structure with acoustic shadowing (*arrowhead*) is identified within the hypoechoic soft tissue. Arrows identify the tract. **C,** Transducer repositioning shows the linear nature of the hyperechoic foreign body (2.29 cm between electronic cursors). Surgical exploration revealed a wooden stick.

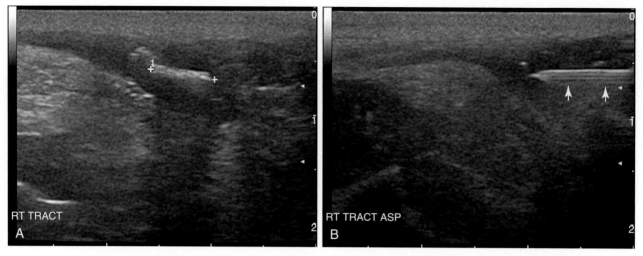

Figure 6-46 **Sequestrum in a dog presented several months after a dog fight with a recurrent draining tract over the right shoulder. A,** A linear hyperechoic structure is present underneath the swelling (0.62 cm between electronic cursors). The structure is surrounded by a hypoechoic area. **B,** A fine-needle aspirate (*arrows*) was obtained and revealed the presence of pus. A sequestrum was found during surgical exploration.

REFERENCES

1. Skanalakis J, Godwin J, Androulakis J, et al. The differential diagnosis of tumors of the neck. *Prog Clin Cancer* 1977;**4**:141–59.
2. Solbiati L, Montali G, Croce F, et al. Parathyroid tumors detected by fine-needle aspiration biopsy under ultrasonic guidance. *Radiology* 1983;**148**:793–7.
3. Simeone J, Daniels G, Mueller P, et al. High-resolution real-time sonography of the thyroid. *Radiology* 1982;**145**:431–5.
4. Wisner E, Nyland T, Mattoon J. Ultrasonographic examination of cervical masses in the dog and cat. *Vet Radiol Ultrasound* 1994;**35**:310–15.
5. Wisner E, Mattoon J, Nyland T, et al. Normal ultrasonographic anatomy of the canine neck. *Vet Radiol* 1991;**32**:185–90.
6. Issing P, Ohmayer T, Schonermark M, et al. Jugular vein thrombosis as incidental ultrasound finding in tumor patients. *HNO* 1995;**43**:672–5.
7. Gaitini D, Kaftori J, Pery M, et al. High-resolution real-time ultrasonography. Diagnosis and follow-up of jugular and subclavian vein thrombosis. *J Ultrasound Med* 1988;**7**:621–7.
8. Hubsch P, Stiglbauer R, Schwaighofer B, et al. Internal jugular and subclavian vein thrombosis caused by central venous catheters. Evaluation using Doppler blood flow imaging. *J Ultrasound Med* 1988;**7**:629–36.
9. Routh CE, Hagen RU, Else RW, et al. Imaging diagnosis—congenital venous aneurysm of the left external jugular vein. *Vet Rad Ultrasound* 2009;**50**:506–8.
10. Jmor S, El-Atrozy T, Griffin M, et al. Grading internal carotid artery stenosis using B-mode ultrasound (in vivo study). *Eur J Vasc Endovasc Surg* 1999;**18**:315–22.
11. Beebe H, Salles-Cunha SX, Scissons R, et al. Carotid arterial ultrasound scan imaging: a direct approach to stenosis measurement. *J Vasc Surg* 1999;**29**:838–44.
12. Hetzel A, Eckenweber B, Trummer B, et al. Colour-coded duplex sonography of preocclusive carotid stenoses. *Eur J Ultrasound* 1998;**8**:183–91.
13. Gooding G, Langman A, Dillon W, et al. Malignant carotid artery invasion: sonographic detection. *Radiology* 1989;**171**:435–8.
14. Taeymans O, Penninck DG, Peters RM. Comparison between clinical, ultrasound, CT, MRI, and pathology findings in dogs presented for suspected thyroid carcinoma. *Vet Radiol Ultrasound* 2013 Jan-Feb;**54**(1):61–70.
15. Fife W, Mattoon J, Drost W, et al. Imaging features of a presumed carotid body tumor in a dog. *Vet Rad Ultrasound* 2003;**44**:322–5.
16. Knappertz VA, Tegeler CH, Hardin SJ, et al. Vagus nerve imaging with ultrasound: anatomic and in vivo validation. *Otolaryngol Head Neck Surg* 1998;**118**:82–5.
17. Reese S, Ruppert C. Ultrasonographic imaging of the vagosympathetic trunk in the dog. *Vet Radiol Ultrasound* 2001;**42**:272–5.
18. Ruppert C, Hartmann K, Fischer A, et al. Cervical neoplasia originating from the vagus nerve in a dog. *J Small Anim Pract* 2000;**41**:119–22.
19. Wisner E, Nyland T. Ultrasonography of the thyroid and parathyroid glands. *Vet Clin North Am Small Anim Pract* 1998;**28**:973–91.
20. Wisner E, Theon A, Nyland T, et al. Ultrasonographic examination of the thyroid gland of hyperthyroid cats: comparison to ^{99m}Tc scintigraphy. *Vet Radiol Ultrasound* 1994;**34**:53–8.
21. Taeymans O, Duchateau L, Schreurs E, et al. Intra- and interobserver variability of ultrasonographic measurements of the thyroid gland in healthy beagles. *Vet Radiol Ultrasound* 2005;**46**:139–42.
22. Brömel C, Pollard RE, Kass PH, et al. Comparison of ultrasonographic characteristics of the thyroid gland in healthy small-, medium-, and large-breed dogs. *Am J Vet Res* 2006;**67**:70–7.
23. King A, Ahuja A, King W, et al. The role of ultrasound in the diagnosis of a large, rapidly growing, thyroid mass. *Postgrad Med J* 1997;**73**:412–14.
24. Taeymans O, Peremans K, Saunders JH. Thyroid imaging in the dog: current status and future directions. *J Vet Intern Med* 2007;**21**:673–84.

25. Reese S, Breyer U, Deeg C, et al. Thyroid sonography as an effective tool to discriminate between euthyroid sick and hypothyroid dogs. *J Vet Intern Med* 2005;**19**: 491–8.

26. Brömel C, Pollard RE, Kass PH, et al. Ultrasonographic evaluation of the thyroid gland in healthy, hypothyroid, and euthyroid golden retrievers with nonthyroidal illness. *J Vet Intern Med* 2005;**19**:499–506.

27. Taeymans O, Daminet S, Duchateau L, et al. Pre- and post-treatment ultrasonography in hypothyroid dogs. *Vet Radiol Ultrasound* 2007;**48**:262–9.

28. Rajatanavin R, Fang S, Pino S, et al. Thyroid hormone antibodies and Hashimoto's thyroiditis in mongrel dogs. *Endocrinology* 1989;**124**:2535–40.

29. Chastain C, Young D, Kemppainen R. Anti-triiodothyronine antibodies associated with hypothyroidism and lymphocytic thyroiditis in a dog. *J Am Vet Med Assoc* 1989;**194**:531–4.

30. Gosselin S, Capen C, Martin S, et al. Autoimmune lymphocytic thyroiditis in dogs. *Vet Immunol Immunopathol* 1982;**3**:185–201.

31. Vollset I, Larsen H. Occurrence of autoantibodies against thyroglobulin in Norwegian dogs. *Acta Vet Scand* 1987;**28**:65–71.

32. Set P, Oleszczuk-Raschke K, von Lengerke JH, et al. Sonographic features of Hashimoto thyroiditis in childhood. *Clin Radiol* 1996;**51**:167–9.

33. Scheible W, Leopold G, Woo V, et al. High-resolution real-time ultrasonography of thyroid nodules. *Radiology* 1979;**133**:413–17.

34. Butch R, Simeone J, Mueller P. Thyroid and parathyroid ultrasonography. *Radiol Clin North Am* 1985;**23**: 57–71.

35. Blum M, Passalaqua A, Sackler J, et al. Thyroid echography of subacute thyroiditis. *Radiology* 1977;**125**:795–8.

36. Yeh H, Futterweit W, Gilbert P. Micronodulation: ultrasonographic sign of Hashimoto thyroiditis. *J Ultrasound Med* 1996;**15**:813–19.

37. Ying M, Brook F, Ahuja A, et al. The value of thyroid parenchymal echogenicity as an indicator of pathology using the sternomastoid muscle for comparison. *Ultrasound Med Biol* 1998;**24**:1097–105.

38. Barbertet V, Baeumlin Y, Taeymans O, et al. Pre- and posttreatment ultrasonography of the thyroid gland in hyperthyroid cats. *Vet Radiol Ultrasound* 2010;**51**: 324–30.

39. Moulton JE, editor. *Tumors in domestic animals*. 3rd ed. Berkeley: University of California Press; 1990.

40. Birchard S, Roesel O. Neoplasia of the thyroid gland in the dog: a retrospective study of 16 cases. *J Am Anim Hosp Assoc* 1981;**17**:369–72.

41. Brodey R, Kelly D. Thyroid neoplasms in the dog. A clinicopathologic study of fifty-seven cases. *Cancer* 1968;**22**:406–16.

42. Zarrin K. Naturally occurring parafollicular cell carcinoma of the thyroid in dogs. A histological and ultrastructural study. *Vet Pathol* 1977;**14**:556–66.

43. Harari J, Patterson J, Rosenthal R. Clinical and pathologic features of thyroid tumors in 26 dogs. *J Am Vet Med Assoc* 1986;**188**:1160–4.

44. Leav I, Schiller A, Rijnberk A, et al. Adenomas and carcinomas of the canine and feline thyroid. *Am J Pathol* 1976;**83**:61–122.

45. Peterson M. Feline hyperthyroidism. *Vet Clin North Am Small Anim Pract* 1984;**14**:809–26.

46. Turrel J, Feldman E, Nelson R, et al. Thyroid carcinoma causing hyperthyroidism in cats: 14 cases (1981-1986). *J Am Vet Med Assoc* 1988;**193**:359–64.

47. Hoenig M, Goldschmidt M, Ferguson D, et al. Toxic nodular goiter in the cat. *J Small Anim Pract* 1982;**23**: 1–12.

48. Peterson M, Ferguson D. Thyroid diseases. In: Ettinger S, editor. *Textbook of veterinary internal medicine*. Philadelphia: WB Saunders; 1989. p. 1632–75.

49. Loar A. Canine thyroid tumors. In: Kirk R, editor. *Current veterinary therapy IX*. Philadelphia: WB Saunders; 1986. p. 1033–9.

50. Leveille R: Unpublished data.

51. Lippi F, Ferrari C, Manetti L, et al. Treatment of solitary autonomous thyroid nodules by percutaneous ethanol injection: results of an Italian multicenter study. The Multicenter Study Group. *J Clin Endocrinol Metab* 1996; **81**:3261–4.

52. Komorowski J, Kuzdak K, Pomorski L, et al. Percutaneous ethanol injection in treatment of benign nonfunctional and hyperfunctional thyroid nodules. *Cytobios* 1998;**95**:143–50.

53. Bennedbaek F, Karstrup S, Hegedus L. Percutaneous ethanol injection therapy in the treatment of thyroid and parathyroid diseases. *Eur J Endocrinol* 1997;**136**: 240–50.

54. Wells AL, Long CD, Hornof WJ, et al. Use of percutaneous ethanol injection for treatment of bilateral hyperplastic thyroid nodules in cats. *J Am Vet Med Assoc* 2001; **218**(8):1293–7.

55. Mallery KF, Pollard RE, Nelson RW, et al. Percutaneous ultrasound-guided radiofrequency heat ablation for treatment of hyperthyroidism in cats. *J Am Vet Med Assoc* 2003;**223**(11):1602–7.

56. Potanas CP, Armbrust L, Klocke EE, et al. Ultrasonographic and magnetic resonance imaging diagnosis of an oropharyngeal wood penetrating injury in a dog. *J Am Anim Hosp Assoc* 2011;**47**:e1–6.

57. Wesche MFT, Tiel-v.Buul MM, Smits NJ, et al. Ultrasonographic versus scintigraphic measurement of thyroid volume in patients referred for I therapy. *Nucl Med Commun* 1998;**19**:341–6.

58. Massaro F, Vera L, Schiavo M, et al. Ultrasonography thyroid volume estimation in hyperthyroid patients treated with individual radioiodine dose. *J Endocrinol Invest* 2007;**30**:318–22.

59. Loevner L. Imaging of the parathyroid glands. *Semin Ultrasound CT MR* 1996;**17**:563–75.

60. Koslin D, Adams J, Andersen P, et al. Preoperative evaluation of patients with primary hyperparathyroidism: role of high-resolution ultrasound. *Laryngoscope* 1997;**107**: 1249–53.

61. Hopkins C, Reading C. Thyroid and parathyroid imaging. *Semin Ultrasound CT MR* 1995;**16**:279–95.

62. Campbell J, Diamond T, North L. Ultrasound-guided parathyroid aspiration to diagnose parathyroid adenomas. *Australas Radiol* 1996;**40**:273–5.

63. Randel S, Gooding G, Clark O, et al. Parathyroid variants: US evaluation. *Radiology* 1987;**165**:191–4.

64. Levin K, Gooding G, Okerlund M, et al. Localizing studies in patients with persistent or recurrent hyperparathyroidism. *Surgery* 1987;**102**:917–25.

65. Liles SR, Linder KE, Cain B, et al. Ultrasonography of histologically normal parathyroid glands and thyroid lobules in normocalcemic dogs. *Vet Radiol Ultrasound* 2010;**51**:447–52.

66. Feldman E, Wisner E, Nelson R, et al. Comparison of results of hormonal analysis of samples obtained from selected venous sites versus cervical ultrasonography for localizing parathyroid masses in dogs. *J Am Vet Med Assoc* 1997;**211**:54–6.

67. Graif M, Itzchak Y, Strauss S, et al. Parathyroid sonography: diagnostic accuracy related to shape, location, and texture of the gland. *Br J Radiol* 1987;**60**:439–43.
68. Karstrup S, Hegedus L, Holm H. Parathyroid ultrasonography in patients with primary hyperparathyroidism. *Dan Med Bull* 1988;**35**:583–5.
69. Lloyd M, Lees W, Milroy E. Pre-operative localisation in primary hyperparathyroidism [see comments]. *Clin Radiol* 1990;**41**:239–43.
70. Long C, Goldstein R, Hornof W, et al. Percutaneous ultrasound-guided chemical parathyroid ablation for treatment of primary hyperparathyroidism in dogs. *J Am Vet Med Assoc* 1999;**215**:217–21.
71. Sample W, Mitchell S, Bledsoe R. Parathyroid ultrasonography. *Radiology* 1978;**127**:485–90.
72. Reading C, Charboneau J, James E, et al. High-resolution parathyroid sonography. *AJR Am J Roentgenol* 1982;**139**:539–46.
73. Simeone J, Mueller P, Ferrucci JJ, et al. High-resolution real-time sonography of the parathyroid. *Radiology* 1981;**141**:745–51.
74. Krubsack A, Wilson S, Lawson T, et al. Prospective comparison of radionuclide, computed tomographic, sonographic, and magnetic resonance localization of parathyroid tumors. *Surgery* 1989;**106**:639–44, discussion 644–6.
75. Abati A, Skarulis M, Shawker T, et al. Ultrasound-guided fine-needle aspiration of parathyroid lesions: a morphological and immunocytochemical approach. *Hum Pathol* 1995;**26**:338–43.
76. Wisner E, Nyland T, Feldman E, et al. Ultrasonographic evaluation of the parathyroid glands in hypercalcemic dogs. *Vet Radiol Ultrasound* 1993;**34**:108–11.
77. Wisner E, Penninck D, Biller D, et al. High-resolution parathyroid sonography. *Vet Radiol Ultrasound* 1997;**38**:462–6.
78. Abati A, Skarulis M, Shawker T, et al. Ultrasound-guided fine-needle aspiration of parathyroid lesions: a morphological and immunocytochemical approach. *Hum Pathol* 1995;**26**:338–43.
79. Takebayashi S, Matsui K, Onohara Y, et al. Sonography for early diagnosis of enlarged parathyroid glands in patients with secondary hyperparathyroidism. *AJR Am J Roentgenol* 1987;**148**:911–14.
80. Attie J, Khan A, Rumancik W, et al. Preoperative localization of parathyroid adenomas. *Am J Surg* 1988;**156**:323–6.
81. Gear RNA, Neiger R, Skelly BJS, et al. Primary hyperparathyroidism in 29 dogs: diagnosis, treatment, outcome and associated renal failure. *J Small Anim Pract* 2005;**46**:10–16.
82. Sueda MT, Stefanacci JD. Ultrasound evaluation of the parathyroid glands in two hypercalcemic cats. *Vet Radiol Ultrasound* 2000;**41**:448–51.
83. Giangrande A, Castiglioni A, Solbiati L, et al. Chemical parathyroidectomy for recurrence of secondary hyperparathyroidism. *Am J Kidney Dis* 1994;**24**:421–6.
84. Karstrup S, Holm H, Glentohj A, et al. Nonsurgical treatment of primary hyperparathyroidism with sonographically guided percutaneous injection of ethanol: results in a selected series of patients. *AJR Am J Roentgenol* 1990;**154**:1087–90.
85. Charboneau J, Hay I, van Heerden JA. Persistent primary hyperparathyroidism: Successful ultrasound-guided percutaneous ethanol ablation of an occult adenoma. *Mayo Clin Proc* 1988;**63**:913–17.
86. Fletcher S, Kanagasundaram N, Rayner H, et al. Assessment of ultrasound guided percutaneous ethanol injection and parathyroidectomy in patients with tertiary hyperparathyroidism. *Nephrol Dial Transplant* 1998;**13**:3111–17.
87. Pollard RE, Long CD, Nelson RW, et al. Percutaneous ultrasonographically guided radiofrequency heat ablation for treatment of primary hyperthyroidism in dogs. *J Am Vet Med Assoc* 2001;**218**:1106–10.
88. Wisner E, Nyland T. Localization of a parathyroid carcinoma using high-resolution ultrasonography in a dog. *J Vet Intern Med* 1994;**8**:244–5.
89. Sawyer ES, Northrup NC, Schmiedt CW, et al. Outcome of 19 dogs with parathyroid carcinoma after surgical excision. *Vet Comp Oncol* 2011;**10**:57–64.
90. Daly B, Coffey S, Behan M. Ultrasonographic appearances of parathyroid carcinoma. *Br J Radiol* 1989;**62**:1017–19.
91. Edmonson G, Charboneau J, James E, et al. Parathyroid carcinoma: high-frequency sonographic features. *Radiology* 1986;**161**:65–7.
92. Evans HE. *Miller's anatomy of the dog*. 3rd ed. Philadelphia, PA: Saunders; 1993. p. 726–7 and 753–4.
93. Burns GO, Scrivani PV, Thompson MS, et al. Relation between age, body weight, and medial retropharyngeal lymph node size in apparently healthy dogs. *Vet Radiol Ultrasound* 2008;**49**:277–81.
94. Ahuja A, Ying M, King W, et al. A practical approach to ultrasound of cervical lymph nodes. *J Laryngol Otol* 1997;**111**:245–56.
95. Sako K, Pradier R, Marchetta F, et al. Fallibility of palpation in the diagnosis of metastasis to the cervical nodes. *Surg Gyneol Obstet* 1964;**118**:989–90.
96. Toriyabe Y, Nishimura T, Kita S, et al. Differentiation between benign and metastatic cervical lymph nodes with ultrasound. *Clin Radiol* 1997;**52**:927–32.
97. Hajek P, Salomonowitz E, Turk R, et al. Lymph nodes of the neck: evaluation with US. *Radiology* 1986;**158**:739–42.
98. Takes R, Knegt P, Manni J, et al. Regional metastasis in head and neck squamous cell carcinoma: Revised value of US with US-guided FNAB [see comments] [published erratum appears in Radiology 202:285, 1997]. *Radiology* 1996;**198**:819–23.
99. Kruyt R, van Putten WL, Levendag P, et al. Biopsy of nonpalpable cervical lymph nodes: selection criteria for ultrasound-guided biopsy in patients with head and neck squamous cell carcinoma. *Ultrasound Med Biol* 1996;**22**:413–19.
100. Atula T, Grenman R, Varpula M, et al. Palpation, ultrasound, and ultrasound-guided fine-needle aspiration cytology in the assessment of cervical lymph node status in head and neck cancer patients. *Head Neck* 1996;**18**:545–51.
101. Atula T, Varpula M, Kurki T, et al. Assessment of cervical lymph node status in head and neck cancer patients: palpation, computed tomography and low field magnetic resonance imaging compared with ultrasound-guided fine-needle aspiration cytology. *Eur J Radiol* 1997;**25**:152–61.
102. Ahuja A, Ying M, Yang W, et al. The use of sonography in differentiating cervical lymphomatous lymph nodes from cervical metastatic lymph nodes. *Clin Radiol* 1996;**51**:186–90.
103. Gooding G. Gray-scale ultrasonography of the neck. *JAMA* 1980;**243**:1562–4.
104. Nyman HT, Lee MH, McEvoy FJ, et al. Comparison of B-mode and Doppler ultrasonographic findings with histologic features of benign and malignant superficial lymph nodes in dogs. *Am J Vet Res* 2006;**67**:978–84.

105. Nyman HT, Kristensen AT, Skovgaard IM, et al. Characterization of normal and abnormal canine superficial lymph nodes using gray-scale B-mode, color flow mapping, power and spectral Doppler ultrasonography: a multivariate study. *Vet Radiol Ultrasound* 2005;**46**: 404–10.

106. Tsunodo-Shimizu H, Saida Y. Ultrasonographic visibility of supraclavicular lymph nodes in normal subjects. *J Ultrasound Med* 1997;**16**:481–3.

107. Som P. Lymph nodes of the neck. *Radiology* 1987; **165**:593–600.

108. Santa DD, Gaschen L, Doherr MG, et al. Spectral waveform analysis of intranodal arterial blood flow in abnormally large superficial lymph nodes in dogs. *Am J Vet Res* 2008;**69**:478–85.

109. Lurie DM, Seguin B, Schneider PD, et al. Contrast-assisted ultrasound for sentinel lymph node detection in spontaneously arising canine head and neck tumors. *Invest Radiol* 2006;**41**:415–21.

110. Nickel R, Schummer A, Seiferle E, editors. *The viscera of the domestic animals.* 2nd ed. New York: Springer-Verlag; 1979.

111. Wittich G, Scheible W, Hajek P. Ultrasonography of the salivary glands. *Radiol Clin North Am* 1985;**23**:29–37.

112. Gooding G. Gray scale ultrasound of the parotid gland. *AJR Am J Roentgenol* 1980;**134**:469–72.

113. Neiman H, Phillips J, Jaques D, et al. Ultrasound of the parotid gland. *J Clin Ultrasound* 1976;**4**:11–13.

114. Gritzmann N. Sonography of the salivary glands. *AJR Am J Roentgenol* 1989;**153**:161–6.

115. Cannon MS, Paglia D, Zwingenberger AL, et al. Clinical and diagnostic imaging findings in dogs with zygomatic sialadenitis: 11 cases (1990-2009). *J Am Vet Med Assoc* 2011;**239**:1211–18.

116. Jubb K, Kennedy P. The upper alimentary canal. In: *Pathology of the domestic animals.* New York: Academic Press; 1970. p. 44–5.

117. Murray M, Buckenham T, Joseph A. The role of ultrasound in screening patients referred for sialography: a possible protocol. *Clin Otolaryngol Allied Sci* 1996;**21**: 21–3.

118. Rudorf H. Ultrasonographic imaging of the tongue and larynx in normal dogs. *J Small Anim Pract* 1997;**38**: 439–44.

119. Bray JP, Lipscombe VJ, White RAS, et al. Ultrasonographic examination of the pharynx and larynx of the normal dog. *Vet Radiol Ultrasound* 1998;**39**:566–71.

120. Rudorf H, Barr F. Echolaryngography in cats. *Vet Radiol Ultrasound* 2002;**43**:353–7.

121. Rudorf H, Brown P. Ultrasonography of laryngeal masses in six cats and one dog. *Vet Radiol Ultrasound* 1998;**39**: 430–4.

122. Rudorf H, Barr FJ, Lane JG. The role of ultrasound in the assessment of laryngeal paralysis in the dog. *Vet Radiol Ultrasound* 2001;**42**:338–43.

123. Rudorf H, Herrtage M, White R. Use of ultrasonography in the diagnosis of tracheal collapse. *J Small Anim Pract* 1997;**38**:513–18.

124. Shih J, Lee L, Wu H, et al. Sonographic imaging of the trachea. *J Ultrasound Med* 1997;**16**:783–90.

125. Doldi S, Lattuada E, Zappa M, et al. Ultrasonographic imaging of neoplasms of the cervical esophagus. *Hepatogastroenterology* 1997;**44**:724–6.

126. Solano M, Penninck DG. Ultrasonography of the canine, feline and equine tongue: normal findings and case history reports. *Vet Radiol Ultrasound* 1996;**37**:206–13.

127. Gooding G, Herzog K, Laing F, et al. Ultrasonographic assessment of neck masses. *J Clin Ultrasound* 1977;**5**: 248–52.

128. Ahuja A, King A, Kew J, et al. Head and neck lipomas: sonographic appearance. *AJNR Am J Neuroradiol* 1998; **19**:505–8.

129. Oates C, Wilson A, Ward-Booth RP, Williams ED. Combined use of Doppler and conventional ultrasound for the diagnosis of vascular and other lesions in the head and neck. *Int J Oral Maxillofac Surg* 1990;**19**:235–9.

130. Lambrects NE, Pearson J. Cervical teratoma in a dog. *J S Afr Vet Assoc* 2001;**72**:49–51.

131. Armbrust LJ, Biller DS, Radlinsky MG, et al. Ultrasonographic diagnosis of foreign bodies associated with chronic draining tracts and abscesses in dogs. *Vet Radiol Ultrasound* 2003;**44**:66–70.

CHAPTER 7
Thorax

Dana A. Neelis • John S. Mattoon • Thomas G. Nyland

ltrasound examination has become a valuable diagnostic procedure for assessment of thoracic disease in small animals.[1-9] The usefulness of thoracic ultrasonography is maximized when it is performed with thoracic radiography and in the presence of pleural fluid. Pleural fluid often masks intrathoracic lesions on radiographs yet serves as an acoustic window into the thorax for ultrasound examinations. Ultrasonography may be used to detect, characterize, and determine the cause of pleural fluid; to diagnose pneumothorax and mediastinal, pleural, and pulmonary diseases; and to assess the integrity of the diaphragm. Ultrasound is invaluable in differentiating cardiac from noncardiac disease. It is routinely used to aid needle placement for thoracentesis and to safely procure needle aspirates or biopsy samples. Ultrasound examination of the thorax when disease is not diagnosed on thoracic radiographs is challenging and often unrewarding because most intrathoracic anatomy is hidden by the lungs. Thoracic ultrasonography is limited by the barriers of the aerated lungs, bony thorax, and pneumothorax.

SCANNING TECHNIQUES

After appropriate clipping of the hair coat and application of acoustic coupling gel, intercostal, parasternal, cardiac, thoracic inlet, and subcostal (abdominal) windows into the thorax may be used. The patient may be positioned in lateral, sternal, or dorsal recumbency, or scanning may be performed while the patient is standing or sitting (Figure 7-1). Sternal recumbency or standing is preferable when significant respiratory compromise or discomfort is present (e.g., severe pleural effusion). Imaging the dependent portion of the thorax through a cardiac table is often ideal. This approach optimizes the use of gravity-dependent pleural fluid as an acoustic window and allows assessment of the heart. In practice, repositioning the patient and using multiple scan windows are routinely required for thorough examination of the thorax.

The acoustic window into the thorax must not be in an area where aerated lung lies between the transducer and the site of disease, because aerated lung effectively reflects the insonating ultrasound beam. The location or type of disease found on thoracic radiographs usually determines the appropriate site to begin the examination. Pleural fluid provides an excellent acoustic window for visualizing most intrathoracic structures. When large effusions are present, virtually every site provides an acoustic window into the thorax. If the effusion is small, the patient may need to be scanned from the dependent portion of the thorax to take advantage of fluid displacement of the lungs. When pleural fluid is absent, selecting an appropriate acoustic window may be challenging.

For the intercostal approach, the transducer is placed between ribs, and the intercostal spaces are scanned from dorsal to ventral (see Figure 7-1, *A, D* to *F*). With the plane of the ultrasound beam directed parallel to the ribs, a transverse (cross-sectional) image of the thorax is produced. Rotating the transducer 90 degrees sections the thorax in a dorsal (frontal) image plane. Ribs interfere with the contact area of transducers that have a large footprint, creating strong acoustic shadows. This is particularly true with linear-array transducers. Transducers with smaller footprints make better contact with the patient, but acoustic shadows from underlying ribs may still compromise the image because of divergence of the ultrasound beam.

From an intercostal approach, the transducer may be positioned ventrally between costal cartilages, adjacent to the sternum, allowing access to the cranial and caudal mediastinum. This is the parasternal window (see Figure 7-1 *A* and *D*). In this position, the ultrasound beam may be ventral to the aerated lung margins and allow a window to mediastinal structures.

The heart may be used as an acoustic window for assessment of noncardiac structures. Access to the cranial and caudal mediastinum and the heart base region in the absence of pleural fluid is sometimes possible. The diaphragm and liver are often seen when the heart is imaged through a standard cardiac window. Scanning the dependent side of the patient in right lateral recumbency provides the most successful acoustic window to the heart when pleural fluid is minimal or absent (see Figure 7-1, *F*). Other useful scanning approaches include left lateral recumbent, sternal recumbent, standing, and sitting positions.

Placement of the transducer in the thoracic inlet allows limited visualization of cranial mediastinal structures (see Figure 7-1, *B* and *C*). It is often a supplementary approach to the more standard imaging windows. The transducer is placed in the thoracic inlet to the right or left of midline or on midline between the manubrium ventrally and the trachea dorsally. The transducer is oriented to produce dorsal, sagittal, or oblique images of the cranial mediastinum and thorax. The patient is usually standing or in sternal recumbency. The thoracic inlet window is most useful in the presence of pleural fluid or mediastinal mass lesions. This technique is also useful for certain cardiac applications.

A subcostal approach uses the liver as an acoustic window into the thorax (see Figure 7-1, *G*). The transducer is positioned caudal to the costal arch, and the patient is positioned in dorsal or lateral recumbency, standing, or sitting. The subcostal window is particularly suited for assessment of the diaphragm and the caudal lung field and when the caudal thorax is of particular interest. In some instances, use of the

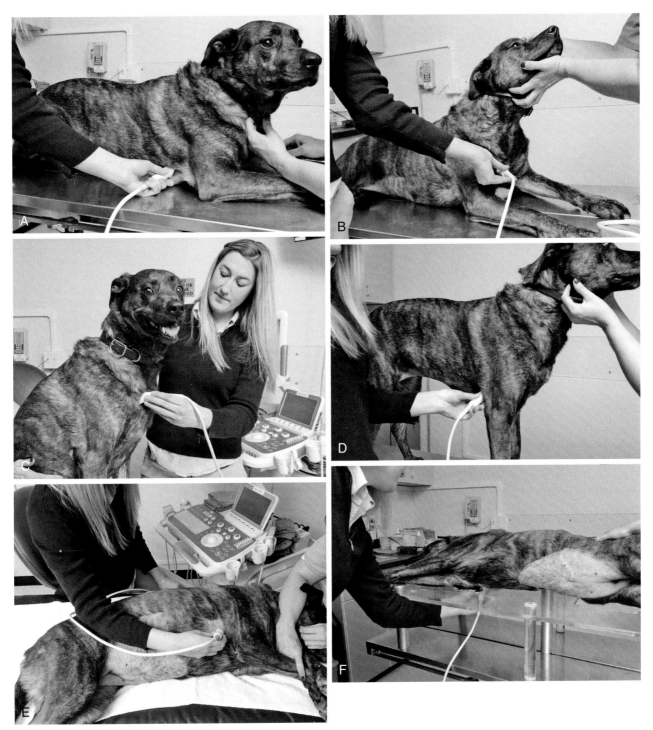

Figure 7-1 **Examples of positioning the patient and transducer for thoracic ultrasound examinations.**
A, Sternal recumbency. The transducer is positioned in a right intercostal space dorsal to the sternum. The patient is frequently positioned in sternal recumbency when pleural effusion is present, which may compromise respiration. **B,** Sternal recumbency with the transducer positioned in the thoracic inlet, a useful, often supplementary window to view the cranial mediastinum. **C,** Sitting position with transducer positioned in the thoracic inlet. **D,** Standing patient. The transducer is in a parasternal position on the right thoracic wall. The standing position is frequently used when the patient is in respiratory distress. **E,** Left lateral recumbency. The transducer is in an intercostal position on the nondependent right thoracic wall. This position is particularly useful for interventional procedures of the thorax. **F,** Right lateral recumbency. The use of a notched table (cardiac table) allows the transducer to be positioned on the dependent right thoracic wall from below. This position allows small amounts of gravity-dependent pleural fluid to be used as an acoustic window into the thorax. It is also a standard position for cardiac imaging.

Continued

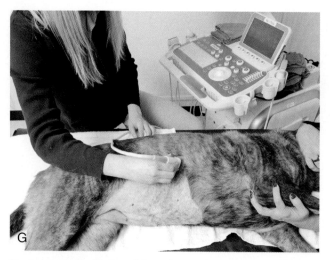

Figure 7-1, cont'd **G,** Left lateral recumbency subcostal window. The transducer is positioned just caudal to the costal arch, and the liver is used as an acoustic window into the thorax. This position is commonly used for assessing the diaphragm and for imaging caudal or accessory lung lobe lesions.

liver as an acoustic window may be the only way to image a lesion (e.g., caudal or accessory lung lobe lesions).

As always, the highest frequency transducer that allows adequate depth penetration is desired for optimal resolution of anatomic structures. When pleural fluid is present, higher frequency transducers may be used despite a patient's large size, because fluid is efficient in propagating ultrasound. In very small patients, it is often helpful or necessary to use a standoff pad to position shallow structures within the focal zone of the transducer.

NORMAL ANATOMY

Ultrasound assessment of normal intrathoracic structures (excluding the heart) is less rewarding than that of most other anatomic regions owing to the limitations created by aerated lung. Nonetheless, it is important for the sonographer to recognize normal structures and to appreciate the inherent limitations of thoracic ultrasound examination.

Body Wall and Lung Surface
Subcutaneous tissue, abdominal wall and intercostal musculature, and pleural lining of the thorax (parietal pleura) and the lung surface (visceral pleura) may be visualized (Figure 7-2). The subcutaneous fat and connective tissue are echogenic, and just deep to this, thin abdominal and intercostal muscles may be seen as relatively hypoechoic tissue with coarse parenchymal texture. Without a standoff pad or high-frequency transducers capable of high near-field resolution (linear-array, convex, and microconvex electronic transducers in the 7.5- to 15-MHz range), extrathoracic tissues will not be satisfactorily imaged. The parietal pleura is rarely recognized as a discrete structure, but when it is resolved from the lung surface, it is seen as a thin, highly echogenic, linear structure (see Figure 7-2, C; see also Figure 7-33, *B*). The parietal pleura is easiest to visualize separately from the visceral pleura in real time as the lung surface glides along it. The lung surface has a characteristic linear echogenic appearance because of it is highly reflective. It glides to and fro along the parietal surface during respiration and is readily identified by respiratory motion (the gliding sign).[10] In patients with shallow and rapid respiration, the gliding sign may be difficult to observe.

The bright linear echoes created by the parietal and visceral pleural surfaces should be thin and smooth. Although a small amount of pleural fluid normally acts as a lubricant between the two pleural surfaces, this is not routinely observed in small animal patients. Careful observation of the pleural surface is important; a roughened or cobblestone appearance usually indicates a pathologic process, such as pleuritis, carcinomatosis, chronic pleural effusions, and some types of pulmonary disease.

Reverberation artifact is created as the ultrasound beam strongly reflects off the surface of the aerated lung. Air has a low acoustic impedance ($Z = 0.0004$ versus 1.70 of muscle), so when the insonating ultrasound beam exits the thoracic wall and interacts with the lung surface, 99% of the sound is reflected. A series of reflections ensue between the lung surface and the transducer, creating a sequence of highly echogenic linear echoes deep to the surface of the lung, known as reverberation artifact. These repeating linear reverberations occur most strongly when the incident ultrasound beam is exactly perpendicular to the surface of the lung. When off-incident ultrasound interacts with the surface of the lung, distinct reverberations may not be seen. Instead, composite echoes are commonly encountered below the lung surface, giving the appearance of actual lung tissue. This image is a form of acoustic shadowing. It has been referred to as dirty shadowing as opposed to clean, distinct anechoic shadowing created by bone or mineral. These artifacts *do not represent lung parenchyma.* Normal lung parenchyma cannot be imaged by ultrasound; only its surface can be imaged.

Because of the acoustic properties of aerated lung, only the lung surface may be imaged in the presence of normal lung. Accordingly, if peripheral lung tissue is aerated, pathologic processes deeper within the pulmonary parenchyma cannot be imaged because of interposition of aerated lung.

Mediastinum
The mediastinum is the space between the right and left pleural sacs and may be divided anatomically into cranial, middle (cardiac), and caudal portions.[11] The mediastinum is difficult to image in normal patients because it is surrounded by lung. It also contains a varying amount of fat, which has a coarse echo texture and does not transmit ultrasound well. Obese patients and breeds in which the cranial mediastinum normally contains abundant fat (e.g., bulldogs) are especially difficult to image. Although fat does not lend itself to high-quality images, it may still provide an acoustic window in some instances. Because normal mediastinal tissue is difficult to image, small lesions such as mild lymphadenopathy may easily be overlooked unless pleural fluid is present to provide a better acoustic window. Fortunately, mediastinal masses large enough to contact the thoracic wall are easily imaged through an intercostal or parasternal acoustic window.

One approach to the cranial mediastinum is through the thoracic inlet. The image plane may be sagittal, sagittal oblique, or dorsal (frontal). Consistent anatomic landmarks on imaging of the thoracic inlet include the trachea, the esophagus, and various caudal cervical and cranial mediastinal vessels (see Chapter 6, Figures 6-6 to 6-13). The trachea is readily identifiable because of its characteristic sonographic pattern created by the tracheal rings and acoustic shadowing, reverberation, and mirror image artifact. The esophagus is to the left of the trachea at the level of the thoracic inlet. The right or left jugular veins are seen as anechoic tubular structures during superficial imaging of the cervical region, leading into the thoracic inlet and joining the right and left brachiocephalic veins, which in turn drain to the cranial vena cava. Careful scanning technique may allow identification of additional venous structures, such as the subclavian and internal jugular veins.

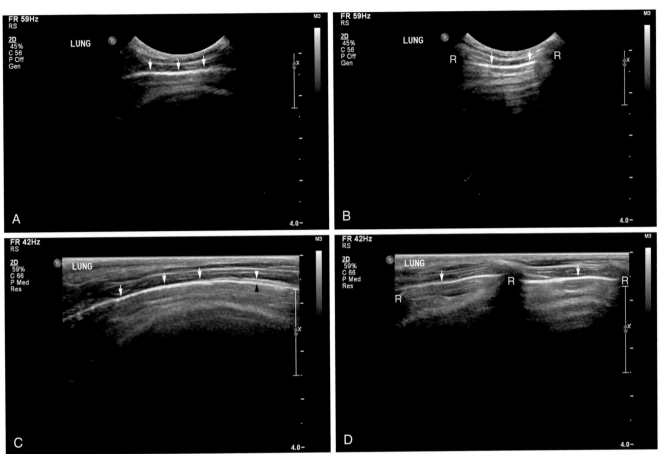

Figure 7-2 **Normal thoracic body wall and lung surface.** *A,* Transverse intercostal image. The thin, smooth echogenic lung surface is indicated by the arrows. Subcutaneous fat and intercostal musculature are seen in the near field as mixed echoes with some striation. The area beneath the lung surface is reverberation artifact and "dirty" acoustic shadowing. A microconvex transducer was used. *B,* Dorsal intercostal image. The thin, smooth echogenic lung surface is indicated by the arrows. Subcutaneous fat and intercostal musculature are seen in the near field as mixed echoes with some striation. Ribs (R) are creating strong ("clean") acoustic shadows. In this example, multiple, repeating horizontally oriented reverberation echo artifacts are noted below the lung surface in addition to dirty acoustic shadowing. A microconvex transducer was used. *C,* Transverse intercostal image. The near-field subcutaneous tissues are better resolved with the use of a linear-array transducer. The lung surface is denoted by *white arrows*. Mild retraction of the lung surface allows visualization of the thin hypoechoic pleural space (*between arrowheads*), between the parietal (*white arrowhead*) and visceral (*black arrowhead*) pleura. *D,* Dorsal intercostal image, linear-array transducer. The echogenic lung surface (*arrows*) is present between ribs (R) creating strong acoustic shadows.

The common carotid arteries can readily be identified in most patients; other arterial vessels are less consistently seen and identified unless pleural or mediastinal fluid is present (Figure 7-3). Arterial structures include the aortic arch, the brachiocephalic trunk, and the left subclavian artery. The right subclavian and the left and right common carotid arteries arise from the brachiocephalic truck.

Arteries can be identified by their pulsatile movement as well as by familiarity with anatomy. Arteries are generally smaller than veins in the mediastinum. Doppler analysis can definitively differentiate arterial from venous blood flow (see Chapter 6, Figure 6-6). Familiarity with normal anatomy may allow identification of individual vascular structures. However, angiography (and computed tomography (CT) angiography) is the gold standard when vascular anatomy must be studied in detail, such as for evaluation of vascular ring anomaly before surgery.

In the normal dog or cat, mediastinal lymph nodes can rarely be imaged, because they are hidden behind mediastinal fat. Normal small, hypoechoic, round to oval mediastinal lymph nodes are occasionally seen in cases of pleural effusion, such as that secondary to heart failure. Reactive lymph nodes may be difficult if not impossible to distinguish from normal lymph nodes in such instances. Neoplastic lymph nodes are generally much larger than reactive lymph nodes. However, size alone cannot be used to reliably differentiate neoplastic from nonneoplastic lymphadenopathy.

The thymus may be seen as mediastinal tissue of moderate echogenicity with a granular, coarse, yet homogeneous echo texture ventral to mediastinal vessels. It is best imaged from a left parasternal window. Because the thymus is positioned obliquely within the ventral cranial mediastinum, it is best imaged in an oblique transverse plane, positioned to approximate thymic orientation. It contacts the cranial margin of the heart (Figure 7-4). The thymus is largest by 4 to 5 months of age and begins involuting shortly thereafter.[12]

Assessment of cranial mediastinal thickness is difficult in most patients without the presence of pleural fluid. A thoracic inlet or parasternal window may occasionally be used to assess the mediastinal structures in the absence of pleural fluid. This is especially applicable for patients with abundant body fat, because a mediastinum that is wider because of fat deposition displaces lung tissue laterally and dorsally. Cranial mediastinal fat is echogenic and has a coarse but homogeneous texture (Figure 7-5). Recognition of the sonographic appearance of normal mediastinal fat is important in differentiating it from lymphadenopathy and other mediastinal disease or fluid, all of which may present radiographically as a widened mediastinum.

A cardiac window may be used to assess the heart base region and to access the cranial and caudal mediastinum. Normal tracheobronchial lymph nodes cannot be imaged transcutaneously because lung interferes with assessment of the heart base region in most patients. In fact, even hilar

lymphadenopathy may be difficult to image unless pleural fluid is present. Once the heart is in view from a parasternal window, the mediastinum may rarely be viewed by tilting the image plane cranially or caudally. Cranial direction of the ultrasound plane may yield a view of the cranial mediastinal structures. Caudal orientation may allow visualization of the diaphragm and liver.

Alternatively, endoscopic ultrasonography can be used to evaluate mediastinal structures that may be difficult to visualize transcutaneously because of the overlying aerated lung. One in-depth report describes the normal appearance of the canine mediastinum by transesophageal ultrasonography.[13] In this description, transesophageal ultrasonography allowed excellent visualization of the heart base region, the major cranial mediastinal vessels, and the descending aorta, yet hilar lymph nodes were inconsistently imaged. However, in another more recent review of endoscopic ultrasound in veterinary medicine, the authors reported that tracheobronchial lymph nodes and heart base lesions were readily identified.[14]

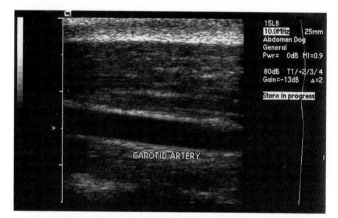

Figure 7-3 Thoracic inlet dorsal plane image of the common carotid artery. The lumen is anechoic and the arterial wall is thicker than the jugular vein wall.

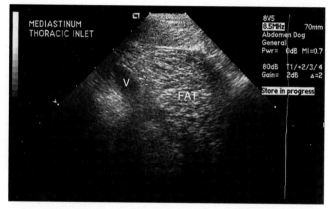

Figure 7-5 Cranial mediastinal fat in a dachshund. Thoracic inlet window shows the mediastinal fat (FAT) as a coarse but homogeneous echogenicity. An anechoic vessel (V) is seen to the left of the mediastinal fat.

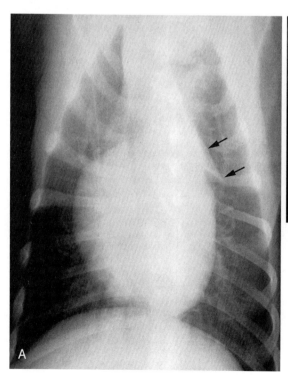

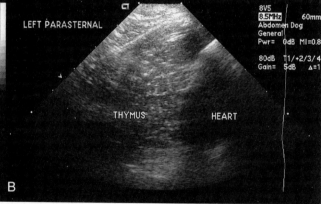

Figure 7-4 Thymus in a 4-month-old German shepherd. A, Ventrodorsal radiograph showing the thymus (*arrows*), often referred to as the "sail sign." **B,** Left parasternal oblique transverse image of the thymus. The thymus has a granular, coarse, and homogeneous parenchyma. The thymus is in contact with the cranial margin of the heart.

Additionally, two clinical cases have been reported using endoscopic ultrasound to help diagnose intrathoracic pathology.[15] In these two cases, endoscopic ultrasound allowed visualization of a caudal mediastinal cavitary mass, enlarged tracheobronchial lymph nodes, and a right caudal lung lobe mass. Unfortunately, this technique uses ultrasound equipment specifically designed for transesophageal application, which is currently not readily available to most veterinarians. Transesophageal ultrasonography may become more common in veterinary practice as used equipment becomes available from human hospitals. One negative aspect of transesophageal ultrasonography in small animal practice is that general anesthesia is required.

In the presence of pleural fluid, the normal mediastinum is seen in a lean animal as a thin, echogenic, and distinct structure (Figures 7-6 and 7-7). Varying amounts of echogenic fat will increase cranial and caudal mediastinal thickness accordingly. Cranial and caudal mediastinal vessels are readily apparent in the appropriate scan plane (Figure 7-8). An intercostal or parasternal window works well with either a dorsal or transverse scan plane, allowing the sonographer to determine whether there is a mediastinal mass or other pathologic process concurrent with pleural effusion.

Diaphragm

The diaphragm is routinely imaged through the abdomen by a subcostal approach using the liver as an acoustic window. In fact, the diaphragm is seen routinely in all thorough ultrasound evaluations of the liver. It is normally difficult to resolve the diaphragm as a discrete structure from the adjacent highly reflective, echogenic lung interface. The diaphragm appears as an echogenic, thin, curvilinear structure bounding the cranial surface of the liver (Figure 7-9). Mirror image artifact is usually seen at this location, with the illusion of liver on the thoracic side of the diaphragm (see Chapter 1, Figures 1-41 and 1-42).

The presence of pleural fluid, abdominal fluid, and especially both allows better resolution of the diaphragm than is otherwise possible. The peripheral to mid portion of the diaphragm is muscular and may be imaged when high-resolution

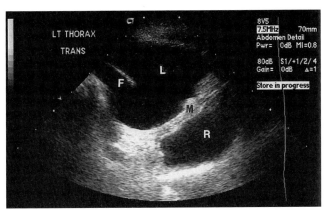

Figure 7-6 Left parasternal transverse image of a normal canine cranial mediastinum (*M*) surrounded by anechoic pleural fluid in the left (*L*) and right (*R*) hemithoraces. A thin echogenic fibrin tag (*F*) is identified. Note in this case of chylothorax that the pleural fluid is anechoic.

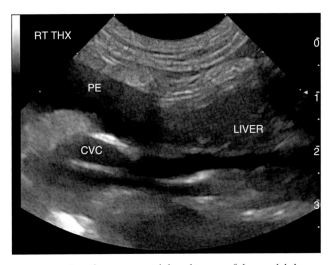

Figure 7-8 Standing intercostal dorsal image of the caudal thorax in a cat with a large amount of anechoic pleural effusion (*PE*) shows the caudal vena cava (*CVC*) coursing from the liver (*LIVER*) toward the right atrium. This patient had pneumonia with collapse of the right middle lung lobe.

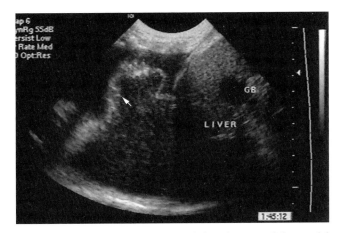

Figure 7-7 Standing right intercostal dorsal image of the caudal thorax showing the caudal mediastinum as a thin and irregular echogenic structure (*arrow*) within hypoechoic to anechoic pleural fluid. Loss of the image of the diaphragm and liver in the mid to far field is an artifact. The liver and gallbladder (*GB*) are seen to the right.

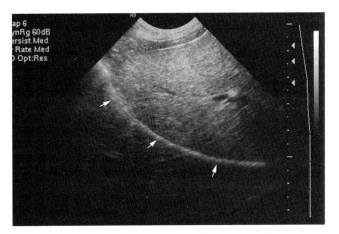

Figure 7-9 Sagittal subcostal image of the liver showing the diaphragm-lung interface as an echogenic curvilinear structure (*arrows*).

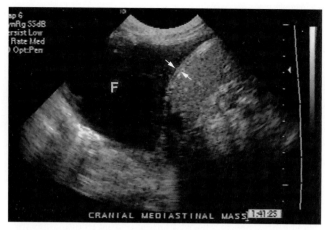

Figure 7-10 Standing left intercostal dorsal image of the caudal thorax in a patient with severe pleural effusion. The peripheral muscular portion of the diaphragm is seen as two parallel curvilinear echogenic structures (*arrows*) separating anechoic pleural fluid (*F*) from the liver.

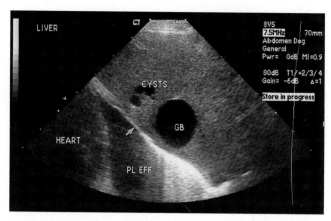

Figure 7-11 Subcostal sagittal image of the liver and cranial abdomen showing hypoechoic pleural effusion (*PL EFF*). The thin echogenic diaphragm (*arrow*) is seen separating the liver from the pleural fluid. Several anechoic hepatic cysts (*CYSTS*) and the gallbladder (*GB*) are seen. The heart is in the lower left of the image.

equipment is used (Figure 7-10). The diaphragm appears as a thin hypoechoic structure sandwiched between two thinner, highly echogenic layers, which represent endothoracic fascia and parietal pleura on the thoracic side and transversalis fascia and peritoneum on the abdominal surface. The central portion of the diaphragm is tendinous and thinner than the peripheral muscular portion; it is seen as a thin, single, echogenic curvilinear structure (see Figure 7-9).

The basic caveat for sonographic assessment of the diaphragm is to visualize it completely. Radiography helps localize the portion of interest in the diaphragm; in most cases, search for a diaphragmatic hernia is done after radiography. When pleural fluid is absent, the diaphragm should be imaged transabdominally, by a subcostal approach supplemented with intercostal imaging. The area should be thoroughly scanned in sagittal body planes from left to right, with the liver used as an acoustic window. It is often necessary to aim the transducer cranially to fully image the diaphragm. The transducer should also be oriented 90 degrees to create a transverse (cross-sectional) image. In this plane, the transducer is slowly directed cranially; the scan plane thus changes from a transverse to a dorsal plane. This technique allows simultaneous assessment of the right and left portions of the diaphragm in small to medium-sized patients. Along the lateral-most margins of the diaphragm, the transducer may need to be rotated nearly 90 degrees to be essentially perpendicular to the body wall. Subcostal herniation may occur here, and it is perhaps the most challenging portion of the diaphragm to assess. Imaging this area from an intercostal approach has proved beneficial. A standoff pad is usually necessary for critical evaluation of these superficial diaphragmatic attachments.

PLEURAL DISEASE

Pleural Effusion

The presence of pleural fluid, particularly moderate or large amounts, greatly enhances the ability to image intrathoracic structures. This is contrary to radiography, in which normal anatomy is obscured. Mediastinal fat and vessels are readily apparent, as are surfaces of the heart, lungs, and diaphragm. The caudal vena cava may be seen, traced into the right atrium (see Figure 7-8). On occasion, the esophagus may be imaged. In rare instances, the trachea and main stem bronchi are seen.

Pleural effusion is recognized as anechoic or echogenic material within the pleural space, between the thoracic wall or diaphragm and lung (Figures 7-11 to 7-15; see also Figures 7-6 to 7-8, and 7-10). The appearance is variable, depending on the amount as well as the type of fluid. Transudates, modified transudates, and chylous effusions are generally anechoic or hypoechoic, whereas exudates (see Figure 7-13), hemorrhage, and carcinomatosis are usually more echogenic. However, as Figure 7-14 illustrates, analysis of fluid based on echogenicity is unreliable. If it is echogenic, movement may readily identify the material as fluid. Chronic effusions can lead to fibrin formation, which may be seen as linear, irregular echogenic strands floating within the fluid (pleural septations). A small amount of fluid, seen as mild separation of the parietal and visceral pleura, may be difficult to detect. This may be noted through intercostal windows with separation of the lung surface from the thoracic wall, or small anechoic spaces between the lung and the diaphragm. Scanning of the dependent thoracic wall may be required. Moderate or large effusions are recognized immediately from virtually any window into the thorax. The heart is recognized by fluid around it, and the lungs may literally be floating. As the amount of fluid increases, lung volume diminishes to the point of total atelectasis.

In the cranial thorax, pleural fluid can be seen as two discrete pockets separated by the mediastinum (see Figure 7-6). The cranial extent of the pleural space is rounded or blunted. The appearance is distinctly different from mediastinal fluid accumulation, in which the boundaries of the mediastinum are widened and the mediastinal vessels are separated from echogenic mediastinal fat by anechoic, irregularly shaped fluid pockets.

Asymmetrical fluid accumulation may be difficult to detect or be missed entirely on an ultrasound examination unless there is direction provided by thoracic radiographs. Examples include focal hemorrhage from trauma, pleural disease such as inflammation secondary to migrating foreign bodies,[16] and neoplastic processes involving the pleura or ribs. The contribution of thoracic radiographs to successful ultrasound examination of the thorax cannot be overemphasized.

Identification of pleural fluid dictates that the sonographer search for a cause within both the thorax and the abdomen. Ultrasound assessment may contribute to the diagnosis of heart failure, neoplasia (mediastinal, pulmonary, pleural,

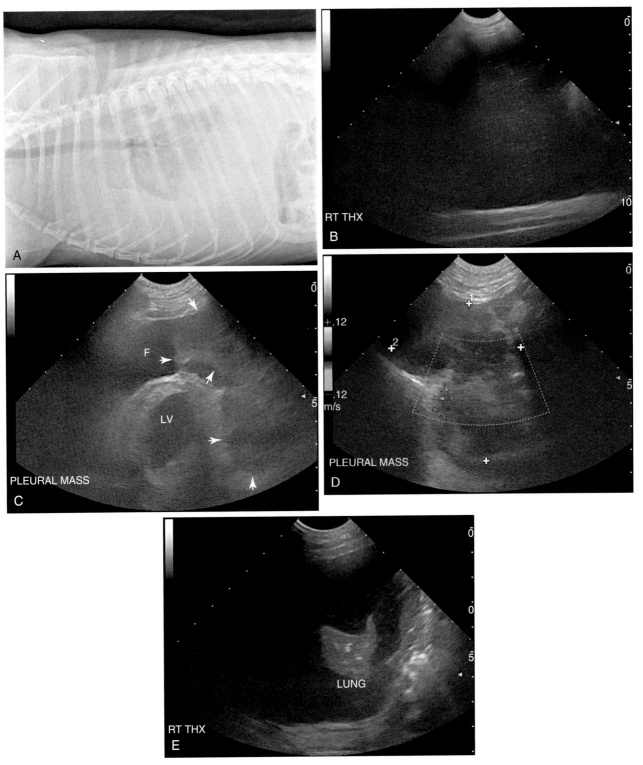

Figure 7-12 **Hemorrhagic pleural effusion secondary to mesothelioma in an 8-year-old dog with a 2-week history of lethargy and inappetence, presented with severe dyspnea. A,** Massive pleural effusion is seen on this lateral thoracic radiograph. Ultrasound is often used in cases such as this to determine an etiology for the effusion. **B,** Ultrasound image of the right hemithorax shows tiny echoes evenly dispersed throughout nearly anechoic fluid. This was a hemorrhagic exudate; malignant cells were not seen on cytology. **C,** A large, lobulated, and solid appearing thoracic mass is visible (*arrows*). Its origin was uncertain but did not contain any residual air that would indicate a lung mass. *F,* Pleural fluid; *LV,* heart. **D,** Color Doppler image of the thoracic mass shows only a small amount of blood flow in the periphery of the mass (between electronic cursors, 6.85 × 5.78 cm). **E,** A completely atelectatic (collapsed) lung lobe (*LUNG*) is seen floating in the pleural effusion. The gross diagnosis at necropsy was a hemangiosarcoma (presumptive) with associated blood clot and hemothorax. However, histologic final diagnosis was mesothelioma, metastatic to pleura and mediastinal lymph nodes.

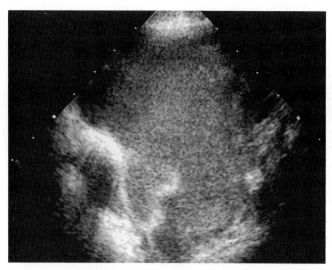

Figure 7-13 Highly echogenic severe pleural fluid accumulation in a dog with pyothorax.

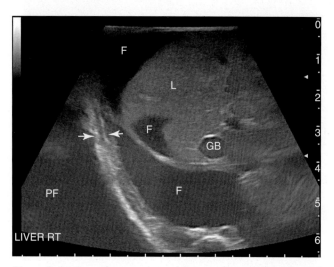

Figure 7-14 Juvenile cat presented for an enlarging abdomen and some respiratory distress, with a prior history of being attacked by a dog 2 months earlier. There was clinical suspicion of a potential diaphragmatic hernia. A sagittal image of the cranial abdomen (L, liver; GB, gallbladder) and caudal thorax shows a large amount of abdominal fluid (F) and pleural fluid (PF). The fluids in the two cavities appear identical and are essentially anechoic. A muscular portion of the diaphragm is seen (between arrows) and could be imaged nearly completely, indicating that a diaphragmatic hernia is unlikely. However, the similarity of the pleural and abdominal effusions suggested potential communication between the thorax and the abdomen and prompted sampling of both. Interestingly, the thoracic fluid was a hemorrhagic exudate, whereas the abdominal fluid was a clear and colorless transudate. This example illustrates the potential errors of "fluid analysis" based on ultrasound appearance. A diaphragmatic hernia was not present.

cardiac), pneumonia, lung torsion, trauma, diaphragmatic hernia, and possible esophageal rupture. Hepatic disease, pancreatitis, glomerulonephritis, pyometra, and systemic effects secondary to parturition may cause pleural effusions, indicating the potential need for abdominal ultrasound examination. Other causes of pleural effusion are infectious agents, foreign

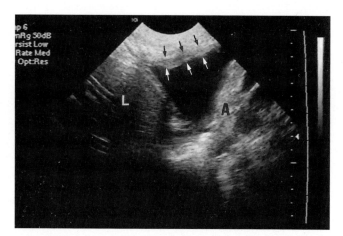

Figure 7-15 Pleural thickening (arrows) in a patient with chronic pleural effusion secondary to pyothorax. Anechoic pleural effusion separates an echogenic atelectatic lung lobe (A) and the liver (L).

body migration, autoimmune disease, coagulopathies, pulmonary thromboembolism, hyperthyroidism, and prior invasive procedures of the thorax and abdomen.[17] Pleural fluid analysis is paramount in reaching a definitive diagnosis and should not be overlooked regardless of the findings of an ultrasound examination.

Pleural Surfaces

Pleural thickening is usually first diagnosed on thoracic radiographs. Ultrasound may be used to characterize the thickening or to more precisely locate the pathologic process. This may include differentiating parietal pleural from visceral pleural disease. Mild pleural fibrosis is seen as smooth, echogenic thickening of the parietal or visceral pleura. Of more concern is when the pleural surfaces are irregularly thickened; this is more indicative of inflammation, as may be seen with empyema, or pleural neoplasia (see Figure 7-15). Active pleuritis generally has some degree of accompanying pleural fluid, which may be echogenic and contain fibrinous strands. Neoplastic pleural disease is also generally effusive.

In cases of thoracic trauma, the pleura may be scanned to assess whether wounds have penetrated the thorax or are confined to the extrathoracic tissues. Integrity of the pleural surface is evaluated by observing the continuous nature of the linear parietal pleura echogenicity. Focal pleural fluid accumulation is usually present with penetrating wounds. Hypoechoic areas beneath the surface of the lung indicate lung disease, such as hemorrhage or inflammation.

Pleural Masses

Pleural masses may be detected radiographically and thus prompt ultrasound evaluation (Figure 7-16). Pleural masses may also be hidden radiographically, silhouetting with pleural fluid and subsequently diagnosed by ultrasound examination (see Figure 7-12). Deciding whether a peripheral thoracic mass is pleural, mediastinal, or pulmonary in origin can be challenging on the basis of radiographic findings alone; multiple tangential views are often required. The two masses can theoretically be distinguished on ultrasound evaluation by observing whether the mass moves with respiratory motion (pulmonary origin) or is stationary with lung motion surrounding it (indicating a parietal pleural origin). However, this is often easier said than done. Figure 7-12 shows an example where a large mass was identified, but the organ of origin could not be confidently determined by ultrasound.

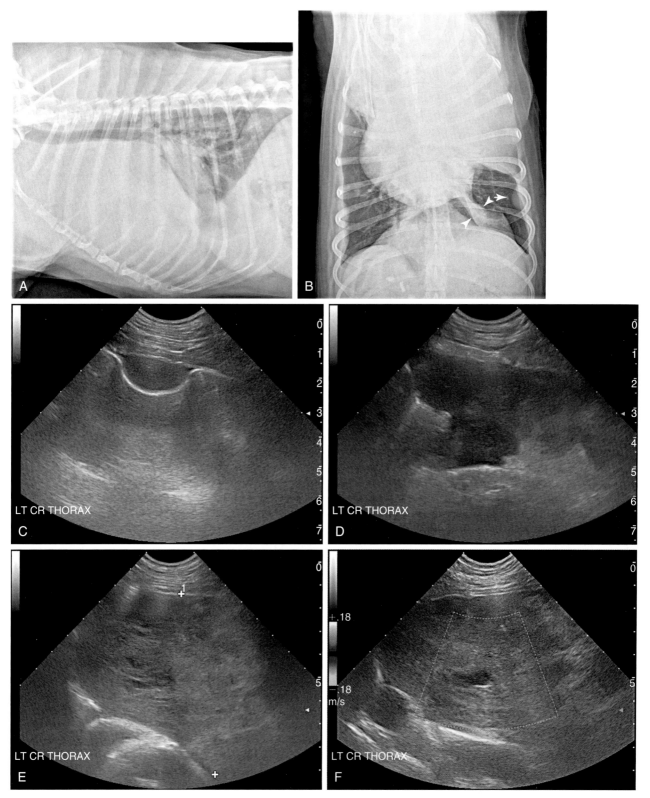

Figure 7-16 **Pleural and mediastinal undifferentiated sarcoma is a 4-year-old Samoyed dog. A,** Right lateral radiograph showing large abnormal soft tissue opacity in the cranial thorax with severe tracheal elevation. **B,** Ventrodorsal view shows large cranial thoracic soft tissue mass. A focal pleural soft tissue nodule is also present along the left thoracic wall (*arrow*). Also note the thickened caudal mediastinum (*arrowheads*). **C,** Ultrasound image of the pleural nodule seen on the ventrodorsal radiograph (**B**). The hyperechoic lung surface provides a smooth contour against the nodule. **D,** Large, hypoechoic, irregularly marginated pleural mass is present. Hyperechoic lung surfaces adjacent to the mass are seen in the far field. **E,** Large, echogenic, complex cranial mediastinal mass (between electronic cursors, 7.95 cm). **F,** Color Doppler image of the cranial mediastinal mass shown in **E,** indicating lack of blood flow within the mass.

A report in the human literature illustrates the appearance of a solitary fibrous tumor arising from the pleural surface of the diaphragm.[18] It was described as a well-circumscribed, relatively hypoechoic structure displacing adjacent lung. The linear echogenic diaphragm was still evident. The appearance is amazingly similar to a caudal lung lobe mass in a dog[1] and illustrates the necessity of observing lung motion to help differentiate pleural from pulmonary lesions.

Pneumothorax

Thoracic radiology is the imaging modality of choice for diagnosis of pneumothorax, although ultrasound is emerging as a tool for pneumothorax detection, especially in veterinary emergency medicine. Ultrasound assessment for the presence of pneumothorax can be useful, particularly after interventional procedures of the thorax or when a patient cannot be transported for a radiographic or CT examination.[19] Accurate diagnosis of pneumothorax (or its absence) using ultrasound takes practice. It a diagnosis made on real-time examination, assessing the presence or absence of lung gliding motion. The sonographer must differentiate a highly reflective normal lung surface that moves with respiration (gliding sign) from a highly reflective stationary parietal pleural air surface, which does not move with respiration. However, ultrasound is comparable to radiography for detection of pneumothorax in humans.[20-22]

With concurrent pleural fluid and pneumothorax, a gas-fluid interface can be detected sonographically. Gas in a dorsal space creates a reverberation artifact, which masks the underlying lung. The characteristic visceral pleural surface of the lung will thus be absent when pneumothorax is present. On imaging of the thorax in a transverse (cross-sectional) plane, the gas-fluid interface may be observed to repetitively move ventral to dorsal, synchronous with respiration. The gas level moves ventrally (drops) at inspiration but moves dorsally (rises) at expiration, owing to differences in thoracic volume during inspiration and expiration. As the dorsally located air moves ventrally during inspiration, it masks underlying structures seen during expiration. This is best observed by imaging just below the gas-fluid level. At this location, only pleural fluid is imaged during exhalation. During inhalation, the reverberation artifact progressively invades the image dorsally, replacing the pleural fluid. The effect has been compared with the lowering of a curtain and is referred to as the "curtain" sign.[10] It is best seen when pleural fluid and consolidated or atelectatic lung are present.

Pneumothorax without concurrent pleural effusion can be difficult to detect sonographically. It may be diagnosed by the absence of the gliding sign in spite of reverberation artifact. The gliding sign is the normal, smooth motion of the lung against the thoracic wall during inspiration and expiration. Free air within the thorax creates the same reverberation artifact that normal lung does, so determining whether the gliding sign is present is paramount. One study compared a FAST (focused assessment with sonography for trauma) scan with thoracic radiographs for detection of pneumothorax in 145 dogs with a history of trauma.[23] This FAST exam was performed bilaterally in the dorsolateral aspect of the 7th to 9th intercostal spaces and ventrally in the 5th to 6th intercostal spaces. Pneumothorax was diagnosed sonographically by the absence of the gliding sign, and when the FAST scan was compared with radiography, it had an overall 78% sensitivity and 93% specificity. The investigator who completed the majority of the scans during the study had the highest sensitivity and specificity, suggesting that detection of pneumothorax with ultrasound requires additional training and expertise.

An important role of sonography is detecting pneumothorax after interventional procedures. Emergence of a gassy pleural effusion (representing hemorrhage and leakage of air) and sonographic disappearance of the lung lesion indicate a pneumothorax.

MEDIASTINAL DISEASE

Mediastinal widening is first detected radiographically. Ultrasound plays a valuable role in differentiating incidental widening secondary to fat accumulation from pathologic conditions of the mediastinum or from pleural fluid accumulation. Mediastinal masses are often accompanied by pleural effusion and may be masked on thoracic radiographs (Figure 7-17; see also Figure 7-16, E and F).

Mediastinal lesions may be small or become large enough to contact the thoracic wall. In the latter instance, imaging is easy from a parasternal or intercostal approach because lung is displaced away from the chest wall by the mass. Mediastinal masses associated with pleural fluid are easily imaged.

Inflammation

Inflammation of the mediastinum is not commonly diagnosed in small animal practice. An inflamed mediastinum is less defined and more heterogeneous than normal mediastinal tissue. The mediastinal vessels may be less distinct. Small anechoic or hypoechoic pockets of fluid may be present, and the thickness of the mediastinum may increase. Lymph nodes may be seen as hypoechoic round to oval structures and are usually not as large as those typically encountered with neoplastic processes (see Figure 7-17, C).

Mass Lesions

Lymphoma is the most common type of mediastinal mass lesion found in dogs and cats. The classic appearance is a hypoechoic nodular mass (or masses) with a thin, distinct echogenic periphery[1,2,7] (Figures 7-18 and 7-19, A; see also Figure 7-17, D). In some cases, the masses may appear to coalesce and become large, with lumpy or irregular margins (see Figures 7-17, E, and 7-19, B and C). In other instances, large smooth, homogeneous, relatively hypoechoic masses may be present. Lymphomas sometimes have a more heterogeneous echo texture.[2,7] Color flow Doppler analysis often indicates little blood flow (see Figures 7-17, E, and 7-19, D), but some cases show extensive vascularity. Pleural effusion, often severe, is a common concurrent finding, especially in cats.[24]

Because ultrasonographic findings alone cannot accurately predict the histologic classification of pathologic tissue, it is not surprising that other types of mediastinal masses, such as mast cell tumor, thyroid carcinomas, melanomas, undifferentiated neoplasia (see Figure 7-16), and even reactive lymphadenopathy (although rare) may appear sonographically identical to advanced lymphoma. Fibrous masses and hemorrhage (Figure 7-20) are benign differential diagnoses for large or complex mediastinal mass lesions.

Large thymomas are usually characterized by an echogenic mass with small anechoic cavitations or larger cystic lesions[2,7] (Figure 7-21), although they may be solid and homogeneous. In one ultrasound case report of a thymoma in a cat, the mass was primarily filled with echogenic, slightly swirling fluid, which was later determined to be cholesterol-rich fluid.[25] A small thymoma diagnosed in a case of myasthenia gravis had a hypoechoic homogeneous appearance resembling a lymph node (Figure 7-22). The radiographic findings suggested differential diagnoses of a cranial mediastinal mass or a focal pulmonary lesion, such as aspiration pneumonia. A mediastinal origin was confirmed on ultrasound assessment by observing the motion of the right and left cranial lung lobes over the

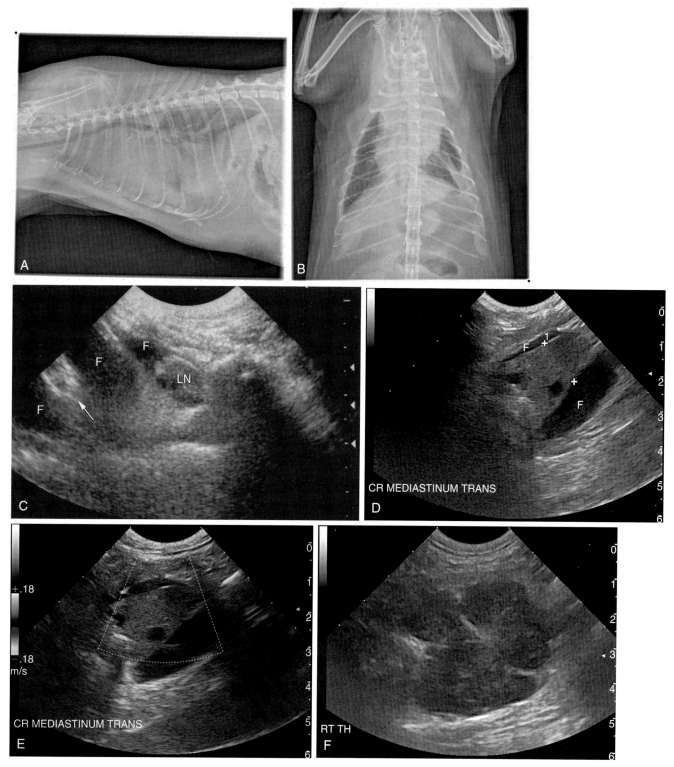

Figure 7-17 **Examples of cranial mediastinal disease in cats causing pleural effusion.** Left lateral (**A**) and dorsoventral (**B**) radiographs of a cat with severe pleural effusion. **C**, Dorsal plane image of the cranial thorax. A small, oval, hypoechoic cranial mediastinal lymph node (*LN*) was identified, but a mediastinal mass was not present. Pleural fluid (*F*) is present, and the tip of an atelectatic lung lobe is seen (*arrow*). This cat had a pyothorax. The relatively small lymph node with retained normal shape is usually a feature of benign inflammatory reaction rather than neoplasia. **D**, Widened cranial mediastinum (between electronic cursors, 1.40 cm) in a cat with mediastinal lymphoma. Pleural fluid (*F*) is present in the right and left hemithorax. **E**, Color Doppler image of **D**, showing characteristic lack of blood flow within the cranial mediastinal lymphoma. **F**, Large, lobulated cranial mediastinal mass in a cat with lymphoma.

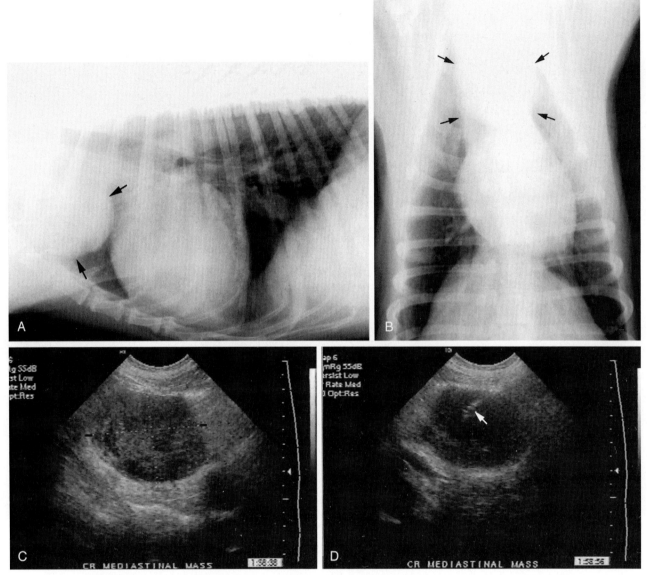

Figure 7-18 Cranial mediastinal lymphoma in a 10-year-old dog. A, Right lateral radiograph showing a well-defined cranial thoracic soft tissue mass (*arrows*). **B,** Dorsoventral radiograph showing a cranial mediastinal soft tissue mass (*arrows*). **C,** Intercostal image of the cranial mediastinal mass. It is slightly inhomogeneous, hypoechoic, and well delineated from the surrounding mediastinal tissue. It measured 4.4 × 3.3 cm. **D,** Biopsy of the cranial mediastinal mass was performed by direct ultrasound guidance with a freehand technique and use of an automated 18-gauge needle (*arrow*).

mass (the gliding sign). Additionally, thymomas may invade the cranial vena cava.[26] Idiopathic thymic hemorrhage has been reported in two littermate puppies but not documented sonographically.[27]

Caudal mediastinal masses are less common than cranial mediastinal lesions. Large masses can usually be imaged through a subcostal approach, using the liver as an acoustic window (Figure 7-23). Smaller lesions can be imaged in the presence of pleural fluid (Figure 7-24). The most frequently encountered caudal mediastinal disease is lymphoma, usually as a manifestation of multicentric lymphoma. Infectious or granulomatous disease from migrating foreign bodies or esophageal perforations and esophageal neoplasia are other infrequently encountered caudal mediastinal diseases.

Cystic Lesions

Thymic branchial cysts develop from remnants of the fetal branchial arch system and present as predominantly cystic mediastinal masses in dogs and cats.[28,29] Thymic branchial cysts are associated with pleural effusion, mediastinal mass lesions, and head and neck swelling. Rupture of cysts can lead to chronic mediastinitis. Thymic branchial cysts may appear identical to the cystic form of thymomas grossly and sonographically.

In cats, idiopathic cysts have been occasionally diagnosed within the mediastinum, most commonly as incidental findings.[30,31] On ultrasound, these cysts appear as small anechoic thin-walled structures that are ovoid to bilobed and have distal acoustic enhancement[31] (Figure 7-25).

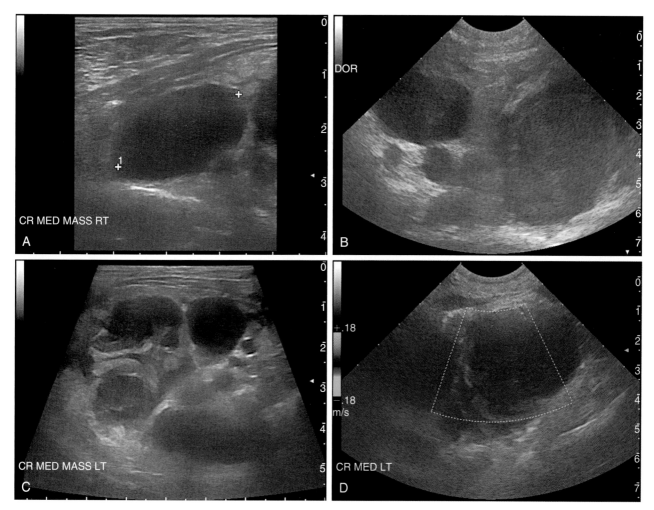

Figure 7-19 **Examples of the various appearances of mediastinal lymphoma in dogs.** A, Solid, homogeneous, nearly anechoic smoothly marginated cranial mediastinal lymphoma (between electronic cursors, 2.64 cm). B, Multilobulated cranial mediastinal lymphoma. C, Multilobulated, complex cranial mediastinal lymphoma. D, Color Doppler of cranial mediastinal lymphoma showing the typical low blood flow associated with these tumors.

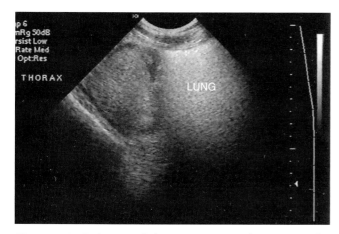

Figure 7-20 Right cranial thorax, transverse plane image of a cranial mediastinal hematoma in a dog hit by a car approximately 36 hours before presentation. An echogenic, homogeneous structure surrounded by a hypoechoic rim is present in the ventral mediastinum. Aerated normal lung is present dorsally.

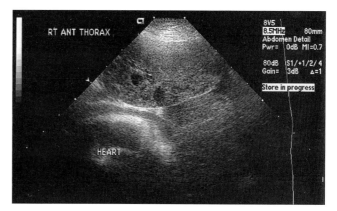

Figure 7-21 Right cranial thorax, transverse image of a large thymoma in a 13-year-old mixed-breed dog presented for edema of the head and neck and coughing. Radiographs showed a large cranial mediastinal mass. Although the mass is primarily homogeneous, small cystic areas can be seen. The heart could be seen beating adjacent to the mass during real-time imaging.

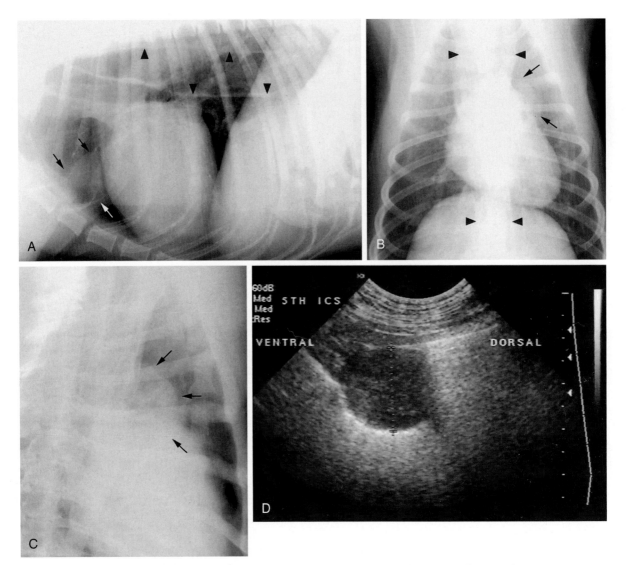

Figure 7-22 Small thymoma in a middle-aged Labrador retriever with megaesophagus and myasthenia gravis. The radiographic appearance warrants consideration of pulmonary or mediastinal origin of the mass. Mediastinal origin was confirmed by observation of both right and left lung movement over the mass. **A,** Right lateral radiograph showing a small soft tissue mass in the cranial thorax (*arrows*). A gas-dilated thoracic esophagus is present (*arrowheads*). **B,** Dorsoventral radiograph. The small cranial thoracic mass is poorly visible adjacent to the heart (*arrows*). Mediastinal widening is caused by the megaesophagus (*arrowheads*). **C,** Left ventrodorsal oblique radiograph better delineates the small cranial thoracic mass (*arrows*). **D,** Left parasternal transverse image showing a round, hypoechoic, homogeneous mass. Observation in real time showed right ventral lung and dorsal left lung motion independent of the mass (gliding sign), confirming its mediastinal location. The mass was 1.85 cm in diameter.

Although uncommon, thyroglossal duct cysts have been reported to develop in the mediastinum in humans[32] and veterinary patients.[33] In one case report of a cat with dyspnea and pleural effusion, a cystic mass was identified with ultrasound within the caudal mediastinum.[33] This mass was determined histopathologically to be an encapsulated thyroglossal duct cyst and inflamed ectopic thyroid tissue. Thyroglossal duct cysts arise from ectopic thyroid tissue, which can be found between the base of the tongue to the diaphragm. These cysts are most commonly found in the cervical region, but can occasionally be identified within the mediastinum.

Esophageal Lesions

In rare instances, the normal esophagus can be identified during liver sonography as a striated structure entering the stomach. The normal esophagus is occasionally identified in cases of severe pleural effusion. It is possible to detect certain esophageal diseases, such as megaesophagus (Figures 7-26 and 7-27), dilation secondary to a vascular ring anomaly, redundant esophagus, and caudal esophageal neoplastic process. However, contrast radiographic procedures should be considered the primary diagnostic imaging modality for the esophagus.

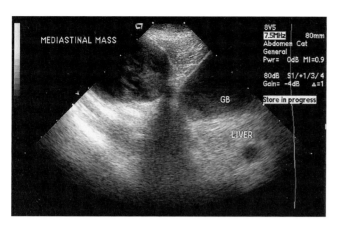

Figure 7-23 Right sagittal subcostal window showing a complex caudal mediastinal mass. The gallbladder (*GB*) and the liver are seen caudal to the mass.

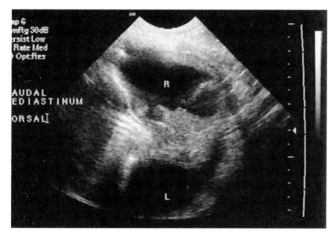

Figure 7-24 Standing right caudal thoracic transverse image in a cat with pleural effusion secondary to multicentric lymphoma. A homogeneous mass with irregular margins is present in the caudal mediastinum between right (*R*) and left (*L*) anechoic pleural fluid. Dorsal is to the right, ventral to the left in this image.

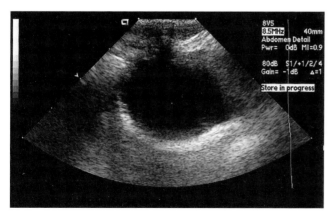

Figure 7-25 Right parasternal transverse image of a solitary cranial mediastinal cyst in a middle-aged cat. The anechoic thin-walled structure contacted the cranial margin of the heart. Aspiration by ultrasound guidance yielded a clear, colorless, low-viscosity fluid. This mediastinal cyst was an incidental finding on thoracic radiographs. The cyst was approximately 2.5 × 2 cm.

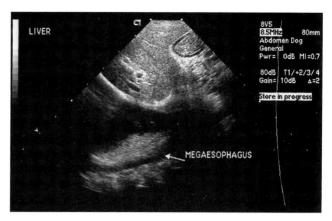

Figure 7-26 Megaesophagus in a 13-year-old dachshund presented for intermittent vomiting. Sagittal subcostal image of the cranial abdomen and caudal thorax. An anechoic fluid distended esophagus with echogenic luminal contents (*MEGAESOPHAGUS*) is present in the far field; the liver and stomach are in the near field.

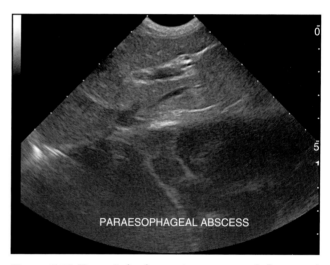

Figure 7-27 Young Labrador retriever presented for several month duration of vomiting and lack of maintained body condition. An abdominal ultrasound was requested. During the examination an abnormal, fluid-filled, septated structure was identified in the caudal thorax. This was later determined to be a paraesophageal abscess. The liver is in the near field.

PULMONARY DISEASE

Because only the visceral pleural surface of normal lung can be imaged, pulmonary disease can only be assessed by ultrasound when mass lesions, nodules, consolidation, or atelectasis are present in peripheral lung tissue. The presence of aerated lung between the transducer and the lesion effectively blocks the transmission of ultrasound, so interior lesions cannot be imaged. As fluid or cellular infiltrate invades the interstitial and air spaces, an acoustic window develops (provided that this occurs in peripheral lung tissue). The lung parenchyma begins to appear as solid tissue owing to the acoustic properties of the fluid or cellular infiltrate. The sonographic appearances of pulmonary lesions vary, depending primarily on the extent of parenchymal involvement. The degree of remaining air-filled alveoli and bronchi and, conversely, the extent to which the air spaces are fluid filled greatly affect the sonographic appearance of diseased lung.

At the lung surface, pulmonary lesions are seen as interruptions of the linear, highly echogenic visceral pleural surface (Figure 7-28). For small lesions, such as metastatic pulmonary nodules, two sonographic appearances occur: small hypoechoic areas directly beneath the visceral pleural surface (see Figure 7-28, *B* to *D*), and minor surface irregularities that create striking comet-tail artifacts (see Figure 7-28, *C* and *E*). As pathologic tissue extends deeper into the pulmonary parenchyma, it displaces aerated lung. Lesions are hypoechoic relative to bordering aerated lung (Figures 7-29 and 7-30). The deep margin of the lesion may be smooth and regular (see Figure 7-29, *C*), irregular and poorly defined (Figure 7-31), or somewhere in between (see Figure 7-30, *D* and *E*). In humans, the majority of neoplastic pulmonary lesions have regular, smooth margins, whereas most cases of nonneoplastic pulmonary consolidation show irregular margins.[34,35] From our experience and that of others, this seems to be the case in dogs and cats as well.[7]

Deep to the distal margin of the lesion, a region of intense hyperechogenicity will be apparent. This artifact is analogous to the strong reverberation artifact created at the surface of normal lung and has been referred to as enhancement artifact.[34] When the margins of the lesions are irregular, comet-tail artifacts will be seen (see Figures 7-29 to 7-31).

Establishing the lateral margins of a pulmonary lesion may be challenging and in some instances impossible. This occurs when the deeper portion of the lesion is wider or larger than the peripheral part contacting the surface of the lung. Sonography cannot entirely delineate the pulmonary lesion because the lateral edges are masked by reverberation artifact produced between the chest wall and the lesion by air within the superficial lung tissue.[35] Acoustic shadows created by ribs can also mask the margins of pulmonary lesions (see Figure 7-30, *E*).

Adhesions of lung to the parietal pleura are referred to as lesion-pleural symphysis, diagnosed when the gliding sign is absent. This finding may represent extension of pulmonary neoplasia to the chest wall or occur with inflammatory lesions. The gliding sign might be barely perceptible or absent for patients with rapid, shallow respiration. Absence of the gliding sign may also result from loss of diaphragmatic excursion, indicating the possibility of phrenic nerve paralysis.

As is true of any ultrasound examination, a histopathologic diagnosis cannot be based solely on the sonographic appearance. Nonetheless, some general statements can be made regarding categories of pulmonary disease.

Pulmonary Neoplasia
Pulmonary neoplasms are often solid and homogeneous (Figure 7-32; see also Figures 7-29 and 7-30). In many instances, the echogenic deep margin of the lesion is smooth, in contrast to many inflammatory pulmonary lesions. Nodular protuberances from the lung surface may be present.[1] Neoplastic masses undergoing necrosis may appear more complex, with pockets of fluid, internal septa, and a heterogeneous internal echo pattern. Sediments may form in centralized fluid. The presence of highly echogenic foci with dirty acoustic shadowing or reverberation indicates gas within the mass. From this description, it is evident that pulmonary neoplasia may present in a manner that is similar to and indistinguishable from inflammatory disease or abscess.

Consolidation
Consolidation is a disease of the lung in which alveolar air has been replaced by fluid, cells, or cellular exudate, including neoplastic cells,[36] usually without significant loss of lung lobe volume. Consolidated areas may be focal or regional, or they may involve an entire lobe or lobes. Lobar pneumonia and

inflammatory conditions such as pulmonary infiltration with eosinophils are more common than lobar neoplasia.

As in most pulmonary pathologic processes, interruptions are seen in the echogenic visceral pleural surface. The parenchyma of consolidated lung is relatively hypoechoic. The earliest sign of consolidation is irregularity of the surface of the lung, created by nonuniform aeration of peripheral lung air spaces.[37-40] Characteristic comet-tail artifacts radiate from the small areas of the peripheral consolidation. Comet-tail artifacts, or similarly appearing ring-down artifacts, are not specific because they may be visualized with edema, exudate, pneumonia, mucus, pleuritis, neoplastic infiltrate, contusions, or interstitial fibrosis.[41-45] These changes are seen in horses with pneumonia, pleuritis, hemorrhage or edema, chronic obstructive pulmonary disease, and granulomatous or neoplastic disease.[40] These early, sometimes subtle peripheral pulmonary consolidations are rarely seen in small animal patients because we do not ordinarily clip the entire thoracic hair coat to scan the entire lung surface, as is routinely done in equine practice.

As pulmonary consolidation progresses, it spreads to the deeper parenchyma. It may be homogeneous (Figure 7-33), but more often the sonographic appearance is that of inhomogeneous tissue (Figure 7-34; see also Figure 7-31). This inhomogeneity occurs when some air spaces are filled with fluid or exudate while others remain air filled. Residual air within alveoli and bronchi creates multiple, echogenic foci. These foci are termed air bronchograms.[46]

Fluid accumulations within air spaces appear as tubular, sometimes branching anechoic or hypoechoic structures, termed fluid bronchograms[47] (Figure 7-35). They are nonpulsatile, which differentiates them from pulmonary vascular structures. They may occasionally taper toward the periphery of the lung when they are longitudinally imaged. Without Doppler evaluation, differentiation of small pulmonary vessels from fluid bronchograms may not be possible. However, the presence of pulmonary vessels or fluid bronchograms is indicative of pulmonary consolidation because neither is seen in normally aerated lung. The superficial portion of consolidated lung may become a homogeneous hypoechoic zone or band without air or fluid bronchograms; this is termed superficial fluid alveologram.[34]

Consolidation of lung is termed hepatization, a gross anatomic description that can sometimes be used to describe the sonographic appearance as well (see Figures 7-29, *C*; 7-32; 7-33, *D* and *E*; and 7-35). The sonographic appearance of consolidated lung can resemble liver tissue, especially when larger bronchi are fluid filled, which mimics hepatic vessels. This appearance is seen with lobar pneumonia, lobar neoplasia, and lung torsion. However, in many cases of lung lobe torsion, scattered reverberating foci are also present. These foci are most consistent with gas that is trapped centrally within the affected lobe.[48] Because of its resemblance to hepatic parenchyma, consolidated lung may be incorrectly identified as herniated liver.

Pulmonary Abscesses
Pulmonary abscesses, although rare, are usually caused by aspiration pneumonia or primary pneumonias in small animals. *Escherichia coli*, *Pseudomonas*, and *Klebsiella* are frequently involved with necrotizing pneumonia in small animals.[17,49] Sterile abscesses secondary to tumor necrosis also occur. Pneumothorax and empyema are potential sequelae.

The classic appearance of a pulmonary abscess is a cavitary lesion. The central cavitary area may contain anechoic or echogenic fluid. Cavitation may be compartmentalized or loculated, with echogenic internal septations separating anechoic or echogenic fluid. Layering can occur, with

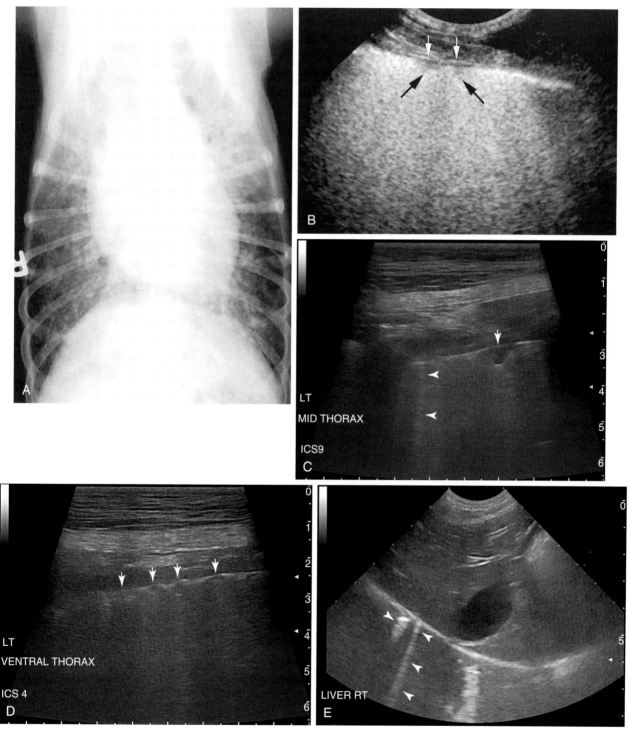

Figure 7-28 **Metastatic pulmonary neoplasia, lung surface nodules, and irregularities. A,** Dorsoventral radiograph showing multiple small coalescing pulmonary nodules. **B,** Two small hypoechoic nodules on the surface of the lung (*black arrows*). The parietal pleural surface is seen as a thin linear hyperechoic structure adjacent to the nodules (*white arrows*). **C,** A small hypoechoic nodule on the surface of the lung is visible (*arrow*). Comet-tail reverberation artifact is also seen arising from the lung surface (*arrowheads*). **D,** Minor surface irregularity is visible on the surface of this lung with widespread pulmonary metastasis (*arrows*). **E,** Comet-tail artifacts (*arrowheads*) arising from the lung surface visible during an abdominal ultrasound examination. It is not uncommon to diagnose lung disease when using ultrasound to examine the abdomen; thoracic radiographs should be considered.

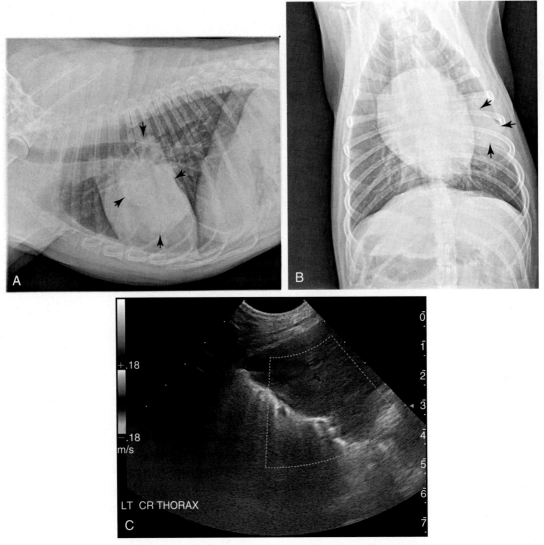

Figure 7-29 Bronchogenic adenocarcinoma in a 10-year-old Labrador retriever dog. The radiographs are diagnostic for a large, lobulated mass within the caudal segment of the left cranial lung lobe. The radiographs provide information necessary for selecting an appropriate window into the thorax, which allowed an ultrasound-guided biopsy to be performed. **A,** Right lateral radiograph showing a large soft tissue mass in the middle lung lobe (*arrows*). **B,** Ventrodorsal radiograph showing the mass located in the caudal segment of the left cranial lung lobe (*arrows*). **C,** Transverse image at the level of the mid left 6th intercostal space showing a homogeneous hypoechoic mass. Color Doppler image shows very little blood flow within the lung mass.

sedimentation of heavy echogenic cellular debris ventrally and less echogenic fluid dorsally.[40] Echogenic gas may be found within the abscess cavity, in the dorsal portion of the lesion. The presence of gas indicates anaerobic or aerobic microbial infection or communication of the lesion with an airway. The lining of the abscess cavity may be rough and irregular or relatively smooth. Fibrous encapsulation, which occurs if the abscess is chronic, is seen as a hyperechoic outer margin. The appearance may be layered or striated. Often, however, there is a less defined hypoechoic periphery to the abscess.

A report describes the ultrasonographic appearance of a wooden foreign body within a pulmonary abscess.[50] In this case, the abscessed lung contained echogenic fluid and was well defined by surrounding pleural fluid. The wooden foreign body was an irregularly shaped elongate echogenic structure that created a strong acoustic shadow.

Pulmonary Cysts

A pulmonary fluid-filled cyst has anechoic or hypoechoic fluid within it and a thin, echogenic wall. A hematoma may appear similar initially, but it will organize internally over time, with fibrin formation, internal septa, and development of a thicker wall. Hematomas in general have a plethora of age-dependent sonographic appearances. Pulmonary hematomas are perhaps most commonly associated with trauma, but they may be seen with coagulopathies and neoplasia (e.g., hemangiosarcoma).

Atelectasis

Atelectasis, or lung lobe collapse, occurs in the presence of pleural fluid or pneumothorax and when an airway is occluded. Atelectatic lung is easily imaged in the presence of pleural fluid but cannot be imaged when a pneumothorax is present. Small amounts of fluid allow excellent assessment of the

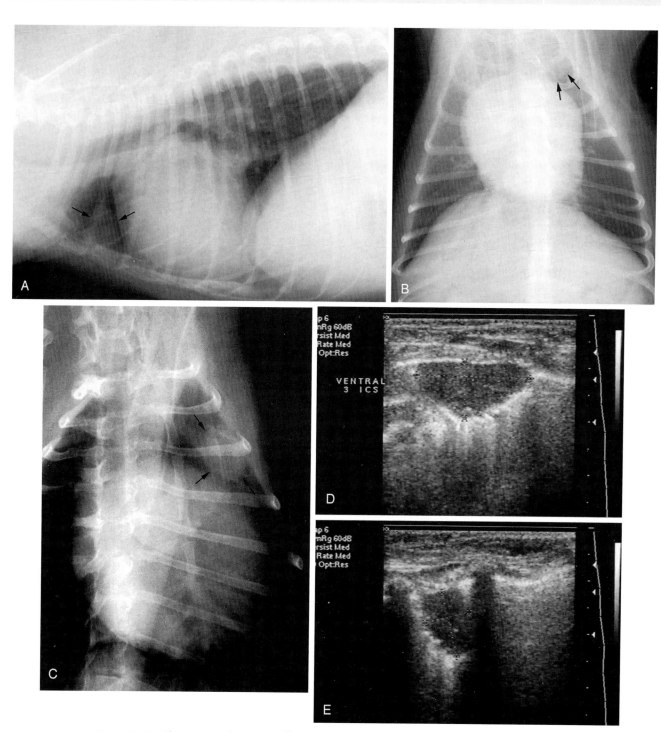

Figure 7-30 Chronic mitral valve insufficiency and tracheal membrane redundancy in a 10-year-old small-breed dog, with an incidental finding of a small bronchogenic adenocarcinoma. Radiographs allowed selection of an appropriate window for ultrasound evaluation of the pulmonary mass and guided fine-needle aspiration. **A,** Right lateral radiograph showing a small soft tissue mass in the ventral thorax just cranial to the heart (*arrows*). The cardiac silhouette is large, including the left atrium. Tracheal membrane redundancy is noted in the thoracic inlet. **B,** Dorsoventral radiograph faintly shows the soft tissue mass to be in the left cranial lung lobe (*arrows*). The cardiac silhouette is large, including both atria. **C,** A ventrodorsal oblique radiograph more clearly shows the left cranial lobar mass (*arrows*). **D,** Transverse image at the left 3rd intercostal space shows a hypoechoic pulmonary mass. The distal margin is hyperechoic and slightly irregular. Comet-tail artifacts are seen radiating from these irregularities, and an enhancement artifact is also present. Dorsal is to the right, ventral to the left. The mass measured 2.3 × 1.1 cm. **E,** Dorsal image at the left 3rd intercostal space. The cranial margin of the lesion is slightly irregular; the caudal margin is obscured by an acoustic shadow from the rib. The lesion measured 1.2 × 0.9 cm.

visceral pleural surface of the lungs. As the amount of fluid increases, the degree of lung collapse increases. As this occurs, the lung becomes less and less air filled, allowing the pulmonary parenchyma to be imaged. Atelectatic lung lobes are identified as small triangular, highly echogenic structures floating within pleural fluid, attached dorsally to the stem bronchi (see Figures 7-12, *E*; 7-15; and 7-17, *C*). The echogenicity is caused by residual air-filled alveoli. In severe effusions, only the caudal lung lobes may be air filled or partially so, sustaining life.

THORACIC WALL LESIONS

Ultrasound assessment of externally evident thoracic wall lesions may provide information about the internal appearance, size, and extent of the lesion; it can determine whether

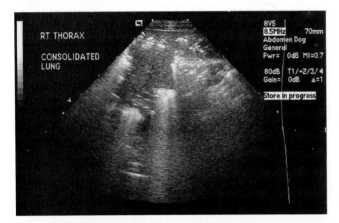

Figure 7-31 **Consolidated lung in a dog with fungal pneumonia.** The hypoechoic consolidation is poorly marginated laterally and distally. Comet-tail artifacts radiate from the interface between consolidated and aerated lung. Multifocal hyperechogenicities represent bronchi, bronchioles, and alveoli that remain aerated, termed air bronchograms.

the lesion has invaded the pleural space or lung and if localized pleural fluid is present. Ultrasound can also be used to assess body wall integrity. A study of human patients with lung cancer showed that ultrasonography had a much higher sensitivity and specificity than CT in detecting tumor invasion of the chest wall.[51] Ultrasonographic findings that are highly suggestive of lung tumor extension into the thoracic wall include disruption of the pleura, extension through the chest wall, and fixation of the tumor during respiration.

Rib neoplasms, abscesses, and granulomas and trauma are commonly encountered pathologic processes of the chest wall. Rib neoplasia is generally diagnosed on thoracic radiographs as a destructive or proliferative process with an accompanying soft tissue mass lesion. Ultrasound assessment in these cases helps establish the extent of the lesion relative to the pleura and pleural space and may provide useful information for surgical intervention (Figure 7-36).

Diagnosis of body wall masses or swelling without radiographic evidence of rib involvement may be more challenging. An area of fluid accumulation centrally within a walled-off periphery is the classic appearance of chronic abscess. Body wall abscesses are often caused by foreign material, and the foreign object can occasionally be identified with the mass. Necrosis within neoplasms may be similar to some abscesses, but a walled-off appearance is usually absent.

DIAPHRAGMATIC HERNIAS

Ultrasound examination of the diaphragm is a fairly reliable technique for the diagnosis of hernias. Subcostal, intercostal, and cardiac windows may be useful. Complete and accurate assessment is augmented by the presence of pleural or abdominal fluid, which serves as a nice backdrop for outlining the smooth contour of the thin echogenic diaphragm. Because it is noninvasive, ultrasound examination may be the next logical diagnostic procedure after survey radiography. Positive contrast peritoneography is more sensitive than ultrasonography, especially if the diaphragmatic defect is small, and may be considered the practical gold standard.

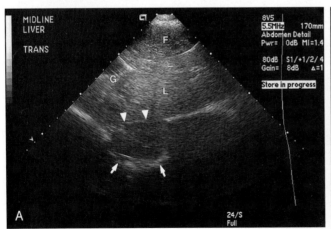
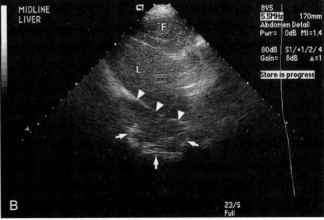

Figure 7-32 Bronchogenic adenocarcinoma in the accessory lung lobe of an older large-breed dog. A subcostal approach using the liver as an acoustic window allowed visualization of the mass, which could not be imaged through an intercostal window because of aerated lung between the transducer and the mass. **A,** Transverse dorsal image of accessory lung lobe mass (*arrows*). The distal margin is smooth in this plane with enhancement artifact. Note the faint echogenic diaphragm (*arrowheads*) that separates the mass from the liver (*L*). Mirror image artifact of the liver is noted to the left of the mass. *F,* Falciform fat; *G,* gallbladder. **B,** Sagittal image of accessory lung lobe mass (*arrows*). The distal margin is more irregular in this image plane. Note the diaphragm (*arrowheads*). *F,* Falciform fat; *L,* liver.

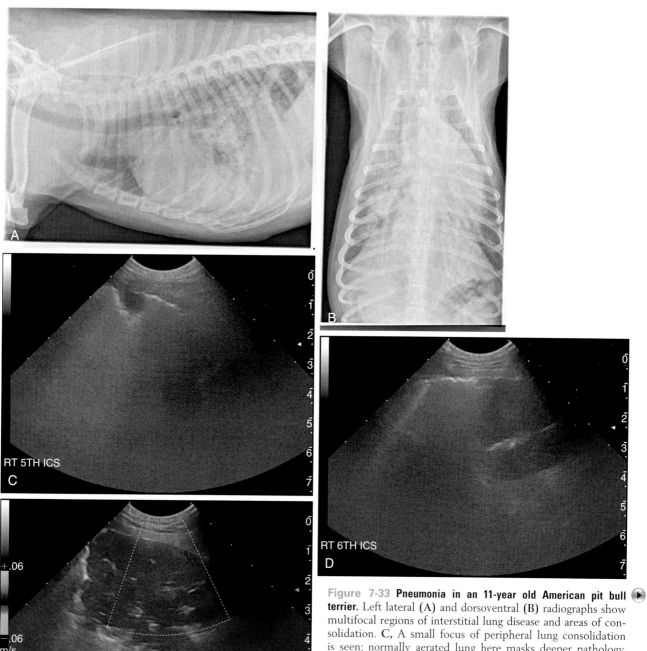

Figure 7-33 **Pneumonia in an 11-year old American pit bull terrier.** Left lateral (**A**) and dorsoventral (**B**) radiographs show multifocal regions of interstitial lung disease and areas of consolidation. **C,** A small focus of peripheral lung consolidation is seen; normally aerated lung here masks deeper pathology. **D,** Aerated lung is seen to transition into consolidated (airless) lung. **E,** Color Doppler examination shows no blood flow within the pneumonic lung (the small red area is motion artifact and not representative of blood flow). Small anechoic tubular areas may represent small fluid-filled bronchi or bronchioles.

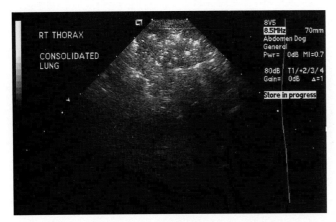

Figure 7-34 Consolidated lung secondary to pneumonia. The consolidated lung is hypoechoic and poorly marginated. Multiple echogenic foci represent residual air-filled alveoli and bronchioles and small bronchi.

Diaphragmatic hernias are often traumatic in origin (Figure 7-37). Accordingly, many patients examined have a history of recent trauma. In some cases, however, the traumatic event may have occurred some time ago or be unknown. True diaphragmatic hernias in which the diaphragm is intact are occasionally seen. The continuous echogenic interface between the liver-diaphragm and lung is the principal landmark (see Figure 7-37, C). Discontinuity of this curvilinear echogenicity may indicate a diaphragmatic hernia. Careful attention to the presence or absence of herniated abdominal contents through the defect is a second consideration. In most instances, herniated liver is easily imaged (Figure 7-38). Falciform fat may herniate and is more difficult to diagnose because of its mottled, indistinct appearance. Other organs, such as the stomach, spleen, small intestines, and occasionally a kidney,[52] may be herniated; these are usually readily identifiable by their characteristic sonographic appearance. Diaphragmatic hernias are often accompanied by pleural and abdominal fluids. When fluid is present, it greatly enhances the diagnostic capacity of ultrasound and confidence in the diagnosis. In one study, ultrasound had an accuracy of 93% (25 out of 27 cases) in diagnosis of diaphragmatic rupture in dogs and cats, with 1 false-positive and 1 false-negative.[53] The most consistent sonographic signs associated with a diagnosis of diaphragmatic rupture were abdominal contents within the thoracic cavity and an irregular or asymmetric cranial liver margin. In another retrospective review of chronic diaphragmatic hernia in dogs and cats, ultrasound diagnosed the hernia in 9 out of 10 animals based on visualization of the abdominal organs within the thoracic cavity and loss of the diaphragmatic line.[54] Omentum was the only herniated tissue in the 1 case not diagnosed with ultrasound.

Ultrasonographers must be able to recognize the difference between the commonly encountered mirror image artifact and the herniated liver. The key distinction is the presence or absence of the characteristic echogenic line representing the diaphragm. If the diaphragm can be seen separating the abdominal and "thoracic" liver, a mirror image artifact is present, not a hernia. A mirror image artifact is convincing evidence that *there is no disruption of the diaphragm at that particular location.*

Congenital peritoneopericardial diaphragmatic hernia (CPDH) occurs in the dog and cat. Ultrasonography is an excellent noninvasive method to confirm the presence of CPDH in most cases. Abnormal development of embryonic midline structures (septum transversum, pleuroperitoneal folds) leads to a defect within the ventral diaphragm with resultant communication between the abdomen and the pericardial space.[55,56] Falciform fat, liver, gallbladder, and intestines may be within the pericardial sac. Not all cases of CPDH are clinically apparent; it may be incidentally diagnosed or suspected on thoracic radiographs obtained for other reasons. Generalized enlargement of the cardiac silhouette is the common radiographic abnormality, prompting differential diagnoses of various cardiac diseases and pericardial effusion. A dorsal peritoneopericardial mesothelial remnant is a radiographic sign indicative of CPDH in cats.[56] Caudal sternal abnormalities are sometimes present along with a reduced number of sternebrae.[55]

The diagnosis of CPDH can be made sonographically by visualization of liver (or other organs) surrounding the heart, contained within the pericardial sac. This may be accomplished by using the heart as an acoustic window or by taking a subcostal (transabdominal) approach through the liver. Observing the diaphragm will reveal the absence of the echogenic diaphragmatic landmark centrally and continuation of the liver parenchyma (or other structures) into the pericardial sac. If only falciform fat is herniated, the diagnosis may be more uncertain because falciform fat is difficult to distinguish from pericardial fat. In this case, careful attention to the continuity of the echogenic diaphragm is essential.

Hiatal hernias, especially if they are intermittent, may be difficult to image with ultrasound and are thus often diagnosed radiographically and possibly fluoroscopically. Stomach wall and rugal folds may be seen crossing the diaphragm into the thorax.

INTERVENTIONAL PROCEDURES OF THE THORAX

Ultrasound-guided interventional procedures of the thorax are now common in veterinary and human medicine.[57-67] Transesophageal ultrasound-guided biopsies are now performed in human patients with mediastinal and pulmonary lesions.[68,69]

Thoracentesis

Thoracentesis is essential for a definitive diagnosis when pleural fluid is present. Although the sonographic appearances of various types of pleural effusion have been described, proper laboratory analysis of the fluid is still required for a definitive diagnosis. The analysis should include cytologic evaluation and culture and sensitivity (aerobic and anaerobic). Ultrasound can be used to safely guide the thoracentesis needle for sample collection and therapeutic drainage. Thoracentesis is usually performed with a freehand technique. On occasion, a biopsy guide may be useful for sampling small fluid accumulations or fluid collections near vital anatomic structures.

Hypodermic needles, spinal needles, and various types of catheters have been used successfully. In cases of viscous pleural fluid (e.g., empyema), larger bore needles (14 to 16 gauge) are necessary. Catheters with multiple side holes may be useful if pleural septations are present, because end-hole catheters are more susceptible to occlusion.

Identification of suitable sites depends on whether the fluid is present in large quantities or in small focal accumulations. In general, the safest windows are ventral and cranial to the heart. Most patients, even cats, tolerate the procedure well. Local anesthesia should be considered and perhaps sedation, if necessary. General anesthesia is seldom required and may be contraindicated.

With proper positioning of the patient, most pleural fluid may be removed safely. There is usually a point at

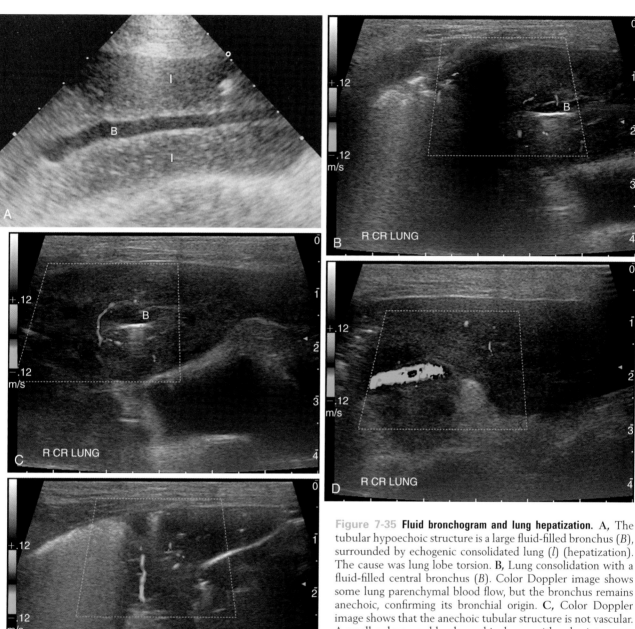

Figure 7-35 **Fluid bronchogram and lung hepatization.** A, The tubular hypoechoic structure is a large fluid-filled bronchus (*B*), surrounded by echogenic consolidated lung (*l*) (hepatization). The cause was lung lobe torsion. **B,** Lung consolidation with a fluid-filled central bronchus (*B*). Color Doppler image shows some lung parenchymal blood flow, but the bronchus remains anechoic, confirming its bronchial origin. **C,** Color Doppler image shows that the anechoic tubular structure is not vascular. A small pulmonary blood vessel is shown with color interrogation. **D,** Consolidated lung with color Doppler evaluation showing the presence of a large lobar blood vessel. **E,** Color Doppler evaluation of hepatized (consolidated) lung shows small vascular blood flow. There is also clear demarcation between consolidated lung and aerated lung to the left.

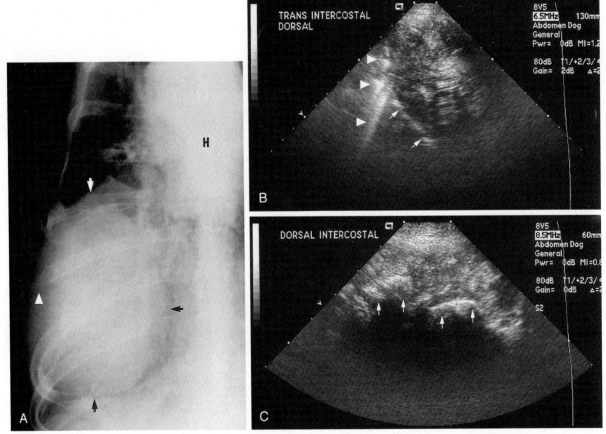

Figure 7-36 **Rib sarcoma. A,** Dorsoventral close-up of right caudal thoracic wall neoplasia (*arrows*), rib destruction (*arrowhead*), and adjacent rib periosteal reaction. *H,* Heart. **B,** Transverse intercostal image shows a complex thoracic wall lesion protruding into the thoracic cavity. Portions of the adjacent lung surface are irregular, and comet-tail artifacts are noted (*arrowheads*). Deeper, the lung surface is smooth (*arrows*). Real-time imaging showed lung movement independent of the thoracic wall mass during respiration. Doral is to the left, ventral to the right. **C,** Dorsal image of the thoracic wall mass. Irregular curvilinear, highly echogenic structures (*arrows*) with acoustic shadowing represent lytic and productive rib lesions noted on the radiographs.

which aspiration of fluid ceases or the amount remaining is minimal and the risk of lung laceration precludes further attempts.

Sonographic quantification of pleural fluid has been reported in dogs,[70,71] cats,[72] and humans.[73,74] In the human studies, measurement of pleural fluid thickness with the patient in a supine position correlated with fluid volume obtained by thoracentesis and was significantly better than measurements made radiographically.[73] In a second study, the angle formed by the lung and diaphragm (right side) or pericardium (left side) with the patient in a sitting position was used to estimate the quantity of pleural effusion.[74] Two studies in veterinary medicine have used cadavers in an attempt to quantify the amount of pleural fluid using sonographic assessment, one using canine cadavers and the other using feline cadavers.[71,72] Both studies used a transsternal approach to determine the amount of pleural fluid present, measuring the distance between the sternum and ventral lung margin with the cadaver positioned in sternal recumbency. Unfortunately, neither study was able to produce a reliable equation to accurately determine the volume of fluid present within the pleural space. However, the method described in these studies for measuring pleural fluid could be useful for monitoring the amount of fluid in a patient over time.

In clinical veterinary practice, subjective assessment of mild, moderate, or severe effusion is generally sufficient. However, when it is important to evaluate fluid recurrence after thoracentesis or therapy, two useful guidelines can be offered. On scanning of the dependent portion of the thorax, the thickness of fluid present between the parietal and visceral surfaces can be measured with electronic cursors and compared with values obtained on follow-up examinations. A second method is to document the pleural fluid level while the patient is standing or in sternal recumbency. Common landmarks include the point of the shoulder and the elbow; or the sternum or spine can be used as a point of reference for quantitative measurement of the fluid level.

Fine-Needle Aspirations and Biopsies of Mass Lesions

Ultrasound-guided fine-needle aspirations, fine-needle biopsies, and tissue-core biopsies are routinely performed on mediastinal masses for a definitive diagnosis (see Figure 7-23, *D*). Special care must be taken to prevent laceration of the mediastinal vessels because fatal hemorrhage is likely to occur. We generally perform fine-needle aspiration first, using freehand ultrasound guidance with a small-gauge needle (22 to 25 gauge). Because the majority of cases are lymphosarcoma, a

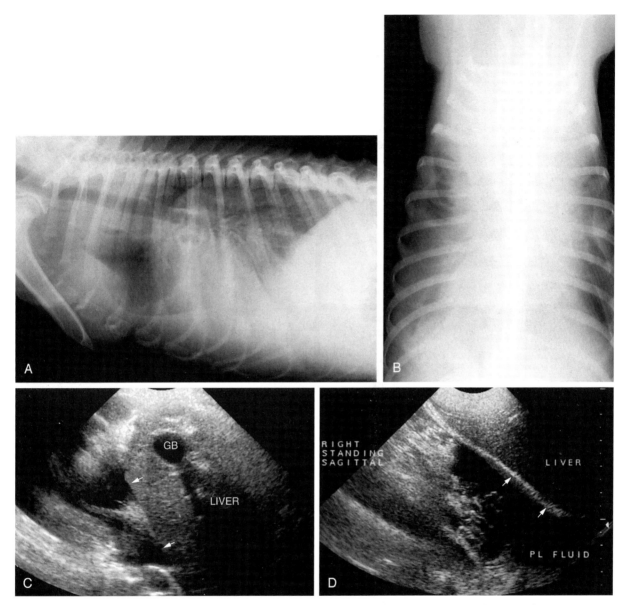

Figure 7-37 Traumatic diaphragmatic rupture. This dog was run over by a tractor and presented in respiratory distress. Thoracic radiographs show the presence of a moderate to severe pleural effusion. A diaphragmatic rupture was diagnosed on ultrasound examination. **A,** Right lateral radiograph shows an increased soft tissue opacity of the thorax, lobar fissures and rounded borders, and nonvisualization of the mid to ventral diaphragm. **B,** Dorsoventral radiograph shows increased soft tissue opacity of the thorax silhouetting the heart and diaphragm, and retraction of lung lobes from the thoracic wall. **C,** Subcostal image obtained while the patient was standing shows discontinuity of the diaphragm (*arrows*) with hypoechoic to anechoic pleural fluid adjacent to the liver. *GB,* Gallbladder. **D,** Subcostal image obtained while the patient was standing shows an intact portion of the diaphragm. Note the continuity of the echogenic diaphragm (*arrows*) in this image plane. Anechoic pleural fluid (*PL FLUID*) is present, and echogenic strands representing fibrin tags are visible.

definitive diagnosis is usually made. Our experience with interventional ultrasonography in small animals is similar to that in humans; both transthoracic needle biopsies and core needle biopsies of anterior mediastinal masses are safe and reliable diagnostic procedures.[60,63]

Sonographic visualization of pulmonary lesions will usually allow ultrasound-guided biopsies or aspirations to be performed. An 18-gauge biopsy needle is generally used, whereas 22- to 25-gauge needles are used for aspirations. A spinal needle may be used. The stylet allows the sonographer access to the lesion without attachment of the needle to a syringe or extension tube. Once the needle is within the lesion, the stylet is removed and the aspiration performed. Core-tissue samples or fine-needle aspirates may be safely obtained from solid masses. Needle aspirates may be the first choice in mixed pulmonary lesions because there is increased risk of pneumothorax if aerated lung is still present. Fortunately this has not been a common sequela of lung biopsies or aspirations in our

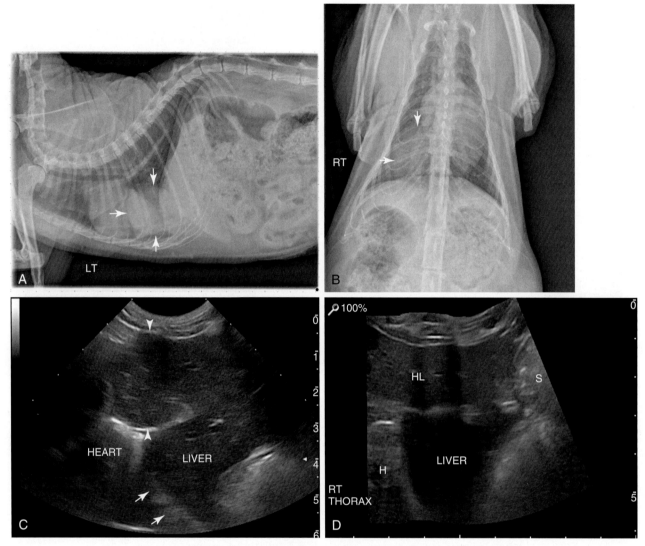

Figure 7-38 Diaphragmatic hernia. Respiratory distress in a kitten. Thoracic radiographs show the presence of a large ventral, caudal, right-sided homogeneous soft tissue mass. **A,** Left lateral radiograph shows a spherical soft tissue mass (*arrows*) summating with the heart and diaphragm/liver. **B,** Dorsoventral radiograph showing the right-sided nature of the mass (*arrows*). **C,** Sagittal ultrasound image made from a subcostal window shows herniated liver (*arrowheads*) between the chest wall and the heart. Normally positioned liver is seen in the far field (*LIVER*) adjacent to the diaphragm (*arrows*). **D,** Extended field of view image shows herniated liver (*HL*) and normally positioned liver (*LIVER*). *H,* Heart; *S,* stomach.

experience or that of others.[59] Whereas solid masses pose little risk of pneumothorax, hemorrhage is still a concern. Avoidance of large anechoic tubular pulmonary vessels is essential. If the lesion is large enough, the procedure may be done with or without sedation in a cooperative patient with a local anesthetic. Smaller patients or small lesions may require the use of heavy sedation or general anesthesia for safety. Biopsy guides offer precise needle placement, especially for the inexperienced practitioner, but they limit accessibility in some instances because of rib interference.

Although very rare, percutaneous aspiration of a tumor can result in seeding of the neoplastic cells along the needle tract. In one case report, a left caudal lung lobe mass, diagnosed as a pulmonary adenocarcinoma, was successfully aspirated using ultrasound guidance in a dog.[75] Approximately 1 year after surgical resection of the lung tumor, a mass was identified along the left dorsolateral thoracic wall, in the region of the previously performed aspirates, with periosteal reaction on the adjacent ribs. This mass along the thoracic wall was cytologically diagnosed as a pulmonary adenocarcinoma.

Immediately after the procedure, the sonographer should examine the patient for signs of hemorrhage. Accumulation of anechoic or echogenic fluid around the biopsy site not noted before the procedure is indicative of hemorrhage. Color flow Doppler interrogation of the biopsy site allows detection of small hemorrhages. Pneumothorax is seen after biopsy as emergence of a gassy pleural effusion and partial or complete loss of visualization of the lung lesion. These cases should be monitored radiographically.[35,76]

The patient's positioning during needle biopsy of the lung does not appear to have a significant effect on the development of pneumothorax in humans,[77,78] although one report found that puncture site–down positioning after lung biopsy reduced the need to place a chest tube.[77]

REFERENCES

1. Stowater JL, Lamb CR. Ultrasonography of noncardiac thoracic diseases in small animals. *J Am Vet Med Assoc* 1989;**195**:514–20.
2. Konde LJ, Spaulding K. Sonographic evaluation of the cranial mediastinum in small animals. *Vet Radiol* 1991;**32**:178–84.
3. Cartee RE. The heart vessels, lungs and mediastinum. In: *Practical Veterinary Ultrasound*. Baltimore: Williams & Wilkins; 1995. p. 68–87.
4. Bahr RJ. Thorax. In: Green RW, editor. *Small Animal Ultrasound*. Philadelphia: Lippincott-Raven; 1996. p. 89–104.
5. Tidwell AS. Ultrasonography of the thorax (excluding the heart). *Vet Clin North Am Small Anim Pract* 1998;**28**:993–1015.
6. Schwartz LA, Tidwell AS. Alternate imaging of the lung. *Clin Tech Small Anim Pract* 1999;**14**:187–206.
7. Reichle JK, Wisner ER. Non-cardiac thoracic ultrasound in 75 feline and canine patients. *Vet Radiol Ultrasound* 2000;**41**:154–62.
8. Saunders HM, Keith D. Thoracic imaging. In: King LG, editor. *Textbook of respiratory diseases in dogs and cats*. Philadelphia: WB Saunders; 2004. p. 72–93.
9. Larson MM. Ultrasound of the thorax (noncardiac). *Vet Clin North Am Small Anim Pract* 2009;**39**:733–45.
10. Targhetta R, Bourgeois JM, Chavagneux R, et al. Ultrasonographic approach to diagnosing hydropneumothorax. *Chest* 1992;**101**:931–4.
11. Evans HE, Christensen GC. The respiratory apparatus. In: *Miller's Anatomy of the Dog*. 2nd ed. Philadelphia: WB Saunders; 1979. p. 507–43.
12. Evans HE, Christensen GC. The lymphatic system. In: *Miller's Anatomy of the Dog*. 2nd ed. Philadelphia: WB Saunders; 1979. p. 802–41.
13. St.-Vincent RS, Pharr JW. Transesophageal ultrasonography of the normal canine mediastinum. *Vet Radiol Ultrasound* 1998;**39**:197–205.
14. Gashen L, Kircher P, Lang J. Endoscopic ultrasound instrumentation, applications in humans, and potential veterinary applications. *Vet Radiol Ultrasound* 2003;**44**:665–80.
15. Gashen L, Kircher P, Hoffman G, et al. Endoscopic ultrasonography for the diagnosis of intrathoracic lesions in 2 dogs. *Vet Radiol Ultrasound* 2003;**44**:292–9.
16. Schultz RM, Zwingenberger A. Radiographic, computed tomographic, and ultrasonographic findings with migrating intrathoracic grass awns in dogs and cats. *Vet Radiol Ultrasound* 2008;**49**:249–55.
17. Bauer T, Woodfield JA. Mediastinal, pleural and extrapleural diseases. In: Ettinger SJ, Feldman EC, editors. *Textbook of Veterinary Internal Medicine*. 4th ed. Philadelphia: WB Saunders; 1995. p. 812–42.
18. Tublin ME, Tessler EN, Rifkin MD. US case of the day. *Radiographics* 1998;**18**:523–5.
19. Husain LF, Hagopian L, Wayman D, et al. Sonographic diagnosis of pneumothorax. *J Emerg Trauma Shock* 2012;**5**:76–81.
20. Dulchavsky SA, Schwarz KL, Kirkpatrick AW, et al. Prospective evaluation of thoracic ultrasound in the detection of pneumothorax. *J Trauma* 2001;**50**:201–5.
21. Kirkpatrick AW, Sirois M, Laupland KB, et al. Hand-held thoracic sonography for detecting post-traumatic pneumothoraces: the Extended Focused Assessment with Sonography for Trauma (EFAST). *J Trauma* 2004;**57**:288–95.
22. Blaivas M, Lyon M, Duggal S. A prospective comparison of supine chest radiography and bedside ultrasound for the diagnosis of traumatic pneumothorax. *Acad Emerg Med* 2005;**12**:844–9.
23. Lisciandro GR, Lagutchik MS, Mann KA, et al. Evaluation of a thoracic focused assessment with sonography for trauma (TFAST) protocol to detect pneumothorax and concurrent thoracic injury in 145 traumatized dogs. *J Vet Emerg Crit Care* 2008;**18**:258–69.
24. Davies C, Forrester SD. Pleural effusion in cats: 82 cases (1987-1995). *J Small Anim Pract* 1996;**37**:217–24.
25. Galloway PEJ, Barr FJ, Holt PE, et al. Cystic thymoma in a cat with cholesterol-rich fluid and an unusual ultrasonographic appearance. *J Small Anim Pract* 1997;**38**:220–4.
26. Hunt GB, Churcher RK, Church DB, et al. Excision of a locally invasive thymoma causing cranial vena caval syndrome in a dog. *J Am Vet Med Assoc* 1997;**210**:1628–30.
27. Coolman BR, Brewer WG, D'Andrea GH, et al. Severe idiopathic thymic hemorrhage in two littermate dogs. *J Am Vet Med Assoc* 1994;**205**:1152–3.
28. Liu S, Patnaik AK, Burk RL. Thymic branchial cysts in the dog and cat. *J Am Vet Med Assoc* 1983;**182**:1095–8.
29. Malik R, Garbor L, Hunt GB, et al. Benign cranial mediastinal lesions in three cats. *Aust Vet J* 1997;**75**:183–7.
30. Ellison GW, Garner MM, Ackerman N. Idiopathic mediastinal cyst in a cat. *Vet Radiol Ultrasound* 1994;**35**:347–9.
31. Zekas LJ, Adams WM. Cranial mediastinal cysts in nine cats. *Vet Radiol Ultrasound* 2002;**43**:413–18.
32. Granato F, Roberts F, West D. A thyroglossal duct cyst of the anterior mediastinum. *Ann Thorac Surg* 2011;**92**:1118–20.
33. Lynn A, Dockins JM, Kuehn NF, et al. Caudal mediastinal thyroglossal duct cyst in a cat. *J Small Anim Pract* 2009;**50**:147–50.
34. Targhetta R, Chavagneux R, Bourgeois JM, et al. Sonographic approach to diagnosing pulmonary consolidation. *J Ultrasound Med* 1992;**11**:667–72.
35. Targhetta R, Bourgeois JM, Marty-Double C, et al. Peripheral pulmonary lesions: Ultrasonic features and ultrasonically guided fine needle aspiration biopsy. *J Ultrasound Med* 1992;**12**:369–74.
36. Suter PF. Methods of radiographic interpretation, radiographic signs and dynamic factors in the radiographic diagnosis of thoracic disease. In: Suter PF, Lord PF, editors. *Thoracic Radiography: A Text Adas of Thoracic Disease in the Dog and Cat*. Wettswil, Switzerland: PF Suter; 1984. p. 77–126.
37. Rantanen NW. Diseases of the thorax. *Vet Clin North Am Equine Pract* 1986;**2**:49–66.
38. Sugama Y, Tamaki S, Kitamura S, et al. Ultrasonographic evaluation of pleural and chest wall invasion of lung cancer. *Chest* 1988;**93**:275–9.
39. Reef VB. Ultrasonographic evaluation. In: Beech J, editor. *Equine Respiratory Disorders*. Philadelphia: Lea & Febiger; 1991. p. 61–88.
40. Reef VB. Thoracic ultrasound: Noncardiac imaging. In: Reef VB, editor. *Equine Diagnostic Ultrasound*. Philadelphia: WB Saunders; 1998. p. 187–214.
41. Lichtenstein D, Mézière G, Biderman P, et al. The comet-tail artifact: An ultrasound sign of alveolar-interstitial syndrome. *Am J Resp Crit Care* 1997;**156**:1640–6.
42. Reissig A, Kroegel C. Transthoracic sonography of diffuse parenchymal lung disease: The role of comet tail artifacts. *J Ultrasound Med* 2003;**22**:173–80.

43. Louvet A, Bourgeois J. Lung ring-down artifact as a sign of pulmonary alveolar-interstitial disease. *Vet Radiol Ultrasound* 2008;**49**:374–477.

44. Sartori S, Tombesi P. Emerging roles for transthoracic ultrasonography in pulmonary diseases. *World J Radiol* 2010;**2**:203–14.

45. Gargani L. Lung ultrasound: A new tool for the cardiologist. *Cardiovasc Ultrasound* 2011;**9**:6.

46. Weinberg B, Diakoumatis EE, Kass EG, et al. The air bronchogram: Sonographic demonstration. *AJR Am J Roentgenol* 1986;**147**:593–5.

47. Dome HL. Differentiation of pulmonary parenchymal consolidation from pleural disease using the sonographic fluid bronchogram. *Radiology* 1986;**158**:41–2.

48. D'Anjou M, Tidwell AS, Hecht S. Radiographic diagnosis of lung lobe torsion. *Vet Radiol Ultrasound* 2005;**46**:478–84.

49. Hawkins EC. Diseases of the lower respiratory system. In: Ettinger SJ, Feldman EC, editors. *Textbook of Veterinary Internal Medicine*. 4th ed. Philadelphia: WB Saunders; 1995. p. 767–811.

50. Radlinsky MG, Homco LD, Blount WC. Ultrasonographic diagnosis-radiolucent pulmonary foreign body. *Vet Radiol Ultrasound* 1998;**39**:150–3.

51. Suzuki N, Saitoh T, Kitamura S. Tumor invasion of the chest wall in lung cancer: Diagnosis with US. *Radiology* 1993;**187**:39–42.

52. Katic N, Bartolomaeus E, Böhler A, et al. Traumatic diaphragmatic rupture in a cat with partial kidney displacement into the thorax. *J Small Anim Pract* 2007;**48**:705–8.

53. Spattini G, Rossi F, Vignoli M, et al. Use of ultrasound to diagnose diaphragmatic rupture in dogs and cats. *Vet Radiol Ultrasound* 2003;**44**:226–30.

54. Minihan AC, Berg J, Evans KL. Chronic diaphragmatic hernia in 34 dogs and 16 cats. *J Am Anim Hosp Assoc* 2004;**40**:51–63.

55. Suter PF. Abnormalities of the diaphragm. In: Suter PF, Lord PF, editors. *Thoracic Radiography: A Text Adas of Thoracic Disease in the Dog and Cat*. Wettswil, Switzerland: PF Suter; 1984. p. 180–204.

56. Berry CR, Koblik PD, Ticer JW. Dorsal peritoneopericardial mesothelial remnant as an aid to the diagnosis of feline congenital peritoneopericardial diaphragmatic hernia. *Vet Radiol* 1990;**31**:239–45.

57. Barrett RJ, Mann FA, Aronson E. Use of ultrasonography and secondary wound closure to facilitate diagnosis and treatment of a cranial mediastinal abscess in a dog. *J Am Vet Med Assoc* 1993;**203**:1293–5.

58. Finn-Bodner ST, Hadicock JT. Image-guided percutaneous needle biopsy: Ultrasound, computed tomography, and magnetic resonance imaging. *Semin Vet Med Surg (Small Anim)* 1993;**8**:258–78.

59. Wood EF, O'Brien RT, Young KM. Ultrasound-guided fine-needle aspiration of focal parenchymal lesions of the lung in dogs and cats. *J Vet Intern Med* 1998;**12**:338–42.

60. Herman SJ, Holub RV, Weisbrocl GL, et al. Anterior mediastinal masses: Utility of transthoracic needle biopsy. *Radiology* 1991;**180**:167–70.

61. Yang PC, Luh KT, Lee YC, et al. Lung abscesses: US examination and US-guided transthoracic aspiration. *Radiology* 1991;**180**:171–5.

62. Hsu WH, Chiang CD, Hsu JY, et al. Impalpable thoracic bony lesions diagnosed by sonographically guided needle aspiration biopsy. *J Ultrasound Med* 1992;**11**:105–9.

63. Heilo A. Tumors in the mediastinum: US-guided histologic core-needle biopsy. *Radiology* 1993;**189**:143–6.

64. Arakawa A, Matsukawa T, Kira M, et al. Value of ultrasound-guided core-needle biopsy for peripheral intrathoracic and mediastinal lesions. *Comput Med Imaging Graph* 1997;**21**:23–8.

65. Sistrom CL, Wallace KK, Gay SB. Thoracic sonography for diagnosis and intervention. *Curr Probl Diagn Radiol* 1997;**26**:1–49.

66. Yang PC. Ultrasound-guided transthoracic biopsy of peripheral lung, pleural, and chest-wall lesions. *J Thorac Imaging* 1997;**12**:272–84.

67. Sheth S, Hamper UM, Stanley DB, et al. US guidance for thoracic biopsy: A valuable alternative to CT. *Radiology* 1999;**210**:710–26.

68. Hunerbein M, Ghadimi BM, Haenschy W, et al. Transesophageal biopsy of mediastinal and pulmonary tumors by means of endoscopic ultrasound guidance. *J Thorac Cardiovasc Surg* 1998;**116**:554–9.

69. Wiersema MJ, Kochman ML, Cramer HM, et al. Preoperative staging of non-small cell lung cancer: Transesophageal US-guided fine-needle aspiration biopsy of mediastinal lymph nodes. *Radiology* 1994;**190**:239–42.

70. Kim JG. Ultrasonographic evaluation of experimentally induced pleural effusion in dogs. *Korean J Vet Clin Med* 1996;**13**:38–41.

71. Newitt ALM, Cripps PJ, Shimali J. Sonographic estimation of pleural fluid volume in dogs. *Vet Radiol Ultrasound* 2009;**50**:86–90.

72. Shimali J, Cripps PJ, Newitt ALM. Sonographic pleural fluid volume estimation in cats. *J Feline Med Surg* 2010;**12**:113–16.

73. Eibenberger KL, Dock WI, Ammann ME, et al. Quantification of pleural effusions: Sonography versus radiography. *Radiology* 1994;**191**:681–4.

74. Miyamoto T, Sasaki T, Kubo T, et al. Non-invasive determination of the quantity of pleural effusion and evaluation of the beneficial effect of pleuracentesis in patients with acute exacerbation of chronic congestive heart failure. *J Cardiol* 1997;**30**:205–9.

75. Warren-Smith CMR, Roe K, de la Puerta B, et al. Pulmonary adenocarcinoma seeding along a fine needle aspiration tract in a dog. *Vet Rec* 2011;**169**:181.

76. Brant WE. Interventional procedures in the thorax. In: McGahan JP, editor. *Interventional Ultrasound*. Baltimore: Williams & Wilkins; 1990. p. 85–99.

77. Moore EH, LeBlanc J, Montesi SA, et al. Effect of patient positioning after needle aspiration lung biopsy. *Radiology* 1991;**181**:385–7.

78. Collings CL, Westcott JL, Banson NL, et al. Pneumothorax and dependent versus nondependent patient position after needle biopsy of the lung. *Radiology* 1999;**210**:59–64.

CHAPTER 8
Echocardiography

John D. Bonagura • Virginia Luis Fuentes

Echocardiography is widely used for the noninvasive evaluation of cardiovascular (CV) diseases in dogs and cats, and is arguably the most significant advance in cardiac diagnosis witnessed over the last 50 years. Cardiac ultrasonography (US) studies complement auscultation, electrocardiography, and thoracic radiography, and represent the clinical gold standard for the diagnosis and staging of most congenital and acquired heart diseases. This chapter provides an introduction to the principles and practice of echocardiography and offers specific guidelines for establishing a cardiac diagnosis and prognosis based on US findings. The authors acknowledge the contributions of Dr. William P. Thomas and Dr. Richard E. Kienle to the field and also thank them for reproduction of some of their figures from the last edition of this textbook.[1]

There are many comparative aspects between veterinary and medical echocardiography, and when general references to human imaging are raised in this chapter, the interested reader can find more detail by consulting appropriate chapters and figures in textbooks of human echocardiography. Some of our specific recommendations and references we used in the preparation of this chapter include the *Textbook of Clinical Echocardiography* by Dr. Catherine Otto[2] (from which some figures for this chapter have been generously provided); *Feigenbaum's Echocardiography* by Drs. Armstrong and Ryan[3]; *The Echo Manual* by Drs. Oh, Seward, and Tajik[4]; and Dr. Nanda's *Comprehensive Textbook of Echocardiography*.[5] For those interested in the physical principles and instrumentation central to echocardiography, the classic textbooks of Drs. Hatle and Angelsen,[6] Dr. Goldberg and colleagues,[7] Drs. Kisslo, Adams and Belkin,[8] and Dr. Weyman[9] remain excellent resources.

As the literature attests, veterinary echocardiography in dogs and cats has progressed dramatically, from early days of dedicated M-mode studies,[10-33] to grayscale two-dimensional (2D) imaging recorded on videotape,[34-43] to an expanding, multimodality digital-ultrasound examination as demonstrated in current reviews[44,45] and reference textbooks on the subject.[46,47] To control the length of this chapter standard cardiology abbreviations have been used throughout (Box 8-1), and the companion website to this textbook is used extensively as a repository for video loops, supplemental images and reference tables. Considering the published literature pertinent to all aspects of veterinary echocardiography now exceeds 2000 original papers, case reports, reviews, and textbook chapters, the authors have been forced to limit citations within the textbook proper. We have attempted to overcome this shortcoming by tabulating additional references by subject in the supplemental web content.

Echocardiography is just a specialized type of US examination, and the concepts of physics and instrumentation detailed in Chapter 1 are also relevant to cardiac examinations. The examiner must appreciate the practical applications of physics

and instrumentation so that artifacts are not misinterpreted and important diagnostic information is not suppressed by inadequate technique.[2,6,9] Veterinarians with experience in other forms of US imaging will find the fundamentals of echocardiography similar to those described for abdominal evaluation (Chapter 4), general thoracic examination (Chapter 7), and peripheral vascular imaging (Chapter 13). Echocardiographic studies are repeatable in experienced hands; however, results can be highly operator and equipment dependent. *Foremost, all clinicians should practice within their level of knowledge, training, experience, and expertise,* and should not hesitate to send patients to cardiac specialists when referral will serve the best interests of the patient and client.

Some aspects of echocardiography are different from abdominal ultrasonography. These include special features of cardiac transducers, acoustic windows used to image the heart, US-signal processing, and the application of postprocessing myocardial image analyses. Although advanced imaging technologies are largely confined to referral practices and research laboratories, many practicing veterinarians already perform echocardiography at entry or intermediate levels of competency.[48,49] Undoubtedly this practice will increase, enhancing opportunities for cardiac diagnosis in the first-opinion setting while highlighting issues of quality control in imaging and clinical management of complicated cardiology patients. Ultimately, the results of any echocardiographic study should contribute to a definitive cardiac diagnosis, delineate the severity of disease, inform the prognosis, and guide medical, interventional, or surgical treatments.

Echocardiography should be placed in clinical context. It is not a substitute for a careful history and physical examination. Cardiac auscultation is still a cost-effective and expedient examination capable of identifying many serious heart diseases. For example, it would be unusual to identify a clinically relevant valvular lesion by echocardiography in the complete absence of a heart murmur. Likewise basic thoracic radiography remains a critical examination in patients with acute or chronic respiratory signs, considering the broad differential diagnosis of cough, abnormal ventilation, and hypoxemia. Additional examinations including electrocardiography (for arrhythmias), serum biochemistries, heartworm tests, and circulating cardiac biomarkers are often contributory to the diagnosis or to patient management.

Echocardiography should be performed and echocardiograms interpreted by examiners with appropriate technical training and who understand the landscape of cardiovascular disease, appreciate the issues pertinent to the specific patient, and recognize the limitations of the study. Furthermore, an individual capable of integrating information from all sources, including the history, physical examination, and laboratory studies, should ultimately direct patient management.

BOX 8-1

Frequently-Used Abbreviations

ECHOCARDIOGRAPHIC ABBREVIATIONS

2D = two dimensional
2DE = two-dimensional echocardiography/ic
3D = three dimensional
4D = real-time 3D
CDI = color Doppler imaging
CWD = continuous wave Doppler
DCM = dilated cardiomyopathy
DE = Doppler echocardiography
ECG = electrocardiogram/electrocardiographic
MHz = megahertz
PWD = pulsed wave Doppler
ROI = region of interest
TDI = tissue Doppler imaging
TEE = transesophageal echocardiography
TTE = transthoracic echocardiography
US = ultrasound

CARDIAC ANATOMY AND FUNCTION

AMV = anterior (cranioventral) mitral valve
AV = aortic valve
A-V = atrioventricular
EF = ejection fraction
(LVEF = left ventricular ejection fraction)
FS = fractional shortening
(LVFS = left ventricular fractional shortening)
FAS = fractional area shortening
IVS = interventricular septum/septal

LA = left atrium/left atrial
LV = left ventricle/left ventricular
LVOT = left ventricular outflow tract
LVW = left ventricular (posterior) wall
MV = mitral valve
RA = right atrium/right atrial
PA = pulmonary artery/pulmonary arterial
RV = right ventricle/right ventricular
RVOT = right ventricular outflow tract
TV = tricuspid valve

CARDIAC DISEASES

AR = aortic regurgitation
ARVC = arrhythmogenic right ventricular cardiomyopathy
AS = aortic stenosis
ASD = atrial septal defect
AVSD = atrioventricular septal defect
CHF = congestive heart failure
DCM = dilated cardiomyopathy
HCM = hypertrophic cardiomyopathy
LVOTO = left ventricular outflow tract obstruction
MR = mitral regurgitation
MS = mitral stenosis
PFO = patent foramen ovale
PDA = patent ductus arteriosus
PS = pulmonic (pulmonary) stenosis
PHT = pulmonary hypertension
SAM = systolic anterior motion (of the mitral valve)
SAS = subvalvular aortic stenosis
TR = tricuspid regurgitation
VSD = ventricular septal defect

Decisions about patient care should not be relegated to a sonographer unless that person has a full understanding of the clinical situation and sufficient expertise in veterinary cardiology to orchestrate comprehensive patient care.

For those clinicians beginning to learn echocardiography, it might be instructive to consider different levels of imaging acuity while gradually building on previously-learned knowledge and skills. For example, although it is inappropriate for a beginner to evaluate a patient with congenital heart disease, US detection of serous cavity effusions, diffuse pulmonary edema, severely-reduced ventricular systolic function, and moderate to severe left atrial enlargement are within the capabilities of most minimally-experienced examiners. A stepped approach, as envisioned by the authors, involves three broad levels of expertise. *Entry Level* (1) and *Intermediate Level* (2) capabilities are broadly outlined in Table 8-1, and specifically detailed in Web Table 8-1. More advanced imaging methods (*Level 3*) are typically held by a cardiac specialist.

This chapter has been written to provide a foundation for understanding and performing echocardiography. The bulk of the chapter deals with general issues of echocardiography pertinent to the evaluation of acquired and congenital cardiac diseases in dogs and cats. There is neither space nor intent to provide an encyclopedic review of echocardiography in all forms of heart disease. The interested reader can find entire textbooks devoted to the subject in both medicine and in veterinary practice.[2-7,9,46,47] While the principles of echocardiographic diagnosis of congenital heart disease are explained in this chapter, this topic is highly specialized and beyond the scope of this review.

OVERVIEW OF ECHOCARDIOGRAPHY

Echocardiography is the application of US imaging to the heart and those blood vessels contiguous with the heart. In current primary and referral practices, virtually all examinations are completed via transthoracic echocardiography (TTE).[46] Endoscopic-mounted probes that place the transducer directly over the heart base are used for transesophageal echocardiography (TEE). These transducers are expensive. Moreover, when compared to the human imaging situation, TEE is rarely needed in dogs or cats for a high quality study. TEE also requires general anesthesia, which significantly depresses cardiac function and poses some degree of patient risk. While there are a small number of papers detailing TEE in the veterinary literature[50-62] only brief mention of this technique will be made in this chapter.

Echocardiographic Formats

The commonly used cardiac modalities are two-dimensional echocardiography (2DE);[35] motion-mode echocardiography (M-mode Echo);[20] 2D color Doppler imaging (CDI);[63] and spectral formats of Doppler echocardiography,[64-67] namely pulsed wave Doppler (PWD) and continuous wave Doppler (CWD) echocardiography. As with CDI, spectral Doppler examinations interrogate blood flow along a specified line or region of interest (ROI), but spectral displays are graphical not overlaid on the 2D image. Both CDI and PWD also can be applied to moving myocardial walls in the form of tissue Doppler imaging (TDI). Different modalities give us complementary information about heart anatomy and function,

TABLE 8-1

Proposed Levels of Competency in Echocardiography: Capabilities of Level 1 & Level 2 Examiners*

Foundational Knowledge	Level 1	Level 2A	Level 2B
1. Understand the role and clinical value of echocardiography in primary care veterinary practice.	✓	✓	✓
2. Understand the limitations of 2D echocardiography in primary care veterinary practice.	✓	✓	✓
3. Understand the physics, instrumentation, examination techniques, and artifacts pertinent to the type of echocardiographic examinations performed.	✓	✓	✓
4. Appreciate supplemental sources of information available to guide diagnosis and management, and understand when referral to a cardiac specialist is the most appropriate course.	✓	✓	✓

Technical Examination Competency	Level 1	Level 2A	Level 2B
5. Obtain a technically-competent, basic 2D echocardiogram from the right thorax of dogs and cats.	✓	✓	✓
6. Obtain a technically-competent M-mode echocardiogram.		✓	✓
7. Obtain a technically-competent, basic 2D echocardiogram from the left thorax.		✓	✓
8. Obtain a technically-competent, basic, Doppler Echocardiogram to record blood flow across the four cardiac valves.		(optional)	✓

Interpretation and Diagnosis	Level 1	Level 2A	Level 2B
9. Develop a consistent approach to interpretation to identify acquired cardiac diseases, cardiac chamber enlargement, ventricular systolic dysfunction, and findings that support or argue against a diagnosis of heart failure.	✓	✓	✓
10. Effectively integrate knowledge of cardiac disease, clinical findings, and results of echocardiography to develop plans for patient management.	✓	✓	✓

*Level 3 Examiners are cardiac specialists. See Web Table 8-1 for detailed characteristics/capabilities of Level 1 and Level 2 Examiners.

cardiac blood flow, diseases, and the hemodynamic burden placed on the heart.

These established methods can be augmented by advanced image processing techniques including three-dimensional (3D) reconstruction and real-time 3D (so-called 4D) echocardiography. A number of emerging post-processing methods track acoustic speckles within myocardium to quantify tissue velocities, displacement, deformation (strain), as well as cardiac rotation, torsion, and twist. A listing of various echocardiographic modalities is found in Box 8-2.

Diagnostic Information

A complete echocardiographic study can reveal detailed information about the heart including morphology and pathology, size and motion, systolic and diastolic ventricular function, atrial function, blood flow, valvular function, and hemodynamics (Web Table 8-2). Complete information only can be obtained by application of complementary modalities that include 2D/3D and M-mode imaging followed by CDI and spectral Doppler formats. Properly gathered and interpreted, this information should lead to a definitive cardiac diagnosis in most cases and illustrate the functional and hemodynamic consequences of cardiac lesions noninvasively. While a complete, multimodality study represents the standard for cardiac US imaging, focused 2D examinations can be useful and cost-effective.[68] Accomplishing a limited, but technically-competent 2DE examination is usually the best first step to learning more advanced procedures of echocardiography (see Web Table 8-1).

Alternative Imaging

Other imaging examinations deliver different, complementary, or more detailed information than echocardiography. For example, while pulmonary US can be successful in identify pulmonary infiltration or edema,[69,70] simple thoracic radiography is often superior for assessing lung pathology or identifying pulmonary edema in cardiac patients. Lung disease is also better assessed by computerized tomography (CT), although heavy sedation or anesthesia is required for this examination. While ventricular and atrial volumes can be estimated by M-mode and 2D/3D echocardiographic techniques, magnetic resonance imaging (MRI) is considered the gold standard for these assessments (although currently impractical for this purpose). Additionally, CT angiography and MRI are better suited for visualizing many vascular anomalies, such as an abnormal aortic arch, and most coronary, pulmonary or systemic vascular lesions, especially when the abnormality is not contiguous with the heart. Cardiac catheterization with angiography also maintains a role for identifying certain vascular malformations, acquired lesions, intrapulmonary shunts, and even some rare cardiac lesions.

Limitations of Echocardiography

Limitations and diagnostic pitfalls of echocardiography must be learned, and some specific examples of these are highlighted in this chapter. Examiners should not overinterpret day-to-day variability. Many echocardiographic measurements can change by 10% or more due to biologic variability, differences in operator technique, and interobserver factors when measuring images. For example, a decrease of 4% or 5% in LV fractional shortening might represent a change of clinical importance or just normal daily variation. Echocardiographic measurements and Doppler findings are also influenced by heart rate, ventricular filling pressures, and by the forces opposing the ejection of blood (collectively termed "afterload"). As examples, systemic hypertension or aortic stenosis worsen mitral regurgitation simply by increasing LV systolic pressure. Similarly, increased or decreased afterload often confounds the assessment of contractile function.

Echocardiographic studies can be misinterpreted when normal physiologic findings are mistaken for evidence of disease. This is common when assessing LV systolic function

---

BOX 8-2

Echocardiography: Overview of Imaging Modalities

BRIGHTNESS MODE (B-MODE) IMAGING— 2D ECHOCARDIOGRAPHY
   Sector Scan
   Real-Time 2D Echocardiography

MOTION MODE IMAGING—M-MODE ECHOCARDIOGRAPHY

THREE-DIMENSIONAL ECHOCARDIOGRAPHY
   Real-Time 3D Echocardiography ("4D")

DOPPLER ECHOCARDIOGRAPHY
Color Doppler Echocardiography
   Color Flow Imaging
   Color M-Mode Imaging
Color Tissue Doppler Imaging
Spectral Doppler Studies of Blood Flow
   Pulsed-Wave Doppler Echocardiography (PW Doppler)
   High Pulse-Repetition Frequency Doppler Echocardiography
   Continuous Wave Doppler Echocardiography (CW Doppler)

TISSUE DOPPLER IMAGING (TDI)
   PW-Doppler Based TDI
   Color Doppler Based TDI

ADVANCED CARDIAC IMAGE PROCESSING
Speckle Tracking-Based Image Processing
Tissue Doppler-Based Image Processing
Cardiac Function Obtained from Advanced Image
   Processing*
   Tissue Displacement (Tissue Tracking)
   Deformation (Strain and Strain Rate) Imaging
      Longitudinal, Radial and Circumferential Strain
   Vector Imaging
   Cardiac (Dys)synchronization
   Rotation, Torsion, and Twist
   Tissue Activation Imaging

*These indices are obtained from proprietary software and can be vendor specific in terms of availability.

in large-breed dogs due to the emphasis placed on minor axis shortening while ignoring apical to basilar contraction. Too often multiple indices of LV systolic function point to entirely different interpretations! Ambiguous echocardiographic results become clearer when serial examinations are obtained and even more definitive when clear trends in heart size or cardiac function are observed.

Another common pitfall involves examination of heart valves using color Doppler echocardiography. As will be discussed later, physiologic valvular regurgitation is common, especially involving right-heart valves. Furthermore, Doppler technology is so sensitive that the blood flow associated with normal valve closure can be mistaken for true valvular regurgitation. Thus the clinician must beware of creating what in medicine has been termed "Doppler disease." When echocardiographic findings are confusing or inconsistent with clinical or other imaging findings, one should reconsider the diagnosis and obtain a second opinion from a cardiologist.

OVERVIEW OF INSTRUMENTATION FOR CARDIAC STUDIES

A technically proficient examination requires appropriate transducer selection, adjustment of operator controls, sufficient imaging skill to record normal and abnormal blood flow, and appreciation of normal findings and variation. An experienced examiner is characterized by knowledge of cardiac diseases, an ability to adjust the examination based on contemporary findings, and an appreciation for common artifacts and technical issues that might lead to errors of interpretation. Stated simply, clinicians unwilling to tackle instrumentation issues should not perform echocardiography, especially those studies involving Doppler applications. *Details of US instrumentation previously described in Chapter 1 are relevant to echocardiography.* Some general comments regarding cardiac instrumentation are considered here, and specific technical information is offered in subsequent sections of this chapter by modality.

With the exception of subspecialty practices, most veterinarians purchase US equipment with the intent of performing abdominal, cardiac, and noncardiac thoracic imaging using that single system. This is feasible considering more similarities than differences are found between these three examinations. Nevertheless, some distinctions between cardiac and abdominal imaging can be highlighted and some of these issues are summarized in Table 8-2. Important departures from abdominal studies involve the cardiac imaging transducers, settings for dynamic range (compression) and grayscale (greyscale) processing, requirements for temporal resolution, and filter and pulse repetition frequency (PRF) settings for color and spectral Doppler imaging.

Transducers

US transducers manufactured for cardiac examinations have a smaller footprint than those used for abdominal scanning. The US is typically emitted as a sector rather than the wider formats used elsewhere in the body. This relates in part to need to access the smaller acoustic windows located between the ribs. The use of an abdominal probe for cardiac work is done as a cost savings but at the expense of processing speed. Additionally, many abdominal transducers cannot perform the full complement of Doppler imaging needed for CV assessment. The assumption that one or even two transducers will suffice for all cardiac studies is another common error, especially when the examiner expects to record quality studies from patients ranging from cats to giant breed dogs.

Optimal feline studies (and those involving toy canine breeds) usually demand transducer frequencies within a 7-12 MHz range. Conversely studies of large-breed dogs require lower frequency transducers in the range of 3 to 4 MHz. Small and mid-sized dogs are often too large to be examined effectively with feline transducers but too small to be imaged clearly with the optimal transducer for the larger canine breeds. The authors use three or four different transducers for small animal cardiac studies. Obviously the trade-off between image quality and cost of equipment becomes important.

For Doppler studies, lower transducer frequencies improve recording sensitivity. Modern systems automatically adjust Doppler-activated crystals to lower frequency vibrations while maintaining 2D imaging at higher frequencies or harmonics. The selection of frequency bands is operator adjustable to some degree, and experimentation is useful to determine the optimal signal to noise ratio for a particular study. Despite the caveat that lower frequencies are more sensitive, many transducers deliver the best CDI and spectral Doppler imaging

TABLE 8-2

Instrumentation Differences between Cardiac and Abdominal Ultrasound Imaging

Imaging Factor	Distinctive Features of the Cardiac Examination
Transducer footprint	Cardiac transducers have a smaller footprint to fit between ribs when compared to abdominal (convex or linear) probes.
Transducer frequencies	Wide range of frequencies needed; for cats (typically >6 or 7 MHz); for large-breed dogs (typically <4 MHz).
	Three or four transducers are generally needed to create high-quality cardiac studies across the typical range of small animal patients.
	Doppler studies are typically done with operator adjustable "dual" frequencies (lower for Doppler activated crystals).
Harmonic imaging	Harmonic or octave imaging is appropriate for cardiology and improves resolution, but some settings/systems might result in "thickening" of valves or reduced frame rates.
Digital playback	Critical for evaluating cardiac motion at slow playback speeds.
	Generally needed to view every frame when acquisition rate is >30 FPS.
Manufacturer presets for imaging	A good starting point but must be optimized for species and patient size. Adult cardiology and pediatric cardiology presets might involve imaging processes that are not operator adjustable and therefore are unique to the application selected. Abdominal presets typically result in acquisition frame rates that are too low.
B-mode line density	Most cardiac presets are adjusted to a 50% line density of that used for abdominal imaging. This improves frame rate and temporal resolution (but at the cost of overall image quality). System specific "switches" can exert a profound effect on frame rate, often leading to $\frac{1}{2}$ or 2× changes.
Temporal (time) resolution and acquisition frame rates	Higher frame rates are more important for cardiac studies than for other forms of grayscale (greyscale) imaging. Frame rates of >30/s (and typically much higher) should be obtained. The width of field might need to be compromised (reduced) to improve temporal resolution.
Grayscale compression (dynamic range); post-processing; reject filters; edge enhancement	Dynamic range influences the contrast and shades of gray. Many systems have both a compression (dynamic range) and postprocessing options for grayscale or spectral image data. Cardiac images are often processed with higher contrast than abdominal scans to facilitate endocardial and vascular wall resolution and color Doppler imaging of the blood pool. During Doppler imaging pixels must be prioritized to either grayscale or Doppler processing.
Frame averaging and image persistence	Generally set to lower values of persistence (or turned "off") to minimize blur artifacts of rapidly-moving cardiac structures. Low persistence is especially important in CDI with faster heart rates.
Adjusting color quality (packet size)	Larger packet sizes ("quality") and lower setting for low-velocity filters can improve Color Doppler "filling" of the blood pool, but at the expense of lower acquisition frame rates.
Low velocity filters and pulse-repetition frequency (PRF) in CDI	Low velocity filters are typically set at higher values than for the abdomen (or automatically adjusted to higher cutoffs by increasing the PRF and aliasing limits). There is a trade-off between low velocity filters and CDI acquisition frame rates.

when activated near their central frequencies. Within a single transducer, extremes of the Doppler frequency band can fail to transmit sufficient power, precluding the delivery of high-quality images.

Temporal Resolution

This relates to the system's ability to accurately characterize motion over time. Temporal resolution is rarely an issue with abdominal studies but is paramount when assessing the heart with 2DE, 3DE, and CDI, and especially challenging in patients with rapid heart rates. As a general guideline 2D real-time echocardiographic studies should be recorded and stored at frame rates of at least 30 per second. Modern systems often record 2D images at frame rates exceeding 150/sec. Stored digital video loops should be reviewed in slow motion to visualize each captured frame. When clinically relevant (as when assessing valve motion, valvular regurgitation, or a ventricle functioning at a rapid heart rate), the image review should occur prior to storing the study because most archived images are forced to DICOM frame rates of 30/s. This important point is further discussed under CDI later in the chapter.

System Controls

The operator should become conversant with US system settings best suited for the different imaging modalities. Certainly application specialists can offer invaluable training and guidance, and modern US systems offer vendor-specific "automated" buttons to quickly optimize 2D and Doppler images. However, the fine-tuning of a US system is ultimately charged to the examiner and if manufacturer presets are the only settings applied, the US system will undoubtedly underperform. The authors advise examiners to "push every button" and "enter every menu" so that optimal presets are established for the wide range of patients examined by veterinarians.

The variety among vendors, systems, and proprietary controls precludes any detailing of US system settings beyond the most general recommendations. Table 8-3 lists some of the steps that might be taken when optimizing cardiac instrumentation and creating imaging "presets" for 2D, M-mode, color Doppler, and spectral Doppler imaging. Some of the settings are instrument- and vendor-specific. Additionally, function controls available on a specific platform might be available on another system but denoted with a completely different label or descriptor.

TABLE 8-3

Optimizing Your Echocardiographic System and Presets: Some Initial Steps

Setting(s)	Comment(S)
Select candidate **Manufacturer Preset**	Transducer specific for most systems. Cardiology vs. general vs. abdominal. Adult cardiology vs. Pediatric applications.
Activate the **ECG**	Insure it works! Determine the best approach for connecting electrodes. Adjust initial ECG lead setting, gain, and trace position. Horizontal speed might be controllable as well.
Select the 2D/Doppler **Transducer**	Tradeoff of penetration vs. resolution. Tradeoff of Doppler sensitivity vs. resolution. Select initial imaging frequency and mode (harmonics or not). Initial imaging frequency depends on size of patient and options for harmonics imaging.
Select the **Image Orientation** Adjust the **Left/Right Invert** switch	The actual image presentation depends on whether the transducer is coming from below (cutout) or above/standing, and how the operator holds the reference "notch" (thumb or index finger). The left/right invert switch allows for appropriate presentation to the viewer (i.e., cranial and dorsal structures to the viewer's right eye except for apical 4-chamber images). Pediatric orientations ("apex down") can be obtained with the up/down invert switch.
Adjust the **Depth of Field**	While a deeper present is useful to detect pleural effusion, presets are easier to "set up" by selecting an optimal depth (cats 4 or 5 cm; small to medium dogs ~ 6 to 8 cm; larger dogs ~ 12 cm).
Adjust the size of the 2D **Sector Angle**	Generally start wide, but it will affect frame rate. Many systems allow the operator to steer the 2D sector.
Preset the size of the 2D **Image Zoom**	Typically an operator-adjustable isosceles trapezoid, but it might be a rectangle in some systems—should be able to focus on a cardiac valve and immediately adjacent chambers.
Move the 2D **Transducer Focus**	Select a single focal zone (unless the frame rate is unaffected by dual focal zones). While system-specific, one typically sets a single focus within the most distant 25% of the imaging field or just at the maximum depth of imaging (interest).
Adjust overall **Transmit Power**	Typically placed near maximum.
Adjust 2D **Gain** Readjust after TGC settings are fixed	Adjust to create a black blood pool. Gain affects all returning echoes—both strong and weak.
Adjust the **Time-Gain-Compensation**	Set to provide a uniform B-mode image from the near to the far field. Most "ramps" are relatively flat in modern equipment with a slightly higher TGC setting for the far-field. When transducer penetration is relatively great for patient size adjust to near center of control settings; when penetration is relatively marginal, adjust to the right.
Adjust the **Frame Rate** (if available)	Generally select fast frame rate minus 1 click (to optimize image).
Check/adjust **2D Line Density**	If the (2D) frame rate is too slow, identify any controls that affect the image quality by doubling B-mode line density (it is rarely called that). Abdominal presets are usually 2X the line density of cardiac presets; some newer Echo systems change line density with different preset applications.
Turn off or minimize **Spatial and Temporal Averaging** (persistence) of the image	In most systems temporal averaging is a "persistence" control. For dogs, a value of 0 or 1 is appropriate (out of 5); or 2 (if >5 settings). For cats, persistence is often best at zero.
Adjust **B-mode Compression (Dynamic Range) and Post-processing Grayscale**	Controls are system dependent and might have different names. Dynamic range (dB) is the difference between the weakest and strongest acoustic signals; these must be processed for display on the imaging monitor. The initial processing (compression) is operator adjustable and affects the length of the grayscale. For 2D processing, aim for the widest grayscale possible that maintains a sonolucent (relatively black) blood pool. Most adjustments of acoustic data are nonlinear and can lead to hardening (more contrast), softening, altering blood pool reflectors, or optimizing borders. The impact of applying different post-processing curves is more difficult to predict and are "trial and error."
Test different **Post-Processing** curves	Experiment with the available gray-scale processing curves in order to optimize the image for that transducer and preset.
Understand **Chroma** (coloring)	In general, use Chroma for specific issues such as identification of borders or echogenic smoke in the atria.

TABLE 8-3

Optimizing Your Echocardiographic System and Presets: Some Initial Steps—cont'd

Setting(s)	Comment(S)
Adjust the **Reject** setting (if available)	Reject removes the weakest echoes from the image.
Adjust **Additional 2D Image Processing Controls** including lateral gain, edge, smoothing (system dependent)	Alter lateral gain controls, contrast, edge enhancement, smoothing, and speckle reduction to personal taste. Sometimes it is quite difficult to appreciate any substantive change when making these adjustments!
Activate the cursor to record an **M-mode Echo** of the left ventricle	Many M-mode settings are tied to the B-mode imaging. Adjust any independent M-mode settings (gain, B-mode processing, edge-enhancement, reject to optimize the image); set the horizontal sweep speed for the display.
Save the B-mode/M-mode preset	After optimizing the images above, name and save the preset.
Turn on **color Doppler Imaging (CDI)**	After optimizing the 2D image plane of interest.
Balance the **Pixel Priorities** for grayscale and color	Insure 2D image has sufficient "black" blood pool but adequate tissue delineation. System adjustments vary (specific color balance or tissue priority settings might be available to optimize pixel display for color encoding).
Adjust the 2D **Sector Angle**	May need to narrow to enhance frame rate
Adjust the CDI **Region of Interest**	Usually some variation of an isosceles trapezoid is selected. Sufficient 2D grayscale imaging should surround the ROI to provide an anatomic template for the image.
Select a **Color Map**	Color maps are usually variations on "BART" (blue away, red toward); consider using an enhanced color map with addition of variance encoding (either green or "split" green/yellow algorithms).
Adjust **Color Gain**	Increase the gain until tiny numbers of stray color "speckles" appear in the blood pool.
Adjust **Pulse Repetition Frequency**	The PRF determines the Nyquist (aliasing) limits and is tied into automated low-velocity filters; generally select the highest or second-highest switch option. Higher PRF (higher velocity scales) result in filtering out of lower velocity signals and therefore less color filling. Lower PRF settings might overwhelm the image with normal flow patterns and bleed into the tissues.
Adjust the **Color Zero Baseline**	Generally, set to mid-point; shift when performing PISA.
Set **Color Packet Size**/Dwell time	This is typically set as a color "quality" setting. Higher quality = slower frame rates ±lower velocity scales.
Adjust the **Color Low-Velocity Filter**	Lower filter settings reveal more low-velocity flow. Settings that are too low overwhelm the image data. Lower settings might tie to lower PRF or frame rates.
Lower **Color Persistence**	Set persistence to off or to a minimal setting
Adjust **Color Smoothing, Averaging,** or **Spatial Filtering**	System specific controls that adjust for the smoothness of the image; personal preference. Don't over-smooth: more "pixelated" color imaging might provide better delineation of flow disturbances.
Readjust image to obtain sufficient **temporal resolution**	Tradeoff between color "quality" and frame rates. Angle width, depth, transducer frequency, color quality, low velocity filters, persistence and PRF all impact temporal resolution or the appearance of real-time CDI.
Activate **Color M-mode** imaging	Observe appearance of flow event timing with current settings (should be satisfactory if 2D CDI is good quality).
Activate **Spectral Doppler** imaging and adjust initial settings.	The manufacturer preset should provide initial spectra for inspection and adjustments.
Set the **Doppler Power** to maximum	Use a lower Doppler power transmit setting when the transducer frequency is somewhat "overpowered" for the patient size.
Set the **Doppler Gain** to a mid-level	Avoid over-gained signals that bloom the peak velocity profile.
Adjust the **Frequency Setting**	Adjust the frequency setting for the Doppler activated crystals distinct from that of the 2D imaging frequency. Remember: extremes of frequency, distant from the central Doppler frequency, are often inferior/weaker.
Adjust the **Sweep Speed**	Faster sweep speeds (e.g., 100 mm/s or more) are used for feline presets and for recording timing events (can be later adjusted during the examination).

Continued

TABLE 8-3

Optimizing Your Echocardiographic System and Presets: Some Initial Steps—cont'd

Setting(s)	Comment(S)
Adjust the **Audio Volume**	Many animals are frightened when hearing audible Doppler frequency shifts; low speaker volumes or the use of headphones are desirable.
Activate the cursor and **Sample Volume size**	The sample volume size depends on the patient and the application: smaller for blood flow detection except in the pulmonary veins; larger for tissue Doppler imaging.
	Typical initial PW "gates" 1-2 mm (cats); 1-3 mm (small dogs); 2-4 mm (larger dogs).
	The CW Doppler cursor displays a focal zone; move zone to distance just far to the flow disturbance of interest.
Assure **angle correction** is **OFF**	You cannot assure alignment to the third plane; danger of over-estimating peak velocity.
Set the **PRF/Scale** for the PW/CW imaging modality. Be aware of high-PRF Doppler	For PW Doppler the highest scale is selected (with high-PRF Doppler imaging turned "off"). Attempt to minimize aliasing. If high-PRF is activated, the Nyquist will increase but at the expense of additional sample volume(s).
Set the **Baseline**	For CW Doppler higher velocity limits are preset (~ 3 to 4 m/s velocity limit in each direction).
	The Doppler baseline is centered or shifted slightly upward (to record higher velocity negative flow signals).
Set the **Low Velocity Filters** for the PW/CW/TDI modality	Also called "wall" filters.
	Typical PW settings are 1-3 "clicks" from the lowest filtering.
	Typical CW settings are higher than PW to filter out low velocity signals; low velocity filter settings are often different between PW and CW Doppler (e.g., 50, 100, 200 Hz for PW Doppler vs 100, 200, 400, 800 Hz for CW Doppler).
	When TIMING of events is critical, or when visible valve noise is desired, low velocity filters should be set to minimal values or to "off." When TDI is performed, the wall filters should be turned "off"—this is done automatically in most TDI modules.
Readjust the **Gain**	Avoid overgained signals that bloom the envelope.
Set **Compression (Dynamic range)** and **Post-processing** Grayscale	Adjust to an optimal velocity spectrum—aim for a spectrum with a clean envelope, clear peak, lack of blooming, and a visible modal velocity within the grayscale of the spectrum.
Activate Chroma maps as desired	Select a post-processing spectral color of choice; for weak signals a black (gray) on white or white (gray) on black might be the best.

As a practical matter to enhance workflow, the authors create separate presets for cats, small dogs, medium-sized dogs, and larger-breed dogs. When both pediatric and adult image processing applications are available, it is worthwhile to create presets for each to see which provides the best imaging and temporal resolution. This is not always predictable! One approach is to optimize 2D and M-mode imaging first and then immediately name and save the preset (such as: Feline_ Std, Canine_Small; Canine_Large; Feline_Ped). Once the 2D imaging is set, move to CDI (optimize and resave); then select the appropriate initial settings for spectral imaging (and save). This is repeated for "adult" and "pediatric" applications to determine which performs better within a defined patient group. Other presets are then created, leveraging the settings from earlier customizations.

EXAMINATION TECHNIQUE

Once the indications for performing echocardiography are understood and the clinical issues identified, the examination can proceed. Initial considerations should include the respiratory status of the patient, temperament, willingness to tolerate restraint, and the examination detail necessary to address the clinical questions.

Patient Preparation

The vast majority of dogs and cats are examined under gentle manual restraint. Some operators place Elizabethan collars on cats to reduce risk of injury to the holders.[71] Sedatives and tranquilizers can reduce heart rate and impair cardiac function but are appropriate when patients will not lie quietly, become overly stressed, or exhibit aggression during the examination. Normotensive cats can be lightly sedated with butorphanol (0.25 mg per kilogram, IM, mixed with acetylpromazine 0.05-0.1 mg per kilogram, IM). Following drug administration the cat should be allowed to rest in its carrier in a quiet room for 20 to 30 minutes before handling. Most dogs can be well-sedated with either butorphanol (0.2-0.3 mg per kilogram, IV or IM) or a combination of butorphanol mixed with acepromazine (0.025-0.03 mg per kilogram, IV or IM). An alternative for dogs is buprenorphine (0.005 to 0.01 mg/kg IV or IM) combined with the aforementioned dose of acetylpromazine. These tranquilizer/sedatives exert minimal effects on cardiac function[72,73] although heart rate often slows following withdrawal of sympathetic tone. When more potent sedation is required, an alpha-2 agonist such as dexmedetomidine can be considered. Drugs in this class can increase ventricular afterload—an advantage for patients with dynamic LVOT obstruction[74]—but also reduce heart rate. When butorphanol and acetylpromazine are insufficient for a cat, either dexmedetomidine or a low intravenous dose of ketamine (5-10 mg/cat, IV) will usually provide sufficient immobilization, but with some influence on heart rate and on cardiac function.[30,73,75] Echocardiography should not be performed under general anesthesia except in extraordinary situations or to allow for TEE or when echocardiographic guidance is used during an interventional catheterization procedure.

The acoustic windows should be identified by palpation of the cardiac apical impulses or intercostal spaces. While sufficient skin contact might be achieved by parting and wetting of the hair with isopropyl alcohol, most examinations are improved after clipping the hair, especially in those with long- or coarse-hair coats. US gel should be recurrently applied to the transducer surface to maintain air-free contact with the thorax and facilitate *minimal* pressure on the chest. With experience most examiners can sense when patient stress is about to compromise the examination. In such cases, remov-

ing the probe and gently reassuring the dog or cat can sometimes extend the time available for the study. Repositioning the patient diagonally can also be helpful, especially if a cat or small dog is sagging into the cutout of the imaging table.

ECG electrodes should be attached whenever possible to record the cardiac rhythm. While this is especially critical when performing Doppler imaging, a simultaneous ECG recording also should be the *routine* for 2D and M-mode echocardiograms. It can be useful to know noninvasive systemic arterial blood pressure, and this can be obtained just prior to the examination.

Small animals can be imaged while they stand, sit, or rest on their sternum (a position especially appropriate for those in respiratory distress). However, most examiners prefer to place the dog or cat in lateral recumbency and use a cutout table to scan from underneath (Figure 8-1, *A*). There is little question that when the dog or cat is placed in lateral

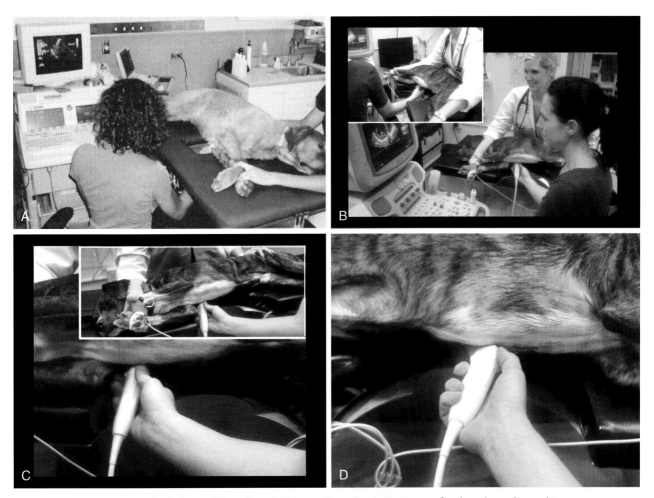

Figure 8-1 **Techniques of Transthoracic Echocardiography. A,** Positioning for the echocardiographic examination. The cutout is inside the table edge. **B,** Examination of a dog using a table with a cutout located at the edge of the table. This method is usually less stressful on the operator's arm and shoulder but requires more attention to patient positioning and restraint. The imaging table can be raised by a hydraulic lift. The chair should be comfortable and some operators prefer an arm-rest for support (inset). The control console is operated with the left hand and is positioned vertically and horizontally if possible to reduce stress on the left arm and shoulder. Limiting the angle between the imaging table and the ultrasound console might also reduce neck and back strain. **C,** Hand placement for obtaining the 4-chamber long-axis image from the right parasternal position. The transducer has been partially removed from thoracic contact to demonstrate the positioning. **D,** Hand placement for obtaining left apical images. The transducer is pointed cranially and dorsally with progressive clockwise rotation used to acquire 4-chamber, 3-chamber, and 2 chamber images. See Box 8-1 for abbreviations for this and subsequent figures.

recumbency, the quality of the images is better when approaching from the dependent side. The vast majority of examiners position the patients so they are facing their limbs. Some operators prefer to face the patient's spine, but this approach can prove more difficult for assistants in terms of manual restraint.

Most operators hold the transducer with their right hand and control the imaging system with their left hand (Figure 8-1, *B*), but while typical, it is not a requirement. Suitable attention should be paid to the comfort of the examination chair, the level and distance of the US control console, and the height and distance of the table imaging cutout from the operator. The risks for repetitive motion injury and neck strain can be reduced with attention to the ergonomics in the examining area. Key aspects have been summarized by Macdonald, King and Scott[76,77] and include: (1) keeping the hands within a near reach zone to reduce shoulder strain; (2) maintaining an upright cervical spine posture and limiting neck rotation to approximately 30 degrees in each direction; (3) minimizing effort to position the US transducer against the thoracic wall; and (4) limiting necessary but awkward maneuvers.

Transducer Management

A raised edge or marker or a small notch is found along the surface of most transducers and corresponds to one edge of the sector image. This reference edge is identified on the screen by an icon. Entry level operators should start by facing this maker and placing it under the thumb (or alternatively rotate the marker 180 degrees to lie under the index finger). Rotation through imaging planes should be accomplished using this tactile and visual reference as a guide. Electronically controlled left-to-right inversion of the image might be required to maintain the imaging conventions that call for displaying most cranial and dorsal structures to the right side of the imaging screen (as viewed by the observer).[78-79] With greater experience, the examiner learns to rotate the transducer while releasing the reference marker. This maneuver considerably reduces strain on the wrists and arms.

Transducer manipulation usually involves the following three main movements: (1) *placement* of the transducer; (2) *rotation* or twisting of the transducer; and (3) *angulation* of the central US beam of the transducer. These major actions are followed by *fine-plane imaging* adjustments: modifying the rotation or tilt to optimize the image. Of these movements, transducer placement and rotation have the greatest impact on the image unless extreme angulation has been engaged.

In this chapter it is assumed that the examiner is imaging from *underneath* the small animal patient using a cut-out table, and the authors define *clockwise* rotation as twisting to the right while looking down the cable with the transducer face pointing away (the same rotation is counter-clockwise if one looks onto the transducer face from above the table). Thus for the right-handed operator, if the thumb is rotated toward the right shoulder, the transducer rotation is considered clockwise. Neutral or zero rotation in this chapter indicates that the sector reference notch is either directly facing the operator (under the thumb) or directly opposite from the operator (under the index finger). Again, depending on how the probe is held, activation of left/right inversion might be needed. As an example of this approach, when obtaining a right parasternal, 4-chamber, long-axis image of the heart with the dog lying on its right side, the examiner will place the transducer at the right fourth intercostal space, rotate the transducer approximately 30 degrees clockwise (to start) and then angulate the axial (central) US beam caudally and dorsally (Figure 8-1, *C*).

When a steeply-angled transducer creates a tenuous contact with the thorax, it can be useful to move the transducer one intercostal space in the direction of the axial (central) beam. To maintain the same structures within the imaging plane, the examiner must then tilt the transducer back toward the direction of prior placement. There are some exceptions to this guideline of avoiding steep angulation. For example the left apical three-, four-, and five-chamber images require steep craniodorsal angulation of the transducer (Figure 8-1, *D*). A steep dorsal angulation also is needed to image the pulmonary artery and its branches.

Thus 2D images are acquired in these steps: (1) moving the transducer to an intercostal (parasternal) acoustic window; (2) rotating or twisting the transducer; (3) applying angulation; and concluding with (4) fine-plane adjustments. With enough training and experience, stereotypical transducer positions can be learned to obtain the standard imaging planes. Owing to differences in the feline thoracic conformation and cardiac position (a thinner thorax and more horizontal heart), there are slight differences between imaging planes used in cats and dogs; however, the same transducer management principles hold. Specific imaging planes and associated transducer movements and pointers are discussed in detail in an upcoming section.

Other Instrument Controls

Image optimization requires the use of appropriate presets and active adjustments on the imaging console.[2,9] Some of the most important controls affecting image processing and quality are discussed in Chapter 1 and in upcoming chapter sections (see "2D Instrumentation"). The M-mode and Doppler examinations also require operator manipulation of a trackball to control discrete elements within the transducer array. In the case of the M-mode study, a linear cursor or M-line is directed across the 2D image to acquire an "icepick" image of the heart. For CDI studies an adjustable ROI is constructed and this trapezoid-shaped sample is positioned within the 2D grayscale image. With PWD the operator steers a cursor containing a small sample volume to focal locations within the blood pool or myocardium. A cursor is also used for CWD; this line indicates the direction of continuous Doppler interrogation and often includes an adjustable marker that controls the US focal zone.

Core Examination

Certain 2D images are routinely selected for evaluation of cardiac anatomy and motion. Other images are suited for estimating LV and RV function. Still others are chosen to optimize the blood flow information obtained from Doppler examinations. Experienced examiners move quickly across these images with an understanding of their utility and the need to archive those still frames and video loops that characterize the study. Of course cardiac lesions are not constrained by standardized imaging planes, and the examiner often obtains the optimal alignment to an abnormal flow pattern with unconventional or modified images. Adapting the examination as new findings appear requires both imaging skill and knowledge of cardiac diseases. One should also be aware of extracardiac findings that might suggest a diagnosis of CHF or contribute to the differential diagnosis even if the cardiac examination is normal. Examples include the findings of pleural effusion, pulmonary edema, or intrapulmonary disease (see Chapter 7). Pulmonary edema is often manifested as multiple, adjacent pulmonary B-lines or "lung rockets".[69,70]

Accepting there is no prescribed standard in veterinary medicine for a core examination, nearly every small animal study begins with 2D long- and short-axis images obtained from the right thorax. Standardized 2D and M-mode image planes have been described for veterinary studies,[79] these are detailed in the next two sections. Most veterinary examiners activate the M-mode cursor to estimate LV size and wall thickness and to characterize valve and wall motion. Complete examinations also include 2D imaging from the left thorax and routine CDI and PWD recordings of transvalvular blood flow.

Whenever structural heart disease is suspected or a heart murmur is under investigation, detailed Doppler images should be recorded. This procedure involves activating CDI to screen for flow disturbances, using color M-mode and spectral Doppler to time flow events, and applying CWD to quantify flow velocities and estimate pressures differences along any path of high-velocity flow. If indicated, PWD examination and TDI are obtained for assessments of ventricular diastolic function and filling pressures. In cats with atrial enlargement a PWD examination of the left auricle is also recommended.

Some centers perform TEE[50,51,53]; however, this is not a standard part of the veterinary examination due to limited availability and cost of transesophageal echocardiographic transducers as well as the need for general anesthesia. TEE is briefly demonstrated in this chapter and videos are available on the companion website.

Lastly, digital reconstruction of orthogonal 2D images (those planes at right angles) can generate 3D colorized images, which can be composed in real-time to yield "4D" Echo. This study can be further advanced by activating CDI to demonstrate complex flow patterns within a 3D architecture. Due to limited availability of these systems in current practice, 3D is but briefly described (with some examples available on the companion website).

Cardiac Imaging: Nomenclature and Display

The 2DE quantifies cardiac size and function and identifies most serious morphologic lesions. Consequently this modality constitutes the foundation of the echocardiographic examination and forms the anatomic template for M-mode and Doppler imaging. Complementary orthogonal and off-angle 2D images are recorded to provide anatomic detail (Box 8-3). The different TTE image planes are identified as long-axis (sagittal); short-axis (transverse); apical (when the transducer is placed near the left apex); or angled (specialized or hybrid imaging planes). The heart can also be evaluated using subcostal or subxiphoid placements that image through the liver.

The various *2D images* are defined by these identifiers: (1) transducer *location* (right or left, parasternal/intercostal, apical, subcostal/subxiphoid); (2) *plane* of the US cut (long-axis, short-axis, apical, or angled); (3) the *number of chambers* or great vessels imaged (2-, 3-, 4- or 5-chamber views); and other tomographic characteristics. With off angled images the view is often named for the main structures imaged, but nomenclature can become confusing when certain structures are imaged in short-axis while others appear in long-axis. There are clear standards for imaging adults, guided by the European and the American Society of Echocardiography (ASE).[2,48,68,80-87] There are also limited 2D Echocardiographic standards for veterinary studies.[79] The examiner should strive to follow these recommendations and emulate the accepted approaches.

In terms of other examinations, *M-mode images* are named for the main structures identified in the imaging plane (see below) while spectral Doppler studies are defined on the interrogated flow; for example, transmitral or aortic blood flow. With *3D imaging*, the acoustic data set is returned as a "blob" and the examiner digitally cuts off parts and colorizes the remaining 3D pixels (called "voxels") to create a 3D image of interest. Although these images can be standardized, as in an apical 2-chamber view of the LV and LA, the volume can

BOX 8-3

Transthoracic Two-Dimensional Imaging Planes

RIGHT PARASTERNAL (INTERCOSTAL) LONG AXIS IMAGES
Long axis four-chamber image optimized for left atrium and left ventricular inlet
  Zoom: Mitral valve
Long axis four-chamber image optimized for the right atrium, atrial septum, and right ventricular inlet
  Zoom: Tricuspid valve
Long axis image optimized for the left ventricular outflow tract
  Zoom: Aortic valve
  Zoom: Tricuspid valve
Long axis left ventricular inlet-LV outflow tract view
  Standard image plane in cats
  Angled image in dogs (ventral placement/dorsal angulation)

RIGHT PARASTERNAL (INTERCOSTAL) SHORT AXIS IMAGES
Papillary muscle level
Chordal level
Mitral valve level
Aortic valve level
  Zoom: Aortic valve
Optimized for the pulmonary artery
  Zoom: Pulmonary valve

LEFT CAUDAL (APICAL) PARASTERNAL IMAGES
Four-chamber image (LA, LV, RA, RV)
Five–chamber image (includes proximal aorta)
Two-chamber image of the LA and LV inlet.
Apical three-chamber (apical long axis) image of the left heart
Angled image optimized for the caudal vena cava and coronary sinus
Modified apical image optimized for the RA and RV inlet

LEFT CRANIAL PARASTERNAL (INTERCOSTAL) IMAGES
Cranial, long axis image optimized for the LV outflow tract and aorta
Cranial image optimized for the pulmonary artery
Cranial image optimized for the right atrium and right auricle

OTHER LEFT-SIDED IMAGES
Left atrial appendage (cats)
Right ventricular inlet—RV outlet—Pulmonary artery
Short axis images optimized for the aortic valve and auricles

be rotated and cut to virtually any plane. As a result, some 3D images have developed utilitarian descriptors such as the "surgeon's view" of the mitral valve (MV). Special displays and viewing glasses also have been developed in some advanced systems to create a more realistic 3D appearance.

Echocardiographic images are usually displayed on the viewing screen with the cranial and dorsal structures to the viewers' right side as they face the monitor. There are some exceptions, notably the left apical 4-chamber image, which is displayed with the LA and LV to the viewer's right side and the RV and RA to the left. Pediatricians commonly use the up/down electronic inversion switch to show "apex down" or "anatomically correct" left apical images. Currently, this display is not standard for veterinary medicine but it is sometimes easier for non-imagers to understand. Although veterinarians often indicate that images were obtained using "ASE guidelines," even our core 2D and M-mode images planes are different than the human standard in a number of ways.* Considering many veterinarians also study from standard medical textbooks, the authors advise keeping these and other relevant anatomic differences in mind.

TWO-DIMENSIONAL ECHOCARDIOGRAPHY

The 2DE is the most frequently recorded and easiest to understand cardiac examination. It is also the launch pad for all other echocardiographic modalities. Synonyms for this examination include the B (brightness)-mode echocardiography and the real-time, B-mode sector scan.[35,79]

These planar images are the composite of scores of adjacent lines of B-mode (for "brightness") US. The 2D image frame is constructed from lines of B-mode, grayscale "dots" as discussed in Chapter 1. Image lines are acquired at extraordinary speed to form a slice-of-pie-shaped image. The frames are displayed within the pixels of a video screen and continually refreshed. By updating the image frame dozens of times each second, relatively smooth cardiac motion can be appreciated.

This section focuses on the most frequently obtained 2D images used for morphologic diagnosis, assessment of cardiac chambers, and guidance of M-mode and Doppler examinations (see Box 8-3). Stereotypical transducer movements needed to obtain these views are suggested. The novice and intermediate examiner can be further guided by the figures and video loops accompanying these descriptions, both in the textbook and web content. Before considering the specific images, some points about 2D instrumentation are addressed.

2D Instrumentation

When performing 2DE the examiner should select the highest transducer frequency that balances demands for sufficient penetration with those of optimal axial and lateral resolutions. In modern systems this often requires tissue harmonic imaging

as opposed to fundamental frequency imaging. With harmonic imaging lower frequency US is emitted in a relatively narrow band and higher frequency vibrations at multiples from the fundamental frequency (octaves) are then received and processed.[82,88,89] This treatment often improves tissue resolution in the mid-to-far imaging fields, although some tissues such as cardiac valves might appear thicker. Harmonic imaging is more variable when dealing with very small patients or at imaging depths of less than five or six cm.

Once an appropriate transducer frequency and imaging mode have been selected, B-mode processing should be addressed. The examiner should first test any automated image adjustments available on the system; these simultaneously modify gain and multiple image processing settings. If more adjustments are needed, the operator can control transmit power, gain, grayscale compression, or postprocessing curves with the goal of obtaining images that are not too dark, bright, or stark in contrast. One approach is aiming for 2D images with the highest range of grayscale across the myocardial walls while preserving a black or sonolucent blood pool. Persistence within pixels should be set to minimal values for cardiac imaging to reduce blurring of real-time images. Endocardial border detection is especially important in cardiology to ensure accurate measurements of chambers and walls. Various postprocessing or system-specific controls can enhance the interface between blood and endocardium. Switching between fundamental and tissue harmonic imaging might also be effective.

Excessive gain or improper grayscale compression is especially problematic during CDI when pixels within the blood pool become miscoded as "tissue" and exclude color-coded Doppler shifts. To prevent this situation, it is common practice to make the 2D image a bit "harder" (more black and white) prior to activating CDI. This might involve an automated image adjustment by the CDI system, having the operator adjust tissue priority settings that preferentially record Doppler shifts, changing postprocessing maps, or simply reducing the overall 2D gain.

During fundamental frequency imaging, those cardiac structures oriented perpendicular to the axial resolution of the US beam yield the clearest images. This explains why right parasternal (intercostal) images are initially chosen to examine the morphology of the heart and to identify cardiac lesions. However, modern equipment with excellent lateral resolution will also generate high quality left apical and angled images, and as a diagnostic principle, examiners should learn to evaluate lesions from complementary image planes. Furthermore, some lesions are best identified from the left side. Common examples include right auricular hemangiosarcoma in the dog, left auricular thrombosis in the cat, and dilated coronary sinus in cases of persistent left cranial vena cava or right-sided congestive heart failure (CHF).

The examiner must be cognizant of temporal resolution. Frame rates of 30 per second should be the minimal acceptable standard, and with digital echocardiographic systems, 2D grayscale image frames exceeding 60/s are anticipated. If 2D frame rates are deemed too slow, a number of adjustments can be applied to improve the situation; these include: reducing the line density of B-mode imaging; avoiding abdominal imaging presets for cardiac studies; adjusting frame rate directly (if available); reducing the 2D sector width; and decreasing signal averaging, which can involve altering settings for harmonic imaging. While the highest frame rates provide optimal temporal resolution of cardiac motion, backing off slightly from the fastest speed should yield a better quality B-mode image at acceptable frame rates. Representative digital video loops are stored for subsequent review, and in most systems are forced to (DICOM) standards of 30 frames per second.

---

*Most human parasternal studies are performed from the *left* side of the thorax; whereas canine and feline long-axis and short-axis images are routinely obtained from the *right* side. This relates in part to differences in thoracic conformation as well as the location and rotation of the heart within the mediastinum. For example, the near field of a human parasternal long-axis image shows the right ventricular *outflow* tract; in contrast, that of dogs and cats contains the RA, RV inlet, and RV. The clear images veterinarians obtain of the atrial septum and fossa ovalis from dogs and cats (using right parasternal positions) can only be obtained in children using a subcostal approach, and the same detail in an adult human often necessitates a TEE examination. Similarly (right) parasternal short-axis views of the dog and cat most often reveal the cranioventral ("anterior") papillary muscle as farthest from the transducer. Just the opposite is the case when standard (left) parasternal images are recorded from humans; thus, the heart is rotated and examined somewhat differently.

Long-Axis Images from the Right Side

The typical starting point is at the fourth (or fifth) intercostal space (ICS), dorsal to the sternum and below the costochondral junction. To obtain a parasternal, 4-chamber, image of the atria and ventricles (Figures 8-2 and 8-3) approximately 30-degree clockwise rotation is initally applied, followed by mild to moderate dorsal and caudal angulation of the central US beam. The image is optimized for the LV inlet and the MV leaflets by completely excluding the aortic valve (AV), visualizing the atrial septum and fossa ovalis, and recognizing the right pulmonary venous ostium adjacent to septum (Video 8-1, A to C). In this image plane the RA and the RV are situated in the near field and the LA and LV in the far field. Adjacent to the left ventricular wall (LVW) is the pericardial/mediastinal/pleural interface, a highly echogenic and important far-field landmark. The aorta is not visualized when the image is optimized for the LV inlet. Both cardiac septa, ventricular inlets, atrioventricular valves, and the proximal LV outflow tract (LVOT) are oriented mostly perpendicular to the axial US beam.

In terms of technical corrections for this image plane, if the examiner holds the reference sector under the thumb, the reference marker should appear to the right of the upper sector as the image monitor is viewed. If the atria are not displayed to the right the electronic left/right inversion switch should be applied. The axial (central) US beam should be positioned somewhere between the tips of the papillary muscles and the mitral annulus. If the axial beam is across the body of the LA or near the ventricular apex, the transducer face should be moved to an adjacent intercostal space. If the long-axis of the heart is not close to perpendicular to the center of the imaging beam, the transducer is too ventrally placed. This can be adjusted by slowly moving the transducer face dorsally while orienting the surface transducer body perpendicular to the thoracic wall. The same optimized LV inlet image can be obtained in cats (Figure 8-3, C) but one might need to place the transducer slightly more dorsally or caudally to exclude the aorta from the view. This image plane offers

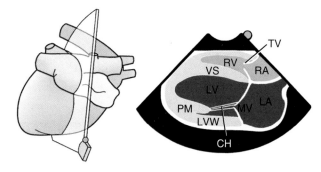

Long axis 4 chamber view

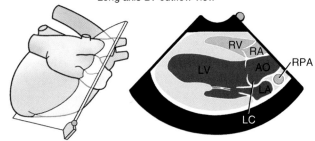

Long axis LV outflow view

Figure 8-2 Long-axis images from the right thorax. Long-axis 4-chamber image (top panel) demonstrates the RA and RV in the near field and LA and LV in the far field. The atrial and ventricular septa are roughly perpendicular to the central US beam. The mitral and tricuspid valve anatomy can be evaluated in this plane with fine-plane imaging. The long-axis LV outflow view (lower panel) is obtained from the 4-chamber long-axis view by applying clockwise rotation (or cranial tilt) of the transducer face. Only the proximal aorta is usually visualized. CH = chordae tendineae; PM = papillary muscle; RPA = right pulmonary artery; LC = left cusp (leaflet) of the aortic valve.

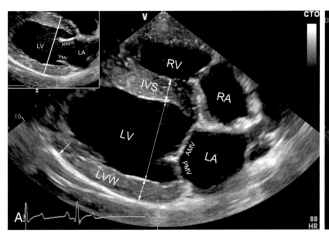

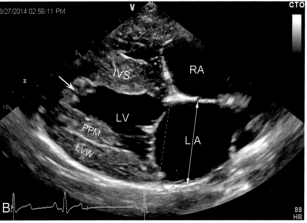

Figure 8-3 Long-axis images. A, Long-axis 4-chamber image optimized for LA, mitral valve, and the LV inlet (canine image). The image was captured during the isovolumetric period before ventricular shortening. Note the aorta is excluded from this image. The pericardial interface creates a highly reflective target (*left arrow*). The general placements for an M-mode cursor or 2D calipers for measurement of the LV cavity and wall thicknesses is shown. The actual diastolic wall measurement should be timed for end-diastole, typically at the onset of the QRS complex (inset) to just before the R-wave. Practically, the first frame showing mitral valve closure prior to wall thickening offers equivalent measurements. Compare to Fig. 8-2 (top panel) and B. **B,** Long-axis 4-chamber image from the dog in 3A frozen in end systole. The frame is immediately before opening of the mitral valve. One method for measuring the LA is shown. The dashed line indicates the approximate hinge points of the mitral valve. Note how the walls have thickened, and the apex has seemingly moved toward the base (*left arrow*) relative to the mitral annulus. Translational movement and rotation have brought the posterior papillary muscle (PPM) into the image plane. *Continued*

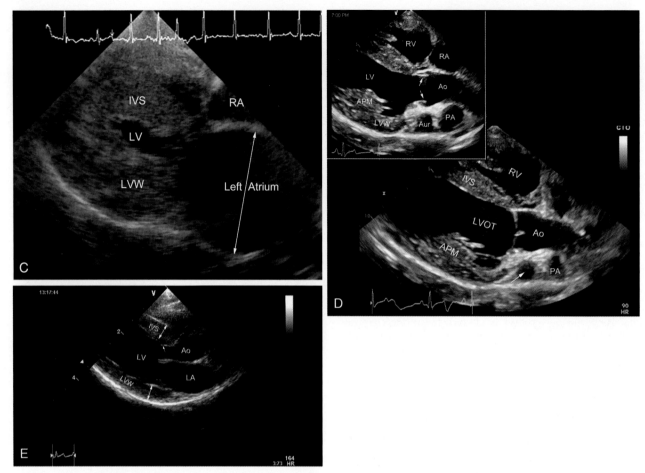

Figure 8-3, cont'd **C,** Long-axis, 4-chamber image frozen in end systole in a cat with hypertrophic cardiomyopathy. One method for measuring the LA is shown (see text for details). **D,** Long-axis image optimized for the left ventricular outflow tract (canine image). Notice the far field now crosses only the junction of the left atrium and auricular appendage (*arrow*). Compare this to Figure 8-2 (lower image). The image was acquired immediately before AV opening and the valve leaflets are closed. Later in systole (inset), two opened AV leaflets are visible (*arrows*). Note the anterior (cranioventral) papillary muscle (APM) is often prominent in the imaging field. **E,** Long-axis diastolic image from a cat optimized for the LV inlet and LV outflow tract. This is one of the most common images used to assess feline cardiac anatomy. One method for measuring the ventricular septum and LVW is shown. The small arrow points to a false tendon (also called LV moderator band or trabecula septomarginalis). This structure often tracks the left surface of the IVS and should not be included in measurements.

the largest measurement of LA internal diameter in both species so long as the aorta is excluded and the measurement is taken at end-systole.

The long-axis image optimized for the LV inlet is the most important imaging plane for evaluating the anatomy and motion of the MV. The anterior (cranioventral or septal) leaflet projects inward from the mitral annulus, extending farther into the LV lumen than the posterior (caudodorsal or parietal) leaflet, which originates near the junction of the caudal LA and LV walls. The leaflets open twice: once in early diastole and immediately after the P-wave of the ECG before closing. Inasmuch as the valve is three-dimensional, only rarely can valvular incompetency be determined by 2D imaging (a principle that holds for all valves). Chordae tendineae are readily imaged in this plane, and gentle rocking of the transducer will reveal one of the two LV papillary muscles, usually the posterior muscle, which is contiguous the LV freewall in this image plane. The papillary muscle must be excluded

when measuring the LVW thickness and particular care is needed to avoid this structure in cats with concentric hypertrophy.

There are some image variations derived from this 4-chamber image. Purposefully sliding the transducer ventrally toward the sternum and angulating the beam dorsally will "tilt" the heart, sometimes to a nearly vertical appearance on the screen. With appropriate clockwise transducer rotation a LV inlet-outlet image can be achieved. This can be a useful maneuver when interrogating the tricuspid valve, atrial septum, and ascending aorta using CDI. It is especially helpful in cats and in deep-chested dogs such as Doberman Pinschers. Conversely, sliding the transducer dorsally from the right parasternal 4-chamber image increases the availability of the RA until lung interference precludes imaging. Thus a good acoustic window can offer a more extensive view of the RA, but at the risk of over-interpreting the size of the chamber. Barring lung interference, placing the transducer even more cranially in this dorsal position can bring the aortic arch into the image plane.

Additional clockwise rotation of the transducer (or a slight cranial tilt of the axial US beam) produces a long-axis image that is optimized for the LVOT, including the AV, sinuses of Valsalva, and ascending aorta (see the lower panel of Figure 8-2 and also Figure 8-3, *D*). In larger breeds this image might require moving the transducer one ICS cranially. In canine studies, the LA is largely rotated out of the image plane once the LVOT is optimized. As the junction of the LA and the left auricular appendage is now recorded, this is an inferior image for measuring LA size. In cats the body of the LA is better recorded; however, the LA size is still underestimated when compared to the LV inlet view.

Long-axis images obtained from cats and dogs are slightly different. *In cats*, the position of the heart permits a more typical parasternal long-axis image showing the entire LVOT and most of the LV inlet (Figure 8-3, *E*). While this image still differs from the human image plane (because the feline RV inlet is located in the near field), it is a standard view for most cardiologists and is often used to measure ventricular septal and LVW thicknesses. As mentioned above, a "tipped" inflow-outflow tract image can be obtained in dogs through ventral transducer placement and steep craniodorsal angulation (see Video 8-1, *D*). However, the left apical long-axis images are normally best to visualize the relationships and blood flow patterns within LV inlet and LVOT.

Color Doppler imaging can be activated but the large angle of incidence between the interrogating US beam and normal blood flow for most of the described planes causes underestimation of red blood cell (RBC) velocity. Consequently if CDI velocity limits are set near 70-90 cm/s, there is minimal signal aliasing or turbulence encoding of normal flow. This means that higher-velocity or turbulent flow patterns are more readily identified. Eccentric high-velocity flow patterns, or "jets," caused by mitral, tricuspid, or aortic valvular regurgitation or by left ventricular outflow tract obstruction (LVOTO) are commonly observed from long-axis images. Abnormal flow across atrial or ventricular septal defects might also be detected.

Short-Axis Images from the Right Side

Nearly orthogonal to the long-axis tomograms are a series of right parasternal, *short-axis* images. These are located by turning the transducer approximately 90 degrees (clockwise) from the 4-chamber, long-axis plane (Box 8-3, Figures 8-4 and 8-5). The typical levels of interrogation include low (ventral) ventricular, papillary muscle, chordal, mitral, and aortic/LA. These images are acquired by beginning with the transducer oriented slightly ventrally, gradually sweeping the sector dorsally, and eventually applying additional clockwise rotation once the subaortic level is reached. The RV cannot be completely evaluated from these images and usually becomes larger as the examination plane scans dorsally (see Video 8-2). These views are also used to guide the cursor for *M-mode studies* in the three main planes: high papillary/chordal (for the LV); mitral; and aortic/LA. It should be noted that the chordal level (Figure 8-4, *C*) is relatively limited in dogs and cats, as the MV is quickly encountered once the US beam is tilted dorsally from the papillary muscles.

One of the most important of all 2D images is obtained in short-axis at the "high" papillary muscle level. In this view both LV papillary muscles project into the LV cavity creating a lumen with a broad-based "toadstool" or "mushroom" contour. In the near field the RV appears as a relatively small crescent. The posterior (dorsocaudal) papillary muscle is normally closest to the transducer in dogs (Figure 8-4, *B* and Figures 8-5, *A* and *B*). The examiner should strive to exclude MV echoes, observe nearly-symmetrical papillary muscles, and achieve a relatively circular ventricular circumference. This image is often used to identify enlargement of the LV, subjectively evaluate circumferential contraction, measure linear and area fractional shortening, and detect regional wall hypertrophy or motion abnormalities.

The anatomy and motion of the MV leaflets can be further assessed from the short-axis image that produces the fish mouth view of the valve. The inflow tract is between the opened leaflets; the outflow tract is between the anterior mitral valve (AMV) and the ventricular septum (Figure 8-4, *D* and Figure 8-5, *D*). When watching the leaflets in real time,

Right short axis views

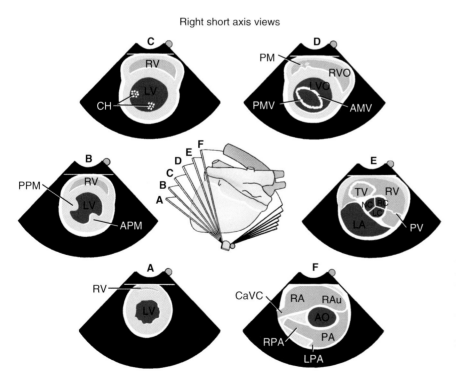

Figure 8-4 **Short-axis images from the right thorax.** The most ventral (apical) cross section is shown in panel **A,** Scanning dorsally the papillary muscle (**B**), chordal (CH, panel C), and mitral valve levels (**D**) are obtained. The LV outflow tract (LVO) shown in panel D is bounded by the anterior mitral valve (AMV) leaflet and the ventricular septum. To image the aorta in short-axis (**E**) the transducer is usually rotated clockwise from the mitral position; alternatively a cranial tilt or and placement might be needed. The pulmonary valve and PA bifurcation are acquired by more dorsocranial tilt of the transducer, often facilitated by more ventral placement. With more clockwise rotation the plane can cross the right auricle (**F**). PMV = posterior mitral valve leaflet; LC = of aortic valve (closer to left auricle); RC = right cusp of aortic valve (close to RV), and NC = noncoronary cusp of aortic valve (which straddles the atrial septum); RPA and LPA = right & left pulmonary arteries; CaVC = caudal vena cava.

both early diastolic and presystolic openings will be seen. The PMV leaflet includes a slightly greater amount of the circumference of the short-axis mitral orifice. Off angle imaging can cause even a normal valve to appear thickened.

Proceeding dorsocranially from the short-axis image of the aorta, the LA/aortic plane is crossed (Figs. 8-4E and 8-5E) and an angled view of the right atrium, tricuspid valve, RV, RVOT, and pulmonary artery (in long-axis) along with its bifurcation is obtained. Steep dorsocranial angulation of the beam aiming toward the patient's left shoulder (or alternatively, clockwise rotation of the transducer) is needed to image the RVOT. The right heart structures extend—like a large "U"—around the circular aorta. This image also reveals parts of the LA, atrial septum, and caudal right atrium (Figure 8-4, *F* and Figure 8-5, *F*; Video 8-3) if the tilt is somewhat caudal. At the opposite edge of the sector from the right atrium are the pulmonic valve and main pulmonary artery, visualized in long-axis. A useful anatomical pointer relates to the relationship of the left auricle and main pulmonary artery. The latter is just cranial so that either slight clockwise rotation or cranial tilt from the

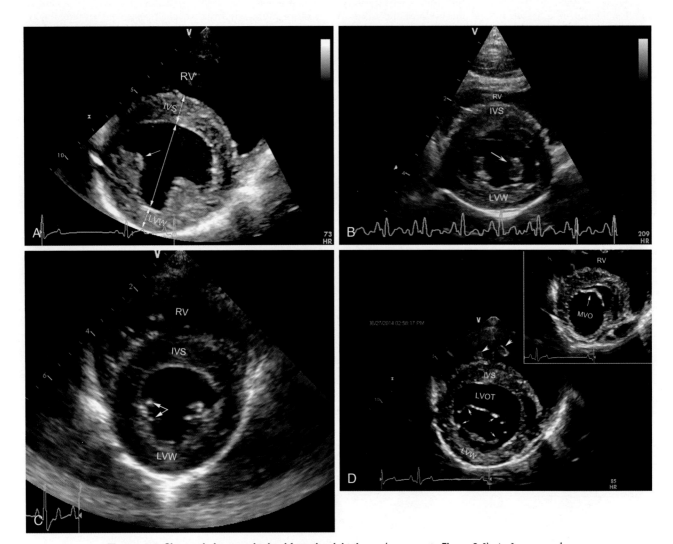

Figure 8-5 **Short-axis images obtained from the right thorax (compare to Figure 8-4).** **A,** Image at the papillary muscle level obtained from a normal dog. The posterior (caudodorsal) papillary muscle is indicated by the arrow. A method for measuring the left ventricle is shown. Compare to Figure 8-4, *B.* **B,** Image at the papillary muscle level recorded from an obese cat with borderline LV hypertrophy to demonstrate the papillary muscles. The anterior (cranioventral) papillary muscle is indicated by the arrow. This structure is usually farthest from the transducer unless the heart is rotated. The interventricular septum is poorly resolved in this image. **C,** Image at the chordal level obtained from a normal dog at end-systole with multiple bright echoes indicating chords imaged in cross section (*arrows*). This level is normally very narrow and can be difficult to capture or distinguish from a "partial" mitral valve view. Compare to Figure 8-4, *C.* **D,** Image at the mitral level of a normal dog illustrating the "fish-mouth" view. The image is acquired during atrial contraction with the valves in a partially-opened position. The AMV (*upper arrows*) and PMV (*lower arrows*) can be seen. The LVOT is between the septum and AMV leaflet. Right ventricular papillary muscles are also evident (*arrowheads*). Inset: The AMV leaflet is fully opened in early diastole (*arrow*). The mitral valve orifice (MVO) is contained within the circumference of the opened leaflets. The PMV is adjacent to the walls and not easily visualized. Compare to Figure 8-4, *D.*

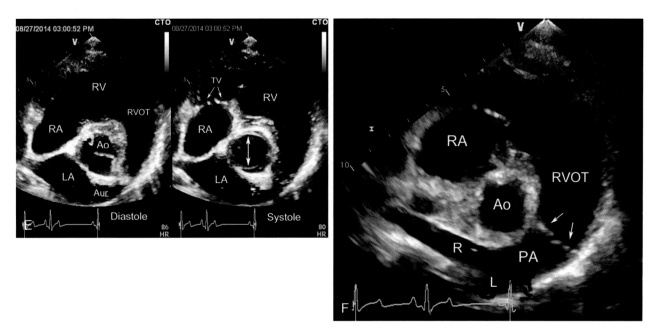

Figure 8-5, cont'd E, Image at the aortic valve level recorded from a normal dog. The aortic valve leaflets are closed in diastole (left) and open during systole (right). Compare to Figure 8-4, *E*. Aur, left auricle. F, Image at the pulmonary valve level obtained from a normal dog and optimized for the pulmonary valve (*arrows*), main pulmonary artery and left (L) and (right) branches.

auricular tip will expose the pulmonary artery and its principal branches. Placing the transducer in a more ventral position will improve the image of the RVOT and branch vessels with the right branch extending leftward across the screen and the left branch orientated away from the transducer and effectively diving into the lung. It is also important to increase the depth of field a few cm. in order to see the bifurcation well.

Short-axis images from the right thorax can be augmented with CDI, which can demonstrate flow abnormalities across the tricuspid valve, ventricular septum, RVOT, and left-sided valves. A large portion of the ventricular septum can be interrogated by Doppler studies from short-axis planes and this view is used to identify and classify ventricular septal defects. Dorsal to the mitral position, the LA and aortic root can be perused for valvular regurgitation. This can also be a useful view for assessing the extent of eccentric mitral regurgitant jets and pinpointing regurgitant lesions to specific AV leaflets (the noncoronary cusp straddles the atrial septum while the right and left coronary leaflets are in the near and far-fields, respectively).

Two-Dimensional Images from the Left Side of the Thorax

After the patient has been turned to the other side, a series of caudal, cranial, and specialized left-sided images are obtained.[79] Imaging from the left side permits the operator to better align the US beam with normal blood flow and to guide spectral Doppler recordings. Additionally, some images from the left are well suited for examining the caudal right atrium, the right and the left auricles, and the heart base.

Left Apical Images

The left apical (caudal intercostal) imaging planes (Figures 8-6 and 8-7 and Video 8-4, *A* and *B*) include the 2-chamber view (showing the LA and LV), 3-chamber view—also called the apical long-axis image (showing the LA, LV, and ascending aorta), 4-chamber view (showing both atria and ventricles), and 5-chamber view (a 4-chamber view that includes the AV and

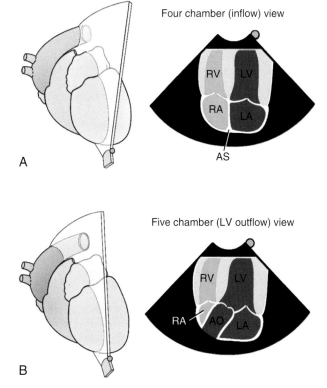

Figure 8-6 **Left Apical images.** The apical 4-chamber (inflow) view and apical 5-chamber (outflow) view are shown. The 5-chamber image is attained by tilting the transducer cranially from the 4-chamber view. A longer segment of the aorta with better alignment to blood flow might require a 3-chamber image as shown in Figure 8-7, *B*.

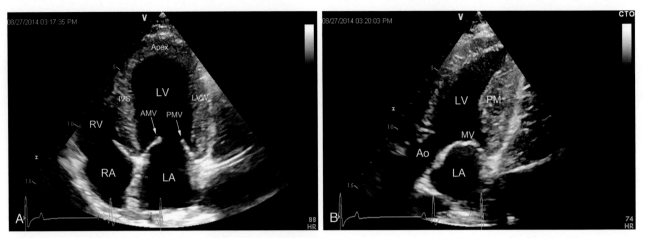

Figure 8-7 Left Apical images (compare to Figure 8-6). **A,** Apical (or left caudal) four-chamber image obtained from a normal dog. The anterior and posterior mitral valve leaflets are evident. Compare to Figure 8-6, *A.* Slight cranial tilt would incorporate the proximal aorta to yield a left apical 5-chamber view (see Figure 8-6, *B*). **B,** Apical 3-chamber image (apical long-axis). The LA, LV, and ascending aorta are imaged by rotating the transducer approximately 85 to 90 degrees from the apical four chamber view and adding cranial and dorsal tilt (see Figure 8-1, *D*). This view is the usually the best apical plane for aligning to aortic blood flow.

supravalvular aorta). These image planes are used for estimating LV and RV size and function and for recording Doppler flow studies across the atrioventricular valves and LVOT. Apical images also guide TDI of longitudinal contraction and relaxation.

Left apical images are obtained with the transducer placed caudoventrally at or slightly caudal to the palpable apical impulse. A common error involves cranial placement of the transducer, which can be mitigated by starting with the transducer over the liver and nudging it forward until the heart appears. At that point the central US beam is minimally rotated clockwise (≈15 degrees) followed by mild to moderate cranial and steep dorsal angulation to reveal the apical, 4-chamber image (see Figure 8-1, *D* and the upper panel of Figure 8-6). The axial (central) US beam should fall to the anatomic left of the ventricular septum (Figure 8-7, *A*). If it falls over the IVS or the RV the transducer placement is too cranial. The aorta should be excluded from this image, and its presence suggests too much cranial tilt or clockwise rotation. To prevent foreshortening, the transducer should be positioned ventrally with steep dorsal angulation applied so that the IVS is vertical on the viewing monitor. Even with optimal placement, "apical" image planes do not cross the true apex of the canine or feline LV, and in many cases, the length of the LV from mitral annulus to the apparent apex is actually greater when measuring from a right parasternal long-axis view.[35,90]

The apical 4-chamber view can be considered "home base" for obtaining subsequent caudal images. Gently tilting the transducer cranially opens the LVOT, AV, and proximal aorta to create a five-chamber view (see the lower panel of Figure 8-6). Greater aortic length can be obtained using a 3-chamber, apical long-axis image plane (Fig. 8-7, *B*). This is achieved by rotating the transducer ≈75-80 degrees clockwise from the 4-chamber view, sliding the transducer even more ventrally, and tilting the transducer craniodorsally with the hand assuming a "hitchhiking" position and the thumb pointed at the patient's head. Fine-plane imaging can position the aorta parallel to the edge of the image sector providing near optimal alignment with normal blood flow in most dogs. This alignment is surpassed only by that achieved from the subxiphoid position. From the 3-chamber image, additional clockwise

rotation and slight caudal tilt will eliminate the ascending aorta and most of the right heart from the image to yield a 2-chamber view of the LA and LV. While poorer in quality and endocardial border resolution, this image plane often produces the best transmitral flow patterns for Doppler assessment of LV diastolic function and filling pressures. From these four complementary left apical images, mitral regurgitation (MR), aortic regurgitation (AR), mitral stenosis (MS), and aortic stenosis (AS) are readily diagnosed and assessed using Doppler modalities. Longitudinal TDI and deformation (strain) imaging of the LV also requires one or more of these apical views.

The left apical image planes just described are also relevant to *feline studies.* However, the feline heart is more horizontal and ideal alignment with aortic blood flow in the 3-chamber image is usually unattainable, resulting in underestimation of peak aortic velocities. The transducer is placed caudally, directed cranially to image the aorta, and then slowly moved from a ventral to dorsal position within the intercostal space until the best alignment is achieved. One must be careful not to erroneously sample the PA, which lies adjacent to the aorta.

Modified Apical Images

In dogs a modified plane can be used to view the caudal right atrium. From the standard left apical 4-chamber image the transducer is slowly rotated clockwise while simultaneously flexing the wrist and pushing the transducer cable away from the examiner. Once the image plane drops below the LA, additional fine plane adjustments are used to visualize of the caudal vena caval entry into the right atrium near the atrioventricular sulcus. Between the vena cava and the heart is the coronary sinus, which becomes more prominent when RA pressures are high and is grossly dilated when receiving blood flow from a persistent left cranial vena cava. This view is shown in Figure 8-8, *A* and in Video 8-5.

The RV is a complicated structure with an inlet, apical region, and outflow tract.[81,91] To obtain a better image of the RV inlet and the tricuspid valve, a modified 4-chamber view is used (Figure 8-8, *B*). From the left apical 4-chamber view, the transducer is advanced one ICS cranially and then angled slightly caudally. This image truncates the LA and LV, but so long as the axial US beam is oriented anatomically to the right

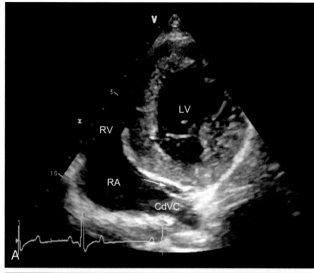

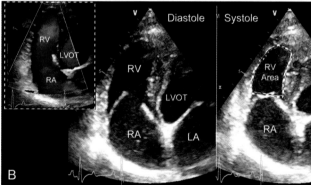

Figure 8-8 **Modified left-apical images. A,** Angled image from a dog optimized for the caudal vena cava (CdVC) and coronary sinus (*arrow*). This image is obtained from the apical four chamber image by applying slow clockwise rotation followed by ventral angulation (pushing the cable away). It is useful for identifying dilation of the coronary sinus as might be observed with persistent left cranial vena cava or elevated right atrial pressure. Caudal vena caval flow can be interrogated using Doppler techniques. Cranial tilt may reveal the right auricle. **B,** Modified left apical 4-chamber image optimized for the right atrium, tricuspid valve, and right ventricle obtained from a normal dog. This image is recorded by placing the transducer one intercostal space cranially from the left apical 4-chamber image and angulating caudally; the left heart is truncated in this plane. Although the LVOT is evident, the aortic valve should be excluded from the image. Trans-tricuspid blood flow (inset) and right ventricular function can be assessed. The right panel shows the end-systolic RV area used to calculate fractional area change.

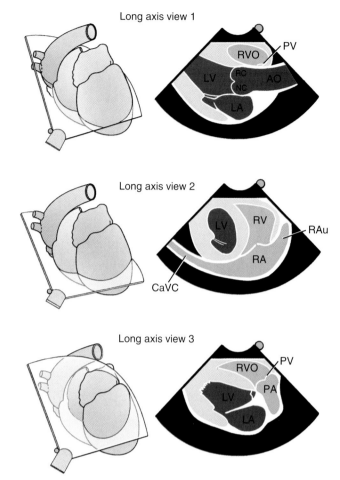

Figure 8-9 **Left cranial parasternal images.** The Long-Axis View 1 shown in the top panel is optimized for the LVOT including the ascending aorta. This image is in the middle of the transition between Long-Axis Views 2 and 3. The reference sector is pointed toward the nose (or tail) and adjusted to optimize the LVOT. View 2 is obtained by flexing the wrist from View 1 and using small amounts of rotation to optimize the right auricle. The caudal vena cava is not always evident. View 3 is obtained from View 1 by extending the wrist (raising the cable upward) until the PA is found. The pulmonary valve is closer to the transducer than for the right-sided image planes. (Examples of left cranial images are found in the supplemental video content.)

side of the IVS and the ascending aorta is not visible, the RV inlet is well demonstrated. The view is especially important for assessing tricuspid regurgitation (TR) or tricuspid stenosis as well as for measuring RV systolic function using tricuspid annular plane systolic excursion (TAPSE), TDI of the lateral wall, and myocardial strain (all discussed later). Additional more cranial image planes are needed to assess the rest of the RV apex and RVOT.

Left Cranial Images
Various standard and off-angle long-axis images can be obtained from the cranial intercostal positions along the left thorax. Some of those most often used are demonstrated in Figures 8-9, 8-10, and 8-11. A series of three cranial long-axis

images can be obtained from a single transducer location. With the transducer rotated ≈90 degrees cranially (and the reference notch directed toward the patient's nose), the beam is centered near the AV and the LVOT and ascending aorta are identified in long-axis projection. The RVOT is in the near field, and either the RA or LA evident in the far field depending on placement and amount of caudal angulation (see the upper panel of Figure 8-9). If the transducer is angulated ventrally from the aortic image, the RA is identified in the mid- and far-fields and fine-plain angulation reveals the right auricle (see the middle panel of Figure 8-9 The opposite maneuver, pulling the cable up and angulating the transducer leftward and dorsally from the cranial image of the LVOT optimizes the RVOT. In this image the aorta is excluded, the RVOT and pulmonary valve are evident in the near field, and the proximal PA extends into the far field (see the lower portion of Figure 8-9). These cranial long-axis images are useful for assessing disorders in the RVOT and pulmonary artery, identifying flow patterns of patent ductus arteriosus,

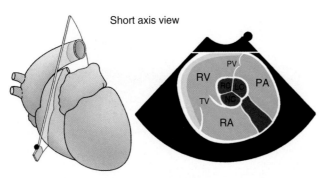

Short axis view

Figure 8-10 Left cranial parasternal image. Left cranial image optimized for the right side of the heart and forms a U-shape around the aorta which is observed in short-axis.

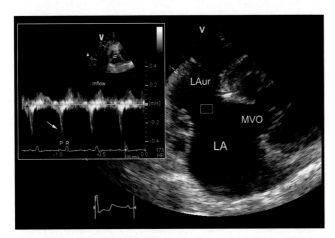

Figure 8-11 Left atrial appendage. Image optimized for the left auricle and left atrium in a cat with hypertrophic cardiomyopathy. This image is obtained by moving the transducer craniodorsal to the left apex until the auricular appendage is directly under the center of the US beam. The LA is displayed in the far-field; the mitral orifice is partially observed in long-axis. This image is used to detect auricular thrombus, echogenic smoke, and to record auricular filling and emptying velocities (see sections on Atrial Function and Cardiomyopathy). Inset: Spectral Doppler recording obtained from another cat with HCM with sample volume positioned at the junction of the LA and its auricular appendage (see rectangle in larger figure). Note the inflow velocity (positive) and the prominent auricular outflow velocity obtained following atrial contraction and timed just after the P-wave of the ECG (*arrow*). The peak velocity is approximately 36 cm/s.

evaluating diseases of the AV and ascending aorta, and visualizing right atrial and heart base tumors.[36]

A cranial RV inflow-outflow tract image is often used to assess the pulmonic valve and RVOT (see Figure 8-10). This image can be obtained by placing the aorta in short-axis within the axial US beam, applying slight counterclockwise rotation to the transducer and tilting the far edge of the transducer dorsally to capture the RVOT and PA. The aorta appears in short-axis and the RA, RV, and RVOT are evident circling the aorta. With further fine plane adjustments the right and left PA branches can be observed or the left PA partially excluded to image a ductus arteriosus.

Other Imaging Positions
Additional 2D images can be obtained with standard transducers from the suprasternal notch, subxiphoid (subcostal) position, and dorsal intercostal positions. Some of these posi-

tions are demonstrated in Video 8-6. Small aperture transducers can be used to examine the cranial great vessels from the *suprasternal notch*; however, most patients object to the procedure unless sedated.

In nearly every dog the *subxiphoid (subcostal) position* offers the best alignment to blood flow in the proximal aorta and this should always be used for patients with suspected AS or increased LVOT ejection velocities.[92,93] At times subcostal positions can be used to record blood flow in the aortic arch and to better align to tricuspid regurgitant jets, especially when the heart is rotated. The US beam first passes through the liver, so deep-chested dogs offer a challenge in terms of image resolution. Cats tolerate this examination position poorly and it does not seem to improve the angle of incidence for Doppler studies.

To obtain 2D and CDI of the *caudal vena cava and hepatic veins*, one approach is placement of the transducer dorsally within the ninth to twelfth ICSs on the right side. A satisfactory long-axis image of the caudal vena cava is obtained and alignment can be achieved to flow in the cranial hepatic veins). More detailed images are attained using standard abdominal techniques (Chapters 4 and 9).

An important image plane when examining cats with LA enlargement is that optimized for the *feline left auricular appendage*. This image is created with the transducer placed between the apical and cranial positions on the left side of the thorax. The transducer is slowly moved upward from the sternum to a more dorsal intercostal location until the left auricle is directly under the transducer and the LA and MV are identified in the far field (see Figure 8-11 and Video 8-6). This image is especially useful for identifying auricular thrombus and spontaneous echocontrast ("smoke"), and for measuring inflow and outflow velocities from the auricle using PWD.[94,95]

M-MODE ECHOCARDIOGRAPHIC IMAGING

The M-mode (motion mode) echocardiogram is generated from a single line of B-mode US.[2,9,46] In the modern transducer containing hundreds of elements, this modality is recorded from an operator-guided M-line that is steered with the trackball across a 2D anatomic template. The US system processes returning sound waves from the moving cardiac tissues with a high sampling rate, usually exceeding 1000 pulses per second. The echocardiograph constantly updates the returning echoes along the line of interrogation and displays the structures as grayscale "dots" in which depth is shown relative to the static transducer artifact at the top of the recording and reflector intensity by the relative grayscale. By sweeping the digital recording surface along this continuously updated output, a graph of cardiac motion is displayed, showing time (in seconds) along the horizontal axis and depth from the transducer face (in cm) along the vertical axis. Typical examples of M-mode studies are shown in Figure 8-12.

M-Mode Recording and Instrumentation
Standard M-mode studies include the following images: (1) the LV cavity and walls at the level of the papillary muscles or the mitral chordae tendineae; (2) at the MV tips, capturing the peak diastolic excursion of the anterior mitral valve (AMV) leaflet; and (3) the level of the closed AV with part of the LA crossed in the far field.

The RV is always traversed during standard M-mode echocardiography. Because of the triangular-shaped of the RV in the right parasternal long-axis views and the crescent-shape in the short-axis views, quantitation of RV size using M-mode studies is inconsistent. In dogs with RV hypertrophy, the

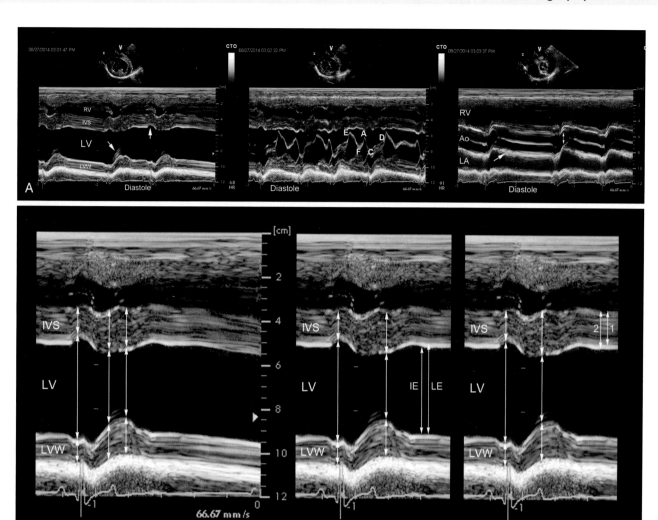

Figure 8-12 **M-mode Echocardiography. A,** M-mode images recorded from the LV level (left), mitral valve level (center) and aortic/left atrial level (right) from a healthy dog. Left: The M-line curser crosses the RV, IVS, LV cavity, and LVW. Chordal echoes are evident in systole (*lower arrow*). Note subtle changes in the imaging texture of the ventricular walls after atrial contraction (*upper arrow*) and during ventricular systole. Center: the curser crosses the RV, IVS, LVOT, AMV, mitral orifice, PMV, and dorsal LV wall. The opening and closing movements of the mitral valve are labeled based on standard nomenclature. Right: the curser crosses the RV, aortic root and aortic valve, and the junction of the left atrium and left auricular appendage. Two opened AV leaflets are evident during systole (*double arrow*) with a single line of closure during diastole. The larger arrow shows where intrapericardial fat might be included in the recording when a "leading edge" method is used the atrial measurement includes this tissue. **B,** Methods for measuring the LV are demonstrated. Left: The leading edge method of wall and cavity measurement is demonstrated with ventricular systole timed at the nadir of ventricular septal motion and then compared to the maximal excursion (apogee) of the LV wall. Alternative methods for measuring the LV dimensions are demonstrated in the center and right panels. Center: The TIL (for trailing, inner, leading) method of wall measurement is shown in the center panel. This includes one endocardial border for measurement of the IVS and LVW and measures the LV cavity at the blood-endocardial interface. The LVW is measured using a leading edge method and includes one endocardial border. In this example, systole is measured from the maximal excursion (apogee) of the LVW. To the right a comparison of an inner edge (IE) vs. leading edge (LE) measurement of the LV cavity is shown. Right: The measurements to the last panel demonstrate how a still 2D image would be measured (also see Figure 8-5, *A*). In this approach both endocardial echoes of the IVS are included in the septal measurement and LV endocardial and epicardial echoes are included in the LVW measurement (the parietal pericardium is excluded). In the present example, systole is measured using a vertical line that coincides with the smallest vertical distance between the septal nadir and maximal excursion of the LVW. The inner endocardial borders delineate the LV cavity. At the far right of this panel the differences in IVS measurements are shown when including two (2) versus one (1) endocardial border. Differences in measurement technique can influence the ultimate diagnosis. See text for details.   *Continued*

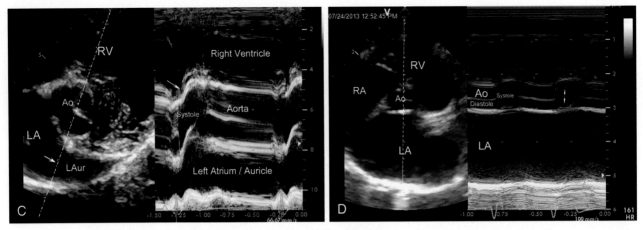

Figure 8-12, cont'd **C,** Split screen image demonstrating the derivation of the M-mode echo of the aortic valve in a dog. Note the M-mode cursor is crossing the junction of the left atrium and left auricular appendage (*left arrow*). In the resultant M-mode study note the vigorous motion of the aortic wall toward the transducer (*right arrow*) observed with normal LV systolic function. **D,** Split screen image demonstrating the derivation of the M-mode echo of the aorta and LA in a cat with enlargement of the LA. The M-mode cursor crosses more of the atrial body in the cat when compared to the dog. The systolic aortic root motion is reduced in this example, a sign of impaired systolic function. The opened aortic valves often form linked "boxcars" when cardiac output is reduced.

M-mode exam can demonstrate increased freewall thickness provided near field resolution is good. RV size is better assessed by tracing the RV inlet, from the modified left apical view or by subjectively comparing it to the LV in the left apical 4-chamber view.

The M-mode exam is informed by 2D imaging and can be guided by either short-axis or long-axis image planes. In practice, both should be used when measuring the LV. Long-axis guidance avoids cursor placements that pass too close to the aortic root in the near field, through the papillary muscle in the far field, or across the body instead of the tips of the AMV leaflet. However, short-axis guidance assures the LV is divided symmetrically at the septal arc, that the cursor crosses between the two papillary muscles, and that the portion of the LA sampled by the M-line is well delineated. The authors first obtain a right parasternal long-axis image and then activate the cursor so the line is at an appropriate level and perpendicular to the IVS and LVW. The transducer is then rotated into the short-axis plane, adjusting the image and M-line until the cursor bisects the LV. Scanning from ventral to dorsal the "high" papillary muscle (or chordal), MV, and AV levels are then recorded. For cats a similar approach can be used, but switching to the long-axis image might be needed to capture the small segment of LVW located between a hypertrophied caudal papillary muscle and the mitral annulus.

M-mode instrumentation issues are minimal so long as the 2D image guiding the study is properly composed and the examiner carefully guides the M-line. Compression and gray-scale processing should highlight endocardium and resolve these borders from the RV trabeculae, the septal tricuspid leaflet, and the trabecula septomarginalis (LV moderator band or false tendons) that track along the left side of the IVS.

Most technical mistakes arise from suboptimal placement of the M-mode cursor and from recordings with poor demarcation of the endocardium. For example, when guiding the LV measurement from the short-axis the M-line should cross the center of the septal crescent, bisect the chamber, and cross the LVW between the two papillary muscles. The optimal cursor angle is often achieved by moving the 2D image to the edge of the sector. This and some common cursor placement errors

are demonstrated in Video 8-7, *A* to *E*. When appropriate guidance cannot be attained, measurements of frozen LV images should be made using 2D calipers, as shown in Figure 8-3, *E* and Figure 8-5, *A*. Another corrective approach involves activation of anatomical M-mode if that functionality is available on the system. This generates a digitally reconstructed M-mode image derived from steering of an operator-controlled line through the 2D image (Video 8-7, *C*).[96,97] The quality of the resultant image is somewhat degraded but generally sufficient for measuring. However, endocardial border resolution can be marginal if the angle is too obtuse to the axial beam.

One of the main uses of the M-mode study is assessment of LV systolic function, and this can be underestimated if the cursor crosses the subaortic portion of the IVS. At that level septal motion is reduced or even paradoxical due to the presence of a "hinge" or transition zone between the aortic root—that moves toward the transducer in systole—and the IVS, which moves in the opposite direction. Adding long-axis guidance of the cursor can prevent this error. Another common mistake when examining cats involves sampling the posterior papillary muscle where it blends into the LVW. This error, as well as including the septal tricuspid apparatus or LV moderator band within the septal measurement, can foster a misdiagnosis of LV hypertrophy.

M-Mode: Normal Findings and Interpretation

Interpretation of the M-mode study requires a preconceived knowledge of normal and an understanding of morphologic and motion abnormalities that might develop with specific diseases (Figure 8-13).[20,21,24,28,33,40,90,96,98-110] Although these patterns are not difficult to learn, the graphical nature of the format, and the limited anatomical reference provided has diminished the importance of the modality. Despite these limitations, the extremely rapid pulse repetition of the M-mode study provides both clarity and temporal resolution of rapidly moving structures sampled by the US beam.[110] M-mode images are useful for measuring LV wall thicknesses, LV chamber size, and systolic function across one minor axis of the LV. This modality is also capable of recording rapid motion, as might be seen with a ruptured chordae tendineae

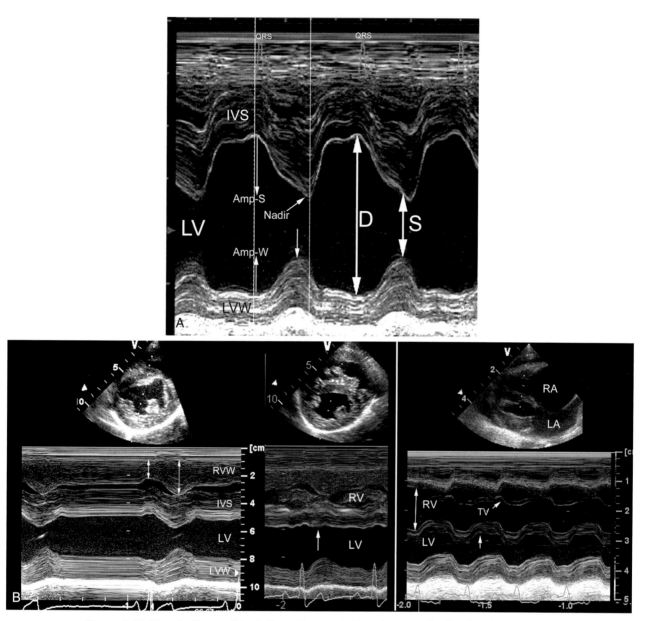

Figure 8-13 **M-mode Abnormalities in Heart Disease.** A, LV volume overload and exuberant septal motion in a small breed dog with heart failure due to chronic, severe mitral regurgitation. The IVS is displaced toward the RV in diastole and begins its systolic motion from an abnormal position. In contrast to normal, the amplitude of the ventricular septum (Amp-S) becomes greater than that of the LVW (Amp-W). Vertical lines indicate the onset of QRS complex (left) and the septal nadir, which is somewhat delayed. The shortening fraction, (D-S)/D is very high despite the presence of congestive heart failure. **B,** Right ventricular overloads. Left: RV pressure overload in a dog with severe pulmonic stenosis. The RV free wall (*arrows*) is hypertrophied and thickens markedly during systole (*arrows*). Septal motion is normal. Center: Another case of RV pressure overload has led to hypertrophy in this dog. A large papillary muscle is crossed within the RV cavity, creating an intraluminal echo. In this case motion of the IVS is flat (*arrow*), typical of severe pressure overload. Right: Volume overload in a cat with pulmonary hypertension and severe tricuspid valve regurgitation. The RV cavity and right atrium are dilated (see 2D reference image). The cursor crosses parts of the tricuspid valve (TV) in the RV. There is paradoxical septal motion (*left arrow*) typical of severe volume overload (*lower arrow*). *Continued*

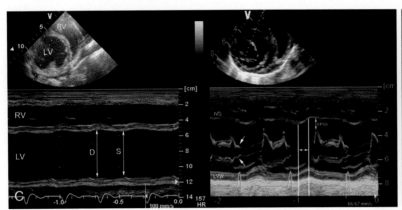
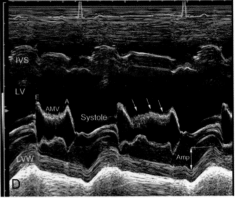

Figure 8-13, cont'd **C,** Dilated cardiomyopathy in two dogs. Left panel: A giant breed dog with DCM demonstrating severe LV dilatation (>60 mm), RV dilatation, and markedly depressed systolic wall motion with low fractional shortening. Right panel: An unusual case of DCM in a beagle dog presented for CHF. There is ventricular dyssynchrony evident (between the vertical lines), increased mitral valve EPSS for a small-breed dog, and delayed mitral valve closure creating a B-shoulder (*arrows*) typical of elevated end-diastolic pressure. **D,** Diastolic fluttering of the aortic valve in a dog with ventricular septal defect, aortic valve prolapse, and aortic regurgitation (AR). During middiastole the anterior mitral valve leaflet appears thicker as a consequence of high-frequency vibrations caused by AR. The EPSS is markedly increased due to impingement of the AMV leaflet by the regurgitant jet; nevertheless, the LVW has normal systolic amplitude (Amp) suggesting normal LV systolic function. Video 8-7, *E* offers a compilation of M-mode echocardiographic abnormalities.

or fluttering valve, findings that could be less obvious when using the slower sampling rate of 2DE. Lastly, M-mode studies can be combined with color-coded Doppler or contrast echocardiography to accurately depict the *timing of flow events.* *Color M-mode echocardiography* is easy to perform and grossly underused relative to its value in timing flow events.

Left Ventricle

The *M-mode study of the LV* (see the left panel of Figure 8-12, *A* and also Figure 8-12, *B*) tracks the wall motion of the LV across a minor axis over the cardiac cycle. After the MV opens in early diastole, the LV walls rapidly move away from each other as the LV undergoes early diastolic filling. A small early diastolic "dip" is observed in the IVS reflecting different rates of ventricular filling. Changes in the respiratory cycle cause the RV cavity to fill relatively more during inspiration and moves the IVS away from the transducer. This likely reflects both increased right heart filling and translational motion with ventilation. Subtle rightward movement of the IVS is often seen at end-diastole after the active atrial contraction and additional small movements in both walls are observed during the QRS from isovolumetric contraction. Immediately after the QRS complex the AV opens and ejection begins. This is characterized by progressive thickening of the ventricular walls and inward movements of the IVS and LVW. There is often a slight timing offset in maximal wall motion characterized by the IVS reaching its nadir just prior to the maximal upward excursion (or apogee) of the LVW[40] that coincides with AV closure. The thickening and excursion of the LVW from end-diastole to its apogee is a useful estimate of systolic function. This LVW amplitude normally exceeds that of the IVS.[100]

LV Measurements. Linear measurements of the LV[111] are demonstrated in Figure 8-12, *B* and include the IVS, LV cavity, and LVW, excluding the parietal pericardium. Measurements are optimally made in expiration. When measuring the walls and chambers, it is helpful to refer to the 2D reference image. This guidance reduces confusion about the precise location of endocardial borders, especially when bright intramural

reflectors are crossed by the US beam. It also can identify moderator bands or papillary muscles within the path of the beam. Plasma volume status can influence LV measurements, especially severe volume depletion, which causes *pseudohypertrophy* of the walls from reduced diastolic stretch.

Diastolic measurements of the LV should be made between the onset of the QRS complex and the peak of the R-wave, before the ventricle shortens. A larger LV diastolic cavity dimension than projected for that patient (based on species, breed, and body-size) indicates ventricular dilatation. In the absence of dehydration or cardiac tamponade, increased LVW or IVS diastolic thicknesses usually relates to myocardial hypertrophy and increased LV mass.

The point in time selected for systolic LV measurement can influence the M-mode estimate of systolic function. Some conventions call for measuring systolic dimension at the septal nadir, although a smaller systolic dimension is often obtained between the septal nadir and the apogee of the LVW. Whatever the individual case, as shown in Figure 8-12, *A,* the measuring cursor should drop *vertically,* never on a diagonal. Nor should the measurement be timed after the apogee of the LVW, which coincides with AV closure. The authors measure the smallest vertical distance between the septal nadir and LVW apogee as the systolic dimension. Failure to identify this point can foster a false-positive diagnosis of "systolic dysfunction," especially when there is considerable dyssynchrony.

The placement of the measuring cursor relative to endocardial borders also influences measurements, especially of the IVS and LVW. At least three approaches are used by different cardiologists (Figure 8-12, *B*) with no clear consensus for veterinary practice. The original ASE standard for dedicated (unguided) M-mode echocardiography called for a "leading edge" approach based on a low-response survey. This method incorporates the thickness of the "leading" endocardial border into the measurements of the IVS, LV cavity, and LVW. An argument can be made for modifying this convention because frozen 2D images are measured differently according to current ASE standards.[82,83,85] The 2D measurement of the IVS includes *both* right and left-sided endocardial borders, the cavity measurement *excludes* both endocardial borders (measuring from the blood-endocardial interface), and the LVW measurement incorporates the endocardial and the epicardial thicknesses (if identified), stopping at the leading edge of the parietal pericardium. An alternative approach involves an inner method (actually a "trailing-inner-leading" edge method). The measurements include the trailing-edge endocardial border for the IVS, the inner LV cavity, and the leading-edge endocardial border for LVW thickness. This method has the benefit of excluding RV muscle trabeculae and septal tricuspid tissue hugging the right surface of the IVS (see Weyman,[9] p. 294 for a discussion of this issue). While these points might seem pedantic, the inclusion of two endocardial borders increases the thickness of the IVS relative to the LVW, and also can change the diagnosis in a small dog or cat from "normal" to "septal hypertrophy" as discussed later under "Cardiomyopathy."

LV Motion. The LV *fractional shortening* (LVFS) is defined as: LVFS = [LVd – LVs]/LVd, where LVd is the inner diastolic dimension and LVs is the inner systolic dimension. Impaired myocardial contractility is reflected in reduced wall motion, less systolic thickening, and depressed LVFS. This variable is also influenced strongly by ventricular loading conditions (see "Ventricular Function" later in the chapter).

Departures from normal wall motion can stem from depressed or enhanced myocardial contractility, disorders of electrical impulse conduction, from pressure or volume overloads, and as a consequence of structural cardiac diseases. Conduction changes associated with bundle branch blocks, ventricular ectopy, cardiac pacing, and myocardial diseases also can alter the activation sequence across the LV. This is another reason why the M-mode study should include a simultaneous ECG. Ventricular *dyssynchrony* is sometimes revealed in the M-mode examination by a larger than normal time offset between the septal nadir and LVW apogee, although more advanced tissue imaging methods are needed to identify many cases.[112-117] With the possible exception of maximal LVW systolic excursion (also called LV amplitude), assessing systolic function in a dyssynchronous ventricle is prone to error.

Volume and pressure overloads of either ventricle also influence cardiac motion and shortening even in the absence of any change in myocardial inotropy (see Figure 8-13, *A* and *B*). Identification of ventricular overload on the M-mode study is both a diagnostic clue and a warning that indices of LV systolic function could be misleading. For example, increased LV diastolic volume pushes the IVS rightward during rapid filling, and this starting position permits exuberant downward septal motion once contraction begins.[118,119] This is an underrecognized sign of moderate to severe LV volume overload. In contrast, moderate to severe right ventricular (RV) volume overload forces the IVS leftward in diastole and encroaches on the LV cavity. During systole the higher developed LV pressure pushes the septum upward, leading to *paradoxical septal motion*.[40] Another example is the influence of concentric LV hypertrophy, which reduces wall stress and increases LVFS. Hyperdynamic LVSF is commonly measured in cases of canine SAS and feline HCM.[24] In contrast, with severe RV pressure overload, the IVS thickens in systole but overall septal excursion is diminished or flat because of near-equal pressures in the two ventricles. Thus, as with dyssynchrony, ventricular overloads can confound the M-mode measurement of LV systolic function. With LV volume and pressure overloads fractional shortening is frequently enhanced; whereas, with RV overloads it is usually diminished.

Pericardial effusion creates abnormal cardiac motion due to translational effects.[15] Moderate to large effusions permit swinging of the heart within the pericardial space. In this setting, wall motion and systolic function become uninterpretable. With cardiac compression the ventricular walls also thicken due to pseudohypertrophy. The manifestations of *constrictive pericarditis* on the M-mode study are slightly different and caused by impediments to normal ventricular filling and increased diastolic pressures. These can induce abnormal diastolic septal movements that include paradoxical septal motion in systole or a series of exuberant early diastolic oscillations termed a "septal bounce."

Mitral Valve
The M-mode study at the MV level displays the opening and closing movements of both leaflets (Figure 8-12, *A*) but focuses on the AMV leaflet. Motion is characterized by an early diastolic opening (E point) that brings the tip of the AMV in close approximation to the ventricular septum. The posterior (caudal) leaflet moves in the opposite direction. Following a period of reduced LV filling and partial valve closure (F), the MV reopens (A) after the P wave and atrial contraction. At the onset of systole, the two mitral leaflets are brought to apposition (C). During systole the entire valve moves toward the transducer and at end-systole (D) the leaflets are poised to separate once again with rapid ventricular filling (E), completing the cycle.[11,17,19]

The distance between the E point and IVS is referred to as E point to septal separation (EPSS) and is inversely related to LV ejection fraction (Figure 8-13, *C*).[120-122] The EPSS increases when there is dilated cardiomyopathy or ventricular dilation with impaired systolic function. In larger breed dogs values exceeding 6 to 7 mm are abnormal. False-positive reasons for increased EPSS include off-angle imaging, stenosis of the MV, and aortic regurgitation (AR) with impingement of the regurgitant jet on the AMV leaflet. The latter condition should also lead to high-frequency diastolic fluttering of the AMV leaflet (Figure 8-13, *E*). The C-point typically occurs during the QRS complex but can be delayed in the setting of increased ventricular filling pressures. This can create a characteristic "B-shoulder" or bump between the A- and C waves of MV excursion. Conversely, in acute and severe AR, increased LV end-diastolic pressure (relative to LA pressure) is recognized by premature closure of the MV with the C-point occurring before the QRS complex.

Abnormal MV motion is often observed in dynamic LVOTO associated with HCM, MV malformations,[123] LV volume depletion, and in some cases of AS.[110] The AMV departs from its normally-parallel movement with the LVW, and suddenly contacts the IVS in mid-to-late systole. This movement, termed *systolic anterior motion* of the MV, creates dynamic LVOTO and initiates an eccentric jet of MR (changes demonstrated later under "Feline Hypertrophic Cardiomyopathy.")

Aortic Valve/Left Atrium
The M-mode image of the AV in dogs generally crosses two leaflets and the junction of the LA and LA appendage. Aortic root size and LA size can be quantified using the M-mode examination, but this is an inferior approach method because the M-mode cursor crosses one sinus of Valsalva on a diagonal and the LA size is grossly underestimated. Although LA size is better assessed with M-mode echocardiography in cats[30,31] (Figure 8-12, *D*), it still fails to capture the maximal chamber diameter. However, fractional shortening of the LA—the percentage change in diameter from filling to emptying—can be measured using the M-mode cursor.[124,125] In terms of motion, the aorta moves toward the transducer in systole (Figure 8-12, *C*) and overall aortic root motion correlates coarsely to stroke volume becoming diminished in DCM. Intervals of

systole (preejection time and ejection time) can be calculated from the M-mode study.[126]

In terms of identifying lesions, the movements related to AV opening and closing can be followed by the M-mode examination, but with the icepick view, the information provided is limited. For example, valvular competency cannot be assessed and in cases of valvular AS, parts of the leaflets can separate while other portions remain fused so careful 2D guidance is needed to capture the restricted motion. With infective endocarditis, the cursor must cross the vegetation to capture the lesion. This is better identified with 2D imaging. Similarly a congenitally bicuspid AV classically leads to an eccentric line of closure within the lumen; however, this can be misdiagnosed if there is a dilated aortic root and an off angle interrogation of the valve.[21]

With the high frequency sampling of this modality, rapid valvular movements can be captured. These include high-frequency systolic fluttering of the valve during ejection,[103] which is a normal finding. Abnormal valvular movements might be observed with dynamic LVOTO including partial, midsystolic AV closure and reopening correlating to the onset of dynamic obstruction. Diastolic fluttering of the AV and of the aortic root has been observed in cases of AR. The extremely rare case of aortic dissection[127] might be recognized by a "double" aortic wall caused by the presence of a true lumen and a false lumen consequent to intimal tearing and dissection with blood.

ADVANCED 2D AND 3D ECHOCARDIOGRAPHIC IMAGING METHODS

Advanced imaging methods include contrast, transesophageal, and 3D echocardiography. This section merely introduces these examinations, and the interested reader is referred to the references and companion website for more details.

Contrast Echocardiography

Contrast echocardiography is performed to identify abnormal patterns of blood flow, delineate endocardial borders, assess myocardial perfusion, enhance Doppler flow signals, and outline lesions such as an atrial thrombus, cardiac mass, or LV non-compaction.[22,88,128-130] The contrast echocardiogram is produced by altering the sonographic characteristics of part of the blood pool with the injection of a fluid that generates microbubbles. The agent is injected in a peripheral vein and followed into the heart using 2DE, often with specified harmonic imaging.[82] These solutions or suspensions alter the acoustic impedance of the blood through the creation of microcavitations or the release of gases that act as powerful US reflectors. A variety of agents have been injected for contrast echocardiography, with agitated saline most often used in veterinary medicine. Most noncommercial agents are filtered within the pulmonary circulation and are therefore confined to the right side of the heart unless there is a right-to-left shunt. Contrast agents developed to outline the LA and LV or demonstrate coronary perfusion must first survive transpulmonary passage. A number of proprietary microsphere suspensions are available for this use in human patients. These contain perfluorocarbon gas, which is released when the outer shell of the microsphere is disrupted by US. Although human contrast agents have been tried in dogs,[129] there has been little movement to adapt microspheres for veterinary patients despite the potential to study myocardial perfusion.

Saline contrast echocardiography is simple to perform and has demonstrated utility in demonstrating right-to-left shunts. One simple method involves the agitating of sterile saline between two syringes that are attached to an IV catheter via

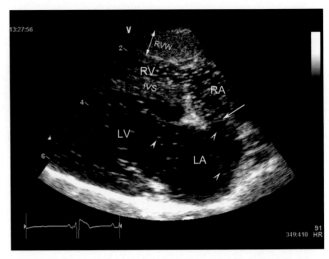

Figure 8-14 **Saline Contrast Echocardiography.** Right to left shunting is demonstrated in a dog with a patent foramen ovale (near the arrow) and increased right-sided pressures caused by pulmonic stenosis. The saline contrast fills the right side of the heart and is also detected in the LA and LV. Discrete "microbubbles" can be identified (*arrowheads*). RVW = hypertrophied RV free wall.

a three-way stopcock. While maintaining a closed-to-air system the saline is vigorously agitated back-and-forth between the syringes about five times and then quickly injected into a peripheral vein. Although agitated saline contains microcavitations of air, visible gas bubbles should *never* be injected into the vascular system. Injection of 3 to 6 ml of agitated saline is usually sufficient to produce a good quality contrast study. Adding ¼ ml of the patient's own blood can improve the contrast effect, but this is rarely needed.

Saline contrast does not endure the pulmonary capillaries; therefore, finding echodense contrast within the left side of the heart suggests a right-to-left shunt (Figure 8-14 and Video 8-8).[†] In the case of patent foramen ovale (PFO) or right-to-left ASD, contrast moves from RA to LA. With the tetralogy of Fallot, contrast can be traced along a path from the RV to the LVOT. Additional diagnostic uses are verification of persistent left cranial vena cava, and reversed PDA with imaging over the abdominal aorta to detect the passage of contrast agent through the descending aorta (Video 8-8, *B* and *C*).

Although Doppler studies have largely replaced contrast echocardiography, the technique is relatively sensitive for right-to-left cardiac shunts and results are often less ambiguous than CDI when identifying an ASD or PFO. At times negative contrast effects are visualized when blood derived from the left heart crosses a shunt and dilutes the positive saline contrast in the right heart. However, normal streaming of systemic venous return into the RA and RV inlet can create false positives. Pulmonary artery transit times, a general estimate of cardiac output, also can be determined using commercial contrast agents.[130] The risk of anaphylactoid reactions with commercial contrast agents should be noted,[131] and that human patients have died suddenly following injection of these products.

[†]An exception is observed in healthy anesthetized patients in whom pulmonary arteriovenous shunts have opened. However, in these cases, the arrival of contrast is delayed and enters the LA through a pulmonary vein.

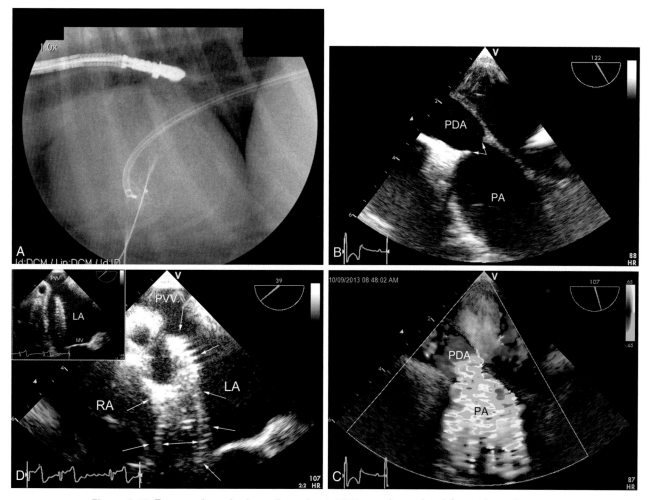

Figure 8-15 Transesophageal echocardiography. A, TEE transducer placed for guidance during an interventional catheterization procedure. Note the position of the transducer relative to the base of the heart. The imaging crystals are positioned near the end of the endoscope. **B,** TEE image of patent ductus arteriosus (PDA) in a dog. The minimal ductal diameter is evident (between arrows). The pulmonary artery is dilated. **C,** Color Doppler TEE image obtained from the dog shown in panel B demonstrating turbulent flow across the patent ductus arteriosus into the PA. **D,** The use of TEE for guidance of a transvenously-delivered atrial septal defect occluder. The device has two retaining discs which are deployed on each side of the atrial septum as outlined by the arrows. Once deployed the disc closed the septal defect. PVV = pulmonary vein. Inset: During manipulation the left-atrial disc is evident, dorsal to the mitral valve (MV).

Transesophageal Echocardiography

The technique of transesophageal echocardiography (TEE) uses transducer crystals mounted near the tip of a flexible endoscope. The transducer is advanced down the esophagus and positioned over the heart base (Figure 8-15, *A*). General anesthesia is required. In contrast to the human experience, the improvement in imaging over standard transthoracic windows is less impressive in dogs and cats. The technique of TEE has been applied to cardiac and vascular imaging of healthy animals.[50-53,55,60] A number of longitudinal and transverse images can be obtained, including good views of the cardiac valves, atrial and ventricular septa, pulmonary veins, and great arteries. Image planes have been categorized as cranial, middle or caudal (relative to the base of the heart) as well as transgastric. Initial reports suggest transgastric images are inferior for imaging the canine heart but more acceptable in cats.

Although TEE can be used for diagnosis of cardiac diseases (Figure 8-15, *B* and C; Video 8-9, *A* and *B*), TEE studies are mainly used for guidance of *interventional catheterization* pro-

cedures (Figure 8-15, *D*; and Video 8-9, C) that include device closure of persistently patent ductus arteriosus (PDA) or defects in the cardiac septa.[54,57,58,61,132] Other potential uses include identification of small heart base tumors, atrial thrombi, and vascular defects. TEE has been used for guidance of heartworm extraction[133] and intracardiac surgery. The instrumentation is costly and impractical for all but subspecialty practices. Sizes of endoscopes are relevant due to the different weights of veterinary patients. Both adult and pediatric transducers are available. The endoscopes can integrate single- or multi-plane crystal arrays with the most advanced TEE probes capable of performing real-time, 3D reconstruction with CDI.

Three-Dimensional Echocardiography

With the advent of 3D echocardiography (3DE) there has been an explosion in imaging technology, mostly designed for imaging human adults. These systems have been applied to dogs and cats with varying degrees of success. The fully sampled matrix array transducers used for 3D imaging contain thousands of piezoelectric elements and are connected to powerful processing systems offering even real-time (4D) imaging.

Currently, the major issues impeding wider 3DE application to veterinary patients include the processing speed of the systems related to the faster heart rates of animals; the requirement for stitching multiple cardiac cycles (ideally with breath holding!) to obtain optimal 3D images; and the large footprint of 3D transducers that limit full transthoracic contact. Nevertheless, if future advances include pediatric transducer designs, we can expect 3D technologies to take wider hold in veterinary medicine regardless of the cost.

Imaging modalities include narrow sector real-time imaging; focused wide sector enlargement of regions of interest; and full volume, ECG-gated, acquisition of the LV and LA useful for calculating ejection fraction and atrial volumes. Images can be manipulated by cropping to highlight specific structures and lesions. Surface rendering can create contours or models of the LV and LA[78,134] and these methods have been applied to dogs and cats on a limited basis.[135-139] Additionally, CDI can be superimposed on the 3D image to better assess abnormal blood flow patterns along with the severity of shunts and regurgitant lesions. Examples of 3D imaging are shown in Figure 8-16 and Video 8-10.

Some potential veterinary uses for 3DE include: quantitation of chamber volumes for detection of cardiac dilatation and estimation of ventricular and atrial function; delineation of congenital shunts and guidance for interventional treatments; and improved visualization of valvular lesions and regurgitant jets to provide more accurate prognostication and guide future catheter-based or open-heart treatments. Some vendors have developed technologies to measure myocardial strain in three dimensions, and there are even off-line analyses systems that outline the pathway of electrical activation, which could be useful in the diagnosis or therapy of arrhythmias. Critical issues involve the increment in clinical informa-tion and the imaging detail provided beyond our current levels of routine transthoracic examinations. Obstacles include quality of images obtainable from cats and smaller dogs as well as the cost-effectiveness of the technologies within the veterinary space.

CARDIAC DOPPLER STUDIES: OVERVIEW

Doppler echocardiography (DE) is a special processing of cardiac US that displays the directional movement and velocity of blood flow or of myocardial tissue during the cardiac cycle.[6-8,63,65-67,140-145] These examinations also can detect turbulent blood flow, sometimes referred to as *variance*. When interpreted alongside other echocardiographic findings, DE can identify shunting, valvular regurgitation, and obstruction to flow. Doppler examinations are also directed for assessment of atrial and ventricular function and for quantifying hemodynamics (pressure, volumetric flow, and resistance to flow).

Doppler Principles

As discussed in Chapter 1, Doppler studies are based on the frequency shift that occurs when US waves are reflected back from a moving object to a stationary observation point. This principle, as embodied in the Doppler equation, indicates that the Doppler frequency shift is directly proportional to the *velocity* and *direction* of the moving targets. When the equation is solved for velocity (V), then: $[V = Fd(C)/2Fo \cos \Theta]$,[8] where Fd is the frequency shift caused by the reflection of US from targets moving at a velocity (V) and calculated as the difference between emitted frequency and returning frequency; Fo is the initial emitted frequency; C is the velocity of US in tissue; and Θ is the angle of incidence (or intercept angle) formed by the path of the moving reflector and the interrogating US beam. The emitted or carrier frequency (Fo) and the velocity of US in tissue (1540 m/s) are known. The angle Θ is assumed to equal either 0 or 180 degrees in cardiac Doppler so the cosine function (plus or minus 1) is noncontributory to velocity calculation. The reflectors in DE are either red blood cells (RBC) within the flow pattern of interest or (for TDI) the movements of myocardial tissue during systole and diastole. The direction of movement—toward the transducer (positive) or away from it (negative)—determines the sign of the Doppler frequency shift. The DE system analyzes the returning Doppler frequency shifts using a fast Fourier transform process, and displays the direction and velocity of blood flow in either a color-coded format (CDI) or in a graphical display called spectral Doppler (for PWD, CWD, and TDI).

Although the angle is ignored in cardiac studies, the US beam-target angle of incidence remains highly relevant to the output. If US returns from reflectors moving at right angles to the emitted US beam, no Doppler shift is recorded (as the cosine of 90 degrees = 0). Because the cosine function is nonlinear, any returning signals associated with angles >22 degrees significantly *underestimate* true velocity.[8] For this reason, cardiology examinations must be performed so that orientation of the US beam to flow is as parallel as possible. The examiner must subtly adjust the transducer and 3D beam angle to achieve maximal velocity estimates. Although the operator could apply subjective angle correction, as commonly performed in peripheral vascular imaging, this adjustment is *never* used in cardiac Doppler because the third plane is unknown. Thus angle correction is turned "off" and a 0 or 180-degree incident angle to flow is implicit. Importantly, one cannot assume that the 2D anatomy tracks the true direction of blood flow, and RBC velocities will probably be overestimated when angle correction is applied based on this presumption.[146]

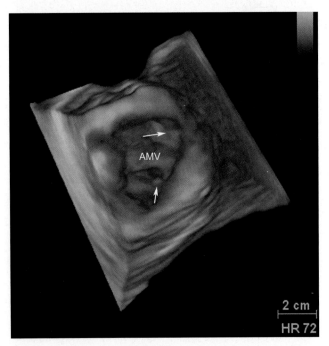

Figure 8-16 **3D Echocardiography.** Still frame of a 3D, en face rendering of a closing canine mitral valve from an apical perspective. The AMV separates the mitral orifice from the LV outflow tract (*upper arrow*). A chordae tendineae on the posterior leaflet is evident (*lower arrow*). Also see Video 8-10.

US is inaudible to examiners but Doppler frequency shifts are really quite small—measured in kilohertz—and therefore fall within the audible range of the human ear. Accordingly, spectral Doppler instruments include an audio channel that allows the operator to listen to the pitch of returning Doppler frequency shifts. These sounds can be helpful when optimizing Doppler studies. Unfortunately, audible Doppler shifts often frighten or agitate animals, so the audio volume must be turned off, set at the lowest level, or monitored with headphones if that output is available.

Overview of Doppler Modalities

Standard Doppler modalities include CDI, PWD, and CWD. Additionally, color M-mode, pulsed-wave TDI, and color TDI applications are available on high-end cardiac systems. The PWD records from a single operator-selected sample volume; whereas, CDI samples Doppler shifts along a series of contiguous lines of US. These sample volumes are processed within an operator adjustable color ROI that is overlaid on the 2D image (Figure 8-17). One line of color-coded Doppler shifts can be activated to generate a color M-mode study.

Spectral Doppler refers to the PWD and CWD studies, which are processed to demonstrate direction and velocity of blood flow or tissue movement graphically (Figure 8-18). When PWD is applied to myocardial tissues, the term *tissue Doppler imaging* (TDI) is used. Whereas the PWD and TDI examinations display a spectrum of velocities recorded within a discrete sample volume, the CWD records all of the Doppler shifts returned along the line of transmitted US. This allows for quantitation of high-velocity flow events. Spectral formats

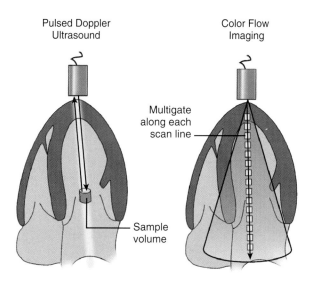

Figure 8-17 **Doppler Echocardiography.** Comparison of pulsed-wave Doppler (PWD) ultrasound and color Doppler Imaging CDI), also called color flow imaging. The PWD study records Doppler shifts only from a single, operator directed sample volume (left). When screening normal LV blood flow the sample is moved from the tips of the opened mitral valve to the ascending aorta between the leaflets of the opened aortic valve. In contrast to PWD, continuous wave Doppler echocardiography (not shown) records and superimpose all Doppler shifts obtained along the entire line of emitted ultrasound. CDI (right) is a form of PWD and records and displays Doppler shifts from multiple sample volumes along each scan line. The process is repeated for adjacent scan lines across the 2D region of interest. (From Otto C. *Textbook of Clinical Echocardiography*. 5th ed. Philadelphia: Saunders/Elsevier; 2013, with permission).

display direction and velocity simultaneously along the y-axis of the recording while the timing of events is correlated to the ECG, displayed along the horizontal axis. Although the various modalities encompass similar Doppler principles, they are different enough to warrant separate discussions in terms of recording principles, examination practices, instrumentation, normal findings, and clinical applications. As discussed later, understanding system instrument controls is also crucial to obtaining quality Doppler studies.

Doppler Examination Techniques

A Doppler examination should include images from both right and left sides of the thorax. Because timing of flow can be misleading when watching real time CDI, digital loops should be captured and reviewed in slow motion or frame-by-frame. The ECG assists in determining the systolic and diastolic periods of the cardiac cycle. Mechanical systole usually begins during the latter half of the QRS complex and ends just after inscription of the T-wave. LV ejection begins after the QRS is fully inscribed (Figure 8-18, A). The ECG interval between the P-wave and QRS complex delineates the time period for events related to atrial contraction. The points where atrial events end relative to QRS are influenced by PR interval, the heart rate, and the LV end-diastolic pressure.

The examiner should observe and capture CDI loops and spectral Doppler recordings of blood flow from the ventricular inlets and ventricular outflow tracts. These recordings are guided from 2D imaging planes. In *normal* dogs and cats all blood flow patterns can be obtained from the left thorax using left apical images (for mitral and AV); the modified left apical image optimized for the tricuspid valve; and one of the left cranial positions aligned to PA flow (see Figures 8-6 through 8-11 and Video 8-11, A). The PA also can be interrogated from the cranial short-axis image from the right thorax; however, the vessel tends to curve away from optimal US beam alignment. Both right- and left-sided short-axis images of the aorta can offer reasonable alignment to a good portion of tricuspid transvalvular flow. Aortic blood flow velocity in dogs is usually the highest when recorded from the subcostal (subxiphoid) position,[93] but for practical purposes, the left apical five or three-chamber image is usually sufficient for recording aortic velocity in the absence of LVOT obstruction. Subcostal (subxiphoid) windows should always be used when measuring LVOT velocities in dogs with aortic stenosis or elevated LVOT velocities.[92]

In addition to "screening" the ventricular inlets and outlets, additional evaluations of blood flow patterns are based on clinical suspicions along with any morphologic lesions or flow disturbances identified as the examination progresses. Timing of pathologic flow events is critical and is assured by recording a simultaneous ECG. Cardiac motion on the 2D image, adjacent blood flow events, and complementary spectral Doppler and color M-mode recordings also inform the assessment. Additional imaging planes complement those used to identify normal blood flow. For example, right-parasternal long- and short-axis images are often best for aligning to a ventricular septal defect (VSD) and a tipped right parasternal long-axis image might optimally record an eccentric jet of mitral regurgitation (MR), aortic regurgitation (AR), or tricuspid regurgitation (TR). For these reasons most examiners also activate CDI to evaluate the mitral, tricuspid, and AV using both long- and short-axis image planes obtained from the right thorax.

Sample volume placements for standard PW Doppler imaging are demonstrated in Video 8-11, B. When measuring systolic velocity profiles in the aorta and PA, the PWD sample volume is placed at the tips or slightly distal to the opened valve leaflets. Diastolic filling velocities are recorded with the sample volume placed within the tips of the opened atrioventricular valves. The peak velocity zone can be identified by the brightest color hues or a signal alias during the CDI study. For the LV inlet, peak velocity might be obtained slightly laterally to the central orifice; the left apical 2-chamber image often provides the cleanest diastolic inflow signals. The CDI images of the RV inlet in the modified apical view are usually truncated and slightly off angle, so there is the most spectral dispersion for these recordings. Additionally, a positive, low-velocity, systolic waveform is observed and this can be confusing if there is no ECG recorded. Discrete sample volume lengths of 1 to 4 mm are typical. For cats and small dogs, 1 to 2 mm is appropriate to start; for larger dogs, 2 to 3 mm is used; for distal structures or pulmonary veins, the sample volume is increased by 1 or 2 mm from the usual. A

wider sample volume improves sensitivity for recording but also leads to greater spectral broadening.

Evaluation of LV diastolic function involves recordings of transmitral flow, TDI of the lateral LV wall, and potentially flow patterns across pulmonary veins (Figure 8-18, *B*, C, and *F*). Although there are seven pulmonary veins (one for each lobe), echocardiographic imaging usually detects only the confluence of multiple veins.[147] Most often pulmonary venous flow is obtained from the common ostium draining the caudal and accessory lung lobes, located at 5 o'clock in the apical 4-chamber image plane.[144] The left cranial lobar veins enter nearer to 3 to 4 o'clock in this image, but the intercept angle to flow is suboptimal. The right cranial and middle lobes enter to the left (anatomically) of the atrial septum, about 7 o'clock

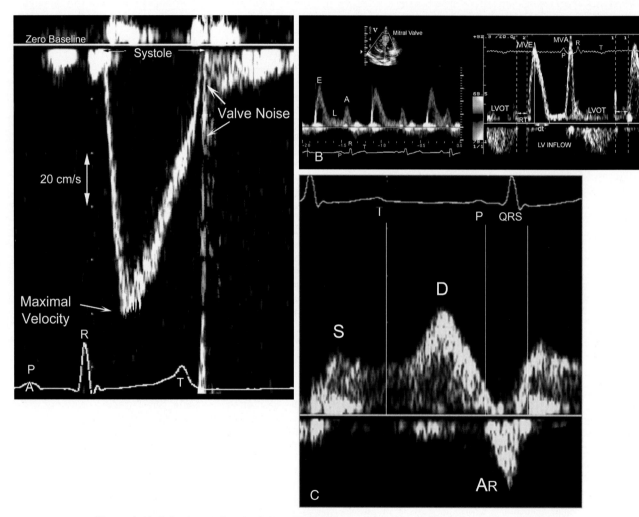

Figure 8-18 **Pulsed-wave Doppler Echocardiography. A,** Aortic blood flow (dog): Note the sharp acceleration and normal amount of deceleration spectral broadening. The maximal velocity is approximately 1 m/s. The valve noise indicates the closure of the aortic valve and is a useful timing clue. Note that minimal zero baseline filtering has been applied. **B,** Trans-mitral flow: Left: A prominent E-wave and a well-defined A-wave are seen in this canine recording. Due to low settings for baseline filters and a relatively slow heart rate, the low velocity, middiastolic flow characteristic of diastasis (L-wave) is also present. Right: This feline recording is recorded to capture both transmitral flow and ejection across the LVOT. Diastolic intervals used to assess ventricular filling are illustrated, including isovolumetric relaxation time (IRT) and mitral deceleration time (dt). The intervals are measured between the valve noise signals (see text for details). **C,** Pulmonary venous flow (dog): The three primary waveforms are labeled in this recording. The timing of the waves is shown relative to the ends of the T-wave, P-wave, and QRS complex. The S-wave begins within the QRS owing to atrial relaxation and suction. The S and D waves are more often equal in size in healthy cats.

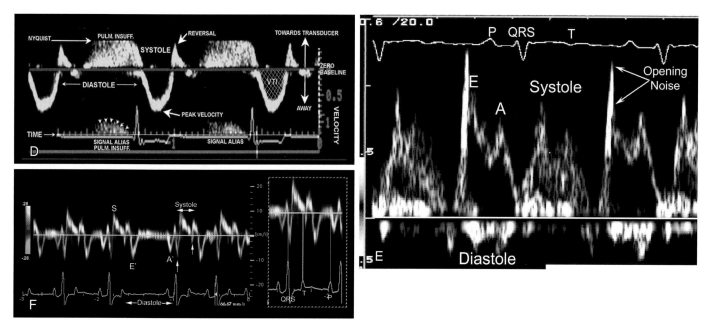

Figure 8-18, cont'd **D,** Pulmonary artery flow (dog): The PA velocity profile accelerates more slowly than flow across the AV and the peak velocity is lower. Low-velocity physiologic pulmonary insufficiency is common and is shown in both diastolic cycles. As the baseline has been shifted up to preferentially record flow away from the transducer (negative), the regurgitant signal exceeds the positive Nyquist limit and aliases at the bottom of the tracing. The area under the curve (VTI) correlates to stroke volume. The end-systolic-early diastolic reversal wave is normal. **E,** Transtricuspid flow (cat): Note the prominent valve noise that confounds the peak velocity of the E-wave. More important is the presence of a low-velocity, positive systolic wave that might be confused with diastolic flow without a corresponding ECG. This common finding is normal in both cats and dogs for this valve. **F,** Tissue Doppler imaging in a small breed dog with the sample volume placed in the dorsolateral LV wall. The early diastolic recoil is normally greater than that caused by atrial contraction (E' > A'). The cycle on the right shows the waves relative to the peaks of the QRS, T, and P-waves. Tissue motion during isovolumetric contraction and relaxation are normal and has been used to time these events.

in the sector image, but translational motion might allow contamination from the adjacent artery, which can be confused with the atrial reversal wave. Good alignment to left pulmonary venous flow is also obtainable from right parasternal short-axis or off-angle images of the left atrium, especially in cats. For each recording a relatively large sample volume is placed just inside the venous entrance to the LA.

Filling and emptying of the left atrial appendage should be obtained when examining cats with cardiomyopathy or left atrial dilatation.[94] The PWD sample volume is placed at the opening into the auricle and the sample volume increased in size to record both inflow velocities and out flow due to active auricular contractions (see Figure 8-11; Videos 8-6, *B* and C). The transducer placement is dorsal, between caudal and cranial intercostal locations, and directly over the appendage. Identification of the curving flow patterns is guided by CDI, but with the velocity limits substantially decreased (to about 20-30 cm/s in each direction).

When performing TDI of the LV or RV myocardium,[113,148-155] the most important location for the sample volumes is just below the A-V junction in the lateral ventricular wall (Video 8-13). The left apical 4-chamber or 3-chamber image planes are used for the LV wall; the modified left apical view of the RV inlet is used for the RV wall. The sample volume should be made larger than for transvalvular flow. It is imperative to minimize the angle of incidence between the apical-basilar movements of the freewall and the cursor. Off angle imaging reduces calculated tissue velocities. If a TDI module is avail-

able, it should be used because it will automate adjustments of frequency, power, gain, velocity scales, clutter filtering, and image processing.

Doppler Transducers

Although stand-alone CWD transducers are available, nearly all modern Doppler systems employ a phased array technology that integrates 2D imaging and CDI with steerable, image-guided PWD and CWD. Advanced units also contain modules for preferentially selecting the strong but low-velocity signals derived from the myocardial tissues. Tissue Doppler imaging can involve a discrete sample volume or a region of interest that must be evaluated using off-line software. Individual transducers offer a range of frequencies to perform simultaneous 2D imaging and Doppler studies. One begins with the transducer most appropriate for B-mode imaging. As a general rule the presets for DE activate lower frequency crystal elements than for grayscale imaging because Doppler signal to noise ratio is improved. Although Doppler transmit frequency can be adjusted, many cardiac transducers work best nearer their central Doppler frequency. Improving Doppler sensitivity often involves *switching* from a higher to a lower frequency transducer during the examination (as opposed to activating a lower frequency band within a single probe).

One of the more common errors made in spectral Doppler imaging is forgetting to "freeze" the 2D image. Time-sharing of the crystals for both real-time 2DE and spectral Doppler studies creates a number of artifacts and distorts the velocity spectra. Only certain high-end systems permit simultaneous 2D imaging and spectral Doppler. Operators learn to toggle between real time imaging, which allows repositioning of the sample volume, and freezing the 2D image. Automated updating of the image every few seconds is frequently available but is best turned off. Once the cursor has been sufficiently guided, the 2D reference image should be frozen while recording the velocity spectra. If the spectral signal is degraded or lost, real time imaging should recommence to reposition the cursor.

PULSED-WAVE DOPPLER ECHOCARDIOGRAPHY

The PWD study quantifies frequency shifts arising from a small, defined anatomic area called a *sample volume*.[65,140,156] This discrete region of interest is positioned by the operator within the anatomic template of the 2D image using a trackball and further guided by visualizing a simultaneous CDI (see Video 8-11, A and B). After each US pulse is emitted, the Doppler system temporarily suspends the sampling of returning signals until that instant when US from the sample volume returns to the transducer face. This process is called *range gating* and is the basis for the precise source localization that characterizes PWD. The sample volume (typically from 1 to 4 mm in length in cats and dogs) is directed within the anatomic/color flow ROI and further modified based on patient size, recording location, and other factors such as the dispersion of the recorded velocity spectrum.[65,67,140,157-161] Systems controls are used to optimize the spectral display as described later.

The graphical time-velocity (x-y) spectra recorded with PWD displays flow characteristics from the sample volume. Even within this tiny area of interest, there will be variations in RBCs velocity. Therefore the generated display is not a thin line, but a wider *spectrum* of velocities (see Figure 8-18). The spectrum is characterized by a position above (positive Doppler shift) or below (negative Doppler shift) the adjustable *zero baseline* (Figure 8-19) that indicates the general direction of flow relative to the transducer. There is a *modal velocity* for the RBCs, and this is displayed in the brightest or most compressed shades of grayscale. Smaller masses of RBCs traveling at lower and higher velocities relative to the modal velocity are displayed less brightly.

Normal or laminar blood flow is characterized by a relatively compact modal velocity spectrum with (darker) velocity variations clustered to either side. In comparison, abnormal blood flow is characterized by spectral broadening, often characterized as "turbulence." Importantly, spectral broadening also can represent an artifact of recording within a structurally-normal heart. Some causes include: introducing a large angle of incidence between the US beam and blood flow; opening the sample volume to record a larger ROI; and high cardiac output states. For example, widening the sample volume from 1 mm to 5 mm will invariably broaden the recorded velocity spectrum when recording diastolic flow within the MV orifice.

Signal Aliasing

Signal Aliasing is one of the important limitations of PWD (and CDI) and explained by the concepts of range gating, pulse-repetition frequency (PRF), and the Nyquist limit (also see Chapter 1). Range gating in PWD dictates that only those Doppler shifts returning from the sample volume are processed. The time interval between US pulse emission and the return of Doppler shifts from the sample volume limits the PRF or total US pulses transmitted per second. The maximal RBC velocity that can be recorded with accuracy is directly proportional to this PRF and also affected by the transducer transmit or carrier frequency (lower frequencies yield higher PRF). Shifting of the baseline increases velocity scale in one direction, but limits the maximum velocity the other (see Figure 8-19). The PRF further decreases as the sample volume is moved farther from the transducer. This is why—with other settings equal—the near-field velocity limits are higher than those obtained during far-field sampling. As higher RBC velocities develop, signal aliasing is observed. More specifically,

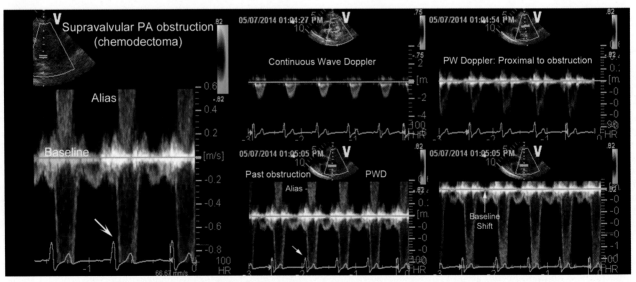

Figure 8-19 Nyquist Limits in Pulsed-wave Doppler. Spectral Doppler recordings are shown from a dog with supravalvular pulmonary stenosis caused by a chemodectoma. Flow distal to the obstruction is turbulent with spectral broadening and as well as increased in velocity (left panel and center lower panel) when compared to flow proximal to the obstruction (upper right). The aliasing velocity is effectively doubled by maximally shifting the baseline up or down (lower right panel). However, high-velocity turbulent flow will continue to alias when a single sample volume is used. The maximal velocity recorded by CW Doppler was approximately 1.9 m/s (center panel, upper).

aliasing occurs when RBC velocity exceeds $\frac{1}{2}$ of the PRF (the *Nyquist limit*).[2,6] Practically speaking, the typical cardiac transducers and depths of field used in small animal practice limit peak RBC velocities to ≈2 m/s in one direction.

The actual alias is characterized by a velocity spectrum that "wraps" around the display and appears on the opposite side of the zero baseline so that flow seemingly originates from the opposite direction. The signal alias has been likened to a movie where the spokes of a wagon wheel seem to move backward because the sampling rate of the video film is too slow to record the true direction of movement. When pathologic blood flow exceeds ≈4 m/s, multiple "wraps" can occur in the PWD tracing, creating a broad, ambiguous velocity spectrum. Aliasing is common in both PWD and in CDI (see later) and forces the examiner to activate a modality capable of high PRF. These are either CWD or high pulse-repetition frequency Doppler (a hybrid of PW and CW methods).

High PRF Doppler Echocardiography
One alternative to CWD is activation of high PRF Doppler if that feature is available on the system. This modality inserts additional, equally-spaced sample volumes as the operator either increases the PRF and velocity scale or moves the sample volume to a greater depth in the imaging field. The PRF and Nyquist limits are essentially doubled by adding a second sample volume. Additional equidistant sample volumes can be inserted to facilitate measurement of even higher velocity flow. Because the sample volumes are evenly spaced, when the recording aperture opens for the closest sample volume, the timing coincides with the arrival of US from the distant sample volumes. For example, the operator interested in ascending aortic flow at 12 cm from the transducer can effectively double the Nyquist limit by placing one sample volume there and increasing the velocity scale (PRF) until another sample volume is inserted 6 cm from the transducer face. The resultant PWD spectrum represents the superimposition of both samples and creates *range ambiguity*; however, the signal is less likely to alias. If the closest sample volume is located in an area of known low-velocity flow, the examiner can be relatively certain the higher velocities within the spectrum arise from the distal sample volume.

High PRF is most useful when sampling mildly-increased flow velocities within the aorta or pulmonary artery, especially when the target is in the far field as occurs with left apical or subcostal imaging. Another use is found when multiple flow streams are crossing and the examiner wants to focus on discrete regions of interest within that complicated pattern.

Instrumentation in PW-Doppler
A technically proficient examination requires appropriate transducer selection, adjustment of the Doppler console, imaging skill, and appreciation of normal variation. Knowledge of cardiac diseases, the ability to alter the examination based on contemporary findings, and an appreciation of technical and interpretation errors are also important.[86]

The transmit power, receiver gain, compression in the dynamic range, and the signal processing (postprocessing grayscale), must be properly set to achieve optimal signal to noise ratio and avoid blooming of the spectrum.[6,7] Some specific suggestions are offered in Table 8-3. Filtering refers to the low-velocity (clutter or wall) filters designed to eliminate high-intensity signals from slowly moving valves and myocardial walls. There is a trade-off between recording low-velocity spectra near the zero velocity baseline (allowed by low filter settings) and the mitigation of extraneous Doppler noise (requiring higher settings). If the exact timing of flow events is not critical, increasing the filter setting often prevents valve

noise (also called "clicks") from contaminating the flow signal. However, when the duration of a flow event is the focus, lower settings must be used and valve noise accepted. Doppler angle is always set to "off" (zero) for cardiac applications. The audio channel is adjusted to "off" or the lowest volume that minimizes patient stress (alternatively: headphones are worn to hear Doppler shifts). The authors set a total (positive and negative) velocity scale for PWD between 1 and 2 m/s initially and then adjust the scale (or PRF control) and the zero baseline position to optimize the display.

The imaging goals for spectral recordings are delineation of a *clean envelope and a clear peak* with some element of grayscale distribution that reflects the number of RBCs contributing to the different velocity bins. Irregular contours at the outer edges of a spectrum and specious expansion of the peak velocities are consequences of suboptimal recording technique or excessively high instrument settings and create a misleading assessment of disease severity.[2,6] Spectral broadening can indicate a too-wide beam angle of incidence, an excessively-large sample volume, or inadvertent activation of high-PRF Doppler when increasing velocity scales. Overgained spectra are caused by using a transducer of too-low frequency, applying excessive transmit power, or setting too much Doppler gain (Figure 8-20). The opposite problems of weak or unapparent Doppler spectra also can occur.

A weak spectrum might indicate a flow disturbance that is trivial or mild and difficult to record even with good technique. Changing to a lower frequency transducer and adjusting the image processing might illuminate the spectrum; additionally, modifying dynamic range (compression), grayscale, colorization, or the background of the spectral tracing will sometimes improve the image.

Instrumentation for TDI
Optimal *instrument settings for TDI* are quite different than for blood flow. The LV and RV tissue velocities are much lower, usually between 5 and 20 cm/s (see Figure 8-18, *F*). Furthermore, the returning Doppler shifts are strong. This reflected US is normally filtered out of spectral Doppler recordings by activating baseline (clutter) filters; however, for TDI these low-frequency Doppler shifts are the focus. Most higher-end systems contain a module for automating TDI that involves colorizing myocardium based on direction and velocity of tissue movement. The operator then guides a sample volume to record PWD spectra within the tissues (see Videos 8-12 and 8-13).

If the examiner hopes to collect TDI without the benefit of an automated module, some recording suggestions include: switching to the next highest-frequency transducer; turning the baseline (wall) filters to lowest settings; adjusting the velocity scales to 20 cm/s in each direction; reducing Doppler transmit power to ~75% of maximum; reducing Doppler gain to ~25% of maximum and adjusting upward as needed; increasing sample volume length to about twice that used for aortic flow measurements; and adjusting dynamic range (compression), postprocessing, and chroma to create optimal spectra.

Physiologic Basis for PW Doppler Velocity Spectra
The movement of blood depends on the development of pressure gradients within the heart and circulation. The cardiac cycle is relevant to understanding the relationship between pressures and normal blood flow patterns (Figure 8-21). Relatively small instantaneous pressure gradients—called impulse gradients[162,163]—drive RBCs across the cardiac valves.[9] Although differences in peak systolic pressures in the LV and aorta are negligible, a small impulse gradient is generated by the rise in LV pressure preceding that in the aorta. Similarly a small difference in LA and LV diastolic pressure is sufficient

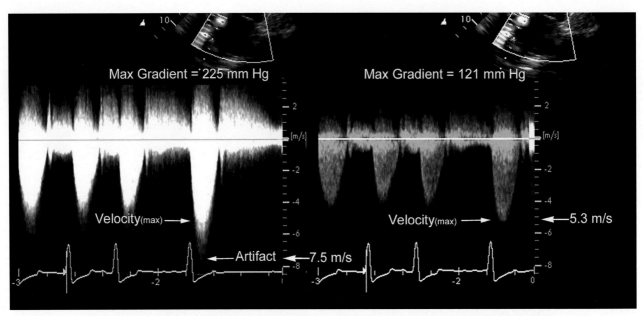

Figure 8-20 Effects of Excessive Transmit Power & Receiver Gain in Spectral Doppler Recordings. Left: This recording shows blooming of the outer envelope (*right arrow*) in a CWD recording from a dog with subaortic stenosis. The Doppler ultrasound transmit power was set too high and the receiver gain was also excessive. If the "maximal" envelope is assumed to equal 7.5 m/s, the estimated maximal pressure gradient is 225 mm Hg. Right: The image is the same as in the left panel but the postprocessing receiver gain was modified (this was a raw data image file) and set at a more appropriate level. While still imperfect, the peak velocities are more clear. In general, the maximum velocity should be measured at the outer edge of the modal velocity spectrum that typically outlines the outer "envelope" in spectral recordings. Because the peak velocity is squared when quantifying pressure gradients (gradient = $4V^2$), measuring the bloomed edge (left) increases the pressure gradient. In the present case the error was ~100 mm Hg compared to the estimate from the maximal envelope on the right (5.3 m/s).

to propel blood across the mitral orifice pressures (see Figure 8-21, right).

Semilunar Valves

Normal blood flow in the ventricular outflow tracts is characterized by PWD velocity spectra with a roughly-triangular profile and a relatively high-pitched, whistling sound in the audio channels of the system.[140] Velocities are highly dependent on ventricular function, stroke volume, and the presence of any lesions in the outflow tracts. There are also relevant issues of biologic and operator variability.[159]

The *aortic velocity profile* has a rapid acceleration, with a thin acceleration envelope and relatively sharp peak (see Figure 8-18, *A*). The deceleration limb of the aortic spectrum is approximately twice the thickness of the acceleration limb and the slope is less steep. Systolic RBC velocities increase substantially, roughly doubling in dogs from about 70 cm/s to 150 cm/s, as the sample volume is mapped from the proximal outflow tract (at the level of the AMV tip) into the ascending aorta. Velocity peaks just distal to the valve. Outflow tract velocity profiles in normal cats are similar to dogs, but peak velocities are lower. It is difficult to align the cursor with aortic blood flow in cats, and peak velocities are usually underestimated. Brief periods of trivial aortic regurgitation (AR) are of uncertain significance in dogs and cats, although trace, holo-diastolic AR is regarded with suspicion. Because maximal aortic velocity strongly depends on ventricular stroke volume, it can be significantly depressed by certain sedatives and is always reduced during anesthesia. Some reported maximum values obtained with PWD (without angle correction) in healthy dogs and cats are reported in Table 8-4.

Ejection velocity is enhanced by heightened sympathetic activity,[164] longer cardiac cycle length, or the presence of obstructive lesions, as with AS. Variation is also observed during ventilation, and the examiner must be aware of effects just due to cardiac translation. An increase in maximal aortic ejection velocity is a salient feature of aortic stenosis. However, peak velocities can exceed 3m/s in healthy dogs subjected to catecholamine infusions in the absence of LVOTO. Similar findings occur in disorders characterized by high stroke volumes, as with patent ductus arteriosus (PDA), severe AR, or complete A-V block, particularly in larger dogs.

When compared to the aorta, the *pulmonary artery velocity profile* is slower to accelerate, more rounded at the peak, and slightly lower in maximum velocity (usually <140 cm/s). Increased PA velocity is identified with pulmonic stenosis (PS) but also observed with high adrenergic states and left-to-right shunting (ASD, VSD). In healthy cats, high ejection velocities sometimes develop from sympathetic tone and dynamic obstruction within the RV infundibulum.[165] This creates a mid-to-late systolic acceleration in blood flow characterized by a dagger-shaped profile with a concave acceleration limb typical of other dynamic obstructions. Additional reasons for dynamic RVOT obstruction include RV concentric hypertrophy from PS and feline HCM. Pulmonary hypertension (PHT) can alter the appearance of the PA flow signal. As the pulmonary vascular resistance comes to resemble that of the systemic circulation, PA acceleration time shortens relative to ejection time; additionally, a prominent deceleration notch is sometimes observed.[2-4]

Physiologic pulmonary regurgitation of low-velocity (<2.2 m/s) is normal and common in healthy dogs and

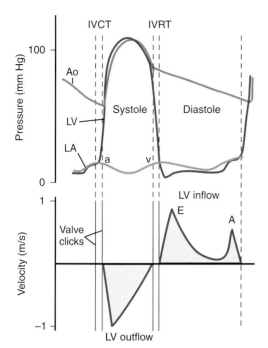

Figure 8-21 Cardiac Cycle—Doppler Correlates. The cardiac cycle: LV, aortic (Ao), and LA pressures are shown with the corresponding Doppler LV outflow and inflow velocity curves. See text for details. Valve clicks are due to opening/closing of cardiac valves. The isovolumic contraction time (IVCT) represents the time between mitral valve closure and aortic valve opening, while the isovolumic relaxation time (IVRT) represents the time between aortic valve closure and mitral valve opening. (From Otto. *Textbook of Clinical Echocardiography*. 5th ed. Philadelphia: Saunders/Elsevier; 2013, with permission).

cats.[63,67,166,167] In the setting of PHT, higher regurgitant velocities are measured because RBCs are driven backward under greater pressure as often observed with pulmonary vascular disease or left-sided CHF.[66,168-174] When pulmonary regurgitation is severe, the contour of the regurgitant envelope is altered, with a steeper descent indicative of pressure equilibration between the PA and RV. This is often observed after balloon valvuloplasty of PS.

Atrioventricular Valves

Ventricular filling is measured in the inflow tracts with a sample volume at the tips of the opened mitral and tricuspid valves (Figure 8-22, *A*). Normal diastolic blood flow has two peaks, an early rapid filling wave (E-wave) and a lower velocity presystolic wave due to atrial contraction (A-wave). The audio signals are multiphasic with two distinct signals (see Figure 8-17, *B* and Figures 8-21 and 8-22). Normal values for spectral Doppler in dogs and in cats are summarized in Table 8-4. Filling patterns in the ventricles are affected by numerous factors, including: myocardial relaxation; ventricular chamber distensibility; heart rate; venous pressures; atrioventricular pressure gradients; ventricular afterload; ventilation; pericardial constraint; ventricular interdependence; and the presence of any cardiac lesions, especially MV disease[119,175] and left-to-right shunts. Additionally, even in healthy animals the transmitral flow velocities depend greatly on heart rate and filling pressures.[148,176-181] Due to these multiple determinants, the assessment of diastolic ventricular function is complicated.[87,182-187]

The typical appearance of *transmitral* flow recorded at the tips of the opened valve is an "M-shaped" waveform, consisting of two triangles, one representing early ventricular filling (E) and the second atrial contraction (A) (see Figure 8-22). The LV filling is initially rapid, usually achieving a maximum

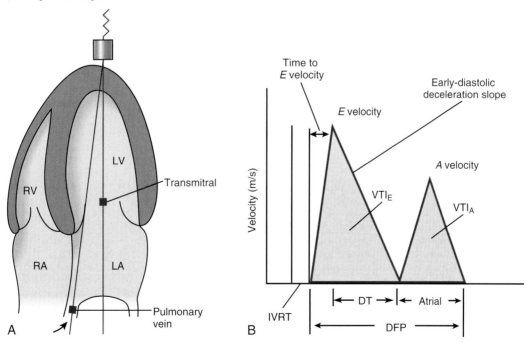

Figure 8-22 Left Ventricular Filling. A, Sample volume placement for recording of transmitral blood flow and pulmonary venous flow. **B,** Schematic diagram of quantitative measurements that can be made from the Doppler LV filling curve. The transmitral flow pattern is comprised of two "triangles" at normal heart rates. With long diastolic cycles, a period of diastasis or slow filling leads to separation of the waves. DFP, diastolic filling period; DT, deceleration time; IVRT, isovolumic relaxation time; VTI, velocity-time integral. (A and B from Otto. *Textbook of Clinical Echocardiography*. 5th ed. Philadelphia: Saunders/Elsevier; 2013, with permission).

TABLE 8-4

Pulsed-Wave Doppler Variables in Healthy Dogs and Cats*

Source (reference) (number) ⇨ / Doppler Variable ⇨	Gaber[1]	Yuill & O'Grady[2]	Brown, et al.[3]	Bonagura & Miller[4]	Schober et al.5,6	Petric, et al.[7]	Distian, et al.[8]	Chetboul, et al.[9]	Santilli & Budsadori[10]	Suggested Canine Reference**
Species (number)	Dogs, n = 28	Dogs, n = 20	Dogs, n = 28	Dogs, n = 15	Dogs, n = 92,5 n = 146	Cats, n = 31 to 53	Cats, n = 87	Cats, n = 100 (51 MCC)	Cats, n = 20	Composite of studies
Aorta	118.9 ± 17.8 cm/s	118.1 ± 10.8 cm/s	106.0 ± 21.0 cm/s	115.4 ± 15.3 cm/s		104 cm/s (77-140 cm/s)		110 ± 20 cm/s		170 cm/s (PW) <200 cm/s (CW) Uncertain: 200-240 cm/s***
Pulmonary artery	99.8 ± 15.3 cm/s	98.1 ± 9.4 95.5 ± 10.3 Right side (top) Left side	84.0 ± 17.0 cm/s	106.0 ± 13.8 cm/s 106.8 ± 10.2 cm/s Right, Left		96 cm/s (65-121 cm/s)		90 ± 20 cm/s		<140 cm/s
Mitral E-wave****	75.0 ± 11.8 cm/s	86.2 ± 9.5 cm/s		73.9 ± 8.9 cm/s	73 ± 116 Means: 69-77 cm/s5 In dogs <10 years old 52, 93 cm/s 10, 90 percentiles^	68 cm/s (48-101 cm/s)	70 ± 14 cm/s	70 ± 10 cm/s	67 ± 13 cm/s	<105 cm/s
Mitral A-wave	53.8 ± 8.7 cm/s			45.9 ± 10.6 cm/s	48 ± 16 cm/s E:A ratio 1.63 ± 0.476 Means: 48-57 cm/s5 In dogs <10 years old 52, 93 cm/s 10, 90 percentiles^	56 cm/s (38-73 cm/s)	65 ± 14 cm/s Ratio of E/A: 1.1 ± 0.2	50 ± 10 cm/s Ratio of E/A: 1.5 ± .3	59 ± 14 cm/s Ratio of E/A: 1.19 ± 0.3	MVE > MVA Decreases with age
Tricuspid E-wave	56.2 ± 16.1 cm/s	68.9 ± 8.4 cm/s		59.7 ± 8.8 cm/s						<90 cm/s
Tricuspid A-wave				45.4 ± 6.8 cm/s						TVE wave > TVA
Pulmonary venous flow Diastolic wave					56 ± 146 Means: 50-57 cm/s5 In dogs <10 years old 36, 82 cm/s 10, 90 percentiles^		47 ± 10 cm/s		44 ± 9 cm/s	S < D typical S:D <1.4
Pulmonary venous flow Systolic wave					39 ± 146 Means: 34-45 cm/s5 In dogs <10 years old 24, 70 cm/s 10, 90 percentiles for all age groups		48 ± 14 cm/s		39 ± 12 cm/s	S < D typical S:D <1.4

Pulmonary venous flow Reversal (A_R) wave (Velocity)	Means: 21-24 cm/s[5] In dogs <10 years old 15, 30 cm/s 10, 90 percentiles^		23 ± 6 cm/s			A_R < 90 cm/s Duration A_R < MVA
Pulmonary vein A_R (Duration)	Means: 67-70 ms[5] In dogs <10 years 53, 103 10, 90 percentiles^		52.9 ± 13.5 ms			
Isovolumetric relaxation time****	60 ms ± 20[6] Means: 43-47 ms[5] In dogs <10 years 31, 65 ms 10, 90 percentiles^	58 ms (35-84 ms)	46.2 ± 7.6 ms	43 ± 9 ms (all cats) 50 ± 11 ms DSH 55 ± 11 ms MCC	55.4 ± 13 ms	>30 ms <65 ms
Mitral deceleration time****	Means: 67-80 ms[5] In dogs <10 years 49, 110 ms 10, 90 percentiles	68 ms (49-113 ms)	59.9 ± 14 ms			

All velocity values are expressed in centimeters per second (cm/s); all time values are expressed in milliseconds (ms)

*Values reported are mean ± 1SD or as a median (range); Doppler data reported have *not* been angle-corrected.

**When dealing with small studies with normal distribution, a suggested normal range is the mean ± 2.5 to 3SD. For samples >120, 2SD are appropriate. Reference limits for dogs suggested by the authors are indicated in this column but are subject to refinement with future studies.

***For feline reference values, the reader is referred to the three studies presented in the table.

****The upper limit defining peak aortic velocities is controversial. Peak aortic velocities using PWD recorded from the left apex are typically <170 cm/s in dogs without cardiac murmurs; CWD increases the signal to noise and records slightly higher peak velocities with values <200 cm/s suggested as normal. The velocity range between 200-240 cm/s is often associated with an ejection murmur and in the absence of any 2D imaging lesions is considered ambiguous or equivocal for aortic stenosis.

In normal dogs, slightly higher maximal velocities are usually recorded from the subxiphoid (subcostal) position using CW Doppler.

See references for further details.

****Mitral valve E-velocity and MVE:MVA normally decrease with increasing age; mitral valve deceleration time and isovolumetric relaxation time normally prolong with increasing age.5,6

^Study involved dogs of varying age groups—the data quoted in ranges are the range of four sets of means for 84 of the healthy study dogs, divided into four arbitrary age groups of n = 30 (<2 years of age), m = 30 (≥2 to <4 years of age), m = 13 (≥4 to <6 years of age), and m = 11 (≥6 to <10 years of age)

MCC = Maine Coon cats; DSH = domestic shorthair cats

Table 8-4 References
1. Gaber C. Doppler echocardiography. *Probl Vet Med* 1991;3:479–99.
2. Yuill CD, O'Grady MR. Doppler-derived velocity of blood flow across the cardiac valves in the normal dog. *Can J Vet Res* 1991;55:185–92.
3. Brown DJ, Knight DH, King RR. Use of pulsed-wave Doppler echocardiography to determine aortic and pulmonary velocity and flow variables in clinically normal dogs. *Am J Vet Res* 1991;52:543–50.
4. Bonagura JD, Miller MW, Darke PG. Doppler echocardiography. I. Pulsed-wave and continuous-wave examinations. *Veterinary Clinics of North America Small Animal Practice* 1998;28:1325–59, vii.
5. Schober KE, Fuentes VL. Effects of age, body weight, and heart rate on transmitral and pulmonary venous flow in clinically normal dogs. *Am J Vet Res* 2001;62:1447–54.
6. Schober KE, Fuentes VL, McEwan JD, et al. Pulmonary venous flow characteristics as assessed by transthoracic pulsed Doppler echocardiography in normal dogs. *Vet Radiol Ultrasound* 1998;39:33–41.
7. Petric AD, Rishniw M, Thomas WP. Two-dimensionally-guided M-mode and pulsed wave Doppler echocardiographic evaluation of the ventricles of apparently healthy cats. *J Vet Cardiol* 2012;14:423–30.
8. Disatian S, Bright JM, Boon J. Association of age and heart rate with pulsed-wave Doppler measurements in healthy, nonsedated cats. *J Vet Intern Med* 2008;22:351–6.
9. Chetboul V, Sampedrano CC, Tissier R, et al. Quantitative assessment of velocities of the annulus of the left atrioventricular valve and left ventricular free wall in healthy cats by use of two-dimensional color tissue Doppler imaging. *Am J Vet Res* 2006;67:250–8.
10. Santilli RA, Bussadori C. Doppler echocardiographic study of left ventricular diastole in non-anaesthetized healthy cats. *Vet J* 1998;156:203–15.

inflow velocity of about 75 to 80 cm/s in dogs. The mitral velocity spectral profile is relatively "tight" around the modal velocity. With increased transmitral flow, the E-wave velocity is higher and spectral dispersion increases. Following the E-wave there is a deceleration of inflow. The deceleration time becomes abbreviated physiologically with vigorous diastolic relaxation (as blood is literally sucked into the ventricle) or pathologically when high atrial pressures are superimposed on a stiff ventricle. During diastasis inflow velocity is low, but if not eliminated by baseline filters, might be evident as a late or L-wave. Atrial contraction produces the second prominent inflow pattern with a peak velocity averaging about 50 to 60 cm/s in dogs.

The relationship of inflow waves in both healthy dogs and cats is E>A. Various components of the E- and A-waves, as well as deceleration time, can be used to assess LV diastolic function and filling pressures as discussed later in the chapter. The E-wave often exceeds 1 m/s in left-to-right shunts, clinically significant anemia, severe MR, left-sided CHF, and with some tachycardias. Preload directly affects the E-wave and A-wave velocities, for example, volume overload or dehydration will increase and decrease the filling velocities, respectively. The A-wave is enhanced when early diastolic atrial emptying is reduced, as with impaired ventricular relaxation or stenosis of an A-V valve. Conversely, in atrial fibrillation the A-wave is lost.

Mitral recordings are influenced by other factors. The E/A ratio decreases in healthy dogs and cats as they age.[180] As one moves the sample volume closer to the LA, the A-wave becomes relatively higher in velocity and this can cause a spurious E/A reversal. Rapid heart rates, which are common in the dog and typical of cats, also can increase the amplitude of the inflow waves (A on E) or result in a single fused filling wave. Premature complexes or short cycles in atrial fibrillation can lead to early closure of the mitral valve with a spurious shortening of mitral deceleration time. These situations can impede Doppler analysis of LV diastolic function.

The *tricuspid* valve recording is qualitatively similar to the MV with some important differences. The peak inlet velocities are usually lower than for the left heart. There is often greater spectral dispersion of the inlet signal that might indicate difficulties in aligning to inflow in all planes. In many studies, a dispersed, positive systolic wave is recorded; this can be confusing if a simultaneous ECG is not recorded (see Figure 8-16, *E*). Physiologic tricuspid regurgitation is extremely common in dogs and cats, evident in over 50% of cases examined from multiple acoustic windows.

Pulmonary Veins

These velocity spectra have been measured from healthy dogs and cats under a variety of conditions using both transthoracic and transesophageal techniques.[141,144,180,188,189] Flow across the pulmonary venous ostia is driven by pressure gradients between the pulmonary venous system and the LA. These gradients reflect diastolic and systolic ventricular function as well as plasma volume status. Pulmonary venous flow profiles are polyphasic, reflecting the various functions of the left atrium over the cardiac cycle and respective changes in LA pressure over the cardiac cycle. There are two positive waves (S, D) and one negative or reversal wave (A_R). Normal values reported for these waveforms in dogs and cats are summarized in Table 8-4.

At the conclusion of atrial contraction, one or two forward waves (S_1S_2) are registered (see Figure 8-18, *A*). The first begins just *before* the QRS complex and is due to suction created by atrial relaxation. This usually blends into the second S wave which follows the QRS complex and occurs while the LA functions as a reservoir for venous return. The genesis of S_2 is the negative pressure created within the LA by descent

of the mitral annulus during ventricular contraction. The RV stroke volume might also contribute to this wave. The S-wave becomes smaller relative to the D-wave in the setting of LV failure and elevated LA pressure, which impedes venous return while the mitral valve is closed. Severe MR often contaminates the S-wave when the regurgitant jet extends into a pulmonary vein.

During protodiastole another forward flow wave is recorded as the LA functions as a conduit (or passageway) for venous return. This D-wave is explained by the pulmonary vein-to-LV pressure gradient that is exposed with opening of the MV. The pulmonary vein D-wave occurs as the transmitral E-wave is filling the LV. Accordingly, conditions that increase the velocity of the transmitral E-wave, especially high pulmonary venous pressures, also enhance the amplitude of the D-wave.

In late diastole, after the P-wave, the LA functions as a pump and causes an atrial reversal wave (A_R). This reflects regurgitation of blood into the pulmonary veins at the same time the LV is filling again (coincident with the transmitral A-wave). Vigorous atrial contraction increases the peak A_R wave while increased LV diastolic pressure prolongs the duration of this event. The ratio of mitral A-wave duration to A_R duration is about 1.2 to 1.5 in healthy dogs but the ratio decreases with reduced distensibility of the ventricle and increased end-diastolic pressures.

Atrial Function

This evaluation is generally confined to feline patients with LA enlargement. The transmitral A-wave and the pulmonary venous A_R waves do relate to atrial function but also to ventricular diastolic function and filling pressures. The function of the LA chamber or the auricular appendage can be assessed by various methods. The LA ejection fraction can be estimated from tracing the 2DE, 3D estimates, or from LA fractional shortening derived from an M-mode examination. Left auricular filling and emptying velocities can be measured near the junction of the LA and left auricle. In healthy cats two or three waveforms are identified.[94] The authors usually focus on the active contraction of the LA appendage: this ejection velocity normally exceeds 25 cm/s in cats (see Figure 8-11). As a general guideline, peak auricular velocities between 20 to 25 cm/s are suspicious for impaired LA function and those <20 cm/s are usually associated with significant atrial disease, increased risk of blood stasis characterized by echogenic "smoke," and an overall higher risk for arterial thromboembolism. The need for antithrombotic prophylaxis is often based on the combined assessment of LA size, left auricular contraction, and the pertinent medical history. Atrial function can also be evaluated by M-mode or 2D methods as discussed below.

Normal Tissue Doppler Imaging

When a PWD sample volume is placed within the myocardium adjacent to the mitral or tricuspid annulus, myocardial motion and velocity are recorded (see Figure 8-18, *F*; Videos 8-12 and 8-13).[190,191] Three waveforms are evident. With the transducer located at the left apex, the TDI profile appears as low-velocity, mirror images of transmitral and aortic blood flow. Early diastolic recoil of the LV results in a negative tissue velocity called E' (called "E-prime" or "Ea", for the mitral annulus). Late diastolic recoil following atrial contraction produces a negative, lower-velocity tissue wave, A' or Aa. A single positive wave is evident during systole, coinciding with ventricular ejection and apical displacement of the annulus. Rapid oscillations are also observed coincident with isovolumetric relaxation and contraction. Peak myocardial velocities are usually <20 cm/s, and as previously discussed, the instrumentation settings must be optimized to record quality signals. Tissue velocities have varied across species, studies, and methodologies (PW TDI versus color-based tissue Doppler);[148-151,153,170,177,192-198] some published reference values are summarized in Table 8-4. As with all echocardiographic variables repeatability can be a concern.[159,177] Similar to transmitral flow, the normal E' is greater than A'. Myocardial (or annular) velocities are used in the assessment of ventricular diastolic function, filling pressures, and evaluation of segmental systolic function. Some of these indices are summarized later under "Ventricular Function".

Clinical Applications of Pulse-Wave Doppler Echocardiography

The most important uses of PWD are confirmation of normal blood flow velocities across the cardiac valves, detection of turbulent or high-velocity blood flow, and applications for assessing ventricular diastolic function. Volumetric flow, including ventricular stroke volume, cardiac output, and shunt fractions, can be estimated using PW methods, but these are infrequently performed in clinical practice. LV and RV longitudinal contraction velocities can be assessed with TDI. Additionally, it is possible to generate a variety of systolic time intervals and indices with spectral Doppler techniques as described later under "Ventricular Systolic Function."

Among the more useful PWD applications are assessments of ventricular filling and diastology. Used together the PWD and TDI examinations constitute the standard for assessing the interactions between ventricular diastolic function and ventricular filling pressures (see "Ventricular Diastolic Function"). The authors also consider the PWD measurement of left auricular filling and emptying of significant clinical value and perform these in every cat with cardiomyopathy or atrial dilatation (see "Atrial Function" earlier and "Feline Cardiomyopathies" later).

CONTINUOUS-WAVE DOPPLER ECHOCARDIOGRAPHY

The CWD examination quantifies blood flow velocity by using two (or more) crystals that independently emit and receive US on a continual basis. High PRFs are attainable, allowing for accurate mapping of high velocities typical of pathologic flow (Figure 8-23). However, this resolution involves the tradeoff of range ambiguity: All returning US along the line of interrogation is sampled and processed simultaneously, superimposing all Doppler frequency shifts onto a single spectrum. As a result spectral broadening is inherent to this modality and is of no diagnostic significance.

The caveat of obtaining clean envelopes with clear peaks is even more critical for this modality, and the examiner must appreciate the characteristics of a quality CWD recording. When high-velocity blood flow is captured by CWD, it is common to see brighter portions of grayscale within the spectrum; these represent the relative number of RBCs traveling at that velocity. The brightest region within the spectrum is usually a lower velocity profile designed as V_1 (Figure 8-23, C). This modal velocity represents the RBCs flowing proximal to the lesion in the case of outflow tract stenosis, valvular regurgitation, or restrictive shunts. Additionally, a second modal velocity is usually evident as a narrow band tracking inside the envelope of the highest velocities. The peak of this envelope is the maximal velocity or V_2 (see Figures 8-20, 8-21, and 8-23) and this velocity is commonly measured when estimating pressure gradients. The outer spectral envelope is affected by the strength of the flow disturbance, the presence of turbulence in the flow stream, and a host of technical factors (see Table 8-3). Assuming good alignment with flow, the greatest pitfall in measuring these spectra involves over-

estimation of the peak velocity and pressure gradient, because these are used to guide prognosis and therapy.[6] Some practical tips for avoiding technical problems with CWD measurements are advanced under the "Bernoulli Equation" in the next section.

Caveats described previously under "Instrumentation" for PWD also apply to CWD. One obvious technical difference relates to the lack of a sample volume; instead CWD systems include a focal zone. This marker should be placed within or just past the flow disturbance of interest. Low-velocity (clutter or wall) filters are set at higher frequency limits than for PWD. Of course overall velocity scales are also set much higher. Both high PRF settings and baseline shifting are needed to accommodate flow that can exceed 6 m/s.

Inherent *limitations* of CWD should be appreciated. It is easy to become confused by a CWD recording if multiple jets are crossed. For example, in the setting of combined subaortic stenosis and mitral regurgitation it would not be uncommon to cross both jets from the left apical position. As another example, when recording blood flow from the RVOT, late diastolic flow signals within the RV caused by atrial contraction often cross the CWD line and are therefore sampled within the spectrum. Owing to the limitation of range ambiguity, with CWD the operator cannot be certain of the precise origin of the returning signals. Practically this limitation is managed by sequentially using CDI, PWD (±high PRF Doppler) and CWD examinations as complementary studies. When a CDI area of high-velocity or disturbed flow is localized by a signal alias or turbulence algorithm, the CWD mode is activated to record the peak velocities within the flow disturbance.

Hemodynamic Quantitation Using CW Doppler

Important quantitative information is derived from CWD measurements.[84,86,199,200] Foremost is the estimation of the pressure gradient, a determination that previously required cardiac catheterization. Normally when systolic pressures are measured on either side of an opened semilunar valve, the peak pressures in the ventricle and its contiguous great vessel are equal though not occurring at precisely the same instant (see Figure 8-21). Similarly diastolic pressures on either side of an opened A-V valve also demonstrate minimal differences between atrium and ventricle. However *instantaneous* pressure gradients across opened valves can be detected with high-fidelity manometers mounted on cardiac catheters. These normal impulse gradients drive blood through the circulation,[162] but are small in magnitude, about 2-12 mm Hg in the outflow tracts and lower (<5 mm Hg) across the ventricular inlets. Impulse gradients generate red blood cell velocities ranging from approximately 0.25-1.6 m/s, depending on location and timing in the cardiac cycle. Such velocities are quantifiable using spectral Doppler methods and are represented in the normal values summarized in Table 8-4.

The situation is quite different in the setting of cardiac pathology, wherein abnormal, high-velocity blood flow is commonly identified. Common examples include aortic stenosis, pulmonary stenosis, dynamic ventricular outflow stenosis (as with hypertrophic cardiomyopathy), A-V valve stenosis, ventricular septal defect, valvular regurgitation, and patent ductus arteriosus (Box 8-4). In each of these conditions, RBCs converge toward the lesion along accelerating, isovelocity shells. These eventually form a high-velocity jet and a distal flow disturbance (turbulence). This dynamic is driven by an abnormal *pressure gradient* that moves the blood across a restrictive orifice at velocities typically ranging from 2.4 m/s to 7 m/s (or rarely higher!). High velocities can arise from the normal intravascular pressure differences that become exposed by a shunt or an incompetent heart valve. Systemic or pulmonary hypertension superimposed on an insufficient heart valve

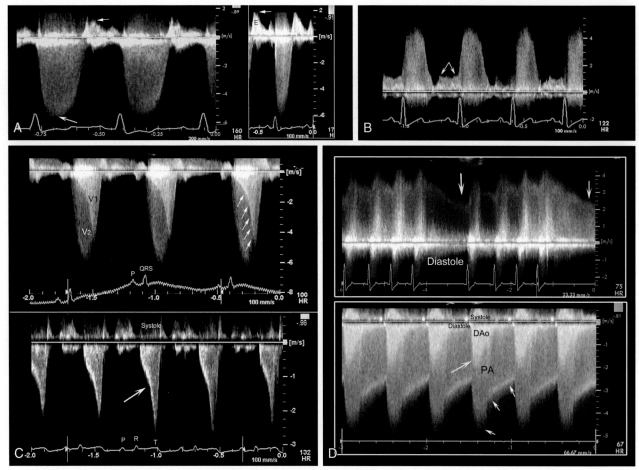

Figure 8-23 Continuous-wave Doppler Echocardiography. A, CW Doppler recordings of MR from two dogs. Left: The MR jet is recorded as fast sweep speed (200 mm/s) and the maximal velocity (arrow) is approximately 5.4-5.5 m/s. The rounded contour suggests left atrial pressure is not very increased. Assuming good alignment with inflow, peak E-wave velocity (*upper arrow*) is about 1.2 m/s, the upper limits of normal. Right: A jet of MR is evident. Accepting the slower recording speed (100 mm/s), the velocity still peaks relatively earlier in systole. Additionally transmitral filling E-wave exceeds 2 m/s. Both of these findings are compatible with higher LA pressure (see text for details). **B,** CW Doppler recording across a ventricular septal defect in a dog. The orifice is likely restrictive based on the estimated pressure difference exceeding 90 mm Hg between the ventricles. The envelope is somewhat ragged, a common finding with VSD jets. Low-velocity, diastolic shunting is also evident (*arrow*). **C,** Outflow tract obstructions recorded by CW Doppler. Top: Recording of flow across pulmonic stenosis in a dog. There are two velocity profiles evident, the peak velocity envelope (V_2) and a slower developing velocity profile (V_1) that is closer to the baseline for most of systole. Note that V_1 suddenly accelerates in late systole (*arrows*), indicating the development of dynamic muscular obstruction to flow within the ventricle secondary to RV hypertrophy. Bottom: Typical mid-to-late systolic ejection profile of LVOT obstruction in a cat with hypertrophic cardiomyopathy. Unlike a fixed subvalvular aortic stenosis, the blood does not accelerate until dynamic obstruction develops between the AMV leaflet and the IVS. **D,** Continuous high-velocity flow recorded in the pulmonary artery from two dogs with patent ductus arteriosus. Top: Transthoracic recording from a sedated dog shows left-to-right shunting throughout the cardiac cycle. The peak velocity occurs near the end of systole. The greater drop in shunt velocity during longer diastolic cycles (arrows) indicates decreasing pressure difference between the aorta and PA. Lower: Transesophageal recording in an anesthetized dog with the transducer positioned to record flow moving out of the descending aorta (DAo) and into the PA (*lower arrows*). Aortic flow can be discerned as a systolic lower velocity profile (*upper arrow*) that is summated on the higher velocity continuous flow entering the PA across the ductus arteriosus (*lower arrows*).

BOX 8-4

Estimation of Pressure Gradients Using CW Doppler

AORTIC STENOSIS (AS, SUBAORTIC STENOSIS)
- Record the maximal velocity profile in m/s across the stenosis.
- Use the simplified Bernoulli equation (pressure gradient = $4V^2$) to determine the maximum instantaneous pressure gradient across the LVOT.
- Measure noninvasive systemic arterial blood pressure.
- Maximal left ventricular systolic pressure = systolic arterial blood pressure + maximal instantaneous pressure gradient.
- Trace the outer envelope of the aortic VTI to determine the mean pressure gradient across the LVOT.
- Mean gradient is usually ≈ 55% to 60% of the peak instantaneous gradient.

PULMONIC STENOSIS (PS)
- Record the peak velocity profile in m/s across the stenosis.
- Use the simplified Bernoulli equation (gradient = $4V^2$) to determine the maximum instantaneous pressure gradient across RVOT.
- Right ventricular systolic pressure = peak gradient + 20 to 25 mm Hg (where 20 to 25 mm Hg is an estimate of pulmonary artery systolic pressure based on catheterization experience).
- Verify RV systolic pressure if there is a tricuspid regurgitant jet available (see Pulmonary Hypertension).
- If a dynamic subvalvular component is identified, also calculate the peak end-systolic dynamic pressure gradient obstructs.
- If there is an increase in the proximal velocity (V_1) before the fixed obstruction that peaks in midsystole, recalculate the distal valvular obstruction using both the PA velocity (V_2) and the proximal velocity, as peak gradient = $4(V_2 - V_1)^2$.
- Trace the outer envelope of the pulmonary artery VTI to determine the mean pressure gradient.
- Mean gradient is usually ≈ 55% to 60% of the peak instantaneous gradient.

PULMONARY HYPERTENSION (PHT)
- Measure the peak velocity of tricuspid regurgitation if present.
- Abnormal TR velocity is >2.6 m/s; >3.0 m/s is typically used to indicate PHT in the absence of any outflow stenosis.
- High velocity tricuspid regurgitation correlates to elevated right ventricular systolic pressure.
- Peak systolic pressure in the PA equals peak right ventricular systolic pressure.
- Peak PA pressure equals the calculated RV to RA instantaneous pressure gradient plus right atrial pressure (usually zero unless there is congestive heart failure).
- To estimate diastolic pulmonary artery pressure, record the maximal velocity of any pulmonary insufficiency and calculate the PA pressure in early and late diastole using the simplified Bernoulli equation. The PA diastolic pressure = right ventricular diastolic pressure + Doppler-derived PA to RV diastolic pressure gradient (in the absence of CHF, RV diastolic pressure is assumed to be zero or is estimated by measuring the venous pressure from inspection of the jugular veins or from a CVP recording).

VENTRICULAR SEPTAL DEFECT
- Determine the peak velocity across the aortic valve. If the aortic velocity is less than 2 m/s, assume LV systolic pressure = the systemic arterial systolic pressure measured simultaneously by noninvasive means. (If the velocity is >2 m/s, calculate the gradient; see aortic stenosis).
- Measure the peak velocity across the VSD. Assuming close parallel alignment with flow, one can use the simplified Bernoulli equation to estimate the peak instantaneous left ventricular to right ventricular pressure gradient.
- RV systolic pressure equals systolic arterial blood pressure minus the pressure gradient between the left and right ventricles.
- Interpretation is difficult if there is concurrent right ventricular obstruction or subaortic stenosis, or if the angle of Doppler interrogation is greater than 20 degrees.

PATENT DUCTUS ARTERIOSUS
- Use the simplified Bernoulli equation to estimate the peak aortic to pulmonary artery pressure gradient and pulmonary artery systolic pressure.
- PA systolic pressure equals systolic arterial blood pressure minus the pressure gradient between the aorta and PA.
- The peak aortic to pulmonary artery systolic gradient should be approximately 80 to 100 mm Hg in normotensive animals with left to right shunting PDA.
- Poor alignment with flow, or a long, narrow ductus may produce a lower gradient despite normal PA pressures.
- Markedly decreased shunting gradients, <20 to 30 mm Hg, suggest moderate to severe pulmonary hypertension.

MITRAL OR TRICUSPID VALVE STENOSIS
- Estimate the transvalvular diastolic gradients from the modified Bernoulli equation.
- Trace the diastolic envelope to measure both maximal diastolic and mean diastolic pressure gradients.
- Also calculate the pressure half-time, the time (in seconds) required for the instantaneous pressure gradient to decrease by ½ as calculated from the Bernoulli equation (see text).
- Results can be altered by a high heart rate (which shortens diastolic flow time), increased transvalvular flow (from a concurrent shunt, atrioventricular valvular regurgitation), or generally-high cardiac output states (sympathetic activity, fever, or anemia).

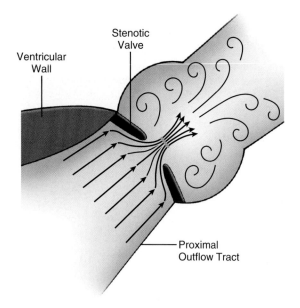

Figure 8-24 **Pattern of Blood Flow Across a Stenotic Semilunar Valve.** Flow in the proximal outflow tract is laminar with a velocity (designated as V_1). Flow accelerates as it converges toward the stenotic valve orifice, attaining a peak velocity (V_2) immediately distal to the obstruction. This high velocity laminar flow is designated the vena contracta (blue line). Distal to the lesion flow is disturbed or turbulent within the proximal great vessel. (Modified from Otto. *Textbook of Clinical Echocardiography*. 5th ed. Philadelphia: Saunders/Elsevier; 2013; and from Judge KW, Otto CM. Doppler echocardiographic evaluation of aortic stenosis. *Cardiol Clin* 1990;8:203, with permission).

is another common cause. High intracardiac pressures are also needed to accelerate blood across a stenotic ventricular outflow tract. These abnormal flow patterns can be quantified and characterized by physical laws. Especially pertinent are the applications of the continuity equation and the Bernoulli relationship.

Continuity Relationship

The *continuity relationship* states that the product of flow velocity x cross-sectional area along a single path is a constant. When the cross-sectional area (CSA) along the path of blood flow decreases abruptly, RBCs progressively accelerate and move across the proximal flow region into the stenotic zone (Figure 8-24). This principle is straightforward when dealing with the stenotic valves or outflow tracts. It is also relevant to regurgitant valve orifices and to restrictive shunts. If the proximal CSA is measured by 2D imaging, the proximal area velocity by PWD, and the stenotic jet velocity by CWD, then a functional cross sectional area of the lesion ($CSA_{stenotic}$) can be estimated as follows: ($CSA_{Stenotic}$) = $CSA_{Proximal}$ * ($V_{Proximal}$ / $V_{Stenotic}$), assuming the same volume of blood crosses both zones. In some ways this approach is more valid than evaluating a lesion by the pressure difference on either side because pressure gradients also depend on the amount of flow. Thus when cardiac output is increased (as with anemia or high sympathetic tone) or diminished (from heart failure or cardiodepressive drugs), the assessment of lesion severity by pressure gradient can be erroneous. The continuity relationship has been used to estimate the severity of LVOT stenosis in dogs.[201] However, limitations to this approach include the need to accurately measure the CSA and velocity in the proximal zone as well as the necessity to consider range of patient sizes encountered in veterinary practice. For example, a ste-

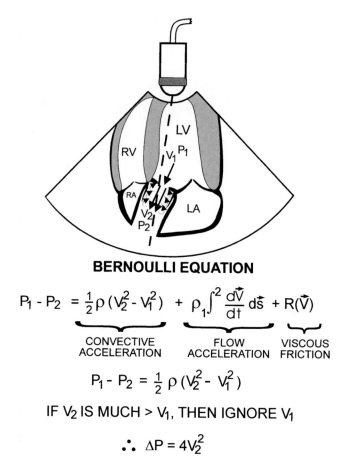

BERNOULLI EQUATION

$$P_1 - P_2 = \tfrac{1}{2}\rho\,(V_2^2 - V_1^2) + \rho_1\!\int_1^2 \frac{d\vec{V}}{dt}\,d\vec{s} + R(\vec{V})$$

$$\underbrace{\phantom{P_1 - P_2 = \tfrac{1}{2}\rho\,(V_2^2 - V_1^2)}}_{\text{CONVECTIVE ACCELERATION}} \quad \underbrace{\phantom{\rho_1\!\int_1^2 \frac{d\vec{V}}{dt}\,d\vec{s}}}_{\text{FLOW ACCELERATION}} \quad \underbrace{\phantom{R(\vec{V})}}_{\substack{\text{VISCOUS}\\\text{FRICTION}}}$$

$$P_1 - P_2 = \tfrac{1}{2}\rho\,(V_2^2 - V_1^2)$$

IF V_2 IS MUCH > V_1, THEN IGNORE V_1

$$\therefore\ \Delta P = 4V_2^2$$

Figure 8-25 **Bernoulli Relationship.** The Bernoulli equation is shown with the relationship between pressure gradient ($P_1 - P_2$) and hydraulic variables of convective acceleration, flow acceleration, viscous friction, and blood density (ρ). The variable $1/2\rho$ simplifies to a value of 4. If the proximal velocity is <1.5 m/s it is ignored, so the relationship simplifies to $\Delta P = 4V^2$. If for example, a maximal flow velocity of 4 m/s is recorded, the predicted pressure gradient across the stenosis equals (4 * 4²) or 64 mm Hg.

notic orifice area of 0.44 cm² would have a different clinical significance in a Maltese dog versus a bull Mastiff.

Bernoulli Relationship

While the continuity relationship emphasizes the interactions between flow velocity and orifice area, the *Bernoulli relationship* (Figure 8-25) relates the flow velocity through a shunt, stenosis, or incompetent valve to the pressure difference that has developed across the lesion. Details of the full Bernoulli relationship are beyond the scope of this chapter.[9,162,163] However, the simplified Bernoulli equation is used in daily practice. Instantaneous pressure gradient (in mmHg) is calculated from the product of $4V^2$ (where maximal velocity is measured in m/s). For example, in a case of pulmonary stenosis, a peak ejection velocity of 4.5 m/s would correspond to an 81 mm Hg (as 4 * 4.5 * 4.5 = 81).

Using the simplified method, proximal blood flow velocity is ignored and only maximal (peak) velocity or the mean velocity (that averaged over time) is considered. The maximal velocity measurement is obtained by placing the cursor at the outer edge of the velocity spectrum; the mean velocity requires tracing the outline of the outer modal envelope of the velocity spectrum (Figure 8-26). Conceptually, the mean gradient can be thought of as the sum of an infinite number

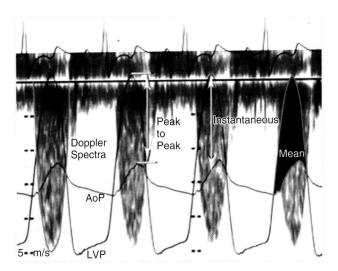

Figure 8-26 **Pressure Gradients Calculated with CW Doppler.** Estimation of maximal instantaneous (peak) and mean pressure gradients in a dog with subvalvular aortic stenosis. Simultaneous LV pressure (LVP) and aortic pressure (AoP) measurements were recorded with superimposed CW Doppler.[92] The highest ejection velocity is used to calculate maximal (peak) instantaneous pressure gradient. The mean pressure gradient (the average over the time period of systole) is obtained by tracing the outer envelope of the velocity spectrum. There is no Doppler correlate to the traditional catheterization peak to peak gradient calculated by subtracting maximal LVP from maximal AoP.

of instantaneous gradients measured over the time period of interest (systole or diastole) and then divided by the number of measurements taken. The echocardiographic system calculates the mean gradient from the area under the time-velocity curve. Experience indicates that mean systolic gradients in the outflow tracts are often ≈55% to 60% of the maximal instantaneous gradient.

There are substantial risks for both under- and overestimating pressure gradients with CWD. Maximal instantaneous pressure gradient will be *underestimated* unless the US beam angle of incidence is close to 0 degrees or 180 degrees and velocity estimates will be significantly underestimated at intercept angles exceeding 22 degrees.[2] Novices often underestimate maximal velocities because they do not record the velocity spectra from the optimal transducer window or fail to optimize the beam relative to flow in three dimensions. The greatest risks for *overestimation* involve application of angle correction (which is *never* done in the heart) and expansion of the velocity spectrum caused by excessive transmit power, an over-gained receiver, or inappropriate compression and grayscale processing (see Figure 8-20). While turbulence and filtering do impart some "feathering" to the outer velocity envelope, any of the following observations should prompt concerns about technical issues: (1) a distorted, erratic envelope; (2) a "bloom" in the peak that does not connect smoothly to the outer velocity envelope; (3) a record with maximal velocities far from the outer dense (bright) edge of the velocity spectrum; or (4) a mirror image spectrum displayed in the opposite direction.[6] This is more than a theoretical issue! As an example, if a mature dog with subaortic stenosis has a peak velocity of 3.6 m/s, the estimated maximal gradient is 52 mm Hg, representing a moderate stenosis with a relatively favorable prognosis. However, if the spectra are overgained and the peak velocity is measured at 4.5 m/s, the calculated gradient becomes [4.5 * 4.5 * 4] = 81 mmHg, or a "severe" AS.

Color Doppler Imaging

Color Doppler Imaging (CDI), also called color-coded Doppler and color flow mapping, is a sophisticated form of PWD imaging that overlays blood flow velocity and directional information onto a two-dimensional, gray-scale image.[46,63] The examiner selects an ROI using the trackball and simultaneously maps blood flow (or tissue movements) while recording 2DE images in real time. The grayscale and Doppler shift data are collected independently and then reconstructed into a single image frame, which is updated multiple times each second. Doppler shift data are depicted in colors, most often in shades of blue and red, and variance from laminar flow is displayed as either a mosaic of colors or in an algorithm-determined encoding of green or yellow (Figure 8-27).

CDI is useful both for documenting normal blood flow and for screening the heart and great vessels for abnormal flow patterns (Videos 8-14 to 8-17). When CDI is combined with M-mode echocardiography a precise temporal resolution of flow events is displayed (Figure 8-28). Advanced CDI technologies, such as color-coded tissue Doppler imaging, have been used to assess ventricular wall motion and systolic and diastolic ventricular function.

The main advantage of CDI is the ability to screen relatively large ROIs for valvular regurgitation, shunting, stenosis, and other flow disturbances. Small shunts and regurgitant flow patterns, muscular ventricular septal defects, and subtle lesions resulting in flow disturbances are more readily visualized with this modality. Furthermore, the color flow study guides placement of PWD sample volumes and steerable CWD cursors across suspicious areas, streamlining the examination. The CDI examination is complemented by spectral Doppler Echo. Analysis of cardiac CDI images is mainly subjective and is only semiquantitative in terms of velocity estimates or application of the proximal isovelocity surface area (PISA). Because larger ROIs are examined, the US beam-flow angle of incidence is variable and also less of a concern than for spectral studies where tight alignment to blood flow is a priority.

Accepting differences in the presentation of Doppler shift information, CDI is simply another format of PWD echocardiography so the same concepts apply, including: angle of incidence between US beam and targets; sample volumes; Nyquist limits; and signal aliasing. Traditional PWD records frequency shifts within a single sample volume and with CDI the Doppler shifts are received from scores of individual, adjacent sample volumes within the defined ROI. The sampled Doppler shifts are computer averaged and filtered to generate a smooth transition of colors and hues adjustable by the operator. The CDI image involves multiple lines of US (see Figure 8-17), which are emitted radially like spokes projecting from the near field. Therefore each sample volume encounters blood flow with a slightly different angle of incidence. While potentially a disadvantage, abnormal CDI studies become easier to interpret because normal flow obtuse to the US beam is depicted as a lower-velocity signal encoded in the darker shades of blue or red. In contrast, even with large angles of incidence, pathologic blood flow will often manifest as variance (turbulence) or at least create a signal alias.

Color Mapping

Recording and interpretation of 2D color imaging is based on an understanding of color flow sample volumes.[2,8,63,202] These indicate Doppler shift information in terms of flow direction, RBC velocities, and detection of turbulence. The clinician must also appreciate the different approach to temporal (time) resolution in CDI and its influence on image analysis.

The 2D color Doppler image is nongraphical and the direction and relative velocities of blood cells across the ROI are determined by comparing the color mapping to a reference map (see Figure 8-27, *A*; Video 8-11, *A*). Positive Doppler shifts are encoded as flow "toward" the transducer and traditionally displayed in red, while negative Doppler shifts are interpreted as flow "away" from the transducer and displayed in blue. Thus BART maps—blue away, red toward—are conventional. Beginners must remember that these colors do not correspond to arterial and venous blood flow, but define the direction of movement along the line of interrogation, within each sample volume. More importantly, even advanced users sometimes forget that CDI is not analogous to an angiogram and while flow is responsible for the Doppler shifts, the image is a map of directions and velocities, not volumes of RBCs. Flow moving at right angles to the US line creates no Doppler shifts and is

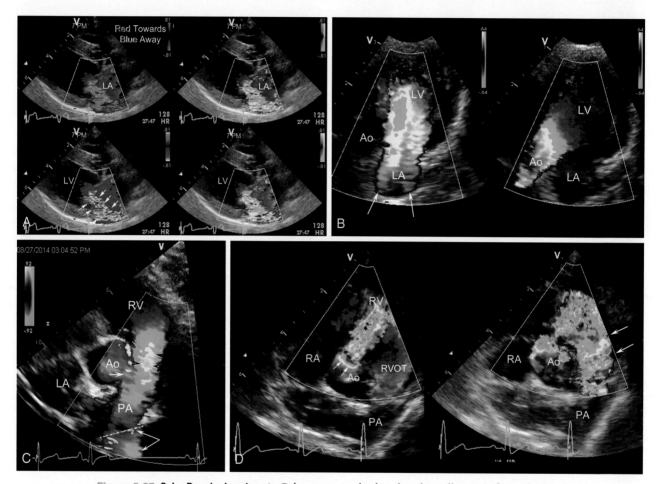

Figure 8-27 Color Doppler Imaging. A, Color maps are displayed in this still image of mitral regurgitation from a dog with degenerative valve disease. Different forms of color encoding are illustrated. Clockwise from upper left: Simple BART (blue away, red toward) map; split variance BART map in which system algorithms encode turbulent blood flow in yellow or green; enhanced BART map showing faster velocities and turbulence in brighter hues; BART map with white added to depict highest velocities. The jet (approximately delineated with small arrows in the lower left panel) is easiest to visualize with the split variance and enhanced variance maps to the right. **B,** Still images of LV filling and ejection in a cat. Left: Transmitral inflow is shown with an enhanced BART map. Blood enters from the pulmonary venous ostia (*arrows*) and crosses the open mitral valve. Note the core of fastest-moving RBCs moving toward the transducer. Accelerated flow leads to encoding in bright yellow which then aliases to cyan (the brightest shade of blue). Blood curling up from the apex codes in dark blue. Angle of incidence also impacts the projected velocity. Right: During systole there is a clear progression in "layers" of accelerated flow changing from the darkest blue to cyan and then aliasing to yellow and continuing to accelerate to encode in dark red. Some turbulence mapping is also seen, which is normal. **C,** Still image of blood flow in the RVOT in systole recorded in a dog. Enhanced BART map with variance. RBCs accelerate and alias (*arrowheads*) as they move across the pulmonic valve. A number of color artifacts are shown. There is "color bleeding" across the walls of the aorta and pulmonary artery (*left arrow*); variance encoding (in green) although the flow is normal; and a mirror image artifact (*right arrows*) in the far field beyond the PA wall that is delineated with the dotted line. **D,** Turbulence mapping of blood flow across a ventricular septal defect in a dog. Left: An early systolic frame shows a signal alias and proximal isovelocity area (*arrows*) prior to flow crossing the VSD. This is followed by turbulent encoding (green and yellow) of blood flow entering the RV across a restrictive defect. Right: later in systole turbulent flow is observed entering both the VSD and in the RV outflow tract (*arrows*).

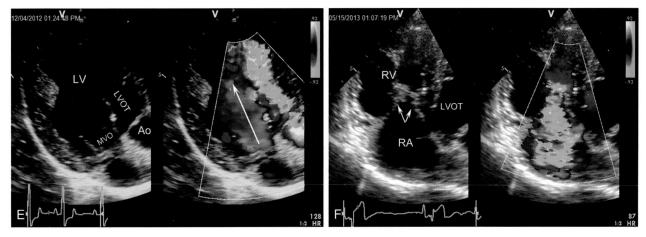

Figure 8-27, cont'd **E,** Aortic regurgitation in a dog with infective endocarditis. A modified apical image plane records transmitral inflow across the mitral valve orifice (MVO), which is coded in dark red as well as a long, wide jet of aortic regurgitation crossing the LVOT and mixing with transmitral flow. The AR is encoded strongly in green to indicate "turbulence." **F,** Tricuspid regurgitation in a young dog with malformation of the tricuspid valve leaflets (*arrows*). A wide origin jet is evidence of severe regurgitation. The turbulence fills much of the right atrial area.

encoded in black. Angle does matter and the highest velocity blood flow might not be encoded accurately if the angle of incidence is large.

The reference color map in CDI can be compared to the vertical axis of the spectral Doppler display. Zero velocity is coded in black and is analogous to the zero baseline in spectral Doppler. Direction of target movement is shown by the colors red and blue. Despite differences among vendors, BART maps are universal and many cardiologists apply enhanced color maps that display higher velocities in progressively brighter hues. For example, flow away would change from black to dark blue to light blue to cyan (see Figures 8-27, *B* and *C*). As with spectral Doppler, the zero baseline in CDI can be shifted up or down to increase the maximum velocity scale in one direction. This is not particularly helpful except when using advanced CDI techniques like PISA to estimate regurgitant or shunt flow. The colors are velocity surrogates and therefore confined by Nyquist limits, which are displayed as velocities at the top and bottom of the color bar. The operator can increase color PRF to a point, but even normal blood flow velocities can exceed the Nyquist limits, wrap around the color bar, and reappear as an aliased signal. The sample volumes affected by signal aliasing are thereby encoded in the color *opposite* that of the real flow direction. Fast-moving targets can create double or triple color wraps, presenting a challenging image analysis (see Figure 8-28). Aliasing is easier to identify when enhanced BART color maps are used: The aliased core is surrounded by brightly encoded flow patterns seemingly moving in the opposite direction. As an example, cyan encoding, surrounded by yellow or bright orange (instead of darker shades of blue) would suggest signal aliasing (see Figure 8-27, *C*).

The main value of CDI for cardiac diagnosis resides in detection of valvular regurgitation, obstruction to flow, and shunting. To this end specialized maps were developed to direct the examiner's eyes to turbulence. BART maps are often overlaid with a *variance* encoding that is based on a vendor-defined algorithm. Variance is displayed as another color (green or yellow) at the edge of the color map (see Figure 8-27, *A* and *D*). Another common convention is the "split variance" map in which turbulence is coded yellow for one direction and green for the opposite. Operator controls allow

for switching between maps or more practically turning "variance" on and off. Many examiners also find that disturbed flow is readily identified with simple enhanced BART maps and inspect the image for aliasing or a mosaic of intermixed colors as guides for further spectral Doppler investigation. There is neither a single best way to color map blood flow nor a standard for turbulence detection algorithms across vendors.

Color Doppler Instrumentation

As summarized in Table 8-3, operator controls strongly influence color image processing. When performing CDI, overall grayscale image gain is reduced or grayscale reject is increased because color coding might not proceed if the video pixel is occupied by tissue density or intraluminal "noise." Color gain is usually increased up to the point where sporadic color artifacts are observed in some pixels. Various low-velocity "flash" artifacts can obscure useful information and present confusing color images. These are reflections from valves, chamber walls, and edges of moving lung that are diminished by applying low-velocity reject and filtering. (The exceptions are examinations focused on tissue based Doppler shifts).

The 2D color frame rate is often degraded by processing that pits color sensitivity versus other Doppler or 2D imaging settings. Many of the operator-control positions that improve color flow mapping also reduce the frame rate. To attain optimal frame rates in CDI the examiner might take the following steps: narrow the sector size; decrease depth of field to the minimum distance required; minimize or turn off any frame averaging/persistence/color smoothing; and filter out low-velocity signals. Velocity scales affect both frame rate and color filling creating a tradeoff between "quality" and temporal resolution. Other operator controls might include modification of US pulse trains (packet sizes) with controls variously called "quality" or "color," or "dwell time"; altering color spatial filters or smoothing; and adjusting other proprietary controls. Despite these adjustments, the examiner might become perplexed when satisfactory color flow mapping is not evident in views that seem anatomically aligned to blood flow. This situation is common, and can generally be corrected by choosing a lower frequency transducer, aligning the US beam more closely to actual flow, or readjusting the aforementioned controls.

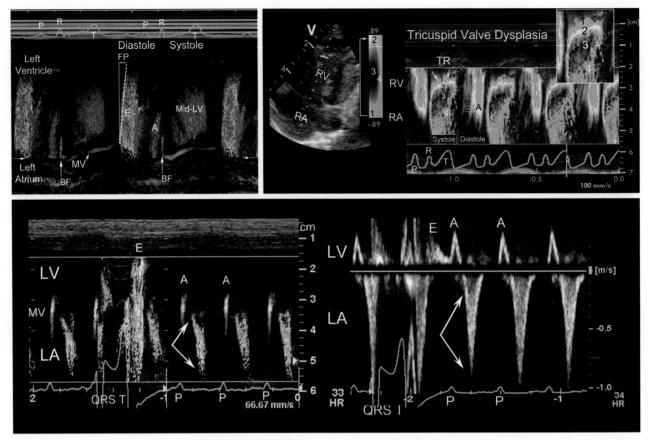

Figure 8-28 Color M-mode Echocardiography. Precise timing and spatial distribution of blood flow is offered by color M-mode echocardiography. Upper left panel: Normal ventricular inflow in a cat recorded from the left apical position is shown. The cursor region of interest was set between the apical LV and the level of the mitral annulus (*horizontal arrows*) near the mitral valve (MV). The direction and relative velocity of flow along the cursor is shown over the cardiac cycle. Note the two inflow patterns filling the LV (labeled "E" and "A") that correspond to normal transmitral flow recorded on PWD. The early diastolic filling wave exceeds the Nyquist limit creating a blue signal alias. The slope of this alias (*dotted line*), termed *flow propagation* (FP), is an advanced variable of LV diastolic function. During systole the cursor captures ventricular outflow in the middle of the LV. This is coded in dark blue and does not alias owing to the large angle of incidence to flow. The small "backflow" signals (BF) seen at the mitral orifice would have intruded into the LA if the ROI had been extended more in the far field. These can be confused with true MR if viewed only in 2D color imaging (see lower panel for an example). Upper right panel: Tricuspid flow patterns recorded from a puppy with tricuspid valve dysplasia. The cursor captures the direction, duration, and turbulence of flow associated with tricuspid regurgitation (TR) and the early and later filling phases of tricuspid inflow (E and A). The flow across a regurgitant valve displays the usual features of pathological regurgitation: acceleration of flow away from the transducer (color map, point 1); signal aliasing to yellow (2); continued acceleration of flow along the map crossing dark red and entering dark blue (3); and finally turbulence encoding in green (4). The "halo" of cyan-light yellow is equivalent to a proximal isovelocity area in the region of flow convergence proximal to the regurgitant orifice. Spatial relationships for the CDI M-cursor are shown as right ventricle (RV) and right atrium (RA). Lower panel: Diastolic mitral regurgitation (*arrows*) recorded from the left apex in a dog with complete AV block and a ventricular escape rhythm (QRS T). Multiple blocked P-waves generate transmitral A-waves in both the color M-mode (left) and PWD studies (right). These increase the LV diastolic pressure leading to diastolic regurgitation (arrows). Note these low velocity signals extend many cm into the LA, activate turbulence encoding in the color study and spectral broadening in the PW examination. This phenomenon is also common during initial valve closure in animals with sinus rhythm and can be confused with systolic MR. The comparably low velocity nature of the events and the precise timing of regurgitation are demonstrated by the complementary color and spectral Doppler studies.

The Nyquist (aliasing) limits should be set by adjusting the control labeled variously velocity, scale, or PRF depending on the system. As a practical goal, CDI settings should encourage sufficient color encoding of the blood pool while also avoiding color bleeding into the tissues or overwhelming the eye with low-velocity or aliased signals. Higher PRF settings automatically activate low-velocity filters. Overall color flow mapping deteriorates if the aliasing velocity is set too high. In practice it is rarely possible to eliminate signal aliasing from the heart, and this not an important goal because these displays bring the eye to the fastest moving (normal or abnormal) blood flow. Accordingly, Nyquist limits of approximately 50 to 100 cm/s in each direction are usually acceptable.

CDI instrument settings have a profound impact on color mapping, aliasing, and variance detection. For example, simply reducing the velocity scale or changing the transducer frequency can lead to "turbulence" encoding. Moreover, as with signal aliasing, the finding of variance by CDI can be completely *normal*. Therefore, any suspicious color flow pattern detected as aliasing or turbulence must be qualified and quantified using a spectral Doppler technique.

Normal Findings

CDI is viewed in real time during the course of the examination and experienced examiners can quickly recognize abnormal flow patterns. However echocardiographic diagnosis should be grounded on review of digital cine loops because interpretation in real time can be confusing, especially if there is low temporal resolution. Most interpretations are subjective, based on examiner training and experience, but are solidified when the lesion is confirmed by complementary echocardiographic modalities. One also must be cognizant of changes occurring over the cardiac cycle.

A simple approach to interpretation involves examining the flow patterns adjacent to the lengths of the ventricular and atrial septa, flow crossing each of the four cardiac valves, and flow in the RVOT and main PA. These evaluations screen for the most common causes of cardiac murmurs. Additional examinations can inspect venous flow in the pulmonary veins and caudal vena cava, and low-velocity flow patterns in the left auricle of cats. One should be cognizant of flash or ghosting artifacts from strong reflectors,[2,5] skeptical of color "bleeding" across grayscale images, and unwilling to accept a regurgitant signal as clinically relevant until it has been timed within the cardiac cycle. The CDI study should be assessed in light of cardiac auscultation considering that right-sided cardiac valves *normally* demonstrate small jets of regurgitation.

Flow observations should be viewed within the context of the cardiac cycle, which can be divided into five arbitrary phases for routine analysis: early diastole (from isovolumetric relaxation through rapid ventricular filling); middiastole (diastasis); atrial contraction (presystole); early systole (from isovolumetric contraction to the peak velocity of ejection); and late systole. High frame rates are needed for discrete timing of flow events when using only 2D color imaging.

The LV and RV inlets shows two major filling phases, coded in red, when viewed from left apical image planes (see Figure 8-27, *B* and Figure 8-28). The first waves begin immediately after the end of the T-wave with opening of the A-V valves and correspond to the PWD E-wave. Following the P-wave, the atrial contraction propels the second filling wave into the ventricle; this corresponds to the PWD A-wave. If the heart rate is slow, a low-velocity inflow signal might be observed in diastasis; conversely, if the heart rate is fast (as in cats) the two inflow patterns merge, similar to E/A fusion in PWD studies. At end-diastole a low-velocity movement of

blood is seen to move toward the semilunar valves (coded dark blue). The semilunar valves are normally closed during diastole; however, physiologic pulmonary valve regurgitation is very common and is considered normal. The signal can be holodiastolic or presystolic in timing and is coded in red in RVOT images from the cranial positions. Whether aortic regurgitation (AR) is ever physiologic in dogs or cats is unresolved, but it is sometimes recognized in young healthy animals, especially after sedation. One of the problems with defining normal limits for CDI of the AV is the lack of timing information (e.g., early-, holo-, or late-diastolic) available in published studies describing normal color flow imaging in dogs and cats. Interpretation is also confounded when young dogs with a breed predisposition to SAS are examined. Many dogs with borderline-high aortic ejection velocities also have trivial (trace) AR. Inasmuch as an AR jet is driven by a far greater pressure gradient than for physiologic PR, the regurgitant signal is often turbulent at the valve with a gradual progression to darker color encoding as the velocity dissipates within the ventricle (Video 8-14).

Blood is rapidly ejected into the aorta and PA, from the last portion of the QRS complex and continuing through the end of the T-wave. The LVOT is encoded in blue when aortic flow is examined from apical imaging planes (see Figure 8-27, C). A similar coding is observed in the RV outlet when cranial long-axis images of the pulmonary artery are taken. Ejection is rapid and signal aliasing is expected even in normal subjects once peak velocities exceed the Nyquist limit. Concurrent with ejection is pulmonary venous return and atrial filling encoded in red.

Atrioventricular valves are normally closed during systole but physiologic tricuspid regurgitation (TR), silent to auscultation, is considered normal. This poses a problem in examining dogs prone to tricuspid valve malformations (e.g., Labrador retrievers), since the distinction between normal variation and abnormal has not been satisfactorily defined. Whether MR can occur as a normal variation is unresolved, but similar to the situation in humans,[2] tiny jets of MR are sometimes identified in healthy, young dogs including athletes and sight hounds. Interpretation of these regurgitant signals becomes confused in breeds prone to mitral dysplasia or after a dog attains an age when myxomatous disease might begin. A true regurgitant signal should begin with mitral closure and extend into the first half of systole (or develop from pure mitral prolapse in mid-to-late systole). This should not be confused with normal presystolic or protosystolic backflow associated with increasing LV pressure and valve closure. In instruments with slow frame rates, physiologic backflow can be misinterpreted as significant valvular regurgitation. In general, these physiologic events are brief (less than 40 or 50 msec) when timed by spectral Doppler or color M-mode and encompass <20% of mechanical systole (see Figure 8-28, top left.).

Interpretation and Quantitation

Flow patterns mapped by CDI are examined for *spatial distribution* relative to other heart structures and *timing* within the cardiac cycle. The 2D image provides the *anatomical reference* and the *simultaneous ECG tracing* delineates time. Inasmuch as significant flow abnormalities usually occur near morphologic lesions, the approach to interpretation is logical. The examiner's eyes are usually drawn to flow acceleration, signal aliasing, or turbulence encoding suggestive of valvular regurgitation, fixed or dynamic stenosis, or abnormal direction of blood flow as might occur with shunting or regurgitant lesions. Many cardiac lesions generate eccentric jets such that long-axis, off-angle and unconventional image planes might be needed to optimally align to flow disturbances. With CDI each

2D image is composed, displayed and updated within fractions of a second so that blood flow can be displayed in real time. As a general guideline, when the frame rate during CDI approaches 50 to 60/s the temporal resolution should be excellent and slow motion video loop and frame-by-frame playback quite reliable for timing. Frame rates near the 30/s DICOM standard for digital storage are also quite acceptable in most cases when reviewed in slow motion.

However, too many examiners rely on just a real time assessment for diagnosing flow disturbances and fail to appreciate the time encompassed by the flow event within the color frames. Some CDI systems demonstrate the time interval per frame as a moving vertical line, rectangle, or break in the ECG tracing. However, this time period might not be obvious on other systems. The problem is also complicated when examinations are recorded without an accompanying ECG. As stated previously, the velocity of any CDI flow disturbance should be quantified by CW Doppler and the duration of the event carefully timed using a spectral study or color M-mode.

Advanced quantitative methods based on the continuity relationship include analysis of the *proximal isovelocity surface area* (PISA) of flow convergence region adjacent to a regurgitant valve or a cardiac shunt.[84] The PISA method combines 2D color and CWD imaging to estimate effective regurgitant or shunt orifice size.[203-206] These are somewhat complicated to perform and like the continuity relationship, require scaling to body size. Additional details are provided under "Valvular Regurgitation."

Limitations and Pitfalls of CDI

Despite the many advantages of CDI, there are some downsides and diagnostic pitfalls including those summarized in Table 8-5. The first issue is the practical matter of equipment cost that includes a need for multiple transducers. Another issue is the time one must spend to gain the training and experience needed for technical proficiency in examination and instrumentation.

Perhaps one of the most important limitations relates to timing of flow events during the CDI examination. Failure to

appreciate this point is a common source of misdiagnosis. Systems with slower processors can provide misleading information if the examiner is unaware of these limitations. For example, in a cat with a heart rate of 240 beats per minute and a CDI examination frame rate of 20/s, each cardiac cycle will be characterized by just five frames. Indeed, it is possible for late systolic and early diastolic flow events to summate in one composed frame. Furthermore, at slower processing speeds, even brief normal valve closure signals (of 20-40 msec duration) can be overemphasized leading to a misdiagnosis of valvular regurgitation during playback analysis. Lack of timing awareness can also lead to mislabeling of diastolic atrioventricular valve regurgitation, a finding so often observed in patients with bradycardias and arrhythmias, as a systolic event (see the lower panel of Figure 8-28). If 2D CDI frame rates cannot be increased by imaging controls, the solution to these temporal resolution issues is application of a rapidly processing examination like color M-mode or spectral Doppler along with simultaneous ECG recordings (Figure 8-29).

ADVANCED IMAGE ANALYSES

In addition to the 3D reconstructions discussed earlier in this chapter, a number of advanced image processing methods are available for cardiac evaluation. These applications can measure global and regional ventricular function, ventricular dyssynchrony, or the sequence of cardiac activation. There is certainly hope that these indices could be more sensitive measures of cardiac function[47] but few have been validated with gold standards or longitudinal studies in veterinary patients. Due to limited current use (and high expense) these will be briefly introduced in this chapter.

Most advanced image processing techniques assess myocardial function in a longitudinal (apical-basilar), radial (epicardial to endocardial), circumferential, or global manner.[207] Some advanced tissue analysis systems combine orthogonal datasets to construct 3D models of heart function. Nearly all are proprietary, vendor-specific, off-line image processing

TABLE 8-5

Doppler Echocardiographic Studies: Pitfalls Associated with Image Acquisition and Interpretation

Pitfall(s)	Possible Consequence(s)
Instrumentation and Examination Errors	
Failure to use appropriate frequency transducer crystals for optimal Doppler sensitivity	Too high: Underestimation of abnormal flow signal strength and spatial resolution. Too low: Overgained Doppler signals.
Inappropriate power, gain, or compression settings	Inability to visualize flow signals in spectral display. Creation of CDI artifacts.
Excessive color flow Doppler gain	Expansion of the color signal overestimating flow patterns and leading to color "bleeding" into areas without flow.
Excessive tissue gain during color flow studies Over-prioritization of the pixel for grayscale or for color (on systems where control is available)	Pixel cannot be occupied by color coding; poor color flow characterization.
Excessive pulse-wave or CW Doppler gain	Expansion and elongation of the flow "envelope" causing overestimation of velocity and lesion severity.
Inadequate filtering of low velocity, strong reflectors (including cardiac valves, chamber walls, and lungs)	Spectral and color flow artifacts. False color Doppler diagnosis of valvular regurgitation.
Excessive filtering of low velocity signals	Failure to identify low velocity flow patterns or normal signals interrogated at a wide angle.

TABLE 8-5

Doppler Echocardiographic Studies: Pitfalls Associated with Image Acquisition and Interpretation—cont'd

Pitfall(s)	Possible Consequence(s)
Excessive angle of interrogation (greater than 22 degrees to flow)	Underestimation of maximum velocity. Increased spectral dispersion in the PW-Doppler mode.
Activating angle correction features for evaluation of cardiac flow disturbances	Overestimation of true velocity and lesion severity.
Failure to use the visual and audio displays to obtain optimal Doppler signals	Inability to record peak velocities in the azimuthal plane.
Lack of familiarity with cardiac disorders	Not understanding the issues that must be addressed during the echocardiographic and Doppler study; incomplete assessment.
Failure to obtain appropriate and complementary images of the heart for Doppler studies	Missed flow disturbance(s) or over-interpretation of flow disturbances such as normal caudal vena caval return as an atrial septal defect
Failure to use appropriate transducer placement sites (e.g. subcostal position to measure aortic velocity; left apex to record mitral or tricuspid regurgitation) and enough tomographic planes	Underestimation of maximal velocity or spatial distribution for jets caused by regurgitant flow, stenosis, or shunting
Failure to recognize the simultaneous interrogation of multiple jets during CW Doppler studies	Erroneous conclusions about lesion severity. Overestimating the severity of valvular stenosis (as with crossing the jets of subaortic stenosis and mitral regurgitation)
Failure to time flow events, relative to the ECG, with spectral Doppler tracings or through color M-mode recordings	Duration of flow events is uncertain. Normal backflow or diastolic regurgitation might be misinterpreted.
Inability to maintain the PW Doppler sample volume or CW-Doppler line of interrogation within the abnormal flow throughout its duration	Limits the faithful recording of the maximal velocity Doppler spectrum during the cardiac cycle. May result in over-estimation of severity in aortic regurgitation (e.g., shortened pressure half-time)
Errors of Interpretation	
Lack of familiarity with cardiac lesions	Missed diagnoses or incomplete assessments
Assuming one can reliably image all minor lesions or definitively identify the source of all murmurs using Doppler methods	Over-interpretation of normal variation or equivocal lesions often leads to false-positive diagnoses and inappropriate therapy.
Failure to appreciate normal variation	Misdiagnosis of normal backflow, physiologic regurgitation, or diastolic regurgitation as clinically significant valve regurgitation
Over-reliance on qualitative information such as spectral dispersion in pulsed wave studies, "acceleration" of flow, or "turbulence" maps in color coded studies	Misdiagnoses such as "aortic stenosis" when the Doppler findings are related to normal flow patterns and color flow encoding; beam angulation errors; too-low settings for PRF; or normal physiology (sympathetic tone)
Over-interpreting color "bleeding"	False-positive diagnosis of atrial and ventricular septal defects and rare aorticopulmonary communications
Relying on a single frame of 2D-color information or the position of a color frame relative to the ECG (without reviewing complementary spectral Doppler or color M-mode studies)	Inadequate temporal resolution of events. Misdiagnosis of presystolic or protosystolic backflow as significant regurgitation. Misinterpreting pulmonary venous return as mitral regurgitation
Failure to appreciate the effects of cardiac output and stroke volume on Doppler derived velocities and estimated pressure gradients	False-positive diagnosis of valvular stenosis. Over or under-estimation of lesion severity. Overestimation of LVOT gradient when there is concomitant left-to-right shunting (PDA), fever, or anemia
Quantifying valvular regurgitation from only 2D color Doppler studies	Analysis of receiving chamber flow patterns in CDI might lead to misinterpretation of severity. Overestimation based on more central jets and technical factors (too much gain; lower nominal frequency; low setting for PRF). Underestimation based on eccentric jets, transducer selection, filters, and PRF
"Sizing" shunts from color Doppler studies	Erroneous estimation of shunt diameter is possible and often overestimated

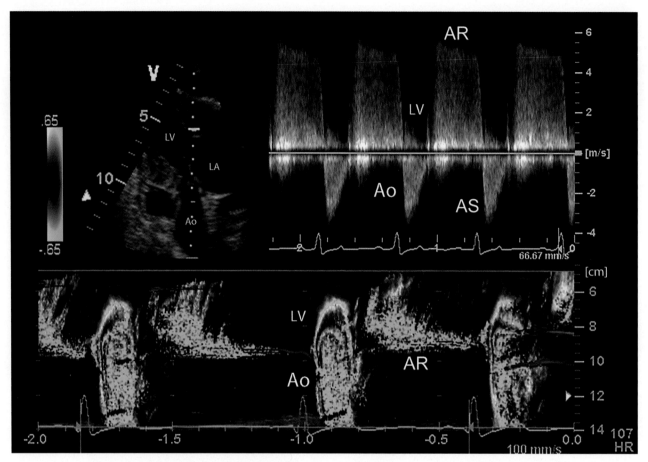

Figure 8-29 **Color M-mode Echocardiography.** The dog has subaortic stenosis and the image was obtained from a subcostal position (upper left). CW Doppler captures a moderately increased velocity profile compatible with SAS. There is also AR (above the baseline). The color M-mode study from the same direction shows a multiple-wrap signal alias within the region of flow acceleration proximal to the stenosis. This is characterized by color changes from blue to cyan to red then again to blue before turbulence encoding supervenes (green). The holodiastolic nature of the AR, encoded in green, is also clear between the second and third cardiac cycles.

computers contained within imaging systems or work stations. Some of the initial versions involved proprietary methods for analyzing Doppler shifts within multiple tissue sample volumes. Newer techniques are based on the concept of *speckle tracking*, in which patterns of myocardial reflectors are identified and tracked over the cardiac cycle. Speckle tracking has the advantage of angle independence; whereas, tissue-based Doppler recordings, like blood flow, are highly affected by angle of incidence to the US beam. Another advantage of speckle tracking relates to its relative independence from tethering. This is relevant because myocardial movements in one part of the heart can "pull" other segments—even those not actively contracting—due to tethering from adjacent myocardium and connective tissue.

Algorithms created for human hearts have been applied to canine and feline studies.[45,113-117,136,154,192,193,197,208-223] Some seem to work well, but others not at all. An overview of these advanced techniques follows. Some examples of 2D tissue-Doppler based imaging and speckle tracking technologies are shown in Figure 8-30 and Video 8-12.

Regional Doppler shifts can be measured for timing of cardiac activation, estimating systolic function, and assessing myocardial relaxation. Regions of interest can incorporate relatively large or discrete comparisons between epicardium and endocardium (myocardial gradients).[192,193,197,209,224-226] Linear tissue movements or displacement also can be measured segmentally. Sometimes called "tissue tracking" this represents a method for automating the base to apex contraction of the LV (similar to M-mode mitral annular motion) or the RV (similar to tricuspid annular plane systolic motion or TAPSE[227]).

When tissue Doppler or speckle tracking is used to measure myocardial deformation, regional or global myocardial strain and rate of deformation (strain rate) can be calculated.[45,114,116,117,207-209,212,213,215-222,228-230] Speckle tracking methods can be applied to dogs and cats, with a number of veterinary studies published on these techniques. Another proprietary method displays myocardial deformation using velocity vectors. While promising in some laboratory and human studies, it has not been determined in spontaneous canine and feline disorders if these methods offer unique functional information or just complement established indices of ventricular performance. Speckle tracking and deformation also can measure rotation of the heart at the apex and base, allowing for calculation of myocardial twist and torsion.[45,116,209,219-222] These variables have been shown to correlate to both systolic and diastolic ventricular function in humans.

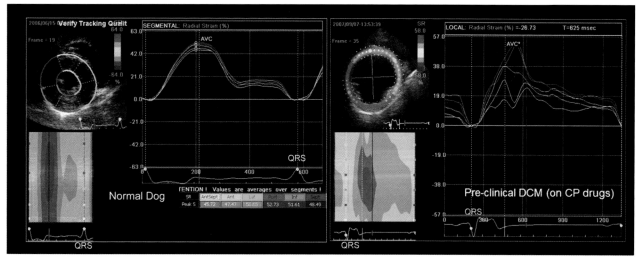

Figure 8-30 **Myocardial Strain.** Normal radial strain measurements in six regions of interest obtained from a healthy dog (left) compared to abnormal radial strain recorded from a dog with preclinical dilated cardiomyopathy (right). There is significant disparity in the peak strain velocities measured across the segments of the myocardium. A human algorithm has been applied with off-line analysis software; therefore the specific segment names are somewhat arbitrary. Nevertheless, marked reductions in deformation and in time to peak strain are evident, indicating impaired systolic function and ventricular dyssynchrony.

ASSESSMENT OF CARDIAC CHAMBER SIZE

One of the major outcomes of echocardiographic examination is measurement of cardiac chamber size. Once cardiomegaly is identified, the enlargement is graded broadly as mild, moderate, or severe. This categorization can inform prognosis, therapy, and follow-up recommendations. Intertwined with measurement of ventricular size is the quantitation of LV systolic function, specifically estimates of ejection fraction. These are calculated from measurements of ventricular diameters, areas, and volumes. Some of the approaches to identifying and assessing cardiac remodeling are considered here, while ventricular function is addressed in the subsequent section.

The literature contains a number of publications about echocardiographic measurement of normal and abnormal heart size in dogs,[34,44,96,105,107,108,111,135,138,231-246] while a smaller number address the subject in cats.[31,75,99,101,107,177,242,247-250] Most canine studies report either *breed-specific* values or combine different breeds and emphasize the importance of *body size* on chamber measurements, modeling this influence into normal reference values. In terms of feline standards, most publications report linear measurements of the LV obtained from mature cats of different breeds. Although the effect of body size is less critical in cats, it is relevant statistically in multibreed studies,[31] and might be considered when imaging the heavier feline patients. It is possible, however, that some of the larger breeds might have chamber sizes that are more dependent on breed characteristics than body size, but this requires further study. Alternative approaches for identifying cardiomegaly are based on *ratios*, especially the indexing of chamber measurements to the aorta.[107,235,237,238] Some approaches and selected values for normal cardiac size are presented in Tables 8-6 to 8-9 and Web Table 8-3.

Limitations and Suggested Approach
Considering that cardiac chamber walls can be delineated by 2D and M-mode echocardiography, the quantitation of heart size would seem straightforward. However, a number of limitations confound current approaches. Whereas physicians can refer to consensus reports and guidelines that inform cardiac mensuration,[82,83] similar standards are lacking in veterinary medicine. Most veterinarians rely on linear measurements for predicting chamber volumes and wall mass. In contrast, the standard in human echocardiography involves volumetric estimates calculated from 3D imaging or bi-plane 2DE, approaches that have been validated against the gold standard of MRI. Normal values for dogs and cats are highly influenced by species, breed, and body weight and further affected by physiologic variation, plasma volume status, heart rate and rhythm, and measurement errors. Disregarding these factors can lead to erroneous conclusions regarding the presence of cardiomegaly or ventricular hypertrophy.

The normal distribution of cardiac measurements in dogs should reflect the influence of bodyweight or surface area. This relationship is only linear within a confined range (typically near the low to middle weight range of the sample). Unfortunately, linear modeling was the standard approach taken in most early studies and still influences some published reference values.[‡] More appropriate modeling for the

---

[‡]When prediction intervals are generated for reference values, the sampling should include about 120 to 140 subjects or more; such studies are rare in veterinary medicine. Most studies, especially those evaluating a single breed, are impacted by small sample sizes or the application of inappropriate statistical methods for estimation of laboratory normals. For example, the use of a mean value plus or minus some estimate of the sample variance (two standard deviations) usually produces a prediction interval that is too narrow or too wide, depending on the sample variability and the sample size. Additional problems with published studies include the use of aortic indices based on blind M-mode recordings and obtained before the development of 2D guidance. These are statistically relevant but induce more uncertainly to reference limits because the precise method of measurement for the aorta has not been standardized or 2D guided). Furthermore, most studies are derived from a single laboratory and lack repeatability data needed to define biologic and interobserver variation.

TABLE 8-6

General Approaches for Identifying Cardiomegaly

General Method	Examples	
Subjective Assessment		
2D Echo*	Left Atrial Dilation	Rounded appearance of the left atrium
		Distended pulmonary venous confluence
		↑ Luminal axis area relative to aortic area (short-axis images)
		Distraction of atrial septum to the right
	Right Atrial Dilation	↑ Area compared to left atrial area in the right parasternal long-axis image or the left apical 4-chamber view.
		Bowing of the atrial septum to the left
	Left Ventricular Dilation & Hypertrophy	↑ Sphericity
		↑ Cross-sectional internal area compared to thickness
		Flattened papillary muscles (dilated)
		↓ Reduced LV internal area compared to wall thickness
		Tall or wide-based papillary muscles (hypertrophy)
	Right Ventricular Dilation & Hypertrophy	↑ RV area compared to LV area (4-chamber views)
		Flattening of ventricular septal motion or paradoxical motion
		↑ RV wall thickness relative to LV freewall
		↑ Thickness and trabeculation to right surface of ventricular septum
		↑ Thickness of the right ventricular papillary muscles
	Great Vessels—Dilation	Comparison of inner diameters of the two great vessels in side-by-side images
Linear Measurements	Measurement of cavity and wall dimensions compared to:	
M-mode or 2D Measurements	• Species- & breed-specific references (see Tables 8-8 and 8-9; Web Table 8-3)	
	• Allometric or logarithmic scaling (see Table 8-7)	
	• Normalized dimensions based on allometry (see Table 8-7)	
	• Reference standards for the specific variable as with long-axis left atrial diameter in cats (see text)	
Area/Volume Measurements	Calculation of atrial and ventricular volumes using:	
	• Calculation of LV volumes based on area-length methods or Simpson's method of discs	
	• Calculation of left atrial volumes based on area-length measurements or on Simpson's method of discs (see Tables 8-8 and 8-9; Web Table 8-3)	
	• Automated estimation of LV and LV volumes using 3D echocardiography with volume rendering	
Ratios	Calculation of ratios that normalize for body size (see Text and Tables 8-8 and 8-9)	
	• Left Atrial:Aorta ratio from M-mode study (cats only)	
	• Left Atrial:Aorta ratio from 2D right parasternal, short-axis image plane	
	• Left Atrial:Aortic Valve ratio from 2D right parasternal, short-axis or long-axis images	
	• Left atrial and left ventricular: Echocardiographic ratio indices (indexed to the diastolic aortic diameter or to the maximal distance between the opened AV leaflets during systole).	
	• Ventricular septal diastolic: LV diastolic wall ratios	
	• Left ventricular sphericity index	
Allometric or Power Scaling	Measuring cardiac dimensions and comparing the results to reference values based on allometry (nonlinear relationships between echocardiographic variables and body-weight)	
Breed or Species Specific References	Measuring cardiac dimensions and comparing the results to reference values based on species specific studies or breed-specific normal values (see Tables 8-8 and 8-9, and Web Table 8-3)	

*See text for details; see Figures for specific examples.

LV involves nonlinear methods or allometric scaling.[233] However, even when mathematical approaches are sound,[108] reference data can be limited by an uneven distribution of body weights within the sample, a paucity of dogs at the extremes of body size, and sampling that is biased by over-representation of certain breeds. Thus the available prediction limits defining "normal" in dogs are probably more *specific* for diagnosing moderate cardiomegaly than sensitive for recognizing mild cardiomegaly. This problem is especially acute in larger-breed dogs. The thoughtful examiner appreciates the limitations of available techniques and reference values and exercises clinical judgment when equivocal measurements are obtained.

Additional problems occur when assessing puppies, kittens and other immature patients where the young age and rate of growth is a factor. There are limited data available on the nonlinear changes observed in cardiac size related to development.[98,101,240]

Accepting these uncertainties in the veterinary landscape, the authors use a *multifaceted approach* for measuring chamber

TABLE 8-7

Identification of Left Ventricular and Left Atrial Enlargement in Dogs

Weight (kg)	LEFT VENTRICLE						LEFT ATRIUM	
	Predicted LVIDd (mm)	LVIDd 95% Prediction Limits (mm)		LVEEND = 1.70	LVWd 95% Prediction Limits (mm)		Left Atrial Size (2D)	Suggested Upper Limits
	Goncalves et al.	Cornell et al.		Based on data from Cornell et al.	Cornell et al.		Rishniw et al.	
Weight (kg)	Average LVIDd	Lower 2.5%	Upper 97.5%	LVID (mm) for Bodyweight	Lower 2.5%	Upper 97.5%	Weight Range	Long Axis Diameter (mm)
1.5	9.5	14.3	20.8	19.2	3.2	6.6	5	21
2	12.2	15.6	22.7	20.8	3.4	7.0	10	26
3	16.0	17.5	25.6	23.5	3.7	7.7	15	31
4	18.7	19.1	27.8	25.6	4.0	8.3	20	34
5	20.8	20.4	29.7	27.3	4.2	8.7	25	37
6	22.5	21.5	31.3	28.8	4.4	9.1	30	40
7	24.0	22.5	32.8	30.1	4.6	9.4	35	42
8	25.2	23.4	34.1	31.3	4.7	9.7	40	43
9	26.3	24.2	35.3	32.4	4.8	10.0	45	44
10	27.3	25.0	36.4	33.5	4.9	10.2	50	44
11	28.2	25.7	37.4	34.4	5.1	10.5	55	54
12	29.1	26.4	38.4	35.3	5.2	10.7		
13	29.8	27.0	39.3	36.1	5.3	10.9		
14	30.5	27.6	40.2	36.9	5.3	11.1		
15	31.2	28.2	41.0	37.7	5.4	11.2		
16	31.8	28.7	41.8	38.4	5.5	11.4		
17	32.3	29.2	42.6	39.1	5.6	11.6		
18	32.9	29.7	43.3	39.8	5.7	11.7		
19	33.4	30.2	44.0	40.4	5.7	11.9		
20	33.9	30.6	44.6	41.0	5.8	12.0		
21	34.3	31.1	45.3	41.6	5.9	12.2		
22	34.8	31.5	45.9	42.2	5.9	12.3		
23	35.2	31.9	46.5	42.7	6.0	12.4		
24	35.6	32.3	47.1	43.3	6.1	12.5		
25	36.0	32.7	47.7	43.8	6.1	12.7		
26	36.3	33.1	48.2	44.3	6.2	12.8		
27	36.7	33.5	48.8	44.8	6.2	12.9		
28	37.0	33.8	49.3	45.3	6.3	13.0		
29	37.4	34.2	49.8	45.7	6.3	13.1		
30	37.7	34.5	50.3	46.2	6.4	13.2		
31	38.0	34.9	50.8	46.7	6.4	13.3		
32	38.3	35.2	51.2	47.1	6.5	13.4		
33	38.6	35.5	51.7	47.5	6.5	13.5		
34	38.9	35.8	52.2	47.9	6.6	13.6		
35	39.1	36.1	52.6	48.4	6.6	13.7		
36	39.4	36.4	53.1	48.8	6.7	13.8		
37	39.7	36.7	53.5	49.1	6.7	13.9		
38	39.9	37.0	53.9	49.5	6.7	14.0		
39	40.1	37.3	54.3	49.9	6.8	14.0		
40	40.4	37.6	54.7	50.3	6.8	14.1		
41	40.6	37.8	55.1	50.7	6.9	14.2		
42	40.8	38.1	55.5	51.0	6.9	14.3		
43	41.1	38.4	55.9	51.4	6.9	14.4		
44	41.3	38.6	56.3	51.7	7.0	14.4		
45	41.5	38.9	56.7	52.1	7.0	14.5		
46	41.7	39.1	57.0	52.4	7.0	14.6		
47	41.9	39.4	57.4	52.7	7.1	14.7		
48	42.1	39.6	57.7	53.1	7.1	14.7		

Rishniw and Erb	
Left Atrium: Aorta	Short-axis, Diastolic LA:Ao
Ratio LA/Ao	1.6

Continued

TABLE 8-7

Identification of Left Ventricular and Left Atrial Enlargement in Dogs—cont'd

		LEFT VENTRICLE					
Weight (kg)	Predicted LVIDd (mm)	**LVIDd 95% Prediction Limits (mm)**		LVEEND = 1.70	**LVWd 95% Prediction Limits (mm)**		
	Goncalves et al.	Cornell et al.		Based on data from Cornell et al.	Cornell et al.		
Weight (kg)	Average LVIDd	Lower 2.5%	Upper 97.5%	LVID (mm) for Bodyweight	Lower 2.5%	Upper 97.5%	
49	42.3	39.9	58.1	53.4	7.2	14.8	
50	42.5	40.1	58.4	53.7	7.2	14.9	

LVIDd = Left ventricular end-diastolic dimension; LVWd = Left ventricular (free-)wall diameter at end-diastole
For LVIDd, predicted value = $BW^{0.294}*1.27$ (lower limit); $BW^{0.294}*1.85$ (upper limit)
For LVWd, predicted value = $BW^{0.232}*0.29$ (lower limit); $BW^{0.232}*0.6$ (upper limit)
Values for LVIDd achieving an LV end-diastolic dimension (normalized) that is equal to 1.7 multipled by the average (normalized) LVIDd from the Cornell meta-analysis. These values appear to identify mild-to-moderate LV dilation and were calculated as: $LVEDDN(1.7) = (1.7 * LVIDd)/(weight^{0.294})$, where weight is in kilograms; or $LVEDDN(1.7) = (1.7 * LVIDd)/(0.45359 * weight^{0.294})$, where weight is in pounds. The multiplier of 1.7 was selected by the authors based on results of published studies that calculated different normalized ratios, (see table reference 6), the use of this factor in ongoing clinical trials, and personal experience.
Although an upper limit of ~1.3 was identified in healthy Cavalier King Charles spaniels (table reference 4), the ratio of LA/Aorta of 1.6 is suggested as an upper limit of normal all breeds (table reference 3).
Alternative approaches include Echocardiographic Ratio Indices and Ventricular: Aortic valve and 2D left atrial: Aortic valve ratios (see text).

Table References
1. Goncalves AC, Orton EC, Boon JA, et al. Linear, logarithmic, and polynomial models of M-mode echocardiographic measurements in dogs. *Am J Vet Res* 2002;63:994–9.
2. Cornell CC, Kittleson MD, Della TP, et al. Allometric scaling of M-mode cardiac measurements in normal adult dogs. *J Vet Internal Med* 2004;18:311–21.
3. Rishniw M, Erb HN. Evaluation of four 2-dimensional echocardiographic methods of assessing left atrial size in dogs. *J Vet Intern Med* 2000;14:429–35.
4. Hansson K, Haggstrom J, Kvart C, et al. Left atrial to aortic root indices using two-dimensional and M-mode echocardiography in cavalier King Charles spaniels with and without left atrial enlargement. *Vet Radiol Ultrasound* 2002;43:568–75.
5. Hall DJ, Cornell CC, Crawford S, et al. Meta-analysis of normal canine echocardiographic dimensional data using ratio indices. *J Vet Cardiol* 2008;10:11–23.
6. Hezzell MJ, Boswood A, Moonarmart W, et al. Selected echocardiographic variables change more rapidly in dogs that die from myxomatous mitral valve disease. *J Vet Cardiol* 2012;14:269–79.

sizes, identifying cardiomegaly, and assessing ventricular function. These recommendations include: (1) *subjective assessment*; (2) use of simple *ratios that* relate chamber sizes to an aortic measurement; (3) reference values indexed to bodyweight by *allometry* or other forms of *non-linear modeling*; and (4) *breed-specific* normal ranges, when available. The situation in cats is considerably simpler as described later in this section.

Taking this approach the authors have advanced specific suggestions for identifying cardiomegaly in dogs in Table 8-6, and have tabulated some of the multi-breed study data from two larger studies in Table 8-7 along with breed-specific canine reports in Web Table 8-3. Suggested normal ranges for feline echocardiographic measurements are presented in Table 8-9. All recommendations need further refinement. Echocardiography is similar to other diagnostic laboratory tests and any cut-off value that defines "abnormal" represents some balance between test sensitivity and specificity, breed variation, and disease prevalence. Accordingly the clinician should expect both false-positive and false-negative results depending on the approach taken.

Left Atrial Size and Function
Quantitation of LA size or volume is perhaps the most important of all echocardiographic measurements.[251] Dilation (dilatation) of the LA develops from anything that increases LA pressure or volume, such as left-to-right shunting, MV disease, cardiomyopathies, and significant systolic or diastolic dysfunction of the LV. High output states, including hyperthyroidism and anemia, also can induce LA dilation, perhaps from volume retention. The LA dilates in response to primary atrial cardiomyopathies, chronic bradyarrhythmias, or persistent tachyarrhythmias with secondary LV dysfunction. When heart disease is *chronic*, the magnitude of LA enlargement relates to the hemodynamic burden of the underlying lesion, whereas normal LA size portends a more favorable short-term prognosis. Notable exceptions are peracute causes of heart failure, such as MR from ruptured chordae tendineae or infective endocarditis. In these situations LA dilation might be minimal even if CHF is severe.

Approaches to measuring LA diameter and estimating LA volume are reasonably developed in dogs and cats but far from standardized.[105,125,135,232,233,235,236,238,239,243,246-248,250,252-255] Quantitation of LA mass is far more difficult because the atrial walls are so thin. Because no standardizations or accepted guidelines are in place, a variety of different diameters, areas, and ratios have been advocated, along with some newer volumetric approaches using bi-plane 2DE or 3D methods. Although there are exceptions,[105,248] most proposed M-mode, 2D and 3D measurements of atrial size are obtained at end-systole, when atrial volumes are maximal. This point occurs just after the end of the T-wave on the ECG and more precisely

TABLE 8-8

Normal M-Mode Echocardiographic Measurements in Cats: Multi-breed Studies

	STUDY (REFERENCE)						
M-Mode Variable	Sisson[1] n = 78*	Moise[2] n = 11	Jacobs[3] n = 30	Fox[4] n = 30**	Smith[5] n = 24*	Mottet[6] n = 30*	Petric[7] n = 50*
Left Atrium (S)	11.7 ± 1.7	12.1 ± 1.8	12. ± 1.4	10.3 ± 1.4		11.0 [10.6-11.5]	
Aorta (D)	9.5 ± 1.4	9.5 ± 1.5	9.5 ± 1.1	9.4 ± 1.1		9.3 [9.1-9.5]	
Left Atrium (S): Aorta (D)	1.25 ± 0.18	1.29 ± 0.23	1.30 ± 0.17	1.10 ± 0.18		1.17 [1.13-1.21]	
Left Ventricular Diameter (D)	15.0 ± 2.0	15.1 ± 2.1	15.9 ± 1.9	14.0 ± 1.3	13.4 ± 0.2	15.0 [14.2-16.7]	13 (8.8-18.9)
Left Ventricular Diameter (S)	7.2 ± 1.5	6.9 ± 2.2	8.0 ± 1.4	8.1 ± 1.6		7.8 [7.2-8.4]	7.4 (4.0-11.4)
LV Fractional Shortening	52.1 ± 7.1	55.0 ± 10.2	49.8 ± 5.3	42.7 ± 8.1	46 ± 12	47.8 [45.5-50.0]	46 (32-68)
Interventricular Septum (D)	4.2 ± 0.7	5.0 ± 0.7	3.1 ± 0.4	3.6 ± 0.8	3.5 ± 0.8	4.0 [3.7-4.3]	4.1 (2.7-5.7)
Left Ventricular Wall (D)	4.1 ± 0.7	4.6 ± 0.5	3.3 ± 0.6	3.5 ± 0.8	3.9 ± 0.6	4.2 [3.9-4.5]	4.1 (2.3-5.7)

All linear measurements are tabulated in millimeters and expressed as mean ±SD; median (range) or mean [95% confidence interval].
See Text for specific suggestions for assessing left atrial and ventricular size.
Abbreviations: D = end-diastole; S = end-systole; LVW = left ventricular wall
*Bodyweights: Sisson: 4.7 ± 1.2 kg; Smith: 4.3 ± 0.7; Mottet: 3.97 [3.6-4.3]; Petric: 5.1 (2.2-8.0)
**Cats sedated with ketamine; heart rate mean(±SD): 255/min (±36)

Table References
1. Sisson DD, Knight DH, Helinski C, et al. Plasma taurine concentrations and M-mode echocardiographic measures in healthy cats and in cats with dilated cardiomyopathy. *J Vet Intern Med* 1991;5:232–8.
2. Moise NS, Dietze AE. Echocardiographic, electrocardiographic, and radiographic detection of cardiomegaly in hyperthyroid cats. *Am J Vet Res* 1986;47:1487–94.
3. Jacobs G, Knight DH. M-mode echocardiographic measurements in nonanesthetized healthy cats: effects of body weight, heart rate, and other variables. *Am J Vet Res* 1985;46:1705–11.
4. Fox PR, Bond BR, Peterson ME. Echocardiographic reference values in healthy cats sedated with ketamine hydrochloride. *Am J Vet Res* 1985;46:1479–84.
5. Smith DN, Schober KE. Effects of vagal maneuvers on heart rate and Doppler variables of left ventricular filling in healthy cats. *J Vet Cardiol* 2013;15:33–40.
6. Mottet E, Amberger C, Doherr MG, et al. Echocardiographic parameters in healthy young adult Sphynx cats. *Schweizer Archiv fur Tierheilkunde* 2012;154:75–80.
7. Petric AD, Rishniw M, Thomas WP. Two-dimensionally-guided M-mode and pulsed wave Doppler echocardiographic evaluation of the ventricles of apparently healthy cats. *J Vet Cardiol* 2012;14:423–30.

immediately before MV opening as visualized by 2D imaging. Again the various methods used for measurement are not interchangeable[135,246] and ultimately agreement will be needed for measurement standards validated against MRI.

Atrial Functional Indices

In addition to the previously described PWD measurement of atrial appendage velocities, a number of atrial *functional indices* can be calculated for the LA. These are not widely used but should gain greater favor with adoption of bi-plane 2D and 3D methods. These indices require measurements taken during the phasic changes of atrial volume including the times of maximal LA filling and immediately after LA emptying. These include percent changes in LA diameter or measured LA area, passive and active atrial emptying fractions, and LA ejection fraction.[125,136,246,248,254,256,257] Approaches include single and bi-plane length-area or Simpson's methods for estimating volumes and application of different M-mode cursor planes to measure fractional change. Impairment of LA function has been shown to correlate with the development of pleural effusion and to prognosis in cats with cardiac disease. However, the value of real time 3D estimation of LA ejection fraction did not correlate as well with disease severity in dogs with primary MR.[136] Deformation imaging has also been used to estimate regional LA motion,[223] but repeatability among laboratories will be needed to insure reliable results can be gleaned from canine or feline atria. The specific techniques used to measure LA function are beyond the scope of this chapter and the interested reader is directed to the references,

with the reminder that the methods used have differed somewhat across laboratories.

M-Mode Methods

Prediction of LA size based on the M-mode examination was discussed previously (see M-mode Echocardiography). The authors reemphasize this assessment severely underestimates maximum LA dimension in dogs. The cursor crosses the junction of the LA body and appendage and also (illogically) incorporates extracardiac fat when the older ASE leading-edge convention for measurement is used. Careless cursor placement can even measure the right pulmonary artery instead of the LA. In cats the body of the LA is more effectively crossed with an M-mode cursor; but still does not quantify the maximal chamber diameter.

Long-Axis Methods

Subjective recognition of LA dilation in the long-axis plane is difficult for mild chamber enlargement but often obvious when moderate to severe enlargement dilatation. In cases of chronic LA enlargement, there is often distraction of the atrial septum toward the right with dilation of the adjacent pulmonary venous ostium. Dilation associated with high LA pressure leads to a more spherical appearance of the chamber; this is especially noticeable in cats.

Maximal LA dimension at end-systole (LAs) can be measured with good repeatability from the right parasternal, 4-chamber, long-axis image optimized for the MV, and this approach is superior to radiography for detecting mild LA

TABLE 8-9

Normal M-Mode Echocardiographic Measurements in Cats: Single Breed Studies

M-Mode Variable	Gundler[1] Maine Coon cats (MCC) n = 42	Drourr[2] Male MCC n = 46	Drourr (Fe)[2] Female MCC n = 59	Chetboul[3] MCC n = 23	Granstrom[4] British Shorthair n = 282	Chetboul[5] Sphinx (Sphynx) n = 53	Mottet[6] Sphinx (Sphynx) n = 72-89	Kayar[7] Turkish Van (n = 40)
Left Atrium (S)	11.6 ± 2.0	14.4 ± 1.4	13.2 ± 1.6		9.5 (6.7-14.4)*		12.1 [11.7– 12.4]	9.4 [6.6-12.4]
Aorta (D)	8.9 ± 1.6	11.7 ± 1.2	10.8 ± 1.1		8.7 (6.1-11.5)*		9.7 [9.5-10]	8.2 [7.9-8.6]
Left atrium: Aorta	1.3 ± 0.3	1.24 ± 0.15	1.23 ± 0.16	1.0 ± 0.2	1.1 (0.9-1.4)*	0.9 ± 0.14	1.24 [1.21-1.28]	1.14 [1.0-1.3]
Left Ventricular Diameter (D)	14.8 ± 2.5	19.4 ± 1.8	17.9 ± 2.2	16.9 ± 1.8	15.0 (11.0-21.2)	15.2 ± 1.6	16.3 [15.9-16.7]	14.8 [14.2-15.4]
Left Ventricular Diameter (S)	8.7 ± 2.4	9.5 ± 1.8	8.5 ± 1.9	9.1 ± 1.5	7.4 (0.5-12.1)	7.2 ± 1.5	8.1 [7.6-8.5]	7.6 [4.6-11]
LV Fractional Shortening	41.8 ± 9.9	51.1 ± 7.6	52.4 ± 7.8	47 ± 6	50 (29-95.8)	53 ± 7	50.7 [48.5-52.8]	48.4 [45.7-51.1]
Interventricular Septum (D)	4.3 ± 1.2	4.2 ± 0.6	3.8 ± 0.7	4.7 ± 0.7	3.8 (2.6-5.2)	4.4 ± 0.4	4 [3.8-4.2]	3.7 [3.5-3.8]
Left Ventricular Wall (D)	4.1 ± 0.8	4.4 ± 0.6	4.1 ± 0.6	4.6 ± 0.6	3.8 (2.6-5.0)	4.2 ± 0.6	4.1 [4.0-4.3]	3.66 [3.4-3.9]
Bodyweight (kg)	4.9 ± 1.3	6.47 ± 0.92	4.86 ± 1.17	5.0 ± 1.0	4.1 (2.2-8.3)	3.76 ± 1.09	3.62 [3.5-3.8]	3.41 kg Females 4.16 kg Males

All linear measurements are tabulated in millimeters and expressed as mean ±SD; median (range) or mean [95% confidence interval].
See Text for specific suggestions for assessing left atrial and ventricular size.
*Left atrial and aortic diameters and ratio were calculated from short-axis, 2D images using method of Hansson.[105]
Abbreviations: D = end-diastole; S = end-systole; LVW = left ventricular wall
Significantly larger LV Internal Diameters are found in male versus female Maine Coon cats and Van cats for some variables.
A 'relatively weak, but statistically significant relationship is identified between body weight and some echocardiographic variables.

Table References
1. Gundler S, Tidholm A, Haggstrom J. Prevalence of myocardial hypertrophy in a population of asymptomatic Swedish Maine Coon cats. *Acta Vet Scand* 2008;50:22.
2. Drourr L, Lefbom BK, Rosenthal SL, et al. Measurement of M-mode echocardiographic parameters in healthy adult Maine Coon cats. *J Am Vet Med Assoc* 2005;226:734–7.
3. Chetboul V, Sampedrano CC, Tissier R, et al. Reference range values of regional left ventricular myocardial velocities and time intervals assessed by tissue Doppler imaging in young nonsedated Maine Coon cats. *Am J Vet Res* 2005;66:1936–42.
4. Granstrom S, Godiksen MT, Christiansen M, et al. Prevalence of hypertrophic cardiomyopathy in a cohort of British Shorthair cats in Denmark. *J Vet Intern Med* 2011;25:866–71.
5. Chetboul V, Petit A, Gouni V, et al. Prospective echocardiographic and tissue Doppler screening of a large Sphynx cat population: reference ranges, heart disease prevalence and genetic aspects. *J Vet Cardiol* 2012;14:497–509.
6. Mottet E, Amberger C, Doherr MG, et al. Echocardiographic parameters in healthy young adult Sphynx cats. *Schweizer Archiv fur Tierheilkunde* 2012;154:75–80.
7. Kayar A, Ozkan C, Iskefli O, et al. Measurement of M-mode echocardiographic parameters in healthy adult Van cats. *Jpn J Vet Res* 2014;62:5–15.

dilation.[255] The measured image must include the atrial septum (and fossa ovale) and the right pulmonary vein but should exclude the aorta. This approach is preferred by the authors. A digital video loop is recorded and played back frame by frame until the MV opens. The midchamber diameter is measured one or two frames prior to mitral opening. The measuring line is drawn approximately parallel to the mitral annulus, extending from the inner edge of the fossa ovale to the internal reflection of the pericardium, which is bright (Figure 8-3, B and C and Figure 8-31, B). If multiple bright echoes are evident, the border can be informed by following the pericardial echo up from the LV. This LA diameter is related to body size, and can be compared to published normals[232] as shown in Table 8-7 or indexed to one or more measurements of the aorta.[232,235,237-239,243,246,248]

One of the authors commonly uses a simple long-axis *ratio* of LAs divided by the distance between the opened AV leaflets in systole (AVs). The ratio LAs/AVs in dogs is normally <2.6.§ The LAs is measured as just described. The maximal opening distance between the AV leaflets (or the valve hinge points) is measured during early- to mid-systole from the right parasternal long-axis image optimized for the AV (Figure 8-31, B). Importantly, this A-V measurement does *not* include the far field sinus of Valsalva. The systolic LA to diastolic LV ratio also can be constructed and this ratio is close to unity in normals, and typically ranges from 0.85 to 1.15. The LV is measured at end-diastole at the chordal level in the same 2D

---

§JDB: personal observations in 50 healthy dogs

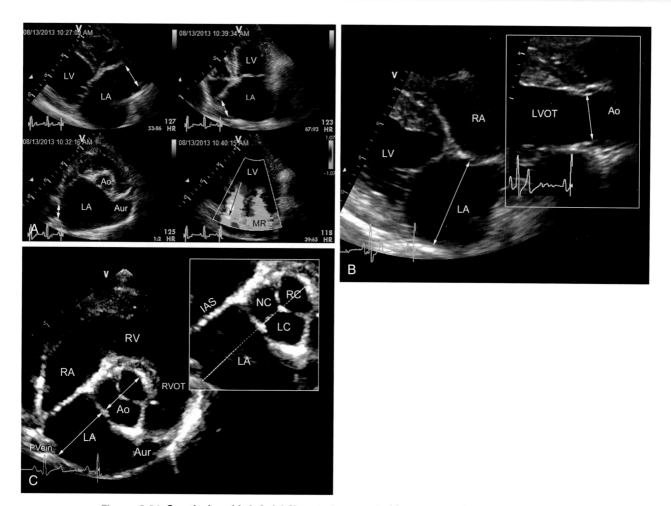

Figure 8-31 Quantitation of Left Atrial Size. A, Severe LA dilatation in a dog with chronic MR. From the lower left, clockwise, the image planes are a short axis image at the level of the aorta and left atrium; an angled right parasternal image, left apical 4-chamber view, and left apical five chamber view. These demonstrates severe dilatation (relative to the aorta); distraction of the atrial septum to the right; dilation of the pulmonary venous ostia (*arrows*), and increased mid-chamber diameter. The color Doppler shows a jet of MR along with flow entering the aorta (*long arrow*). **B,** Measurement of distance between the aortic valve leaflets during systole (inset) taken from the right parasternal, long-axis image. A measurement can be taken between the maximally opened leaflets (*arrows*) or the valve hinge points during early to mid-systole. The LA is measured as shown previously in Fig. 8-3B. The usual ratio of long-axis LA diameter to AV distance in dogs is <2.6. See text for details. **C,** Measurement of LA size in a dog according to the method of Hansson[105] using the diastolic LA/Aortic ratio from the right parasternal short-axis image of the aorta. The aortic diameter is drawn along the commissure of the left (LC) and noncoronary (NC) cusps and often include the sinus of Valsalva of the right coronary cusp (RC). The atrial measurement is taken by continuing the aortic line to the edge of the pulmonary, which should not be entered. An alternative method for measuring aortic size draws the line across the commissure of the right and noncoronary cusps of the aortic valve (see Rishniw and Erb[232]). See text for details.

long-axis plane used to measure the LA (or alternatively, obtained from conventional M-mode echocardiography). Disproportional LV dilatation (with less LA enlargement) is observed in some early cases of dilated cardiomyopathy or with isolated AR; this usually results in LA/LV <0.85. Conversely severe LA dilatation associated with MR often leads to both increased LAs/AVs and LAs/LVd >1.15 when using this specific method of measurement.

The same long-axis diameter of the LA can be measured in cats, but again the aorta must be *excluded* from the image so at least the fossa ovale is evident. The upper limit of normal for LA diameter in a mature cat is ≈16 mm,[94,255] but adjustments must be made for a kitten or small adult, or when dealing with a larger feline breed (for which 17 to 18 mm is a more appropriate upper limit). As a clinical guideline, an LA long-axis diameter of 20 mm is considered at least moderate LA dilation and represents a higher risk for atrial thrombosis and arterial thromboembolism. LA diameter exceeding 24 mm in the long axis represents a severe state of dilatation.

Short-Axis Methods

It is somewhat easier to develop a subjective impression of LA dilatation using the short-axis image, provided the image plane is consistent and includes a clear picture of the aorta and the left atrial appendage (auricle). The auricle becomes especially prominent in cats with LA dilatation. This image plane also has been used to trace end-systolic LA area, but LA area seems to offer no greater sensitivity for detecting LA enlargement in cats than the simpler long-axis diameter previously described.[255]

Other LA dimensions can be derived from a short-axis image at the level of the AV. Because the precise image planes can vary with transducer positioning and angulation, it can become difficult to standardize these approaches. As one example, the largest short-axis dimension can be obtained in *end-systole* by drawing a line that extends from the right-caudal edge of the aortic root to the LA wall near the entry of the pulmonary venous ostium. Normal values are similar to the long-axis diameter described above.

A more popular short-axis approach involves calculating the *ratio* of an LA measurement to a diameter of the aortic root, with both measurements obtained in early *diastole***.[105,232] The measurements are made from a frozen 2D image from the first frame in which closed AV leaflets are identified. The aortic line is drawn along the closed commissure formed by the noncoronary and left coronary cusps and extended the inner aortic walls to include one sinus of Valsalva (Figure 8-31, C). This aortic measurement line is used to guide a second diagonal line that crosses the LA to record an internal LA dimension. The LA/Ao ratio in most normal dogs and cats is <1.3 to 1.4 (varying with authors), and values exceeding 1.5 to 1.6 in dogs are suggestive of LA enlargement, especially if long-axis imaging and measurements support the diagnosis of LA dilation. Despite widespread use, there are some drawbacks to this approach. First, the maximal LA diameter is not measured compared to a long-axis method. The atrial plane is not standardized among investigators so some use a short-axis image that excludes the pulmonary venous ostium, while others include the vein as a landmark. Perhaps most importantly, if closed AV leaflets cannot be identified until mid- or late-diastole, the LA continues to empty and LA size is underestimated. While the method is consistent in the hands of experienced examiners, differences in the image plane or the timing of measurement can lead to variable results.

Volume Estimates
The estimation of LA volumes is the ultimate goal in assessing LA size and will undoubtedly increase as 3D imaging becomes more available. In humans 3D echo provides the best estimate of LA volumes compared to MRI.[251] The approach is also well-suited to assess phasic changes in LA function. Some recent papers have evaluated LA volumes using either 3D or bi-plane 2D approaches in dogs.[135,241] Specific maximal volumes reported as upper limit values for dogs are 0.92 mL/kg[254] and 1.1 mL/kg[46] depending on the method.

Left Ventricular Chamber Size
The diseased LV can undergo a number of morphologic adaptations, including: simple dilation (dilatation); dilation with a normal wall thickness (eccentric hypertrophy); wall thickening at the expense of the ventricular lumen (concentric hypertrophy); and concentric hypertrophy with chamber dilatation (mixed hypertrophy). Simple dilatation is seen in the worst cases of dilated cardiomyopathy or myocarditis. Eccentric hypertrophy is typical of volume overload (valvular regurgitation, left-to-right shunts) and compensated dilated cardiomyopathy. Concentric hypertrophy is most often seen with aortic stenosis, hypertrophic cardiomyopathy, systemic hypertension, and in some cases of hyperthyroidism and obesity.[258] Mixed hypertrophy is observed in combined aortic stenosis/insufficiency, with aortic stenosis or hypertrophic cardiomyopathy complicated by myocardial failure, and in some cases of chronic hyperthyroidism.

Linear, area, and volumetric methods can be used for analysis of LV size. Traditionally veterinarians have focused on linear measurements, from the M-mode examination or frozen 2D image. Such measurements are really surrogates of ventricular volume, which represents a better standard for the identification of cardiomegaly (and the estimation of LV ejection fraction). Some of the volumetric approaches used for examinations of people are applicable to animals; these are mentioned below and summarized in Figure 8-32, A. Ventricular hypertrophy refers to an increase in ventricular mass, not simply to an increase in wall thickness. As indicated, a dilated ventricle with normal wall thickness would represent an eccentrically-hypertrophied chamber. With concentric hypertrophy, cardiac mass is also increased but characterized mainly by wall thickening with a normal to reduced luminal size. Although it is possible to estimate overall ventricular mass by combining various wall and area measurements, linear determinations of wall thicknesses represent a more practical approach. As discussed below, *multiple* measurements of the same wall segment should be averaged to reduce the influence of measurement errors.

There is a tendency to perform serial echocardiograms in patients to "follow heart size." However, once moderate to severe ventricular remodeling has been identified, follow-up studies should probably be focused on other more pertinent issues such as Doppler estimates of ventricular filling pressures, PA pressures, and risk factors for atrial thrombosis (in cats). Once cardiomegaly is obvious, serial measurements of LV internal diameter or volume are unlikely to change patient management unless the values offer useful prognostic information or dictate a specific treatment plan. Such guidelines must be based on clinical trial data, and currently these are limited.[259,260]

Models for Estimating Left Ventricular Volume
The various approaches used when measuring the LV involve some geometric assumptions about the chamber and its volume. The simplest models view the chamber as a sphere or ellipsoid and these assumptions generate the volumes and ejection fraction values reported by echocardiographic analysis packages. Most M-mode estimates of volume are based on the LV as a sphere in which volume (V) is a function of the cube of the radius (r), as $V = 4/3\pi r^3$.[2,9] This radius (diameter/2) is obtained from the frozen 2D image or from the M-mode study (see Figures 8-3, A; 8-3, E; 8-5, A; and 8-12, B). Most veterinary echocardiographic reporting systems modify these volumes using the Teichholz correction (where volume = 7/[2.4 + diameter] * diameter^3). While simple linear measurements for estimating LV volumes are easy to obtain and therefore attractive, characterizing the volume and function of the LV from one minor dimension can be inaccurate. This is especially true in the settings of ventricular dilatation or segmental motion abnormality. While the Teichholz correction might yield reasonable volume estimates in a normal ventricle,[27,244,261] this has not always been found.[138] More importantly, both LV diastolic and end-systolic volumes are reportedly overestimated in dogs when there is ventricular dilation, likely related to geometric changes in the mid-ventricle.[241,262] Volume overestimation can interfere with calculation of an end-systolic volume index from the M-mode study; the results might indicate impaired systolic function even while other functional indices point the opposite way.

Area-length and ellipsoid models of the LV combine 2D area traces with linear measurements of LV length to estimate ventricular volumes. Contraction in multiple short-axis segments and in the apical to basilar direction are incorporated and volumes then estimated with formulae that model the LV as a prolate ellipsoid, a truncated (cut off) ellipsoid, or a bullet

---

**Other echocardiography laboratories have modified the timing of the measurement and use different normal values

LV VOLUME

Method of Discs (modified Simpson's rule)

Two chamber view   Four chamber view

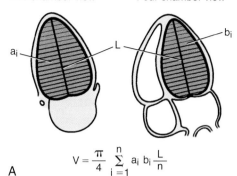

Single Plane Area Length Method

Two or four chamber view

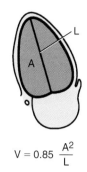

$$V = \frac{\pi}{4} \sum_{i=1}^{n} a_i \, b_i \, \frac{L}{n}$$

A

$$V = 0.85 \, \frac{A^2}{L}$$

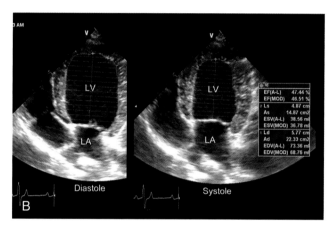

EF(A-L)   47.44 %
EF(MOD)   46.51 %
Ls   4.87 cm
As   14.87 cm2
ESV(A-L)   38.56 ml
ESV(MOD)   36.78 ml
Ld   5.77 cm
Ad   22.33 cm2
EDV(A-L)   73.36 ml
EDV(MOD)   68.76 ml

Diastole   Systole

B

Figure 8-32 **Quantitation of Left Ventricular Size.** **A,** Methods for measuring LV volumes using 2D imaging are shown. The method of discs (Simpson's rule) requires a tracing of the endocardial borders and the apical to basilar length in diastole and systole. The left apical four chamber image is used for one measurement and for a "bi-plane" estimate (that averages values from orthogonal planes), either the right parasternal long-axis image (the authors' preference) or the left apical two chamber view (shown here) is also measured. A single plane method can also be used either from a 4- or 2-chamber image or from the right parasternal long–axis image plane, whichever provides the greatest length. Alternative formulae are available for volume calculations, including the area-length method shown in the lower figure. The software analysis package is usually preset for the method preferred by the clinician. **B,** Measurements of LV internal area and length using the left apical 4-chamber view. Diastole is shown on the left; systole on the right. Once the areas and lengths are traced, the echocardiographic software estimates volume using an area-length formula or fills the chamber with discs for estimation of ventricular volume using a modified Simpson's rule. In this example, the two results provide nearly identical values for LV ejection fraction (EF), about 47%.

(see Weyman's textbook,[9] pp. 588-590, for an expansive list). The approach of choice among the area–length methods is the method of discs (Simpson's rule), which models the LV chamber as a series of circular plates extending from the mitral orifice to the apex (Figure 8-32). LV volumes in dogs can be obtained by measuring right parasternal long-axis images optimized for the LV inlet and the left apical 4- and 2-chamber images. Incorporation of LV area and length should more accurately predict the EDV (and therefore LV enlargement) as well as the ESV (and LV systolic function) but at the expense of requiring more time for image acquisition and measurement. Other impediments to these approaches in dogs relate to truncation of the long-axis plane (foreshortened length), poor endocardial border resolution (especially at the apex), and translational motion of the LV. Examples of the latter are the sudden appearance of the posterior papillary muscle into the systolic image frame and translation of the heart out of the image plane resulting in apparent apical-basilar contraction. The accuracy of different 2D volumetric approaches compared to a gold standard (MRI) still must be determined.

Either a bi-plane (Simpson's) method of discs or a 3D volumetric rendering is used for LV volume measurements in human echocardiography laboratories. Both approaches have been applied to dogs[241,245,263] and will likely become the standard for measurement in the future. For the Simpson's method, the echocardiographic analysis package must be programed to apply either a single or bi-plane approach. The method of discs (see the top of Figure 8-32) adjusts for geometric remodeling, apical to basilar shortening, and segmental dysfunction. The greatest limitation to wider application of 2D methods, especially for detection of LV dilation, is the need for more extensive reference values. Obviously the introduction of 3D methods will lag further based on the costs of equipment. Estimation of ventricular EF using volumetric approaches is further discussed in the section on "Ventricular Function".

Subjective Methods

Experienced examiners have little difficulty subjectively recognizing moderate to severe LV enlargement (Figure 8-33; Video 8-18). In the long-axis plane an increased sphericity of the chamber with rounding of the apex is suggestive of cardiomegaly. In short-axis images, a "squashing" of the mushroom-shaped LV lumen at the papillary muscle level is indicative of significant chamber enlargement. Concentric hypertrophy is usually recognized as a relatively greater area encompassed by the ventricular walls and papillary muscles in the short-axis image planes. Imaging too apically can lead to false-positive subjective diagnosis of LV hypertrophy.

Ratios in Dogs

As with the left atrium, a number of relatively simple ratios have been suggested that incorporate linear measurements of the LV and aorta.[107,238] Assuming aortic size is normal, or a breed-specific aortic measurement is available (as would be needed for breeds like boxers and bull terriers),[237,264] these aortic-based ratios are potentially more sensitive for detecting mild cardiomegaly. Aortic size can be measured from the patient under study or obtained from a published nomogram

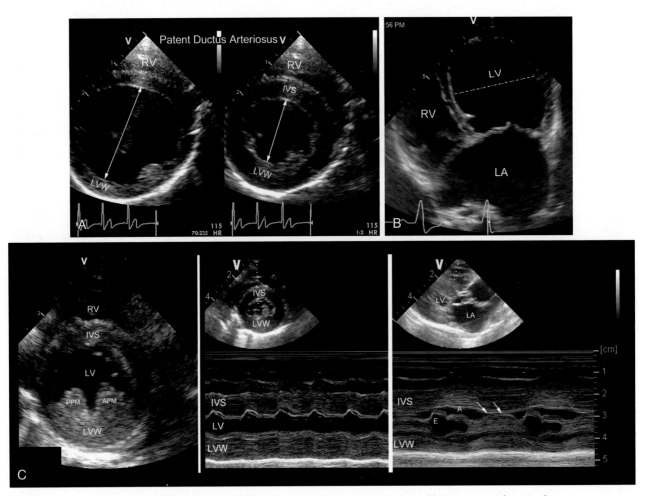

Figure 8-33 **Left Ventricular Enlargement. A,** Moderate to severe LV dilatation is evident in the end-diastolic frame (left) obtained from a dog with left-to-right shunting patent ductus arteriosus. Compare the overall size and shape of the cavity in this short-axis image to that of a normal ventricle (Fig. 8-5, *A*). Global systolic function appears preserved in this case as evidenced by the appearance of the LV at end-systole (right). **B,** Increased sphericity in a dog with dilated cardiomyopathy. Rounding of the chamber and expansion across the midventricle leads to a reduced sphericity index ratio. Note that the M-mode examination would preferentially sample this midventricular region. See text for details. **C,** Concentric hypertrophy in feline hypertrophic cardiomyopathy. Left: LV wall thickening is shown in the short-axis 2D image. The papillary muscles are affected and "blend" into the LV wall. Center: The M-mode study from the same cat at the level of the papillary muscles shows the marked thickening of both the IVS and the LVW. Wall motion is also diminished, indicating a high risk for development of congestive heart failure or arterial thromboembolism. Right: Interventricular septal and LV wall hypertrophy are evident and with mitral-septal contact (*arrows*) during systole. The mitral valve also appears thickened during opening movements (E and A). Note that at this level the cursor crosses the more dorsal aspect of the LVW and thickness is much less than that at the level of the papillary muscles.

related to body weight.[235,237,238] As discussed under LA measurements previously, the technique used for aortic measurement—M-mode vs. short-axis (diastolic) vs. distance between opened AV leaflets—significantly affects the calculated ratios and cannot be used interchangeably. For example, if the aortic root measurement that includes one sinus of Valsalva is used, the ratio of LVd/Ao will be smaller than for a ratio of LVd/AV where the sinus is excluded. There is simply no accepted veterinary standard. Some of the various ratios used for detecting LV dilatation in dogs are summarized in Table 8-6. The authors have used a simple ratio of LV *diastolic* dimension (from 2D or M-mode) divided by the maximal *systolic* distance between the opened aortic leaflets in a long-axis view. This is used mainly to identify mild LV dilation when multi-breed confidence intervals are too wide to detect mild cardiomegaly. This LVd/AVs ratio is usually <1.6 in dogs <20 kg. The major pitfalls of this approach involve identifying the opened valve leaflets and excluding the left sinus of Valsalva from the measurement (see previous discussion and Figure 8-31, *B*). This method requires independent validation. The *diastolic* ratio of LV to short-axis aortic root diameter was a predictor of first onset of CHF in one trial of dogs with severe, chronic MR.[260] In that study the median LVd/Ao ratio was 2.8 versus a median of 2.0 in dogs with MR but without CHF. In another study the change in LV diameter to LV wall ratio, among other variables, was a predictor of cardiac mortality.[259]

Another ratio reported in dogs is the ventricular sphericity index, which is probably influenced by combined effects of LV remodeling, systolic ventricular function, and ventricular filling pressures. This is a diastolic ratio of LV length (from mitral annulus to LV apex) divided by the LV minor dimension (from M-mode or 2D measurement). With cardiomegaly from DCM or from advanced mitral valve disease, the LV becomes more spherical, and the sphericity index becomes smaller.[118,122,135] Some normal values for sphericity index have been published for certain breeds and have been used to predict a diagnosis of DCM. For example, a value <1.65 was considered diagnostic of DCM in the Doberman pinscher breed,[122] a value similar to that suggested in a consensus report on DCM.[265] This index should progressively decrease with incipient or overt CHF. The value of this index for identifying *preclinical* DCM in different breeds remains to be determined.

Measurements Indexed to Body Size in Dogs

The use of *multi-breed canine reference values* based on *allometric* or another form of nonlinear modeling to body weight is another recommended approach for evaluating the LV. As indicated in the introduction to this topic, most of the published multibreed data sets are based are relatively small samples; furthermore, measured values have often been compared to body weight only with linear regression.

Selected data for LV diastolic diameter and LV diastolic wall thickness, derived from two of the larger multi-breed studies,[108,233] are shown in Table 8-7. In each study a nonlinear modeling of LV diastolic dimension to body weight provided a superior fit to the data for LV internal dimension, although the mean values are somewhat different between the two studies. The metaanalysis of 494 dogs[108] was well powered and conducted with rigorous statistical methods and as a result these study data are widely used to diagnose cardiomegaly. However, as discussed by the authors, the retrospective nature of the data collection, different sampling methods, and interobserver differences resulted in relatively wider reference limits than might have been anticipated from prospectively-collected data. Additionally, this metaanalysis included a preponderance of sight-hounds and Irish Wolfhounds (nearly 40% of the sample). The practical relevance of this is that mild or even mild-to-moderate cardiac enlargement might be missed using these prediction intervals.

However, another potentially useful variable derived from this canine meta-analysis is so-called LV end-diastolic normalized dimension. This is a single value that relates the LV end-diastolic dimension to a specific body size using the formula LVEDND/(body weight [kg])$^{0.294}$ Once values for this index exceed 1.7 at least mild to moderate LV enlargement is likely.[108] Clinical experience indicates this cutoff relates to cardiomegaly based on vertebral heart size and presence of concurrent LA enlargement. In one clinical trial, dogs that survived had a median normalized LVEDD of 1.8 whereas those that died within 6 months of their last examination had a median value of 2.2.[259] Calculated "cutoffs" this for index for increasing body weight are also presented in Table 8-7. Note that these values actually fall *within* the prediction limits for the LV internal dimension, again suggesting the meta-analysis data are likely better for identifying moderate to severe cardiac enlargement. Based on clinical experience, values of LVEDND ≥1.7 represent a relatively specific cutoff for LV dilation but perhaps not a sensitive one.

Canine Breed-Specific Reference Values

If a *breed-specific* reference range is available for comparison it should be consulted, accepting that most of these studies are based on small samples, come from a single laboratory, and lack estimates of repeatability. Nevertheless, such references can be quite useful because in addition to bodyweight, both the somatotype[266] and breed[102,121,231,252,253,264,267-276] appear to influence normal LV size. The authors have tabulated some of the published, breed-specific reference values and have posted this information in the on-line textbook content in Web-Table 8-3.

In addition to linear measurements of LV internal dimensions and wall thicknesses, there are some breed-specific studies evaluating 2D-based estimates of LV volume. Studies of boxers and Doberman pinschers have been published along with some comparisons of linear vs. length area approaches for volume estimation in other breeds. In normal boxers end-diastolic volumes indexed to body surface area was 49 to 93 ml/m^2 for diastole and 22 to 50 ml/m^2 for end-systole.[245] In Doberman pinschers, cutoffs suggested by the authors were end-diastolic and end-systolic volume indices greater than 95 ml/m^2 and 55 ml/m^2, respectively.[263]

Left Ventricular Measurements in Cats

Reference values reported for cats have been slightly more uniform, probably related to the smaller dispersion in body size; however, LV internal dimension does demonstrate a weak statistical correlation to body size[31] and also might be influenced by breed. Minor LV internal diameter in healthy cats averages about 15 to 16 mm in diastole, and is generally less than 19 to 20 mm (Tables 8-8 and 8-9). Diastolic LV diameters as large as 21 or 22 mm are sometimes observed in larger breeds like the Maine Coon cat; however, the ventricular walls do not appear any thicker than domestic cats despite the luminal size (see below).[247,249] The reported LV end-systolic dimension in cats averages about 7 to 8 mm[99] and relates to contractility and ventricular loading. The internal diameter will be underestimated (and wall thickness overestimated) if the measurement fails to exclude the papillary muscles.

Left Ventricular Mass in Dogs and Cats

Measurement of the ventricular walls and identification of LV hypertrophy can be obtained through measurements of M-mode or frozen 2D images (see Figures 8-3, *A*; 8-5, *A*; and 8-12, *B*). These measurements are obtained at end-diastole, roughly between the onset or the QRS complex and peak of the R-wave. Systolic measurements of wall thickness are strongly affected by myocardial contractile function and ventricular afterload, and are therefore inappropriate for diagnosing ventricular hypertrophy. Most reference ranges are based on linear measures of LV and septal wall thicknesses across the chordal level as recorded with M-mode techniques (See prior section on M-mode Echocardiography). While M-mode measurements are appropriate in the setting of uniform ventricular wall thickness, the measurements become misleading if the cursor fails to sample the thickest parts of the ventricular walls. For this reason the exam should first be guided by 2D inspection of the ventricle for any regional hypertrophy (Figure 8-33, C). If asymmetry is evident, 2D measurements of affected segments should be included along with the standard M-mode dimensions. Additionally the report should include a *narrative describing the distribution* of any wall thickening (or thinning), as this information can hold diagnostic or prognostic significance. For example, in a cat with HCM, diffuse LV freewall hypertrophy is more likely to progress to CHF as compared to focal, subaortic hypertrophy, even if both situations are labeled "hypertrophic." As a practice guideline, the authors recommend routinely measuring the thickest segments of the IVS and LVW identified from both right parasternal long- and short-axis planes. This is especially relevant to cats.

The interpretation of LV wall thicknesses in dogs must be done within the context of bodyweight or surface area (Table 8-7). The ratio of diastolic dimensions of the IVS and LVW is approximately 1:1 in dogs, although the septum will be slightly thicker if both RV and LV endocardial borders are included in the measurement. In contrast to the dog, a slightly thicker dimension for the IVS than LVW is common in cats, especially if both endocardial borders are included. The upper limits of normal for the septum is uncertain in breeds like the Bengal cat where asymmetrical measurements might be the norm. Papillary muscles should also be inspected for gross hypertrophy. Cats with increased LV wall thickness often have papillary muscle thickening, but there is substantial overlap between affected and normal cats for papillary muscle measurements rendering these of limited value for detection of mild disease.[277] In the Maine coon cat papillary muscle thickening has been reported as an early finding of HCM.[278]

Most cardiologists select between 5.5 to 5.9 mm as an upper limit of normal for diastolic wall thicknesses in cats (measured on frozen 2D images). As a guideline, the authors use a diastolic thickness exceeding ≥5.5 mm as a relatively sensitive cutoff for ventricular hypertrophy and a value of ≥6 mm specific for LV hypertrophy.[279] However, not all cardiologists agree with these limits and some contend that an upper limit of 5 mm might be more reasonable.[249] Experience has taught that M-mode wall measurements can be thinner than ones obtained from frozen 2D images in the same cat, perhaps related to better temporal resolution and border delineation. This may be a practical factor to consider. Additionally, many older cats have focal dorsal upper septal hypertrophy (DUST in humans). The pathogenesis and clinical importance of this subaortic thickening is unresolved but could be related to dilatation in the proximal aorta, as is observed in both cats and in people.[2] Linear and area measures of wall segments also can be used to calculate ventricular mass, but these methods are beyond the scope of this discussion.[††]

A number of pitfalls are relevant to measurement of LV wall thickness. Cats are frequently misdiagnosed with LV hypertrophy due to these errors of recording or interpretation. Overgained or powered studies can cause blooming of bright ventricular walls. Allowing an M-mode cursor to cross a papillary muscle by failing to delineate the caudal papillary muscle from the LV freewall commonly leads to inaccuracies of measurement.[280] As discussed previously, the latter problem can be minimized by using the long-axis image to identify the dorsal extent of the posterior papillary muscle. Including the tricuspid septal leaflet or the LV trabecula septomarginalis (the false tendons or moderator bands that track along the left septal surface) in measurements of septal thickness is another common error. Additionally, caution must be exercised when diagnosing ventricular hypertrophy in volume-depleted patients because hemorrhage or the loss of plasma volume from dehydration or diuretic therapy can reduce LV cavity size and filling.[179,281] The loss of intraluminal distending pressure at end-diastole increases the wall thickness, sometimes dramatically. This pseudohypertrophy mimics hypertrophic cardiomyopathy and other causes of concentric hypertrophy.

The depth of field and size of the patient can increase the chance of an erroneous diagnosis. For example, at an imaging depth of 4 to 5 cm, the inclusion of one versus two endocardial border thicknesses for the IVS (or about 2 pixels!) can change the septal measurement by up to 0.5 mm, tipping the diagnosis in a cat from normal to HCM. It is important to measure wall thicknesses using 2D images in cats; however, the anatomic clarity provided during real-time, 2D imaging is degraded once the image is frozen. Still frames from systems (or instrument setting) with slow 2D processing can substantially blur the endocardial borders of the rapidly-beating feline heart. Even the separation of end-diastole from early-systole can be confused, especially when ECG leads are unattached. The latter problem can be circumvented by leveraging the high temporal resolution of the M-mode study, provided the M-line can be directed across the zone of *representative* wall thickness and the endocardial borders are *clear*. High quality 2D images, endocardial border resolution and careful M-mode cursor placements, as well as averaging three or more measurements of the same segment, can circumvent many mistakes.

Right-Sided Chambers

The right atrial and RV cavities are more complex geometrically and are therefore more difficult to quantify. The acoustic windows available for imaging of right heart structures are also limited. The RV cavity is difficult to assess subjectively or measure consistently because it appears as either a rapidly tapering triangle when viewed from the right parasternal long-axis view or a crescent adjacent to the LV or aorta when viewed in the short-axis planes (see Figures 8-3, A; 8-5, A, D and E; and 8-8, B). The size of the RA from the right parasternal windows depends in part on how dorsally one places or angulates the transducer and a good acoustic window can lead to overestimation of RA size. The left apical four chamber view (see Figures 8-6, A and 8-7, A) is probably better for subjective identification of moderate to severe RA enlargement, as both atria are relatively circular in this plane and the LA normally appears slightly larger than the right atrium when the two atria are viewed side-by-side.

The RV freewall diastolic and systolic thickness can be measured with a higher frequency transducer from the right parasternal windows. Diastolic thickness is typically about 1/3 of the LVW and should be <50% of the LV measurement if pericardial echoes are excluded. Reported RV internal dimensions are smaller than for the LV when measured by M-mode from the right thorax. There are no definitive studies

---

[††]The general approach involves measuring internal endocardial area, external epicardial area, and calculating the difference. Myocardial tissue volume is then calculated based on a mathematical model of the ventricle and multiplied by 1.05 (the specific gravity of myocardial tissue) to obtain ventricular mass.[3]

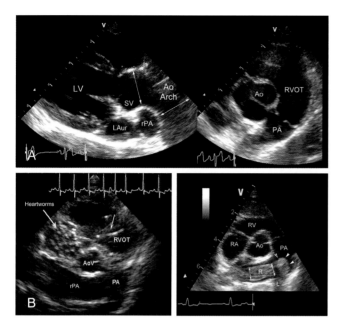

Figure 8-34 Dilatation of the Great Vessels. A, Idiopathic aortic dilatation in a dog. Left: The aortic root is dilated and a portion of a dilated aortic arch also can be seen. Right: The short axis image from the same dog shows relatively larger aortic root than pulmonary artery at the levels of the semilunar valves. Blood pressure and the aortic valve were normal with no evidence of subaortic stenosis or dynamic LVOT obstruction. **B,** Left panel: Dilation of the main and right PA in a dog with severe dirofilariasis, pulmonary hypertension, and caval syndrome. A mass of echogenic heartworms can be identified in the right atrium (*left arrow*) and adult parasite with a distinctive acoustic signature of paired hyperchoic lines surrounding a sonolucent center is present in the RVOT (*right arrow*). Right panel: Similar short axis view from another dog, a Cavalier King Charles spaniel, with a large pulmonary artery thrombosis (*double arrows*) extending from the main PA and into both main branches. The thrombus is believed to have formed in situ. The edge is rounded, typical of a chronic thromboses exposed to blood flow (*arrowheads*).

of internal right atrial or RV measurements, and the clinician is frequently forced to use experience and multiple image planes to identify right-sided cardiomegaly. Defining mild RV enlargement is especially challenging.

Great Vessels
Cardiomegaly might be accompanied by dilation of the aorta or the pulmonary artery (Figure 8-34; Video 8-19). Dilation of the pulmonary artery is usually associated with three major abnormalities: left-to-right shunts, PHT (including dirofilariasis), and pulmonic stenosis. Idiopathic PA dilation is encountered infrequently. The differential diagnosis for dilation of the aorta is more extensive and includes: (sub)aortic stenosis, patent ductus arteriosus, malformations of the conotruncal septum (tetralogy of Fallot, pulmonary atresia), systemic hypertension, idiopathic aortopathy, and hypertrophic obstructive cardiomyopathy. Middle aged to older cats often develop idiopathic dilation sometimes with tortuosity of the aorta. Idiopathic aortic dilatation is also identified regularly in dogs and falls within the differential diagnosis when radiography suggests a craniodorsal heart base mass. Leonberg dogs have been reported to have familial aneurysm of the aorta.[282]

Dilatation of a great vessel is often evident from subjective evaluation. Normal values for aortic root dimension (at the level of the AV), aortic sinuses, and the ascending aorta have

been reported for dogs in multibreed studies and also in some specific breeds with a high prevalence of heart disease, including the boxer and Cavalier King Charles spaniel.[105,283] Most of the aortic measurements reported—whether from M-mode examinations or 2D images—include one sinus of Valsalva. Many examiners perform a subjective assessment or compare the aorta in cross-section to the PA in long-axis (see Figure 8-5, *F*). Importantly, dimensions across the aortic sinuses are significantly wider than those measured between the attachment (hinge) points of the AV, the opened valve leaflets, or the sinotubular junction.[41] As a guideline, the normal main PA just distal to the pulmonic valve appears no wider than the short-axis aorta at the same level. Assuming normal aortic dimensions, this rule of thumb can be used to identify a dilated or attenuated pulmonary artery (Fig. 8-34).

VENTRICULAR FUNCTION

Noninvasive quantitation of ventricular systolic and diastolic function can inform diagnosis, prognosis, and therapy. The ventricles can be assessed globally, as in estimation of ejection fraction (EF), or regionally, as with tissue-based calculations of myocardial velocities and strain. While most published studies of ventricular function refer to the LV, recent investigations have focused on the RV as well.[81,139,227,284-286] At least fifty measured, calculated, or derived echocardiographic variables have been proposed to assess how the heart fills and pumps.[2,3,9] Some of these function studies are summarized in Table 8-10.

The clinical priority is for a limited number of indices that are impactful, reliable, and relatively efficient to obtain. An understanding of ventricular function tests requires some knowledge of the underlying concepts of myocardial contraction and chamber shortening, including: (1) inotropic state prior to the influence of ventricular loading; (2) ventricular preload (related to filling volume); (3) ventricular afterload (forces opposing shortening and ejection); and (4) electrical activity of the heart. The technical aspects of measuring and interpreting echocardiographic measures of ventricular function involve: (1) identifying the images, specific measurements, and formulae used for a given index; (2) technical issues related to image acquisition and signal processing; (3) validation of the echocardiographic variable against a gold standard; (4) repeatability related to acquisition, measurement, and day-to-day variability; (5) data suggesting an impact on diagnosis, prognosis, or therapy; (6) a focus on specific patient groups where the measurement is most relevant; (7) availability of suitable reference values; and (8) appreciation of the limitations of the echocardiographic variable.

Systolic Ventricular Function
Even with the introduction of newer technologies such as myocardial strain imaging, it is important to emphasize that echocardiographic variables tell us about global or regional systolic function, not myocardial contractility *per se*. The effects of autonomic tone, loading conditions, and heart rate and rhythm on functional indices are all relevant. Drug intervention can also affect ventricular function, either by directly altering inotropic state, or by modifying the loading conditions or heart rate.

Overview and Practical Considerations
Most of the commonly used estimates of ventricular function are classified as *ejection phase indices* and involve measuring changes in ventricular volume or dimensions from end-diastole to end-systole. The most popular are linear, area, and volumetric estimates of LV ejection fraction (EF), defined as the stroke

TABLE 8-10

*Indices of Ventricular Systolic Function**

Name of Index	Units	Measurement or Calculation	General Interpretation/Comments
LV Fractional Shortening (LVFS)	Percent or fraction	$$\frac{LVIDd - LVIDs}{LVIDd}$$	Minor axis, linear correlate to LV ejection fraction Directly related to contractility Highly affected by preload, afterload, synchrony Only a single minor axis is sampled
LV Fractional Area Change (FAC)	Percent or fraction	$$\frac{LVAd - LVAs}{LVAd}$$	Short-axis area correlate to LV ejection fraction Directly related to contractility Highly affected by preload and afterload Does not include longitudinal LV contraction
RV Fractional Area Change (FAC)	Percent or fraction	$$\frac{RVAd - RVAs}{RVAd}$$	Modified left apical image optimized for the RV inlet Correlates to global RV systolic function Directly related to RV contractility Highly affected by preload and afterload Does not evaluate all segments of the RV

LV End-systolic Volume LVESV (index)	Volume in ml Index: ml/m^2	Volume estimates from:
		  Teichholtz (m-mode)
		  Simpsons method of discs
		  Area-length formulae
		  Automated (software toolkit)
			End-systolic volume following ejection
			Used in calculation of ejection fraction
			Inversely related to contractility
			ESV is overestimated by M-mode in dilated ventricles
			Best estimated by 3D or bi-plane 2D methods

Ejection Fraction	Percent or fraction	$$\frac{EDV - ESV}{EDV}$$ See above for volume estimates	"Gold standard" of global LV systolic function Directly related to contractility Highly affected by preload and afterload Optimally measured by bi-plane 2D or 3D methods
Mitral Valve Annulus Motion	Amplitude (mm)	Direct measurement using M-line or speckle tracking software	Measures longitudinal displacement of the LV annulus Normal values directly related to body size Mainly used to evaluate dogs with equivocal LVFS
Tricuspid Plan Annular Excursion (TAPSE)	Amplitude (mm)	Direct measurement using M-line or speckle tracking software	Measures longitudinal displacement of the RV annulus Records along the major plane of RV contraction Normal values directly related to body size Used to evaluate RV systolic function in dogs
E-point to Septal Separation (EPSS)	Distance (mm)	Direct measurement the distance between the mitral E-point and ventricular septum Measured with M-mode calipers	Inversely related to LV ejection fraction Smaller values are normal; related to breed False positives: aortic regurgitation; mitral stenosis

TABLE 8-10

Indices of Ventricular Systolic Function*—cont'd

Name of Index	Units	Measurement or Calculation	General Interpretation/Comments
Tissue Doppler Imaging (S') Systolic Myocardial Velocity (TDI)	Velocity (cm/s)	Direct measurement of peak systolic tissue velocity measured with pulsed-wave Doppler (TDI) Maximal mean tissue velocity measured from color Doppler encoding of the ventricle using proprietary software tool kit	Correlate to contractility; affected by preload and afterload Usually measured in the lateral wall of the LV or the RV near the annulus of the atrioventricular valves Velocities are directly related to body size Single, PWD sample volume method records higher velocity Color-Doppler based methodologies record mean tissue velocities within regions of interest; values are not interchangeable with PWD-based TDI
Tei Index of Myocardial Performance (IMP)	Fraction	$$\frac{\text{Isovolumetric time periods}}{\text{Ventricular ejection time}}$$ Typically measured by PW Doppler	Combined index of systolic and diastolic function Alternative method of measurement with TDI Impaired ventricular function prolongs the isovolumetric contraction and relaxation times relative to ejection time Smaller values indicate better ventricular function
Systolic Time Intervals	Time (ms) or Ratio	$$\frac{\text{Pre-ejection Period (PEP)}}{\text{Ejection Time (ET)}}$$	The ratio of PEP/ET is inversely related to contractility. The index is significantly affected by preload and afterload Widening of the QRS complex prolongs the PEP
Myocardial Strain Myocardial Strain Rate	Percent deformation Units/second	Proprietary software analysis of deformation of myocardial segments based on apical long axis or parasternal short-axis grayscale images. Longitudinal, radial, circumferential	Higher values of deformation and higher strain rates correlate with greater contractility Affected by preload and afterload Older methods used TDI based technology Current methods use speckle tracking technology
LV Twist and Torsion	Degrees	LV rotation is measured at the base and at the apex of the LV Twisting or Torsion are calculated from the differences in rotation	Correlates to both systolic function and diastolic function Greater twist correlates to improved global systolic function Timing of events also correlate to ventricular function

*Selected indices are presented.
**Some Echo system analysis packages, or off-line software products, can automatically recognize borders or myocardial speckles and calculate the index.
***Can be reported as a fraction or percentile.

volume/end-diastolic volume and calculated as EF = [EDV − ESV] / EDV, where EDV = end-diastolic volume and ESV = end-systolic volume (in ml). Left ventricular fractional shortening (LVFS) and fractional area change (or shortening) are simply linear and area-based variations on this same formula. The accuracy of any volume estimate depends on how faithfully the geometric model selected represents the size of the normal or diseased chamber. Various approaches to modeling of the LV and the difficulty of modeling the RV chamber volume have been previously discussed (see "Assessment of Cardiac Chamber Size"). In general, the more complicated the model and more detailed the measurements, the better the approximation of volumes and therefore systolic function.

As indicated earlier the EF indicates the combined effects of myocardial inotropy, loading condition, and wall stress. Importantly, the increased preload and reduced afterload of severe MR, typical of advanced degenerative MV disease in dogs, usually masks any depression in contractility. Similarly in both hypertrophic cardiomyopathy (HCM) and in aortic stenosis (AS) thicker LV walls reduce wall stress and can generate a normal EF even in the setting of depressed myocardial inotropy. Despite such limitations, EF is still considered a standard for the assessment of global systolic function. Other ejection phase indices including end-systolic ventricular volume (or diameter) index, LV fractional shortening, and LV fractional area change are merely simpler measurements intended to track ejection fraction. However, these variables carry more limitations as discussed below.

Functional indices based on time intervals include pre-ejection period, flow acceleration, and ejection time, along with the hybrid estimate of the (Tei) index of myocardial performance (Table 8-10). These indices are calculated from spectral Doppler modalities with simultaneous ECG, optimally at a fast sweep speed of 100 mm/s or greater. Spectral Doppler and 2DE methods can be combined to estimate ventricular stroke volume (ml/beat) and cardiac output (ml/minute) because mean flow velocity × cross sectional area equals volumetric flow.[158,287] A host of regional and segmental systolic indices also have been studied; these include: measuring tissue velocities; calculating myocardial velocity gradients; assessing myocardial deformation or strain in orthogonal planes, and recording LV torsion and twist.[45,114,116,117,154,192,197,208,211,212,214-218,220-223,286,288,289]

Overt LV systolic dysfunction is most often observed with idiopathic DCM in dogs and cats, but can also develop from myocarditis, drug toxicosis, taurine/L-carnitine deficiency, relentless tachycardia, or as a cardiomyopathy secondary to chronic volume or pressure overload. Conversely, heart failure in the setting of normal systolic function suggests a cardiac disorder either dominated by diastolic dysfunction as occurs with HCM, or compensated by reduced wall stress as observed with advanced MR.

Echocardiographic assessments of systolic function are used for clinical diagnosis, research studies, and phenotype screening of breeding populations. The "significance" of reduced LV systolic function can differ across these situations. Marked depression of LVEF in the setting of CHF is almost certainly an indication of impaired systolic function that demands treatment. Conversely, statistically significant depression of LV function reported between research study groups might be of no clinical significance when assessing an individual patient, perhaps falling within day-to-day variation. Problems often arise during "screening clinics," where subtle decreases in LV function—typically measured by LVFS—are sought and often overemphasized. The consequences can include questioning the breeding soundness of a dog or advancing a recommendation for treatment. A better approach to ambiguous findings would involve a comprehensive battery of LV function tests and a recheck examination at a suitable interval to identify any serial changes in size or function.

Tests of systolic function are often insensitive for detecting mild reductions in contractility such that precise cutoffs separating normal from abnormal often lack sensitivity or specificity for the diagnosis of LV dysfunction. In comparison most experienced examiners can reliably "eyeball" moderate to severe ventricular dysfunction. This lack of sensitivity for identifying mild LV dysfunction has fostered other approaches. Exercise echocardiography is sometimes used in people, but the value and safety of this approach in dogs has not been determined. Tissue-based methods based on TDI or speckle tracking have developed and evaluate a small segment of the LV (or RV) with the hope of enhancing sensitivity for detection of ventricular dysfunction. However, these newer techniques lack standardization in veterinary patients and most variables have not been validated by MRI or cardiac catheterization in patients with spontaneous disease. Lacking this information, advanced tissue-based analyses require longitudinal studies that might verify their superiority over conventional estimates like EF or LVFS. These are rare in our literature.

Indices of ventricular function are affected by biologic variation, disease, heart rate and rhythm, drug therapy, and a host of technical factors. Two specific limitations of tissue Doppler based assessments of ventricular function are the influence of tethering of adjacent segments on tissue motion and the angle dependence of the velocity estimates. The influence of abnormal heart rhythms, varying cardiac cycle lengths, conduction disturbances (bundle branch block), and ventricular dyssynchrony[112,290] also must be appreciated. For example, most measures of LV systolic function are reduced by premature complexes but increased by a long preceding cycle length as occurs with post-extrasystolic beats, atrial fibrillation, and even pronounced sinus arrhythmia. Protracted tachyarrhythmias can create transient LV systolic dysfunction that may persist for days or even weeks following reestablishment of sinus rhythm, so-called tachycardia-induced cardiomyopathy. Considering that day to day variation of a single examiner often approaches 10% (or more) for many echocardiographic variables, it might be difficult to identify subtle changes in ventricular function even within a single patient. Thus it is probably incorrect to apply rigid benchmarks and cutoffs for "normal" systolic function, especially when focusing on a single index such as LVFS or end-systolic volume index.[††] The importance of an "abnormal" designation is emphasized because a diagnosis of "systolic dysfunction" will prompt additional investigations, more frequent follow-up examinations, and possibly life-long therapy.

Specific Systolic Function Indices

In this section echocardiographic tests of ventricular systolic function are categorized based on imaging modality, beginning with the M-mode and 2D approaches and followed by systolic time intervals, Doppler based methods, and advanced tissue focused methods. The studies of ventricular systolic function are summarized in Table 8-10.

M-Mode Measurements and Indices. The LV fractional shortening (LVFS) is still the most popular linear estimate of EF (see Figure 8-12, B; Video 8-7) and measures the fractional change of the LV inner diameter (LVID) along one minor axis. This variable is measured with the cursor crossing either the high papillary muscle level or the chordal level and is calculated as LVFS = [LVIDd–LVIDs]/LVIDd (where d = diastole and s = systole). When both LV size and FS fall within the normal reference ranges for the species and breed, global LV systolic function is considered "normal" and most examiners will be satisfied with that result. However, *no single cut-off value* has proven to offer optimal sensitivity/specificity for the recognition of LV dysfunction or prediction of heart failure across the various canine breeds. While most examiners consider LVFS ≥25% as normal, many healthy dogs exhibit values closer to 20% and demonstrate these "slightly low" values for years without a cardiac event. This might relate to a reliance on more shortening along the apical-basilar (long) axis,[104] a lack of specificity for this index, or alternatively indicate a

---

[††]It is quite common to perform 8 or 10 different estimates of LV function in a single dog only to find that half of these variables point in one direction and the others the opposite way.

protracted period of preclinical DCM in some dogs. Interpretation of LVFS is especially problematic in the presence of dyssynchrony because the offset in timing of wall motion has no accepted adjustment, aside from the eye of a practiced examiner. In dogs with early DCM, marked dyssynchrony of the LV can produce a substantially lower LVFS, while other estimates such as LV fractional area change or bi-plane LVEF reveal minimal dysfunction. Thus, while the determination of LVFS is efficient, the clinician must appreciate the limitations, particularly in healthy dogs. The M-mode situation in *cats* seems less confusing. Although lower values have been reported most normal cats exceed a LVFS of 40%.[99] Anesthetic agents and some sedative combinations can markedly depress these values.

Among many other M-mode derived indices of LV systolic function are the amplitudes of septal and LVW excursion, E-point to septal separation (EPSS), end-systolic diameter and volume indices, and EF. The interpretation of wall amplitudes and EPSS has been previously discussed in the introduction to M-mode echocardiography. When dyssynchrony is evident, LV wall amplitude is often normal and this finding suggests LV systolic function is not impaired. The normal range for EPSS varies across breeds and body sizes, and increases in the setting of myocardial failure (see Figure 8-13, C).[108,121,122] The use of M-mode derived calculation of LV end-systolic volume, indexed to body size, has been proposed as a method of identifying LV systolic dysfunction in dogs.[27] This volume should be larger if contractility is impaired and ejection fraction decreased. Although theoretically sound, the value of this index is uncertain because, as discussed below, the end-systolic volume of a dilated LV is probably overestimated by M-mode methods. Additional concerns include the use of nonvalidated human angiographic benchmarks for classifying various grades of LV dysfunction in dogs with MR (with a value of 30 ml/m^2 often quoted as the upper limit of normal). Additionally, there is a collinear relationship between end-diastolic and end-systolic diameters[27,260] meaning as one gets bigger so does the other. Thus while the concept appears sound, the authors are unsure if this popular index of ventricular systolic function, as currently calculated by M-mode, should be used at all. Indeed values of end-systolic volumes indexed for body size exceed 30 ml/m^2 in some normal dogs when estimated from bi-plane 2D methods.[245] Perhaps 3D methods with MRI validation will address this issue more definitively. In a similar vein, the use of M-mode data to calculate an LVEF is also suspect, and should be supplanted by 2D or 3D methods.

The aforementioned M-mode indices are focused on cardiac motion across one minor axis, but if the transducer is placed near the cardiac apex and the beam directed toward the atria, systolic basilar to apical movements of the mitral and tricuspid annuli can be captured. Either the M-mode cursor or advanced tissue-tracking techniques can be used to track this motion. Mitral annular motion in dogs[104] correlates to global LV systolic function and represents another way to assess the LV, especially when results of LVFS are ambiguous. A related estimate of RV systolic function is *tricuspid annular plane systolic excursion* or TAPSE (Figure 8-35).[227] Because RV shortening is mainly in the apical to basilar plane,[81] TAPSE can provide an objective estimate of RV systolic function. For both mitral annular motion and for TAPSE the cursor is placed to record the downward movement of the lateral annulus from end-diastole to end-systole. It is important to place the cursor across the appropriate lateral annulus with its path as parallel as possible to the long-axis of the ventricular wall. The A-V valve itself must be avoided as early diastolic opening can be confused with basilar to apical shortening. Values for mitral annular motion and for TAPSE are related to body size. Normal reported 95% confidence intervals for mitral annular

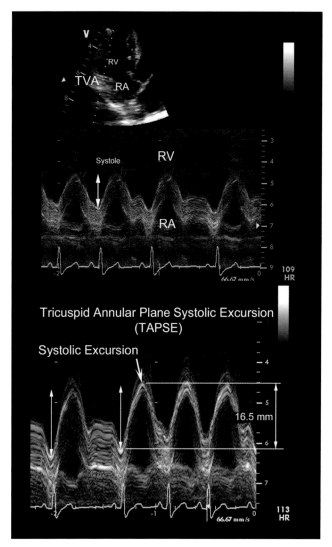

Figure 8-35 Tricuspid Annular Plane Systolic Excursion. Measurement of TAPSE using the M-mode cursor. The M-line should cross the tricuspid valve annulus and measure maximal systolic excursion toward the apex. It should not cross the parietal leaflet. Displacement is measured in mm and is demonstrated in the lower panel. A single bright annular echo (*arrow*) should be tracked from end-diastole to peak excursion. Normal values can be predicted by allometric scaling.

motion104 in dogs were: 6.5 to 7.5 mm (in dogs <15 kg) with <4.5 mm considered too low; 10.3 to 11.3 mm (in dogs 15 to 40 kg) with <8 mm considered too low; and 12.1 to 18.1 mm (in dogs >40 kg) with <12 mm considered too low. Preliminary data suggest that average values for TAPSE are approximately 14 mm in dogs of all sizes but values in dogs <5 kg are about half as great as values in dogs >40 kg. Reference values in dogs of different body size have been published and demonstrate the curvilinear relationship of TAPSE to body-weight,[227] and additional studies (Visser, et al.) are in press.

Two-Dimensional Indices. The 2D echocardiogram can be used to estimate global and regional myocardial function in dogs. Evaluation begins with subjective assessment and experienced examiners can usually identify normal systolic function. However, less experienced observers tend to underestimate LV systolic function in dogs when viewing real-time video loops, especially from the right parasternal long-axis plane. Focusing on the apical movement of the mitral annulus in this image plane can be instructive and represents an estimate of mitral annular motion. A very useful subjective assessment is obtained by reviewing a slow motion loop at the high papillary muscle level (see Figure 8-5, *A*; Video 8-20). If the internal LV chamber area decreases by at least 50% over the cardiac cycle, global systolic function will be normal. This change can be quantified by calculating the fractional area change (see below). As a practical measure, when a normal LVFS is accompanied by subjectively normal mitral annular motion and fractional area change, the examiner can be reasonably assured that global LV systolic function is normal.

When additional 2D measurements of the LV are indicated, the *fractional area change* (FAC) can be calculated. Similar to LVFS, this variable assesses minor-axis shortening and is calculated as the percent reduction in internal ventricular area from end-diastole to end-systole. The LV-FAC is derived from frozen 2D short-axis images recorded at the high papillary muscle level. The two areas are traced along the internal blood-endocardial interface but excluding the papillary muscles (Figure 8-36). This technique has some advantage over LVFS because it considers wall motion across the entire minor-axis plane and somewhat less sensitive to IVS and LVW dyssynchrony. The disadvantage is that LV-FAC does not include shortening in the apical-basilar direction. Furthermore the image can be difficult to measure, especially in systole when the path through the base of the papillary muscles is less obvious. Values exceeding 45% (0.45) appear to represent normal contraction in dogs with values <40% suggesting impaired systolic function or a need to further evaluate the LV, especially in terms of apical-basilar shortening. Right ventricular systolic function also can be assessed this way with the internal areas obtained from the modified left apical image optimized for the RV inlet. Areas are measured at end-diastole and end-systole by tracing the "triangle" formed by the apex, lateral wall, IVS, and tricuspid valve annulus (see Figure 8-8, *B* and Videos 8-4, *B* and 8-5). Preliminary data suggest that average RV FAC in healthy dogs is close to 45% but varies widely with a range extending from 30% to 70%.

The standard for estimation of global LV function in human laboratories is the LVEF obtained from either a bi-plane 2D or a 3D method. The estimation of end-diastolic and end-systolic volumes using 2D imaging has already been discussed (see "Models for Estimating Left Ventricular Volumes"). The calculation of EF requires tracing LV internal areas and measuring the ventricular lengths at end-diastole and end-systole (see Figure 8-32). The authors recommend using the right parasternal long-axis image optimized for the LV inlet and the left apical 4-chamber image optimized for LV length when performing a single- or bi-plane method of discs (Simpson's rule) for determination of LV volumes. When EF is estimated in dogs using these approaches, normal values usually exceed 45% with single plane and 50% with bi-plane approaches.[262]

Regional and global estimates of LV function also can be obtained with 2D echo, using "speckle" imaging modalities (see Figure 8-30; Video 8-12). Unique grayscale signatures (speckles) are followed by the software algorithm to calculate regional myocardial deformation or strain. This approach may have some benefits—including less angle dependency—when compared to TDI. An introduction to speckle tracking and myocardial deformation imaging was presented earlier in this chapter, but the subject is generally beyond the scope of the introductory review.

Intervals of Systole. The time intervals encompassed by the isovolumetric periods, the preejection period, and the duration of ventricular ejection relate to systolic or diastolic ventricular function and factors influencing contraction and ejection. Briefly, the isovolumetric periods are those short intervals when ventricular pressure is either rising or falling while all four cardiac valves are closed (see Figure 8-21). Isovolumetric contraction time (ICT) relates inversely to rate of change of pressure over time (dp/dt), which is highest immediately prior to ejection. The *pre-ejection period* (PEP) is measured from the onset of the QRS complex to the beginning of ventricular ejection. This PEP period encompasses both the interval of electromechanical delay and the ICT, the period of rapid pressure rise prior to aortic valve opening. The PEP prolongs with decreased contractility. The QRS complex must be clearly delineated or else the PEP will be inaccurate and the duration is influenced by the width of the QRS. For example, a bundle branch block will prolong the electromechanical delay and PEP. The left and right ventricular *ejection times* (ET) span the intervals between opening and closing of the aortic and pulmonary valves, respectively. These time intervals can be determined with M-mode methods,[126] but spectral Doppler approaches are preferred (Figure 8-37). Recording sweep speeds should be fast, at least 100 mm/s and preferably ≥150 mm/s. Like ejection phase indices, systolic time intervals are influenced by ventricular preload and afterload and by extremes of cardiac cycle length. Furthermore, these periods are difficult to interpret in the setting of significant MR. However, when evaluating dogs for preclinical DCM or other causes of impaired contractility, systolic time intervals provide another means of assessing global ventricular function. The ratio of PEP/LVET relates inversely to LV contractility, increasing as myocardial function deteriorates. This can be explained by the greater time needed by the failing LV to develop pressure and the delivery of a smaller stroke volume during a shorter ejection time. Normal values in healthy dogs of varying sizes range from 0.24-0.42, with small dogs generally <0.3 and larger dogs generally <0.42. For the RV, normal values of PEP/ET between 0.23 to 0.34 have been reported.[284] Other laboratories have reported similar or quite different values, demonstrating the need to standardize methods or better define reference populations. Based on human studies, these systolic times intervals are probably inaccurate in the setting of significant mitral or aortic valvular disease or when tachycardia is present. Assuming a consistent QRS duration, serial increases in PEP or PEP/ET could potentially track changes in LV function in dogs with preclinical DCM or those with doxorubicin-induced cardiomyopathy.

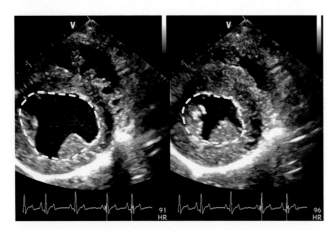

Figure 8-36 LV Fractional Area Change. The fractional change in the short-axis LV area can be measured by tracing the inner endocardial borders in diastole and systole. Per the convention in human echocardiography laboratories, the papillary muscles are ignored and a circular to oval area recorded. In many cases subjective evaluation of the frozen end-diastolic and end-systolic frames efficiently provide evidence of normal systolic function.

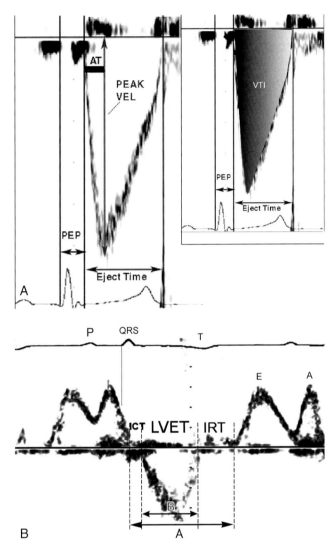

Figure 8-37 **Intervals of Systole. A,** The pre-ejection period and ejection time can be measured with a high-fidelity recording of aortic blood flow that shows the onset and end of ejection. Either PWD (shown in this canine recording) or CWD can be used. The area under the curve (velocity-time integral or "stroke-distance") correlates to ventricular stroke volume. **B,** (Tei) Index of Myocardial Performance for the LV. The calculation is shown for this feline recording. Both transmitral filling and LVOT flow signals must be recorded. The index equals the sum of the isovolumetric periods divided by the ejection time and is calculated as the time period A minus the time period B divided by B. This is a combined index of diastolic and systolic function. See text for details.

An *index of myocardial performance* (IMP) combines both ventricular systolic and diastolic function within a single ratio. As developed by Tei who used spectral Doppler for the timing of flow signals, IMP = (ICT + IRT) / ET. The (Tei) IMP is obtained from the LV by using either a CWD cursor to capture flow and valve noise, or a large PW sample volume that records both inflow and outflow tract signals (Figure 8-37, *B*). Peak velocities are not important for these timings, but baseline filtering must be minimal so the start and stop of velocity spectra can be accurately timed. Myocardial disease prolongs both isovolumetric periods and shortens ejection time, so larger values indicate *worse* ventricular function. In one study of Newfoundland dogs, IMP was 0.28 +/− 0.12 in the normal dogs studied but higher values were recorded

in those with DCM.[291] In a multibreed study of healthy dogs, IMP had a wide range of 0.32 to 0.50 for the LV, similar to some other reports.[292,293] A Tei index of RV function also can be calculated, but it requires two different recordings (tricuspid inflow and PA outflow) of similar cardiac cycle length.[293] Within the same dog, values for the RV-IMP are nearly always lower than those obtained from the left side.[284]

Doppler Methods for Assessment of LV Function. Beyond systolic time intervals, the aortic velocity profile recorded by PWD or CWD can yield additional estimates of LV function (Figure 8-37, *A*). Myocardial function must be significantly depressed before these variables are obviously altered. Instantaneous peak *aortic acceleration* and to a lesser extent peak aortic velocity relate positively to myocardial inotropy. However, it is difficult to calculate maximal aortic acceleration with conventional echocardiographic systems as these measure only average outflow acceleration.

Doppler estimates of ventricular *stroke volume* also can be recorded from the aortic time-velocity profile, but the measurements have limited practical use because the range of normal values is so great. Stroke volume and cardiac output are usually of greatest interest in the short-term, serial evaluation of patients in critical care and anesthetic situations or when assessing cases of congenital heart disease. Stroke volume calculations are based on the concept that the area under the aortic (or pulmonic) flow velocity signal—termed the velocity-time integral or stroke distance—correlates directly to the ventricular stroke volume. The velocity time integral has units of cm/s on the y-axis and sec on the x-axis resulting in "stroke distance" units measured in centimeters. To calculate LV stroke volume, the needed recordings are a spectral (PWD or CW) tracing of blood flow taken between the opened AV leaflets and a diameter (d) obtained from the site of sample volume placement. Stroke volume (in cc or ml) is calculated by tracing the modal velocity of the aortic flow signal and multiplying the resultant stroke distance (in cm) by the calculated cross-sectional area of the aorta or PA (in cm^2; where CSA = $\pi[d/2]^2$). Cardiac output (ml/min) equals ventricular stroke volume (in ml per beat) * heart rate/min. Measurements of stroke volume index and cardiac index relate favorably to invasive indicator dilution techniques when changes are tracked within a single animal, but individual point measurements show unacceptably large standard errors of the estimate and limits of agreement between the methods.[287]

When MR is present, the rate of LV pressure rise or *LV dP/dt* can be estimated by recording the time interval (in seconds) needed for a regurgitant jet to change from 1 to 3 m/s. This time value is then divided by 32 mm Hg, the pressure increment (from 4 mm Hg to 36 mm Hg) calculated from the simplified Bernoulli equation. The result is a "mean" dp/dt or average pressure rise over that part of the pre-ejection period. The method has been validated with simultaneous, high-fidelity intracardiac catheter recordings.[294-296] The greatest application for this technique is probably as an adjunct for the diagnosis of preclinical DCM or when following changes in LV systolic function over time as might be done during doxorubicin therapy. In awake catheterized dogs peak LV dp/dt is ≈3000 mm Hg/s or more, but the values obtained using the Doppler method are can be lower because of the average time period pressure change is measured. Measurements taken over time are probably more instructive than results of a single point-in-time measurement.

When Doppler examination is applied to the myocardium, the measured tissue velocities can be used as indices of LV or RV systolic function. Normal TDI has already been discussed. The plane of examination must be specified when reporting TDI results and the methodology also indicated (postanalysis color Doppler based or standard PWD with a single sample volume). Longitudinal (apical-basilar) and radial (short-axis) velocities are most often measured. As per conventional Doppler, obtaining parallel alignment with tissue movements is critical. Longitudinal velocities obtained with TDI in healthy dogs range from about 12 to 20 cm/s near the lateral mitral annulus and are influenced by body size and heart rate. The values obtained from a single sample volume using TDI are higher than those generated by proprietary applications that use tissue CDI[285] or speckle strain imaging to measure mean velocities within a defined wall segment. The authors have been disappointed by tissue velocity measurements of the LV for systolic function, which can be normal even in the setting of reduced EF. Importantly, TDI velocities are often enhanced in the setting of primary MR, even in dogs with CHF. These methods offer better diagnostic value when assessing diastolic heart function, as described later. Readers interested in various methods of assessing the LV in systole using TDI are directed to the references.

Myocardial Strain, Twist, and Dyssynchrony. Calculation of regional myocardial deformation—strain and strain rate—is a recent application of TDI and of 2D speckle tracking technologies. Longitudinal strain is calculated as a negative value because segments shorten during systole, while radial strain is positive (as the wall thickens). Circumferential strain and segmental rotation are also available from a number of vendors. Global 3D strain can be calculated from 3D images of the LV. Strain recorded by speckle tracking is purported to overcome the TDI limitations of angle and tethering. Limited veterinary publications have described strain imaging for the ventricles.[45,114,116,117,154,192,197,208,211,212,214-218,220-222,228-230,286,288,289] Standardization and reference values are needed before widespread veterinary application can be recommended beyond the research setting. Unfortunately, deformation imaging does not appear to be any more sensitive than conventional methods for detecting myocardial dysfunction in dogs with MR and thus far has not been evaluated sufficiently in longitudinal studies of dogs with preclinical DCM that eventually develop overt myocardial failure.

Speckle tracking can also measure the rotation of the heart at the base and apex to allow estimation of ventricular torsion or twist. The apex and base rotate in opposite directions in normal hearts and their calculated differences can be used to assess ventricular systolic function (twisting) and diastolic function (untwisting). It should be noted that the values obtained for ventricular twist are calculated from disparate segments that reach their maximal rotations at different points of time.[116,209,219]

A number of methods are used to measure ventricular dyssynchrony and some of the more advanced include multisegment TDI or deformation (strain) analyses. Variables such as time to peak strain across different myocardial wall segments or the standard deviation of time differences to peak strain can be used to quantify the delays in ventricular activation associated with prolonged QRS complexes, cardiomyopathy, or ventricular pacing. Dyssynchrony is believed to further impair LV function.[45,112-117,154,223,229]

Examples of these advanced, tissue-based approaches for assessing ventricular function are illustrated in Figure 8-30 and Video 8-17.

Diastolic Ventricular Function
Diastole extends from closure of the AV to closure of the MV. Active myocardial relaxation begins even before ejection is complete, and this initiates a complicated process that allows the A-V valves to open and normal ventricles to fill under low venous pressures during rest and exercise. Severe diastolic dysfunction is considered a negative prognostic finding. Of course pericardial diseases are characterized by diastolic dys-

function, but myocardial diseases, volume overloads, and pressure overloads are also impacted by diastolic abnormalities. For example, heart failure in feline HCM is usually initiated by diastolic dysfunction. Diastolic abnormalities are also evident in aortic stenosis, systemic hypertension, and dilated cardiomyopathy, but are often overshadowed by other findings. As with tests of systolic function, the diastolic assessment is *confounded by moderate to severe mitral regurgitation* in the setting of preserved or hyperdynamic ventricular systolic function. Some echocardiographic indices of ventricular diastolic function relative to categories of diastolic dysfunction are summarized in Table 8-11.

Overview and Practical Considerations
Diastolic function is complicated and no single index incorporates all the determinants of ventricular filling.[119,176,182,185,187,190,297,298] Some relevant factors include active myocardial relaxation, ventricular fiber restoring forces (recoil), myocardial stiffness, chamber compliance, pericardial restraint, ventricular interaction, and LA contractility. Additional influences include ventricular loading, inotropy, heart rate, and coronary blood flow. The interplay among these factors is dynamic and complex. Although invasive indices such as the relaxation constant Tau and the ventricular pressure-volume loop are considered invasive gold standards for assessing diastolic function, echocardiography is the only practical method for evaluating diastolic performance in patients. Different echocardiographic approaches have been used to assess how ventricles fill, with most attention directed to the LV. In humans diastolic dysfunction might not be present at rest but can become evident during exercise. Presumably this is also true in animals, but the influence of exercise on diastolic function has not been reported. The literature on diastolic function is expansive in medicine[87,119,175,176,182-187,190,298-301] and a significant number of studies have also been performed in veterinary medicine.[45,143,145,151,176,180,181,188,189,191,193,208,225,302-310] The concepts are advanced, and the details are beyond the scope of this introductory chapter. The authors have tried to explain some of the more practical aspects used in their cardiology practices without emphasizing the research applications.

Perhaps the single most important concept underlying echocardiographic methods for assessing diastolic filling is this: Most indices measure the *combined effects* of diastolic heart function and ventricular filling pressures. Filling pressures relate to mean LA pressure—the average atrial pressure over the cardiac cycle and strongly influenced by pulmonary venous pressure—and to the LV end-diastolic pressure, which is also affected by LV compliance and the strength of atrial contraction. For example, transient increases in atrial pressure during a vigorous atrial contraction can compensate for impaired ventricular relaxation and recoil, so long as the instantaneous heart rate is not so fast as to abbreviate diastole. Conversely, chronic elevations in mean LA pressures are usually related to severe impairment of ventricular function, including decreased chamber compliance or distensibility and neurohormonal-renal compensations leading to volume retention. The identification of high pulmonary venous pressures during the diastolic assessment often indicates a need for drug therapy to prevent or to treat CHF. Conversely, mild diastolic dysfunction associated with lower mean LA pressure recommends a more favorable short-term prognosis (or indicates that previous therapy for CHF has been successful).[2] Of importance to veterinarians is the point that diastolic function can appear normal or even hyperdynamic when the ventricular has moderate to severe volume overload with relatively preserved systolic function. This limits the value of the value of diastolic assessment in most small breed dogs with chronic

TABLE 8-11

Ventricular Diastolic Function and Filling Pressures

FUNCTIONAL DESIGNATION	LA size	Mitral: E/A	TDI: E'/A'	IVRT	Mitral:DT	E/E'	E/IVRT	PVF: S D	PVF-A_R
								ESTIMATES OF LEFT VENTRICULAR DIASTOLIC FUNCTION & VENTRICULAR FILLING	
Normal / Normal diastolic function	Normal	E > A	E' > A'	Ref	Ref	Ref	Ref	S < D (dog) / S ≈ D (cat)	Duration MVA > A_R
Grade 1 dysfunction / Relaxation abnormality	Normal to ↑	E < A	E' < A'	↑	↑	Ref to ↓	Ref to ↓	S > D	Duration MVA > A_R ↑A_R Vel
Grade 2 dysfunction / Pseudonormal filling	↑	E > A	E' < A'	Normalizes	Normalizes	Ref to ↑	Ref to ↑	Variable	Duration MVA: A_R Variable; ↑A_R Vel
Grade 3 dysfunction / Restrictive filling: reversible	↑↑	E ≫ A	↓E', ↓A'	↓	↓	↑	↑	S < D	Duration MVA < A_R
Grade 4 dysfunction / Restrictive filling: irreversible	↑↑	E ≫ A	↓E', ↓A'	↓	↓	↑	↑	S < D	Duration MVA < A_R

Notes
(1) The patterns shown here are generalizations, and it is uncommon for each variable to change in the manner shown in the table.
(2) Diastolic function is very difficult to assess in primary mitral regurgitation (see text). Higher end-systolic left atrial pressure develops due to the regurgitant volume and this has a disproportionate influence on early diastolic filling. Additionally, both systolic and early diastolic motion tend to increase in primary mitral valve disease. Compared to cardiomyopathies, much higher ratios of mitral E-wave to TDI E' and mitral E-wave to IVRT are needed before increased filling pressures can be identified.
(3) Sinus tachycardia can lead to fusion of E and A waves and uninterpretable patterns; atrial fibrillation eliminates the A-wave and short cycles can reduce MV-DT.
Abbreviations: LA, left atrial size; Transmitral E, A: Filling velocity in early diastole, Filling velocity after atrial contraction; TDI-E', A': Longitudinal tissue velocity in early diastole, Longitudinal tissue velocity after atrial contraction, Late diastolic longitudinal tissue velocity related to atrial contraction; IVRT, isovolumetric relaxation time; DT, mitral valve deceleration time; PVF, pulmonary venous flow: A_R, atrial reversal wave; D, diastolic wave; S, systolic wave; Var, variable; Vel, velocity; ↓ = decreased; ↑ = increased; ↑↑ = moderate to severe LA enlargement; Ref = within reference range for species (see Table 8-4)

MR in which hyperdynamic diastolic function is often observed.

The mainstays for assessment of LV diastolic function are the analysis of transmitral inflow patterns and TDI of the LV wall.[3,4,200] Pulmonary venous flow patterns, isovolumetric time intervals, the pattern of color flow propagation into the LV, and advanced tissue analyses offer additional avenues for exploring diastolic function. Normal patterns of transmitral and pulmonary venous flow and of Doppler imaging of the LV wall have been described previously in this chapter, and these should be reviewed before reading through this section (see Figure 8-18, *B* and *F*). Diastolic dysfunction is usually classified into three (or four) broad categories, which are summarized in the upcoming paragraphs and in Table 8-11 and demonstrated in Figures 8-38, 8-39, and 8-40.

Evidence of *delayed ventricular relaxation* is probably the most common finding of diastolic dysfunction and can be

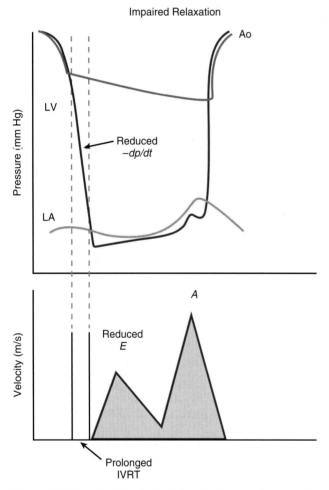

Impaired Relaxation

Figure 8-38 **Impaired Ventricular Relaxation.** Impaired ventricular relaxation decreases the rate of pressure decline in the LV, prolonging the IVRT and reducing the E-wave velocity. More of ventricular filling is shifted to late diastole with greater dependency on active atrial contraction. The higher pressure gradient between the LA and LV during atrial contraction increases the amplitude of the mitral A-wave. Parallel changes are observed in tissue Doppler recordings from the LV wall, while the pulmonary venous waveform is characterized by decreased D-wave amplitude and an enhanced A_R wave (not shown). (Figure from Otto C. *Textbook of Clinical Echocardiography*. 5th ed. Philadelphia: Saunders/Elsevier; 2013, with permission).

identified even in healthy dogs and cats as an aging change.[180] In general relaxation abnormalities are embodied in indices that depend on isovolumetric relaxation, restoring forces, and mean pressure within the LA. When delayed relaxation is evident the following changes are observed: (1) isovolumetric relaxation time is prolonged; (2) the amplitude of the mitral E-wave is reduced with E<A; (3) the deceleration time of the E-wave is prolonged; (4) the early diastolic recoil in the LV wall is diminished with a lower velocity E' wave and decreased E'/A'; and (5) the pulmonary venous flow D-wave decreases relative to the S-wave. So long as heart rate is normal, impaired early filling is compensated by shifting ventricular filling fractions to late diastole. This is evident as increased amplitudes of the mitral A wave, tissue Doppler A' wave, and pulmonary venous A_R wave. Collectively these findings are typical of *Grade 1 diastolic dysfunction* and are rarely associated with CHF unless fluid therapy, protracted tachycardia, or acute volume overload supervenes to increase filling pressures (so-called *Grade 1a diastolic dysfunction*). The most obvious changes during real-time examination are E-wave to A-wave reversal in both the transmitral and tissue Doppler recordings. The reduced transmitral E-wave indicates that filling pressures are not high and therefore the likelihood of CHF is relatively low at this stage: it is a favorable prognostic finding.

Abnormalities in diastolic function are less apparent once mean venous and atrial pressures increase. Higher ventricular filling pressures mask Doppler findings of impaired relaxation because the MV opens sooner under higher pressure and the LA empties more quickly. This compensation produces pseudonormal mitral inflow velocities, mitral E/A ratio, mitral deceleration time, and isovolumetric relaxation time (see Table 8-11). However, the early diastolic recoil measured with TDI does not normalize and TDI demonstrates that E'<A'. The pulmonary venous flow is characterized by an S wave that still exceeds the D wave and in some cases the duration of the pulmonary venous A_R wave will be greater than the transmitral A-wave. Collectively these findings define *Grade 2 diastolic dysfunction* and indicate a patient at higher risk for CHF. Thoracic radiographs are obtained, home respiratory rate monitoring implemented, and the potential for lowering venous pressures with drug therapy at least considered.

Progressive ventricular disease is usually associated with a loss of ventricular distensibility and represents a severe form of diastolic dysfunction. The reduced chamber compliance can only be overcome by increased venous pressures. Although these can partially mitigate the resistance to cardiac filling, capillary pressures also increase predisposing to pulmonary edema or to pleural effusion. Both myocardial relaxation and distensibility of the ventricle are impaired at this stage, and most ventricular filling is limited to early diastole. The result is the so-called *restrictive filling pattern* evident in the transmitral flow pattern and termed *Grade 3 diastolic dysfunction*. Typical Doppler findings include a high-velocity E-wave, shortened deceleration time, and attenuated A-wave so that E≫A. The precise E/A ratios used in human patients have not been sufficiently defined for dogs and cats, but the diminutive A-wave is often filtered out by the low-velocity (wall) filter setting. The changes in the E-wave are caused by the combination of initial filling under high LA pressure and increased ventricular stiffness that causes the atrioventricular pressure gradient to rapidly approach zero, stopping further ventricular inflow (Figure 8-39, C). The small A-wave is explained by the reduced LA to LV end-diastolic pressure gradient and possibly by concurrent atrial myocardial failure. In most cases of cardiomyopathy, the early diastolic tissue recoil (E') is not normalized by high filling pressures. Thus with restricted filling mitral E/A and mitral E/E' ratios are greatly increased. The precise E/E' value that predicts

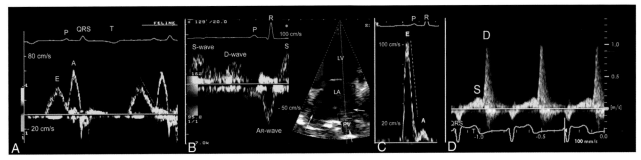

Figure 8-39 **Diastolic Dysfunction: Transmitral and Pulmonary Venous Flow. A,** Relaxation abnormality (Grade 1 diastolic dysfunction) in a healthy, aged cat. There is E/A reversal and a prolonged MV deceleration time (note slope of E-wave deceleration). **B,** Relaxation abnormality in the pulmonary venous velocity profile in a dog. The pattern is characterized by reduced D-wave (normally D>S in canine recordings) and a prominent atrial reversal (A$_R$) wave suggesting active atrial contraction as compensation. The three venous confluences typically seen in the apical 4-chamber image are indicated by arrows. The sample volume is in the confluence of the veins draining the left and right caudal and the accessory lung lobes. **C,** Restrictive filling abnormality (Grade 3 diastolic dysfunction) in a cat with cardiomyopathy and CHF. The E-wave is markedly increased and the A-wave decreased in amplitude resulting in a high E/A ratio. The MV deceleration time is abbreviated indicating high LA pressure and a noncompliant ventricle (compare the slope to that in 8-39A). **D,** Restrictive filling abnormality in the pulmonary venous velocity profile in another cat with CHF due to cardiomyopathy. The D-wave is increased in amplitude and S-wave reduced. The genesis of the small negative wave during the QRS is uncertain; there is no obvious atrial electrical activity.

pulmonary edema is subject to some debate, and clearly depends on the underlying heart disease (for example, DCM versus MR), the acuteness of the heart failure, and the influence of any therapy such as diuretics, which decrease the E-wave as the pressures decline.[176,190] The isovolumetric relaxation time actually *shortens* in restrictive filling because high venous pressures initiate earlier filling. This is characterized by an increase in the E/IVRT ratio.[175,311] Complementary changes are observed in the pulmonary veins, characterized by a small systolic filling wave (due to high atrial pressure and reduced LA compliance), pronounced D-wave from high pulmonary venous pressure (Figure 8-39, *D*)—a situation paralleling the tall MV E-wave—and sometimes a prolonged A$_R$ waves (as pulmonary veins offer less resistance to flow than the noncompliant LV). These changes should be reversed by cardiac drug therapy and returned to the Grade 2 pseudonormal pattern; however, if the diastolic abnormalities do not improve, *Grade 4 diastolic dysfunction* is said to be present.

Specific Variables in Diastolic Dysfunction

Some additional points and reference values for diastolic function indices are included in the upcoming sections. Reference values and ratios can assist in both the recognition of diastolic dysfunction and prediction of CHF (see Tables 8-4 and 8-11). However, as suggested earlier, while the aforementioned grades of diastolic dysfunction are often observed in cats and dogs, the exact ratios used to predict pulmonary edema depend on the type and the acuteness of heart disease. Some of the ratios suggested by models of cardiac failure might not translate directly to the natural occurring diseases and the clinical arena.

The clinician is especially cautioned about interpreting diastolic function tests when examining dogs with primary MR, secondary volume overload, and hyperdynamic global systolic function. The increased LA volume associated with MR increases the end-systolic LA pressure and improves early diastolic filling (as the extra blood returns to the LV), but often without the expense of increasing mean LA pressure significantly. Moderate to severe MR normalizes or increases the E-wave velocity and also can shorten the mitral deceleration and isovolumetric relaxation times. The LV is often hyperdynamic in early diastole as well as in systole.[119,175,299] Consequently, most diastolic indices show normal to hyperdynamic function in dogs with moderate to severe MR due to endocardiosis. Clearly more clinical studies are needed.

Isovolumetric Relaxation Time. The IVRT is largely affected by ventricular relaxation, aortic and LA end-systolic pressures, and intrinsic myocardial factors. Doppler derived reference values for isovolumetric relaxation time are summarized in Table 8-4. Isovolumetric relaxation time is lengthened with impaired LV relaxation, but is also prolonged by advancing age in healthy dogs and cats. Elevated LV filling pressures normalize or shorten this variable and the ratio of transmitral E-wave to IVRT increases. In one small study of dogs with left-sided CHF due to MR,[311] the ratio of mitral E/IVRT exceeding 1.88 was both sensitive and specific for a radiographic diagnosis of pulmonary edema.

Mitral Inflow Velocities. Mitral inflow velocities are determined by the instantaneous LA to LV pressure gradient and tall E-waves suggest either an extremely healthy heart with vigorous diastolic suction or increased LA pressure as described above under Grade 3 diastolic dysfunction. Filling velocity is decreased by volume depletion and increased by volume expansion. Additionally, severe MR can increase the E-wave velocity even when radiographs do not indicate CHF. Mitral deceleration time is prolonged by impaired relaxation, normalized under the influence of increasing filling pressures, and abbreviated in Grade 3 diastolic dysfunction. A short deceleration should not be diagnosed in atrial fibrillation when an abbreviated cardiac cycle suddenly closes the MV. Some normal values for transmitral flow are summarized in Table 8-4. In general, left-sided CHF is more likely when MV E-wave ≥1.3 m/s,[312,313] especially if accompanied by an abbreviated deceleration time that indicates reduced LV distensibility.

The ratio of E/A is most often used for assessing diastolic function, and a reduced E/A ratio with prolonged mitral deceleration times is usually a straightforward indication

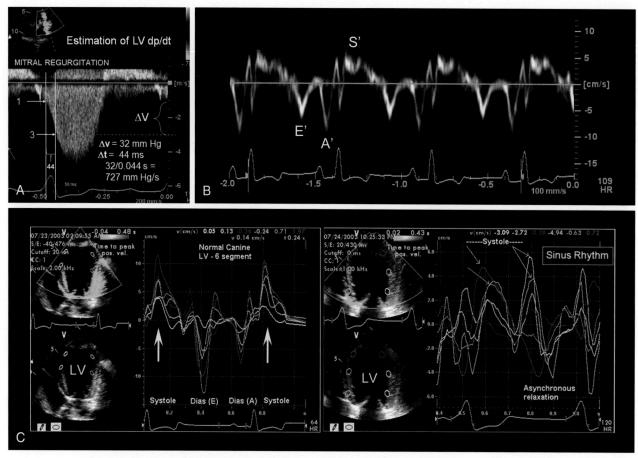

Figure 8-40 Ventricular Dysfunction: Other Echocardiographic Indices. A, Estimation of LV dp/dt in a large-breed dog with myocardial failure due to chronic MR. The rate of pressure change is very low (727 mm Hg/s), compatible with impaired systolic function. This index is especially affected by inotropic state and preload. **B,** Tissue Doppler imaging of the LV wall from a cat with mild HCM. The cat is receiving a beta-blocker and the heart rate is slow. Notice the slight reversal in E'/A' typical of a relaxation abnormality. **C,** Ventricular dyssynchrony demonstrated using color based TDI with six regions of interest placed in the lateral LV wall and the ventricular septum. Left: Data from a healthy dog demonstrates good timing synchronization of the wall segments in both systole and diastole. It is normal for basilar segments to contract at a higher velocity and to demonstrate a greater excursion toward the apex. Right: A dog with left bundle branch block and a dilated LV shows both systolic and diastolic dyssynchrony of the ventricle. This evaluation also can be performed using myocardial deformation (strain).

of Grade 1 diastolic dysfunction (relaxation abnormality). However, this ratio in isolation is of little diagnostic utility once ventricular filling pressures have increased and normalized the index. A more integrated assessment is required when Grade 2 through Grade 4 diastolic dysfunction is present. This should include TDI of the LV wall, pulmonary venous flow patterns (especially in cats), IVRT, and of course overall left atrial size, because moderate to severe diastolic dysfunction would be highly unlikely in a patient with a normal LA diameter or volume. There are other pitfalls to assessing E/A, for example, both E-wave and A-wave amplitudes are sensitive to cursor positioning, and the ratio decreases when the sample volume is moved into the mitral annulus or LA. High heart rates also create problems as diastasis is obliterated and the E and A waves fuse. The interpretation of fused waves is confusing and strongly discouraged (Figure 8-41). Transient E and A wave separation can occur with sinus arrhythmia or after a premature beat. High heart rates with E and A fusion are especially common in cats, and a vagal maneuver (from gentle, steady pressure on the nasal planum for ~10 seconds) might be successful in transiently slowing the heart rate.[155] Volume

depletion can reduce E/A ratio. In a similar way, effective diuresis in CHF usually decreases the E/A ratio restoring either a pseudonormal filling pattern (Grade 2 dysfunction) or a relaxation abnormality (Grade 1 dysfunction). These changes can occur quickly and might be confusing when an echocardiogram is performed in a dyspneic patient that previously received furosemide. In this situation, the findings of Grade 2 or Grade 1 diastolic dysfunction might (incorrectly) argue against the clinical diagnosis of CHF.

The admonition about assessing dogs with moderate to severe primary MR is repeated as increased transmitral flow volume in the setting of LV volume overload with preserved systolic function *increases* both the E wave and the E' wave amplitudes in dogs and therefore E/A and E/E' ratios do not impart the same information about LV compliance and filling pressures when compared to patients with cardiomyopathies or impaired systolic function. Certainly a normal E-wave velocity in the setting of MR supports mild disease. Conversely a MV E-wave ≥1.3 m/s suggests significant MR especially when the E/E' ratio is high. The ratio of E to IVRT might be a better estimate of elevated filling pressures in smaller

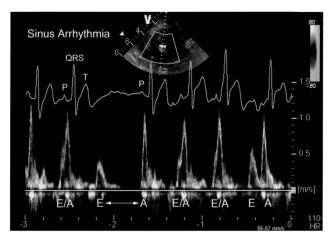

Figure 8-41 Fusion of Mitral E- and A-waves. A common error involves interpreting fused E and A waves, especially when the A wave begins near the peak of the E-wave. In this example from a dog with pronounced sinus arrhythmia, most of the filling waves are fused (E/A) until the heart rate slows (between arrows) allowing for separation of E and A waves. The last cycle demonstrates a typical relaxation abnormality of the LV. Note the marked difference in appearance with the preceding waveforms. A similar situation occurs commonly in cats with sinus tachycardia. A vagal maneuver can sometimes slow the rate transiently.

dogs with myxomatous MR, but this requires further confirmation.

Tissue Doppler Imaging. *Tissue Doppler imaging* (TDI) is most useful for diastolic assessment when combined with other variables. Normal E' and A' velocities demonstrate a similar relative ratio to that of mitral inflow with E'>A'. Unfortunately the message is sometimes mixed, with some segments showing normal ratios and others the inverse of normal. The authors generally concentrate on the TDI of the LVW obtained from the left apical image planes. The cursor is placed within the myocardium as close to the mitral annulus as possible, but not including any of the inward "curve" that is sometimes seen in the freewall. Long cardiac cycles with protracted diastasis sometimes reduce the A' and increase the E'/A' ratio. Finding a consistent E'/A' reversal in a patient with normal MV E/A suggests pseudonormal ventricular filling (Grade 2 dysfunction). With restrictive filling patterns in cardiomyopathy both E' and A' velocities are attenuated and ratio of tissue velocities becomes less important than the absolute value of the E' wave relative to the transmitral E-wave. The ratio of increased transmitral E to tissue E' predicts elevated ventricular filling pressures and CHF. While E/E' ratios exceeding 9 to 10 are likely to predict venous congestion in cardiomyopathy, the ratio probably should exceed 13 to 15 before CHF is diagnosed in a dog with primary MR and preserved systolic function.[148,181,308,311,314]

Other Variables. Subtle, regional abnormalities in myocardial relaxation might be observed as early signs of myocardial disease in some patients, especially in cats with hypertrophic cardiomyopathy[145,193,304,315] and in dogs with certain genetic cardiomyopathies.[228,316-318] Indeed, regional or segmental diastolic dysfunction is probably underappreciated in many cardiac diseases and could have diagnostic utility. Myocardial strain rate derived from TDI or 2D speckle tracking can also be used to assess early and late diastolic deformation (see Figure 8-40, C). As previously mentioned, ventricular untwisting can be calculated as an estimate of LV diastolic function.

The rate of LV filling can be further assessed with color M-mode by placing the cursor through the path of ventricular

filling in a left apical view and measuring the slope of early diastolic inflow along the edge of the signal alias. This slope, called the *LV flow propagation* (Figure 8-28, top), relates to LV relaxation and is thought to be is less load-dependent than transmitral flow patterns. Thus far this method has not been easy to measure or interpret in dogs and cats due to the appearance of multiple slopes and anatomic differences between humans and animals.

Estimates of *RV diastolic function* are far behind those of the LV, but it is quite common to observe E/A reversal in both trans-tricuspid inflow and in the RV freewall using TDI in dogs with pulmonic stenosis or other severe forms of RV disease. TDI and strain rate are readily measured in the RV segments, but further studies are needed to demonstrate prognostic utility of these variables.

VALVULAR REGURGITATION

The diagnosis and assessment of valvular regurgitation (insufficiency) is one of the most common uses of echocardiography. The approach is multimodal. For example, while Doppler studies are needed to confirm valvular insufficiency, an analysis of cardiac chamber size often provides the most important information about the hemodynamic significance of the flow disturbance, especially in veterinary medicine where surgical options for valve repair are very limited. Advanced Doppler techniques also can be used to further assess the hemodynamic situation and the current risk of CHF. The examiner should appreciate the common pitfalls associated with the diagnosis and assessment of severity (see Table 8-5 and below). Most of the principles of diagnosis have already been illustrated in prior sections of this chapter.

Overview and Practical Considerations
The examination should be informed by clinical findings, especially cardiac auscultation. Considering that both pulmonic and tricuspid valves leak by CDI in the majority of healthy dogs and cats, it is important to ask if the flow disturbance(s) detected are reasonable explanations for any murmurs auscultated in the patient. The 2D examination is contributory to the diagnosis because lesions of the valve apparatus are often evident along with predictable changes in cardiac chamber or great vessel size associated with valvular regurgitation. The pivotal Doppler finding is the detection of misdirected, high-velocity, turbulent blood flow timed to a period of the cardiac cycle when the valve should be closed. Pathologic regurgitant flow recorded by PWD creates a signal alias and a broadly-disturbed velocity band (Figure 8-42, *A*). Abnormal transvalvular flow encoded by CDI shows one or more signal aliases (or color bar wraps) with the activation of turbulence algorithms (Videos 8-16 and 8-17). Multiple imaging planes might be required to accurately identify the origin and extent of a regurgitant flow pattern (Video 8-21). The examiner should quantify the velocity profile and pressure gradient with CWD, aiming to record velocity spectra with well-defined envelopes and peaks while avoiding overgained signals. It is also *critical to time the duration* of the regurgitant event within the cardiac cycle using the ECG and cardiac motion along with spectral Doppler or color M-mode. This prevents the misinterpretation of the physiologic backflow signals closing the valve and also helps to define other clinically-insignificant flow patterns such as swirling venous return or valvular regurgitation that could be unrelated to valve disease. Examples of the latter are systolic MR associated with premature ventricular complexes and diastolic MR and TR observed in cases of bradycardia, A-V block (see Figure 8-28), or elevated ventricular end-diastolic pressure. Doppler

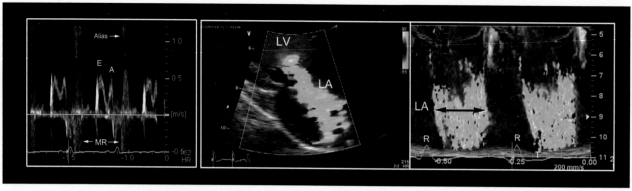

Figure 8-42 Timing of Mitral Valvular Regurgitation. Spectral Doppler and color M-mode are the most accurate ways to time flow events. While high frame rate 2D color Doppler can be accurate, many ultrasound systems are hampered by slow frame rates during CDI. Left: A PWD study from a cat with a brief systolic murmur illustrates the points. There is a high velocity signal with spectral broadening and signal aliasing that lasts about 50% of systole. The flow disturbance is accurately depicted. Diastolic flow (E and A waves) are also evident. Center: A still frame of MR recorded from a dog with myxomatous valve disease (endocardiosis) with sinus tachycardia and heart rate of 215/minute. Turbulence encoding is evident extending to the back wall of the LA. Temporal resolution of flow events is more difficult to attain in a dog at this heart rate. Right: Color M-mode study from the same dog demonstrating the holosystolic nature of the flow event. The red signal at the top represents the fused early and late filling waves (E/A fusion) moving into the mitral orifice. Diastole is abbreviated due to the fast heart rate. While CW Doppler also can be used effectively to time flow events (see Fig. 8-23, *A*) color M-mode is underused and easy to perform when available.

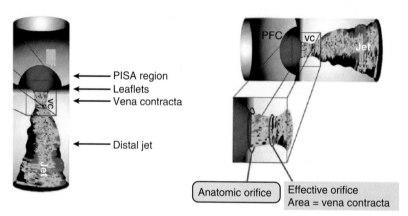

Figure 8-43 The Components of a Regurgitant Jet. These include a proximal isovelocity surface area (PISA) beginning in a region of proximal flow convergence (PFC); the vena contracta (VC); and the jet distal to the regurgitant orifice along with associated turbulence. The effective regurgitant orifice area, which is equivalent to the vena contracta in three dimensions, occurs distal to the anatomic regurgitant orifice defined by the valve leaflets. (Figure from Otto C. *Textbook of Clinical Echocardiography.* 5th ed. Philadelphia: Saunders/Elsevier; 2013; and Roberts BJ, Grayburn P. Color flow imaging of the vena contracta in mitral regurgitation: Technical considerations. *J Am Soc Echocardiogr* 2003;16:1002–6, with permission.)

studies display *direction and velocity* of blood driven by instantaneous pressure gradients into a receiving chamber, not the actual regurgitant *volume*. Thus CDI is not equivalent to a "color angiogram."

Although Doppler studies are highly sensitive for detection of abnormal flow, quantitating the severity of valvular regurgitation is far more difficult. When there is 2D evidence of cardiac remodeling, the situation is relatively obvious because at least mild-to-moderate regurgitation should be present. Conversely, while there are schemes for grading valvular regurgitation based solely on CDI, using standards of veterinary practice, "severe" or even "moderate" MR would be incongruous with normal LA and LV sizes. There are four

commonly-used Doppler methods for semi-quantitation of regurgitation; these involve: (1) assessing the *strength* of the regurgitant signal using CWD provided "standard settings" are used; (2) mapping the *length or area of the regurgitant jet* within the receiving chamber; (3) measuring the diameter or area of the *vena contracta* (the most narrow portion of the jet just distal to the regurgitant orifice); and (4) estimating regurgitant flow rate from analysis of the *proximal isovelocity area (PISA)* that develops in the region in front of the regurgitant orifice (Figure 8-43).[2,5]

Technical aspects of the color Doppler examination can profoundly alter the appearance of regurgitant blood flow in the lower-pressure receiving chamber. Important factors include transducer selection, color and grayscale gain settings, color quality or packet size settings, frame rates, spatial and low-velocity filtering, and PRF or velocity scale. One can completely alter the "severity" of regurgitation by manipulating these CDI settings (Video 8-22).

Mitral Regurgitation

Mitral regurgitation (MR) is one of the most common disorders evaluated by echocardiography.[27,105,117-120,135,136,139,148,154,166,171,172,174,175,202-206,210,217,219,222,229,230,235,241,259,260,262,294,295,306,311,313,319-337] The most important reason for MR in dogs is myxomatous (degenerative) valvular disease, also called valvular endocardiosis. Other etiologies in dogs include MV malformation, infective endocarditis, ruptured mitral chordae tendineae, dilated cardiomyopathy, and other causes of left ventricular (LV) dilatation (such as patent ductus arteriosus). In cats, mitral dysplasia and hypertrophic cardiomyopathy—along with other forms of primary and secondary myocardial diseases—represent the most frequent etiologies. There is no primary literature report of endocardiosis in cats; infective endocarditis is also rare in this species. Regardless of the cause, the principles of echocardiographic evaluation for MR are similar, accepting that the underlying etiology will strongly influence the onset of regurgitation, trajectory of the disease, and associated imaging and clinical findings.

Echocardiographic findings of importance in the assessment of MR include[229,329]: (1) understanding the nature and etiology of the valvular regurgitation; (2) quantifying cardiac remodeling; (3) grading the severity of regurgitation; (4) identifying systolic or diastolic ventricular dysfunction; and (5) detecting Doppler findings indicative of increased pulmonary venous or arterial pressures. As discussed in the previous section of this chapter, in the setting of primary MR, the evaluation of both LV systolic and diastolic function is challenging, and there are no load independent indices available. Examples of mitral valve disease are presented in Figures 8-13, A and 8-42 and also in Figures 8-44 and 8-45; and Videos 8-7, E; 8-17 and Videos 8-21 to 8-27).

Morphologic Lesions and Motion Abnormalities

The normal MV has two leaflets and two papillary muscles from which chordae tendineae extend to each leaflet.[332] The longer anterior (cranioventral) leaflet is closer to the IVS and forms one boundary of the LVOT. The posterior (caudodorsal) leaflet appears shorter in the right parasternal long-axis image but covers a greater part of the annular circumference in short-axis views. The 2D and 3D examinations are used to recognize abnormalities in mitral valvular anatomy, including developmental lesions, changes in valve thickness, valve motion abnormalities, and chordal rupture. The M-mode study might identify abnormalities of valve motion, accepting the limits of this icepick view.

Mitral valve *malformation or dysplasia* (see Figure 8-45, A and B; Video 8-23) can involve any aspect of the valve apparatus including the leaflets, chordae tendineae and papillary muscles.[59,123,338-347] Malformation of the anterior leaflet with either a cleft or a common bridging septal leaflet is also a feature of some atrioventricular septal defects (see "Atrial Septal Defect"). In some cases of mitral valvular dysplasia there is also stenosis of the MV, ranging from mild tethering of otherwise mobile leaflets to severe stenosis with thickened, fused valve cusps. If the valve is stenotic, M-mode examination shows concordant valve motion during diastole, meaning the posterior leaflet follows the anterior leaflet instead of separating from it. Stenotic supravalvular mitral rings have also been identified as a cause of inflow stenosis in cats and dogs and are part of the differential diagnosis for obstruction to LV inflow.[348,349] Atrioventricular valvular stenosis is considered in a subsequent section.

Myxomatous mitral valve disease (see Figure 8-45, D) is characterized by focal to diffuse thickening of the leaflets with changes ranging from subtle to severe. The valve may appear clublike and be confused with a vegetative lesion. Valve thickening in large-breed dogs is often less prominent, and leaflets may appear just mildly thickened or more scalloped and redundant. Ruptured chords are common in degenerative valve disease, and are best observed with high frame rate imaging replayed in slow motion or by application of 3D imaging techniques. Valve prolapse and flail leaflet are also commonly observed (see Video 8-24). In one large study both leaflets exhibited prolapse in 44.5% of dogs studied with some breed differences evident.[331] With prolapse due to myxomatous change, chordal stretch, or minor chordal rupture, there is bulging dorsal to the MV annulus on the right parasternal long-axis view, or one leaflet (usually the anterior one) overrides the other while remaining roughly parallel to the opposing leaflet.[206,320,322,331] In an obvious flail leaflet, the loss of support is evident by bending of the leaflet tip into the LA during systole, the appearance of a double line of closure of that leaflet, or eversion of the anterior mitral leaflet toward the AV in early diastole.[120] Due to the paucity of postmortem studies the precise distinction between prolapse and flail leaflets is unresolved[327] and likely differs among centers.

M-mode studies might demonstrate a thickened mitral leaflet or chaotic, nonpatterned motion of a flail leaflet. In the setting of musical mitral murmurs ("whoops"), careful screening of the valve with an M-mode cursor will often identify high-frequency systolic fluttering of the leaflet and sometimes a chaotic motion suggesting a tear of a smaller chord.

The murmur of MR is often related to dilated or hypertrophic forms of *cardiomyopathy*, so scrutiny of the ventricular chamber and support apparatus is also important to search for morphologic changes. For example, apical displacement of the valvular coaptation point is common with DCM whereas systolic anterior motion is typical of cats with hypertrophic cardiomyopathy (see "Cardiomyopathy" later). In large-breed dogs it can be difficult to distinguish chronic MR with secondary systolic dysfunction from MR caused by DCM. Finding valvular thickening or leaflet prolapse suggests primary valvular disease is either the underlying cause or at least a contributing factor.

The MV is the most commonly affected valve in *infective endocarditis* (see Figure 8-44, D; Video 8-25).[350-353] Because myxomatous MV disease also leads to valvular thickening, the two disorders can be confused, especially in small dogs with severe myxomatous MV disease. Most dogs affected with endocarditis have multisystemic clinical signs that include polyarthritis and features of systemic inflammation. Examiners should also appreciate that epidemiologically, infective endocarditis is uncommon relative to degenerative endocardiosis. If endocarditic lesions are small, they are often visualized as discrete, focal elevations located on the atrial surface of the valve. Acute endocarditis is associated with thrombosis over the ulcerated endocardium and soft thrombus that might oscillate during systole. Infrequently a mobile thrombus is observed stemming from the valve. More severe and larger lesions also can be seen with evidence of tissue destruction across the width of the stroma. Sometimes changes affect one leaflet; whereas with degenerative disease both leaflets are usually involved. Tissue injury from endocarditis can sever chordal attachments and lead to a flail leaflet. Chronic mitral endocarditis lesions, especially in cats, might be indistinguishable from a malformation or severe degenerative changes. Valve calcification with shadowing is uncommon and valve scarring sufficient to cause mitral stenosis is also rare.

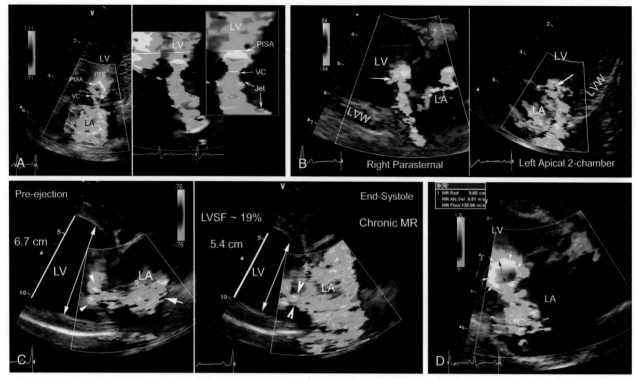

Figure 8-44 **Mitral Regurgitation in Myxomatous Mitral Valve Disease. A,** The components of a regurgitant jet are shown in these images obtained from two dogs with chronic MR due to myxomatous valve disease. Left: The receiving chamber "spray" is well outlined and contaminated by a pulmonary venous return encoded in red (*) See Fig 8-43 for other abbreviations. Right: A relatively flat isovelocity hemisphere and a clearer example of a vena contracta is shown in the right panel. Both the PISA and the VC can be used for advanced analyses of regurgitant severity (see text for details). **B,** Close-up images of an eccentric jet of MR in a dog with severe valvular disease. Note the relatively small area consumed by the "wall-hugging" jet in the right parasternal and left apical images. Eccentric jets infrequently occupy more than 50% of the LA area, emphasizing the importance on not overrelying on receiver chamber assessments. LVW = left ventricular lateral wall. **C,** Measurement of the vena contracta in long axis in a large breed dog with chronic MR and secondary LV systolic dysfunction. Left: Isovolumetric contraction showing preejection MR. Flow moving into the proximal isovelocity area is encoded in both red and blue (*arrowheads*) suggesting the US beam is at close to a right angle to the regurgitant flow. Right: End-systolic frame shows a wide MR jet (with substantial color bleeding into tissues) with a relatively-clear vena contracta between the arrowheads. Thick lines on the left and right depth scales indicate the end-diastolic and end-systolic dimensions, respectively. See text for details. **D,** Proximal isovelocity area in a dog with MR (*small arrows*). The baseline has been shifted down to identify an approximate hemisphere of signal aliasing. The hemisphere is not ideally "flat" on the valvular surface. This "ball on a jet" appearance is common and might be explained by lack of encoding of flow moving at right angles to the ultrasound beam or the complexity of the flow relative to the interrogating beam. The regurgitant jet is also evident in green turbulence encoding within the LA. A software application can be used to estimate the regurgitant flow rate. The radius of the PISA to the regurgitant orifice is shown and is approximately 6 mm (*double arrows*) at an aliasing velocity of 51 cm/s. This finding implies severe MR in this small breed dog despite the relatively small "jet area".

Cardiac Remodeling in Mitral Regurgitation

The diameters and volumes needed for estimation of LA and LV size and for calculation of ejection and shortening fractions can be gleaned from the M-mode, 2D, or 3D studies. Blood regurgitated into the atrium leads to LA dilatation, and the return of this regurgitant volume back to the ventricle—along with the normal venous return—promotes progressive LV dilatation and eccentric hypertrophy. Progressive LA dilatation is often associated with distraction of the atrial septum to the right and dilatation of the pulmonary venous ostia, which can also be caused by MR jets entering the pulmonary veins. Determination of atrial and ventricular dimensions and volumes and the calculation of LV systolic function have been detailed previously in this chapter. The reader is encouraged to review these sections because this information is pertinent to the assessment of cardiac size and to LV function in dogs with chronic MR.

As the severity of MR increases, both LA the LV expand compatible with a state of volume overload. It would be surprising to identify normal LA and LV dimensions in a patient with moderate to severe MR. Exceptions to this rule include cases of peracute MR from endocarditis, of primary chordal rupture, and perhaps of overzealous diuresis (although remodeling should still be evident). With progressive MR the ratios

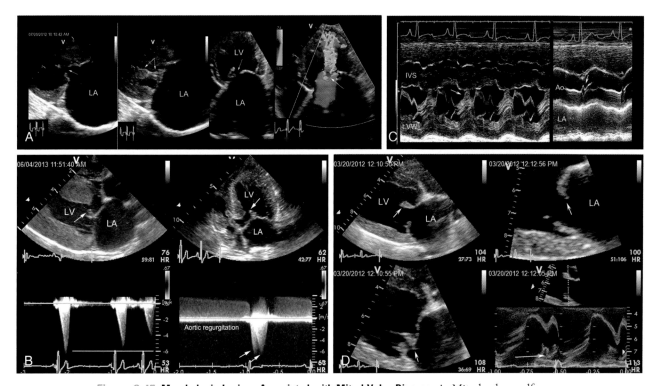

Figure 8-45 Morphologic Lesions Associated with Mitral Valve Disease. A, Mitral valve malformation demonstrating stenosis of the valve from long axis and left apical image planes. The thickened leaflets do not open fully and bow (dome) during diastole. The maximal opening diameter is markedly reduced and forces blood to accelerate through the valve orifice (*single arrows*). The second frame from the left is captured in systole and shows short chordae tendineae and abnormal papillary muscles connecting to the mitral valve (*double arrow*). There is severe LA dilation with marked rounding of the chamber indicating high pressure. The far right panel demonstrates a signal alias as flow approaches the stenotic orifice. Transmitral flow is high velocity and turbulent. **B,** Mitral valve malformation in a dog characterized functionally by systolic anterior motion of the mitral valve (*arrows*) with dynamic LVOT obstruction and mitral regurgitation. These findings are evident in the right parasternal long axis image (upper left) and apical image plane (upper right) along with LV concentric hypertrophy due to outflow obstruction and LA dilation due to MR. Lower left: The LVOT velocity signal is markedly increased in velocity (>6 m/s) and has a late systolic peak due to dynamic obstruction. The first cycle is after a long pause; the last after a short R-R interval. Note how long preceding cycle length influences LVOT velocity related to increased preload and reduced aortic diastolic pressure. Lower right: The effect of crossing two jets with a CW cursor line is evident. Flow patterns of both an eccentric MR jet and the LVOT obstruction are superimposed (*arrows*). There is also aortic regurgitation. The LVOT gradient and MR are often reduced with beta-adrenergic blockade. **C,** Mitral valve malformation in a puppy with systolic anterior motion of the anterior leaflet (*left arrow*) resulting in dynamic LVOT obstruction, secondary LV hypertrophy, and mid-systolic closure of the aortic valve (*right arrow*). These changes were largely reversible with beta-blockade and the LV reverse-remodeled with little residual cardiac problems. **D,** Myxomatous canine valvular disease. Four images obtained from an asymptomatic dog with myxomatous disease of the mitral valve and mitral regurgitation are shown. Thickening of the mitral valve is evident in the three 2D images, especially involving the AMV leaflet (*arrows*). Systolic prolapse is evident during systole (lower left). There is some chaotic motion of the posterior leaflet on the M-mode study (*arrow*), suggestion a chordal rupture.

of LA/AV and LV/AV increase. Once LV size exceeds upper limits based on scaling to body size (see Table 8-7) the degree of remodeling can be considered at least mild-to-moderate. The diastolic LV wall thickness is usually normal, but it has been reported that insufficient hypertrophy, as assessed by the wall thickness to chamber radius ratio, could be a risk factor for development of heart failure in dogs with MR.[259,313] This finding has not been yet been documented prospectively with necropsy studies, and the observation might relate in part to the single, midchamber diameter measurement so often taken. The RV is often compressed in diastole by displacement of the IVS, and in many dogs the size of this chamber appears

relatively normal, even in the presence of CHF. With severe TR, the development of atrial fibrillation, or in the setting of significant PHT, the RV does enlarge.

Color Doppler Assessment of Mitral Regurgitation

The recognition of MR using CDI is straightforward as a turbulent flow signal entering the left atrium during systole (see Figure 8-44; Videos 8-21 to 8-24). At least three different imaging planes (right parasternal long-axis, left apical 4-chamber, and left apical 2 or 3-chamber) should be obtained to confirm (or refute) the diagnosis and assess the severity. The direction of the jet of MR within the LA is most commonly *opposite* to the source. In other words, if the anterior leaflet is prolapsed the jet will likely be directed posteriorly (dorso-laterally) and to the left. Leaks in the posterior leaflet send the regurgitant jet toward the atrial septum. Multiple jets are common and central jets can be observed with primary valve disease (as well as with other causes such as DCM). As noted in the introduction, the assessment of MR severity by CDI can involve receiving chamber analysis (jet length or jet area relative to LA area), measurement of the vena contracta (the jet width close to the regurgitant orifice), or analysis of the proximal isovelocity area in the region of flow convergence proximal to the valve.[319,329] However, grading of MR severity using only CDI is not straightforward, and in the absence of any cardiac remodeling a diagnosis of moderate or severe MR should be made with caution.[330] The heart rate and cycle length also can influence the apparent severity and grading of MR on a beat-to-beat basis.[337]

The length and area of the *regurgitant jet* in the LA is commonly used and misused for grading the severity of MR. The precise definition of the "jet" is also subject to discussion because of differences between system algorithms and displays of turbulence along with influences of instrument settings. It should be noted that the off-cited study comparing jet area to angiography in human patients calls for the use of two or three orthogonal image planes;[5,319] however, most veterinary examinations use a single plane for jet area analysis and rarely describe the technical details of the color Doppler study that so profoundly influence the color encoding (see Video 8-22). Assuming proper flow alignment and correct instrumentation, the finding of a narrow central jet of MR that extends no more than ½ of the distance into the atrium would be typical of trivial or mild MR. Similarly, a long skinny jet that extends >50% of the length into the atrium could indicate more significant MR or simply a higher ventricular driving pressure as encountered in an excited patient or one with systemic hypertension. In contrast, a wide-origin regurgitant jet that extends to the dorsal LA wall or into the pulmonary veins[354] generally indicates moderate or severe MR. The regurgitant jet can entrain other RBCs within the atrium such that a central spray with a wide distribution of turbulence or aliasing can be misleading. Such flow patterns do not always indicate severe MR, especially when lower PRF (velocity scale) settings or a lower frequency transducer is used for the examination. Jet area is also misleading for those regurgitant streams carried along an atrial wall. These are grossly underestimated in terms of severity of regurgitation,[84,86] and even when <25% of the LA area is encompassed by the jet the regurgitation can still be severe (see Figure 8-44, *B*; Video 8-21).

The *width of the vena contracta* corresponds to lesion severity (see Figures 8-43 and 8-44, *A*), but different canine breeds make analysis problematic as jet width must be interpreted relative to the patient's size. In the authors' experience a jet diameter of ≥3 mm in a dog <20 kg usually indicates "significant" MR and measurements exceeding 5 mm are usually indicated of severe disease. These crude clinical observations are similar to those identified in a recent retrospective study of canine MR.[355] If the jet diameter is normalized to the long axis, systolic aortic diameter (measured between opened AV leaflets), a ratio >2.4 predicts increased risk of cardiac mortality (Sargent, et al., in press 2014). When measuring the vena contracta at right angles to regurgitant flow it is helpful to identify a negative (blue) and positive (red) flow pattern converging into the jet, which then can be sampled at right angles to the axial US beam. This image is often obtained from a right parasternal long-axis view (see Figure 8-44, *C*). It is also possible to measure the jet width extending from the "ball" or hemisphere of a PISA obtained from a left apical view (see Figure 8-44, *A*). Some examiners prefer to turn off tur-

bulence encoding when measuring the PISA and the vena contracta. When there are multiple regurgitant jets, this method is problematic; furthermore, 3D imaging in human patients has demonstrated the anatomic complexity of the vena contracta, a characteristic largely missed when using 2DE.

Hydraulic analysis of regurgitant jets[9] indicates that RBCs accelerate in isovelocity, hemispheric surfaces within a region of flow convergence proximal to the regurgitant orifice. The *proximal isovelocity surface area* (PISA) method of analysis[203,204,206,355-357] involves shifting the zero baseline down to create a signal alias until a hemisphere or measurable radius is observed approaching the regurgitant orifice (see Figures 8-43 and 8-44, *D*). This technique can be used to calculate regurgitant flow rates and an effective regurgitant orifice area and has also been described in the veterinary literature. Interested readers are referred to the references for details of this advanced approach. For the most part, the PISA method has not been validated in dogs or cats except by comparing it to measurements of ventricular remodeling; as such, this simply offers redundant information and prospective studies are needed. Physicians mainly use this technique to identify patients with significant MR so that surgical valve repair can be staged *prior* to the development of significant remodeling. Experience and good technique are needed, and the value it might offer to veterinary practice now or in the future requires further definition.

The PISA also can be assessed in a subjective manner. If the zero baseline is shifted down to an aliasing velocity of ~30 to 40 cm/s, a hemisphere representing a PISA (or a ball on a jet) is often seen. If the PISA is relatively far from the vena contracta at this Nyquist limit, and especially if the radius exceeds 5 mm or more, it is likely that MR is moderate to severe in a dog. In contrast, a tiny, somewhat flattened PISA within 1-2 mm of the orifice often suggests trivial to mild MR. Of course this crude analysis should be interpreted in light of other assessments including LV and LA size.

A fascinating finding in some dogs is the development of an atrial septal tear within the fossa ovale.[335,358] This leads to an acquired atrial septal defect with left-to-right shunting (Video 8-26). The condition is probably caused by high LA pressure, stretching of the fossa ovale, and possibly jet injury caused by eccentric jets of MR.

Systolic Function in Mitral Regurgitation

More than half of the total LV stroke volume can be ejected retrograde (into the LA), so any change in LV volume over the cardiac cycle is not equivalent to ejection into the aorta or to cardiac output. Both LVFS and LVEF increase in smaller-breed dogs with chronic MR (see Figure 8-13, *A*; Video 8-27). The enhanced systolic function can be explained by the increased preload and reduced afterload fostered by moderate to severe MR. By the time the AV opens, the LV has already emptied and thickened undergoing morphologic changes that reduce wall stress (afterload). Thus in myxomatous MV disease, standard indices of LV systolic function are unreliable for assessing myocardial contractility. Importantly most *dogs with overt* CHF caused by MR exhibit *hyperdynamic* function based on most indices of LV systolic and diastolic function.[27,119,139,148,210,217,222,230,262,294,326,329]

The finding of a normal LVEF or LVFS in the presence of severe MR does suggest LV myocardial failure, but this is uncommonly observed except in larger breed dogs exceeding ≈20 kg body weight. The reason for these differences in LV function in dogs of different body size is uncertain. Despite its apparent popularity, the use of an end-systolic volume index derived from an M-mode echocardiogram is problematic as a test of systolic function as discussed previously (see

"Ventricular Function"). To reiterate: although end-systolic indices do increase with progressive MR, M-mode techniques overestimate the end-systolic ventricular volume and also do not account for effects of mid-chamber remodeling.[118,154,241] Similarly most of the cited studies of advanced tissue-based methods for assessing LV systolic function in dogs with chronic MR have also shown hyperdynamic segmental contraction of this chamber.[154,217] One exception was a study of dogs with myxomatous MV disease in which ventricular torsion became hyperdynamic in mild-moderate heart failure but then normalized in the dogs with severe CHF.[219]

Right-sided enlargement can be observed in cases of MR when there is concurrent PHT[171,172,174,324] or following the appearance of AF; however, in most cases of chronic MR enlargement of the RV and RA is not obvious. Rightward displacement of the IVS can lead to a hyperdynamic systolic excursion of the IVS that is relatively greater than the systolic amplitude of the LVW (the opposite of normal). This finding is common in dogs with moderate to severe MR and has also been produced experimentally in dogs and shown to be reversible.[119,359] Thus this observation is more likely a feature of moderate to severe LV volume overload than of impaired LV freewall function.

Spectral Doppler Findings in Mitral Regurgitation

Continuous wave (CW) Doppler studies of MR are used to confirm the regurgitant timing and to identify elevated LA pressures. MR is characterized by high-velocity, turbulent, systolic jets recorded at the valve orifice and within the left atrium (see Figures 8-23, A and 8-42). The duration of MR varies, though typical cases are holosystolic, preceding ejection and extending into isovolumetric relaxation. Early-to midsystolic regurgitation is often observed in mild MR and must be differentiated from normal, low-velocity backflow that closes the MV and usually ends within the QRS complex. Delayed onset of regurgitation is typical of MR caused by systolic anterior motion of the MV. The RBC velocity at the envelope of the jet relates to the instantaneous pressure difference between LA and LV (and in the absence of aortic stenosis the ascending aorta). The peak regurgitant velocity in normotensive dogs usually falls into the approximate range of 5.2 to 6.2 m/s. In cases of systemic hypertension (or LVOTO), the peak regurgitant velocity exceeds ≈6.5 m/s owing to elevated LV systolic pressure. Conversely, the peak MR velocity can be decreased when there is systolic dysfunction, systemic hypotension, or high LA pressures, reflecting reductions in the instantaneous pressure gradient.[325] The subjective contour of the MR jet can also change from a rounded peak to an earlier, abrupt peak with a rapid velocity deceleration. This finding indicates an abrupt increase in LA pressure associated with severe MR. As mentioned under "Ventricular Function," the first derivative of LV pressure change, dp/dt, can be obtained from measurement of the MR jet.[295] This value does decline in some dogs with advanced MR, but these are usually larger breed dogs with obvious systolic dysfunction.

As described in the section on "Diastolic Function," the diastolic assessment of the LV in chronic MR is often characterized by hyperdynamic function (increased E') in the walls.[119,175,210] This probably relates to the rapid restoration of a large LV diastolic volume that follows a hyperdynamic contraction. Moderate to severe MR also produces an abrupt increase in LA pressure related to the simultaneous arrival of the regurgitant stroke volume and pulmonary venous return. This prominent v-wave in the LA pressure profile *transiently* increases end-systolic LA pressure (but not necessarily the mean LA pressure), and contributes somewhat disproportionately to early LV diastolic filling, a period often used to assess diastolic function. The finding of a relaxation abnormality

with E/A reversal (Grade 1 diastolic dysfunction) is good evidence for mild MR and normal LA pressures in a dog with endocardiosis, and it indicates a low imminent risk of CHF. However, with increasing regurgitant volume, the increase in LA pressure normalizes the transmitral flow pattern and eventually the E-wave becomes quite tall. In the authors' experience, and based on a retrospective study,[333] once the peak E-wave velocity reaches 1.2 to 1.4 m/s, the likelihood of elevated filling pressures and left-sided CHF is greater. The E/E' ratio apparently does correlate with mean LA pressure based on model studies.[181,306] However, the ratio of E/E' that predicts CHF is probably higher than for cardiomyopathy, likely in the range of 13 to 15 in chronic, spontaneous disease,[148] similar to values observed in people with primary MR.[299] Lower ratios (>9.1) predicted a mean LA pressure of >20 mm Hg in experimental MR of acute onset,[308] emphasizing the need to tailor the "ratios" for the underlying disease and chronicity when attempting to predict elevated pulmonary venous pressures. In addition to a large E/E', a shorted IVRT and abbreviated MV deceleration time support a diagnosis of increased mean LA pressure in the setting of a poorly compliant LV. In one study of dogs with CHF due to MR, abbreviation of IVRT <45 ms (from high LA pressures) and a ratio of E:IVRT >2.5 in dogs predicted radiographic signs of CHF.[311]

Tricuspid Regurgitation

Tricuspid regurgitant jets may stem from valve malformation, tricuspid valvular endocardiosis, cardiomyopathy, RV hypertrophy from other causes (such as pulmonic stenosis), dirofilariasis (including the caval syndrome), and PHT. Infective endocarditis of this valve is rare in small animals. The general echocardiographic approach to patients with TR is similar to those used for MR although there are some specific differences. The examiner should remember that the tricuspid valve of the dog and cat consists of two leaflets, a smaller septal leaflet and a parietal (lateral) leaflet with only a partial commissure. Chords to the septal leaflet are relatively short and the insertion point of the septal tricuspid leaflet is normally slightly apical to that of the anterior mitral leaflet (with the tissue between this offset called the *atrioventricular septum* because it constitutes atrial septum along the right surface and ventricular septum along to the left). There are three to five RV papillary muscles of varying prominence in dogs.

Morphologic Lesions

Dysplasia of the tricuspid valve is a relatively common malformation of larger breeds of dogs and especially of the Labrador retriever.[360-365] In fully-formed tricuspid valve dysplasia the 2D imaging lesions are dramatic. These can include: malformed and thickened leaflets; excessively long or short chordae tendineae; ventral displacement of the annulus with leaflets inserting beyond the normal apical offset (Ebstein's anomaly); and prominent bridging between the medial and lateral papillary muscles (near the apex). In such cases massive RA dilation is expected along with significant RV eccentric hypertrophy. Depending on the leaflet and chordal arrangements there may also be stenosis or rarely atresia of the tricuspid valve. These lesions have also been observed in cats. In contrast, mild tricuspid valve malformations are associated with more subtle abnormalities in the valve apparatus structure and motion and there is more controversy about these diagnoses because some "dysplastic" valves might simply be variations on normal. Imaging features of tricuspid valve disease are emphasized in Figures 8-27, F; 8-28, Top; and Videos 8-14, J, 8-15, I, 8-16, D and E, 8-24, B, and 8-28.

Myxomatous degeneration of the tricuspid valve is probably the most common reason for TR in dogs. Often there is septal leaflet prolapse, creating a bowing appearance to the valve in mid-to-late systole. This is associated with an eccentric jet of TR directed at the lateral RV wall. In comparison to myxomatous MV disease, leaflet thickening is less obvious, ruptured chordae tendineae rare, and the severity of right heart remodeling far less. The development of PHT[171,172,174,229,324] from chronic MR or from concurrent lung or pulmonary vascular disease can worsen TR and lead to right-sided CHF.

Doppler Assessment of Tricuspid Regurgitation

The diagnosis of pathologic TR is hampered by the frequent presence of *physiologic* TR, silent to auscultation and identified by CDI in the majority of healthy dogs and cats when they are examined carefully.[63,67,140,166] The precise features distinguishing physiologic and pathologic TR in breeding dogs without auscultable tricuspid murmurs are a source of contention.

The CDI patterns observed in tricuspid valve regurgitation are qualitatively similar to those described for MR. It is likely that TR jets are underrecognized because transthoracic imaging planes are less available for examining the normal sized RA and the tricuspid orifice is wider and more complicated to interrogate. The principal Doppler finding of TR is the detection of turbulent, high-velocity flow jet exiting the valve orifice and extending into the RA. The retrograde blood flow converging toward the tricuspid orifice can be mapped using PWD and appears as a triangular signal with progressively higher velocity and spectral dispersion as the regurgitant orifice is approached. In cases of "wide-open" TR associated with high RA pressures the spectral appearance before and after the orifice are similar. The RA is more complicated to map than is the circular LA and orientation of TR jets is inconsistent. Regurgitant velocity is directly influenced by the peak RV systolic pressure and can vary with PA pressure, cardiac arrhythmias, and erratic cardiac filling. The velocity of the regurgitant flow generally peaks at less than 2.6 m/s unless there is an elevation in the RV pressure that forces blood into the atrium at a higher velocity. Common reasons for high-velocity TR (that exceeding 3 m/s) are PHT, pulmonic stenosis, and complex congenital heart disease. Pulmonary hypertension is discussed later in this chapter. Sometimes florid TR is associated with a mild increase in regurgitant velocity; the reasons for this are uncertain.

Aortic Regurgitation

Aortic regurgitation is encountered in a number of situations including: subvalvular aortic stenosis; systemic hypertension; infective endocarditis of the AV; malformations of the aortic valve; and with some ventricular septal defects.[17,351,366-370] Trivial aortic regurgitation, silent to auscultation, is often observed in older dogs using CDI and presumably represents age-related valve thickening or endocardiosis. Older cats also develop AR in association with idiopathic dilatation of the aorta (aortoannular ectasia).

Imaging lesions in aortic regurgitation vary with the etiology. In infective endocarditis (see Video 8-25) discrete lesions tend to localize to the ventricular surface of the valve with the principles of diagnosis similar to that discussed above for the MV. In other cases there might be 2D and Doppler evidence of subaortic stenosis or systemic hypertension to suggest the probable cause of AR. Aortic root dilatation should not be overlooked as it is relatively common (Video 8-19). Diastolic fluttering of the mitral valve is a common finding (see Figure 8-13, *D*) and if a large jet impinges on the AMV the EPSS can increase even with normal systolic function.

Doppler diagnosis of AR is straightforward. CDI demonstrates a jet originating from the aortic valve leaflets; it is often eccentric in its path into the LVOT (see Figure 8-27, *E* and Videos 8-17 and 8-29). Placement of the PW sample volume and CW line below the closed AV demonstrates a high-velocity, turbulent, diastolic signal that ends abruptly with ventricular ejection (see Figures 8-29, 8-45, *B*; and 8-46). The regurgitant jet is often eccentric and may contaminate transmitral flow in the LV inlet. The timing of the regurgitant signal can be verified with spectral Doppler or color M-mode (see the right of Figure 8-46).

Grading the amount of regurgitation is more complicated. Certainly LV remodeling can be used as an indicator of severity in chronic AR, provided there are no other reasons for LV enlargement. Compared to equally severe MR, long-standing AR is more likely to impair LV systolic function since the added volume must be ejected back into the high-pressure aorta. Doppler methods of assessment are available but more challenging. Thin regurgitant jets on CDI that extend minimally from the valve orifice are rarely significant. Longer or wider jets may indicate significant AR; however, as discussed

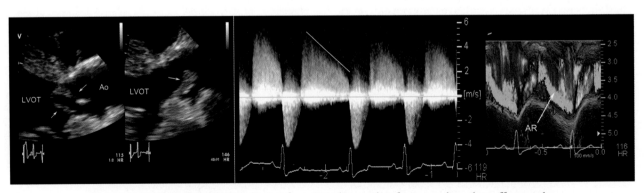

Figure 8-46 Aortic Regurgitation. Images from two dogs with infective endocarditis affecting the aortic valves. Left: Mobile, infected valve with thrombus that oscillated in real time. The leaflet falls into the LV in diastole indicating a tear and lack of support. The marked increase in thickness was evident in systole as well (*right arrow*). Center & Right: CW Doppler and color M-mode recordings from a dog with severe aortic regurgitation and moderate, acquired aortic valvular stenosis due to infective endocarditis. Note the relatively strong regurgitant signal relative to the outflow signal and the steep slope (line) indicating a short pressure half-time and more-rapid equilibration between the aorta and LV diastolic pressures. Compare this to the AR signal in Figure 8-45, *B*. The color M-mode study shows the holodiastolic nature of the flow disturbance.

for MR, the length and area of the jet in the LV is likely to correlate poorly to regurgitant volume. The width of the AR jet at the vena contracta obtained from a long-axis and a short-axis image plane better relates to regurgitant flow volume. Often the color *spray* in the LVOT is prominent in the long-axis or apical images but the *origin* of the jet is small. Assuming the CWD cursor is well-aligned with the regurgitant jet *throughout* diastole, the severity of aortic regurgitation also can be evaluated using CW Doppler by calculating the pressure drop from the beginning to the end of diastole using the simplified Bernoulli equation. Severe aortic regurgitation increases LV diastolic pressure, reducing the pressure gradient, and leading to a sudden drop off in velocity (indicating near equilibration of aortic and ventricular end-diastolic pressures). This can be formally measured by calculating the pressure half-time, which is the duration (in msec) needed for the aortic to LV pressure gradient to decrease by 50%. Short pressure half-times indicate worse AR. Practically the severity of regurgitation can be gauged by the comparing the spectral strength of the regurgitant signal to the grayscale density of the outflow signal and by estimating the pressure half-time by inspecting the slope of the regurgitant signal (see Figure 8-46).

Pulmonary Insufficiency

Pulmonary insufficiency (regurgitation), silent to auscultation, is normal[167] and is encountered in 80% or more of healthy dogs examined by PW Doppler (see Figure 8-18, *D*). It is also common in healthy cats[166] and is often preceded by a prominent reversal wave at end systole that is coded in red by CDI but is low in velocity on the spectral examination. Pulmonary insufficiency is rarely a clinical problem, even when severe. It is a common feature of pulmonary valve dysplasia (before and after balloon valvuloplasty), PHT, and patent ductus arteriosus (see Video 8-17). The main value of identifying pulmonary insufficiency during a Doppler examination resides in the information gained about pulmonary arterial pressures. Increasing pulmonary arterial pressure is associated with progressively higher regurgitant velocities as predicted by the Bernoulli relationship. This is discussed later under "Pulmonary Hypertension."

VALVULAR STENOSIS

Overview and Practical Considerations

Stenosis of the A-V valves is relatively uncommon, typically congenital in nature, and usually associated with valve dysplasia and regurgitation as described in the previous section of this chapter. Obstruction to ventricular or atrial inflow also can occur due to supravalvular mitral rings or from partitioning of the atria through persistence of fetal structures. Examples of the latter are cor triatriatum dexter and sinister[371-380] (Video 8-30). Obstruction to blood flow in the LVOT and RVOT is far more common, especially in dogs where subaortic stenosis (SAS), valvular AS, and pulmonic stenosis (PS) are genetically predisposed diseases of many breeds. Cases of SAS and PS are sporadically identified in cats.

The flow pattern across a stenosis is characterized by conversion of potential (pressure energy) to kinetic energy leading to rapid acceleration of flow, increased peak ejection velocity, and flow disturbance distal to the obstruction (see Figures 8-24 and 8-25; Videos 8-13 and 8-31). In mild cases of AS or SAS, this must be distinguished from the normal impulse gradients that propel blood across the LVOT and into the aorta and are exaggerated by sympathetic tone.[162,163] Identifying and quantifying the severity of moderate to severe outflow tract stenosis is relatively straightforward so long as the exam-

iner obtains good alignment to the jet and does not over-gain the velocity spectrum. Additionally, serious obstructive lesions are accompanied by abnormalities of 2D imaging along with cardiac remodeling. However the identification of mild outflow tract stenosis is more problematic. Normal transvalvular flows frequently alias and activate turbulence mapping in CDI; thus, spectral Doppler studies must be used to confirm any suspected obstruction. The absolute limit of normal outflow tract velocities in various breeds under differing hemodynamic conditions is unresolved. In our experience, most ejection murmurs are associated with peak flow velocities that exceed 1.6 to 1.7 m/s. However, these limits can be exceeded in normal dogs subjected to sympathetic stimulation or when stroke volume is increased. Furthermore, mild increases in ejection velocity are also associated with functional murmurs in breeds not known to develop outflow tract stenosis. Ultimately the examiner has to decide whether more sensitive or more specific limits of outflow velocities are used. An arbitrary up or down adjustment in the cut-off for a normal outflow velocity can change the "diagnosis" from one of stenosis to that of a functional murmur. In either case, the health of the dog is rarely impacted by either designation, but the results can alter recommendations in breeding animals.

Aortic Stenosis

Subvalvular aortic stenosis (SAS) is among the most common congenital heart defect of dogs[381,382] and there is an extensive literature about this disorder.[24,55,92,104,106,128,201,283,365,370,383-392] Typical SAS is characterized by a subvalvular ridge or tunnel that develops after birth; this is very evident on TEE examinations. The aorta is often abnormal with what has been termed *poststenotic dilation*, but a primary aortopathy might also be pertinent to the further development of this defect and abnormal ventricular septal to aortic angles have been identified in Boxers and golden retrievers, even in very young dogs.[389,392] Flow and pressure abnormalities in AS can be defined by the continuity equation and the Bernoulli relationship, which were presented earlier in this chapter.[9,393] Acceleration of blood flow is generated by an increased ventricular systolic pressure and supported by concentric LV hypertrophy. Maximal ejection velocity is reached immediately distal to the obstruction (in the vena contracta) and this velocity is directly proportional to the pressure gradient across the stenosis, simplified as $\Delta P = 4V^2$ (where V is the velocity in m/s). The Doppler-derived maximal instantaneous pressure gradient is somewhat higher than a peak LV-to-peak aortic pressure gradient measured at catheterization (Figure 8-26). Distal to the obstruction there is flow disturbance characterized by a dissipation of kinetic energy and velocity in the form of heat and friction. Some of this energy can be recovered in the form of pressure further explaining why the Doppler estimate of pressure gradient is somewhat higher, even when both gradients are recorded simultaneously.[9]

Anatomic lesions are evident with 2D imaging in moderate to severe cases of SAS (Figure 8-47, *A*). Findings include a subaortic ridge or tunnel, aortopathy and concentric LV hypertrophy. In uncommon cases of valvular AS the leaflets are typically mobile but fused, and dome in systole (Videos 8-9, *A* and 8-31). Compared to humans, stenotic, bicuspid AV leaflets are rarely encountered. With tunnel like obstructions the AMV leaflet is enveloped and can appear thickened. Concurrent MV dysplasia also can be present, creating the bad combination of an incompetent A-V valve with an obstructed outflow tract. Anatomic abnormalities are much less obvious in mild SAS, and their absence often confounds the diagnosis. Post stenotic dilation of the aorta is common (Figure 8-47, *A*; Videos 8-19 and 8-31) along with abnormal ventricular septal to aortic angle.

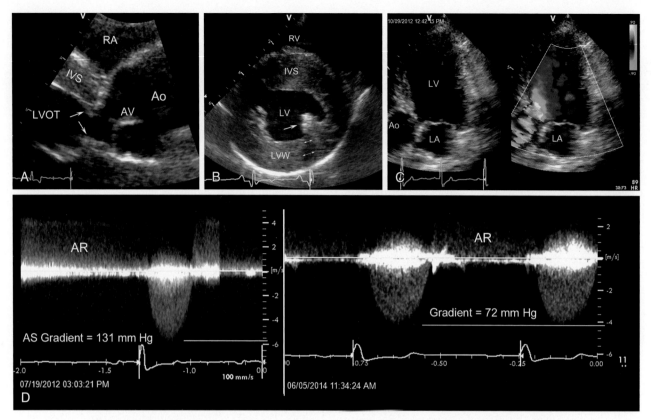

Figure 8-47 **Aortic Stenosis.** A, Close up 2D image of a relatively discrete subvalvular aortic stenosis in a dog (arrows). The aortic valve (AV) is closed. B, Concentric LV hypertrophy shown in the short axis plane in a dog with SAS. The subendocardium is somewhat hyperechoic, especially in the anterior papillary muscle (*arrow*) resulting in an acoustic shadow in the far field (*double arrows*). This is often a sign of ischemic injury to the myocardium with replacement fibrosis. C, Color Doppler imaging of the LVOT in a dog with aortic valvular stenosis. The LVOT contains high velocity turbulent flow. D, Peak LVOT velocity recorded about two years apart in a dog with SAS and progressive LV systolic dysfunction. The difference in the estimated maximal pressure gradients across the stenosis is explained by reduced ventricular stroke volume in the later recording associated with heart failure.

2D and M-mode studies reveal concentric LV hypertrophy (see Videos 8-18 and 8-31) that is usually, though not always, commensurate with the pressure gradient across the obstruction. Subendocardial ischemia in this disease causes myocardial cell death with replacement by fibrous tissue. Sometimes this change is evident as a zone of hyperechogenicity involving the LV subendocardium or papillary muscles; it indicates severe disease (Figure 8-47, *B*). A hyperdynamic EF is often observed in severe AS during the compensated phase of disease. Eventually systolic function becomes normal and then decreased predisposing to ventricular dilatation and left-sided CHF. Diastolic dysfunction is observed in long-standing cases of moderate to severe obstruction[386] and can involve any of the grades previously discussed under "Ventricular Function."

Pulsed-wave Doppler studies and CDI detect proximal acceleration of blood flow and turbulence distal to the stenosis (see Figure 8-29, Videos 8-16 and 8-31). The spectrum usually forms a signal alias, requiring CW Doppler (or high PRF techniques) to faithfully record the maximal velocity in the vena contracta. The examiner should obtain recordings from the subcostal position since this provides the best alignment with flow in most dogs.[92] At least five cardiac cycles should be averaged and there might be value in tracing the outer envelope of the spectrum to obtain a mean pressure gradient (see Figure 8-26). Mean gradients are typically 50% to 60% of maximal gradients, and provide a check on overgained velocity spectra. In patients with concurrent MR, the CWD cursor might cross both jets, contaminating the AS jet and raising the chance the pressure gradient will be overestimated. Concurrent AR is usually evident but in most cases trivial to mild and silent to auscultation. Moderate to severe AR, concurrent MR, or clinical signs of systemic illness should prompt consideration of infective endocarditis, a recognized complication of SAS in dogs.

Although the diagnosis of moderate to severe AS is straightforward, difficulties are encountered in the recognition of mild disease. Different PWD findings such as "spectral dispersion" or "acceleration" of flow across the LVOT are largely subjective, and in our experience 2D imaging lesions are inconsistently identified in mild cases. It is normal for the velocity profile to accelerate (at least double) when velocities are mapped from the apical portion of the outflow tract into the ascending aorta. Peak PWD velocities of >1.7 m/s recorded from the left apex and CWD velocities >2 m/s from subcostal imaging fall outside the "normal range" established for dogs *without any cardiac murmurs*. However, these cutoffs are probably too conservative and do not account for the large number of dogs with apparently benign, functional ejection murmurs in which velocities often exceed 2 m/s. Nor has the influence of relatively small aortic size compared to the LV size been much discussed in veterinary medicine, but this combination should result in acceleration of flow into the ascending aorta,[162,163] as so often observed in the boxer dog and bull terriers. Other "cutoffs" for the diagnosis of AS in dogs have been proposed,[128,201,392,394-396] including peak velocities exceeding 2.2 m/s, 2.25 m/s and 2.4 m/s. Sometimes these values are separated by just a few pixels on the measuring screen, and *none of these recommendations is based on any longitudinal study with necropsy validation.* Fortunately these fine lines are mostly relevant to breeding decisions and do not recommend any therapy or negative prognosis for a dog kept solely for companionship. It has been suggested that holodiastolic AR and an abnormal septal to aortic angle can also be used to predict the likelihood of SAS in dogs, and perhaps these findings will prove useful. Many cardiologists have accepted that there are many dogs with soft ejection murmurs that fall into a maximal aortic velocity range of 2.0 to 2.4 m/s, and in the absence of other imaging findings, simply label the dogs as "equivocal". As mentioned earlier, SAS can progress in puppies,[370,384,389] so a follow-up examination near maturity can sometimes clarify the situation.

Disease severity is often based on the CWD derived maximal pressure gradient (see Figures 8-26 and 8-29). Instantaneous gradients exceeding about 80 mm Hg are generally graded as "severe"[106] accepting some dogs tolerate gradients of 80 to 100 mm Hg reasonably well while others do not and are at risk for sudden cardiac death or CHF. Gradients exceeding 200 mm Hg are sometimes identified, corresponding to peak LV systolic pressures of more than 300 mm Hg. The Doppler gradient obtained in a conscious dog cannot be compared to that obtained during heavy sedation or general anesthesia. These differences relate mainly to effects of general anesthesia that severely depresses stroke volume and reduces the gradient by about 50%. When invasive and Doppler pressure gradients are recorded simultaneously under anesthesia, and mean pressure gradients are calculated and compared, there is little difference between the two methods.[383] This highlights the importance of considering the effect of stroke volume on the pressure gradient. As an example, the maximal pressure gradient decreases over time as LV function deteriorates (see Figure 8-47, C). Varying cycle lengths encountered in sinus arrhythmia or atrial fibrillation also exert a substantial influence on stroke volume and gradient. In giant breeds such as the Newfoundland, the health of the dog can become jeopardized by substantial gradient and disease progression during the first year of life.[384] Presumably this relates to a disproportionate increase in LV stroke volume, relative to the size of the LVOT. Lastly, diagnosing and assessing mild to moderate AS by Doppler methods only is nearly impossible in cases of uncorrected patent ductus arteriosus because outflow velocities are generally increased from the increased LV stroke volume and can even exceed 3.0 m/s.

The special situation of *dynamic left ventricular outflow obstruction* (LVOTO) is associated with hypertrophic obstructive cardiomyopathy, certain MV malformations, other causes of LV concentric hypertrophy, and reduced LV volume associated with congenital RV disease.[124,339,343,346] Dynamic LVOTO is characterized by high-velocity systolic blood flow beginning in the LV outflow tract near the point of mitral-to-septal contact. The peak outflow tract velocity and flow disturbances are labile, increased by sympathetic drive, and attenuated by esmolol or atenolol. A typical "dagger-shaped" signal is expected, with the sudden acceleration of velocity beginning in early to mid-systole, coincident with the onset of dynamic ventricular obstruction (see Figure 8-45, B). This is discussed further under "Hypertrophic Cardiomyopathy." Importantly both dogs and cats have been reported in which there was partial or complete resolution of obstruction and LV hypertrophy subsequent to treatment with beta-adrenergic blockers.

Other relatively rare causes of LVOT obstruction include mass lesions in the LVOT[397] infective endocarditis,[351] and tumors in the proximal aorta.

Pulmonic Stenosis

The prevalence of PS is high among cases of congenital heart disease and echocardiography is a key aspect of diagnosis and assessment.[388,390,396,398-403] Abnormalities observed by 2D imaging include valvular thickening (dysplasia), fusion along the commissural edges, and varying degrees of annular hypoplasia. Additional relevant findings might include a supravalvular tethering or stenosis of the valve leaflets, subvalvular thickening, anomalous single coronary artery (especially in English bulldogs), RV hypertrophy, and changes in the main PA that range from hypoplasia to poststenotic dilatation (Figure 8-48, A and B; Video 8-32). There is some controversy among cardiologists about the criteria for the diagnosis of subvalvular or infundibular pulmonary stenosis[400] versus double chambered right ventricle,[371,404-409] especially in cats (Videos 8-32 and 8-33). Both of these conditions lead to outflow obstruction well below the pulmonic valve. While not strictly a cardiac disease, hypoplasia, stenosis, or obstruction of the main pulmonary artery or a principal branch can lead to many imaging features similar to those caused by congenital PS.[410-413]

The response of the RV to outflow obstruction is hypertrophy of the chamber (see Video 8-18, G) especially concentric thickening when the obstruction is congenital in origin. Similar to severe AS, hyperechoic myocardium is observed in some dogs with marked RV hypertrophy, compatible with subendocardial ischemic fibrosis. The hypertrophy usually includes the right side of the IVS and the increased RV pressure flattens the septum and reduces the LV size (see Figure 8-13, B). Severe RV hypertrophy often leads to a second level of functional, dynamic obstruction in the infundibulum. This secondary obstruction is often relieved by beta-blockade. Diastolic dysfunction is common and can be detected by PWD, TDI, or advanced tissue methods.

The diagnosis of PS can be established by identifying lesions mentioned above through 2D imaging. The valve is often mobile and systolic doming might be seen. The origin of the coronary arteries should be sought in views just off the short-axis. Any RV hypertrophy is generally proportionate to the pressure gradient. Dilation of the main PA is variable and less clearly related to the severity of obstruction. Saline contrast echocardiography should be performed to exclude a PFO that can allow right-to-left shunting (see Figure 8-14; Videos 8-8, A and 8-32). The typical PWD findings include acceleration of RBC velocity across the infundibulum, increased maximal PA velocity (>1.6 m/s), flow disturbance distal to the stenotic valve, and frequently prominent pulmonary insufficiency. These qualitative flow abnormalities are often evident with CDI (see Video 8-32). Peak ejection velocity can be used to quantify the severity of obstruction using the Bernoulli equation in the manner described for AS. Frequently CWD imaging uncovers a velocity profile proximal to the valvular stenosis that is substantially augmented from dynamic, RVOT obstruction (see Figure 8-23, C). This situation creates a subvalvular velocity profile (V_1) superimposed on the peak velocity envelope (V_2). If the second peak is late in systole it should have little effect on the maximal pressure gradient estimate based on squaring the peak velocity (V_2); however, if the velocity is >2 m/s in mid-systole, the simplified Bernoulli equation should not be used as it will overestimate the valvular obstruction. The mean pressure difference across the stenotic valve can be estimated by tracing each profile and subtracting the mean gradient of V_1 from the mean gradient of the peak envelope. Additionally, the longer form of the

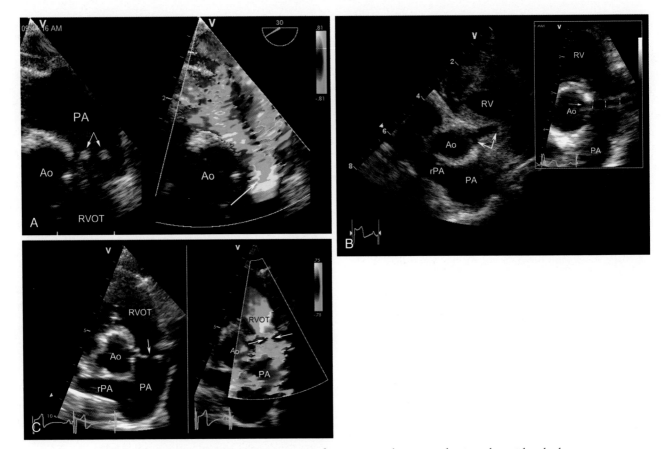

Figure 8-48 Pulmonic Stenosis. A, Doming of a stenotic pulmonary valve in a dog with valvular PS and concurrent PDA. The TEE image shows thick valve leaflets opened into the proximal PA. The CDI (right) shows flow moving toward the transducer which aliases (arrow) and then forms a bifurcating jet (green). Positive flow into the PA (coded in red) is contaminated by flow coming from the ductus arteriosus (coded in blue). **B,** Anomalous (single origin) right coronary artery (R2A type) in an English bulldog. The image is off angle from the short axis to follow the large, single coronary vessel. Inset: Close-up image from another English bulldog with an R2A single origin coronary artery. The vessel originates from the right coronary ostium (arrow) and courses across the RV outflow tract (small arrows). **C,** Valvular/sub valvular PS. A small valve orifice is evident in the left panel. The color Doppler image (right) shows an "apple core" narrowing (arrows) and distal flow disturbance in the post-stenotic dilatation.

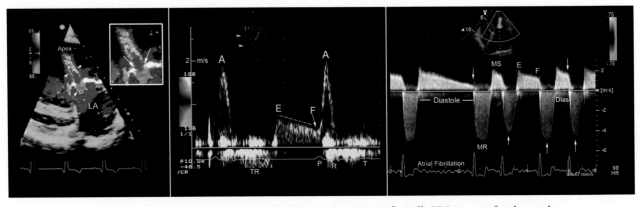

Figure 8-49 Doppler Findings in Mitral & Tricuspid Stenosis. Left: Still CDI image of a dog with mitral stenosis. Note the signal converge to a proximal isovelocity area with a red to blue alias developing proximal to the valve. A jet in evident within the mitral orifice sometimes referred to as a "candle-flame sign" (inset). Center: Prolonged pressure half-time (note the slope between E and F) and prominent A-wave approaching 2m/s in velocity in a young dog with tricuspid stenosis with compensatory RA hypertrophy. A faint aliased jet of TR is also evident (arrowheads). Right: Appearance of mitral inflow velocity profile in mitral dysplasia with stenosis. Note the absence of an A-wave in the setting of atrial fibrillation and effects of cardiac cycle length on the end-diastolic velocity (upper arrows), which is lower with longer cycles. The mean diastolic pressure gradient—calculated as the area under the diastolic velocity curve, divided by time—is higher when diastole (Dias) is brief. There is also MR evident with varying peak velocities related to effects of diastolic intervals on preload and ventricular systolic function.

Bernoulli equation can be used that subtracts from the peak velocity (V_2) the instantaneous V_1, before squaring. It is re-emphasized that Doppler gradients recorded from unsedated dogs are substantially higher than those recorded by cardiac catheterization during general anesthesia. The two cannot be meaningfully compared unless recorded simultaneously.

Dynamic Right Ventricular Outflow Tract Obstruction

Dynamic RVOT obstruction that is not related to RV hypertrophy is commonly associated with high sympathetic tone, especially in cats. It is usually considered a physiologic finding, not an anatomical stenosis. Hypovolemia and hypertrophy of the ventricular septum (with HCM) are also associated with this functional situation. Slow motion playback of 2D images reveals no anatomic obstruction in the outflow tract during diastole, but a strong inward movement of the RV freewall toward the IVS becomes evident in mid-to-late systole. Examination using CDI reveals a signal alias near the supraventricular crest of the ventricular septum and distally turbulence encoding in the subpulmonic RV. A dagger-shaped RVOT signal is recorded with CWD. The peak ejection velocity is typically >1.6 and <3 m/s, but the velocity is probably underestimated due to difficulty in aligning to blood flow in the proximal RVOT where the obstruction originates. This condition is important because it explains many of the functional systolic murmurs heard in cats.[165] Rare causes of dynamic or fixed obstruction of the RVOT include thoracic deformities and neoplasia.[414-416]

Atrioventricular Valve Stenosis

Stenosis of an atrioventricular valve is uncommon in dogs and cats and is usually explained by a valve malformation or obstruction immediately above the valve. Very rare causes include endocarditis, a large intracardiac neoplasm,[417] chronic feline cardiomyopathy,[418] or a congenital supravalvular ring.[348,349] Echocardiographic findings are compatible with anatomic obstruction to ventricular diastolic filling and demonstrated in Figure 8-49 and Videos 8-16, 8-23 and 8-28. The salient 2D features are imaging lesions of the valve such as thickening, commissural fusion, doming, and reduced diastolic excursion, along with atrial dilatation.[123,338,340,342,347] There is often direct insertion of a leaflet into a papillary muscle or very short or stout chordae tendineae. Doppler studies show acceleration of the diastolic flow signal (flow convergence) at the atrial side of the A-V orifice, increased ventricular filling velocities with high-velocity E- and A-waves, and a prolongation of the pressure half-time (as described for aortic regurgitation). A classic CDI appearance[363] of an aliased inflow core with a bright, turbulent rim has been called the "candle flame sign" in people and also has been observed in animals. Some cases of A-V valve stenosis are associated with extremely high-velocity mitral or tricuspid A-waves (>1.5 m/s), presumably representing incomplete atrial emptying in the setting of atrial hypertrophy with preserved atrial function. Frequently there is concurrent valvular regurgitation. The pressure halftime is prolonged,[345] and if there is sinus rhythm the A-wave often exceeds the E-wave unless there is atrial fibrillation (see Figure 8-49, right). These changes distinguish mitral and tricuspid stenosis from other causes of high inflow velocity such as severe A-V valve regurgitation or left-to-right shunts.

PULMONARY HYPERTENSION

Pulmonary hypertension (PHT) is an increase in systolic, diastolic, or mean blood pressure measured within the PA. In resting dogs the normal PA pressures are between 20 and 25 mm Hg in systole and about 8 to 12 mm Hg in diastole, with a mean PA pressure of approximately 14 to 16 mm Hg. Once systolic pressures at rest exceed approximately 35 mm Hg, a diagnosis of PHT is made. There are various classification systems for the causes of PHT in people, but veterinary echocardiographers can simplify the differential diagnosis by considering three general causes: (1) postcapillary PHT due to left-sided heart disease; (2) pre-capillary PHT due to narrowing or obstruction of pulmonary arteries, and (3) PHT associated with severe, parenchymal lung disease. Some disorders likely involve more than one mechanism. Because PHT is not a specific disease (aside from idiopathic or primary PHT), understanding the general causes of elevated PA pressures can help the sonographer restructure the examination once elevated PA pressures have been identified. Echocardiography is the major diagnostic test for confirmation of PHT in dogs and cats.[66,168-174,227,419,420]

Chronic MV disease, cardiomyopathy, and left-sided CHF should only cause mild to moderate PHT if the mechanism is solely from retrograde transmission of left atrial pressure.[172] In human patients, elevated LA pressure can lead to reactive pulmonary arterial vasoconstriction,[2] but while suspected in dogs or in cats it is not yet proven. Left-to-right shunts such as PDA or high cardiac output states such as thyrotoxicosis can contribute to development of PHT, but increased flow should affect PA pressures minimally if recruitment of pulmonary arteries and capillaries is normal. For practical purposes, moderate to severe PHT always indicates a precapillary component associated with some injury or reactivity in the pulmonary arteries. This can stem from heartworm infection,[42,133,421-424] angiostrongylosis, pulmonary thromboembolism, Eisenmenger's physiology, or idiopathic vascular disease. Primary lung diseases such as pulmonary fibrosis usually cause mild to moderate increases in pulmonary vascular resistance from the loss of vascular elements.[420] Reactive pulmonary artery vasoconstriction might contribute when there is low alveolar pO_2, but dogs and cats are not highly reactive compared to other species.

The imaging findings in PHT depend on the etiology, duration, and severity of pulmonary arterial disease. In moderate to severe PHT of any cause, 2D imaging of the PA shows symmetrical dilation of the right and left branches of the PA as well as the main PA (see Figure 8-34, B; Video 8-19). When PHT is due to persistence of fetal vascular resistance or secondary to a large shunt (Eisenmenger's physiology), the concentric RV hypertrophy identified is similar to that seen with pulmonary stenosis. In contrast, when PHT develops after maturity from acquired lung or pulmonary vascular disease, the secondary RV enlargement (cor pulmonale) is variable (see Figure 8-13, B; Video 8-34). The response to acute PHT is often a marked increase in chamber volume with thinning of the ventricular walls. However, with chronic pressure overload the RV develops a mixed type of hypertrophy characterized by increased wall thickness with RV dilatation.

Heartworm infection is an important cause of PHT in some parts of the world. Mature parasites on 2D imaging appear as paired, elongated, hyperechoic lines with a hypoechoic space between (see Figure 8-34, B; Video 8-34). Adult parasites are most often visualized in the right PA; however, in many cases adult filaria cannot be imaged at all. The parasites typically move outward in systole and recoil back toward the heart in diastole; this motion can help distinguish the filaria from reverberation or side-lobe artifacts. Cats with heartworm infection typically have a small number of relatively large adult parasites coiled in the pulmonary artery and sometimes these are observed within the right side of the heart. The right heart is normal to minimally enlarged in most cases of

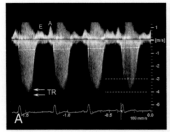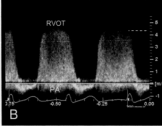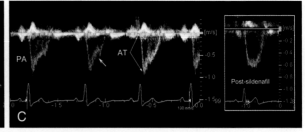

Figure 8-50 Doppler Findings in Pulmonary Hypertension. A, Tricuspid regurgitation in a dog with mild to moderate PHT due to mitral regurgitation. Although the peak velocity is clearly >3 m/s, the envelope is suboptimal and falls somewhere between 3 and 4 m/s (*arrows*)This is a common problem with signal strength and alignment to TR jets, especially if the regurgitant volume is small. Although the tricuspid A-wave is greater than the E wave velocity, it cannot be interpreted because the CW cursor samples in the atrium where the atrial velocity tends to be higher than at the valve tips. **B,** High-velocity jet of pulmonary regurgitation recorded from a dog with bidirectionally shunting patent ductus arteriosus. The maximal PR velocity is approximately 4.3 m/s, indicating a substantial increase in pulmonary vascular resistance. **C,** Altered PA ejection profile in a dog with idiopathic PHT recorded using PWD echocardiography. The acceleration time (AT) is shortened relative to the ejection time. Subjectively, the PA flow signal appears more like an aortic profile. Additionally there is a subtle deceleration notch in the velocity profile, another finding of increased pulmonary vascular resistance (see text). Inset: A more-normal appearing PA velocity profile is recorded from the same dog after initiating sildenafil therapy to reduce pulmonary vascular resistance.

heartworm disease, but severe cor pulmonale with marked PA dilatation is possible. The caval syndrome in dogs is characterized by severe cor pulmonale, a significant jet of TR on CDI, high-velocity TR on CWD, and a mass of adult parasites within the tricuspid valve orifice.[421]

The most common method for confirming PHT uses the simplified Bernoulli equation and applies it to a tricuspid regurgitant jet. When peak TR velocities exceed >3 m/s (in the absence of RVOT obstruction) PHT should be suspected (Figure 8-50, *A*). When TR is not available, a jet of pulmonary regurgitation should be sought (Figure 8-50, *B*). An early diastolic PR velocity >2.2 m/s is suggestive of PHT (Figure 8-50, *B*). Other methods for identifying PH, such as the ratio of PA acceleration time to ejection time can be useful when valvular regurgitation is not present. This ratio decreases as pulmonary artery resistance increases (Figure 8-50, *C*): a ratio of <0.31 was 73% sensitive and 87% specific for the diagnosis of PHT in one canine study[420] and in another report PA acceleration time/ejection time ratio averaged 0.46 in controls but only 0.37 in dogs with moderate to severe PHT. Following this ratio might be useful in identifying onset of significant[170] PHT and in evaluating its treatment. Of course the finding of PA dilation relative to the aorta is also suggestive of PHT and is simpler to identify and measure.

CARDIOMYOPATHY

Cardiomyopathy is an important cause of cardiac morbidity and is especially important in cats, constituting the most common category of diagnosis in this species. As explained later, diseases of the heart muscle encompass different combinations of morphologic and functional abnormalities of the ventricles. This makes the diagnosis mainly an echocardiographic exercise involving the measurement of heart chamber size, quantitation of global and regional ventricular function, and the exclusion of other causes of ventricular dilatation and hypertrophy such as hypertension, congenital heart disease, and valvular regurgitation. From the clinician's perspective, etiologies responsible for cardiomyopathies can be divided somewhat crudely into genetic and idiopathic causes (*primary*

cardiomyopathies) and myocardial diseases of known cause in which there are effects of the disease elsewhere in the body (*secondary* cardiomyopathies). Although cardiomyopathies can be well-tolerated in cats and dogs, potential *clinical outcomes* are serious and include heart failure, arrhythmia, syncope, sudden cardiac death, and (in cats) arterial thromboembolism.

Overview and Practical Considerations

Despite the availability of genetically-based (human) classifications,[425] cardiomyopathies are usually categorized by echocardiography into five general phenotypes: (1) hypertrophic; (2) dilated; (3) restrictive; (4) right ventricular; and (5) unclassified. These diagnostic categories are largely distinguished by five major echocardiographic findings: (1) LV chamber volume or size; (2) LV mass and wall thickness; (3) LV ejection fraction and wall motion; (4) LV diastolic function; and (5) the size of the RV and RA. Functional abnormalities that further refine the diagnosis include: (1) systolic dysfunction; (2) atrial dysfunction; (3) dynamic obstruction to ventricular outflow (including systolic anterior motion of the MV); (4) secondary valvular regurgitation; and (5) elevated ventricular filling pressures. In cats with cardiomyopathy the LA is further examined for the presence or absence of thrombus or echogenic smoke.

While all this might sound quite precise, the reality is *there is considerable overlap among different phenotypes* and the exact criteria used when categorizing the feline cardiomyopathies have largely been extrapolated from human patients. For example, there are legitimate disagreements about the diagnostic criteria for restrictive cardiomyopathy, and the role of myocardial infarction in progressive feline myocardial disease requires greater explanation. In many ways the more important issue for an individual patient with cardiomyopathy is the identification of negative or positive prognostic factors. Without doubt CHF, arterial thromboembolism, and symptomatic ventricular tachycardia each represents a negative prognostic finding in a cat with *any form of cardiomyopathy*. There are also echocardiographic findings that can adversely affect prognosis in myocardial disease. For example, cats with *severe classic HCM, end-stage HCM, RCM, DCM, and UCM will all have an enlarged LA and a poorer prognosis* for life. Additional prognostic indicators are considered below.

Essential Imaging Characteristics

The aforementioned imaging features of cardiomyopathy create significant heterogeneity, even for patients falling in the same diagnosis category. These variations are considered in more detail in the sections that follow. But as a starting point for understanding these disorders, the essential imaging features of each phenotype can be outlined. For classical hypertrophic cardiomyopathy (HCM) these are a hypertrophied, non-dilated LV with normal to increased ejection fraction, often with dynamic LVOTO. Patients with dilated cardiomyopathy (DCM) are characterized by LV (or four-chamber) dilatation with low LV ejection fraction. Cats with restrictive cardiomyopathy (RCM) have striking LA (or bi-atrial dilatation), relatively normal LV wall thickness, normal to reduced LV systolic function, and Doppler findings indicating high filling pressures superimposed on restricted LV filling. The echocardiographic diagnosis of arrhythmogenic RV cardiomyopathy (ARVC) is characterized by focal RV wall thinning or generalized enlargement of the RV and RA. However, right-sided enlargement is more typical of cats, with most canine cases exhibiting a normal echocardiogram or a DCM phenotype. Unclassified cardiomyopathies cannot be readily pigeonholed into the aforementioned descriptors. In practice, there are cases that change from one phenotype to another over time and there are persistent questions about the diagnostic criteria used for *every* form of myocardial disease, especially early or mild cases.

Other Assessments

While the recognition of a classic hypertrophic and dilated cardiomyopathy phenotypes can seem straightforward using echocardiography, the examiner and the primary clinician should also perform any *clinical* and *laboratory* assessments needed to exclude congenital heart disease, acquired valvular degeneration, systemic hypertension, endocrinopathies, and other known causes of ventricular remodeling in cats or dogs as summarized in Table 8-12. Cardiac arrhythmias are an important aspect of cardiomyopathy; therefore, the ECG should be recorded during the echocardiographic study. Isolated atrial and ventricular premature complexes can confound the assessment of ventricular systolic and diastolic function while also inducing transient A-V valve regurgitation. Relentless tachyarrhythmia can over a number of days induce *tachycardia-induced cardiomyopathy*,[426] a reversible disorder readily mistaken for idiopathic DCM. Even those tachyarrhythmias of recent onset impair ventricular function and its echocardiographic assessment through erratic cardiac cycle length, loss of atrial contribution to filling, and ventricular dyssynchrony. Rhythms such as ventricular tachycardia and atrial fibrillation with uncontrolled rate response also require urgent therapy.

Etiologies of Cardiomyopathy

In cats hypertrophic cardiomyopathy (HCM) is the most important cause of myocardial disease and is a frequent echocardiographic diagnosis.[125,145,149,150,193,194,198,249,257,277-280,315,427-436] Most cases are presumed to have a genetic basis, but only a small number of mutations have thus far been elucidated. HCM must be distinguished from LV wall thickening due to dehydration (pseudohypertrophy), systemic hypertension (hypertensive heart disease),[109,127,149,431,437-439] hyperthyroidism (see below), aortic stenosis, AV endocarditis, and isolated MV dysplasia with dynamic LVOTO and secondary LV hypertrophy. Pseudohypertrophy should not be associated with LA enlargement and should resolve with rehydration. The other

causes of LV hypertrophy can be diagnosed based on other clinical, laboratory, or imaging findings. Because HCM is also associated with MV abnormalities, the diagnosis of mitral dysplasia with secondary LV hypertrophy can be challenging if not impossible. Regression of LV hypertrophy after treatment with a beta blocker (or spontaneously, with no therapy) supports that diagnosis. Rare cases of an "HCM phenotype" might be due to myocardial infiltration (e.g., lymphosarcoma) or edema from acute myocarditis.

The etiology of RCM in cats is unknown, but healed myocarditis or repeated bouts of myocardial infarction are possible explanations for some cases. Additionally, end-stage, chronic HCM—the so-called "burned-out" form of HCM—might well be the major cause of the RCM phenotype.[427,428] This is further supported by microscopic features of myofiber disarray in cats with the RCM phenotype.[440] However, it is difficult to diagnose end-stage HCM with certainty unless there is some residual hypertrophy or a prior examination demonstrated HCM.

Dilated cardiomyopathy (DCM) in cats[99,441,442] is relatively uncommon today, with most cases considered idiopathic. Sporadic cases of taurine-deficiency are encountered in cats eating off-brand diets (or exclusively dog food). Diffuse myocarditis can lead to a DCM phenotype but cannot be diagnosed without myocardial histology.

Unlike humans, coronary artery disease is not considered an important diagnostic consideration for DCM, but myocardial ischemia and infarction do seem relevant to the progression of feline cardiomyopathies as noted later. Tachycardia-induced[443] DCM has been observed in the cat. Other types of cardiomyopathy or injury in cats include RV cardiomyopathy[443-445] and various unclassified forms of cardiomyopathy (UCM) including atrial cardiomyopathies and cardiomyopathy associated with repositol corticosteroid treatment. These disorders are either idiopathic in etiology or of uncertain pathogenesis. As mentioned earlier, ventricular remodeling can stem from systemic hypertension (concentric hypertrophy) or various endocrinopathies. Hyperthyroidism, often complicated by high blood pressure, causes a mixed or concentric form of LV hypertrophy, although a DCM phenotype has rarely been seen. Cats with diabetes mellitus, acromegaly,[446,447] or both disorders should be screened for cardiomyopathy, which appears to be an important comorbidity or consequence of these endocrine disorders. Affected cats usually look similar to burned out HCM, but there is potential reversibility following hypophysectomy. It should also be emphasized that in some cases these diverse conditions could simply exacerbate or decompensate a previously stable case of HCM.

Cardiomyopathy in dogs is neither common nor varied. Many giant breeds and spaniels are genetically predisposed to DCM, although the disorder is certainly not confined to these breed types. Secondary DCM can develop in susceptible dogs from micronutrient deficiency such as taurine and L-carnitine depletion that can occur when fed entirely vegan diets or "off-brands" of dog foods. Myocarditis, tachycardia-induced cardiomyopathy, and doxorubicin-induced cardiomyopathy are other diagnostic considerations for a DCM phenotype in dogs. Morbid hypothyroidism depresses LV contractile function, but rarely results in chamber dilatation. Catecholamine excess associated with pheochromocytoma can also injure the myocardium and impair LV systolic function in dogs.[448] Cases of ARVC are especially frequent in the boxer and English bulldog,[449] although as in humans,[91,450] echocardiographic abnormalities are often subtle or absent (cardiac arrhythmias are the main feature). Sporadic cases of HCM are observed in dogs,[451,452] but the etiology is unknown. Systemic hypertension[196,453] from renal disease or pheochromocytoma;

TABLE 8-12

Diagnostic Considerations in Feline Myocardial Diseases

Possible Diagnosis	Potential Cardiovascular Findings	Diagnostic Examinations	Comments
Congenital Heart Disease	Cardiac Murmur Systolic click Heart Failure Arterial thromboembolism Sudden cardiac death	Auscultation Echocardiography with Doppler Radiography NT-pro BNP	Younger cats Uncommon cause in a mature cat with substantiated history of normal cardiac auscultation as a kitten
Functional Murmur* (Innocent; Physiological)	No clinical outcome Signs from underlying causes of the murmur Iatrogenic from inappropriate drug therapy for suspected heart disease	Auscultation NT-pro BNP[†] Rectal temperature PCV or CBC[‡] Serum Thyroxine Echocardiography with Doppler	A low NT-proBNP supports a diagnosis of functional murmur. Blood pressure is usually measured in older cats at higher risk for chronic kidney disease or other causes of hypertension. Measure serum thyroxin in cats ≥7 years old. Hyperthyroidism is a potential cause of functional murmurs. Hyperdynamic RV or LV might be noted.
Secondary cardiomyopathies Anemia-related Corticosteroid (repositol) Acromegaly Diabetes Mellitus Hyperthyroidism Taurine deficiency	Murmur Gallop sound Cardiac arrhythmia Cardiomegaly Heart Failure Arterial thromboembolism Sudden cardiac death	Auscultation NT-proBNP Cardiac troponin I (cTnI) PCV or CBC[‡] Biochemical profile for renal disease or diabetes mellitus in cats at risk Serum Thyroxine Abdominal Ultrasound (US) 2D Echocardiography Doppler Echocardiography	High levels of NT-proBNP or cTnI indicate a greater risk for structural cardiac disease. Taurine deficiency now a rare cause of dilated cardiomyopathy in cats; evaluate dietary history Moderate to severe anemia associated with secondary cardiomegaly and volume retention Hypertensive heart disease and hyperthyroidism can lead to LV hypertrophy. Hyperthyroid cats should also be screened for systemic HTN. Hyperaldosteronism from an adrenal tumor is a rare but treatable cause of systemic HTN. Abdominal US is useful for diagnosis of adrenal tumors. Acromegaly ± diabetes mellitus is associated with cardiomyopathy in older cats.
Vascular Diseases Systemic hypertension (HTN) Idiopathic aortic dilatation (aortoannular ectasia) Pulmonary hypertension	Murmur or gallop Signs due to underlying disease Secondary cardiomegaly Heart Failure (uncommon) Coughing I Tachypnea (lung disease or heartworm disease) Sudden death (heartworm disease)	Examination of ocular fundus for hypertensive retinopathy or retinal degeneration. Noninvasive measurement of systemic arterial blood pressure NT-proBNP Biochemical profile for renal disease Serum Thyroxin Abdominal Ultrasound (US) 2D Echocardiography Doppler Echocardiography	Target organs injured by HTN: brain, eyes, left ventricle, kidneys, small arteries of body Aortic dilatation is sometimes associated with systemic HTN; aortic dissection is a rare complication. Aortoannular ectasia is common in older cats and often associated with discrete upper septal hypertrophy. Feline heartworm disease is a consideration in endemic areas of infection. Cor pulmonale from primary bronchopulmonary diseases is occasionally identified.
Myocarditis	Arrhythmia	Electrocardiography	Myocarditis is most common in young cats.
Myocardial infarction	Heart Failure Sudden Cardiac Death	Cardiac troponin I Tests for infectious disease (geographical considerations) 2D Echocardiography Doppler Echocardiography	Can lead to anesthetic-related death Echocardiographic features are poorly defined. Myocardial infarction often complicates HCM; often leads to increased cTnI and regional wall motion abnormality.

TABLE 8-12

Diagnostic Considerations in Feline Myocardial Diseases—cont'd

Possible Diagnosis	Potential Cardiovascular Findings	Diagnostic Examinations	Comments
Primary cardiomyopathies Hypertrophic Restrictive Unclassified Dilated Right ventricular	Murmur, gallop or click Arrhythmia Cardiomegaly Heart Failure Sudden Cardiac Death Arterial thromboembolism	Auscultation NT-proBNP Cardiac troponin I (cTnI) Radiography Electrocardiography 2D Echocardiography Doppler Echocardiography	An elevated NT-pBNP increases the risk of disease. Echocardiography is the diagnostic test of choice. 6-Lead electrocardiogram has relatively high specificity for cardiac disease but low sensitivity. Routine thoracic radiography has low sensitivity but high specificity for heart disease when there is moderate to severe chamber enlargement; most useful to investigate suspect congestive heart failure.

*Functional murmurs are those developing in a structurally normal heart. Physiologic murmurs are functional murmurs with an identifiable cause of altered physiology. Functional murmurs are typically associated with sympathetic activation, vasodilation, or both. Examples include fever, anemia, thyrotoxicosis, and ketamine administration. Innocent murmurs have no obvious explanation.

†N –terminal, prohormone of B-type natriuretic peptide (feline specific assay or ELISA test)

‡Packed cell volume (or hematocrit); complete blood count

subaortic stenosis; MV malformations with dynamic LVOTO; and chronic, iatrogenic hyperthyroidism fall into the differential diagnosis. Diffuse neoplastic infiltration of the myocardium is rarely observed in dogs but can lead to myocardial thickening. A similar finding has been observed in cases of canine myocarditis.

Feline Hypertrophic Cardiomyopathy

Similar to the condition in people, feline HCM is believed to represent an adult-onset, genetic disease.[278] In its classic form HCM is characterized by a nondilated, hypertrophied LV. The pattern of hypertrophy can be generalized, segmental, or focal.[280] The papillary muscles are often involved in the hypertrophic process.[277] The disease functionally is characterized by LV diastolic dysfunction and progressive increases in LV chamber stiffness and LA size. Systolic anterior motion of the MV is a common feature and predisposes to dynamic LVOTO and to an eccentric jet of MR. The differential diagnosis has been discussed in the previous section. Although normal to enhanced systolic LV function is typical of HCM, it is reduced in a subgroup of affected cats often with replacement fibrosis of the myocardium. In humans with *end-stage HCM* there is myocardial wall thinning and progressive LV dilatation, and these findings have also been observed in cats. Nearly all features of HCM observed in human echocardiography have been observed in cats with the disease.[74,125,145,149,150,153,193,194,198,249,255,257,278,281,315,418,427-433, 435,436,454] Detailed studies of diastolic and regional myocardial function have been performed in the assessment of HCM in cats, mainly in an attempt to identify early disease. The interested reader is referred to the references for details.

Diagnostic Criteria

The *diagnosis of HCM* is predicated on identification of increased ventricular septal, freewall, or papillary muscle thickness or LV mass.[§§] The heterogeneous and asymmetri-

cal patterns of hypertrophy so often found in feline HCM necessitate using both 2D and M-mode measurements for characterizing the ventricle (see Figure 8-51). Moderate or severe cases of HCM with generalized LVH present a straightforward picture, but cats with mild or focal disease are problematic, and many are misdiagnosed. The precise "cutoffs" for LV hypertrophy in cats are still debated. A diastolic wall dimension of 6 mm is generally considered too thick,[279] but values of 5.5 mm (and lower) have also been advanced as abnormal. For these reasons, the authors consider diastolic wall measurements of 5.5-5.9 mm as "suspicious" or "equivocal," and values of 6 mm or more as abnormal. For some of the commonly-affected breeds such as the Maine Coon cat or the Norwegian Forest cat specific breed normals are probably needed along with genetic and longitudinal studies of "mildly-affected" cats. Lastly, as discussed previously, subtle errors in measurement technique— even one or two pixels on the measuring screen—can change the ultimate diagnosis and mislabel a cat as "HCM", potentially leading to a lifetime of follow-up examinations, treatment, and related expense.

2D and M-Mode Examinations

Typical 2D and M-mode findings in HCM include symmetrical thickening of the LVW and IVS and hypertrophy of the papillary muscles (see Figures 8-33, C and 8-51, A; Videos 8-7, E, 8-18 and 8-35). The latter structures might appear taller at the tips or wider across their base, often blending into the LVW. However, asymmetric LV hypertrophy is also common with either the IVS or LVW predominating. When the LVW thickness is significantly greater than septal thickness, the risk of progressive LA dilation, thromboembolism, and CHF are higher. Focal HCM involving the septum is also common, especially in the dorsal subaortic ventricular septum in older cats. This is referred to as discrete upper septal hypertrophy ("DUST") and included in the spectrum of human HCM, but it could also represent a tissue response to aortic dilation and malalignment with resultant flow disturbances promoting growth of the dorsal septum. Focal septal hypertrophy is usually benign.

§§The reader is referred back to the prior section on "Left Ventricular Mass" as it is highly relevant here.

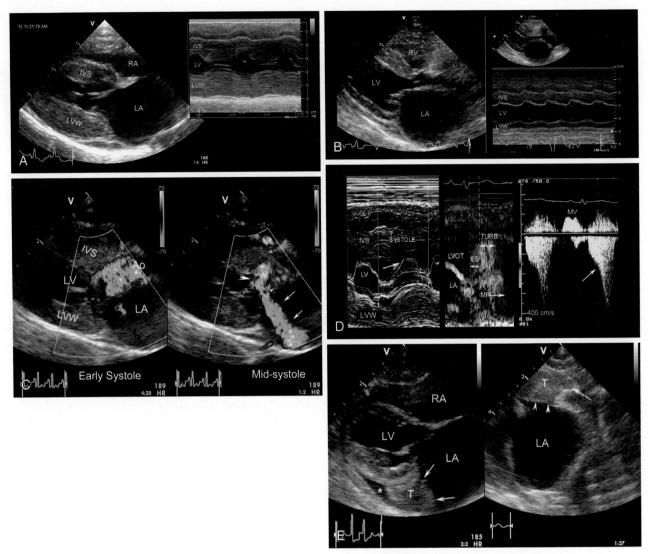

Figure 8-51 Feline Hypertrophic Cardiomyopathy. A, Long axis image demonstrating hypertrophic cardiomyopathy in a cat. There is generalized LV wall thickening with some free-wall predominance, and moderate to severe LA dilatation. Inset: The M-mode study of the LV is shown. **B,** End-stage HCM in a Maine Coon cat. There is residual hypertrophy of the IVS and severe LA dilatation. Right: M-mode study from the same cat shows asymmetrical LV hypertrophy and some impairment of LV systolic function. **C,** Still image showing color flow mapping of dynamic LVOT obstruction and an eccentric jet of MR in a cat with hypertrophic cardiomyopathy. Left: Early systolic frame shows ejection into the aorta. There is turbulence in the LVOT due to developing systolic anterior motion of the mitral valve. Right: An eccentric jet of MR is evident (arrows) beginning near the point of septal mitral contact (arrowhead). **D,** Dynamics of hypertrophic obstructive cardiomyopathy in one cat are shown using the M-mode examination (left), color M-mode (center), and CWD imaging (right). Left: Systolic anterior motion of the mitral valve (arrow) is evident. Center: The color M-mode shows non-turbulent early systolic ejection (ES) coded in red, but at the moment of dynamic obstruction there is turbulence (TURB) in the LVOT and mid-to late systolic mitral regurgitation (MR). Right: There is a typical CW Doppler jet of mid to late-systolic, acceleration due to dynamic obstruction in the LVOT caused by mitral-septal contact. Note the dagger shape in the velocity profile (arrow) from sudden acceleration of flow at the time of systolic anterior motion of the mitral valve. The weak peak velocity signal is typical of HOCM and related to the small amount of blood flowing into the LVOT at end-systole. (Also see Fig. 8-45C for a more clear example of systolic anterior motion.) **E,** Organized left auricular thrombus in a cat with HCM. Left: long axis image shows a dilated LA and the left auricle filled with thrombus (T). The arrows indicate the entrance to the atrial appendage. The auricle is more visible due to a small pericardial effusion (*). Right: Image plane from the left craniodorsal position shows the thrombus extending to the auricular tip (arrow) and the entry to the appendage (arrowheads).

LV chamber diastolic dimensions are either reduced or normal ("nondilated" LV) unless there is end-stage HCM. Systolic function measured by LVFS is normal to hyperdynamic and often induces systolic, mid-ventricular obstruction,[431] or typical dynamic LVOTO with concurrent MR (Figure 8-51, C to D). Impaired ventricular contraction is typical of advanced and end-stage disease although systolic dysfunction might be detectable earlier with advanced tissue imaging methods. The findings of reduced LV systolic function, regional or global wall thinning with hypokinesis, and LA dilatation are markers of a poor prognosis in HCM and in every other form of feline cardiomyopathy. These echocardiographic changes usually indicate replacement fibrosis or myocardial infarction, abnormalities identified by histopathology in cats affected with all forms of cardiomyopathy at high risk of CHF or atrial thrombosis (Figure 8-51, E; Videos 8-7, E and 8-35).

Other 2D findings are less consistent but many are similar to those reported in people.[4,5] In some cats there is marked anticlockwise rotation of the 2D image, such that the anterior papillary muscle moves much closer to the transducer. While not specific for cardiomyopathy or disease, it is relatively common to observe this rotation when there is LV enlargement. Cats with HCM often have a more prominent trabecula septomarginalis (also called false tendons or LV moderator bands; Video 8-18, E). This is a normal structure that tracks along the left surface of the IVS before bridging the lumen to the papillary muscle. Occasionally a network of prominent trabecula is identified. Abnormal muscle bundles have been observed crossing the LV, and these can be confused with MV or papillary muscle malformations. Sphinx cats might be predisposed. Left apical aneurysms have also been described. The ascending aorta is sometimes mildly dilated, presumably from poststenotic flow disturbances. The RV is usually normal in thickness but hypertrophy is sometimes observed (note: pseudonormal hypertrophy also should be considered). The RA might dilate in the face of volume retention from CHF or PHT. Because a small pericardial effusion could indicate imminent heart failure,[455] exposure of thoracic radiographs is recommended when effusion is observed (Video 8-35, F). Larger pericardial effusions and variable-sized pleural effusions are common when HCM has been complicated by CHF. These often decrease or resolve after successful therapy for heart failure.

Moderate to severe LA dilation is the strongest predictor of future clinical complications in all forms of cardiomyopathies, including HCM (see Figure 8-51, B; Video 8-18).[125,257] Experience indicates that when the *maximal* 2D diameter exceeds 20 mm, the risk is greatest and coexistent abnormalities of LA function might be identified. Findings of increased pulmonary venous pressure can be substantiated with careful Doppler studies (or radiography). The risk of thromboembolism is greatest when LA dilation is accompanied by spontaneous echo contrast (smoke), which indicates stasis of blood (Videos 8-6, C and 8-35). Decreased atrial ejection fraction[256] and low left auricular emptying velocity (<22 cm/s)[94,95] point to impaired LA function and also a heightened risk for thrombosis. Careful scrutiny of the left auricle from both the right short-axis and angled left-craniodorsal image planes can identify a mural thrombus (see Figure 8-51, E; Video 8-6, C). When an atrial thrombus has an oval shape, well-delineated borders, and is firmly attached to the auricular wall, it is probably quiescent and of lower immediate concern. In contrast, a thrombus that appears soft, with ill-defined borders and mobile edges, poses a high risk of breaking off from the auricular wall. These different echocardiographic findings can demand aggressive antiplatelet or anticoagulation therapies such as clopidogrel or heparins.

As found in humans, the anatomy and motion of the MV can be abnormal in cats with HCM. Systolic anterior motion of the MV (SAM) is a classic finding on 2D and M-mode imaging and characterized by mid-to-late systolic mitral to septal contact (see Figure 8-51, C and Video 8-7, E). The precise mechanism for SAM is undetermined but could relate to deformed mitral leaflets or abnormal mitral valve position due to changes in the papillary muscles, or chordae tendineae.[429] Once the valve is pulled toward the septum, Venturi effects might maintain the motion abnormality.[9] This event dynamically obstructs the LVOT while also causing MR. Abnormal chordal motion also is common. Midsystolic closure of the AV on M-mode echocardiography is another marker for sudden obstruction to blood flow. Dynamic LVOTO in cats with HCM is labile, enhanced with excitement or stress, and often reduced or eliminated by beta-adrenergic blockade or heavy sedation. While moderate to severe LVOTO is an independent, negative predictor of outcome in people,[456] the prognostic significance of SAM and LVOTO in cats is still undetermined. Its mitigation with atenolol was not associated with better survival in a small, prospective study of cats with HCM.

Doppler Studies

Doppler studies are used to identify midventricular or LVOTO, diastolic dysfunction, valvular regurgitation, and auricular filling and emptying velocities.[145,150,153,193,194,315,431,433] Systolic turbulence in the midventricle, LVOT and ascending aorta along with an eccentric jet of MR are usual findings on CDI. When dynamic outflow obstruction is recorded from the left apical position, a "dagger-shaped" signal is recorded with CWD (see Figure 8-51, C to D; Video 8-35). The spectrum of the fastest blood flow crossing the obstruction is fainter than that comprising the proximal V_1 envelope. This indicates a smaller volume of RBCs and a need to process the spectrum carefully to record the maximal LVOT velocities. In some cats a right dorsocranial transducer placement can reasonably capture the high-velocity signal moving toward the transducer. Within the LV, a sudden acceleration in velocity is recorded after the AV has opened, coincident with the onset of dynamic LVOTO. Similarly, the onset of MR is delayed until SAM has occurred. The MR jet originates at the interface of the ventricular septum and the malpositioned AMV leaflet, and tracks along the posterior leaflet into the LA. While it is simple to distinguish the jets of MR and dynamic LVOTO with CDI, when using CWD the flow disturbances overlap and careful imaging is needed to distinguish the two. In HOCM, the jet of MR is not holosystolic, because initiation depends on the development of SAM. Trace or mild AR is another regular observation in cats with dynamic LVOTO. Color and spectral Doppler recordings often demonstrate dynamic RVOT obstruction. Seemingly ventricular septal hypertrophy predisposes to dynamic RVOT obstruction in cats. Although this is a benign flow disturbance, it might explain some systolic murmurs in cats with HCM.

Asymptomatic HCM is characterized by grade I or grade II diastolic dysfunction (relaxation abnormality or pseudonormal filling; see Figures 8-39, B and 8-40, A and B and the section on "Diastolic Ventricular Function" earlier in this chapter). Typical features are E/A reversal in the mitral inflow profile, E'/A' reversal in TDI of the LVW, prolonged isovolumetric relaxation time, and altered pulmonary venous flow patterns. Mean LA pressure can increase with progressive disease, leading to grade III diastolic dysfunction and left-sided CHF. This situation also can develop suddenly after persistent stress-induced tachycardia (which impairs diastolic function), general anesthesia, or intravenous fluid therapy. Diastolic dysfunction may revert to a lower grade after diuretic therapy, especially if a precipitating cause is identified and reversible.

Serial echocardiograms can be useful when following the course of HCM in an individual cat, accepting the risk that the stress of a veterinary visit can precipitate cardiac decompensation. Although the vast majority of affected cats remain asymptomatic, some do progress substantially. The identification of LA enlargement on follow-up examination indicates a much higher risk for the development of clinical signs and the need to initiate antiplatelet therapy (clopidogrel ± aspirin) and begin home respiratory rate monitoring. Recheck examination is also warranted when a heart murmur disappears in a cat with previously documented LVOTO (and not receiving atenolol) as this could indicate changes in LV morphology or LV function. Reasonable examination intervals might vary from six to 12 months in asymptomatic cats, depending on the disease severity, results of prior examinations, and the clinical situation. Regression of hypertrophy with any therapy is very uncommon. Mild reduction is wall thickness can be observed after plasma volume status has been restored to a cat previously treated with high dosages of diuretics. When dramatic regression of hypertrophy is seen in a young cat with dynamic LVOTO, a suspicion of MV malformation with secondary LV hypertrophy should be higher.[346] Slowing of HR with atenolol often reduces SAM, LVOTO, and the attendant murmurs, but myocardial depression and bradycardia can induce some LV and LA dilation. These changes are acceptable if mild, but in cats with moderate LA dilation or impaired atrial function, beta-blockers should be decreased or discontinued (and therapy with clopidogrel initiated).

Dilated Cardiomyopathy

Dilated cardiomyopathy (DCM) is characterized by LV dilatation and reduced LV ejection fraction. The loss of myocardial contractility is unrelated to a definable valvular lesion, hypertension, or a congenital cardiac defect. Impaired cardiac output often leads to heart failure while myocardial disease and chamber enlargement predispose to arrhythmias. The differential diagnosis of DCM in dogs and in cats has been considered earlier in this section. Additionally, high cardiac output states (moderate to severe anemia[457,458] and hyperthy-

roidism) can lead to sodium retention and four-chamber cardiac dilatation, especially after fluid therapy. Ventricular systolic function is typically normal in these cases, helping to distinguish them from true DCM.

In some canine cases of preclinical DCM (Video 8-37), there is minimal LV dilation and the diagnosis is advanced mainly from complementary and serial evaluations of LV function (see "Ventricular Function" earlier in this chapter). An ECVIM consensus panel has outlined typical features of preclinical (occult) DCM and proposed a scoring system for the diagnosis.[265] While reasonable, this system has not yet been validated with longitudinal (follow-up) studies.

The "classic" diagnosis is the appearance of a dilated, hypocontractile LV unexplained by any other cause. Generalized "4-chamber" dilatation is often seen on 2D and M-mode echocardiography (Figure 8-52; Video 8-36), but LA and LV chamber dilation can predominate in some breeds (especially Doberman pinschers).[115,122,197,263,459,460] Plasma volume status influences overall chamber size with fluid retention increasing and diuretic therapy reducing intracavitary dimensions. In both dogs and cats the LV is more spherical (see Figure 8-33, A). Objectively, linear, area, and volumetric estimates of LVEF are decreased as are indices of myocardial deformation or strain and LV dp/dt estimated by an MR jet (see Figures 8-30 and 8-52). Morphologic and functional changes of the RV in DCM have not undergone rigorous assessments and are variable.

In addition to decreased LVFS, the M-mode examination often reveals regional LV wall dysfunction, arrhythmias, and dyssynchrony (see Figure 8-13, C).[122,442,459,461-467] These can negatively influence the calculation of LVFS even beyond the inherent depression due to underlying myocardial disease. The MV EPSS is increased and a "double diamond" MV sign is evident within the dilated LV. Finding a B-shoulder of delayed mitral valve closure suggests elevated ventricular end-diastolic pressure and CHF.

Doppler studies in DCM can illustrate a number of functional changes.[115,192,263,307,311,312,468-472] Atrioventricular valve insufficiency is usually present (see Figure 8-52; Video 8-36), although the regurgitation is often mild when compared to dogs with primary valvular disease or to cats with

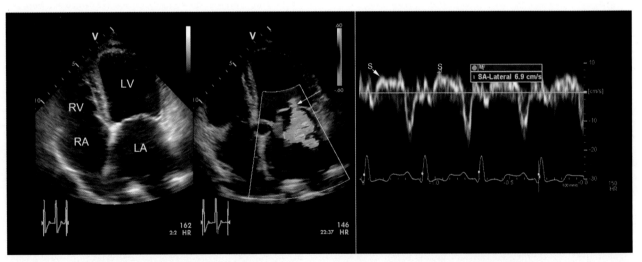

Figure 8-52 Dilated Cardiomyopathy. Left, Center: Two still images from a dog with DCM examined from the left apex. There is four-chamber dilatation. On 2D and M-mode studies systolic function was markedly reduced. There is a central jet of MR in the center panel. The right panel is recorded from another dog with DCM. The TDI of the lateral wall shows reduced systolic wave velocity for a large breed dog. The E' and A' waves are fused due to the relatively fast heart rate (HR 150/min). Other examples of DCM can be found in Figs. 8-13, C, 8-30, and 8-33, B).

HCM. Mild MR is frequently silent to auscultation. However, more severe MR is sometimes evident and this can mask the severity of myocardial failure by unloading the LV. In some dogs it can be difficult to determine if there is primary MR with secondary LV dysfunction, DCM with secondary MR, or both conditions. Tricuspid regurgitation can develop from right heart enlargement and the peak velocity of the TR jet sometimes reveals PHT secondary to left-sided heart failure. Diastolic abnormalities are similar to those discussed earlier in the chapter[307,469] and under feline HCM. An elevated E/E' ratio is more predictive of CHF risk in DCM than in primary MR or HCM where global systolic function is better preserved. A high-velocity mitral E-wave with abbreviated deceleration time (restrictive physiology or Grade 3 diastolic dysfunction) indicates a poor prognosis as this finding is characteristic of left-sided CHF in a noncompliant ventricle. One must be mindful of the effects of heart rate and rhythm since tachycardias and short cycle lengths (from premature complexes or atrial fibrillation) can abbreviate an E-wave by causing the MV to close during the premature contraction.

Once a diagnosis of DCM with CHF is established in a dog, serial echocardiography is not especially useful for following the patient and rarely changes the treatment plan. Although potent medications can modify LV systolic function slightly, there is no practical way to guide CHF therapy using LVSF or LVEF and changes in systolic function have not been shown to constitute a meaningful clinical endpoint. The exception is to document reversible DCM due to taurine deficiency[473-475] or relentless tachyarrhythmia.[426,476-479] Demonstrating improvement in diastolic function indices might be useful, but echocardiography seems to offer little over home respiratory rate monitoring, auscultation, and routine thoracic radiography for monitoring pulmonary edema. When cats are reevaluated for DCM the focus of the examination is often on identification of any LA thrombosis or pleural effusion. However, cats with DCM should always be placed on antiplatelet therapy—regardless of LA size—and serial echocardiographic evaluations probably offer little over careful home monitoring of appetite, respiratory rate, and activity. The clinician must weigh the stress of travel versus any benefits that might be attained from reevaluation.

Restrictive Cardiomyopathy

Restrictive cardiomyopathy (RCM) is a poorly defined myocardial disease of the cat. In human patients the disease includes an endomyocardial form and an infiltrative form, the latter type usually due to amyloid or iron deposition in the myocardium. The disease in cats is characterized by extensive myocardial fibrosis that can be endomyocardial or transmural in distribution.[315,440] Antecedent myocarditis, end-stage ("burned out") HCM, recurrent injury from myocardial ischemia, or myocardial infarctions might be operative mechanisms for this change. The role of chronic neurohormonal activation is undetermined. The features of this disease indicate severe myocardial disease and most cats are symptomatic with clinical findings of CHF, arrhythmia or thromboembolism. Pleural effusions including chylothorax are common (Video 8-38). The presumptive pathophysiology of RCM relates to additive effects of LV systolic failure, regional wall dysfunction, LV diastolic failure, and very likely a noncompliant LA. These functional changes predispose to biventricular CHF, atrial and ventricular ectopy, and thrombus formation. In general the prognosis is poor, regardless of the underlying cause.

The 2DE findings are dominated by severe LA dilatation unexplained by mitral disease, a left-to-right shunt, DCM, or primary atrial disease. There are varying degrees of RA dila-

tion, likely from an elevated central venous pressure and PHT. The LV diastolic diameter is usually normal. High definition 2D imaging might demonstrate: a hyperechoic endomyocardial interface or bright myocardium; normal to thin ventricular walls; a misshapen (U-shaped) LV cavity; or rigid-appearing papillary muscles (Video 8-38). These are usually accompanied by biatrial dilation. A bridging scar spanning the LV is sometime observed. The LVFS is typically in the low normal range, with segmental wall motion abnormalities present. Intracardiac thrombi are often identified. Finding pericardial or pleural effusions can indicate CHF. Doppler patterns are characteristic of grade 3, restrictive filling (see Figure 8-39, C); but as with most cats in CHF, the pattern is not specific for RCM. Other possible findings include MR or TR, evidence of PHT, and regional wall thinning or apical aneurysm suggesting prior myocardial infarction.

If the cat is from a breed often affected by HCM, such as a Maine Coon cat, and if there is some residual IVS or LVW thickening, the diagnosis of "burned out" or end-stage HCM is tenable instead of RCM. But practically, once HCM reaches this stage the disorders are managed no differently unless some reversible underlying etiology can be identified. A failure to identify abnormalities in the LV suggestive of myocardial fibrosis can prompt the ambiguous designation of "unclassified cardiomyopathy." In these cats it is appropriate to simply define the morphologic and functional abnormalities of the heart in order to guide therapy, since a precise diagnosis is unlikely to matter and the therapy (antiplatelet and treatment of CHF if present) will be the same.

Arrhythmogenic Right Ventricular Cardiomyopathy

This disorder is characterized by fibrofatty replacement of RV myocardium with progressive RV failure. Right ventricular ectopy is the most characteristic feature ARVC of dogs; whereas it is more variable in cats and less dominant in the disease presentation.[440,443,444,480] The frequency of echocardiographic abnormalities in ARVC also differs between dogs and cats. The majority of dogs have normal 2D imaging. Detailed 2D imaging of the RV from multiple windows sometimes reveals focal zones of myocardial thinning or aneurysm, but an imaging diagnosis is often elusive. This is similar to human patients with ARVC in whom an MRI is the diagnostic test method of choice. A subset of boxers and perhaps a relatively higher percent of affected English bulldogs manifest overt right-sided cardiac enlargement with dilated RV and RA (Video 8-39). Some of these dogs are predisposed to atrial flutter and fibrillation as well as ventricular ectopy. Dog with CHF can also present with imaging features that are indistinguishable from giant breed DCM,[245,449] aside from more RV dilatation than usual.

In contrast to dogs, nearly every cat with ARVC presents with significant RA and RV dilatation and most have clinical signs of CHF in the form of pleural effusion (Video 8-39, F). The cardiomyopathy in these cases is often confined to the RA and RV, but if there is atrial standstill or atrial fibrillation, the LA and LV can also enlarge. RV systolic function is subjectively decreased in these cats.

Severe RV and RA dilatation can foster TR so severe that the regurgitant velocity spectrum resembles a retrograde PA flow signal from near equilibration of RV and RA pressures. The atrial septum can be distracted toward the LA and the foramen ovale may appear thin, but it is not typically patent. The differential diagnosis for isolated right-sided heart enlargement in these cases includes chronic bradycardia, atrial septal defect (common in boxers), congenital and acquired right-sided valve diseases, PHT with cor pulmonale, and obstruction of the main or branch pulmonary artery. The tricuspid and pulmonary valves are structurally normal in

ARVC and the PA is usually normal in size; these findings are pertinent to the differential diagnosis.

PERICARDIAL DISEASES AND CARDIAC MASSES

Some of the earliest veterinary uses of echocardiography in medicine involved the detection of pericardial effusions and mass lesions, and this persists as an important application of cardiac US.[481-501] Pericardial effusion in cats is most often associated with CHF,[455] and will be found alongside imaging abnormalities of cardiomyopathy or congenital heart disease. Congenital peritoneopericardial diaphragmatic hernia, intrapericardial cysts, and partial absence of the pericardium are considered congenital disorders of the pericardial space in dogs and cats.[43,481,485-487] Small pericardial effusions can be observed with hernias, especially when a liver lobe is entrapped or strangulated. Lymphosarcoma, feline infectious peritonitis, bacterial empyema, and acquired cysts are relatively rare causes of pericardial disease in cats.[482-484,488-490].

The etiology of pericardial effusion in a dog depends very much on age. In younger dogs, intrapericardial cysts,[485] congenital hernias, and bacterial and fungal infections (including foreign bodies) must be considered. With the possible exception of regions endemic for coccidiomycosis, the vast majority of younger dogs with pericardial effusion are affected by idiopathic pericardial hemorrhage. This condition might occur just once and resolve with pericardiocentesis, or present itself recurrently until the pericardium is removed. In contrast, pericardial effusion in dogs older than seven years of age is usually caused by a cardiac-related tumor. The most important of these are hemangiosarcoma, aortic body tumor (chemodectoma, paraganglioma), ectopic thyroid carcinoma, and mesothelioma. In additional to causing hemorrhage, some cardiac-related tumors invade the atrium and obstruct venous return. On rare occasions, pulmonary or mediastinal masses can cause acquired supravalvular pulmonic stenosis.[412] An infrequent cause of acute cardiac tamponade is splitting of the left atrium in dogs with chronic MR.[323,491] This leads to hemopericardium and systemic hypotension.

Pericardial Effusion

The salient 2D and M-mode imaging features of pericardial effusion are the presence of a sonolucent space between the epicardium and pericardial/mediastinal interface, an influence of gravity on the localization of fluid (Figure 8-53, *A*; Video 8-40), altered ventricular filling dynamics, and the frequent association of cardiac neoplasia.[14,15,26,36,38,492-499] Scant effusions are only evident during systole when the epicardium pulls away from the parietal pericardium (systolic separation). Large effusions in dogs can contain more than a liter of fluid and are associated with exuberant motion and swinging of the heart within the pericardial space. The latter is the mechanism for electrical alternans. If multiple long, short, and apical 2D images are obtained, the extent of the effusion and its confinement within the circular pericardial space can be confirmed. The parietal pericardium can appear tense, rigid, and somewhat circular in shape once it reaches its limits of distensibility. Most pericardial effusions are anechoic, and a mixed echoic fluid is compatible with a highly-cellular fluid, an exudate, or active hemorrhage. Concurrent pleural effusions are common in pericardial diseases and will surround the lung and be evident in the near- and far-fields of the thorax (see Chapter 7).

Compression of the right atrium and right ventricle will develop with increasing intrapericardial pressure and can be confirmatory of clinical signs of *cardiac tamponade*. Prolonged diastolic collapse of the RV and inversion of the right atrial wall are typical features of cardiac compression (Video 8-40). In the presence of preexistent right-sided hypertension (e.g., PHT or severe TR), diastolic collapse of the cardiac walls might not be seen. As in humans, large pleural effusions can also induce right atrial or ventricular freewall collapse in dogs causing a false-positive diagnosis of cardiac tamponade.[500] In peracute hemopericardium, as occurs when a tumor bleeds or the LA splits, the volume of effusion can be relatively small yet the impairment of cardiac filling and the resultant hypotension quite severe (Video 8-40). Blood clots are sometimes evident on the heart. In contrast to cardiac rupture, with chronic cardiac tamponade compensated by fluid retention and high systemic venous pressures, a large effusion might barely compress the atrial and ventricular walls.

The diagnosis of *constrictive pericardial disease* is a very difficult one, but is a consideration for clinical signs of severe right-sided CHF, often with a prominent pleural effusion. The most common causes are chronic pericarditis due to infection and recurrent idiopathic pericardial hemorrhage. Effective treatment requires pericardiectomy. In some situations a prior diagnosis of pericardial effusion will suggest constrictive pericardial disease as a possibility. Typical imaging findings include: either absent or small pericardial effusion (constrictive-effusive disease); pericardial thickening; marked ventricular septal fluttering during early ventricular filling; sudden attenuation of early diastolic filling; and marked respiratory variation in ventricular filling recorded by PWD. Guidelines for normal respiratory variation in transmitral and transtricuspid flow have not been established, but the authors suggest that at least a 50% variation would be needed. It should be noted that marked variation in ventricular filling can also be observed in respiratory distress due to other causes.

Cardiac Related Neoplasms in Dogs

Echocardiography has relatively good sensitivity and specificity for the diagnosis of hemangiosarcoma and heart base tumors in dogs,[497] but up to 20% of neoplasms can be missed even in experienced centers.[498] Tumors must be sought from a variety of image planes on *both* sides of the thorax, including the left cranial image positions.[36] The putative diagnosis of a tumor type is often based on findings that include location of the tumor on 2D imaging and breed predilection. Unfortunately, most cardiac tumors do not exfoliate into the effusion so that a cytologic diagnosis infrequently available. Thus echocardiographic localization is critical to decision making and management. Examples of cardiac-related mass lesions are illustrated in Figure 8-53, C and Video 8-40.***

A tumor originating from the RA is usually a *hemangiosarcoma*.[497,498] These masses have a mixed echoic appearance and a classic location at the tip of the right auricle and along the A-V groove. Intracardiac spread can predominate and lead to atrial arrhythmias, venous obstruction and ascites. Invasion into the ventricular wall is also common. *Chemodectomas* (aortic body tumor or paraganglioma) arise from the aortic bodies located within the walls of the aorta, just beyond the AV. These tumors usually spread along the path of least resistance and can become extremely large. The typical chemodectoma extends from the base of the aorta, often circumferentially but also cranially and to the right, where it can be confused with a hemangiosarcoma. These neuroendocrine tumors can envelop the great vessels and extend into the mediastinum,

---

***There are numerous single case reports of cardiac tumors that include rare instances of cardiac fibrosarcoma, chondrosarcoma, extraskeletal osteosarcoma, myxosarcoma, rhabdomyoma, and other tumors. See Web content for additional references.

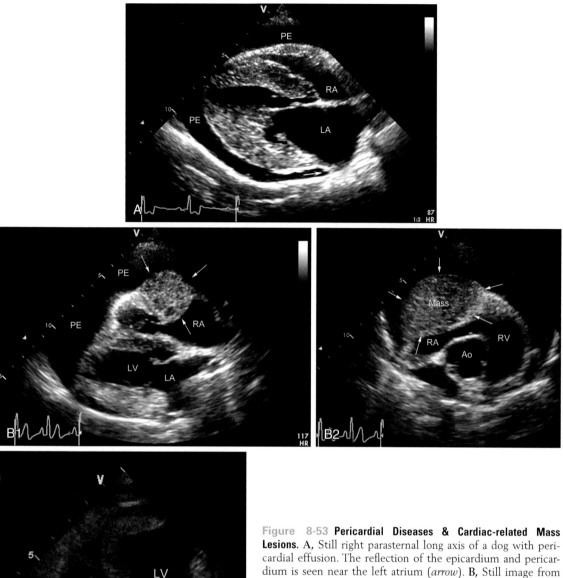

Figure 8-53 Pericardial Diseases & Cardiac-related Mass Lesions. A, Still right parasternal long axis of a dog with pericardial effusion. The reflection of the epicardium and pericardium is seen near the left atrium (*arrow*). **B,** Still image from the right thorax of a dog with right atrial hemangiosarcoma (*arrows*). There is a pericardial effusion (PE) due to prior hemorrhage with gravitational effects evident in this right-side down examination. Right: Right parasternal short axis image from the same dog showing infiltration of the tumor into the myocardium along the atrioventricular groove.) **C,** Left apical image obtained from a dog with a large chemodectoma or aortic body tumor (ABT). The mass has impinged on the pulmonary venous return to the left atrium (*arrows*). The aorta is not visible in this plane.

surrounding the branch vessels off the aorta. Ectopic thyroid carcinomas can also impinge on the heart base in this area and be especially aggressive in terms of local spread into the heart.[501] The imaging characteristics of mesothelioma have not been critically evaluated. Often there is no evidence of neoplasia aside from the pericardial effusion. Occasionally, tumors are observed on the surface of the pericardium or epicardium. These must be distinguished from blood clots or metastatic lesions. The normal fat pad located at the PA and ascending aorta can also be confused for a heart base tumor. This tissue often exhibits the bright US signature of fat as opposed to the mixed echoic soft tissue appearance typical of a tumor. Finally, while 2D imaging is the predominant modality for diagnosis of cardiac related neoplasms, the consequences of venous, intracardiac, or pulmonary arterial obstruction can be quantified using spectral Doppler imaging. The findings would be similar to changes observed with stenosis of an A-V valve or of supravalvular PS.

CONGENITAL SHUNTS

Common congenital defects associated with shunting are atrial septal defect (ASD), ventricular septal defect (VSD), and persistently patent ductus arteriosus (PDA) as demonstrated in Videos 8-41 to 8-43. These lesions are evaluated in dogs and cats using echocardiography, which has largely replaced cardiac catheterization for their diagnosis and assessment. Color Doppler examinations also can identify flow disturbances of other shunts, including aorticopulmonary window, coronary artery fistula, coronary arterial malformation, and systemic to pulmonary arterial communication.[502-506]

Considering even experienced examiners can equivocate or become confused when assessing a dog or cat with congenital heart disease, as a general recommendation, these patients should be referred to a cardiologist for further evaluation. While some cases seem simple or straightforward, many have concurrent lesions or pathophysiologic alterations that require the input of a subspecialist for optimal management. This section only considers basic diagnostic points surrounding ASD, VSD, and PDA but relegates subtleties and complex malformations to textbooks of cardiology and echocardiography.[46,47]

Overview and Practical Considerations

Most intracardiac and many extracardiac shunts can be identified by 2D imaging. The absolute and relative sizes of abnormal communications are relevant to prognosis, as are remodeling changes in the ventricles, atria and great vessels. Along with auscultation, identification of cardiac enlargement is often a clue to the presence and type of congenital shunting lesion. Shunting across an anatomic defect can be verified and further defined with Doppler studies.

The development of CDI facilitated the diagnosis of shunts, especially smaller defects that eluded routine 2D imaging. The flow crossing most left-to-right shunts registers as turbulence in CDI so long as a substantial pressure gradient drives the blood across a "restrictive" orifice. In comparison larger communications with little resistance to flow allow for near-equilibration of pressures across the defect, and the resultant shunting demonstrates minimal turbulence. The same principle applies to defects characterized by right-to-left shunting. These are most often due to severe pulmonary vascular disease and PHT (Eisenmenger's physiology) or to stenosis of the pulmonic or tricuspid valves in association with a VSD or ASD, respectively. In most right-to-left shunts flow across the defect is bidirectional, shunt velocity is low, and turbulence encoding is minimal.

Any shunting detected by CDI should be verified by imaging across orthogonal planes and further confirmed by spectral recordings. Furthermore, confusion caused by color "bleeding" must be avoided. This occurs when grayscale gain is set too low so that colorized Doppler shifts fill the pixels where a chamber or vessel wall should be located. The most important spectral Doppler findings in left-to-right shunts relate to: (1) detection of abnormal, often turbulent, flow across the defect; (2) the calculation of pressure drops across the shunt; (3) the identification of secondary changes in transvalvular flow caused by shunting; (4) detection of secondary

mitral, aortic, or tricuspid regurgitation; (5) estimation of pulmonary arterial pressures and detection of PHT; and (6) recognition of concurrent lesions affecting blood flow.

When the PWD sample volume is placed in the path of a VSD or PDA, a disturbed or aliased flow signal is recorded, often superimposed on an otherwise-normal velocity signal within the receiving chamber (see Figures 8-23, *B* and 8-27, *D*). The pressure difference across a defect can be determined through CWD imaging and application of the simplified Bernoulli relationship. When maximal flow velocity crossing a PDA or VSD exceeds 4.5 to 5 m/s (provided systemic arterial blood pressure is normal), the diagnosis of a restrictive defect is supported. Restrictive defects maintain near-normal pressures on either side of the shunt, portending a better prognosis.

Left-to-right shunting PDA and VSD increase venous return to the LA and LV, augmenting the velocities recorded across the pulmonary veins and mitral orifice in diastole. With ASD and VSD the velocity of ejection into the PA is also increased due to the greater flow entering the right side of the heart. The same situation occurs across the LVOT in PDA. These increases in velocities correlate at least crudely with the magnitude of the shunt. For example, shunting across a PDA would be assessed as mild if both the mitral E-wave velocity and the aortic ejection velocity are within normal limits (in an unsedated patient). One can actually quantify shunt fraction (Qp /Qs) by measuring the flow across the cardiac valves on opposite sides of the shunt,[161,507] but these methods are fraught with technical problems and discrepancies. Any estimates of severity suggested by spectral Doppler examination should be congruous with 2D imaging and the severity of volume overload.

Atrial Septal Defects

An ASD is classified by location within the atrial septum. Specific designations include: (1) persistent patency of the foramen ovale (see Figure 8-14; Video 8-8, *A*); (2) ostium secundum defects located in the fossa ovale caudal to the intervenous tubercle (Figure 8-54, *A*); (3) sinus venosus defects adjacent to pulmonary venous entry; and (4) ostium primum defects located in the ventral atrial septum (Figure 8-54, *B*). A number of small case series and reports describe the imaging features in dogs and cats.[321,364,372,508-516] Typical features of ASDs are shown in Videos 8-41 and below. An additional reason for an ASD in dogs is atrial rupture associated with chronic, severe MR, LA dilatation, and transmural splitting (see Video 8-26).[335,358]

Persistent patency of the foramen ovale is usually associated with a cardiac defect that maintains increases RA pressures, as with PHT, PS, and tricuspid valve malformations. Less appreciated is persistent patency of the foramen from stretching caused by severe LA dilation. An ostium primum ASD can occur as an isolated defect or as a component of a partial or complete atrioventricular septal defect (AVSD). The complete AVSD includes a primum ASD, a VSD located in the ventricular inlet septum, and a bridging septal leaflet shared by the mitral and tricuspid valves. The anticipated offset between the insertion points of the (normally dorsal) septal mitral leaflet and (normally ventral) septal tricuspid leaflet is not present and is replaced by a common leaflet that bridges the space between the ASD and the VSD.

The anatomic diagnosis of an ASD often is made from 2D echocardiography. The salient features are a dropout of septal echoes, evident in more than one imaging plane, and localized to an anticipated site for an ASD. When imaging in the right parasternal short-axis plane, the atrial septum is truncated, and any visualized defect is more likely to be a secundum defect (Video 8-41). It is easier to distinguish a primum from

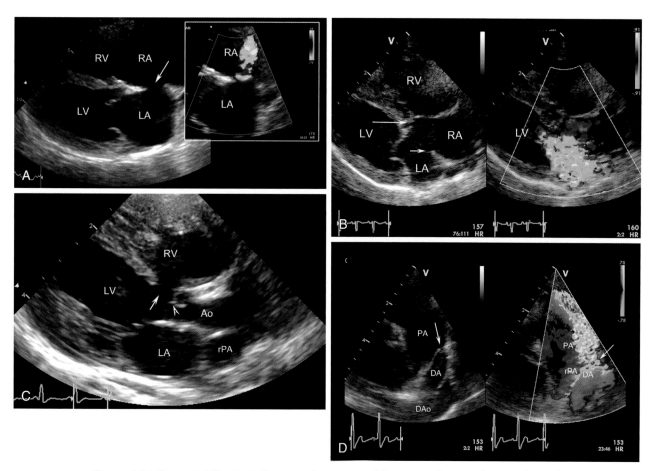

Figure 8-54 **Congenital Shunts. A,** Frozen right parasternal long axis of a secondum atrial septal defect in an older dog with preclinical dilated cardiomyopathy. Inset: Color Doppler imaging across the defect. **B,** Right parasternal image of a primum atrial septal defect and common (straddling) septal leaflet in a young dog. A large gap is evident in the ventral atrial septum (to the left of the upper arrow). This is an ostium primum ASD. The septal tricuspid and mitral leaflets are shared and the two parts of the valve attach at the same level (*long arrow*) instead of following the normal offset. The valve is incompetent (right panel) and in real time studies the regurgitant jet started in the LV and crossed the ASD to enter both atria. **C,** Frozen right parasternal long axis image of a membranous ventricular septal defect in a dog (*arrow*) located below the aortic valve (*arrowhead*) and septal tricuspid leaflet (not seen). See Fig. 8-27D for an example of color Doppler imaging across a VSD. **D,** Frozen left cranial image of a patent ductus arteriosus in a dog. Inset: Color Doppler imaging across the defect.

a secondum ASD in the parasternal long-axis and in the left apical 4-chamber image planes. When imaging a patent foramen ovale the most prominent finding is a small slit between ventral primum septum and the dorsal septum secondum. In some cases the septum primum will move, flapping into the left atrium at discrete points of the cardiac cycle. The use of TEE improves the imaging assessment of an ASD, better delineates the rim of the lesion, and is also used to guide device closure of the atrial septal defects (see Figure 8-15, *D*).

Right-sided volume overload and dilation of the main PA and its principle branches are expected with simple left-to-right shunting ASD (Videos 8-18 and 8-19). The LA does not enlarge, because it immediately decompresses into the RA. Paradoxical motion of the IVS indicates moderate to severe volume overload. The findings with a complete AVSD or an acquired ASD from atrial tearing are somewhat different and the left heart chambers also can be enlarged.

Shunting across an ASD can be visualized with CDI and is predominately left-to-right (see Videos 8-15 and 8-41).

However, right-to-left or bidirectional shunting is observed in the settings of PHT, PS, or tricuspid valve disease. As right-to-left shunting is of low-velocity, either saline contrast or CDI with low-velocity scales must be used to see the abnormal flow. Despite the sensitivity of CDI, establishing the presence of shunting across an atrial septal defect using only color or spectral Doppler imaging can promote false-positive diagnosis. Normal venous return to the RA is derived from cranial and caudal vena cava as well as the coronary sinus, which enters just dorsal to the caudal vena cava. Venous return from the caudal vena cava tracts along the atrial septum and can be readily confused with a left-to-right shunting ASD. Because atrial pressures are so close, turbulent encoding is not often visualized in the RA (with the exception of an acquired ASD caused by severe MR or another cause of increased LA pressure). In cases of AVSD, concurrent valvular malformation can cause MR or TR. Since the atrioventricular septum is imperforate, mitral regurgitation might enter the contralateral atrium (Video 8-41).

Ventricular Septal Defects

The most common VSD is subaortic in location, centered between the right and noncoronary cusps of the AV, and communicates with the RV adjacent to the edge of the tricuspid valve. Such defects are classified as perimembranous (or paramembranous) defects. Other types of VSD include defects located immediately beneath both semilunar valves (variously termed subpulmonic, subarterial, doubly committed, and supracristal); defects within the muscular septum (muscular or trabecular); and defects of the ventricular inlet septum immediately ventral to the septal tricuspid leaflet (part of a complete AVSD). In the case of tetralogy of Fallot, pulmonary atresia, and truncus arteriosus, the VSD is perimembranous but so large that it extends into the supraventricular crest (the so-called conotruncal septal defect). The term "malalignment VSD" indicates that there is some overriding or malpositioning of the aorta over the plane of the IVS. This is a component of the tetralogy of Fallot but also observed in some isolated but large perimembranous defects.

Most VSDs can be recognized as a dropout in echoes using 2D imaging (Figure 8-54, C).[61,517,518] The optimal image planes include the: (1) right-sided parasternal long-axis image optimized for the left ventricular outflow tract and septal tricuspid valve leaflet; (2) right parasternal four chamber image of the ventricular inlets (which includes the cardiac septa); (3) the right and left parasternal short-axis image of the aorta that includes the U-shaped RV inlet and outlet and the tricuspid and pulmonic valves; and (4) left apical 4- and 5 chamber image planes. The exception to this guideline is the muscular VSD located in the ventricular apex, which is difficult to identify without CDI. Examples of these are shown in Video 8-42.

In addition to identifying the defect, attention should be directed to the relative size of the VSD compared to the aortic diameter at the valve hinge points, the size of the cardiac chambers, and the diameter of the PA and its branches. Although it is very difficult to measure the diameter of the defect accurately without TEE or 3D imaging, if the largest diameter is <30% to 40% of the aortic diameter, the defect is probably restrictive. Defects exceeding 50% of the aortic diameter are usually large. With an isolated defect, the magnitude of shunting should correlate at least crudely with enlargement of the LA and LV. The RV is mostly a conduit for shunt flow and minimally enlarged. In the presence of a large shunt, PHT, concurrent PS, or in apically-located defects, the RV diastolic volume and wall thickness are more likely to be increased. Dilation of the PA supports a significant shunt or development of PHT. In staging lesion severity it should be appreciated that pulmonary to systemic flow shunt ratios of 1.5:1 are well tolerated. Thus the finding of LA and LV dilatation does not necessarily indicate a poor prognosis or dictate a surgical procedure such as PA banding. A cardiologist experienced in congenital heart disease should be consulted when formulating a prognosis and multiple imaging findings must be evaluated when rendering an opinion.

The 2D examination should also evaluate systolic LV function (it is generally normal) and search for concurrent lesions that might influence longevity, clinical signs, and treatment options. An obvious lesion is subvalvular PS, a component of tetralogy of Fallot and a lesion that promotes RV hypertrophy, right-to-left shunting, hypoxemia, and secondary polycythemia. Valvular PS can impact an isolated VSD, creating a similar pathophysiology. Another important finding is aortic malalignment when this lesion fosters prolapse of an AV leaflet into the defect. While such prolapse can reduce the functional size of the hole, it also predisposes to AR. When AR is severe (and detectable as an audible diastole murmur), LV failure is more likely to occur in the future. Yet another 2D finding is identi-

fication of hyperechoic tissue along the RV septal surface. This can be caused by fibrous proliferation in response to the high-velocity jet. When confined to the ventricular septum or septal tricuspid leaflet, the rim of the defect can become smaller or the defect can even close over, creating a ventricular septal aneurysm.[519] However, if the RV freewall is enveloped in the process, a *double-chambered RV* might develop (Video 8-33). This midventricular obstruction constitutes a pressure overload on the proximal RV, reducing the severity of the left-to-right shunt but predisposing to right-to-left shunting, exercise intolerance, and right heart failure.[371,404-409,520]

Doppler imaging both verifies the shunt and helps to assess the severity of the lesion. Provided the shunt is restrictive, both CDI and PWD should reveal signal aliasing with holosystolic turbulence within the RV and adjacent to the septal defect (see Figure 8-27, D; Videos 8-15 and 8-41). The PWD examination demonstrates a normal transtricuspid inflow pattern that is ended abruptly by an aliased and turbulent jet. High-velocity systolic shunting is evident in a restrictive defect; low-velocity diastolic shunting might also be observed (see Figure 8-23, B). The path of the shunt flow can be eccentric, especially if the tricuspid valve has adhered to the rim of the defect and acts like a baffle. In apical VSDs the turbulence arises from the RV apex and can be missed unless the entire septum is screened by CDI. If the right coronary cusp of the aorta prolapses into the VSD, holodiastolic AR is seen; the regurgitant jet can extend into the LVOT or cross the VSD and enter the RV.

When shunt flow across a highly restrictive VSD is recorded by CW Doppler, the peak velocity should exceed 4.5 to 5 m/s, assuming good transducer alignment to flow. The pressure drop should be interpreted within the context of a simultaneous, non-invasive measurement of systolic blood pressure, which can be depressed by sedatives and tranquilizers. For example, assume the peak velocity across a VSD is 4.8 m/s and the noninvasive systemic blood pressure in the patient is 125 mm Hg. Using the simplified Bernoulli equation (pressure difference = $4V^2$), the instantaneous pressure gradient across the defect is estimated as $4(4.8)^2 = 4(23) = 92$ mm Hg. Assuming the AV is normal, the noninvasive systolic arterial blood pressure is an estimate of peak LV systolic pressure. From this, the RV and PA systolic pressures can be estimated (provided there is no obstruction to flow across the RV or the RVOT) by subtracting the pressure drop from the LV systolic pressure. In this example, PA systolic pressure = 125 − 92 = 32 mm Hg; a near-normal PA pressure and compatible with a restrictive and well-tolerated defect. Conversely, if RV systolic pressure approaches systemic pressures due to PHT or an obstructive RV lesion, the peak left-to-right systolic flow velocity will be lower velocity (<2 m/s) and turbulence minimal. This is the usual situation with large, unrestrictive septal defects such as those associated with tetralogy of Fallot or when a VSD is complicated RV obstruction or PHT. These complicated patients present a less certain prognosis.

Patent Ductus Arteriosus

This defect is one of the most common cardiac malformations in dogs.[54,56-58,62,521-526] It is relatively rare in cats. Diagnosis is suspected from auscultation of a continuous murmur over the pulmonary artery and confirmed by echocardiography. Aortic pressures in PDA range from about 5 to 8 times higher than those in the PA over the duration of the cardiac cycle. These pressures gradients serve as the driving force for continuous shunting. Definitive treatment is possible with surgery or a catheter-delivered occlusion device, and the prognosis for a normal life is excellent in >95% of properly managed patients.

A small percent of canine cases with PDA develop severe PHT from pulmonary vascular injury early in life. This results in nearly equal pressures across the great arteries and allows for bidirectional shunting, the so-called "reversed PDA." This occurs somewhat abruptly in younger dogs although it might not be recognized until later in life. More gradual onset of PHT is seen in some cats with PDA.[527]

Owing to the extracardiac location of the defect—between the descending aorta and the origin of the left PA—routine 2D imaging is less valuable for diagnosis of the shunt (Figure 8-54, D). Certainly a large PDA can be visualized in many dogs and cats from a right parasternal or a left cranial parasternal image optimized for the PA. Unfortunately artifacts created by lung tissue can obscure the lesion. When there is doubt, TEE can confirm the 2D diagnosis as it provides a clear image of the ductus (see Figure 8-15, B and C). Both 2D and M-mode imaging are used to quantify the anticipated secondary responses of left-to-right shunting. These include LA and LV dilatation, enlargement of the ascending aorta, and dilation of the main PA. Both LA and LV enlargement occur in direct relationship to the shunt size and pulmonary blood flow (see Figure 8-33, A; Video 8-18). The LA can become extremely enlarged when there is moderate to severe MR secondary to cardiac remodeling or from concurrent valvular malformation. Systolic LV function is usually in the low-normal range but in some dogs it is reduced and persists as subnormal following ligation.[522,524] Mild depressions in LV systolic function are sometimes observed, but for the most part do not seem to influence long term survival.[522,524] When PDA is complicated by atrial fibrillation or CHF in a larger breed dog, a secondary DCM phenotype is often found presumably due to chronic volume overload. The RV is normal in PDA except in the situation of "reversed" PDA (Video 8-42).

The diagnosis of PDA is established by examining the PA from cranial imaging positions and observing a turbulent flow pattern that enters near the bifurcation of the PA and extends back toward the pulmonary valve (Videos 8-15 and 8-42). Flow coming from the descending aorta, but still confined to the ductal ampulla, is encoded in red but abruptly changes to a turbulent signal as it reaches the low pressure side of the defect. The appearance of the shunt flow is quite variable: it might track eccentrically along the arterial wall; adopt a serpentine path that leaves and reappears within the imaging plane; or completely fill the PA with turbulence encoding. When a PWD sample volume is advanced from the pulmonary valve toward the ductus the signal becomes turbulent, aliased, and continuous and exhibits a greater intensity and duration in the audio channel, not unlike the sound of moving the stethoscope from the left apex to the left base in this disease. Turbulent flow signals in the main PA are disrupted briefly in early systole because of pulmonary artery ejection. The CWD examination demonstrates continuous, high-velocity flow directed mainly above the baseline, but often including a negative component (see Figure 8-23, D). The peak velocity occurs at the end of systole, just after the T-wave and trails off slightly during late diastole. Good alignment with the ductal flow will yield a peak velocity of 4.5 to 5 m/s, indicating preservation of the nearly-normal aortic to PA pressure difference (and ruling out significant PHT). The pressure gradient can be estimated using the Bernoulli relationship. Velocities <4 m/s are most often from suboptimal alignment or lower systolic pressure due to tranquilizers or physiologic hypotension encountered in some in young animals. Dilation of the main PA often leads to pulmonary regurgitation which is of low-velocity in left-to-right shunting PDA. Most cases also demonstrate MR and AR to varying degrees, related to the LV and aortic dilatation. As flow across the mitral and AV is increased, the peak flow velocities become higher and exceed the normal range. The aortic ejection velocity can exceed 3 m/s simply from high flow volume in the ascending aorta. This makes the diagnosis of concurrent, mild SAS difficult in predisposed breeds such as Newfoundland dogs.

Reversed PDA is not very common and for practical purposes can be excluded with certainly if the cardiac murmur is continuous and the RV cavity is not hypertrophied. When severe PHT does complicate PDA, the LA and LV appear normal to small in size while the RV is thickened, the RA enlarged, and the PA and its main branches dilated (Video 8-42). As a reverse PDA is generally large and unrestrictive, the duct is often imaged by 2DE as it extends from the base of the left PA into the descending aorta. Shunting in this syndrome is bidirectional, very low in velocity, and often difficult to delineate. With careful PWD mapping and imaging from each side of the thorax, the diagnosis is usually straightforward. Placing the sample volume on the ventricular side of the pulmonary valve will yield a positive diastolic flow signal of high-velocity pulmonary insufficiency (see Figure 8-50, B) while placement of the sample volume at the PA bifurcation records low-velocity (<2 m/s), bidirectional flow signals. As mentioned earlier in this chapter, it can be helpful to perform saline contrast echocardiography using a cephalic venous injection while recording images over the abdominal aorta (Video 8-8, C). The appearance of saline contrast in the aorta, but not in the RA or RV, points to right-to-left shunting at the level of the great vessels.

REFERENCES

1. Nyland TG, Mattoon JS. *Small Animal Diagnostic Ultrasound*. 2nd cd. Philadelphia: Saunders/Elsevier; 2002.
2. Otto CM. *Textbook of Clinical Echocardiography*. 5th ed. Philadelphia: Elsevier/Saunders; 2013.
3. Armstrong WF, Ryan T. *Feigenbaum's echocardiography*. 7th ed. Philadelphia: Wolters Kluwer Health/Lippincott Williams & Wilkins; 2010.
4. Oh JK, Seward JB, Tajik AJ. *The Echo Manual*. 3rd ed. Philadelphia: Lippincott Williams & Wilkins; 2007.
5. Nanda NC. *Comprehensive Textbook of Echocardiography*. New Delhi, India: Jaypee Brothers Medical Publishers; 2013.
6. Hatle L, Angelsen B. *Doppler Ultrasound in Cardiology: Physical Principles and Clnical Applications*. 2nd ed. Philadelphia: Lea & Febiger; 1985.
7. Goldberg SJ, Allen HD, Marx GR, et al. *Doppler Echocardiography*. 2nd ed. Philadelphia: Lea & Febiger; 1988.
8. Kisslo J, Adams DB, Belkin RN. *Doppler Color Flow Imaging*. New York: Churchill Livingstone; 1988.
9. Weyman AE. *Principles and Practice of Echocardiography*. 2nd ed. Philadelphia: Lea & Febiger; 1994.
10. Mashiro I, Nelson RR, Cohn JN, et al. Ventricular dimensions measured noninvasively by echocardiography in the awake dog. *J Appl Physiol* 1976;**41**:953–9.
11. Dennis MO, Nealeigh RC, Pyle RL, et al. Echocardiographic assessment of normal and abnormal valvular function in Beagle dogs. *Am J Vet Res* 1978;**39**:1591–8.
12. Pipers FS, Andrysco RM, Hamlin RL. A totally noninvasive method for obtaining systolic time intervals in the dog. *Am J Vet Res* 1978;**39**:1822–6.
13. Pipers FS, Reef V, Hamlin RL. Echocardiography in the domestic cat. *Am J Vet Res* 1979;**40**:882–6.
14. Pipers FS, Hamlin RL. Clinical use of echocardiography in the domestic cat. *J Am Vet Med Assoc* 1980;**176**:57–61.

15. Bonagura JD, Pipers FS. Echocardiographic features of pericardial effusion in dogs. *J Am Vet Med Assoc* 1981;**179**:49–56.

16. Miller CW, Wingfield WE. Applications of ultrasound to veterinary diagnostics in a veterinary teaching hospital. *Biomed Sci Instrum* 1981;**17**:85–90.

17. Pipers FS, Bonagura JD, Hamlin RL, et al. Echocardiographic abnormalities of the mitral valve associated with left sided heart diseases in the dog. *J Am Vet Med Assoc* 1981;**179**:580–6.

18. Miller CW, Wingfield WE, Boon JA. Applications of ultrasound to veterinary diagnostics in a veterinary teaching hospital. *ISA Trans* 1982;**21**:101–6.

19. Wingfield WE, Boon J, Miller CW. Echocardiographic assessment of mitral valve motion, cardiac structures, and ventricular function in dogs with atrial fibrillation. *J Am Vet Med Assoc* 1982;**181**:46–9.

20. Bonagura JD. M-mode echocardiography. Basic principles. *Vet Clin North Am Small Anim Pract* 1983;**13**:299–319.

21. Bonagura JD, Pipers FS. Echocardiographic features of aortic valve endocarditis in a dog, a cow, and a horse. *J Am Vet Med Assoc* 1983;**182**:595–9.

22. Bonagura JD, Pipers FS. Diagnosis of cardiac lesions by contrast echocardiography. *J Am Vet Med Assoc* 1983;**182**:396–402.

23. Jacobs G, Bolton GR, Watrous BJ. Echocardiographic features of dilated coronary sinus in a dog with persistent left cranial vena cava. *J Am Vet Med Assoc* 1983;**182**:407–8.

24. Wingfield WE, Boon JA, Miller CW. Echocardiographic assessment of congenital aortic stenosis in dogs. *J Am Vet Med Assoc* 1983;**183**:673–6.

25. Yamaguchi RA, Pipers FS, Gamble DA. Echocardiographic evaluation of a cat with bacterial vegetative endocarditis. *J Am Vet Med Assoc* 1983;**183**:118–20.

26. Berg RJ, Wingfield WE, Hoopes PJ. Idiopathic hemorrhagic pericardial effusion in eight dogs. *J Am Vet Med Assoc* 1984;**185**:988–92.

27. Kittleson MD, Eyster GE, Knowlen GG, et al. Myocardial function in small dogs with chronic mitral regurgitation and severe congestive heart failure. *J Am Vet Med Assoc* 1984;**184**:455–9.

28. Lombard CW. Normal values of the canine M-mode echocardiogram. *Am J Vet Res* 1984;**45**:2015–18.

29. Sisson D, Thomas WP. Endocarditis of the aortic valve in the dog. *J Am Vet Med Assoc* 1984;**184**:570–7.

30. Fox PR, Bond BR, Peterson ME. Echocardiographic reference values in healthy cats sedated with ketamine hydrochloride. *Am J Vet Res* 1985;**46**:1479–84.

31. Jacobs G, Knight DH. M-mode echocardiographic measurements in nonanesthetized healthy cats: effects of body weight, heart rate, and other variables. *Am J Vet Res* 1985;**46**:1705–11.

32. Moise NS, Dietze AE. Echocardiographic, electrocardiographic, and radiographic detection of cardiomegaly in hyperthyroid cats. *Am J Vet Res* 1986;**47**:1487–94.

33. Bond BR, Fox PR, Peterson ME, et al. Echocardiographic findings in 103 cats with hyperthyroidism. *J Am Vet Med Assoc* 1988;**192**:1546–9.

34. Wyatt HL, Heng MK, Meerbaum S, et al. Cross-sectional echocardiography. I. Analysis of mathematic models for quantifying mass of the left ventricle in dogs. *Circulation* 1979;**60**:1104–13.

35. Thomas WP. Two-dimensional, real-time echocardiography in the dog: Technique and anatomic validation. *Vet Radiol Ultrasound* 1984;**25**:50–64.

36. Thomas WP, Sisson D, Bauer TG, et al. Detection of cardiac masses in dogs by two-dimensional echocardiography. *Vet Radiol Ultrasound* 1984;**25**:65–72.

37. Yamaga Y, Too K. Diagnostic ultrasound imaging in domestic animals: two-dimensional and M-mode echocardiography. *Jap J Vet Sci* 1984;**46**:493–503.

38. Bonagura JD, Herring DS. Echocardiography. Acquired heart disease. *Vet Clin North Am Small Anim Pract* 1985;**15**:1209–24.

39. Bonagura JD, Herring DS. Echocardiography. Congenital heart disease. *Vet Clin North Am Small Anim Pract* 1985;**15**:1195–208.

40. DeMadron E, Bonagura JD, O'Grady MR. Normal and paradoxical ventricular septal motion in the dog. *Am J Vet Res* 1985;**46**:1832–41.

41. O'Grady MR, Bonagura J, Powers JD, et al. Quantiative cross-sectional echocardiography in the normal dog. *Vet Radiol Ultrasound* 1986;**27**:34–49.

42. Badertscher RR 2nd, Losonsky JM, Paul AJ, et al. Two-dimensional echocardiography for diagnosis of dirofilariasis in nine dogs. *J Am Vet Med Assoc* 1988;**193**:843–6.

43. Hay WH, Woodfield JA, Moon MA. Clinical, echocardiographic, and radiographic findings of peritoneopericardial diaphragmatic hernia in two dogs and a cat. *J Am Vet Med Assoc* 1989;**195**:1245–8.

44. Oyama MA. Advances in echocardiography. *Vet Clin North Am Small Anim Pract* 2004;**34**:1083–104.

45. Chetboul V. Advanced techniques in echocardiography in small animals. *Vet Clin North Am Small Anim Pract* 2010;**40**:529–43.

46. Boon J. *Veterinary Echocardiography*. 2nd ed. Ames, IA: John Wiley & Sons; 2011.

47. deMadron E, Chetboul V, Bussadori C. *Echocardiographie Clinique du Chien et du Chat: Techniques et Applicaitons Pratiques*. Issy-le-Moulineaux: Elsevier Masson; 2012.

48. Spencer KT, Kimura BJ, Korcarz CE, et al. Focused cardiac ultrasound: recommendations from the American Society of Echocardiography. *J Am Soc Echocardiogr* 2013;**26**:567–81.

49. Tse YC, Rush JE, Cunningham SM, et al. Evaluation of a training course in focused echocardiography for non-cardiology house officers. *J Vet Emerg Crit Care* 2013;**23**:268–73.

50. Loyer CG, Thomas WP. Biplane transesophageal echocardiography in the dog: Technique, anatomy and imaging planes. *Vet Radiol Ultrasound* 1995;**36**:212–26.

51. Kienle RD, Thomas WP, Rishniw M. Biplane transesophageal echocardiography in the normal cat. *Vet Radiol Ultrasound* 1997;**38**:288–98.

52. St-Vincent RS, Pharr JW. Transesophageal ultrasonography of the normal canine mediastinum. *Vet Radiol Ultrasound* 1998;**39**:197–205.

53. Chetboul V, Pouchelon JL. Transesophageal echocardiography: principles, technique and potential indications in veterinary medicine. *Schweiz Arch Tierheilkd* 2004;**146**:321–6.

54. Pariaut R, Sydney MN, Kraus MS, et al. Use of transesophageal echocardiography for visualization of the patent ductus arteriosus during transcatheter coil embolization. *J Vet Cardiol* 2004;**6**:32–9.

55. Quintavalla C, Pradelli D, Domenech O, et al. Transesophageal echocardiography of the left ventricular outflow tract, aortic valve and ascending aorta in Boxer dogs with heart murmurs. *Vet Radiol Ultrasound* 2006;**47**:307–12.

56. Szatmari V, Stokhof AA. Use of simultaneous fluoroscopic and echocardiographic guidance during

transarterial coil placement for embolization of patent ductus arteriosus in dogs. *J Am Vet Med Assoc* 2006; **228**:881–4.

57. Saunders AB, Miller MW, Gordon SG, et al. Echocardiographic and angiographic comparison of ductal dimensions in dogs with patent ductus arteriosus. *J Vet Intern Med* 2007;**21**:68–75.

58. Saunders AB, Achen SE, Gordon SG, et al. Utility of transesophageal echocardiography for transcatheter occlusion of patent ductus arteriosus in dogs: influence on the decision-making process. *J Vet Intern Med* 2010; **24**:1407–13.

59. Trehiou-Sechi E, Behr L, Chetboul V, et al. Echoguided closed commissurotomy for mitral valve stenosis in a dog. *J Vet Cardiol* 2011;**13**:219–25.

60. Domenech O, Oliveira P. Transoesophageal echocardiography in the dog. *Vet J* 2013;**198**:329–38.

61. Saunders AB, Carlson JA, Nelson DA, et al. Hybrid technique for ventricular septal defect closure in a dog using an Amplatzer(R) Duct Occluder II. *J Vet Cardiol* 2013; **15**:217–24.

62. Porciello F, Caivano D, Giorgi ME, et al. Transesophageal echocardiography as the sole guidance for occlusion of patent ductus arteriosus using a canine ductal occluder in dogs. *J Vet Intern Med* 2014.

63. Bonagura JD, Miller MW. Doppler echocardiography. II. Color Doppler imaging. *Vet Clin North Am Small Anim Pract* 1998;**28**:1361–89, vii.

64. Moise NS. Doppler echocardiographic evaluation of congenital cardiac disease. An introduction. *J Vet Intern Med* 1989;**3**:195–207.

65. Brown DJ, Knight DH, King RR. Use of pulsed-wave Doppler echocardiography to determine aortic and pulmonary velocity and flow variables in clinically normal dogs. *Am J Vet Res* 1991;**52**:543–50.

66. Uehara Y. An attempt to estimate the pulmonary artery pressure in dogs by means of pulsed Doppler echocardiography. *J Vet Med Sci* 1993;**55**:307–12.

67. Bonagura JD, Miller MW, Darke PG. Doppler echocardiography. I. Pulsed-wave and continuous-wave examinations. *Vet Clin North Am Small Anim Pract* 1998;**28**: 1325–59, vii.

68. Via G, Hussain A, Wells M, et al. International evidence-based recommendations for focused cardiac ultrasound. *J Am Soc Echocardiogr* 2014;**27**(683):e1–33.

69. Lisciandro GR, Fosgate GT, Fulton RM. Frequency and number of ultrasound lung rockets (B-lines) using a regionally based lung ultrasound examination named vet blue (veterinary bedside lung ultrasound exam) in dogs with radiographically normal lung findings. *Vet Radiol Ultrasound* 2014;**55**:315–22.

70. Rademacher N, Pariaut R, Pate J, et al. Transthoracic lung ultrasound in normal dogs and dogs with cardiogenic pulmonary edema: a pilot study. *Vet Radiol Ultrasound* 2014.

71. Cote E. Echocardiography: common pitfalls and practical solutions. *Clin Tech Small Anim Pract* 2005;**20**:156–63.

72. Stepien RL, Bonagura JD, Bednarski RM, et al. Cardiorespiratory effects of acepromazine maleate and buprenorphine hydrochloride in clinically normal dogs. *Am J Vet Res* 1995;**56**:78–84.

73. Ward JL, Schober KE, Fuentes VL, et al. Effects of sedation on echocardiographic variables of left atrial and left ventricular function in healthy cats. *J Feline Med Surg* 2012;**14**:678–85.

74. Lamont LA, Bulmer BJ, Sisson DD, et al. Doppler echocardiographic effects of medetomidine on dynamic left ventricular outflow tract obstruction in cats. *J Am Vet Med Assoc* 2002;**221**:1276–81.

75. Jacobs G, Knight DH. Change in M-mode echocardiographic values in cats given ketamine. *Am J Vet Res* 1985;**46**:1712–13.

76. MacDonald K, King D. Work-related musculoskeletal disorders in veterinary echocardiographers: A cross-sectional study on prevalence and risk factors. *J Vet Cardiol* 2014;**16**:27–37.

77. Macdonald K, Scott P. Scanning through the pain: ergonomic considerations for performing echocardiography of animals. *J Vet Cardiol* 2013;**15**:57–63.

78. Lang RM, Badano LP, Tsang W, et al. EAE/ASE recommendations for image acquisition and display using three-dimensional echocardiography. *J Am Soc Echocardiogr* 2012;**25**:3–46.

79. Thomas WP, Gaber CE, Jacobs GJ, et al. Recommendations for standards in transthoracic two-dimensional echocardiography in the dog and cat. Echocardiography Committee of the Specialty of Cardiology, American College of Veterinary Internal Medicine. *J Vet Internal Med* 1993;**7**:247–52.

80. Lai WW, Geva T, Shirali GS, et al. Guidelines and standards for performance of a pediatric echocardiogram: a report from the Task Force of the Pediatric Council of the American Society of Echocardiography. *J Am Soc Echocardiogr* 2006;**19**:1413–30.

81. Rudski LG, Lai WW, Afilalo J, et al. Guidelines for the echocardiographic assessment of the right heart in adults: a report from the American Society of Echocardiography endorsed by the European Association of Echocardiography, a registered branch of the European Society of Cardiology, and the Canadian Society of Echocardiography. *J Am Soc Echocardiogr* 2010;**23**:685–713, quiz 86–8.

82. Lang RM, Bierig M, Devereux RB, et al. Recommendations for chamber quantification. *Eur J Echocardiogr* 2006;**7**:79–108.

83. Lang RM, Bierig M, Devereux RB, et al. Recommendations for chamber quantification: a report from the American Society of Echocardiography's Guidelines and Standards Committee and the Chamber Quantification Writing Group, developed in conjunction with the European Association of Echocardiography, a branch of the European Society of Cardiology. *J Am Soc Echocardiogr* 2005;**18**:1440–63.

84. Zoghbi W. Recommendations for evaluation of the severity of native valvular regurgitation with two-dimensional and doppler echocardiography. *J Am Soc Echocardiogr* 2003;**16**:777–802.

85. Lopez L, Colan SD, Frommelt PC, et al. Recommendations for quantification methods during the performance of a pediatric echocardiogram: a report from the Pediatric Measurements Writing Group of the American Society of Echocardiography Pediatric and Congenital Heart Disease Council. *J Am Soc Echocardiogr* 2010; **23**:465–95, quiz 576–7.

86. Quiñones MA, Otto CM, Stoddard M, et al. Recommendations for quantification of Doppler echocardiography: A report from the Doppler quantification task force of the nomenclature and standards committee of the American Society of Echocardiography. *J Am Soc Echocardiogr* 2002;**15**:167–84.

87. Nagueh SF, Appleton CP, Gillebert TC, et al. Recommendations for the evaluation of left ventricular diastolic function by echocardiography. *J Am Soc Echocardiogr* 2009;**22**:107–33.

88. Ziegler L, O'Brien RT. Harmonic ultrasound: a review. *Vet Radiol Ultrasound* 2002;**43**:501–9.

89. Turner SP, Monaghan MJ. Tissue harmonic imaging for standard left ventricular measurements: fundamentally flawed? *Eur J Echocardiogr* 2006;**7**:9–15.

90. Bonagura JD, O'Grady MR, Herring DS. Echocardiography. Principles of interpretation. *Vet Clin North Am Small Anim Pract* 1985;**15**:1177–94.

91. Yoerger DM, Marcus F, Sherrill D, et al. Echocardiographic findings in patients meeting task force criteria for arrhythmogenic right ventricular dysplasia: new insights from the multidisciplinary study of right ventricular dysplasia. *J Am Coll Cardiol* 2005;**45**:860–5.

92. Lehmkuhl LB, Bonagura JD. Comparison of transducer placement sites for Doppler echocardiography in dogs with subaortic stenosis. *Am J Vet Res* 1994;**55**:192–8.

93. Abbott JA, MacLean HN. Comparison of Doppler-derived peak aortic velocities obtained from subcostal and apical transducer sites in healthy dogs. *Vet Radiol Ultrasound* 2003;**44**:695–8.

94. Schober KE, Maerz I. Assessment of left atrial appendage flow velocity and its relation to spontaneous echocardiographic contrast in 89 cats with myocardial disease. *J Vet Intern Med* 2006;**20**:120–30.

95. Schober KE, Maerz I. Doppler echocardiographic assessment of left atrial appendage flow velocities in normal cats. *J Vet Cardiol* 2005;**7**:15–25.

96. Oyama MA, Sisson DD. Assessment of cardiac chamber size using anatomic M-mode. *Vet Radiol Ultrasound* 2005;**46**:331–6.

97. Chetboul V, Lichtenberger J, Mellin M, et al. Within-day and between-day variability of transthoracic anatomic M-mode echocardiography in the awake bottlenose dolphin (Tursiops truncatus). *J Vet Cardiol* 2012;**14**:511–18.

98. Sisson D, Schaeffer D. Changes in linear dimensions of the heart, relative to body weight, as measured by M-mode echocardiography in growing dogs. *Am J Vet Res* 1991;**52**:1591–6.

99. Sisson DD, Knight DH, Helinski C, et al. Plasma taurine concentrations and M-mode echocardiographic measures in healthy cats and in cats with dilated cardiomyopathy. *J Vet Intern Med* 1991;**5**:232–8.

100. Hanton G, Geffray B, Lodola A. Echocardiography, a non-invasive method for the investigation of heart morphology and function in laboratory dogs: 1. Method and reference values for M-mode parameters. *Lab Anim* 1998;**32**:173–82.

101. Schille S, Skrodzki M. M-mode echocardiographic reference values in cats in the first three months of life. *Vet Radiol Ultrasound* 1999;**40**:491–500.

102. Schober KE, Baade H. Comparability of left ventricular M-mode echocardiography in dogs performed in long-axis and short-axis. *Vet Radiol Ultrasound* 2000;**41**:543–9.

103. Rishniw M. Systolic aortic valve flutter in 6 dogs. *Vet Radiol Ultrasound* 2001;**42**:446–7.

104. Schober KE, Fuentes VL. Mitral annulus motion as determined by M-mode echocardiography in normal dogs and dogs with cardiac disease. *Vet Radiol Ultrasound* 2001;**42**:52–61.

105. Hansson K, Haggstrom J, Kvart C, et al. Left atrial to aortic root indices using two-dimensional and M-mode echocardiography in cavalier King Charles spaniels with and without left atrial enlargement. *Vet Radiol Ultrasound* 2002;**43**:568–75.

106. Oyama MA, Thomas WP. Two-dimensional and M-mode echocardiographic predictors of disease severity in dogs with congenital subaortic stenosis. *J Am Anim Hosp Assoc* 2002;**38**:209–15.

107. Brown DJ, Rush JE, MacGregor J, et al. M-mode echocardiographic ratio indices in normal dogs, cats, and horses: a novel quantitative method. *J Vet Intern Med* 2003;**17**:653–62.

108. Cornell CC, Kittleson MD, Della TP, et al. Allometric scaling of M-mode cardiac measurements in normal adult dogs. *J Vet Internal Med* 2004;**18**:311–21.

109. Henik RA, Stepien RL, Bortnowski HB. Spectrum of M-mode echocardiographic abnormalities in 75 cats with systemic hypertension. *J Am Anim Hosp Assoc* 2004;**40**:359–63.

110. Feigenbaum H. Role of M-mode technique in today's echocardiography. *J Am Soc Echocardiogr* 2010;**23**:240–57, 335–7.

111. de Oliveira VM, Chamas PP, Goldfeder GT, et al. Comparative study of 4 echocardiographic methods of left ventricular measurement in German Shepherd dogs. *J Vet Cardiol* 2014;**16**:1–8.

112. Bank AJ, Gage RM, Burns KV. Right ventricular pacing, mechanical dyssynchrony, and heart failure. *J Cardiovasc Transl Res* 2012;**5**:219–31.

113. Estrada A, Chetboul V. Tissue Doppler evaluation of ventricular synchrony. *J Vet Cardiol* 2006;**8**:129–37.

114. Griffiths LG, Fransioli JR, Chigerwe M. Echocardiographic assessment of interventricular and intraventricular mechanical synchrony in normal dogs. *J Vet Cardiol* 2011;**13**:115–26.

115. Lopez-Alvarez J, Fonfara S, Pedro B, et al. Assessment of mechanical ventricular synchrony in Doberman Pinschers with dilated cardiomyopathy. *J Vet Cardiol* 2011;**13**:183–95.

116. Takano H, Fujii Y, Ishikawa R, et al. Comparison of left ventricular contraction profiles among small, medium, and large dogs by use of two-dimensional speckle-tracking echocardiography. *Am J Vet Res* 2010;**71**:421–7.

117. Zois NE, Tidholm A, Nagga KM, et al. Radial and longitudinal strain and strain rate assessed by speckle-tracking echocardiography in dogs with myxomatous mitral valve disease. *J Vet Intern Med* 2012;**26**:1309–19.

118. Ljungvall I, Hoglund K, Carnabuci C, et al. Assessment of global and regional left ventricular volume and shape by real-time 3-dimensional echocardiography in dogs with myxomatous mitral valve disease. *J Vet Intern Med* 2011;**25**:1036–43.

119. Zile MR, Tomita M, Ishihara K, et al. Changes in diastolic function during development and correction of chronic LV volume overload produced by mitral regurgitation. *Circulation* 1993;**87**:1378–88.

120. Jacobs GJ, Calvert CA, Mahaffey MB, et al. Echocardiographic detection of flail left atrioventricular valve cusp from ruptured chordae tendineae in 4 dogs. *J Vet Intern Med* 1995;**9**:341–6.

121. Voros K, Hetyey C, Reiczigel J, et al. M-mode and two-dimensional echocardiographic reference values for three Hungarian dog breeds: Hungarian Vizsla, Mudi and Hungarian Greyhound. *Acta Vet Hung* 2009;**57**:217–27.

122. Holler PJ, Wess G. Sphericity index and E-point-to-septal-separation (EPSS) to diagnose dilated cardiomyopathy in Doberman Pinschers. *J Vet Intern Med* 2014;**28**:123–9.

123. Lehmkuhl LB, Ware WA, Bonagura JD. Mitral stenosis in 15 dogs. *J Vet Intern Med* 1994;**8**:2–17.

124. Paige CF, Abbott JA, Pyle RL. Systolic anterior motion of the mitral valve associated with right ventricular systolic hypertension in 9 dogs. *J Vet Cardiol* 2007;**9**:9–14.

125. Payne JR, Borgeat K, Connolly DJ, et al. Prognostic indicators in cats with hypertrophic cardiomyopathy. *J Vet Intern Med* 2013;**27**:1427–36.
126. Atkins CE, Snyder PS. Systolic time intervals and their derivatives for evaluation of cardiac function. *J Vet Intern Med* 1992;**6**:55–63.
127. Wey AC, Atkins CE. Aortic dissection and congestive heart failure associated with systemic hypertension in a cat. *J Vet Intern Med* 2000;**14**:208–13.
128. Hoglund K, Bussadori C, Domenech O, et al. Contrast echocardiography in Boxer dogs with and without aortic stenosis. *J Vet Cardiol* 2007;**9**:15–24.
129. Crosara S, Ljungvall I, Margiocco ML, et al. Use of contrast echocardiography for quantitative and qualitative evaluation of myocardial perfusion and pulmonary transit time in healthy dogs. *Am J Vet Res* 2012;**73**:194–201.
130. Streitberger A, Hocke V, Modler P. Measurement of pulmonary transit time in healthy cats by use of ultrasound contrast media "Sonovue(R)": feasibility, reproducibility, and values in 42 cats. *J Vet Cardiol* 2013;**15**:181–7.
131. Yamaya Y, Niizeki K, Kim J, et al. Anaphylactoid response to Optison(R) and its effects on pulmonary function in two dogs. *J Vet Med Sci* 2004;**66**:1429–32.
132. Stern JA, Tou SP, Barker PC, et al. Hybrid cutting balloon dilatation for treatment of cor triatriatum sinister in a cat. *J Vet Cardiol* 2013;**15**:205–10.
133. Arita N, Yamane I, Takemura N. Comparison of canine heartworm removal rates using flexible alligator forceps guided by transesophageal echocardiography and fluoroscopy. *J Vet Med Sci* 2003;**65**:259–61.
134. Yang HS, Bansal RC, Mookadam F, et al. Practical guide for three-dimensional transthoracic echocardiography using a fully sampled matrix array transducer. *J Am Soc Echocardiogr* 2008;**21**:979–89, quiz 1081–2.
135. Tidholm A, Bodegard-Westling A, Hoglund K, et al. Comparisons of 2- and 3-dimensional echocardiographic methods for estimation of left atrial size in dogs with and without myxomatous mitral valve disease. *J Vet Intern Med* 2011;**25**:1320–7.
136. Tidholm A, Hoglund K, Haggstrom J, et al. Left atrial ejection fraction assessed by real-time 3-dimensional echocardiography in normal dogs and dogs with myxomatous mitral valve disease. *J Vet Intern Med* 2013;**27**:884–9.
137. Jung S, Orvalho J, Griffiths LG. Aortopulmonary window characterized with two- and three-dimensional echocardiogram in a dog. *J Vet Cardiol* 2012;**14**:371–5.
138. Meyer J, Wefstaedt P, Dziallas P, et al. Assessment of left ventricular volumes by use of one-, two-, and three-dimensional echocardiography versus magnetic resonance imaging in healthy dogs. *Am J Vet Res* 2013;**74**:1223–30.
139. Young AA, Orr R, Smaill BH, et al. Three-dimensional changes in left and right ventricular geometry in chronic mitral regurgitation. *Am J Physiol* 1996;**271**:H2689–700.
140. Gaber C. Doppler echocardiography. *Probl Vet Med* 1991;**3**:479–99.
141. Chiang CH, Hagio M, Yoshida H, et al. Pulmonary venous flow in normal dogs recorded by transthoracic echocardiography: techniques, anatomic validations and flow characteristics. *J Vet Med Sci* 1998;**60**:333–9.
142. Santilli RA, Bussadori C. Doppler echocardiographic study of left ventricular diastole in non-anaesthetized healthy cats. *Vet J* 1998;**156**:203–15.
143. Schober K, Fuentes VL. Doppler echocardiographic assessment of left ventricular diastolic function in dogs.

Tierarztl Prax Ausg K Kleintiere Heimtiere 1998;**26**:13–20.
144. Schober KE, Fuentes VL, McEwan JD, et al. Pulmonary venous flow characteristics as assessed by transthoracic pulsed Doppler echocardiography in normal dogs. *Vet Radiol Ultrasound* 1998;**39**:33–41.
145. Bright JM, Herrtage ME, Schneider JF. Pulsed Doppler assessment of left ventricular diastolic function in normal and cardiomyopathic cats. *J Am Anim Hosp Assoc* 1999;**35**:285–91.
146. Kirkberger RM, Bland-van den Berg P, Grimbeek RJ. Doppler Echocardiography in the Normal Dog: Part II. *Vet Radiol Ultrasound* 1992;**33**:380–6.
147. Brewer FC, Moise NS, Kornreich BG, et al. Use of computed tomography and silicon endocasts to identify pulmonary veins with echocardiography. *J Vet Cardiol* 2012;**14**:293–300.
148. Teshima K, Asano K, Sasaki Y, et al. Assessment of left ventricular function using pulsed tissue Doppler imaging in healthy dogs and dogs with spontaneous mitral regurgitation. *J Vet Med Sci* 2005;**67**:1207–15.
149. Carlos SC, Chetboul V, Gouni V, et al. Systolic and diastolic myocardial dysfunction in cats with hypertrophic cardiomyopathy or systemic hypertension. *J Vet Intern Med* 2006;**20**:1106–15.
150. Koffas H, Dukes-McEwan J, Corcoran BM, et al. Pulsed tissue Doppler imaging in normal cats and cats with hypertrophic cardiomyopathy. *J Vet Intern Med* 2006;**20**:65–77.
151. Hori Y, Sato S, Hoshi F, et al. Assessment of longitudinal tissue Doppler imaging of the left ventricular septum and free wall as an indicator of left ventricular systolic function in dogs. *Am J Vet Res* 2007;**68**:1051–7.
152. Hori Y, Ukai Y, Hoshi F, et al. Volume loading-related changes in tissue Doppler images derived from the tricuspid valve annulus in dogs. *Am J Vet Res* 2008;**69**:33–8.
153. Simpson KE, Gunn-Moore DA, Shaw DJ, et al. Pulsed-wave Doppler tissue imaging velocities in normal geriatric cats and geriatric cats with primary or systemic diseases linked to specific cardiomyopathies in humans, and the influence of age and heart rate upon these velocities. *J Feline Med Surg* 2009;**11**:293–304.
154. Tidholm A, Ljungvall I, Hoglund K, et al. Tissue Doppler and strain imaging in dogs with myxomatous mitral valve disease in different stages of congestive heart failure. *J Vet Intern Med* 2009;**23**:1197–207.
155. Smith DN, Schober KE. Effects of vagal maneuvers on heart rate and Doppler variables of left ventricular filling in healthy cats. *J Vet Cardiol* 2013;**15**:33–40.
156. Grenadier E, Oliveira Lima C, Allen HD, et al. Normal intracardiac and great vessel Doppler flow velocities in infants and children. *J Am Coll Cardiol* 1984;**4**:343–50.
157. Yuill CD, O'Grady MR. Doppler-derived velocity of blood flow across the cardiac valves in the normal dog. *Can J Vet Res* 1991;**55**:185–92.
158. Uehara Y, Koga M, Takahashi M. Determination of cardiac output by echocardiography. *J Vet Med Sci* 1995;**57**:401–7.
159. Dukes-McEwan J, French AT, Corcoran BM. Doppler echocardiography in the dog: measurement variability and reproducibility. *Vet Radiol Ultrasound* 2002;**43**:144–52.
160. Riesen SC, Doherr MG, Lombard CW. Comparison of Doppler-derived aortic velocities obtained from various transducer sites in healthy dogs and cats. *Vet Radiol Ultrasound* 2007;**48**:570–3.

161. Serres F, Chetboul V, Tissier R, et al. Quantification of pulmonary to systemic flow ratio by a Doppler echocardiographic method in the normal dog: Repeatability, reproducibility, and reference ranges. *J Vet Cardiol* 2009; **11**:23–9.

162. Bird JJ, Murgo JP, Pasipoularides A. Fluid dynamics of aortic stenosis: subvalvular gradients without subvalvular obstruction. *Circulation* 1982;**66**:835–40.

163. Pasipoularides A, Murgo JP, Miller JW, et al. Nonobstructive left ventricular ejection pressure gradients in man. *Circ Res* 1987;**61**:220–7.

164. Sohn S, Kim HS, Han JJ. Doppler flow velocity measurement to assess changes in inotropy and afterload: a study in healthy dogs. *Echocardiography* 2002;**19**:207–13.

165. Rishniw M, Thomas WP. Dynamic right ventricular outflow obstruction: a new cause of systolic murmurs in cats. *J Vet Intern Med* 2002;**16**:547–52.

166. Adin DB, McCloy K. Physiologic valve regurgitation in normal cats. *J Vet Cardiol* 2005;**7**:9–13.

167. Rishniw M, Erb HN. Prevalence and characterization of pulmonary regurgitation in normal adult dogs. *J Vet Cardiol* 2000;**2**:17–21.

168. Johnson L. Diagnosis of pulmonary hypertension. *Clin Tech Small Anim Pract* 1999;**14**:231–6.

169. Johnson L, Boon J, Orton EC. Clinical characteristics of 53 dogs with Doppler-derived evidence of pulmonary hypertension: 1992-1996. *J Vet Intern Med* 1999;**13**:440–7.

170. Serres F, Chetboul V, Gouni V, et al. Diagnostic value of echo-Doppler and tissue Doppler imaging in dogs with pulmonary arterial hypertension. *J Vet Intern Med* 2007;**21**:1280–9.

171. Chiavegato D, Borgarelli M, D'Agnolo G, et al. Pulmonary hypertension in dogs with mitral regurgitation attributable to myxomatous valve disease. *Vet Radiol Ultrasound* 2009;**50**:253–8.

172. Stepien RL. Pulmonary arterial hypertension secondary to chronic left-sided cardiac dysfunction in dogs. *J Small Anim Pract* 2009;**50**(Suppl. 1):34–43.

173. Chatterjee NA, Lewis GD. What is the prognostic significance of pulmonary hypertension in heart failure? *Circ Heart Fail* 2011;**4**:541–5.

174. Kellihan HB, Stepien RL. Pulmonary hypertension in canine degenerative mitral valve disease. *J Vet Cardiol* 2012;**14**:149–64.

175. Diwan A, McCulloch M, Lawrie GM, et al. Doppler estimation of left ventricular filling pressures in patients with mitral valve disease. *Circulation* 2005;**111**:3281–9.

176. Choong CY, Abascal VM, Thomas JD, et al. Combined influence of ventricular loading and relaxation on the transmitral flow velocity profile in dogs measured by Doppler echocardiography. *Circulation* 1988;**78**:672–83.

177. Simpson KE, Devine BC, Gunn-Moore DA, et al. Assessment of the repeatability of feline echocardiography using conventional echocardiography and spectral pulse-wave Doppler tissue imaging techniques. *Vet Radiol Ultrasound* 2007;**48**:58–68.

178. Disatian S, Bright JM, Boon J. Association of age and heart rate with pulsed-wave Doppler measurements in healthy, nonsedated cats. *J Vet Intern Med* 2008;**22**:351–6.

179. Fine DM, Durham HE Jr, Rossi NF, et al. Echocardiographic assessment of hemodynamic changes produced by two methods of inducing fluid deficit in dogs. *J Vet Intern Med* 2010;**24**:348–53.

180. Schober KE, Fuentes VL. Effects of age, body weight, and heart rate on transmitral and pulmonary venous flow in clinically normal dogs. *Am J Vet Res* 2001;**62**:1447–54.

181. Schober KE, Bonagura JD, Scansen BA, et al. Estimation of left ventricular filling pressure by use of Doppler echocardiography in healthy anesthetized dogs subjected to acute volume loading. *Am J Vet Res* 2008;**69**:1034–49.

182. Zile MR. New Concepts in diastolic dysfunction and diastolic heart failure: Part I: Diagnosis, prognosis, and measurements of diastolic Function. *Circulation* 2002;**105**:1387–93.

183. Angeja BG. Evaluation and management of diastolic heart failure. *Circulation* 2003;**107**:659–63.

184. Hatle L. How to diagnose diastolic heart failure a consensus statement. *Eur Heart J* 2007;**28**:2421–3.

185. Paulus WJ, Tschope C, Sanderson JE, et al. How to diagnose diastolic heart failure: a consensus statement on the diagnosis of heart failure with normal left ventricular ejection fraction by the Heart Failure and Echocardiography Associations of the European Society of Cardiology. *Eur Heart J* 2007;**28**:2539–50.

186. Wang J, Nagueh SF. Current perspectives on cardiac function in patients with diastolic heart failure. *Circulation* 2009;**119**:1146–57.

187. Borlaug BA, Paulus WJ. Heart failure with preserved ejection fraction: pathophysiology, diagnosis, and treatment. *Eur Heart J* 2011;**32**:670–9.

188. Hori Y, Kanai K, Nakao R, et al. Assessing diastolic function with Doppler echocardiography using a novel index: ratio of the transmitral early diastolic velocity to pulmonary diastolic velocity. *J Vet Med Sci* 2008;**70**:359–66.

189. Hori Y, Ukai Y, Uechi M, et al. Relationships between velocities of pulmonary venous flow and plasma concentrations of atrial natriuretic peptide in healthy dogs. *Am J Vet Res* 2008;**69**:465–70.

190. Firstenberg MS, Greenberg NL, Main ML, et al. Determinants of diastolic myocardial tissue Doppler velocities: influences of relaxation and preload. *J Appl Physiol* 2001;**90**:299–307.

191. Chetboul V. Tissue Doppler Imaging: a promising technique for quantifying regional myocardial function. *J Vet Cardiol* 2002;**4**:7–12.

192. Chetboul V, Gouni V, Sampedrano CC, et al. Assessment of regional systolic and diastolic myocardial function using tissue Doppler and strain imaging in dogs with dilated cardiomyopathy. *J Vet Intern Med* 2007;**21**:719–30.

193. Koffas H, Dukes-McEwan J, Corcoran BM, et al. Colour M-mode tissue Doppler imaging in healthy cats and cats with hypertrophic cardiomyopathy. *J Small Anim Pract* 2008;**49**:330–8.

194. Carlos SC, Chetboul V, Mary J, et al. Prospective echocardiographic and tissue Doppler imaging screening of a population of Maine Coon cats tested for the A31P mutation in the myosin-binding protein C gene: a specific analysis of the heterozygous status. *J Vet Intern Med* 2009;**23**:91–9.

195. Wess G, Killich M, Hartmann K. Comparison of pulsed wave and color Doppler myocardial velocity imaging in healthy dogs. *J Vet Intern Med* 2010;**24**:360–6.

196. Misbach C, Gouni V, Tissier R, et al. Echocardiographic and tissue Doppler imaging alterations associated with spontaneous canine systemic hypertension. *J Vet Intern Med* 2011;**25**:1025–35.

197. Simak J, Keller L, Killich M, et al. Color-coded longitudinal interventricular septal tissue velocity imaging, strain and strain rate in healthy Doberman Pinschers. *J Vet Cardiol* 2011;**13**:1–11.

198. Chetboul V, Petit A, Gouni V, et al. Prospective echocardiographic and tissue Doppler screening of a large Sphynx cat population: reference ranges, heart disease prevalence and genetic aspects. *J Vet Cardiol* 2012;**14**:497–509.

199. Evangelista A, Flachskampf F, Lancellotti P, et al. European Association of Echocardiography recommendations for standardization of performance, digital storage and reporting of echocardiographic studies. *Eur J Echocardiogr* 2008;**9**:438–48.

200. Baumgartner H, Hung J, Bermejo J, et al. Echocardiographic assessment of valve stenosis: EAE/ASE recommendations for clinical practice. *J Am Soc Echocardiogr* 2009;**22**:1–23, quiz 101–2.

201. Belanger MC, Di FR, Dumesnil JG, et al. Usefulness of the indexed effective orifice area in the assessment of subaortic stenosis in the dog. *J Vet Intern Med* 2001;**15**:430–7.

202. Uehara Y, Takahashi M. Quantitative evaluation of the severity of mitral insufficiency in dogs by the color Doppler method. *J Vet Med Sci* 1996;**58**:249–53.

203. Kittleson MD, Brown WA. Regurgitant fraction measured by using the proximal isovelocity surface area method in dogs with chronic myxomatous mitral valve disease. *J Vet Intern Med* 2003;**17**:84–8.

204. Choi H, Lee K, Lee H, et al. Quantification of mitral regurgitation using proximal isovelocity surface area method in dogs. *J Vet Sci* 2004;**5**:163–71.

205. Falk T, Jonsson L, Olsen LH, et al. Associations between cardiac pathology and clinical, echocardiographic and electrocardiographic findings in dogs with chronic congestive heart failure. *Vet J* 2010;**185**:68–74.

206. Paiva RM, Garcia-Guasch L, Manubens J, et al. Proximal isovelocity surface area variability during systole in dogs with mitral valve prolapse. *J Vet Cardiol* 2011;**13**:267–70.

207. Mor-Avi V, Lang RM, Badano LP, et al. Current and evolving echocardiographic techniques for the quantitative evaluation of cardiac mechanics: ASE/EAE consensus statement on methodology and indications endorsed by the Japanese Society of Echocardiography. *J Am Soc Echocardiogr* 2011;**24**:277–313.

208. Chetboul V, Serres F, Gouni V, et al. Radial strain and strain rate by two-dimensional speckle tracking echocardiography and the tissue velocity based technique in the dog. *J Vet Cardiol* 2007;**9**:69–81.

209. Chetboul V, Serres F, Gouni V, et al. Noninvasive assessment of systolic left ventricular torsion by 2-dimensional speckle tracking imaging in the awake dog: repeatability, reproducibility, and comparison with tissue Doppler imaging variables. *J Vet Intern Med* 2008;**22**:342–50.

210. Bonagura JD, Schober KE. Can ventricular function be assessed by echocardiography in chronic canine mitral valve disease? *J Small Anim Pract* 2009;**50**(Suppl. 1):12–24.

211. Margiocco ML, Bulmer BJ, Sisson DD. Doppler-derived deformation imaging in unsedated healthy adult dogs. *J Vet Cardiol* 2009;**11**:89–102.

212. Marwick TH, Leano RL, Brown J, et al. Myocardial strain measurement with 2-dimensional speckle-tracking echocardiography: definition of normal range. *JACC Cardiovasc Imaging* 2009;**2**:80–4.

213. Geyer H, Caracciolo G, Abe H, et al. Assessment of myocardial mechanics using speckle tracking echocardiography: fundamentals and clinical applications. *J Am Soc Echocardiogr* 2010;**23**:351–69, quiz 453–5.

214. Wess G, Sarkar R, Hartmann K. Assessment of left ventricular systolic function by strain imaging echocardiography in various stages of feline hypertrophic cardiomyopathy. *J Vet Intern Med* 2010;**24**:1375–82.

215. Culwell NM, Bonagura JD, Schober KE. Comparison of echocardiographic indices of myocardial strain with invasive measurements of left ventricular systolic function in anesthetized healthy dogs. *Am J Vet Res* 2011;**72**:650–60.

216. Wess G, Keller LJ, Klausnitzer M, et al. Comparison of longitudinal myocardial tissue velocity, strain, and strain rate measured by two-dimensional speckle tracking and by color tissue Doppler imaging in healthy dogs. *J Vet Cardiol* 2011;**13**:31–43.

217. Smith DN, Bonagura JD, Culwell NM, et al. Left ventricular function quantified by myocardial strain imaging in small-breed dogs with chronic mitral regurgitation. *J Vet Cardiol* 2012;**14**:231–42.

218. Silva AC, Muzzi RA, Oberlender G, et al. Longitudinal strain and strain rate by two-dimensional speckle tracking in non-sedated healthy cats. *Res Vet Sci* 2013;**95**:1175–80.

219. Suzuki R, Matsumoto H, Teshima T, et al. Noninvasive clinical assessment of systolic torsional motions by two-dimensional speckle-tracking echocardiography in dogs with myxomatous mitral valve disease. *J Vet Intern Med* 2013;**27**:69–75.

220. Suzuki R, Matsumoto H, Teshima T, et al. Effect of age on myocardial function assessed by two-dimensional speckle-tracking echocardiography in healthy beagle dogs. *J Vet Cardiol* 2013;**15**:243–52.

221. Westrup U, McEvoy FJ. Speckle tracking echocardiography in mature Irish Wolfhound dogs: technical feasibility, measurement error and reference intervals. *Acta Vet Scand* 2013;**55**:41.

222. Zois NE, Olsen NT, Moesgaard SG, et al. Left ventricular twist and circumferential strain in dogs with myxomatous mitral valve disease. *J Vet Intern Med* 2013;**27**:875–83.

223. Baron Toaldo M, Guglielmini C, Diana A, et al. Feasibility and reproducibility of echocardiographic assessment of regional left atrial deformation and synchrony by tissue Doppler ultrasonographic imaging in healthy dogs. *Am J Vet Res* 2014;**75**:59–66.

224. Koffas H, Dukes-McEwan J, Corcoran BM, et al. Peak mean myocardial velocities and velocity gradients measured by color M-mode tissue Doppler imaging in healthy cats. *J Vet Intern Med* 2003;**17**:510–24.

225. Chetboul V, Sampedrano CC, Concordet D, et al. Use of quantitative two-dimensional color tissue Doppler imaging for assessment of left ventricular radial and longitudinal myocardial velocities in dogs. *Am J Vet Res* 2005;**66**:953–61.

226. Chetboul V, Sampedrano CC, Tissier R, et al. Quantitative assessment of velocities of the annulus of the left atrioventricular valve and left ventricular free wall in healthy cats by use of two-dimensional color tissue Doppler imaging. *Am J Vet Res* 2006;**67**:250–8.

227. Pariaut R, Saelinger C, Strickland KN, et al. Tricuspid annular plane systolic excursion (TAPSE) in dogs: reference values and impact of pulmonary hypertension. *J Vet Intern Med* 2012;**26**:1148–54.

228. Takano H, Fujii Y, Yugeta N, et al. Assessment of left ventricular regional function in affected and carrier dogs with Duchenne muscular dystrophy using speckle tracking echocardiography. *BMC Cardiovasc Disord* 2011;**11**:23.

229. Chetboul V, Tissier R. Echocardiographic assessment of canine degenerative mitral valve disease. *J Vet Cardiol* 2012;**14**:127–48.

230. Suzuki R, Matsumoto H, Teshima T, et al. Clinical assessment of systolic myocardial deformations in dogs with chronic mitral valve insufficiency using two-dimensional speckle-tracking echocardiography. *J Vet Cardiol* 2013;**15**:41–9.

231. della Torre PK, Kirby AC, Church DB, et al. Echocardiographic measurements in greyhounds, whippets and Italian greyhounds–dogs with a similar conformation but different size. *Aust Vet J* 2000;**78**:49–55.

232. Rishniw M, Erb HN. Evaluation of four 2-dimensional echocardiographic methods of assessing left atrial size in dogs. *J Vet Intern Med* 2000;**14**:429–35.

233. Goncalves AC, Orton EC, Boon JA, et al. Linear, logarithmic, and polynomial models of M-mode echocardiographic measurements in dogs. *Am J Vet Res* 2002;**63**: 994–9.

234. Chetboul V, Concordet D, Pouchelon JL, et al. Effects of inter- and intra-observer variability on echocardiographic measurements in awake cats. *J Vet Med A Physiol Pathol Clin Med* 2003;**50**:326–31.

235. Brown DJ, Rush JE, MacGregor J, et al. Quantitative echocardiographic [corrected] evaluation of mitral endocardiosis in dogs using ratio indices. *J Vet Intern Med* 2005;**19**:542–52.

236. Hetyey C, Voros K, Reiczigel J. Comparison of two-dimensional echocardiographic measurements of the left atrium in healthy dogs. *Acta Vet Hung* 2005;**53**:23–33.

237. Cunningham SM, Rush JE, Freeman LM, et al. Echocardiographic ratio indices in overtly healthy Boxer dogs screened for heart disease. *J Vet Intern Med* 2008;**22**:924–30.

238. Hall DJ, Cornell CC, Crawford S, et al. Meta-analysis of normal canine echocardiographic dimensional data using ratio indices. *J Vet Cardiol* 2008;**10**:11–23.

239. Dudas-Gyorki Z, Bende B, Hetyey C, et al. Two-dimensional echocardiographic measurements of the left atrium in dogs with cardiac disease. *Acta Vet Hung* 2009;**57**:203–15.

240. Diez-Prieto I, Garcia-Rodriguez MB, Rios-Granja MA, et al. M-mode echocardiographic changes in growing beagles. *J Am Anim Hosp Assoc* 2010;**49**:31–5.

241. Tidholm A, Westling AB, Hoglund K, et al. Comparisons of 3-, 2-dimensional, and M-mode echocardiographical methods for estimation of left chamber volumes in dogs with and without acquired heart disease. *J Vet Intern Med* 2010;**24**:1414–20.

242. Petric AD, Rishniw M, Thomas WP. Two-dimensionally-guided M-mode and pulsed wave Doppler echocardiographic evaluation of the ventricles of apparently healthy cats. *J Vet Cardiol* 2012;**14**:423–30.

243. Georgiev R, Rishniw M, Ljungvall I, et al. Common two-dimensional echocardiographic estimates of aortic linear dimensions are interchangeable. *J Vet Cardiol* 2013;**15**: 131–8.

244. Lee M, Park N, Lee S, et al. Comparison of echocardiography with dual-source computed tomography for assessment of left ventricular volume in healthy Beagles. *Am J Vet Res* 2013;**74**:62–9.

245. Smets P, Daminet S, Wess G. Simpson's method of discs for measurement of echocardiographic end-diastolic and end-systolic left ventricular volumes: breed-specific reference ranges in Boxer dogs. *J Vet Intern Med* 2014; **28**:116–22.

246. Wesselowski S, Borgarelli M, Bello NM, et al. Discrepancies in identification of left atrial enlargement using left atrial volume versus left atrial-to-aortic root ratio in dogs. *J Vet Intern Med* 2014.

247. Drourr L, Lefbom BK, Rosenthal SL, et al. Measurement of M-mode echocardiographic parameters in healthy adult Maine Coon cats. *J Am Vet Med Assoc* 2005;**226**: 734–7.

248. Abbott JA, MacLean HN. Two-dimensional echocardiographic assessment of the feline left atrium. *J Vet Intern Med* 2006;**20**:111–19.

249. Gundler S, Tidholm A, Haggstrom J. Prevalence of myocardial hypertrophy in a population of asymptomatic Swedish Maine coon cats. *Acta Vet Scand* 2008;**50**:22.

250. Kayar A, Ozkan C, Iskefli O, et al. Measurement of M-mode echocardiographic parameters in healthy adult Van cats. *Jpn J Vet Res* 2014;**62**:5–15.

251. Abhayaratna WP, Seward JB, Appleton CP, et al. Left atrial size: physiologic determinants and clinical applications. *J Am Coll Cardiol* 2006;**47**:2357–63.

252. Muzzi RA, Muzzi LA, de Araujo RB, et al. Echocardiographic indices in normal German shepherd dogs. *J Vet Sci* 2006;**7**:193–8.

253. Lobo L, Canada N, Bussadori C, et al. Transthoracic echocardiography in Estrela Mountain dogs: reference values for the breed. *Vet J* 2008;**177**:250–9.

254. Hollmer M, Willesen JL, Tolver A, et al. Left atrial volume and phasic function in clinically healthy dogs of 12 different breeds. *Vet J* 2013;**197**:639–45.

255. Schober KE, Wetli E, Drost WT. Radiographic and echocardiographic assessment of left atrial size in 100 cats with acute left-sided congestive heart failure. *Vet Radiol Ultrasound* 2013.

256. Johns SM, Nelson OL, Gay JM. Left atrial function in cats with left-sided cardiac disease and pleural effusion or pulmonary edema. *J Vet Intern Med* 2012;**26**:1134–9.

257. Linney CJ, Dukes-McEwan J, Stephenson HM, et al. Left atrial size, atrial function and left ventricular diastolic function in cats with hypertrophic cardiomyopathy. *J Small Anim Pract* 2014;**55**:198–206.

258. Mehlman E, Bright JM, Jeckel K, et al. Echocardiographic evidence of left ventricular hypertrophy in obese dogs. *J Vet Intern Med* 2013;**27**:62–8.

259. Hezzell MJ, Boswood A, Moonarmart W, et al. Selected echocardiographic variables change more rapidly in dogs that die from myxomatous mitral valve disease. *J Vet Cardiol* 2012;**14**:269–79.

260. Reynolds CA, Brown DC, Rush JE, et al. Prediction of first onset of congestive heart failure in dogs with degenerative mitral valve disease: the PREDICT cohort study. *J Vet Cardiol* 2012;**14**:193–202.

261. Henjes CR, Hungerbuhler S, Bojarski IB, et al. Comparison of multi-detector row computed tomography with echocardiography for assessment of left ventricular function in healthy dogs. *Am J Vet Res* 2012;**73**:393–403.

262. Serres F, Chetboul V, Tissier R, et al. Comparison of 3 ultrasound methods for quantifying left ventricular systolic function: correlation with disease severity and prognostic value in dogs with mitral valve disease. *J Vet Intern Med* 2008;**22**:566–77.

263. Wess G, Maurer J, Simak J, et al. Use of Simpson's method of disc to detect early echocardiographic changes in Doberman Pinschers with dilated cardiomyopathy. *J Vet Intern Med* 2010;**24**:1069–76.

264. O'Leary CA, Mackay BM, Taplin RH, et al. Echocardiographic parameters in 14 healthy English Bull Terriers. *Aust Vet J* 2003;**81**:535–42.

265. Dukes-McEwan J, Borgarelli M, Tidholm A, et al. Proposed guidelines for the diagnosis of canine idiopathic dilated cardiomyopathy. *J Vet Cardiol* 2003;**5**:7–19.

266. Morrison SA, Moise NS, Scarlett J, et al. Effect of breed and body weight on echocardiographic values in four

breeds of dogs of differing somatotype. *J Vet Intern Med* 1992;**6**:220–4.

267. Misbach C, Lefebvre HP, Concordet D, et al. Echocardiography and conventional Doppler examination in clinically healthy adult Cavalier King Charles Spaniels: Effect of body weight, age, and gender, and establishment of reference intervals. *J Vet Cardiol* 2014;**16**: 91–100.

268. Marinho Costa de Oliveira V, Pereira Costa Chamas P, Teixeira Goldfeder G, et al. Comparative study of 4 echocardiographic methods of left ventricular measurement in German Shepherd dogs. *J Vet Cardiol* 2014;**16**: 1–8.

269. Gugjoo MB, Saxena AC, Hoque M, et al. M-mode echocardiographic study in dogs. *Afr J Agric Res* 2014; **9**:387–96.

270. Locatelli C, Santini A, Bonometti GA, et al. Echocardiographic values in clinically healthy adult dogue de Bordeaux dogs. *J Small Anim Pract* 2011;**52**:246–53.

271. Bavegems V, Duchateau L, Sys SU, et al. Echocardiographic reference values in whippets. *Vet Radiol Ultrasound* 2007;**48**:230–8.

272. Lazaro Muzzi RA, Lopes Muzzi LA, Araujo RB, et al. Echocardiographic indices in normal German shepherd dogs. *J Vet Sci* 2006;**7**:193–8.

273. Kayar A, Gonul R, Or ME, et al. M-mode echocardiographic parameters and indices in the normal German shepherd dog. *Vet Radiol Ultrasound* 2006;**47**:482–6.

274. Vollmar AC. Echocardiographic measurements in the Irish wolfhound: reference values for the breed. *J Am Anim Hosp Assoc* 1999;**35**:271–7.

275. Stepien RL, Hinchcliff KW, Constable PD, et al. Effect of endurance training on cardiac morphology in Alaskan sled dogs. *J Appl Physiol* 1998;**85**:1368–75.

276. Crippa L, Ferro E, Melloni E, et al. Echocardiographic parameters and indices in the normal beagle dog. *Lab Anim* 1992;**26**:190–5.

277. Adin DB, Diley-Poston L. Papillary muscle measurements in cats with normal echocardiograms and cats with concentric left ventricular hypertrophy. *J Vet Intern Med* 2007;**21**:737–41.

278. Kittleson MD, Meurs KM, Munro MJ, et al. Familial hypertrophic cardiomyopathy in maine coon cats: an animal model of human disease. *Circulation* 1999;**99**: 3172–80.

279. Fox PR, Liu SK, Maron BJ. Echocardiographic assessment of spontaneously occurring feline hypertrophic cardiomyopathy. An animal model of human disease. *Circulation* 1995;**92**:2645–51.

280. Peterson EN, Moise NS, Brown CA, et al. Heterogeneity of hypertrophy in feline hypertrophic heart disease. *J Vet Intern Med* 1993;**7**:183–9.

281. Campbell FE, Kittleson MD. The effect of hydration status on the echocardiographic measurements of normal cats. *J Vet Intern Med* 2007;**21**:1008–15.

282. Chetboul V, Tessier D, Borenstein N, et al. Familial aortic aneurysm in Leonberg dogs. *J Am Vet Med Assoc* 2003; **223**:1159–62, 29.

283. Koplitz SL, Meurs KM, Bonagura JD. Echocardiographic assessment of the left ventricular outflow tract in the Boxer. *J Vet Intern Med* 2006;**20**:904–11.

284. Baumwart RD, Meurs KM, Bonagura JD. Tei index of myocardial performance applied to the right ventricle in normal dogs. *J Vet Intern Med* 2005;**19**:828–32.

285. Chetboul V, Sampedrano CC, Gouni V, et al. Quantitative assessment of regional right ventricular myocardial velocities in awake dogs by Doppler tissue imaging: repeatability, reproducibility, effect of body weight and breed, and comparison with left ventricular myocardial velocities. *J Vet Intern Med* 2005;**19**:837–44.

286. Motoki H, Borowski AG, Shrestha K, et al. Right ventricular global longitudinal strain provides prognostic value incremental to left ventricular ejection fraction in patients with heart failure. *J Am Soc Echocardiogr* 2014;**27**:726–32.

287. Scansen BA, Bonagura JD, Schober KE, et al. Evaluation of a commercial ultrasonographic hemodynamic recording system for the measurement of cardiac output in dogs. *Am J Vet Res* 2009;**70**:862–8.

288. Chetboul V, Sampedrano CC, Gouni V, et al. Ultrasonographic assessment of regional radial and longitudinal systolic function in healthy awake dogs. *J Vet Intern Med* 2006;**20**:885–93.

289. Marwick TH. Measurement of strain and strain rate by echocardiography: ready for prime time? *J Am Coll Cardiol* 2006;**47**:1313–27.

290. Abraham WT, Hayes DL. Cardiac resynchronization therapy for heart failure. *Circulation* 2003;**108**:2596–603.

291. Lee BH, Dukes-McEwan J, French AT, et al. Evaluation of a novel doppler index of combined systolic and diastolic myocardial performance in Newfoundland dogs with familial prevalence of dilated cardiomyopathy. *Vet Radiol Ultrasound* 2002;**43**:154–65.

292. Teshima K, Asano K, Iwanaga K, et al. Evaluation of left ventricular Tei index (index of myocardial performance) in healthy dogs and dogs with mitral regurgitation. *J Vet Med Sci* 2007;**69**:117–23.

293. Teshima K, Asano K, Iwanaga K, et al. Evaluation of right ventricular Tei index (index of myocardial performance) in healthy dogs and dogs with tricuspid regurgitation. *J Vet Med Sci* 2006;**68**:1307–13.

294. Asano K, Masui Y, Masuda K, et al. Noninvasive estimation of cardiac systolic function using continuous-wave Doppler echocardiography in dogs with experimental mitral regurgitation. *Aust Vet J* 2002;**80**:25–8.

295. Chen C, Rodriguez L, Guerrero JL, et al. Noninvasive estimation of the instantaneous first derivative of left ventricular pressure using continuous-wave Doppler echocardiography. *Circulation* 1991;**83**:2101–10.

296. Suzuki R, Matsumoto H, Teshima T, et al. Dobutamine stress echocardiography for assessment of systolic function in dogs with experimentally induced mitral regurgitation. *J Vet Intern Med* 2014;**28**:386–92.

297. Popovic ZB, Richards KE, Greenberg NL, et al. Scaling of diastolic intraventricular pressure gradients is related to filling time duration. *Am J Physiol Heart Circ Physiol* 2006;**291**:H762–9.

298. Gaasch WH, Cole JS, Quinones MA, et al. Dynamic determinants of left ventricular diastolic pressure-volume relations in man. *Circulation* 1975;**51**:317–23.

299. Bruch C, Stypmann J, Gradaus R, et al. Usefulness of tissue Doppler imaging for estimation of filling pressures in patients with primary or secondary pure mitral regurgitation. *Am J Cardiol* 2004;**93**:324–8.

300. Min PK, Ha JW, Jung JH, et al. Incremental value of measuring the time difference between onset of mitral inflow and onset of early diastolic mitral annulus velocity for the evaluation of left ventricular diastolic pressures in patients with normal systolic function and an indeterminate E/E. *Am J Cardiol* 2007;**100**: 326–30.

301. Masutani S, Little WC, Hasegawa H, et al. Restrictive left ventricular filling pattern does not result from increased left atrial pressure alone. *Circulation* 2008; **117**:1550–4.

302. Chetboul V, Athanassiadis N, Carlos C, et al. Assessment of repeatability, reproducibility, and effect of anesthesia on determination of radial and longitudinal left ventricular velocities via tissue Doppler imaging in dogs. *Am J Vet Res* 2004;**65**:909–15.

303. Chetboul V, Athanassiadis N, Carlos C, et al. Quantification, repeatability, and reproducibility of feline radial and longitudinal left ventricular velocities by tissue Doppler imaging. *Am J Vet Res* 2004;**65**:566–72.

304. Chetboul V, Sampedrano CC, Tissier R, et al. Reference range values of regional left ventricular myocardial velocities and time intervals assessed by tissue Doppler imaging in young nonsedated Maine Coon cats. *Am J Vet Res* 2005;**66**:1936–42.

305. Hori Y, Kunihiro S, Kanai K, et al. The relationship between invasive hemodynamic measurements and tissue Doppler-derived myocardial velocity and acceleration during isovolumic relaxation in healthy dogs. *J Vet Med Sci* 2009;**71**:1419–25.

306. Ishikawa T, Fukushima R, Suzuki S, et al. Echocardiographic estimation of left atrial pressure in beagle dogs with experimentally-induced mitral valve regurgitation. *J Vet Med Sci* 2011;**73**:1015–24.

307. O'Sullivan ML, O'Grady MR, Minors SL. Assessment of diastolic function by Doppler echocardiography in normal Doberman Pinschers and Doberman Pinschers with dilated cardiomyopathy. *J Vet Intern Med* 2007;**21**:81–91.

308. Oyama MA, Sisson DD, Bulmer BJ, et al. Echocardiographic estimation of mean left atrial pressure in a canine model of acute mitral valve insufficiency. *J Vet Intern Med* 2004;**18**:667–72.

309. Schober KE, Fuentes VL, Bonagura JD. Comparison between invasive hemodynamic measurements and noninvasive assessment of left ventricular diastolic function by use of Doppler echocardiography in healthy anesthetized cats. *Am J Vet Res* 2003;**64**:93–103.

310. Woolley RM, Devine CB, French AT. Left ventricular flow propagation using color M-mode echocardiography in the diagnosis of effusive-constrictive pericardial disease. *Vet Radiol Ultrasound* 2006;**47**:366–9.

311. Schober KE, Hart TM, Stern JA, et al. Detection of congestive heart failure in dogs by Doppler echocardiography. *J Vet Intern Med* 2010;**24**:1358–68.

312. Borgarelli M, Santilli RA, Chiavegato D, et al. Prognostic indicators for dogs with dilated cardiomyopathy. *J Vet Intern Med* 2006;**20**:104–10.

313. Borgarelli M, Tarducci A, Zanatta R, et al. Decreased systolic function and inadequate hypertrophy in large and small breed dogs with chronic mitral valve insufficiency. *J Vet Intern Med* 2007;**21**:61–7.

314. Schober KE, Stern JA, DaCunha DN, et al. Estimation of left ventricular filling pressure by Doppler echocardiography in dogs with pacing-induced heart failure. *J Vet Intern Med* 2008;**22**:578–85.

315. Gavaghan BJ, Kittleson MD, Fisher KJ, et al. Quantification of left ventricular diastolic wall motion by Doppler tissue imaging in healthy cats and cats with cardiomyopathy. *Am J Vet Res* 1999;**60**:1478–86.

316. Moise NS, Valentine BA, Brown CA, et al. Duchenne's cardiomyopathy in a canine model: electrocardiographic and echocardiographic studies. *J Am Coll Cardiol* 1991;**17**:812–20.

317. Kane AM, DeFrancesco TC, Boyle MC, et al. Cardiac structure and function in female carriers of a canine model of Duchenne muscular dystrophy. *Res Vet Sci* 2013;**94**:610–17.

318. Chetboul V, Blot S, Sampedrano CC, et al. Tissue Doppler imaging for detection of radial and longitudinal myocardial dysfunction in a family of cats affected by dystrophin-deficient hypertrophic muscular dystrophy. *J Vet Intern Med* 2006;**20**:640–7.

319. Helmcke F, Nanda NC, Hsiung MC, et al. Color Doppler assessment of mitral regurgitation with orthogonal planes. *Circulation* 1987;**75**:175–83.

320. Pedersen HD, Haggstrom J. Mitral valve prolapse in the dog: a model of mitral valve prolapse in man. *Cardiovasc Res* 2000;**47**:234–43.

321. Santamarina G, Espino L, Vila M, et al. Partial atrioventricular canal defect in a dog. *J Small Anim Pract* 2002;**43**:17–21.

322. Olsen LH, Martinussen T, Pedersen HD. Early echocardiographic predictors of myxomatous mitral valve disease in dachshunds. *Vet J* 2003;**152**:293–7.

323. Prosek R, Sisson DD, Oyama MA. What is your diagnosis? Pericardial effusion with a clot in the pericardial space likely caused by left atrial rupture secondary to mitral regurgitation. *J Am Vet Med Assoc* 2003;**222**:441–2.

324. Serres FJ, Chetboul V, Tissier R, et al. Doppler echocardiography-derived evidence of pulmonary arterial hypertension in dogs with degenerative mitral valve disease: 86 cases (2001-2005). *J Am Vet Med Assoc* 2006;**229**:1772–8.

325. Tou SP, Adin DB, Estrada AH. Echocardiographic estimation of systemic systolic blood pressure in dogs with mild mitral regurgitation. *J Vet Intern Med* 2006;**20**:1127–31.

326. Lee R, Marwick TH. Assessment of subclinical left ventricular dysfunction in asymptomatic mitral regurgitation. *Eur J Echocardiogr* 2007;**8**:175–84.

327. Serres F, Chetboul V, Tissier R, et al. Chordae tendineae rupture in dogs with degenerative mitral valve disease: prevalence, survival, and prognostic factors (114 cases, 2001-2006). *J Vet Intern Med* 2007;**21**:258–64.

328. Borgarelli M, Savarino P, Crosara S, et al. Survival characteristics and prognostic variables of dogs with mitral regurgitation attributable to myxomatous valve disease. *J Vet Intern Med* 2008;**22**:120–8.

329. O'Gara P, Sugeng L, Lang R, et al. The role of imaging in chronic degenerative mitral regurgitation. *JACC Cardiovasc Imaging* 2008;**1**:221–37.

330. Thomas N, Unsworth B, Ferenczi EA, et al. Intraobserver variability in grading severity of repeated identical cases of mitral regurgitation. *Am Heart J* 2008;**156**:1089–94.

331. Terzo E, Di MM, McAllister H, et al. Echocardiographic assessment of 537 dogs with mitral valve prolapse and leaflet involvement. *Vet Radiol Ultrasound* 2009;**50**:416–22.

332. Borgarelli M, Tursi M, La RG, et al. Anatomic, histologic, and two-dimensional-echocardiographic evaluation of mitral valve anatomy in dogs. *Am J Vet Res* 2011;**72**:1186–92.

333. Borgarelli M, Crosara S, Lamb K, et al. Survival characteristics and prognostic variables of dogs with preclinical chronic degenerative mitral valve disease attributable to myxomatous degeneration. *J Vet Intern Med* 2012;**26**:69–75.

334. Kurt S, Kovacevic A. Atrial rupture and pericardial effusion as a complication of chronic mitral valve endocardiosis. *Schweiz Arch Tierheilkd* 2012;**154**:397–401.

335. Lake-Bakaar GA, Mok MY, Kittleson MD. Fossa ovalis tear causing right to left shunting in a Cavalier King Charles Spaniel. *J Vet Cardiol* 2012;**14**:541–5.

336. Nakamura RK, Zuckerman IC, Yuhas DL, et al. Postresuscitation myocardial dysfunction in a dog. *J Vet Emerg Crit Care* 2012;**22**:710–15.

337. Reimann MJ, Moller JE, Haggstrom J, et al. R-R interval variations influence the degree of mitral regurgitation in dogs with myxomatous mitral valve disease. *Vet J* 2014;**199**:348–54.

338. Fox PR, Miller MW, Liu SK. Clinical, echocardiographic, and Doppler imaging characteristics of mitral valve stenosis in two dogs. *J Am Vet Med Assoc* 1992;**201**:1575–9.

339. Connolly DJ, Boswood A. Dynamic obstruction of the left ventricular outflow tract in four young dogs. *J Small Anim Pract* 2003;**44**:319–25.

340. Tidholm A, Nicolle AP, Carlos C, et al. Tissue Doppler imaging and echo-Doppler findings associated with a mitral valve stenosis with an immobile posterior valve leaflet in a bull terrier. *J Vet Med A Physiol Pathol Clin Med* 2004;**51**:138–42.

341. O'Leary CA, Mackay BM, Taplin RH, et al. Auscultation and echocardiographic findings in Bull Terriers with and without polycystic kidney disease. *Aust Vet J* 2005;**83**:270–5.

342. Matsuu A, Kanda T, Sugiyama A, et al. Mitral stenosis with bacterial myocarditis in a cat. *J Vet Med Sci* 2007;**69**:1171–4.

343. Loureiro J, Smith S, Fonfara S, et al. Canine dynamic left ventricular outflow tract obstruction: assessment of myocardial function and clinical outcome. *J Small Anim Pract* 2008;**49**:578–86.

344. Mitchell EB, Hawkins MG, Orvalho JS, et al. Congenital mitral stenosis, subvalvular aortic stenosis, and congestive heart failure in a duck. *J Vet Cardiol* 2008;**10**:67–73.

345. Oyama MA, Weidman JA, Cole SG. Calculation of pressure half-time. *J Vet Cardiol* 2008;**10**:57–60.

346. Kuijpers NW, Szatmari V. Mitral valve dysplasia in a cat causing reversible left ventricular hypertrophy and dynamic outflow tract obstruction. *Tijdschr Diergeneeskd* 2011;**136**:326–31.

347. Otoni C, Abbott JA. Mitral valve dysplasia characterized by isolated cleft of the anterior leaflet resulting in fixed left ventricular outflow tract obstruction. *J Vet Cardiol* 2012;**14**:301–5.

348. Fine DM, Tobias AH, Jacob KA. Supravalvular mitral stenosis in a cat. *J Am Anim Hosp Assoc* 2002;**38**:403–6.

349. Campbell FE, Thomas WP. Congenital supravalvular mitral stenosis in 14 cats. *J Vet Cardiol* 2012;**14**:281–92.

350. Malik R, Barrs VR, Church DB, et al. Vegetative endocarditis in six cats. *J Feline Med Surg* 1999;**1**:171–80.

351. Miller MW, Fox PR, Saunders AB. Pathologic and clinical features of infectious endocarditis. *J Vet Cardiol* 2004;**6**:35–43.

352. Peddle G, Sleeper MM. Canine bacterial endocarditis: a review. *J Am Anim Hosp Assoc* 2007;**43**:258–63.

353. Macdonald K. Infective endocarditis in dogs: diagnosis and therapy. *Vet Clin North Am Small Anim Pract* 2010;**40**:665–84.

354. Diana A, Guglielmini C, Pivetta M, et al. Radiographic features of cardiogenic pulmonary edema in dogs with mitral regurgitation: 61 cases (1998-2007). *J Am Vet Med Assoc* 2009;**235**:1058–63.

355. Di Marcello M, Terzo E, Locatelli C, et al. Assessment of mitral regurgitation severity by Doppler color flow mapping of the vena contracta in dogs. *J Vet Intern Med* 2014;**28**:1206–13.

356. Doiguchi O, Takahashi T. Examination of quantitative analysis and measurement of the regurgitation rate in mitral valve regurgitation by the "proximal isovelocity surface area" method. *J Vet Med Sci* 2000;**62**:109–12.

357. Gouni V, Serres FJ, Pouchelon JL, et al. Quantification of mitral valve regurgitation in dogs with degenerative mitral valve disease by use of the proximal isovelocity surface area method. *J Am Vet Med Assoc* 2007;**231**:399–406.

358. Peddle GD, Buchanan JW. Acquired atrial septal defects secondary to rupture of the atrial septum in dogs with degenerative mitral valve disease. *J Vet Cardiol* 2010;**12**:129–34.

359. Carlsson C, Haggstrom J, Eriksson A, et al. Size and shape of right heart chambers in mitral valve regurgitation in small-breed dogs. *J Vet Intern Med* 2009;**23**:1007–13.

360. Hoffmann G, Amberger CN, Seiler G, et al. Tricuspid valve dysplasia in fifteen dogs. *Schweiz Arch Tierheilkd* 2000;**142**:268–77.

361. Takemura N, Machida N, Nakagawa K, et al. Ebstein's anomaly in a beagle dog. *J Vet Med Sci* 2003;**65**:531–3.

362. Chetboul V, Tran D, Carlos C, et al. Congenital malformations of the tricuspid valve in domestic carnivores: a retrospective study of 50 cases. *Schweiz Arch Tierheilkd* 2004;**146**:265–75.

363. Nicolle A, Chetboul V, Escoffier L, et al. What is your diagnosis? Tricuspid valve stenosis (TS). *J Small Anim Pract* 2005;**46**:157–8.

364. Diana A, Guglielmini C, Acocella F, et al. Chylothorax associated with tricuspid dysplasia and atrial septal defect in a bullmastiff. *J Am Anim Hosp Assoc* 2009;**45**:78–83.

365. Ohad DG, Avrahami A, Waner T, et al. The occurrence and suspected mode of inheritance of congenital subaortic stenosis and tricuspid valve dysplasia in Dogue de Bordeaux dogs. *Vet J* 2013;**197**:351–7.

366. Wingfield WE, Boon JA, Wise LA, et al. Diagnostic ultrasound unknown. Aortic valvular insufficiency secondary to valvular endocarditis. *J Vet Intern Med* 1989;**3**:175–7.

367. Sisson D, Riepe R. Congenital quadricuspid aortic valve anomaly in two dogs. *J Vet Cardiol* 2000;**2**:23–6.

368. Kettner F, Cote E, Kirberger RM. Quadricuspid aortic valve and associated abnormalities in a dog. *J Am Anim Hosp Assoc* 2005;**41**:406–12.

369. Serres F, Chetboul V, Sampedrano CC, et al. Quadricuspid aortic valve and associated abnormalities in the dog: report of six cases. *J Vet Cardiol* 2008;**10**:25–31.

370. French A, Luis F V, Dukes-McEwan J, et al. Progression of aortic stenosis in the boxer. *J Small Anim Pract* 2000;**41**:451–6.

371. Lopez-Alvarez J, Dukes-McEwan J, Martin MW, et al. Balloon dilation of an imperforate cor triatriatum dexter in a Golden Retriever with concurrent double-chambered right ventricle and subsequent evaluation by cardiac magnetic resonance imaging. *J Vet Cardiol* 2011;**13**:211–18.

372. Nakao S, Tanaka R, Hamabe L, et al. Cor triatriatum sinister with incomplete atrioventricular septal defect in a cat. *J Feline Med Surg* 2011;**13**:463–6.

373. Johnson MS, Martin M, De Giovanni JV, et al. Management of cor triatriatum dexter by balloon dilatation in three dogs. *J Small Anim Pract* 2004;**45**:16–20.

374. Tanaka R, Hoshi K, Shimizu M, et al. Surgical correction of cor triatriatum dexter in a dog under extracorporeal circulation. *J Small Anim Pract* 2003;**44**:370–3.

375. Tobias AH, Thomas WP, Kittleson MD, et al. Cor triatriatum dexter in two dogs. *J Am Vet Med Assoc* 1993;**202**:285–90.

376. Wander KW, Monnet E, Orton EC. Surgical correction of cor triatriatum sinister in a kitten. *J Am Anim Hosp Assoc* 1998;**34**:383–6.

377. Adin DB, Thomas WP. Balloon dilation of cor triatriatum dexter in a dog. *J Vet Intern Med* 1999;**13**:617–19.

378. Koie H, Sato T, Nakagawa H, et al. Cor triatriatum sinister in a cat. *J Small Anim Pract* 2000;**41**:128–31.

379. Mitten RW, Edwards GA, Rishniw M. Diagnosis and management of cor triatriatum dexter in a Pyrenean mountain dog and an Akita Inu. *Aust Vet J* 2001;**79**:177–80.

380. Hoffmann DE, Tobias AH. What is your diagnosis? Cor triatriatum dexter. *J Am Vet Med Assoc* 2003;**223**:951–2.

381. Tidholm A. Retrospective study of congenital heart defects in 151 dogs. *J Small Anim Pract* 1997;**38**:94–8.

382. Oliveira P, Domenech O, Silva J, et al. Retrospective review of congenital heart disease in 976 dogs. *J Vet Intern Med* 2011;**25**:477–83.

383. Lehmkuhl LB, Bonagura JD, Jones DE, et al. Comparison of catheterization and Doppler-derived pressure gradients in a canine model of subaortic stenosis. *J Am Soc Echocardiogr* 1995;**8**:611–20.

384. Nakayama T, Wakao Y, Ishikawa R, et al. Progression of subaortic stenosis detected by continuous wave Doppler echocardiography in a dog. *J Vet Intern Med* 1996;**10**:97–8.

385. Oyama MA, Sisson DD. Evaluation of canine congenital heart disease using an echocardiographic algorithm. *J Am Anim Hosp Assoc* 2001;**37**:519–35.

386. Schober KE, Fuentes VL. Doppler echocardiographic assessment of left ventricular diastolic function in 74 boxer dogs with aortic stenosis. *J Vet Cardiol* 2002;**4**:7–16.

387. Koplitz SL, Meurs KM, Spier AW, et al. Aortic ejection velocity in healthy Boxers with soft cardiac murmurs and Boxers without cardiac murmurs: 201 cases (1997-2001). *J Am Vet Med Assoc* 2003;**222**:770–4.

388. Jenni S, Gardelle O, Zini E, et al. Use of auscultation and Doppler echocardiography in Boxer puppies to predict development of subaortic or pulmonary stenosis. *J Vet Intern Med* 2009;**23**:81–6.

389. Quintavalla C, Guazzetti S, Mavropoulou A, et al. Aorto-septal angle in Boxer dogs with subaortic stenosis: an echocardiographic study. *Vet J* 2010;**185**:332–7.

390. Menegazzo L, Bussadori C, Chiavegato D, et al. The relevance of echocardiography heart measures for breeding against the risk of subaortic and pulmonic stenosis in Boxer dogs. *J Anim Sci* 2012;**90**:419–28.

391. Stern JA, Meurs KM, Nelson OL, et al. Familial subvalvular aortic stenosis in golden retrievers: inheritance and echocardiographic findings. *J Small Anim Pract* 2012;**53**:213–16.

392. Belanger MC, Cote E, Beauchamp G. Association between aortoseptal angle in Golden Retriever puppies and subaortic stenosis in adulthood. *J Vet Intern Med* 2014.

393. Brown DJ, Smith FW Jr. Stenosis hemodynamics: from physical principles to clinical indices. *J Vet Intern Med* 2002;**16**:650–7.

394. Hoglund K, Haggstrom J, Bussadori C, et al. A prospective study of systolic ejection murmurs and left ventricular outflow tract in boxers. *J Small Anim Pract* 2011;**52**:11–17.

395. Bussadori C, Pradelli D, Borgarelli M, et al. Congenital heart disease in boxer dogs: results of 6 years of breed screening. *Vet J* 2009;**181**:187–92.

396. Bussadori C, Amberger C, Le BG, et al. Guidelines for the echocardiographic studies of suspected subaortic and pulmonic stenosis. *J Vet Cardiol* 2000;**2**:15–22.

397. Fernandez-del Palacio MJ, Talavera LJ, Bayon del RA, et al. Left ventricular outflow tract obstruction secondary to hemangiosarcoma in a dog. *J Vet Intern Med* 2006;**20**:687–90.

398. Hopper BJ, Richardson JL, Irwin PJ. Pulmonic stenosis in two cats. *Aust Vet J* 2004;**82**:143–8.

399. Minors SL, O'Grady MR, Williams RM, et al. Clinical and echocardiographic features of primary infundibular stenosis with intact ventricular septum in dogs. *J Vet Intern Med* 2006;**20**:1344–50.

400. Schrope DP. Primary pulmonic infundibular stenosis in 12 cats: natural history and the effects of balloon valvuloplasty. *J Vet Cardiol* 2008;**10**:33–43.

401. Locatelli C, Domenech O, Silva J, et al. Independent predictors of immediate and long-term results after pulmonary balloon valvuloplasty in dogs. *J Vet Cardiol* 2011;**13**:21–30.

402. Fujii Y, Nishimoto Y, Sunahara H, et al. Prevalence of patent foramen ovale with right-to-left shunting in dogs with pulmonic stenosis. *J Vet Intern Med* 2012;**26**:183–5.

403. Visser LC, Scansen BA, Schober KE. Single left coronary ostium and an anomalous prepulmonic right coronary artery in 2 dogs with congenital pulmonary valve stenosis. *J Vet Cardiol* 2013;**15**:161–9.

404. Koie H, Kurotobi EN, Sakai T. Double-chambered right ventricle in a dog. *J Vet Med Sci* 2000;**62**:651–3.

405. MacLean HN, Abbott JA, Pyle RL. Balloon dilation of double-chambered right ventricle in a cat. *J Vet Intern Med* 2002;**16**:478–84.

406. Martin JM, Orton EC, Boon JA, et al. Surgical correction of double-chambered right ventricle in dogs. *J Am Vet Med Assoc* 2002;**220**:770–4, 68.

407. Tanaka R, Shimizu M, Hirao H, et al. Surgical management of a double-chambered right ventricle and chylothorax in a Labrador retriever. *J Small Anim Pract* 2006;**47**:405–8.

408. Koffas H, Fuentes VL, Boswood A, et al. Double chambered right ventricle in 9 cats. *J Vet Intern Med* 2007;**21**:76–80.

409. Fukushima R, Tanaka R, Suzuki S, et al. Epidemiological and morphological studies of double-chambered right ventricle in dogs. *J Vet Med Sci* 2011;**73**:1287–93.

410. MacGregor JM, Winter MD, Keating J, et al. Peripheral pulmonary artery stenosis in a four-month-old West Highland White Terrier. *Vet Radiol Ultrasound* 2006;**47**:345–50.

411. Szatmari V, Freund MW, Veldhuis Kroeze EJ, et al. Juxtaductal coarctation of both pulmonary arteries in a cat. *J Vet Diagn Invest* 2010;**22**:812–16.

412. Scansen BA, Schober KE, Bonagura JD, et al. Acquired pulmonary artery stenosis in four dogs. *J Am Vet Med Assoc* 2008;**232**:1172–80.

413. Schrope DP, Kelch WJ. Clinical and echocardiographic findings of pulmonary artery stenosis in seven cats. *J Vet Cardiol* 2007;**9**:83–9.

414. Fournier TE. Dynamic right ventricular outflow tract (infundibular) stenosis and pectus excavatum in a dog. *Can Vet J* 2008;**49**:485–7.

415. Bright JM, Toal RL, Blackford LA. Right ventricular outflow obstruction caused by primary cardiac neoplasia. Clinical features in two dogs. *J Vet Intern Med* 1990;**4**:12–16.

416. Bracha S, Caron I, Holmberg DL, et al. Ectopic thyroid carcinoma causing right ventricular outflow tract

obstruction in a dog. *J Am Anim Hosp Assoc* 2009;**45**: 138–41.

417. Fernandez-del Palacio MJ, Sanchez J, Talavera J, et al. Left ventricular inflow tract obstruction secondary to a myxoma in a dog. *J Am Anim Hosp Assoc* 2011;**47**: 217–23.

418. Takemura N, Nakagawa K, Machida N, et al. Acquired mitral stenosis in a cat with hypertrophic cardiomyopathy. *J Vet Med Sci* 2003;**65**:1265–7.

419. McQuillan BM, Picard MH, Leavitt M, et al. Clinical correlates and reference intervals for pulmonary artery systolic pressure among echocardiographically normal subjects. *Circulation* 2001;**104**:2797–802.

420. Schober KE, Baade H. Doppler echocardiographic prediction of pulmonary hypertension in West Highland white terriers with chronic pulmonary disease. *J Vet Intern Med* 2006;**20**:912–20.

421. Atkins CE, Keene BW, McGuirk SM. Pathophysiologic mechanism of cardiac dysfunction in experimentally induced heartworm caval syndrome in dogs: an echocardiographic study. *Am J Vet Res* 1988;**49**:403–10.

422. DeFrancesco TC, Atkins CE, Miller MW, et al. Use of echocardiography for the diagnosis of heartworm disease in cats: 43 cases (1985-1997). *J Am Vet Med Assoc* 2001; **218**:66–9.

423. Atkins CE, Arther RG, Ciszewski DK, et al. Echocardiographic quantification of Dirofilaria immitis in experimentally infected cats. *Vet Parasitol* 2008;**158**:164–70.

424. Shibata T, Wakao Y, Takahashi M. A clinical study on velocity patterns of pulmonary venous flow in canine heartworm disease. *J Vet Med Sci* 2000;**62**:169–77.

425. Maron BJ. The 2006 American Heart Association classification of cardiomyopathies is the gold standard. *Circ Heart Fail* 2008;**1**:72–5, discussion 6.

426. Schober KE, Kent AM, Aeffner F. Tachycardia-induced cardiomyopathy in a cat. *Schweiz Arch Tierheilkd* 2014; **156**:133–9.

427. Baty CJ, Malarkey DE, Atkins CE, et al. Natural history of hypertrophic cardiomyopathy and aortic thromboembolism in a family of domestic shorthair cats. *J Vet Intern Med* 2001;**15**:595–9.

428. Cesta MF, Baty CJ, Keene BW, et al. Pathology of end-stage remodeling in a family of cats with hypertrophic cardiomyopathy. *Vet Pathol* 2005;**42**:458–67.

429. Schober K, Todd A. Echocardiographic assessment of left ventricular geometry and the mitral valve apparatus in cats with hypertrophic cardiomyopathy. *J Vet Cardiol* 2010;**12**:1–16.

430. Trehiou-Sechi E, Tissier R, Gouni V, et al. Comparative echocardiographic and clinical features of hypertrophic cardiomyopathy in 5 breeds of cats: a retrospective analysis of 344 cases (2001-2011). *J Vet Intern Med* 2012; **26**:532–41.

431. MacLea HB, Boon JA, Bright JM. Doppler echocardiographic evaluation of midventricular obstruction in cats with hypertrophic cardiomyopathy. *J Vet Intern Med* 2013;**27**:1416–20.

432. Fujii Y, Masuda Y, Takashima K, et al. Hypertrophic cardiomyopathy in two kittens. *J Vet Med Sci* 2001;**63**: 583–5.

433. Chetboul V, Carlos Sampedrano C, Gouni V, et al. Two-dimensional color tissue doppler imaging detects myocardial dysfunction before occurrence of hypertrophy in a young Maine Coon cat. *Vet Radiol Ultrasound* 2006;**47**:295–300.

434. Chetboul V, Sampedrano CC, Gouni V, et al. Two-dimensional color tissue Doppler imaging detects myocardial dysfunction before occurrence of hypertrophy in a young Maine Coon cat. *Vet Radiol Ultrasound* 2006; **47**:295–300.

435. MacDonald KA, Kittleson MD, Kass PH, et al. Tissue Doppler imaging in Maine Coon cats with a mutation of myosin binding protein C with or without hypertrophy. *J Vet Intern Med* 2007;**21**:232–7.

436. Brizard D, Amberger C, Hartnack S, et al. Phenotypes and echocardiographic characteristics of a European population of domestic shorthair cats with idiopathic hypertrophic cardiomyopathy. *Schweiz Arch Tierheilkd* 2009;**151**:529–38.

437. Snyder PS, Sadek D, Jones GL. Effect of amlodipine on echocardiographic variables in cats with systemic hypertension. *J Vet Intern Med* 2001;**15**:52–6.

438. Nelson L, Reidesel E, Ware WA, et al. Echocardiographic and radiographic changes associated with systemic hypertension in cats. *J Vet Intern Med* 2002;**16**:418–25.

439. Chetboul V, Lefebvre HP, Pinhas C, et al. Spontaneous feline hypertension: clinical and echocardiographic abnormalities, and survival rate. *J Vet Intern Med* 2003; **17**:89–95.

440. Fox PR, Basso C, Thiene G, et al. Spontaneously occurring restrictive nonhypertrophied cardiomyopathy in domestic cats: a new animal model of human disease. *Cardiovasc Pathol* 2014;**23**:28–34.

441. Pion PD, Kittleson MD, Rogers QR, et al. Myocardial failure in cats associated with low plasma taurine: a reversible cardiomyopathy. *Science* 1987;**237**:764–8.

442. Novotny MJ, Hogan PM, Flannigan G. Echocardiographic evidence for myocardial failure induced by taurine deficiency in domestic cats. *Can J Vet Res* 1994; **58**:6–12.

443. Fox PR, Maron BJ, Basso C, et al. Spontaneously occurring arrhythmogenic right ventricular cardiomyopathy in the domestic cat: A new animal model similar to the human disease. *Circulation* 2000;**102**:1863–70.

444. Harvey AM, Battersby IA, Faena M, et al. Arrhythmogenic right ventricular cardiomyopathy in two cats. *J Small Anim Pract* 2005;**46**:151–6.

445. Quintavalla C, Bossolini E, Rubini G, et al. Uhl's anomaly in a domestic shorthair cat. *J Am Anim HospAssoc* 2010;**46**:444–8.

446. Niessen SJ, Petrie G, Gaudiano F, et al. Feline acromegaly: an underdiagnosed endocrinopathy? *J Vet Intern Med* 2007;**21**:899–905.

447. Myers JA, Lunn KF, Bright JM. Echocardiographic findings in 11 cats with acromegaly. *J Vet Intern Med* 2014;**28**:1235–8.

448. Edmondson EF, Bright JM, Halsey CH, et al. Pathologic and cardiovascular characterization of pheochromocytoma-associated cardiomyopathy in dogs. *Vet Pathol* 2014.

449. Baumwart RD, Meurs KM, Atkins CE, et al. Clinical, echocardiographic, and electrocardiographic abnormalities in Boxers with cardiomyopathy and left ventricular systolic dysfunction: 48 cases (1985-2003). *J Am Vet Med Assoc* 2005;**226**:1102–4.

450. Scheinman MM, Crawford MH. Echocardiographic findings and the search for a gold standard in patients with arrhythmogenic right ventricular dysplasia. *J Am Coll Cardiol* 2005;**45**:866–7.

451. Marks CA. Hypertrophic cardiomyopathy in a dog. *J Am Vet Med Assoc* 1993;**203**:1020–2.

452. Washizu M, Takemura N, Machida N, et al. Hypertrophic cardiomyopathy in an aged dog. *J Vet Med Sci* 2003;**65**:753–6.

453. Nicolle AP, Carlos SC, Fontaine JJ, et al. Longitudinal left ventricular myocardial dysfunction assessed by 2D

colour tissue Doppler imaging in a dog with systemic hypertension and severe arteriosclerosis. *J Vet Med A Physiol Pathol Clin Med* 2005;**52**:83–7.

454. Olivotto I, Cecchi F, Poggesi C, et al. Patterns of disease progression in hypertrophic cardiomyopathy: an individualized approach to clinical staging. *Circ Heart Fail* 2012;**5**:535–46.

455. Hall DJ, Shofer F, Meier CK, et al. Pericardial effusion in cats: a retrospective study of clinical findings and outcome in 146 cats. *J Vet Intern Med* 2007;**21**:1002–7.

456. Maron MS, Olivotto I, Zenovich AG, et al. Hypertrophic cardiomyopathy is predominantly a disease of left ventricular outflow tract obstruction. *Circulation* 2006;**114**:2232–9.

457. Spotswood TC, Kirberger RM, Koma LM, et al. Changes in echocardiographic variables of left ventricular size and function in a model of canine normovolemic anemia. *Vet Radiol Ultrasound* 2006;**47**:358–65.

458. Yaphe W, Giovengo S, Moise NS. Severe cardiomegaly secondary to anemia in a kitten. *J Am Vet Med Assoc* 1993;**202**:961–4.

459. Calvert CA, Brown J. Use of M-mode echocardiography in the diagnosis of congestive cardiomyopathy in Doberman pinschers. *J Am Vet Med Assoc* 1986;**189**:293–7.

460. Minors SL, O'Grady MR. Resting and dobutamine stress echocardiographic factors associated with the development of occult dilated cardiomyopathy in healthy Doberman pinscher dogs. *J Vet Intern Med* 1998;**12**:369–80.

461. Freeman LM, Michel KE, Brown DJ, et al. Idiopathic dilated cardiomyopathy in Dalmatians: nine cases (1990-1995). *J Am Vet Med Assoc* 1996;**209**:1592–6.

462. Koch J, Pedersen HD, Jensen AL, et al. M-mode echocardiographic diagnosis of dilated cardiomyopathy in giant breed dogs. *Zentralbl Veterinarmed A* 1996;**43**:297–304.

463. Tidholm A, Jonsson L. A retrospective study of canine dilated cardiomyopathy (189 cases). *J Am Anim Hosp Assoc* 1997;**33**:544–50.

464. Vollmar A. Cardiomyopathy in the Irish wolfhound. A clinical study of 393 dogs by electro- and echocardiography and radiology. *Vet Q* 1998;**20**(Suppl. 1):S104–5.

465. Vollmar AC. Use of echocardiography in the diagnosis of dilated cardiomyopathy in Irish wolfhounds. *J Am Anim Hosp Assoc* 1999;**35**:279–83.

466. Vollmar AC. The prevalence of cardiomyopathy in the Irish wolfhound: a clinical study of 500 dogs. *J Am Anim Hosp Assoc* 2000;**36**:125–32.

467. Kirberger RM. Mitral valve E point to ventricular septal separation in the dog. *J S Afr Vet Assoc* 1991;**62**:163–6.

468. Chetboul V, Sampedrano CC, Testault I, et al. Use of tissue Doppler imaging to confirm the diagnosis of dilated cardiomyopathy in a dog with equivocal echocardiographic findings. *J Am Vet Med Assoc* 2004;**225**:1877–80, 64.

469. Garncarz MA. Echocardiographic evaluation of diastolic parameters in dogs with dilated cardiomyopathy. *Pol J Vet Sci* 2007;**10**:207–15.

470. Moneva-Jordan A, Luis F V, Corcoran BM, et al. Pulsus alternans in English cocker spaniels with dilated cardiomyopathy. *J Small Anim Pract* 2007;**48**:258–63.

471. Simpson KE, Devine BC, Woolley R, et al. Timing of left heart base descent in dogs with dilated cardiomyopathy and normal dogs. *Vet Radiol Ultrasound* 2008;**49**:287–94.

472. Stephenson HM, Fonfara S, Lopez-Alvarez J, et al. Screening for dilated cardiomyopathy in Great Danes in the United Kingdom. *J Vet Intern Med* 2012;**26**:1140–7.

473. Gavaghan BJ, Kittleson MD. Dilated cardiomyopathy in an American cocker spaniel with taurine deficiency. *Aust Vet J* 1997;**75**:862–8.

474. Fascetti AJ, Reed JR, Rogers QR, et al. Taurine deficiency in dogs with dilated cardiomyopathy: 12 cases (1997-2001). *J Am Vet Med Assoc* 2003;**223**:1137–41.

475. Belanger MC, Ouellet M, Queney G, et al. Taurine-deficient dilated cardiomyopathy in a family of golden retrievers. *J Am Anim Hosp Assoc* 2005;**41**:284–91.

476. O'Brien PJ, Ianuzzo CD, Moe GW, et al. Rapid ventricular pacing of dogs to heart failure: biochemical and physiological studies. *Can J Physiol Pharmacol* 1990;**68**:34–9.

477. Komamura K, Shannon RP, Pasipoularides A, et al. Alterations in left ventricular diastolic function in conscious dogs with pacing-induced heart failure. *J Clin Invest* 1992;**89**:1825–38.

478. Roche BM, Schwartz D, Lehnhard RA, et al. Changes in concentrations of neuroendocrine hormones and catecholamines in dogs with myocardial failure induced by rapid ventricular pacing. *Am J Vet Res* 2002;**63**:1413–17.

479. Nishijima Y, Feldman DS, Bonagura JD, et al. Canine nonischemic left ventricular dysfunction: a model of chronic human cardiomyopathy. *J Card Fail* 2005;**11**:638–44.

480. Stern JA, Meurs KM, Spier AW, et al. Ambulatory electrocardiographic evaluation of clinically normal adult Boxers. *J Am Vet Med Assoc* 2010;**236**:430–3.

481. Chapel E, Russel D, Schober K. Partial pericardial defect with left auricular herniation in a dog with syncope. *J Vet Cardiol* 2014;**16**:133–9.

482. Brummer DG, Moise NS. Infiltrative cardiomyopathy responsive to combination chemotherapy in a cat with lymphoma. *J Am Vet Med Assoc* 1989;**195**:1116–19.

483. Zoia A, Hughes D, Connolly DJ. Pericardial effusion and cardiac tamponade in a cat with extranodal lymphoma. *J Small Anim Pract* 2004;**45**:467–71.

484. Shih JL, Brenn S, Schrope DP. Cardiac involvement secondary to mediastinal lymphoma in a cat: regression with chemotherapy. *J Vet Cardiol* 2014.

485. Sisson D, Thomas WP, Reed J, et al. Intrapericardial cysts in the dog. *J Vet Intern Med* 1993;**7**:364–9.

486. Less RD, Bright JM, Orton EC. Intrapericardial cyst causing cardiac tamponade in a cat. *J Am Anim Hosp Assoc* 2000;**36**:115–19.

487. Loureiro J, Burrow R, Dukes-McEwan J. Canine intrapericardial cyst—complicated surgical correction of an unusual cause of right heart failure. *J Small Anim Pract* 2009;**50**:492–7.

488. Parra JL, Mears EA, Borde DJ, et al. Pericardial effusion and cardiac tamponade caused by intrapericardial granulation tissue in a dog. *J Vet Emerg Crit Care (SanAntonio)* 2009;**19**:187–92.

489. Scruggs SM, Bright JM. Chronic cardiac tamponade in a cat caused by an intrapericardial biliary cyst. *J Feline Med Surg* 2010;**12**:338–40.

490. Hodgkiss-Geere HM, Palermo V, Liuti T, et al. Pericardial cyst in a 2-year-old Maine Coon cat following peritoneopericardial diaphragmatic hernia repair. *J Feline Med Surg* 2014.

491. Sadanaga KK, MacDonald MJ, Buchanan JW. Echocardiography and surgery in a dog with left atrial rupture and hemopericardium. *J Vet Intern Med* 1990;**4**:216–21.

492. Lombard CW. Pericardial disease. *Vet Clin North Am Small Anim Pract* 1983;**13**:337–53.

493. de Madron E, Prymak C, Hendricks J. Idiopathic hemorrhagic pericardial effusion with organized thrombi in a dog. *J Am Vet Med Assoc* 1987;**191**:324–6.

494. Berry CR, Lombard CW, Hager DA, et al. Echocardiographic evaluation of cardiac tamponade in dogs before and after pericardiocentesis: four cases (1984-1986). J Am Vet Med Assoc 1988;192:1597–603.
495. Gidlewski J, Petrie JP. Pericardiocentesis and principles of echocardiographic imaging in the patient with cardiac neoplasia. Clin Tech Small Anim Pract 2003;18:131–4.
496. Stafford JM, Martin M, Binns S, et al. A retrospective study of clinical findings, treatment and outcome in 143 dogs with pericardial effusion. J Small Anim Pract 2004;546–52.
497. MacDonald KA, Cagney O, Magne ML. Echocardiographic and clinicopathologic characterization of pericardial effusion in dogs: 107 cases (1985-2006). J Am Vet Med Assoc 2009;235:1456–61.
498. Rajagopalan V, Jesty SA, Craig LE, et al. Comparison of presumptive echocardiographic and definitive diagnoses of cardiac tumors in dogs. J Vet Intern Med 2013;27:1092–6.
499. Fraga Veloso G, Fraga Manteiga E, Trehy M, et al. Septic pericarditis and myocardial abscess in an English Springer spaniel. J Vet Cardiol 2014;16:39–44.
500. Little AA, Steffey M, Kraus MS. Marked pleural effusion causing right atrial collapse simulating cardiac tamponade in a dog. J Am Anim Hosp Assoc 2007;43:157–62.
501. Kang MH, Kim DY, Park HM. Ectopic thyroid carcinoma infiltrating the right atrium of the heart in a dog. Can Vet J 2012;53:177–81.
502. Yamane T, Awazu T, Fujii Y, et al. Aberrant branch of the bronchoesophageal artery resembling patent ductus arteriosus in a dog. J Vet Med Sci 2001;63:819–22.
503. Fujii Y, Aoki T, Takano H, et al. Arteriovenous shunts resembling patent ductus arteriosus in dogs: 3 cases. J Vet Cardiol 2009;11:147–51.
504. Jacobs GJ, Calvert CA, Hall DG, et al. Diagnosis of right coronary artery to right atrial fistula in a dog using two-dimensional echocardiography. J Small Anim Pract 1996;37:387–90.
505. Guglielmini C, Pietra M, Cipone M. Aorticopulmonary septal defect in a German shepherd dog. J Am Anim Hosp Assoc 2001;37:433–7.
506. Scollan K, Salinardi B, Bulmer BJ, et al. Anomalous left-to-right shunting communication between the ascending aorta and right pulmonary artery in a dog. J Vet Cardiol 2011;13:147–52.
507. Valdes-Cruz LM, Horowitz S, Mesel E, et al. A pulsed Doppler echocardiographic method for calculating pulmonary and systemic blood flow in atrial level shunts: validation studies in animals and initial human experience. Circulation 1984;69:80–6.
508. Guglielmini C, Diana A, Pietra M, et al. Atrial septal defect in five dogs. J Small Anim Pract 2002;43:317–22.
509. Akiyama M, Tanaka R, Maruo K, et al. Surgical correction of a partial atrioventricular septal defect with a ventricular septal defect in a dog. J Am Anim Hosp Assoc 2005;41:137–43.
510. Kraus MS, Pariaut R, Alcaraz A, et al. Complete atrioventricular canal defect in a foal: Clinical and pathological features. J Vet Cardiol 2005;7:59–64.
511. Nicolle AP, Chetboul V, Namba H, et al. Echocardiographic and Doppler diagnosis: first case of atrial septal aneurysm in a cat. Vet Radiol Ultrasound 2005;46:230–3.
512. Chetboul V, Charles V, Nicolle A, et al. Retrospective study of 156 atrial septal defects in dogs and cats (2001-2005). J Vet Med A Physiol Pathol Clin Med 2006;53:179–84.
513. Chetboul V, Trolle JM, Nicolle A, et al. Congenital heart diseases in the boxer dog: A retrospective study of 105 cases (1998-2005). J Vet Med A Physiol Pathol Clin Med 2006;53:346–51.
514. Gordon SG, Nelson DA, Achen SE, et al. Open heart closure of an atrial septal defect by use of an atrial septal occluder in a dog. J Am Vet Med Assoc 2010;236:434–9.
515. Yamano S, Uechi M, Tanaka K, et al. Surgical repair of a complete endocardial cushion defect in a dog. Vet Surg 2011;40:408–12.
516. Schrope DP. Atrioventricular septal defects: natural history, echocardiographic, electrocardiographic, and radiographic findings in 26 cats. J Vet Cardiol 2013;15:233–42.
517. Rausch WP, Keene BW. Spontaneous resolution of an isolated ventricular septal defect in a dog. J Am Vet Med Assoc 2003;223:219–20, 197.
518. Margiocco ML, Bulmer BJ, Sisson DD. Percutaneous occlusion of a muscular ventricular septal defect with an Amplatzer muscular VSD occluder. J Vet Cardiol 2008;10:61–6.
519. Thomas WP. Echocardiographic diagnosis of congenital membranous ventricular septal aneurysm in the dog and cat. J Am Anim Hosp Assoc 2005;41:215–20.
520. Dirven MJ, Szatmari V, Cornelissen JM, et al. Case report: double-chambered right ventricle (DCRV), ventricular septal defect, and double caudal vena cava in a cat. Tijdschr Diergeneeskd 2010;135:180–8.
521. Van Israel N, French AT, Dukes-McEwan J, et al. Review of left-to-right shunting patent ductus arteriosus and short term outcome in 98 dogs. J Small Anim Pract 2002;43:395–400.
522. Van Israel N, Dukes-McEwan J, French AT. Long-term follow-up of dogs with patent ductus arteriosus. J Small Anim Pract 2003;44:480–90.
523. Jacquet J, Nicolle AP, Chetboul V, et al. Echocardiographic and Doppler characteristics of postoperative ductal aneurysm in a dog. Vet Radiol Ultrasound 2005;46:518–20.
524. Jeong YH, Yun TJ, Song JM, et al. Left ventricular remodeling and change of systolic function after closure of patent ductus arteriosus in adults: device and surgical closure. Am Heart J 2007;154:436–40.
525. Schneider M, Hildebrandt N, Schweigl T, et al. Transthoracic echocardiographic measurement of patent ductus arteriosus in dogs. J Vet Intern Med 2007;21:251–7.
526. Falcini R, Gaspari M, Polveroni G. Transthoracic echocardiographic guidance of patent ductus arteriosus occlusion with an Amplatz(R) canine duct occluder. Res Vet Sci 2011;90:359–62.
527. Connolly DJ, Lamb CR, Boswood A. Right-to-left shunting patent ductus arteriosus with pulmonary hypertension in a cat. J Small Anim Pract 2003;44:184–8.

CHAPTER 9
Liver

Thomas G. Nyland • Martha Moon Larson • John S. Mattoon

Ultrasonography has become an essential imaging tool for evaluating the liver. A complete examination requires a systematic evaluation of the hepatic parenchyma, portal and hepatic veins, and the gallbladder and biliary system. The most common indications for hepatic ultrasonography are hepatomegaly or masses in the liver region, possible metastases, icterus, fever of unknown origin, unexplained weight loss or pain, ascites, and trauma. Ultrasound can also be used to direct percutaneous liver biopsies or follow treatment response for inflammatory or neoplastic conditions. Doppler ultrasonography adds important information about blood flow hemodynamics within the liver and may help differentiate benign from malignant disease by the vascular patterns.

TECHNIQUE

A complete abdominal examination is recommended for each animal, although hepatic imaging is emphasized in this chapter. Hair should be clipped from the 10th intercostal space caudally over the ventral abdomen and halfway down the lateral abdominal walls. Acoustic coupling gel is applied liberally to the skin and worked into the stubble of the hair coat. Alcohol can also be used to clean and wet the skin surface.

Gas in the stomach is a barrier to successful ultrasound examination of the liver. Therefore feeding or procedures that result in struggling or aerophagia should be avoided. The animal should be restrained on a table in dorsal or lateral recumbency (Figure 9-1; see also Chapter 4, Figure 4-8, A). Tranquilization is used as needed.

Imaging while the animal is standing, sitting, or in sternal recumbency may also help to reposition stomach gas if there is poor visualization of the liver. If there is excessive stomach gas, the animal can also be positioned on a Plexiglas table in which a hole has been cut to allow access to the abdomen from underneath. Fluid in the dependent portion of the stomach facilitates liver evaluation by acting as an acoustic window.

A 5.0-MHz sector or curvilinear transducer is most commonly used for beginning the ultrasound examination of the liver in medium to large sized dogs. A 7.5-MHz or higher transducer is adequate for small dogs and cats. In large or giant breed dogs, a 3.0-MHz transducer may be necessary to penetrate to the dorsal aspects of the liver.

Evaluation of the liver is begun by placing the transducer in the subxiphoid position and angling the sound beam craniodorsally in a midsagittal plane (Figure 9-1, A and B; see also Figure 4-8, Aa). This places the transducer cranial to the stomach in most cases and helps avoid interference from stomach gas. Scans of the liver are then made by sweeping the beam in an arc from left to right through the entire liver (see Figure 4-8, Ab and Ac). The transducer should remain in the subxiphoid position as much as possible during the entire sweep. The beam is angled dorsally or ventrally in successive sweeps to make sure the entire liver is imaged. The beam is then oriented in a midtransverse plane and swept in an arc through the liver from ventral to dorsal. Successive sweeps are made by angling the transducer to the left and right of midline to make sure the entire liver is imaged. The liver is also imaged in both planes by moving the transducer laterally along the caudal aspect of the costal arch to the left and right of midline if stomach gas does not interfere with imaging. The liver should also be imaged through an intercostal approach to optimize detection of lesions (Figure 9-1, C). Scanning the liver through the 10th to 12th left and right intercostal spaces may be especially useful in patients that have a small liver, excessive bowel gas, or a deep chest. The right intercostal view is frequently required to optimally view the caudal vena cava, hepatic veins, portal veins, common bile duct, and lymph nodes in the region of the porta hepatis.[1] A sector transducer is necessary to fit in the small contact area between ribs, and it is placed transversely (parallel to the ribs) at about the 11th intercostal space, 5 to 10 cm ventral to the spine. The porta hepatis is usually located at this level, but you may have to "walk" the transducer to a cranial or caudal intercostal space, and slide dorsally to ventrally, to find the best window. If lung gas in encountered, the transducer should be moved one or two intercostal spaces caudally. If the right kidney is seen, the transducer should be moved cranially. The porta hepatis is located when the liver and the cross-sectional views of the aorta, caudal vena cava, and portal vein are seen in a single window.

After evaluation of the dorsal intercostal window, the transducer is moved cranially and ventrally, toward the sternum. The gallbladder can be visualized from this window, along with the cystic duct and left hepatic and portal vein branches.

ANATOMY

Landmarks

The liver is bounded cranially by the diaphragm, ventrally by falciform fat, and caudally by the right kidney on the right, the stomach centrally, and the spleen on the left. The curvilinear echogenic line seen cranial to liver on sonograms is commonly referred to as the diaphragm, but it is really the interface between the diaphragm and lung. This echogenic

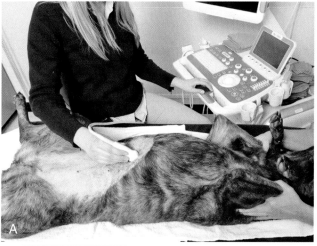
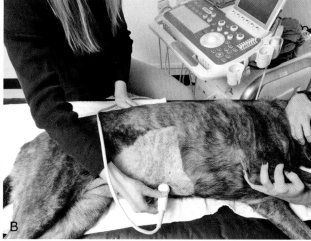
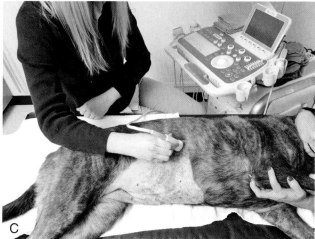

Figure 9-1 **Positioning for ultrasound examination of the liver.** **A,** Dorsal recumbency with subxiphoid positioning for liver examination. **B,** Left lateral recumbency with the transducer placed subcostal on midline. **C,** Left lateral recumbency with the transducer placed for a transverse view at the 10th to 12th right intercostal space.

line is referred to as the diaphragm throughout this chapter for convenience. The actual diaphragm is only seen when there is adjacent peritoneal or pleural fluid, or both. Falciform fat lies ventral to the liver, and in the dog it has a variable echogenicity that may be isoechoic, hypoechoic, or hyperechoic to liver parenchyma. In the cat, falciform fat is typically isoechoic to hyperechoic to liver parenchyma.

Lobation and Vascular Anatomy

The liver is divided into the left, right, quadrate, and caudate lobes (Figure 9-2). The left lobe lies to the left of midline and is divided into the left lateral and left medial sublobes; the right lobe lies to the right of midline and is divided into the right medial and right lateral sublobes. The quadrate lobe lies in the median plane and is partially fused to the right medial sublobe. The gallbladder is located between these two lobes and, along with the portal vein, divides the liver into the left and right lobes. The caudate lobe consists of the caudate and papillary processes, which are connected by a short isthmus bounded ventrally by the portal vein and dorsally by the caudal vena cava. The papillary process, located more centrally, is sometimes mistaken for the body or left limb of the pancreas as the transducer is fanned caudally through the liver in transverse image planes. The cranial pole of the right kidney is situated in the renal fossa of the caudate process of the caudate lobe. The divisions between liver lobes are not well seen ultrasonographically except when peritoneal fluid is present. The branches of the hepatic artery and bile ducts are also poorly seen within the

liver. However, the location of hepatic arteries can be determined by their characteristic arterial signals using Doppler ultrasonography.

The ultrasonographic identification of liver lobes and of the hepatic and portal venous vascular anatomy has been described in detail and compared with angiographic and postmortem examination findings in normal dogs.[2-5] Knowledge of the venous anatomy helps identify specific regions of the liver on ultrasound scans (see Figure 9-2).

Portal veins are identified by their bright, echogenic walls. Hepatic veins lack these prominent walls and appear as anechoic tubular structures. The distinct composition of hepatic vein walls results in more of a specular reflector, becoming hyperechoic only when the sound beam is perpendicular to the vessel wall.[6] Because of its composition, the portal vein wall appears hyperechoic from many angles. Hepatic veins can be traced to their termination in the caudal vena cava at the level of the diaphragm (Figure 9-3). The hepatic veins to the left lobe, quadrate lobe, and right medial lobe are best located in a transverse plane from a subxiphoid location. These veins converge to enter the left ventral caudal vena cava at a single location near the diaphragm. The quadrate hepatic vein, located to the left of the gallbladder, joins the right medial hepatic vein, located to the right of the gallbladder. The left lobe hepatic vein forms from the confluence of the left medial and left lateral portions farther to the left. More caudally, the right lateral hepatic vein and right caudate hepatic vein enter the caudal vena cava separately. These veins are more difficult to see, especially from the ventral abdomen.

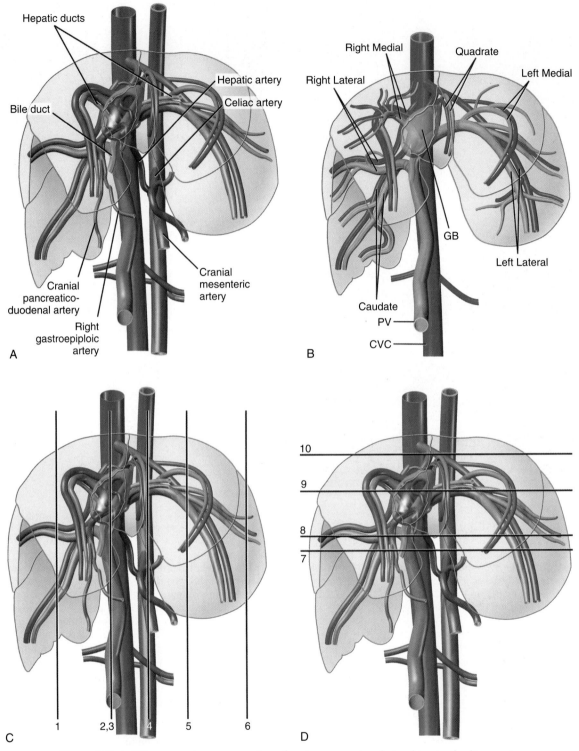

Figure 9-2 **A,** Diagrammatic representation of major anatomic relationships in the liver region showing the aorta and hepatic arterial supply (red), caudal vena cava and hepatic veins (blue), portal veins (purple), and biliary tract (green). **B,** Diagrammatic representation of the major hepatic and portal venous branches to the liver lobes. *CVC,* Caudal vena cava; *GB,* gallbladder; *PV,* portal vein. **C,** Sagittal scan planes 1 to 6 corresponding to ultrasound images in Figure 9-3, A to F. **D,** Transverse scan planes 7 to 10 corresponding to ultrasound images in Figure 9-3, G to J.

The caudate vein enters slightly more caudally than the right lateral hepatic vein, and both are best traced from the caudal vena cava by a right lateral approach through the 9th to 11th intercostal spaces in a longitudinal plane cranial to the right kidney.

Portal vein distribution differs slightly from that of the hepatic veins (see Figures 9-2 and 9-3). The left portal vein,

best viewed in a transverse plane from a subxiphoid or a ventral right intercostal location, is seen caudal and dorsal to the neck of the gallbladder between the gallbladder and hepatic veins. The left portal vein branches into the left lateral and left medial portions slightly caudoventral to the gallbladder. The left lateral portal vein can be traced farther peripherally into the liver than the left medial portal vein. The portal

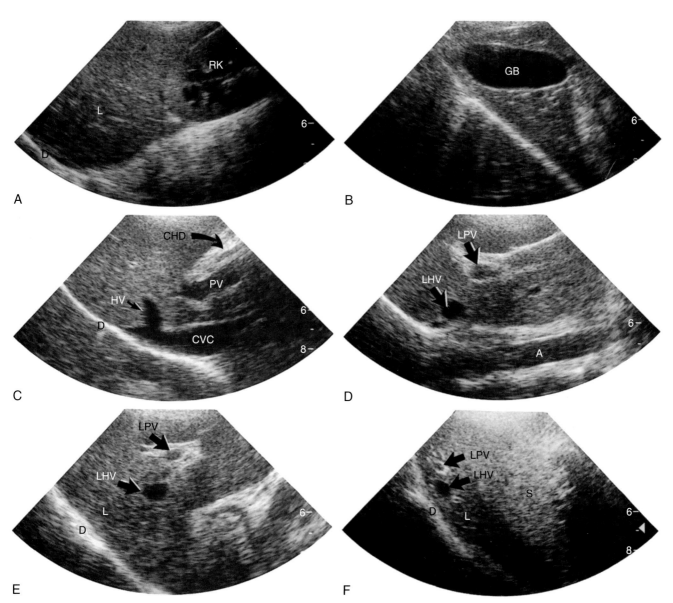

Figure 9-3 **Ultrasound scans of the liver corresponding to the sagittal and transverse planes in Figure 9-2, C and D. A,** Plane 1, right kidney (*RK*) and right liver lobes (*L*). Echogenicity of the liver parenchyma is normally equal to or slightly greater than that of right kidney cortex. *D*, diaphragm. **B and C,** Plane 2 and plane 3. Depending on the exact scan plane, the gallbladder (*GB*), portal vein (*PV*), and caudal vena cava (*CVC*) may be imaged separately or together. The gallbladder appears as an anechoic structure with a thin, poorly visualized wall. The common hepatic duct (*CHD*) may be visualized ventral to the portal vein. Hepatic veins (*HV*) can be seen entering the caudal vena cava near the diaphragm (*D*). **D,** Plane 4, aorta. In this plane, the aorta (*A*), left hepatic vein (*LHV*), and left portal vein (*LPV*) are visualized. **E,** Plane 5, left hepatic lobes (*L*). The left portal vein (*LPV*) can be distinguished from the left hepatic vein (*LHV*) by the echogenic peripheral echoes surrounding all portal structures. *D*, Diaphragm. **F,** Plane 6, left lateral hepatic lobe (*L*). Terminal branches of the left portal vein (*LPV*) and left hepatic vein (*LHV*) can be visualized. The head of the spleen (*S*) is also visualized caudal to the liver. The spleen is normally more echogenic than the liver. *D*, Diaphragm. *Continued*

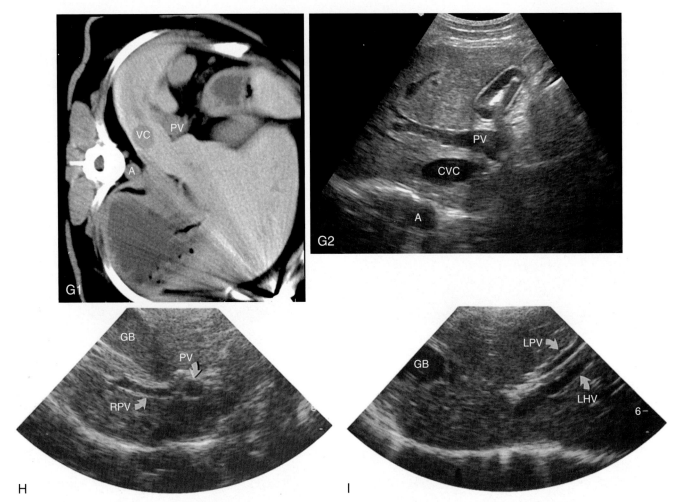

Figure 9-3, cont'd G, Plane 7, computed tomographic (CT) image (**G1**) and corresponding ultrasound image (**G2**) of the right lateral transverse view at the 11th intercostal space. This transducer position allows visualization of the aorta (*A*), caudal vena cava (*VC* or *CVC*), and portal vein (*PV*) by using the caudate and right liver lobes as an acoustic window. The top of the ultrasound image represents the right side of the dog, and ventral is to the right because of the transducer's orientation (see Figure 9-1, C). Visualization of this region from the ventral abdomen is difficult because of interference from gas in the stomach. **H,** Plane 8, right portal vein. The right portal vein (*RPV*) can be seen branching from the portal vein (*PV*) at this level. Cranial to this point, the portal vein continues ventrally and to the left as the left portal vein. *GB,* Gallbladder. **I,** Plane 9, left portal vein (*LPV*) and left hepatic vein (*LHV*). The left portal and left hepatic veins are now parallel to the scan plane. A portion of the gallbladder (*GB*) is also visible.

quadrate vein arises from the portal vein itself or branches from the left medial portal vein. This is in contrast to the hepatic venous system, in which the quadrate hepatic vein usually joins the right medial hepatic vein. The right medial portal vein arises from the portal vein to enter the right medial lobe to the right of the gallbladder. Portal vein branches to the right lateral and caudate lobes are more difficult to identify and cannot be seen in the same plane as the left portal vein. These branches can be seen either from the ventral abdomen or from a right intercostal approach through the 9th to 11th intercostal spaces. The right lateral and caudate portal vessels usually arise together from the portal vein.

The intrahepatic branches of the hepatic arteries are not normally seen within the liver. However, the main hepatic artery may occasionally be identified dorsal to the portal vein and common bile duct, especially on a right lateral intercostal window. It is best distinguished from the common bile duct or portal veins by Doppler ultrasonography.

Size

Determination of liver size is based on subjective assessment. Radiographic criteria of liver margin extension beyond the costal arch may be used for ultrasound assessment. Breed and body conformation must be taken into account. For example, deep-chested dogs may appear to have smaller livers than other breeds even though there is no clinical or biochemical evidence of liver disease. Cats have less variability because of more uniform body size but liver size determination can sometimes be confounded by isoechoic falciform fat.

Liver enlargement should be suspected when there is (1) increased distance between the diaphragm and stomach, (2) increased extension of the liver ventral to the stomach or

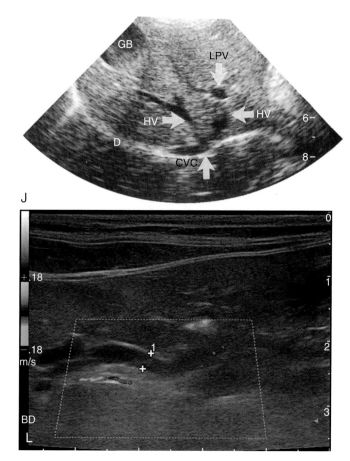

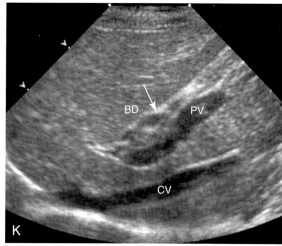

Figure 9-3, cont'd **J,** Plane 10, left portal vein (*LPV*), caudal vena cava (*CVC*), and hepatic veins (*HV*). The left portal vein and the entrance of the hepatic veins into the caudal vena cava are clearly seen. The diaphragm (*D*) and a portion of the gallbladder (*GB*) are also visible. **K,** Longitudinal image of normal cat liver with portal vein (*PV*), caudal vena cava (*CV*) and bile duct (*BD, arrow*). **L,** Longitudinal image of the bile duct in cat. It is seen as an anechoic tube between the electronic cursors (0.27 cm). Color Doppler imaging shows lack of flow within the bile duct, which distinguishes it from the portal vein. The hepatic artery is seen just dorsal to the bile duct in the far field.

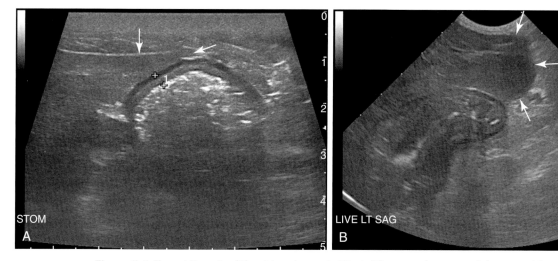

Figure 9-4 **Normal liver size (A) and hepatomegaly (B). A,** The ventral margin of the normal liver (*arrows*) is thin, has a sharp margin, and does not extend much beyond the stomach (between electronic cursors, 0.29 cm) ventrally or caudally. **B,** Sagittal image shows an enlarged liver with thick, rounded caudoventral margins (between arrows) and a diffuse hyperechoic, finely textured parenchyma. An empty stomach is noted in the far field. This dog had hepatic lipidosis.

ventral to the right kidney, and (3) rounded liver margins (Figure 9-4).

Reduced liver size should be suspected when there is (1) poor visualization of the liver even without excessive stomach gas, (2) decreased distance between the diaphragm and stomach, and (3) decreased extension of the liver ventral to the stomach or poor visualization of the liver cranial to the right kidney. Abdominal radiographs should be used to

evaluate liver size in questionable cases, and the ultrasound interpretation should always be correlated with the clinical signs and laboratory work.

Hepatic Parenchyma

The normal hepatic parenchyma has a uniform, medium level of echogenicity (see Figure 9-3). Only the hepatic and portal veins interrupt this uniform echo pattern. The hepatic arteries and bile ducts run adjacent to the portal veins as described previously, but usually they cannot be seen in the normal animal. The parenchymal texture of the liver is coarser than that of the spleen. At the same scanning depth and instrument gain settings, echogenicity of the liver is normally equal to that of the cortex of the right kidney or slightly more or less echogenic (see Figure 9-3, A).[7] The spleen has a somewhat higher echo intensity than the liver, but direct comparisons in the normal animal are difficult at the same depth except in the cranial abdomen near the head of the spleen (see Figure 9-3, F). There is usually a greater difference in echogenicity between the left kidney cortex and spleen than between the right kidney cortex and liver. This indirectly supports the observation that the spleen is slightly more echogenic than the liver in normal animals. In practice, there seems to be enough individual variability to make it difficult to recognize subtle changes in the diffuse echogenicity of the liver, spleen, or kidney that would consistently assist with diagnosis. Therefore changes in echogenicity must be substantial to confidently conclude that one or more of these organs is abnormal.

Gallbladder and Biliary System

The gallbladder is seen as an anechoic, round to oval structure just to the right of midline in most liver scans (see Figure 9-3, B, H to J). The size is variable, depending on when the animal was fed, with as much as 53% of newly produced bile accumulating within the gallbladder during prolonged withholding of food.[8] Normal gallbladder volume is reported to be 1.0 mL/kg or less after food is withheld for 12 hours.[9] A small amount of mobile, dependent echogenic, nonshadowing sediment (biliary sludge) may be present within the lumen in normal dogs.[10] More recent reports indicate that any biliary sludge may be abnormal.[11] The gallbladder wall is poorly seen or appears as a thin (1 to 2 mm) echogenic line in dogs.[12] In cats, normal gallbladder wall thickness is considered to be less than 1 mm.[13]

Distal acoustic enhancement is commonly seen deep to the gallbladder. The intrahepatic bile ducts are not visualized in normal dogs and cats. The extrahepatic biliary ducts are also poorly visualized because of overlying bowel gas, although the proximal common bile duct may be seen under optimal conditions to have parallel echogenic walls approximately 2 to 3 mm apart, ventral to the main portal vein (see Figure 9-3, C). The diameter of the common bile duct in normal dogs is reported to be less than 3 mm.[14] The common bile duct and extrahepatic bile ducts are more easily visualized in cats.[15] The diameter of the common bile duct in normal cats has been reported to be 4 mm or less (see Figure 9-3, K and L).[15] The common bile duct can be identified immediately dorsal to the portal vein, surrounded by hyperechoic tissue, and distinguished from the proper hepatic arteries that are also sometimes seen in the region of the porta hepatis by use of Doppler ultrasonography.

DOPPLER EVALUATION OF THE NORMAL LIVER

A description of general Doppler techniques can be found in Chapter 1. Doppler evaluation of the normal liver is presented here, and the abnormal findings associated with specific liver diseases are presented in their appropriate sections. Doppler ultrasonography of the liver may be used to evaluate flow velocity, flow direction, and spectral patterns of the hepatic arteries, caudal vena cava, and the hepatic and portal veins (Figure 9-5). Flow velocity is usually determined by the uniform insonation method in which a large Doppler sample volume is used to overlap the walls of the vessel.[16,17] The

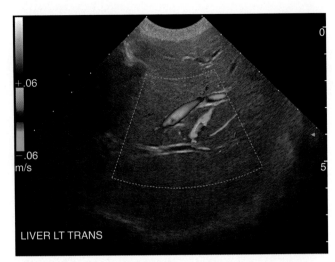

Figure 9-5 Color Doppler image of a normal dog liver. Transverse image of the left side of the liver showing the hepatic veins (blue, blood flow coursing away from transducer toward the caudal vena cava) and portal veins (red, blood flow toward the transducer, away from the porta hepatis into the periphery of the liver).

maximal velocity method can also be used; in this method, maximal velocity measured in the center of the vessel lumen is multiplied by 0.57 to determine mean flow velocity.[18] This method may be preferable if there is considerable artifact due to wall motion with the uniform insonation method. Ideally, incident angles of less than 60 degrees should be used with both methods to obtain reliable measurements. These two Doppler techniques for determining flow velocity, if used properly, show no significant difference in reliability.[16]

Caudal Vena Cava and Hepatic Veins

The Doppler spectral patterns of the caudal vena cava and hepatic veins are complex and depend on changes in cardiac activity, respiration, and intraabdominal pressure.[19,20] Therefore the caudal vena cava and hepatic vein waveforms should be obtained at normal end-expiration in a quiet animal whenever possible. The vena cava is visualized by use of either a ventral or right intercostal approach. It is first localized in a transverse view, ventral and to the right of the aorta and slightly dorsal and to the right of the portal vein (see Figure 9-3, G). Doppler measurements of the caudal vena cava in the liver region are obtained with the vena cava in a long-axis view and the transducer positioned cranially to obtain an incident angle of less than 60 degrees (see Figure 9-3, C).

The normal caudal vena cava and hepatic venous pulsed Doppler waveform demonstrates marked variation in the direction and velocity of flow because of right atrial activity when viewed under ideal conditions.[19,20] (Figure 9-6). Hepatic venous flow is retrograde into liver during right atrial contraction (A wave). After right atrial contraction, there is a rapid flow of blood from the hepatic veins and caudal vena cava toward the right atrium during rapid atrial filling (S wave). Flow slows as the right atrium becomes filled, and velocity starts to return toward baseline (V wave). When the tricuspid valve opens and the right ventricle fills, a second wave of rapid flow out of the hepatic veins toward the right atrium (D wave); this wave is slightly smaller than the first. The right atrium contracts again, and the cycle is repeated. Therefore the pulsatile flow within the hepatic veins and caudal vena cava is referred to as triphasic because there are two antegrade pulses (S and D waves) and one retrograde pulse (A wave).

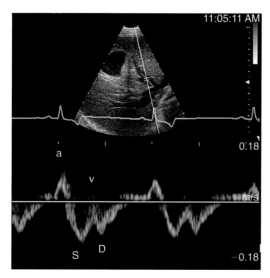

Figure 9-6 Pulsed wave Doppler image of a normal hepatic vein. Here is an example of a duplex image showing the B-mode image, ECG, and spectral tracing. The B-mode image shows the gallbladder, right medial and quadrate liver lobes, hepatic veins and the sample gate with angle correction, placed in the common tributary of these two veins. The waveform consists of two retrograde waves (*a* and *v*), which represent blood flow away from the heart, and two antegrade waves (*S* and *D*), which represent blood flow towards the heart. The various wave components are a result of pressure differences within the right atrium and the hepatic veins. The **a wave** occurs after the P-wave on the ECG. It results from elevated right atrial pressure caused by right atrial contraction that creates a burst of reversed flow into the hepatic veins. The **S wave** occurs after the QRS complex. It results from a negative pressure in the right atrium with corresponding flow from the hepatic veins to the heart. This negative pressure is created by right atrial relaxation and movement of the tricuspid annulus towards the cardiac apex. The **v wave** occurs toward the end of the T wave on the ECG tracing. It results from increased right atrial pressure secondary to overfilling against a closed tricuspid valve. The **D wave** is a diastolic wave that results from negative pressure created in the right atrium secondary to blood flowing into the right ventricle (away from the hepatic veins) through an open tricuspid valve.

The A wave is so named because it occurs during atrial systole, whereas the S and D waves are named because they occur during ventricular systole and diastole, respectively.

Normal respiratory activity also affects flow velocity in the hepatic veins and caudal vena cava. During inspiration, there is increased flow toward the heart because of decreased intrathoracic pressure and increased intraabdominal pressure. These effects are reversed with expiration. Contraction of the abdominal muscles against a closed glottis after inspiration, known as a Valsalva maneuver, raises intrathoracic pressure and causes flow to diminish or stop within the caudal vena cava. This can occur in animals during straining or vocalization.

Portal Vein

The portal vein is visualized by either a ventral or right intercostal approach, whereby it can be seen entering the liver at the porta hepatis. It is ventral and slightly to the left of the caudal vena cava. The relationship of the aorta, caudal vena cava, and portal vein is easiest to recognize in the transverse view (see Figure 9-3, *G*). However, Doppler measurements of the main portal vein at the porta hepatis are obtained with the portal vein in a long-axis view, and the transducer directed cranially to obtain an incident angle of less than 60 degrees (see Figure 9-3, *G*). A scanning protocol for systematic ultrasound evaluation of the portal system in dogs has been proposed.[21] An additional report describes the use of the right portal vein branch rather than the main portal vein for Doppler evaluation.[22]

Doppler ultrasonography has been used to assess the appearance and closure time of the ductus venosus in neonatal Irish Wolfhounds.[23] In this study, the ductus venosus was closed at 9 days after birth. This is slightly longer than reported using more invasive techniques.[24] Assessment of closure of the ductus venosus in other breeds has not been reported but is expected to be similar. Until further studies are available, a patent ductus venosus detected after the first few weeks of life should be considered abnormal. However, confirmation by other means, such as lab work, scintigraphy, or other imaging studies, is essential.

Normal portal blood flow velocity (PBFV) in the main portal vein is relatively slow and nearly uniform with small undulations in the Doppler spectral pattern (Figure 9-7). The portal vein has intestinal capillaries at one end and hepatic sinusoids at the other, so it is insulated from the variable pressures and flow that normally exist in arteries and systemic veins. The small undulations in velocity are thought to be due to respiratory motion of the diaphragm, with velocity increasing during expiration and decreasing during inspiration.[16,18]

Mean PBFV in the main portal vein in normal unsedated dogs has been reported to be 18 ± 7.6 cm/sec,[18] 14.7 ± 2.5 cm/sec,[16] and 19.2 ± 0.5 cm/sec[25]; In another study, mean PVFV was determined based on weight: 16.95 ± 5.79 cm/sec in dogs weighing up to 10 kg; 16.98 ± 3.04 cm/sec in dogs weighing between 10.1 and 20.0 kg; and 17.39 ± 4.77 cm/sec in dogs weighing 20.1 kg or more.[22] Thus the normal range of PBFV is approximately 10 to 25 cm/sec (see Figure 9-7, *A*). The mean PBFV in healthy, unsedated cats has been reported to be 10 to 12 cm/sec[26] or 17.1 cm/sec (range, 9.7 to 18.1 cm/sec) (see Figure 9-7, *B*).[27] Mean portal blood flow (PBF) in dogs has been reported to be 31 ± 9 mL/min/kg,[18,28] 40.9 ± 13 mL/min/kg,[16] and 33.8 ± 1.2 mL/min/kg[25]; 51.7 ± 20.55 mL/min/kg in dogs weighing up to 10 kg; 38.28 ± 8.15 mL/min/kg in dogs weighing between 10.1 and 20.0 kg; and 32.19 ± 13.23 mL/min/kg in dogs weighing 20.1 kg or more[22] by four different investigators. Mean PBF (mL/min/kg) is calculated by multiplying the cross-sectional area (cm²) of the portal vein by the mean PBFV (cm/sec) and dividing by body weight (kg). Eating is known to increase normal portal flow, whereas exercise and upright posture may decrease normal portal flow. These considerations should be taken into account in interpreting PBFV and PBF, but the magnitude and variability of these effects as they apply to clinical cases are still largely unknown. Therefore it is important to perform PBFV and PBF Doppler evaluations in a consistent manner (e.g., unsedated animals, before feeding, in lateral or dorsal recumbency) to reduce variability and provide meaningful results.

The portal vein congestion index (CI, cm × sec) is a measure of vascular resistance and may increase with hepatic cirrhosis and other liver diseases.[18] The CI is determined by dividing the portal vein cross-sectional area (cm²) by the average blood flow velocity (cm/sec). The CI for normal, unsedated dogs is approximately 0.04 ± 0.015 cm × sec.[18] A second report lists CI as 0.022 ± 0.01 cm × sec for dogs weighing up to 10 kg, 0.039 ± 0.009 cm × sec for dogs weighing between 10.1 and 20.0 kg, and 0.043 ± 0.009 cm × sec for dogs weighing at least 20.1 kg.[22]

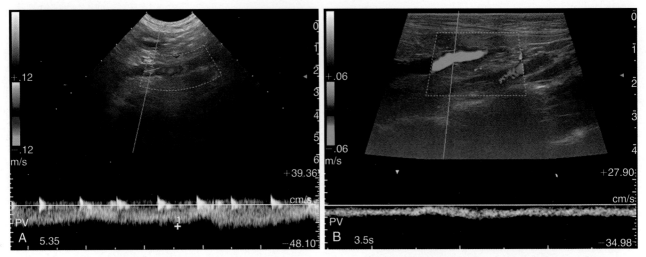

Figure 9-7 **Doppler evaluation of normal portal veins in a dog (A) and cat (B). A,** This triplex image shows a sagittal B-mode image of a dog portal vein with color Doppler and a pulse-wave (PW) spectral image tracing. The color Doppler image depicts portal blood flow as blue (away from transducer, toward the liver to the left). The PW spectral image shows a fairly uniform portal vein blood flow at –23.0 cm/sec (at the point of the electronic cursor, +). The blood flow is below the baseline (away from transducer). The small positive waveforms depict adjacent arterial blood flow. **B,** Cat portal vein triplex image shows a portal vein velocity of approximately –10 cm/sec.

Hepatic Arteries

Normal hepatic arterial blood flow has a typical low resistance arterial waveform with a distinct systolic and diastolic component. The resistive index (RI) is a unitless measure of the resistance of blood flow through an organ. It is calculated by subtracting the end-diastolic velocity from the peak systolic velocity and then dividing the result by the peak systolic velocity. The mean peak systolic velocity and RI of the hepatic artery in normal, fasted dogs was reported to be 1.5 ± 0.4 m/sec and 0.68 ± 0.04, respectively.[17]

In humans, the RI is thought to be a reliable indicator of hepatic vascular resistance, which is unaffected by blood pressure.[29] However, the RI may be affected by heart rate. An increased heart rate was found to decrease RI in the renal arteries, although the effect was small unless the heart rate was markedly abnormal.[30] Hepatic arterial RI has been used to evaluate diseases causing increased resistance to hepatic arterial blood flow (increased RI) such as cirrhosis.[31-33] RI is also useful for detecting increased hepatic arterial flow (decreased RI) in certain types of viral hepatitis[34,35] and portal vein thrombosis.[36] RI may also be used to evaluate outcome of liver transplants.[37-39]

In dogs, the importance of hepatic arterial RI measurements in clinical cases remains to be determined. Two dogs with congenital arterioportal fistulas had a lower mean RI than normal, but in three dogs with portal vein thrombosis and two dogs with acquired hepatic insufficiency, the RI was normal.[17] RI in dogs with congenital portosystemic shunts has not been reported, but hepatic arterial flow was shown to increase after side-to-side portosystemic shunts were created experimentally.[40] Therefore hepatic arterial RI determinations may potentially be useful for diagnosing congenital portosystemic shunts or for serially evaluating changes in hepatic arterial flow after surgical intervention. However, differences in hepatic blood flow in dogs of different ages or breeds may limit the usefulness of the procedure; thus additional studies are indicated.[17]

FOCAL OR MULTIFOCAL DISEASE

Focal lesions in the liver as small as 5 mm or less can be visualized on ultrasound exam, especially when the image is optimized for spatial resolution by using high frequencies and careful setting of the beam focus. However, the ultrasound appearance of focal disease is nonspecific, with a long list of potential etiologies.

Nodular Hyperplasia

Nodular hyperplasia has a variable appearance and cannot be differentiated on the basis of ultrasonography alone (Figures 9-8 and 9-9). It may occur in up to 70% of older dogs,[41] but it is not detected this frequently during hepatic ultrasound examinations because the lesions are often isoechoic to surrounding liver parenchyma. The earliest age that nodules were found was between 6 and 8 years in a series of 50 consecutive postmortem examinations of dogs, whereas all dogs older than 14 years had nodules.[41] These benign lesions may appear isoechoic, hypoechoic, moderately hyperechoic, cavitary, or target-like, or have mixed echogenicity.[42-47] Mixed patterns result when there are dilated venous sinusoids, central necrosis, or hemorrhage. One study reported that hematomas may occur in approximately 35% of the cases.[48] Target lesions have a hypoechoic rim with an isoechoic or hyperechoic center (see Figure 9-9, *A*). A target lesion is an uncommon finding with nodular hyperplasia and is more often associated with neoplasia.[47] Clinical experience indicates that nodular hyperplasia may appear similar to some forms of vacuolar hepatopathy and extramedullary hematopoiesis. When larger, nodular hyperplasia may resemble hematomas, abscesses, necrosis, and primary or metastatic liver neoplasia. A liver biopsy (or FNA for cytology) is indicated, but the histologic appearance may be nondiagnostic or difficult to distinguish from hepatocellular adenoma or well-differentiated hepatocellular carcinoma.[49] Metastatic neoplasia can usually be ruled out on the basis of the biopsy results. Therefore a liver biopsy primarily

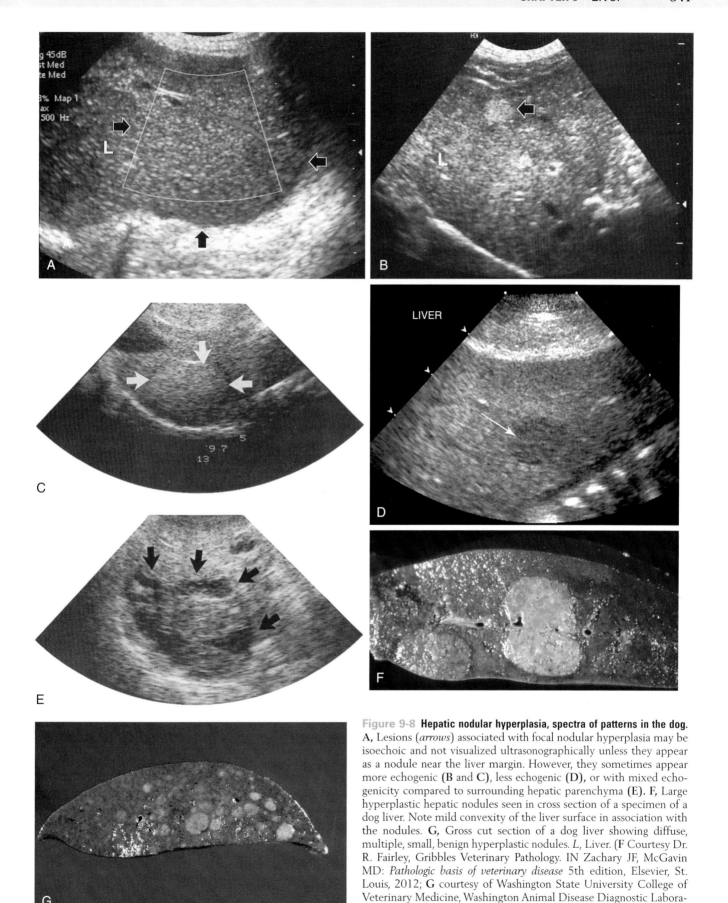

Figure 9-8 Hepatic nodular hyperplasia, spectra of patterns in the dog.
A, Lesions (*arrows*) associated with focal nodular hyperplasia may be isoechoic and not visualized ultrasonographically unless they appear as a nodule near the liver margin. However, they sometimes appear more echogenic (**B** and **C**), less echogenic (**D**), or with mixed echogenicity compared to surrounding hepatic parenchyma (**E**). **F,** Large hyperplastic hepatic nodules seen in cross section of a specimen of a dog liver. Note mild convexity of the liver surface in association with the nodules. **G,** Gross cut section of a dog liver showing diffuse, multiple, small, benign hyperplastic nodules. *L,* Liver. (F Courtesy Dr. R. Fairley, Gribbles Veterinary Pathology. IN Zachary JF, McGavin MD: *Pathologic basis of veterinary disease* 5th edition, Elsevier, St. Louis, 2012; G courtesy of Washington State University College of Veterinary Medicine, Washington Animal Disease Diagnostic Laboratory, Pullman, WA.)

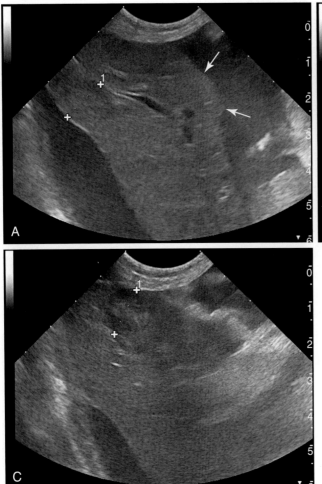

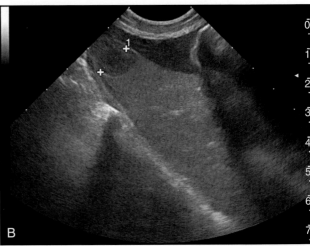

Figure 9-9 **Benign hepatic hyperplasia in a geriatric greyhound presented for ascites; a spectra of patterns in same patient.** **A,** Isoechoic to hypoechoic hyperplastic nodule (1.32 cm between electronic cursors), slightly protruding from the liver surface. Truly isoechoic nodule protrudes from the caudal liver margin (*arrows*). **B,** Hypoechoic hyperplastic nodule (1.20 cm between electronic cursors) in the cranioventral liver. **C,** Mixed echogenicity hyperplastic nodule (1.39 cm between electronic cursors).

serves to rule out neoplasia or other diseases, not to confirm nodular hyperplasia.

Contrast harmonic ultrasound has shown promise for differentiating benign from malignant hepatic nodules.[50] All malignant nodules were hypoechoic to liver parenchyma at peak contrast enhancement, whereas benign nodules were isoechoic to the surrounding normal contrast-enhanced liver.

The ultrasonographic appearance of hepatic nodular hyperplasia in the cat has not been described to our knowledge. However, multiple nodular lesions found during exploratory laparotomy in one young cat were evaluated histopathologically and found to resemble focal nodular hyperplasia in humans.[51]

Cysts

Hepatic cysts are usually detected incidentally. However, clinical signs may be present if widespread polycystic disease replaces the liver parenchyma, mechanical compression of a vital structure occurs, or the cyst becomes secondarily infected. Typical hepatic cysts are characterized by thin and well-defined walls, absence of internal echoes, sharp distal borders, peripheral reflective and refractive zones, and strong distal acoustic enhancement[52] (Figure 9-10, *A*). Reverberation artifacts may be present at the proximal portion of the cyst and should not be mistaken for an irregular wall or internal debris. Cysts may be congenital or acquired and may be solitary (Figure 9-11; see also Figure 9-10, *B* and *C*) or multiple (see Figure 9-10, *A*). They may affect the parenchyma or biliary tract. Acquired cysts (bilomas or biliary pseudocysts) that

form outside the biliary tract may result from trauma or inflammatory disease, but this diagnosis requires a compatible history.[53] Cystlike structures may originate from the biliary tract in Cairn Terriers,[54] West Highland White Terriers,[55] and other breeds.[56-58] The kidneys should always be evaluated because polycystic renal disease may accompany hepatic cysts in both the dog and cat.[54,55,57-61] Careful scanning sometimes suggests communication of the cystlike structure with the biliary tract if localized ductal ectasia is present. Cysts smaller than 1 cm may be recognized because there is a marked change of acoustic impedance at the liver-cyst interface. In our experience, a large number of very small cysts may also produce a hyperechoic lesion because of the presence of multiple reflecting interfaces.

On occasion, cysts do not meet all of these criteria (Figure 9-12; see also Figure 9-10, C and D). They may possess irregular walls, septations, internal debris, or solid elements. In this case, the differential diagnosis must be widened to include traumatic, toxic, inflammatory, or neoplastic disease. Complex cystic lesions include hematoma, abscess, cystic metastasis, hemorrhage, or necrotic tumors. Biliary cystadenomas, seen primarily in older cats, are benign liver tumors that also have a characteristic cystic appearance.[62] Vascular lesions such as portacaval shunts and arteriovenous fistulas may also appear cystlike, but these can be readily identified using Doppler evaluation. The history, physical findings, and laboratory work are used to narrow the differential diagnosis. Percutaneous aspiration of the cyst under ultrasound guidance and cytologic evaluation with bacteriologic culture are advisable. Serial

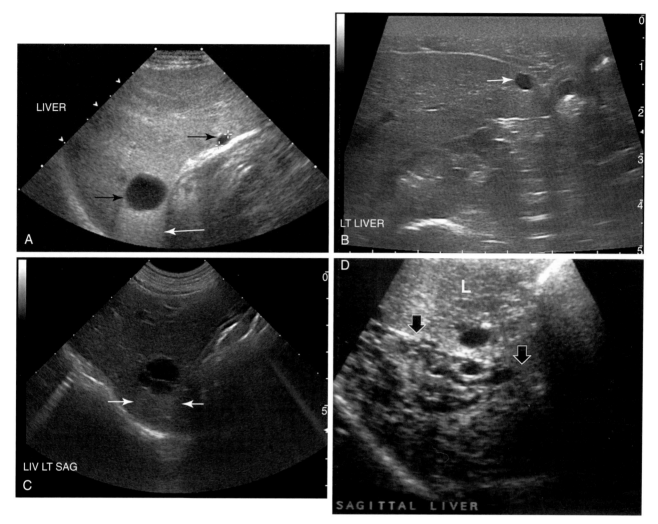

Figure 9-10 **Hepatic cysts. A,** A typical hepatic cyst (*black arrows*) has a thin and well-defined far wall, no internal echoes or septations, and strong distal acoustic enhancement (*white arrow*). **B,** This small hepatic cyst (approximately 5 mm, *arrow*) has anechoic fluid, far wall enhancement, but little distal acoustic enhancement because it is small. The liver is enlarged, based on a thickened, rounded caudoventral margin. **C,** Atypical hepatic cysts do not meet all of the criteria of a typical cyst and may have septations, walls that are irregular or thickened, or echogenic internal contents even though there is distal acoustic enhancement (*arrows*). **D,** Multiple, small hepatic cysts as seen here (*arrows*) may be difficult to differentiate from hepatic neoplasia. Distal acoustic enhancement is poor. Benign hepatic tumors, such as hepatic cystadenomas, and some malignant primary or metastatic hepatic tumors may have a similar appearance. An ultrasound-guided aspiration is indicated in questionable cases. *L,* Liver.

examinations also aid diagnosis because there is little or no change in the cyst on serial examinations compared with cyst-like masses produced by trauma, inflammation, necrosis, or neoplasia.

Hematoma

The internal appearance of a hematoma changes as it ages (Figure 9-13; see also Figure 9-12). Acute parenchymal hemorrhage less than 24 hours old is echogenic.[63] Within the first week, a hematoma becomes more hypoechoic and better defined, with a mixture of solid and fluid components. Over the next several weeks, the hematoma becomes increasingly less distinct as fluid is resorbed and spaces are filled with granulation tissue.

The variable appearance of a hematoma over time is similar to that of necrosis, abscess, or tumor and cannot be differentiated by ultrasonographic appearance alone. Hematomas have also been reported to occur in approximately 35% of cases of nodular hyperplasia, which may give them a complex appearance.[48] Other important factors, such as history of trauma or coagulation disorder, age of the animal, presence of fever and leukocytosis with a left shift, serum biochemical abnormalities, and change in appearance on serial examinations, must be considered. Without a history of trauma, bleeding disorder, or laboratory findings suggestive of other diseases, the lesion should be percutaneously aspirated for culture and cytology to obtain a definitive diagnosis.

Abscess

Hepatic abscesses are relatively uncommon in dogs and cats, and the cause of spontaneously occurring hepatic abscesses is unknown. Two retrospective studies in dogs reported the

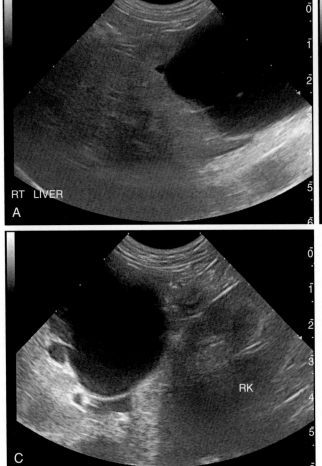

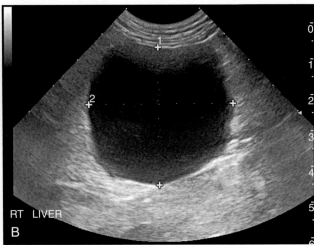

Figure 9-11 Large simple, solitary hepatic cyst in a 14-year old neutered male diabetic Shiba Inu with presenting symptom of vomiting. Liver enzymes were elevated and a mucocele (not shown) was found. This cyst was felt to be incidental to the presenting signs. **A,** Sagittal image of a large anechoic cyst arising from the right caudal margin of the liver showing acoustic enhancement of the far field tissues. **B,** Transverse image of the cyst (3.84 × 4.07 cm, between electronic cursors) shows strong acoustic enhancement. Note the reverberation artifact in the near field of the cyst, mimicking internal debris. **C,** Sagittal image shows the cyst's relationship to the right kidney and adjacent liver blood vessels. Near-field artifact is seen, as in **B.**

diagnosis of hepatic abscesses in 14 dogs during a 12-year period and in 13 dogs during a 6.5-year period.[64,65] The hepatic abscesses were often associated with infection of other organs or organ systems, and bacteria were cultured from the abscesses in the majority of cases. More than one organism was often involved; the most common is *Escherichia coli.*[64] Diabetes mellitus has also been suggested as a predisposing condition associated with hepatic abscessation.[66] Other predisposing conditions, such as biliary disease, pancreatitis, neoplasia, and long-term steroid administration, have likewise been implicated.[64,65] Hepatic abscesses have been reported in dogs with penetrating foreign objects, liver lobe torsion, and hepatic neoplasia.[67,68] A retrospective study reported the diagnosis of hepatic abscesses in 14 cats.[69] Many of the clinical features and ultrasound findings were similar to those of dogs. For example, hepatocellular carcinoma with secondary abscessation was reported in a cat.[70] However, compared with dogs, fewer cats with hepatic abscess were febrile and many were hypothermic. In addition, affected cats were less likely to have elevated liver enzymes than dogs, making the diagnosis in cats more difficult.

A liver abscess may produce lesions that run the spectrum of anechoic, hypoechoic, hyperechoic, and mixed patterns, depending on the age of the abscess and the appearance of the centralized necrosis[65,67] (Figures 9-14, to 9-16). In some cases, the contents are isoechoic, which makes the differentiation from normal or a solid mass extremely difficult. If gas is present within the abscess because of gas-producing bacteria, a hyperechoic pattern is found (see Figures 9-14, *B* to *D,* and 9-15, *A* and *B*).[65,67] Distal acoustic enhancement is variable, depending on the contents of the abscess.[65,67] Diagnosis depends on correlation with the history and ultrasound-guided aspiration of the lesion for culture and cytology. Once a hepatic abscess is diagnosed, ultrasonography is ideal for serially monitoring the response to therapy.

Liver abscesses in the dog usually have a centralized anechoic to hypoechoic region with an irregular, poorly defined hyperechoic margin.[64,65,67] There may be small echogenic clumps within the abscess. Distal acoustic enhancement may be seen if liquefaction necrosis is present (see Figure 9-14, *A*). Abscesses containing gas may be diffusely hyperechoic or have multifocal areas of increased echogenicity; they may also have acoustic shadowing.[65,67]

Liver abscesses may be safely aspirated for diagnosis and culture with a thin needle (such as a spinal needle), especially if they are deep within the parenchyma or surrounded by a thick rim that prevents leakage.[65] Firm transducer pressure is required to displace overlying viscera and reduce the distance of needle passage. The sonographer should choose the shortest possible route that avoids vital structures. To prevent contamination of the pleural cavity, an intercostal route should not be chosen. Multifocal or multilocular abscesses or those not easily accessible percutaneously must be drained surgically, and a sample for culture can be obtained at that time. A study in humans compared ultrasound-guided percutaneous catheter drainage with needle aspiration in the management of pyogenic liver abscess.[71] The authors concluded that

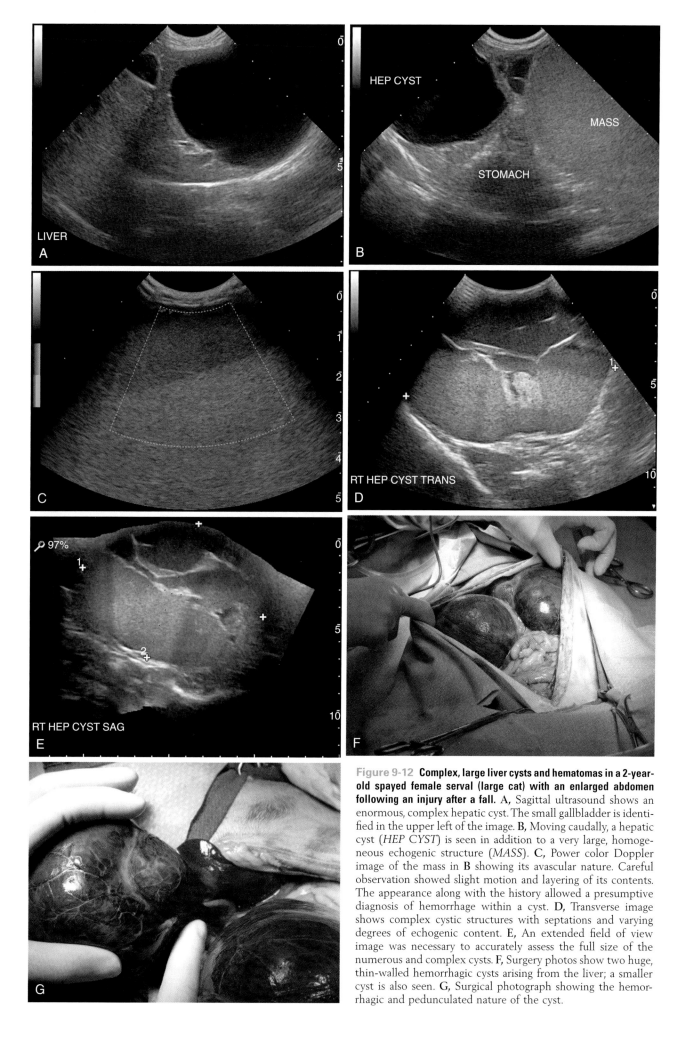

Figure 9-12 **Complex, large liver cysts and hematomas in a 2-year-old spayed female serval (large cat) with an enlarged abdomen following an injury after a fall.** **A,** Sagittal ultrasound shows an enormous, complex hepatic cyst. The small gallbladder is identified in the upper left of the image. **B,** Moving caudally, a hepatic cyst (*HEP CYST*) is seen in addition to a very large, homogeneous echogenic structure (*MASS*). **C,** Power color Doppler image of the mass in **B** showing its avascular nature. Careful observation showed slight motion and layering of its contents. The appearance along with the history allowed a presumptive diagnosis of hemorrhage within a cyst. **D,** Transverse image shows complex cystic structures with septations and varying degrees of echogenic content. **E,** An extended field of view image was necessary to accurately assess the full size of the numerous and complex cysts. **F,** Surgery photos show two huge, thin-walled hemorrhagic cysts arising from the liver; a smaller cyst is also seen. **G,** Surgical photograph showing the hemorrhagic and pedunculated nature of the cyst.

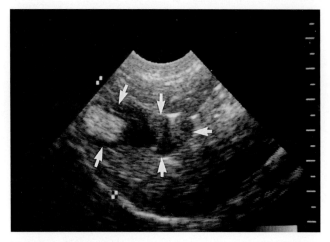

Figure 9-13 Hematoma. A sagittal view through the left liver lobes in this cat revealed a lesion with mixed anechoic and echogenic contents (*arrows*). This represents a hematoma from a liver biopsy performed 2 weeks previously.

percutaneous catheter drainage was more effective than needle aspiration, but that percutaneous needle aspiration was a valid alternative in simple abscesses with a diameter of 5 cm or less. Percutaneous needle drainage in combination with appropriate antibiotic administration for treatment of hepatic abscess has been reported in four dogs without complications.[65]

Necrosis

Chemical, viral, toxic, or immune-mediated insults may cause hepatic necrosis, as may liver lobe torsion (see later). The pattern may be multifocal or diffuse and is similar to that of hepatitis, multifocal abscess formation, or neoplasia (Figure 9-17). Doppler evaluation may be helpful to confirm its avascular nature, but in practice necrosis cannot be reliably differentiated from abscessation. The history may suggest the agent responsible, but a biopsy is required to eliminate a diagnosis of necrosis associated with other conditions.

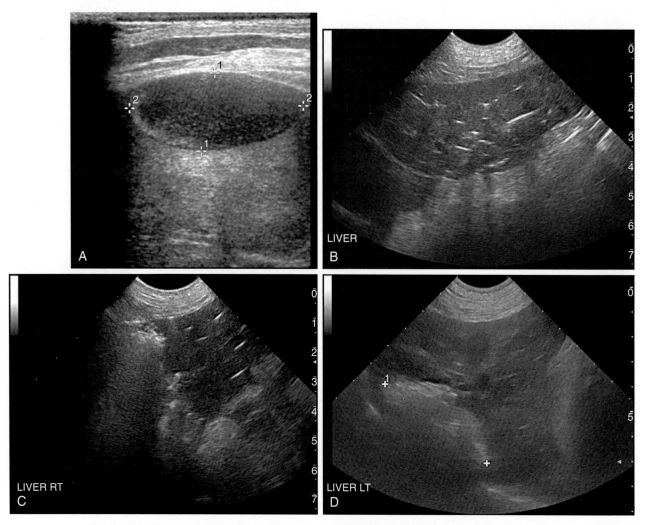

Figure 9-14 Liver abscesses appearing in a spectrum of patterns. A, This liver abscess (between electronic cursors) has echogenic contents produced by necrotic debris and no obvious rim. It would be difficult to differentiate this lesion from an organizing hematoma or focal neoplastic process without a compatible history and clinical signs. An abscess was confirmed at necropsy, and was likely secondary to adjacent pancreatitis. **B,** Multifocal hyperechoic foci represent gas within the liver. **C,** Same case as **B,** a large, irregular hyperechoic interface is present within the liver, representing the boundary of a large abscess. The large amount of gas is creating a "dirty" acoustic shadow. **D,** A large echogenic interface represents the boundary of a large liver abscess (between electronic cursors).

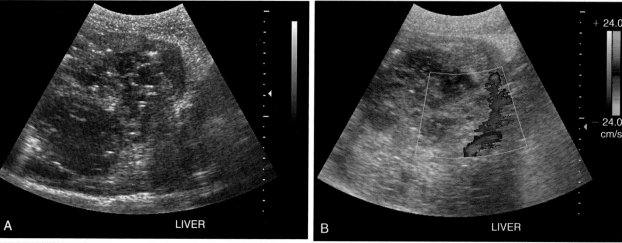

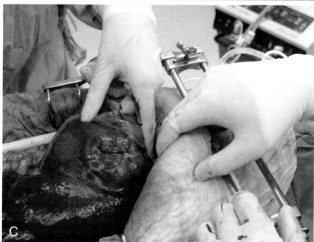

Figure 9-15 **Liver abscess in a 10-year old neutered male golden retriever with sever lethargy. A,** A heterogeneous, poorly demarcated mass is present within the liver, characterized by hypoechoic areas mixed with smaller, very echogenic foci, representing gas pockets. **B,** Color Doppler image shows good peripheral blood flow, but no flow within the abscess. **C,** Photograph of the hepatic abscess taken during surgery. The abscess bulges out from the surface of the liver. Severe suppurative hepatitis and abscessation were found on histology. Extensive peliosis hepatis, nodular regeneration, and biliary hyperplasia were also found.

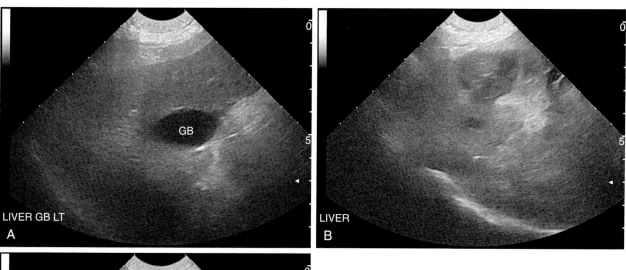

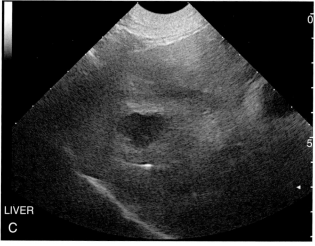

Figure 9-16 **Liver abscess, characterized by cavitation, hyperechoic liver parenchyma, and generally poor hepatic detail. A,** Image of the liver showing the gallbladder (GB). **B,** Heterogeneous liver parenchyma with a lobulated hypoechoic lesion in the near field and poor overall detail. **C,** Hypoechoic area surrounded by a thick hyperechoic wall, representing the liquefactive portion of the liver abscess.

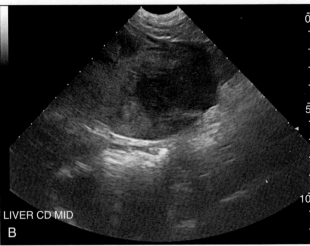

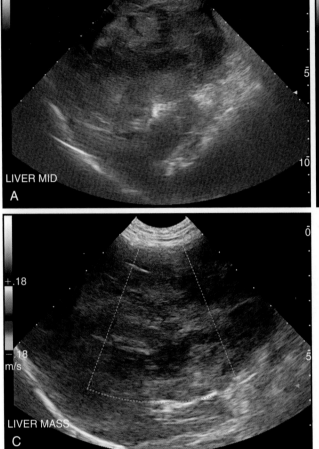

Figure 9-17 Hepatic necrosis from liver lobe torsion. A, Sagittal image of the central portion of the liver shows a heterogeneous, complex mass. **B,** Sagittal image of the caudal margin of the liver shows a hypoechoic mass and a swollen, rounded liver margin. **C,** Color Doppler image of the mass shows no blood flow. The final diagnoses were massive necrotizing bacterial hepatitis of the left lateral and caudate liver lobes, a result of localized ischemia due to lobar torsion.

Trauma

Laceration of the liver can occur with blunt abdominal trauma. The laceration can be small or large, accompanied by a hematoma. Subcapsular hematomas or capsular disruption can also occur (Figure 9-18). The need for surgery depends on the size of the laceration, the amount of blood in the peritoneal cavity, and the patient's clinical status. Computerized tomography (CT) is considered the gold standard for evaluating blunt abdominal trauma in humans. However, ultrasound still has an important role in the initial triage of patients who are not hemodynamically stable and cannot undergo CT. Contrast-enhanced ultrasonography was found to improve the initial detection of liver lesions in patients with blunt abdominal trauma and also help with follow-up healing assessment.[72-77] Liver lesions may appear hyperechoic, mixed echogenic, or hypoechoic with non–contrast-enhanced ultrasound. These patterns change after administration of contrast material. The normal liver parenchyma becomes hyperechoic after contrast administration, but the area of injury appears anechoic or hypoechoic, with well-defined margins. Active bleeding or extravasation can also be visualized.[78] Use of contrast agents enhances visualization of liver injuries relative to what can be achieved without their use. Contrast-enhanced sonography may also eventually prove useful in animals for evaluating solid organ injuries from blunt abdominal trauma.

Liver Lobe Torsion

Although rare, liver lobe torsion may lead to tissue infarction and necrosis, resulting in formation of a liver mass that is hypoechoic or has mixed echogenicity (see Figure 9-17).[68,79-81] Echogenic foci with reverberation artifact or shadowing may be seen within the mass if gas-producing organisms are present. Absent or reduced blood flow within the mass can be demonstrated using Doppler ultrasonography. Abdominal fluid may accumulate secondary to necrosis, venous congestion, or bacterial peritonitis. Torsion may be more likely to occur in large breed dogs[68] and involve the left lateral liver lobe.[79,82] Liver lobe torsions usually occur in dogs, but one case has also been described in a cat.[82]

Neoplasia

Detection of parenchymal lesions compatible with hepatic neoplasia is one of the most important diagnostic and prognostic uses of ultrasonography. Computed tomography is considered the gold standard for detecting small liver lesions in humans. However, ultrasonography is preferred in animals because it is more readily available and rarely requires sedation or anesthesia. In dogs, metastatic liver tumors are more common than primary tumors, typically arising from primary tumors of the pancreas, spleen, and gastrointestinal tract.[83,84,85] Primary hepatobiliary tumors are more common than metastatic disease in cats.[83,86]

Primary liver tumors may appear as solitary masses that are confined to one lobe (Figure 9-19). Multifocal nodules involving several lobes, and diffuse, coalescing nodules involving all lobes are additional patterns that have been identified. Primary hepatic neoplasias are hepatocellular adenoma and carcinoma; bile duct adenoma (cystadenoma) and carcinoma

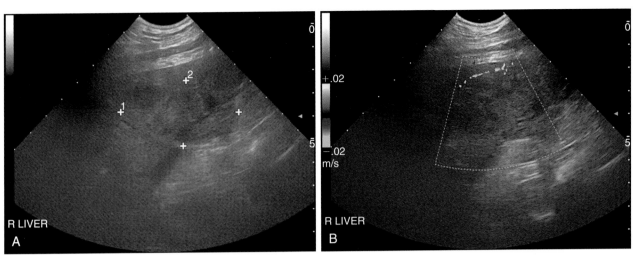

Figure 9-18 Liver laceration in a dog that fell from a truck. A, Heterogeneous area within the liver that protrudes from the liver capsule (5.20 × 2.83 cm, between electronic cursors). **B,** Color Doppler image of the area shows peripheral blood flow only. This patient had a hemoabdomen (not shown) and was later determined to have immune-mediated anemia and thrombocytopenia.

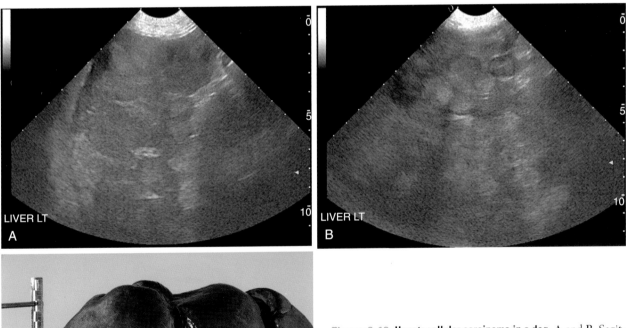

Figure 9-19 Hepatocellular carcinoma in a dog. A and **B,** Sagittal images of the left side of the liver show a very abnormal, nodular appearance of the liver parenchyma. **C,** Specimen photograph of the liver tumor within the left lateral lobe. (C, courtesy of Washington State University College of Veterinary Medicine, Washington Animal Disease Diagnostic Laboratory, Pullman, WA.)

(cholangiocarcinoma); and sarcomas, including hemangiosarcoma, leiomyosarcoma, and fibrosarcoma (Figure 9-20). The liver is frequently involved in dogs with disseminated histiocytic sarcoma (lymphosarcoma, mast cell tumor).[83] Metastatic tumors are commonly sarcomas of the spleen (hemangiosarcoma, fibrosarcoma, leiomyosarcoma) (Figure 9-21); carcinomas originating from the stomach, bowel, pancreas, thyroid, anal gland, or mammary gland (Figure 9-22); and lymphosarcoma. Focal or diffuse involvement of the liver is possible with either primary or metastatic tumor,

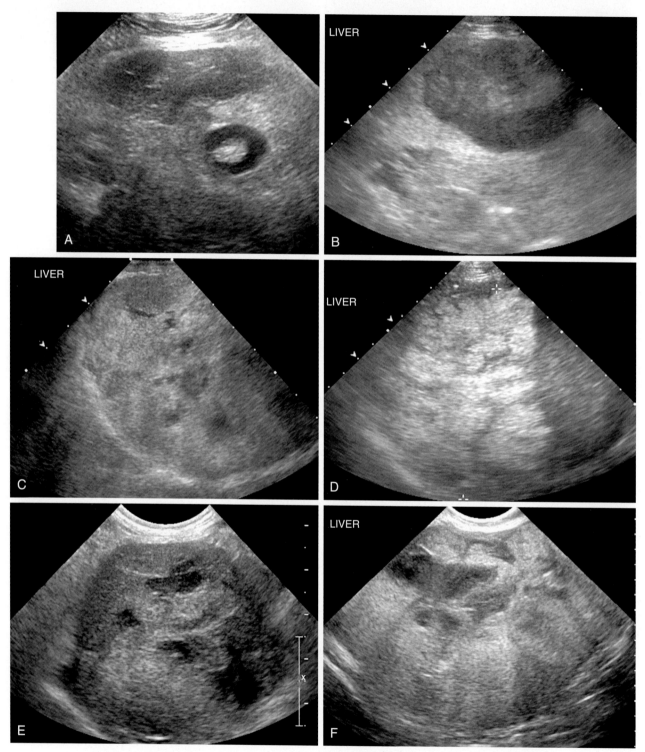

Figure 9-20 **Primary hepatic neoplasia in a variety of appearances in the dog and cat. A to F: Hepatocellular carcinoma. A,** Target lesion (hypoechoic rim and hyperechoic center) associated with hepatic carcinoma. Target lesions commonly indicate malignancy, but have also been associated with benign disease. **B,** Focal hypoechoic mass. **C,** Diffuse hepatic involvement, with both hyperechoic and hypoechoic areas. **D,** Focal, irregular hyperechoic mass. **E,** Focal mass with hypoechoic and anechoic areas. **F,** Large hyperechoic mass with focal hypoechoic nodular areas.

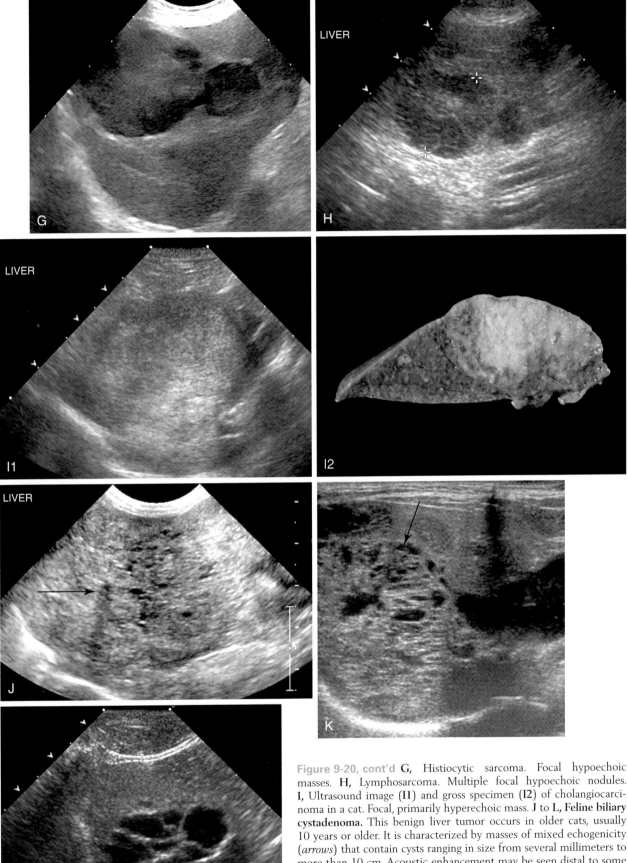

Figure 9-20, cont'd G, Histiocytic sarcoma. Focal hypoechoic masses. **H,** Lymphosarcoma. Multiple focal hypoechoic nodules. **I,** Ultrasound image (**I1**) and gross specimen (**I2**) of cholangiocarcinoma in a cat. Focal, primarily hyperechoic mass. **J** to **L, Feline biliary cystadenoma.** This benign liver tumor occurs in older cats, usually 10 years or older. It is characterized by masses of mixed echogenicity (*arrows*) that contain cysts ranging in size from several millimeters to more than 10 cm. Acoustic enhancement may be seen distal to some of these masses. Lesions with very small diameter cysts may appear hyperechoic because of the increased number of acoustic interfaces. (**I2,** courtesy of Washington State University College of Veterinary Medicine, Washington Animal Disease Diagnostic Laboratory, Pullman, WA.)

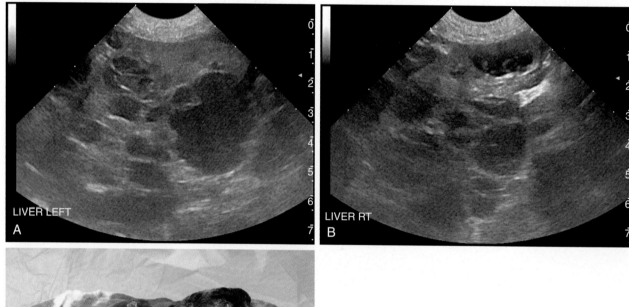

Figure 9-21 Liver hemangiosarcoma in a dog. A, Multiple hepatic nodules are present in the left side of the liver. **B,** Multiple nodules are present in the right side of the liver. **C,** Surgical photograph of widespread hepatic hemangiosarcoma, which may be primary or metastatic. It may be a diffuse, nodular, or focal/multifocal mass lesion.

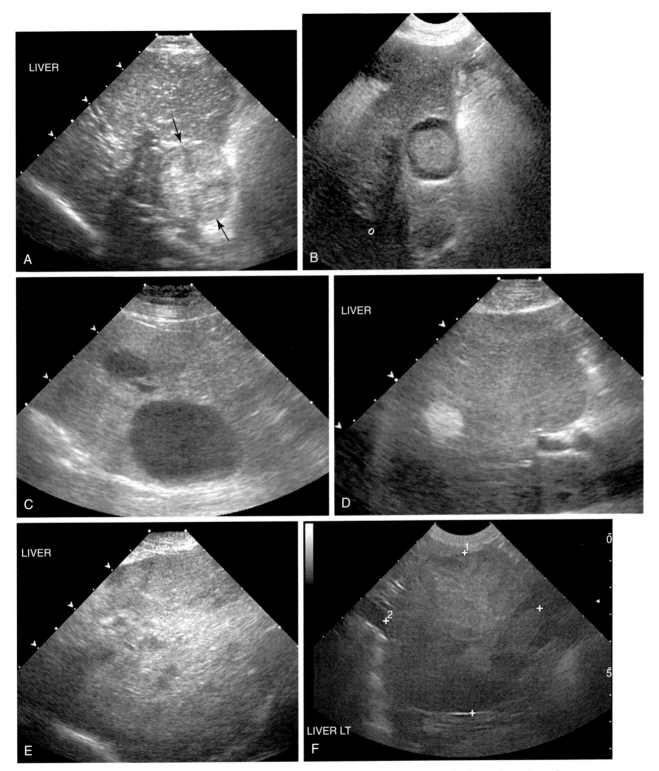

Figure 9-22 **Metastatic hepatic neoplasia with a variety of appearances in the dog and cat.** A to C, Splenic hemangiosarcoma. **A,** Solitary mixed echogenic nodule (*arrows*). **B,** Target lesion. **C,** Focal hypoechoic nodule. **D,** Thyroid carcinoma, focal hyperechoic lesion. **E,** Colon carcinoma. Multifocal, hypoechoic lesions. **F,** Large, solid, heterogeneous anal gland carcinoma.

Continued

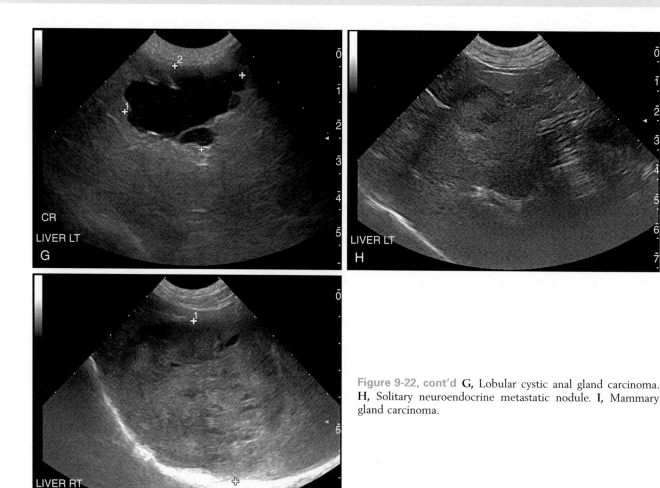

Figure 9-22, cont'd G, Lobular cystic anal gland carcinoma. H, Solitary neuroendocrine metastatic nodule. I, Mammary gland carcinoma.

and they cannot be differentiated solely with ultrasound examination.[42,43,45,46,52,83,87-91]

The ultrasound appearance of hepatic neoplasia is variable, and in some cases, diffuse forms of the disease may show no ultrasound abnormalities. The same tumor may have a variety of appearances, even within the same animal (Figures 9-23 and 9-24). Furthermore, different histologic types of primary or metastatic tumors may appear remarkably similar ultrasonographically. Tumors may abscess, altering their appearance because of necrosis or bacterial gas formation.[70] Ultrasound alone cannot be used to distinguish benign from malignant focal disease. However, ultrasonographically detected larger focal hepatic masses in the presence of peritoneal effusion were associated with malignant liver disease in dogs.[92,93] Hepatic neoplasia may appear as solitary masses that are confined to one lobe, multifocal nodules involving several lobes, or diffuse, coalescing nodules involving all lobes. Nodules and masses can be hypoechoic or hyperechoic, or have mixed echogenicity. Target lesions (nodules with a hypoechoic rim and echogenic or isoechoic center) are commonly, though not exclusively, associated with neoplasia. In one report, one or more target lesions in the liver or spleen had a positive predictive value of 74% for malignancy, whereas finding multiple target lesions in one organ had a positive predictive value of 81% for malignancy.[47] Multifocal target lesions are commonly encountered with carcinomas but are not limited to them.[47] Hemangiosarcoma, lymphosarcoma, and benign conditions such as nodular hyperplasia, pyogranulomatous hepatitis, chronic active hepatitis, and cirrhosis may also produce target lesions.[47]

Although the ultrasonographic appearance of hepatic neoplasia is extremely variable, the visual characteristics of some common hepatic tumors have been described. Hepatic lymphosarcomas have a variety of ultrasound appearances.[94-98] They may be associated with no change from normal, hepatomegaly, coarse parenchyma, ill-defined hypoechoic areas, hypoechoic nodules, target lesions, diffuse hypoechogenicity, and diffuse hyperechogenicity (see Figures 9-23 and 9-24). Abdominal lymphadenopathy is often present (see Figure 9-24, E). Hepatocellular carcinomas are often solitary or multifocal masses, with some reports indicating a trend toward hyperechogenicity.[83,89,93,99] Yet another study indicates no correlation of hepatocellular carcinoma with a particular echogenicity.[93]

Mast cell tumor (MCT) infiltration into the liver does not seem to have a distinctive ultrasound appearance. The liver can appear normal, or it may be enlarged and exhibit subjectively increased echogenicity, with or without hypoechoic nodules (Figure 9-25).[100-102] The liver may appear normal because there is an inherent difficulty in detecting mild changes in hepatic size and echogenicity. Normal, diffusely hypoechoic, or mottled livers have been described with mast cell tumors in cats.[101] However, the sensitivity of ultrasound for detecting mast cell infiltration in the liver was 0%, with a

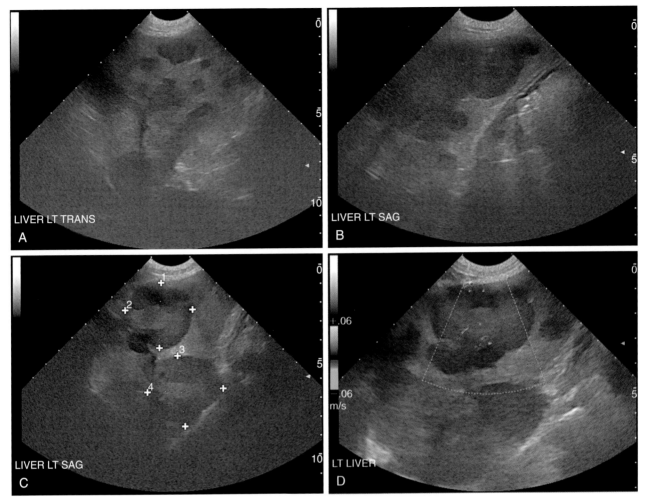

Figure 9-23 **Spectrum of appearances of canine hepatic lymphosarcoma in a 7-year-old male Doberman pinscher with hypercalcemia. A,** Discrete hypoechoic nodules. Note that some of the nodules are not truly round (spherical), appearing almost fusiform. **B,** Large, coalescing hypoechoic nodule. **C,** Discrete target lesions, with thick hypoechoic periphery surrounding more echogenic centers. **D,** Color Doppler assessment of target lesions shows minimal blood flow. In this patient, the spleen was normal and abdominal lymph node enlargement was not present.

specificity of 95% in a recent report. Alteration in the ultrasonographic appearance of the liver was not a reliable predictor of mast cell infiltration.[103]

Malignant histiocytosis can affect multiple organs, including the liver. Generalized hepatomegaly with decreased echogenicity, and hepatic parenchymal nodules (hypoechoic, hyperechoic, and mixed echogenic) have been reported in the liver with this disease process (Figure 9-26).[104,105] Because mesenteric and medial iliac lymph nodes are often involved with malignant histiocytosis, lymphosarcoma is a differential diagnosis for this appearance.

Biliary cystadenomas of cats are benign liver tumors that most often appear as focal or multifocal thin-walled cystic lesions in animals that are usually 10 years of age or older[62,106-108] (see Figure 9-19, *J* to *L*). Cystadenomas may also appear as hyperechoic lesions or have mixed echogenicity. This is possibly due to the variable size and number of cystic components within the tumor and the amount of fibrous tissue stroma present.[62]

As described previously, few neoplastic lesions have specific sonographic features. Describing the ultrasonographic appearance of various liver tumors (or any focal lesion other than a classic cyst) probably serves little purpose because of the marked variability and inconsistency of the image. There is poor correlation between the ultrasound appearance of hepatic disease and cytology and histopathology.[92,93,109,110] A liver that appears normal on ultrasonography does not rule out disease. Ultrasonography primarily serves to detect hepatic lesions, to obtain the required cytologic or histologic samples, and to monitor the course of the disease if therapy is initiated. Cytological analysis of fine-needle aspirates may have serious limitations when used to identify the primary disease process in dogs and cats with clinical evidence of liver disease.[111] Histopathologic samples are preferred for a more accurate and complete diagnosis.

Doppler Evaluation of Focal Neoplasia

Doppler ultrasound evaluation of focal liver lesions has been used previously in an effort to distinguish benign from malignant disease and to characterize various tumor types in humans.[112-117] Vessel morphology characteristics of malignancy include irregular lumen, branching patterns, intervascular shunts, and blind-ended vessels. Nonmalignant vascular patterns consist of a more orderly arrangement of branching

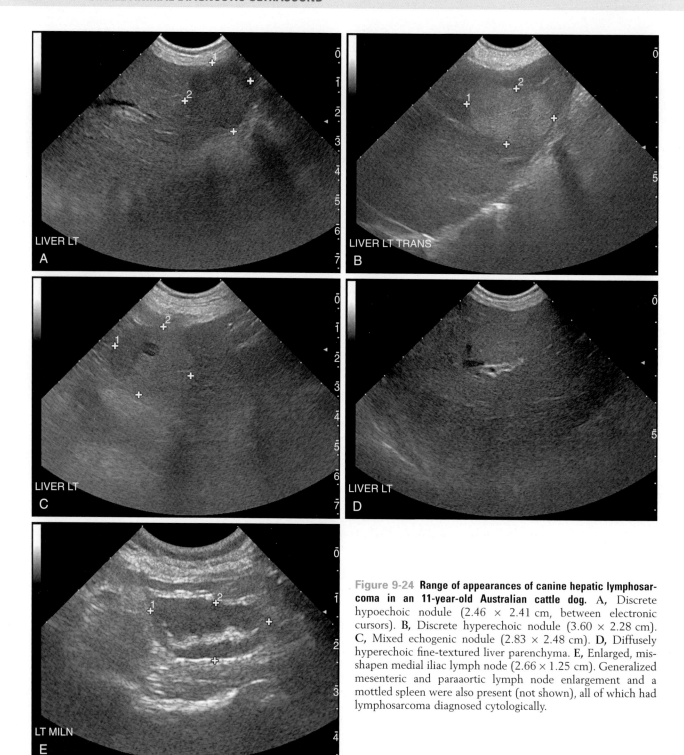

Figure 9-24 **Range of appearances of canine hepatic lymphosarcoma in an 11-year-old Australian cattle dog. A,** Discrete hypoechoic nodule (2.46 × 2.41 cm, between electronic cursors). **B,** Discrete hyperechoic nodule (3.60 × 2.28 cm). **C,** Mixed echogenic nodule (2.83 × 2.48 cm). **D,** Diffusely hyperechoic fine-textured liver parenchyma. **E,** Enlarged, misshapen medial iliac lymph node (2.66 × 1.25 cm). Generalized mesenteric and paraaortic lymph node enlargement and a mottled spleen were also present (not shown), all of which had lymphosarcoma diagnosed cytologically.

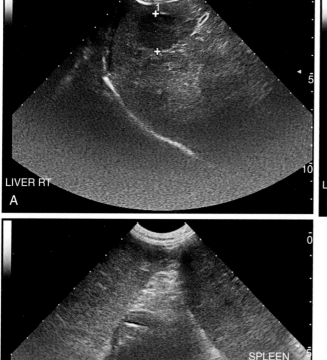

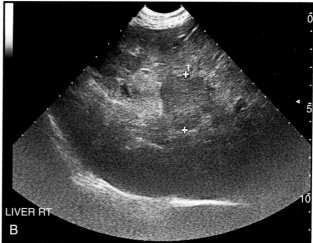

Figure 9-25 **Hepatic mast cell disease in a 9-year-old Labrador retriever. A,** Discrete hypoechoic nodule (2.11 cm, between electronic cursors). A small amount of peritoneal fluid is present between the liver and the diaphragm. **B,** Irregular hypoechoic nodules (3.08 cm, between electronic cursors) surrounded by mottled liver parenchyma. **C,** The liver is hyperechoic and finely textured, slightly more so than the adjacent spleen. The spleen was diffusely enlarged. Fine-needle aspirates of both organs and the peritoneal fluid were diagnostic for mast cell disease.

arteries. High-frequency shifts (5 kHz or greater) compatible with neovascularity and high-velocity arteriovenous (AV) shunts were noted with hepatocellular carcinomas and some highly vascular metastatic tumors. Although not seen with all malignant tumors, these types of signals were not detected with benign disease (Figure 9-27).

Color Doppler imaging has also been used to assess tumor vascularity and help characterize hepatic lesions as benign or malignant.[118,119] However, power Doppler imaging has recently shown higher sensitivity to flow and better edge definition and depiction of continuity of flow compared with conventional color Doppler imaging in humans.[120-124] An excellent review of the sonographic assessment of tumor metastases has been published.[125] The use of ultrasound contrast has enhanced visualization of these abnormal vessels.

Contrast Evaluation of Focal Neoplasia

The liver is likely the most commonly studied organ in the use of ultrasound contrast agents.[126-129] Both metastatic disease and benign nodular hyperplasia commonly cause focal hepatic nodules, especially in older dogs. There are no significant conventional ultrasound characteristics to accurately differentiate benign from malignant etiologies. Multiple studies indicate that contrast-enhanced ultrasound is very accurate in the differentiation of benign from malignant hepatic nodules.[50,130-134] Most benign hepatic nodules are isoechoic to the liver during the arterial phase, and maintain isoechogenicity during the portal venous phase at peak contrast enhancement. Most malignant nodules have early arterial phase enhancement, but

are hypoechoic to the surrounding liver parenchyma during peak contrast enhancement in the portal venous phase (early wash-in, early wash-out phenomenon). Hepatic nodules not identified on conventional ultrasound are more easily visualized after contrast enhancement. Some ultrasound contrast agents (Sonozoid, Levovist) have a parenchymal phase in addition to the arterial and portal venous phase.[133-135] This is thought to be due to phagocytosis of the contrast agent by the reticuloendothelial system (Kupffer cells). The parenchymal phase can last for several minutes (7 to 30 minutes postinjection), and also appears to be equally useful in identifying malignant lesions that are typically hypoechoic during this phase.[133,134] This is presumed to be due to a lack of Kupffer cells in malignant lesions. Contrast-enhanced ultrasound allows the creation of standardized time-intensity curves from selected regions of interest in organs that represent the signal intensity in relation to time, and increased contrast gives a more quantitative assessment of perfusion analysis.[136]

Reports in humans[137,138] also describe the use of microbubble contrast agents in combination with power Doppler imaging to improve detection and diagnosis of focal liver lesions.[137-143] This technique has not been described for liver imaging in dogs or cats, but it has been used to evaluate sentinel lymph nodes in dogs.[144-146]

In summary, the use of power Doppler ultrasound, ultrasound contrast media, and harmonic ultrasound improves the detection and characterization of smaller liver tumors and those that are isoechoic compared to conventional ultrasound

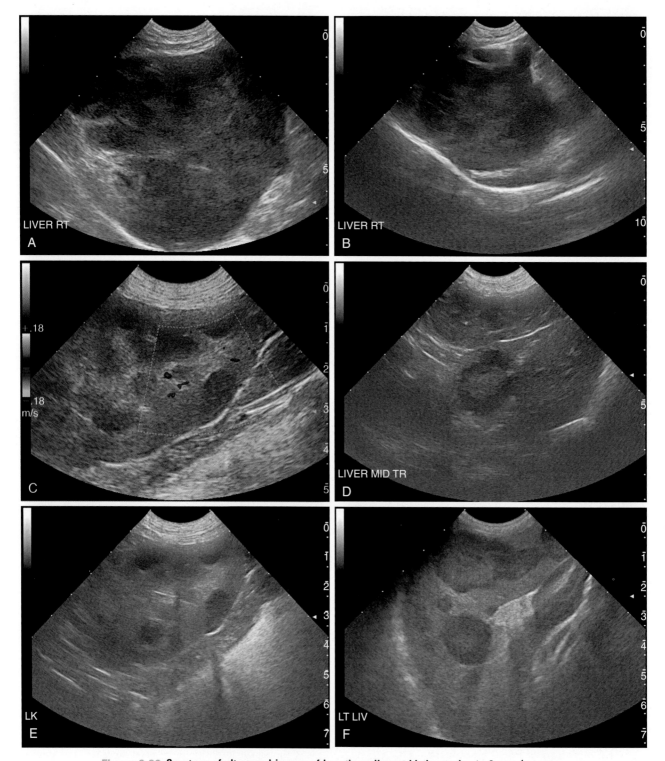

Figure 9-26 Spectrum of ultrasound images of hepatic malignant histiocytosis. A, Large heterogeneous mass. **B,** Discrete hypoechoic nodules of various sizes and shapes. **C,** Multiple hypoechoic nodules of similar sizes, with color Doppler evaluation. **D,** Target lesion with hyperechoic central region surrounded by thick hypoechoic periphery. A smaller hypoechoic nodule is present in the near field. **E,** Two target lesions with hypoechoic centers and thin hyperechoic rims surrounded by thicker hypoechoic tissue. Two discrete hypoechoic nodules are also present. **F,** Discrete, hypoechoic nodules of various sizes and shapes. Subtle, slightly hyperechoic central regions are noted.

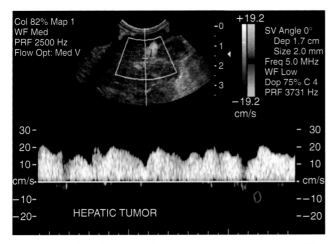

Figure 9-27 Doppler evaluation of hepatocellular carcinoma. The Doppler sample volume is used to detect abnormal high-frequency shifts associated with neovascularization and arteriovenous anastomoses. In this animal with hepatocellular carcinoma, nearly continuous frequency shifts with some pulsatility was noted. Unfortunately, these "tumor signals" are not present in all tumors. It is usually difficult to obtain any spectral tracings from normal hepatic parenchyma and benign lesions.

imaging. This should result in earlier recognition of neoplasia and help narrow the differential diagnosis of focal liver lesions. However, definitive diagnosis still requires a biopsy with cytopathologic or histopathologic evaluation.

DIFFUSE DISEASE

Diffuse hepatic disease can result in changes in size, shape, and echogenicity (Figure 9-28). Ultrasound assessment of these changes is highly subjective, especially when the changes are mild. Diagnosing various types of diffuse liver disease on the basis of the ultrasonographic appearance should be done with caution.[109,147] As a result, ultrasonography is less valuable for recognizing or differentiating diffuse liver disease, and a biopsy is almost always necessary for diagnosis.

Liver echogenicity must be compared with that of the kidneys and spleen at similar depth and instrument gain settings. The liver is normally similar to the right kidney cortex in echogenicity, but can be slightly increased or decreased in normal dogs and cats.[7,148] The liver is usually less echogenic than the spleen in normal dogs (Figure 9-29), though this is not always the case in normal cats. The possibility of a combination of liver, kidney, and spleen abnormalities must always be considered. Therefore relative comparisons of echogenicity may suggest an abnormality in one or more organs, but this must be confirmed by other clinical information or biopsy. The sonographer must always remember that machine settings greatly affect parenchymal echogenicity.

Decreased Echogenicity
Diffuse liver diseases may produce hypoechogenicity of the liver, in which the hepatic parenchyma appears less echogenic than the renal cortex, and the portal vein walls appear more prominent than usual. Diffusely hypoechoic liver parenchyma is not a common finding, but in our experience hepatitis is probably the most common etiology. Liver echogenicity is usually normal in cases of acute suppurative hepatitis, but it may be decreased with enhancement of periportal echoes[110,149] (Figure 9-30; see also Figure 9-28, *A*). Normal or decreased

liver echogenicity has been reported in dogs and cats with diffuse infiltrative processes such as lymphoma, leukemia, and amyloidosis.[42,43,46,52,89,94,110,149-151] But most diffuse lymphoma cases exhibit normal echogenicity or are more echogenic than expected. Passive congestion of the liver may also result in decreased echogenicity accompanied by hepatomegaly and hepatic venous enlargement. This observation usually indicates a cardiac rather than a hepatic abnormality.

Increased Echogenicity
An increase in hepatic echogenicity is considered definitive when it is significantly higher relative to the right renal cortex or spleen. The margins of the portal veins are decreased in prominence because of an overall increase in hepatic echogenicity. There is often increased sound attenuation resulting in incomplete visualization of deeper aspects of the liver (Figure 9-31). In these cases, the sonographer may need to use a transducer with a frequency lower than what would be expected for the size of the patient. The inexperienced sonographer may adjust the time-gain compensation and increase the power output of the ultrasound machine and thus miss this change. Uniformly increased liver echogenicity has been reported with fatty infiltration of the liver (Figure 9-32),[152,153] steroid hepatopathy (Figure 9-33; see also Figure 9-31),[149,154-156] chronic hepatitis,[157] cirrhosis,[149] mast cell tumor (Figure 9-34, *A* and *B*)[100,102,103] (see Figure 9-16, *B* to *E*), and, less commonly, lymphosarcoma (see Figure 9-34, *D* to *G*).[46,89,110] Liver size is usually increased with fatty infiltration (see Figures 9-4, *B*, and 9-32, *G*), steroid hepatopathy, mast cell tumor, and lymphosarcoma. Decreased liver size, sometimes with irregular liver margins, regenerative nodules, and ascites may be seen with chronic hepatitis or cirrhosis (see Figure 9-28, *H1*).

Hepatic lipidosis is the most common form of liver disease diagnosed in cats, and it occurs most consistently in obese cats that become anorexic.[153,158,159] There is usually concurrent hepatomegaly in these cases, and the echogenicity of the liver is normal to increased (see Figure 9-32, *B* to *I*). In severe feline hepatic lipidosis, the liver may be hyperechoic relative to falciform fat and isoechoic or hyperechoic relative to omental fat.[152,153] However, it is reported that normal obese cats may have a hyperechoic liver relative to falciform fat, similar to cats with hepatic lipidosis.[153] In addition, cats affected by hepatic lipidosis may have nonspecific changes in echogenicity. In one study, the calculated accuracy of ultrasound in the diagnosis of hepatic lipidosis was only approximately 70%.[147] Diabetes mellitus can also result in diffuse fatty infiltration of the liver. In dogs, vacuolar hepatopathy is the most common diffuse hyperechoic liver disease we encounter, nonspecific for hyperadrenocorticism and other endocrinopathies. Differentiation between types of vacuolar hepatopathy may require special histologic stains (for glycogen and fat). Although hepatic lipidosis is nearly always diffusely normoechoic to hyperechoic with homogeneous echotexture, vacuolar hepatopathy is often characterized by a mottled texture (see the next section, Inhomogeneous Echogenicity).

Chronic hepatitis or cirrhosis may result in less distinct portal vessel margins because of hyperechogenicity secondary to fibrosis.[149] The liver size may be normal to small with irregular margins, and ascites may be present (see Figure 9-28, *G*). Regenerative nodules accompanying chronic cirrhosis in humans have been reported to be less echogenic or of the same echogenicity as adjacent liver. In dogs with cirrhosis, these nodules, when seen, possess a distinctly rounded contour and are accompanied by an otherwise small, echogenic liver. Focal increases in hepatic echogenicity due to fibrosis or dystrophic calcification are also possible.

Text continued on p. 366

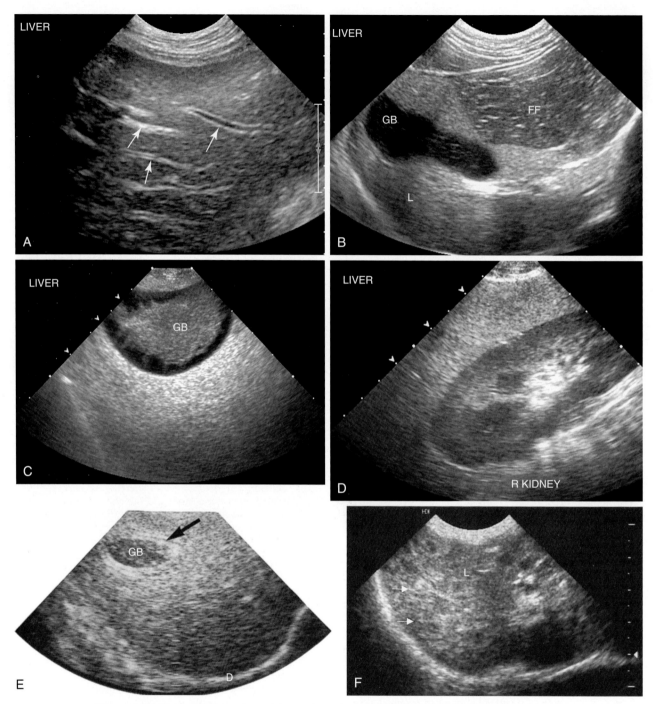

Figure 9-28 Changes in liver echogenicity. A, Acute hepatitis. Reduced hepatic parenchymal echogenicity with enhanced visualization of portal vessels (*arrows*) is evident in this dog with acute hepatitis. In many cases, however, there is no detectable change in hepatic echogenicity with acute hepatitis. **B,** Fatty infiltration. Uniformly increased hepatic parenchymal echogenicity is present in this cat with hepatic lipidosis. The liver parenchyma is hyperechoic to adjacent falciform fat (*FF*). Other signs of hyperechoic hepatic parenchyma include less distinct visualization of portal structures and reduced beam penetration. It is sometimes helpful to compare echogenicity of the liver with that of the right kidney cortex. The liver is normally the same as or slightly more or less echogenic than the kidney. Increased hepatic echogenicity produces a more pronounced difference between the two organs. **C and D,** Steroid hepatopathy. **C,** There is increased hepatic echogenicity diagnosed by reduced visualization of portal structures, increased attenuation of the ultrasound beam, and a fine, dense parenchyma. Centralized, nondependent biliary sludge is noted in the gallbladder lumen, consistent with a biliary mucocele. **D,** The liver is hyperechoic to the right kidney. **E and F,** Chronic hepatitis. **E,** Increased hepatic echogenicity, reduced visualization of hepatic blood vessels, and gallbladder wall thickening (arrow) are present. **F,** Patchy areas of increased hepatic echogenicity (arrows) with poor visualization of hepatic blood vessels were associated with chronic hepatitis in this dog.

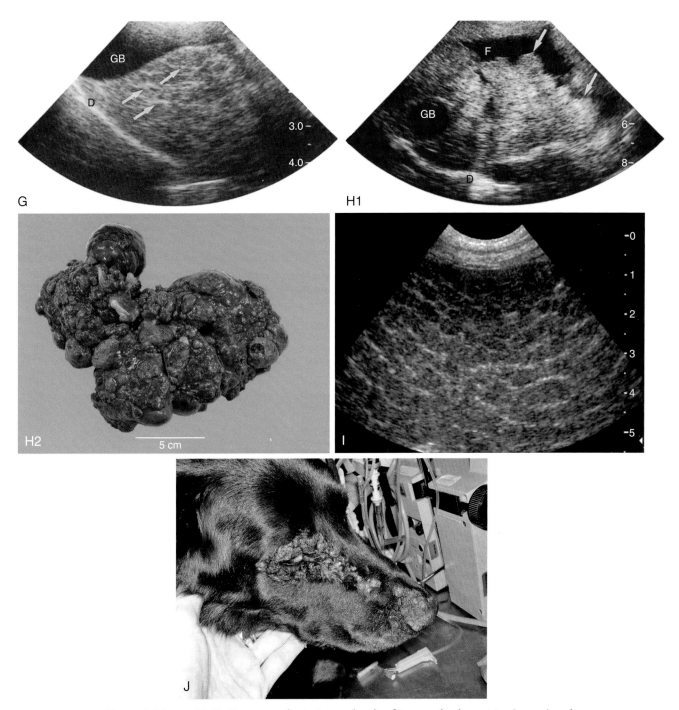

Figure 9-28, cont'd **G,** Hepatic cirrhosis. Linear bands of increased echogenicity (*arrows*) and reduced visualization of portal walls were noted in this dog with chronic hepatitis and cirrhosis of the liver. The size of the liver was also reduced, and the margins were irregular. **H,** Ultrasound **(H1)** and gross specimen **(H2)** of hepatic cirrhosis, with regenerative nodules. **I,** Canine superficial necrolytic dermatitis (hepatocutaneous syndrome). A unique honeycomb or Swiss cheese–like hepatic parenchymal pattern resembling cirrhosis is noted in the liver of this dog with canine superficial necrolytic dermatitis. The skin lesions, unique honeycomb parenchymal pattern, and normal to increased liver size differentiate this syndrome from hepatic cirrhosis **(G),** which may have a similar parenchymal pattern. **J,** Hepatocutaneous syndrome lesion on the muzzle of a dog. This dog also had lesions on the pads of his feet. *D,* Diaphragm; *GB,* gallbladder; *L,* liver. **(H2,** courtesy of Washington State University College of Veterinary Medicine, Washington Animal Disease Diagnostic Laboratory, Pullman, WA.)

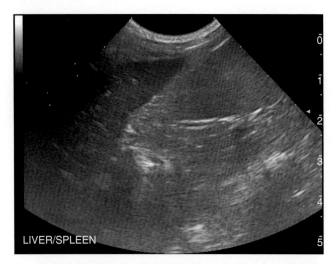

Figure 9-29 Comparison of a normal liver and spleen in a dog. The liver (*left*) is expected to be less echogenic and slightly more coarse in texture than the spleen (*right*). This comparison does not always hold true in cats.

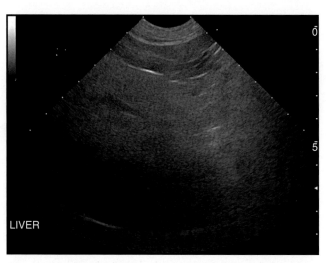

Figure 9-31 Hyperattenuating liver parenchyma in a dog with vacuolar hepatopathy (diabetic ketoacidosis). Noted the very fine texture and echogenicity in the near to middle portion of the liver, with rapid attenuation of the deeper liver tissue. In this small dog, operating at the low end of the transducer frequency range was insufficient to penetrate to a depth of 10 cm.

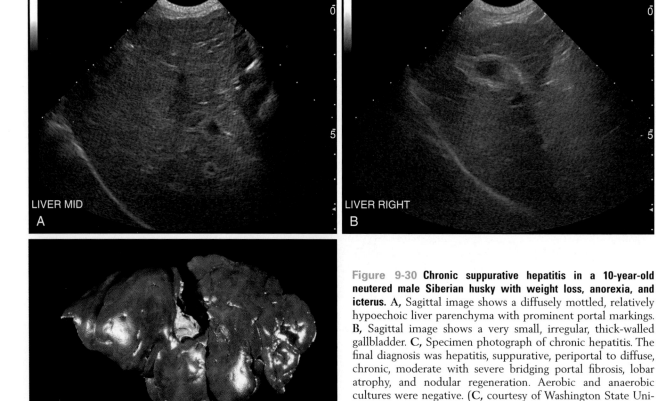

Figure 9-30 Chronic suppurative hepatitis in a 10-year-old neutered male Siberian husky with weight loss, anorexia, and icterus. A, Sagittal image shows a diffusely mottled, relatively hypoechoic liver parenchyma with prominent portal markings. **B,** Sagittal image shows a very small, irregular, thick-walled gallbladder. **C,** Specimen photograph of chronic hepatitis. The final diagnosis was hepatitis, suppurative, periportal to diffuse, chronic, moderate with severe bridging portal fibrosis, lobar atrophy, and nodular regeneration. Aerobic and anaerobic cultures were negative. (**C,** courtesy of Washington State University College of Veterinary Medicine, Washington Animal Disease Diagnostic Laboratory, Pullman, WA.)

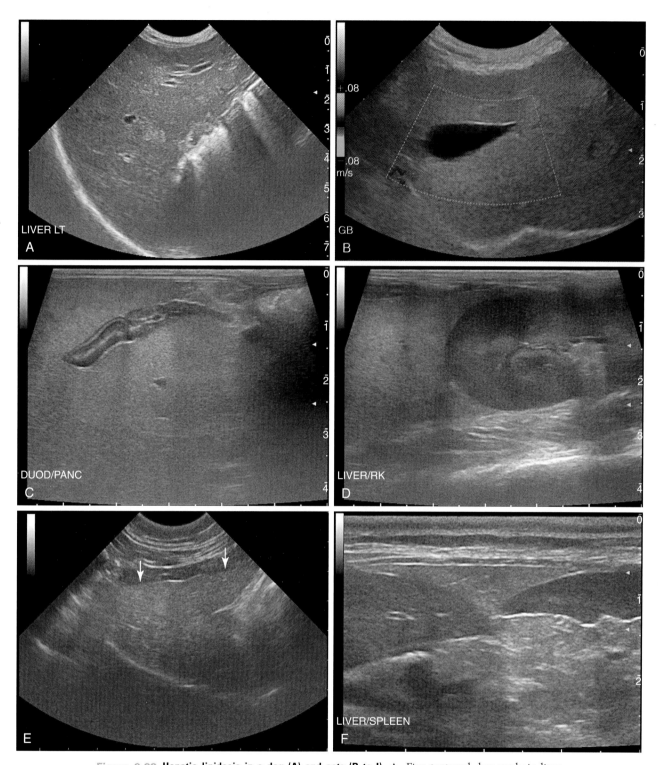

Figure 9-32 **Hepatic lipidosis in a dog (A) and cats (B to I).** **A,** Fine-textured, hyperechoic liver parenchyma in an elderly beagle with third-degree heart block. **B,** Very hyperechoic liver in a cat with severe lipidosis. Normal hepatic vasculature is not seen and not demonstrated with color Doppler analysis. **C,** Severe lipidosis in a cat, showing the enlarged liver wrapping around the duodenum ventrally and dorsally. **D,** Severe lipidosis showing very hyperechoic liver compared to the right kidney. **E,** Hyperechoic liver (*arrows*) contrasts nicely with hypoechoic adjacent near field falciform fat. **F,** Hyperechoic liver has become isoechoic to the adjacent spleen.

Continued

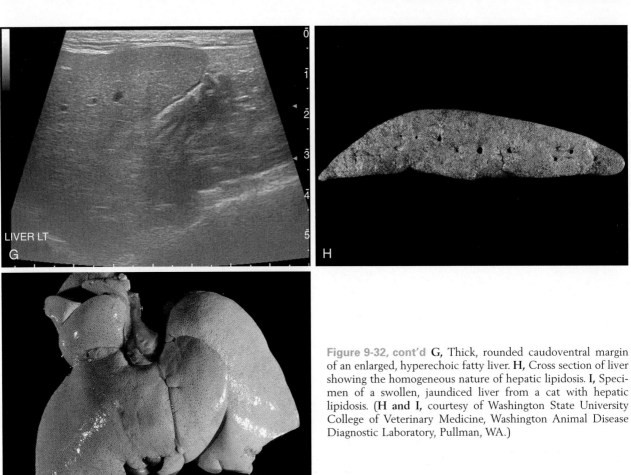

Figure 9-32, cont'd G, Thick, rounded caudoventral margin of an enlarged, hyperechoic fatty liver. H, Cross section of liver showing the homogeneous nature of hepatic lipidosis. I, Specimen of a swollen, jaundiced liver from a cat with hepatic lipidosis. (H and I, courtesy of Washington State University College of Veterinary Medicine, Washington Animal Disease Diagnostic Laboratory, Pullman, WA.)

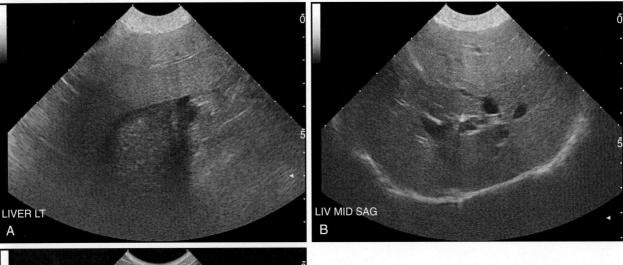

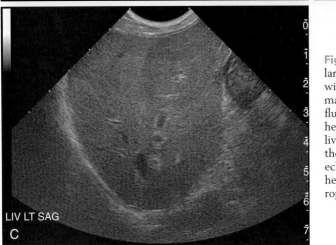

Figure 9-33 Steroid hepatopathy (vacuolar hepatopathy). A, Enlarged, hyperechoic, homogeneous hepatic parenchyma in a dog with a cortisol-secreting adrenal tumor. The thick ventral margin of the liver extends well beyond the stomach (echogenic fluid filled, central image). B, Transverse image of vacuolar hepatopathy in pituitary-dependent hyperadrenocorticism. The liver is diffusely hyperechoic. Note the anisotropism between the two liver lobes, in which the lobes are slightly different echogenicity. C, Sagittal image of liver from a dog with vacuolar hepatopathy showing a hyperechoic, fine texture. Note anisotropism of the two liver lobes.

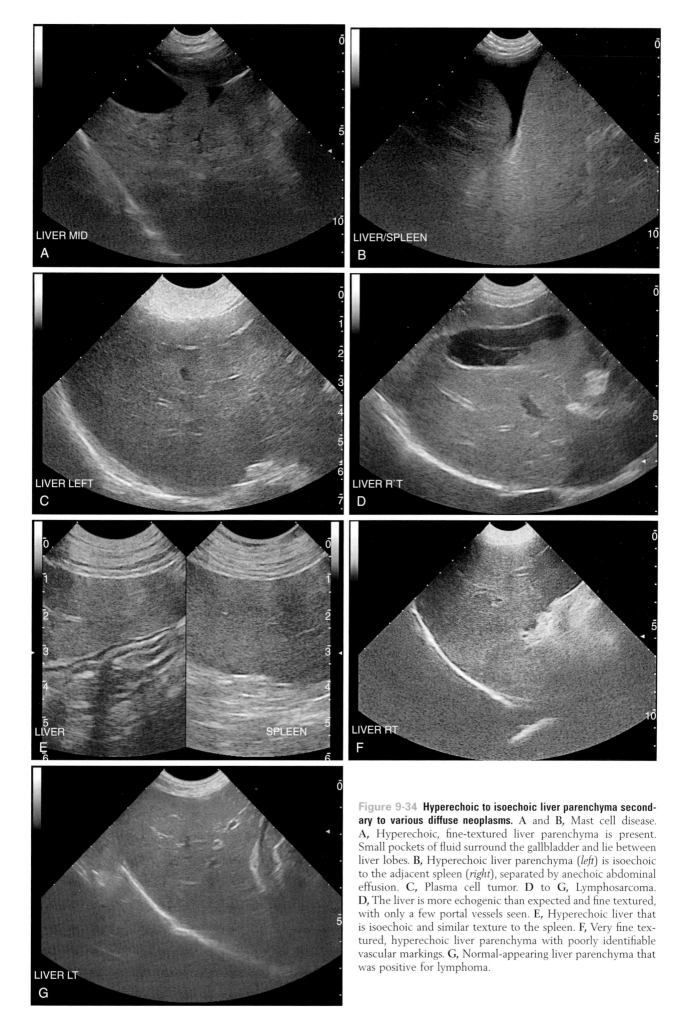

Figure 9-34 **Hyperechoic to isoechoic liver parenchyma secondary to various diffuse neoplasms.** A and B, Mast cell disease. A, Hyperechoic, fine-textured liver parenchyma is present. Small pockets of fluid surround the gallbladder and lie between liver lobes. B, Hyperechoic liver parenchyma (*left*) is isoechoic to the adjacent spleen (*right*), separated by anechoic abdominal effusion. C, Plasma cell tumor. D to G, Lymphosarcoma. D, The liver is more echogenic than expected and fine textured, with only a few portal vessels seen. E, Hyperechoic liver that is isoechoic and similar texture to the spleen. F, Very fine textured, hyperechoic liver parenchyma with poorly identifiable vascular markings. G, Normal-appearing liver parenchyma that was positive for lymphoma.

Inhomogeneous Echogenicity

A diffuse heterogeneous or mottled appearance to the liver is usually characterized by a hyperechoic parenchyma with poorly defined, hypoechoic nodules (Figure 9-35, A to C, E, and F), but hyperechoic nodules (see Figure 9-35, D) or both (see Figure 9-35, G) are also common. Discrete borders cannot be identified in many cases, and it may be difficult to determine whether the more echogenic or less echogenic areas, or both, are abnormal. This appearance is very common in our experience, perhaps even more so than a truly normal liver. This may be a result of using higher resolution equipment, but nonetheless it has afforded the opportunity to routinely sample the liver for cytology. Differential diagnoses for this appearance include vacuolar hepatopathy (see Figure 9-35, A to D) (including steroid hepatopathy and less commonly hepatic lipidosis), nodular hyperplasia, extramedullary hematopoiesis (see Figure 9-35, E and F), chronic hepatitis, fibrosis, toxic hepatopathy, and storage diseases.[147] Often, more than one disease process is present, such as chronic active hepatitis and nodular hyperplasia. The presence of abnormal bile, including sludge and mucoceles, is commonly associated with vacuolar hepatopathy in dogs. Diffuse neoplasia, such as lymphosarcoma, should also be considered, but it is a less common cause of this appearance; the liver in many hepatic lymphosarcoma cases appears perfectly normal. Figure 9-35, H, shows the appearance of a barely perceptible metastatic mammary adenocarcinoma. Hepatic size may be normal or enlarged. A liver biopsy is required for an accurate diagnosis.

Cholangitis/cholangiohepatitis complex in cats can result in hepatic parenchyma that is normal, hyperechoic, hypoechoic, or heterogeneous, and with hepatic size that is normal or increased.[160-162] Biliary abnormalities (thickened gallbladder wall; thickened, dilated, or tortuous bile duct) may also be present.

In cats with systemic amyloidosis, hepatomegaly with irregular liver margins and spontaneous liver rupture has been reported.[163] The hepatic parenchyma has a diffuse, heterogeneous echogenicity with highly echogenic (sparkling) areas and hypoechoic foci. In one report of a shar-pei diagnosed with amyloidosis, the liver appeared enlarged and hypoechoic.[164]

Superficial necrolytic dermatitis, also known as hepatocutaneous syndrome or metabolic epidermal necrosis, causes a unique honeycomb or Swiss cheese–like ultrasound pattern within the liver (see Figure 9-28, I) and characteristic skin lesions in older dogs.[165-168] Findings similar to superficial necrolytic dermatitis in dogs have also reported in cats.[169-171] The hepatic pattern consists of variably sized, hypoechoic regions in the liver, measuring 0.5 to 1.5 cm in diameter and surrounded by highly echogenic borders. Parakeratosis, superficial necrolysis, and basilar hyperplasia of the epidermis accompany the liver lesions. The cause of the disease is unknown, but skin lesions have been associated with diabetes mellitus, pancreatic atrophy and fibrosis, pancreatitis, and pancreatic glucagonoma. Hypoaminoacidemia appears to be a consistent finding.[166] The skin lesions, the unique honeycomb pattern in the liver parenchyma, and the normal to increased liver size help differentiate this syndrome from chronic cirrhosis. Cirrhosis is commonly characterized by a normal to small irregular liver and does not have the characteristic skin lesions or unique hepatic parenchymal pattern seen with superficial necrolytic dermatitis.

Pulsed Doppler Evaluation

Pulsed duplex Doppler ultrasound has also become more commonly used to assess diffuse liver disease in an attempt to partially overcome the shortcomings of conventional imaging. Doppler studies have been especially useful in evaluating the hemodynamics of portal venous flow associated with hepatic cirrhosis.[18,24] Portal blood flow velocity and portal blood flow were measured in dogs with experimentally induced hepatic cirrhosis and found to be approximately 50% of normal. Doppler ultrasound has the potential to provide functional information that may assist the clinician in determining the diagnosis, prognosis, and management of hepatic cirrhosis. The technique requires further evaluation in naturally occurring cases of cirrhosis (as well as in other diffuse liver diseases) before the clinical usefulness of the procedure can be assessed.

Quantitative Contrast Enhanced Imaging

Detecting diffuse liver disease with conventional ultrasound has always been very difficult. In most cases an ultrasound-guided liver aspiration or tissue-core biopsy is required. However, liver perfusion dynamics can be measured using ultrasound contrast agents with conventional ultrasonography or harmonic ultrasound. These procedures may eventually prove useful for evaluating dogs with various types of diffuse liver disease. The general principles and veterinary clinical applications of contrast-enhanced sonography have been recently reviewed.[127] Generation of time-intensity perfusion curves of the liver with assessment of a variety of parameters has been reported in normal dogs.[126,136,172,173] Diseases of the liver that affect the balance of hepatic arterial and portal venous blood flow should theoretically affect one or more of these baseline parameters and eventually prove useful for evaluation of diffuse liver disease.

GALLBLADDER AND BILIARY TRACT

Ultrasound can be used to evaluate structural abnormalities of the gallbladder, biliary inflammation, extrahepatic biliary obstruction, choleliths and choledocholiths, and neoplasia.

Congenital Disorders

Bilobed gallbladders are rare but have been reported most commonly in the cat[174] (Figure 9-36; see also Figure 4-8, D). A bilobed gallbladder is partially divided but has one cystic duct. Two types of bilobed gallbladders have been described. The first consists of a longitudinal septum dividing the gallbladder into two chambers that communicate at the proximal end with one cystic duct. This type appears normal when viewed externally. In the second type, the fundus of the gallbladder is completely divided, but the portions are fused at the neck. This type of bilobed gallbladder appears V-shaped externally. A duplex gallbladder having two cystic ducts may also occur but appears to be less common.[175]

Nonobstructive cystic dilatation of intrahepatic bile ducts has been described in dogs.[57,58] This disorder generally causes saccular biliary ductal dilatation and may predispose the patient to bacterial cholangitis and stone formation. Polycystic kidney disease may also be present.

The absence of a gallbladder is a rare condition that has been reported in dogs.[176,177] This abnormality must be differentiated from severe fibrosis of the gallbladder wall preventing normal distention. With fibrosis, the gallbladder is extremely small and the lumen is not seen. However, the thickened wall can usually be visualized as a small, hypoechoic oval in the normal location of the gallbladder.

Gallbladder Wall Thickening

The normal gallbladder wall is poorly visualized or appears as a thin echogenic line (Figure 9-37; see also Figure 9-3, B). The thickness of the wall depends on angulation of the sound beam and degree of distention. Measurement is most accurate when the beam is directed at right angles to the near wall.

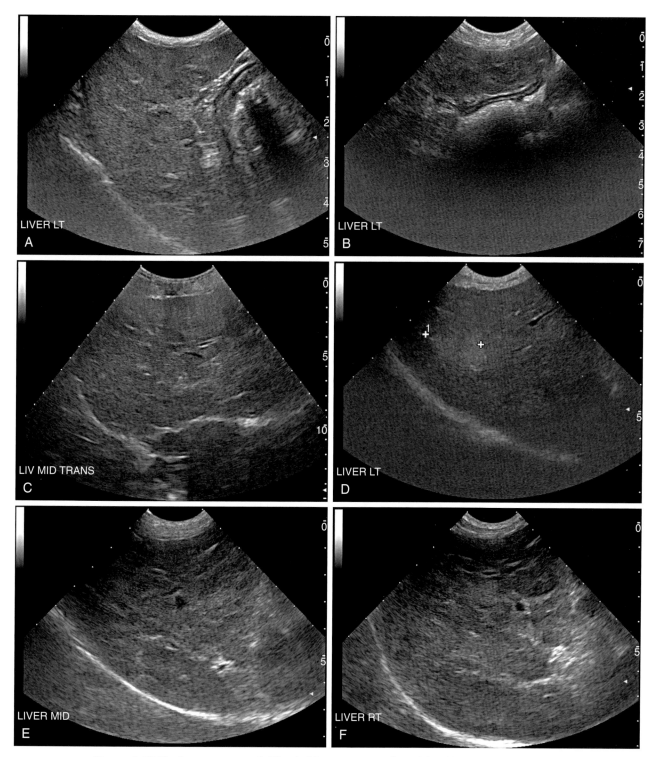

Figure 9-35 **Varying appearance of diffusely inhomogeneous echogenicity of liver parenchyma: vacuolar hepatopathy (A to D), extramedullary hematopoiesis (E to G), and metastatic mammary carcinoma (H to I). A,** Inhomogeneous hepatic parenchyma characterized by multiple poorly defined hypoechoic nodules within otherwise hyperechoic liver tissue. **B,** Sagittal image of the caudoventral liver margin showing multiple hypoechoic nodules and an enlarged liver extending ventral and caudal to the stomach. **C,** Transverse image showing multiple poorly defined hypoechoic nodules. **D,** A hyperechoic nodule is denoted by the electronic cursors (2.14 cm). **E,** Inhomogeneous liver parenchyma with multiple poorly defined areas of hypoechogenicity in a dog with extramedullary hematopoiesis (EMH). **F,** Poorly defined hypoechoic nodules and a lumpy, irregular margin are present in this dog with EMH.   *Continued*

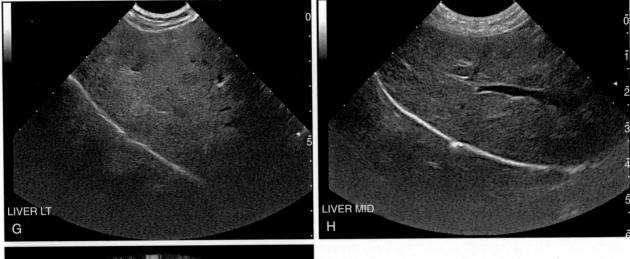

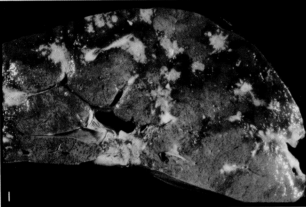

Figure 9-35, cont'd G, Against a backdrop of hyperechoic, fine-textured liver parenchyma, there are multiple poorly defined hypoechoic and hyperechoic nodules in this dog with EMH. H, Essentially normal appearance of liver parenchyma in a dog with proven metastatic mammary carcinoma in the liver, spleen, and lymph nodes. I, Liver specimen shows metastasis with irregular margins, different from the more common smoothly marginated nodules. This may be one explanation for poor conspicuity of some parenchymal lesions, as in this case. (I, courtesy of Washington State University College of Veterinary Medicine, Washington Animal Disease Diagnostic Laboratory, Pullman, WA.)

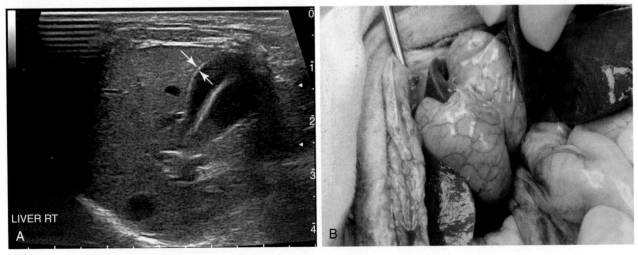

Figure 9-36 Bilobed normal gallbladder in a cat. A, Transverse image of the bilobed gallbladder. Note the very thin wall (<1 mm between arrows) and the thick echogenic septum dividing the gallbladder. B, Photograph of the gallbladder during surgery.

Normal thickness in dogs is reported in one study[12] as 2 to 3 mm; in another, it was found to be approximately 1 to 2 mm.[178] In cats, normal wall thickness is reported to be less than 1 mm (see Figures 9-36, *A*, and 4-8, *C* and *D*).[13] In our experience, most normal gallbladders in both dogs and cats are less than 1 mm. When using a high resolution transducer under ideal conditions, thickened gallbladder walls may appear layered, with a hypoechoic central layer surrounded by thin hyperechoic layers (double rim). This should be differentiated from a halo appearance that can occur when a small amount of perigallbladder fluid accumulates (Figure 9-38). Closer inspection usually reveals a thin wall surrounded by fluid. The sonographer should be careful not to mistake this artifact with true wall thickening.

Diffuse thickening of the gallbladder wall is a nonspecific abnormality, caused by both primary gallbladder disease and secondary involvement of the gallbladder by systemic disease.[12,13,42,43,52,179-185] Primary gallbladder diseases resulting in increased wall thickness include acute and chronic cholecystitis, and cholangiohepatitis (Figure 9-39). In almost all cases there is concurrent abnormal echogenic bile. Systemic disease, including hepatitis (with cirrhosis), right-sided congestive heart failure (increased central venous pressure), portal hypertension, hypoproteinemia, and anaphylaxis, can also result in diffuse wall thickening (Figure 9-40). Adjacent inflammation, such as pancreatitis, may result in a secondary gallbladder involvement and wall thickening.

The pathophysiology of gallbladder wall thickening is most likely a combination of decreased intravascular osmotic pressure and increased portal venous pressure resulting in edema of the gallbladder wall.[12,183] Lymphatics in the gallbladder may be grossly visible during portal hypertension, chronic passive congestion, or hepatobiliary inflammation. Fluid leaked from these lymphatics can contribute to the ultrasonographic appearance of gallbladder wall thickening. More chronic gallbladder inflammation may result in a thickened, less layered, hyperechoic, irregular wall. Diffuse hyperechogenicity of the gallbladder wall can occur with mineralization secondary to inflammatory disease (see Figure 9-39, *G*), hypoalbuminemia, (see Figure 9-40, *B* and *C*), right-sided heart failure (see Figure 9-40, *D*), and neoplasia.[12,13,179-181,186-188] A small amount of free fluid around the gallbladder may mimic gallbladder wall thickening (see Figure 9-38).

Biliary Sludge and Calculi

Biliary sludge is echogenic material that accumulates within the gallbladder lumen; it consists of conglomerates of calcium bilirubinate and cholesterol suspended in mucin-rich bile.[185,189] The amount of sediment or echogenic bile within the gallbladder is variable and is seen in apparently healthy, nonfasting animals or those with biliary stasis from fasting or illness. The cause and clinical significance of sediment are not fully understood. One study concluded that sludge was not particularly related to hepatobiliary disease and should be considered an incidental finding.[10] However, sludge can occur in association with hepatobiliary disease and may indicate biliary stasis. This seems to be particularly true in cats. Gallbladder motility can be determined by measuring the gallbladder volume (length × width × height at largest dimension × 0.53). If the

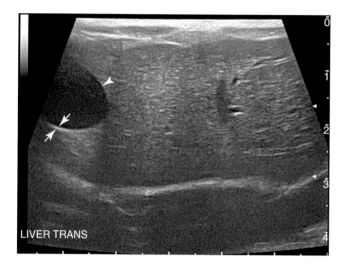

Figure 9-37 Normal gallbladder in a dog. Transverse image of the liver and gallbladder in a dog. The near field gallbladder wall cannot be seen as a discrete entity because it is normally very thin (*arrowhead*). In the far field, it is seen a very thin echogenic curved line (between arrows), visualized because of through transmission of bile (cystlike behavior).

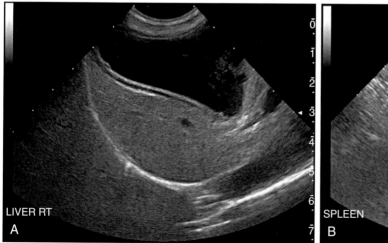
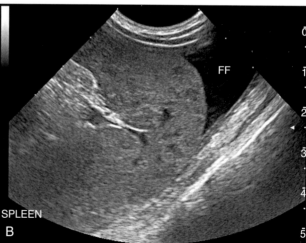

Figure 9-38 Perigallbladder fluid mimicking gallbladder wall thickening. A, Thin anechoic rim around the gallbladder should not be mistaken for gallbladder wall thickening. **B,** Image of the same dog with anechoic peritoneal fluid (*FF*) surrounding the spleen, adjacent to the left body wall. This dog had splenic and hepatic lymphoma.

gallbladder volume is less than 1 mL/kg body weight, normal gallbladder contractility is assumed. If the volume is greater than this, contractility can be determined by measuring the ejection fraction using gallbladder volumes before and at timed intervals after a test meal. Normal percent contractility is higher than 25%.[9,11,184] In a recent study, dogs with biliary sludge (mobile, nonmobile, and mucocele) had a reduction in gallbladder ejection fraction and elevation of gallbladder volume compared to normal healthy dogs without biliary

sludge.[11] These dogs had diminished gallbladder motor function and cholestasis. Impaired gallbladder emptying with subsequent cholestasis may have pathologic effects on the gallbladder through prolonged exposure to concentrated bile.[11] In the majority of cases, biliary sediment does not shadow (Figures 9-41, *A* to *E*, and 9-42, *A*). On occasion, some shadowing is present, but discrete calculi are not identified. Shadowing sediment can be evaluated for calculi by repositioning the animal or using gentle transducer agitation

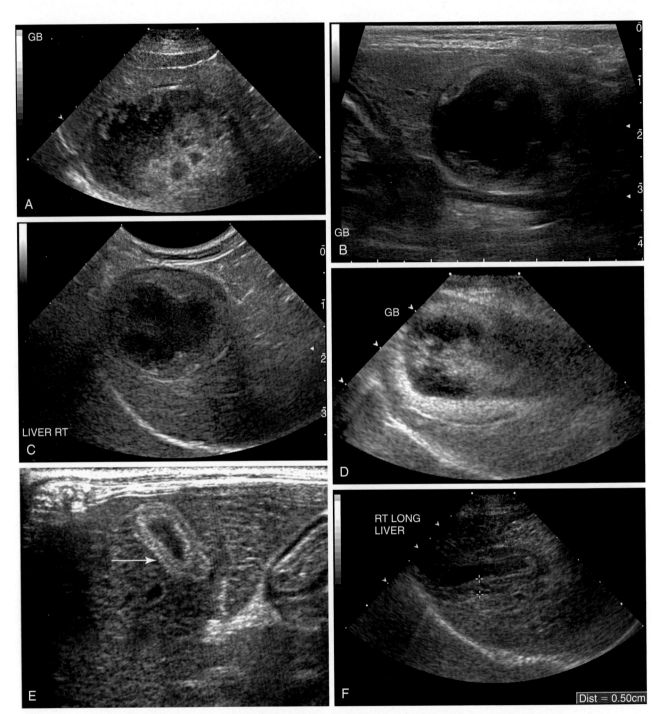

Figure 9-39 **Gallbladder wall changes with cholecystitis.** **A,** Irregular, thickened gallbladder wall, with a polypoid appearance. A large amount of echogenic bile has settled out, obscuring the far-field wall. **B** and **C,** Irregular gallbladder wall thickening with *Escherichia coli* cholecystitis. **D** to **F,** Chronic cholecystitis. In severe chronic cholecystitis or cholangiohepatitis, fibrosis of the gallbladder wall (arrow in **E**) may prevent normal distention (**F**).

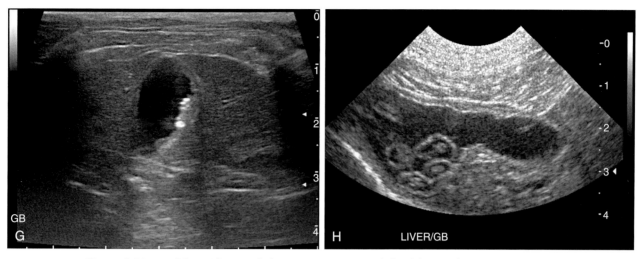

Figure 9-39, cont'd G, Chronic cholecystitis in a cat. Multifocal hyperechoic areas represent minerals, either as lodged calculi or mineralization within the wall. **H,** Gallbladder wall thickening secondary to presence of liver flukes.

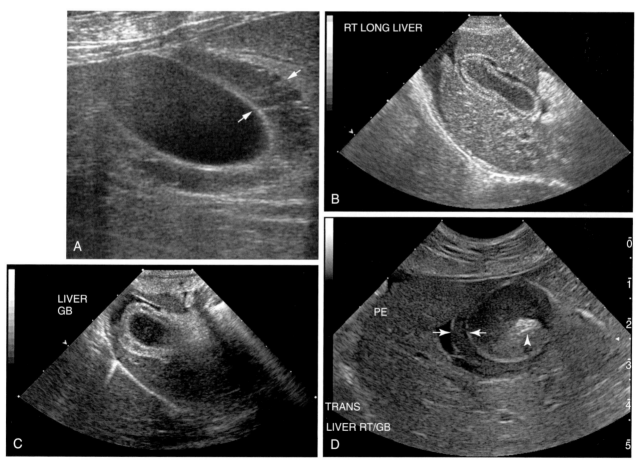

Figure 9-40 Gallbladder wall thickening from edema. A, Hypoechoic gallbladder wall thickening (*arrows*) in experimentally induced acute right-sided heart failure. **B** and **C,** Hyperechoic gallbladder wall thickening in two cases of hypoalbuminemia. Peritoneal fluid is noted. **D,** Thickened gallbladder wall (between arrows) in a patient with a large cholelith (*arrowhead*) and pericardial effusion with resultant right-sided heart failure.

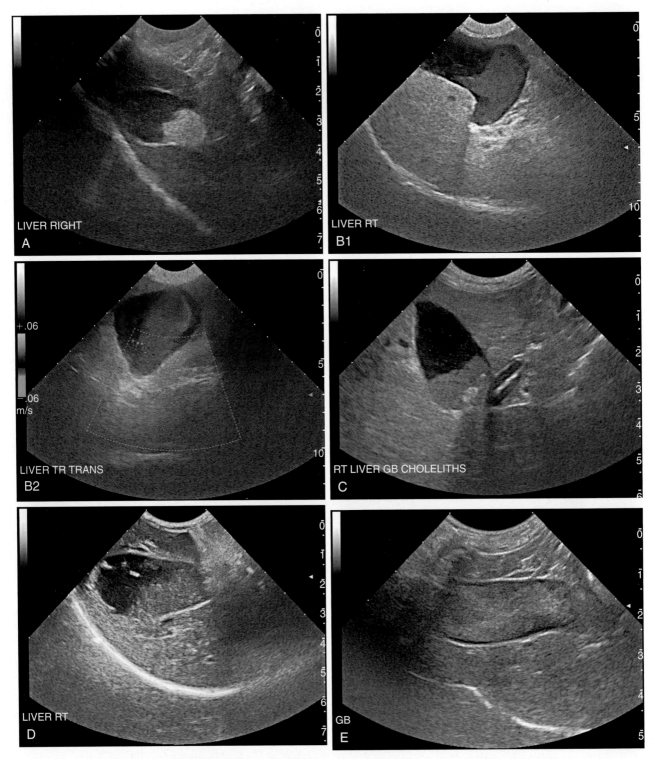

Figure 9-41 Various appearances of gallbladder sediment (sludge). A, Gravity dependent, highly echogenic gallbladder sludge, often termed a sludge ball if it does not disperse upon repositioning or ballottement. **B1** and **B2, Biliary sludge. B1,** Echogenic, gravity dependent biliary sludge. **B2,** Erroneous color Doppler signal within the sludge, caused by high sensitivity of Doppler setting and patient motion. This should not be mistaken for a vascularized gallbladder mass. **C,** Biliary sludge and calculus in a 13-year-old neutered male miniature schnauzer undergoing abdominal ultrasound screening because of a grade III cutaneous mast cell tumor. Note mild acoustic shadowing created by the calculus. **D,** Gravity dependent hyperechoic biliary sludge with small strands of echogenic, nondependent bile in an older beagle with hepatic lipidosis. **E,** Echogenic bile fills the gallbladder lumen in this older Pomeranian. Ballottement induced a slow swirling motion of the bile. Hepatic lipidosis was diagnosed via cytology of the liver.

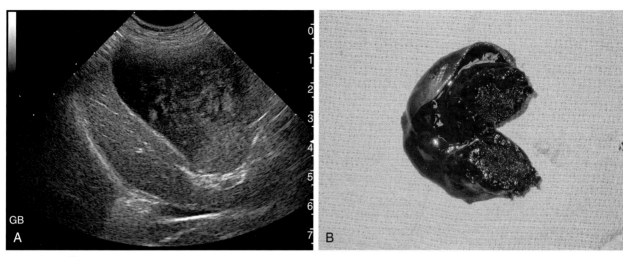

▶ **Figure 9-42 Biliary sludge and cholecystitis in a dog with persistent elevation of liver enzymes.**
A, Sagittal image shows gravity dependent nature of the echogenic, heterogeneous bile, resembling a mucocele. **B,** Surgical specimen obtained after cholecystectomy shows the unhealthy appearance of the gallbladder wall and inspissated bile (not a mucocele). *Escherichia coli* was cultured.

on the ventral abdomen to suspend the sediment. So-called sludge balls have been observed within dog gallbladders. These balls, which may disappear on subsequent examinations or persist for prolonged periods (Figure 9-43, *A*; see also Figure 9-41, *A*), are round, mobile, nonshadowing echogenicities of uncertain cause and significance. Multiple views or examinations are sometimes required to demonstrate their mobility. Unless there is movement to the dependent portion of the gallbladder, they cannot be reliably distinguished from attached polyps or pedunculated tumors.[13] Fortunately, sessile or polypoid lesions caused by mucous gland hyperplasia or adenocarcinomas are extremely rare in the dog and cat. The entire gallbladder occasionally becomes full of sludge and simulates a solid parenchymal mass (see Figure 9-41, *E*). The correct diagnosis is facilitated when the normal gallbladder cannot be identified in this region.

Cholelithiasis (gallbladder calculi) and choledocholithiasis (calculi in the bile duct) are often incidental findings. However, biliary obstruction secondary to cholelithiasis can occur, especially in cats. Etiologies for cholelithiasis and choledocholithiasis include biliary stasis, altered bile composition, cholecystitis, dietary factors, biliary parasites, and bacterial infections.[185,190-196] Cholangiohepatitis is often associated with feline cholelithiasis and may be a predisposing factor in the pathogenesis.[190]

In both dogs and cats, choleliths commonly contain mixtures of calcium (calcium carbonate, calcium bilirubinate), cholesterol, and bilirubin.[185,191,197] This may allow them to be visible on survey abdominal radiographs.[198] Dogs or cats with cholelithiasis may have clinical signs of vomiting, anorexia, weakness, polyuria and polydipsia, weight loss, icterus, fever, and abdominal pain.[185,190,194-196] Gallbladder perforation can occur secondary to cholecystitis and cholelithiasis.[175,199,200] The stones shift to the dependent portion of the gallbladder when the animal is repositioned (see Figure 9-43). Distal acoustic shadowing is present and becomes more evident as the size and calcium content of the calculus increase (see Figure 9-43, *C*, *D*, and *F*). Placing the stone within the focal zone of the transducer and using a high-frequency transducer maximize shadowing. Choledocholiths may be difficult to detect because of interference from bowel gas. Bile duct calculi in cats are more easily visualized, because this anatomy is more consistently identified compared to the dog.[201] Differential diagnosis of shadowing lesions within the liver must include fibrosis,

dystrophic calcification, foreign bodies, and gas. Abdominal radiography or computed tomography may be necessary for a final determination.

Cholecystitis

Acute cholecystitis may have a variety of sonographic appearances (Figure 9-44, see also Figures 9-39 and 9-42). The gallbladder wall may thicken, and the presence or absence of cholelithiasis and the character of biliary sludge are variable. Pain may be detected in the gallbladder region during scanning.[202,203] This has been referred to as the sonographic Murphy sign.[204,205] The use of color Doppler sonography for the evaluation of acute cholecystitis in the dog has been reported in an animal model.[206] Lack of flow was seen early in acute cholecystitis in some animals, but flow later returned and even increased in some of the more severe cases.

Cholangitis/cholangiohepatitis complex is the second most common form of hepatic disease in cats and the most common inflammatory disease.[185,207] In many feline cases, no ultrasound abnormalities are present. However, when present, ultrasound findings include thickened gallbladder wall, biliary sludge, choleliths or choledocholiths, and thickened, tortuous, and sometimes dilated bile duct (Figure 9-45).[110,161,185,190,208,209] These changes can accompany all forms of feline cholangitis/cholangiohepatitis. Dilation may be due to obstruction secondary to a bile duct calculus (choledocholith), biliary sludge, or may simply be bile stasis secondary to inflammation. The liver parenchyma may be normal, enlarged, hypoechoic, heterogeneous, or hyperechoic (possibly due to lipidosis). Pancreatitis and inflammatory bowel disease are often present concurrently, and they may occur because of the unique feline biliary anatomy, where the bile duct and pancreatic duct enter the duodenum together at the major duodenal papilla.

Emphysematous cholecystitis (gas secondary to gas-forming organisms within the wall, lumen of the gallbladder, or pericholecystic tissues) is a form of acute cholecystitis associated with diabetes mellitus, traumatic ischemia, mucocele formation, and neoplasia (see Figure 9-44, *D*).[185,210,211] Gallbladder wall thickening, with increased echogenicity of the wall or lumen, and "dirty" shadowing with reverberation echoes secondary to intraluminal or intramural gas formation can be seen. Intraluminal gas rises to the nondependent portions of the gallbladder, allowing differentiation from shadowing

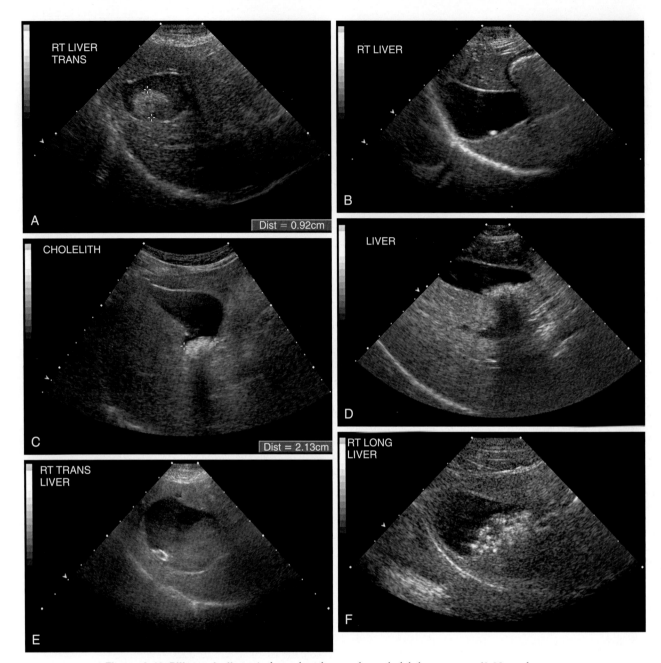

Figure 9-43 Biliary calculi. A, A dependent hyperechoic cholelith is present (0.92 cm between electronic cursors). Note that there are echoes present within the entire calculus and there is no acoustic shadowing. This indicates lack of calcium and probably a high cholesterol content. **B,** A small, solitary cholelith is identified, without acoustic shadowing (due to small size and lack of calcium content). **C,** A large cholelith (2.13 cm between electronic cursors) is seen in the dependent portion of the gallbladder, with acoustic shadowing. This could also represent a collection of smaller calculi. The patient should be repositioned to differentiate the two. **D,** Collection of multiple small choleliths, with acoustic shadowing. These were dispersible on repositioning the patient. **E,** A small cholelith with a thin echogenic rim is present within echogenic gravity dependent sediment. There is no acoustic shadowing. **F,** A collection of multiple small choleliths with acoustic shadowing in a cat. In all of these examples the gallbladder wall was considered to be of normal thickness.

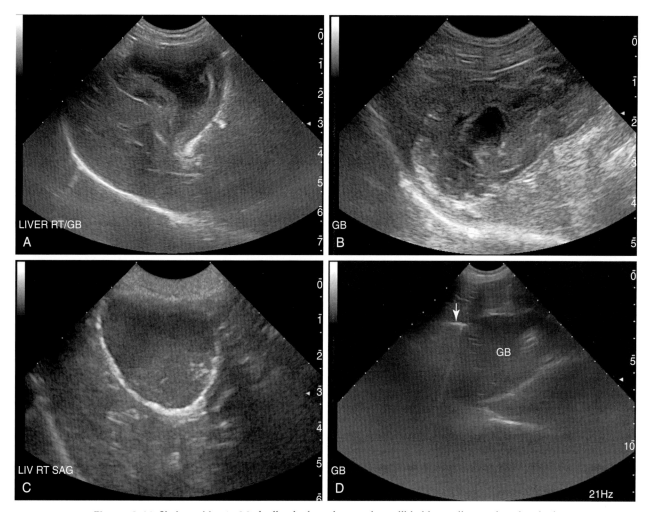

Figure 9-44 Cholecystitis. A, Markedly thickened, irregular gallbladder wall in a dog that had surgery several days prior for gastric torsion. *Serratia marcescens* was cultured following cholecystectomy. **B,** Severely thickened gallbladder and echogenic bile. Cholecystectomy was performed. Culture was negative for both aerobic and anaerobic bacteria. Histology showed chronic, severe fibrosis with histiocytic inflammation and hemorrhage, and moderate diffuse muscosal hyperplasia. The liver was also abnormal with centrilobular hepatitis and biliary hyperplasia. **C,** *Escherichia coli* cholecystitis in an 8-year-old Lhasa apso with lethargy and decreased appetite for several months and increased liver enzymes. **D,** Emphysematous gallbladder from *E. coli* infection, with a gas cap noted (*arrow*).

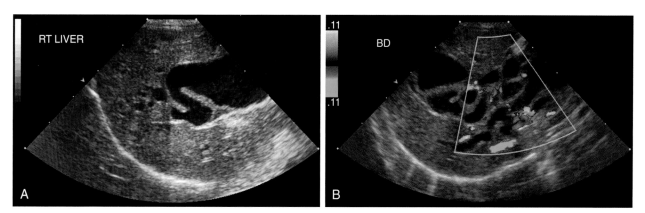

Figure 9-45 Feline cholangitis/cholangiohepatitis complex. A, Dilated gallbladder and cystic duct with surrounding hyperechoic liver parenchyma. **B,** Color Doppler analysis was used to verify the presence of dilated intrahepatic bile ducts, seen as anechoic tubular structures among normal hepatic blood vessels.

sludge or calculi that gravitate to the dependent portion. The presence of gas in the gallbladder region can be confirmed on abdominal radiography or computed tomography.[212-214]

Gangrenous or necrotizing cholecystitis is a form of acute cholecystitis characterized by marked wall irregularity, thickening (may be asymmetric), or discontinuous wall with pericholecystic fluid accumulation. Necrotizing cholecystitis may be secondary to ischemia, ulceration, hemorrhage, or necrosis of the gallbladder wall.[185,215,216] Intraluminal membranes resulting from fibrinous strands or exudate may also be present, but the amount of biliary sludge is variable. Perforation may occur in up to 10% of human cases,[217] and perforation has also been reported in dogs.[200,218] The surgical treatment for this disorder has been described in the dog.[215]

Chronic cholecystitis usually presents in a less acute form than acute cholecystitis, but symmetric or asymmetric thickening of the gallbladder wall is still seen (see Figures 9-39, D

to F, and 9-44, B and C). Permanent thickening occurs in chronic disorders because of inflammation and fibrosis. Mineralization of the gallbladder wall has also been described (see Figure 9-39, G).[146] Polyps may also occur with chronic inflammation.[187] (see Figure 9-39, A to E). In severe cases, fibrosis may prevent normal distention of the gallbladder (see Figure 9-39, E and F). This may make the gallbladder extremely difficult to locate. Calculi may be present in the gallbladder or biliary tract.

Gallbladder Mucocele

Gallbladder mucoceles are an important cause of hepatobiliary disease in dogs, and they have been recognized with increased frequency over the past several years (Figures 9-46 to 9-48). The etiology of gallbladder mucocele in dogs is unknown, but numerous mechanisms are likely involved. These include impairment of a protective mechanism on the

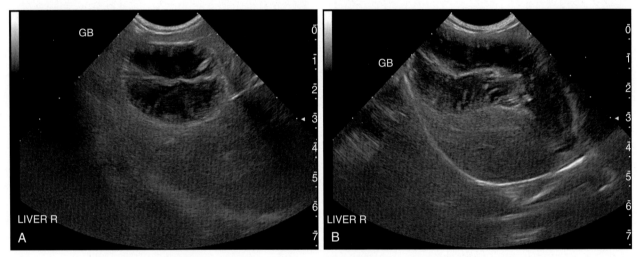

Figure 9-46 **Gallbladder mucocele in a 13-year-old neutered male cockapoo with nonspecific signs and elevated liver enzymes. A,** Transverse image shows echogenic, radiating striations of bile interspersed with anechoic areas. The gallbladder wall is echogenic but thin. No motion of the bile was detected and the contents remained suspended. **B,** Sagittal image of the gallbladder mucocele in **A.**

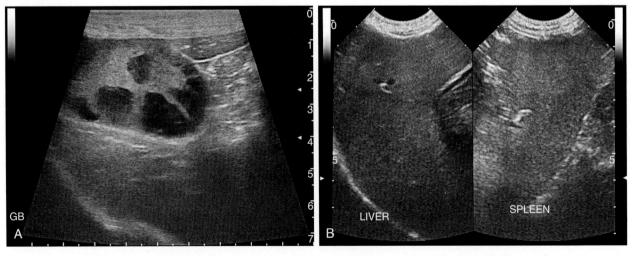

Figure 9-47 **Gallbladder mucocele in a dog with hepatic lipidosis. A,** Mucocele. **B,** Dual ultrasound images show the liver parenchyma (*left*) to be abnormally hyperechoic, fine textured, and homogeneous. Its appearance is identical to that of the spleen (*right*).

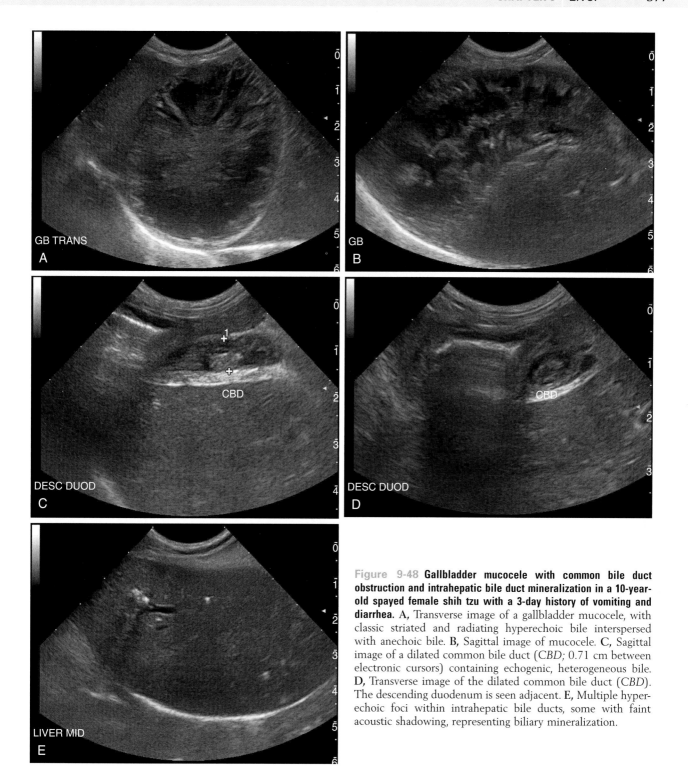

Figure 9-48 **Gallbladder mucocele with common bile duct obstruction and intrahepatic bile duct mineralization in a 10-year-old spayed female shih tzu with a 3-day history of vomiting and diarrhea. A,** Transverse image of a gallbladder mucocele, with classic striated and radiating hyperechoic bile interspersed with anechoic bile. **B,** Sagittal image of mucocele. **C,** Sagittal image of a dilated common bile duct (*CBD*; 0.71 cm between electronic cursors) containing echogenic, heterogeneous bile. **D,** Transverse image of the dilated common bile duct (*CBD*). The descending duodenum is seen adjacent. **E,** Multiple hyperechoic foci within intrahepatic bile ducts, some with faint acoustic shadowing, representing biliary mineralization.

gallbladder epithelium against bile acids, with secondary mucinous hyperplasia and increased mucin secretion; primary or secondary disorders of gallbladder motility with retention of bile; a secondary complication of dyslipidemias; and primary disorders of mucus-secreting cells with prolonged contact of the gallbladder mucosa to abnormal bile.[11,185,219-221] The odds of a biliary mucocele developing in dogs with hyperadrenocorticism are 29 times that of dogs without hyperadrenocorticism.[222] Some reports have suggested that mucoceles are associated with cholecystitis,[219,223,224] whereas others have

reported minimal evidence of a bacterial or inflammatory etiology, or necrosis of the gallbladder wall as the primary abnormality.[225,226] Mucoceles may be associated with extrahepatic biliary obstruction (see Figure 9-48), gallbladder wall necrosis, and perforation (Figure 9-49).[219,223-225,227] Clinical signs, although sometimes absent, include abdominal pain, inappetence, fever, vomiting, and icterus. Cats have fewer mucus-secreting glands in their gallbladder, which may explain why mucoceles do not develop.[228] However, one case of a possible feline gallbladder mucocele has been reported.[229] On

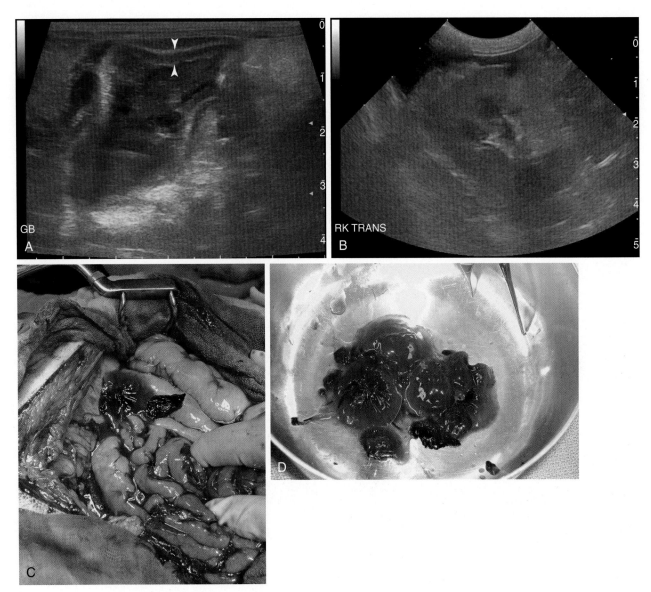

Figure 9-49 Gallbladder rupture from mucocele formation and peritonitis in a 17-year-old spayed female cocker spaniel mix that was severely debilitated and having seizures. **A,** Nearly unrecognizable gallbladder is present, misshapen, with heterogeneous echogenic bile, an irregular wall (between arrowheads), and perigallbladder fluid accumulation. There is acoustic enhancement and poor detail of the surrounding tissue. **B,** Peritoneal fluid surrounds the right kidney, covered with thick echogenic tissue. **C,** Intraoperative photograph of a ruptured gallbladder and bile peritonitis. **D,** Mucocele recovered from peritoneal cavity.

ultrasound examination, mucoceles are characterized by the presence of granular, organized, and centralized non–gravity dependent biliary sludge or intraluminal masses that do not move with changes in the patient's position (see Figures 9-46 to 9-48). There is often a stellate or kiwi-like pattern to the sludge (transverse image) caused by fracture lines between mucus collections. Gallbladder distention, with a hypoechoic rim adjacent to the gallbladder wall or thickening of the gallbladder wall is typically present. Biliary obstruction secondary to extension of abnormal mucus into the cystic duct, extrahepatic ducts, and common bile duct is often identified (see Figure 9-48).[219,223-227] Exploratory surgery for possible cholecystectomy, with or without lavage of the biliary tree, or cholecystoduodenostomy has been recommended. Nonsurgical resolution of gallbladder mucocele has also been reported.[225,227,230]

Gallbladder Rupture

Gallbladder rupture may occur secondary to a variety of gallbladder diseases (Figure 9-50; see also Figure 9-49). Ultrasound detection of wall rupture in dogs with mucocele is reported to have a 85.7 % sensitivity, with a specificity of 100% (see Figures 9-49 and 9-50, *A*).[225] In dogs with more inclusive types of gallbladder disease, ultrasound had a sensitivity of 94.4% and a specificity of 44.4%. It appears to be more difficult to identify a rent in the gallbladder wall without an extruding mucocele or mucocele free in the peritoneum.[226] Ultrasonographic signs of gallbladder rupture include echogenic fluid around the gallbladder, diffuse echogenic peritoneal fluid, adjacent hyperechoic fat, inability to confirm gallbladder wall continuity, and the presence of a mucocele, either protruding from the gallbladder wall or free in the peritoneal cavity.[224-226]

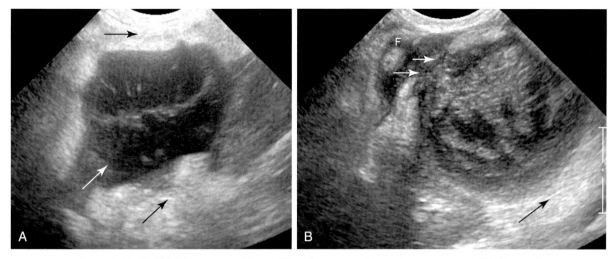

Figure 9-50 Gallbladder rupture (**A** and **B**) is characterized by a discontinuous gallbladder wall (*white arrows*), hyperechoic inflamed surrounding fat (*black arrows*), and associated free fluid (*F*). **A**, Rupture secondary to mucocele formation. **B**, Rupture secondary to necrotizing cholecystitis.

Cholecystocentesis

Ultrasound-guided cholecystocentesis can be performed to obtain bile samples for culture and cytology, and has been used to relieve gallbladder distension caused by pancreatitis-induced extrahepatic biliary obstruction.[185,209,231-233] Both transhepatic and direct fundic (transperitoneal) approaches to the gallbladder have been reported. A small amount of fluid was noted adjacent to the gallbladder after a direct fundic approach in one study in normal cats, but no significant complications were noted with either approach.[232] A transhepatic approach to the gallbladder is preferred by many to attempt to isolate any potential bile leakage. One report from the human medical literature indicated that a transhepatic approach was preferred if ascites was present or there were superimposed bowel loops. This approach can also be used to increase stability of the needle.[234] A transperitoneal approach was preferred if a coagulopathy or liver disease was present. Typically a 22-gauge needle is used, and an effort should be made to empty the gallbladder completely, again to minimize bile leakage. A lethal vasovagal response is a potential complication, along with bile leakage, hemorrhage, hemobilia, and bacteremia.[185,235] We commonly aspirate bile for cytology and culture, without complications. However, we do not aspirate bile in cases of suspect gallbladder mucocele for fear of rupture because of the often thin, friable gallbladder wall.

Extrahepatic Biliary Obstruction

Biliary obstruction is reliably detected by ultrasonography, scintigraphy, MRI, or CT.[193,196,236-241] However, ultrasonography is more commonly used to diagnose extrahepatic biliary obstruction in animals because it is more widely available. Ultrasonography is useful in distinguishing biliary obstruction from hepatocellular disease in clinically icteric animals when the serum biochemical findings are equivocal.[15,42,43,185,193,201,223,242-245] Causes of biliary obstruction are numerous and include pancreatitis, biliary calculi (Figure 9-51), gallbladder mucocele, and neoplasia of the liver, biliary system, or adjacent organs. Granulomas, abscesses, or lymphadenopathy in adjacent structures may obstruct the common bile duct. Biliary obstruction has resulted from duodenal foreign bodies.[246] The ultrasound findings depend on the duration and completeness of obstruction. A normal ultrasound examination finding does not necessarily rule out obstruction.

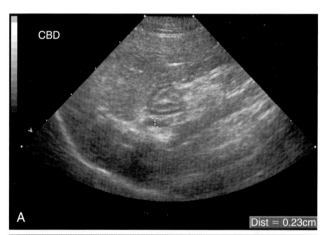
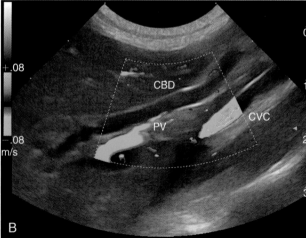

Figure 9-51 **Normal cat common bile duct. A,** Transverse image of the descending duodenum is shown with a cross-section of the common bile duct (*CBD*) seen between electronic cursors (0.23 cm). **B,** Sagittal image of the common bile duct (*CBD*). The use of color Doppler analysis allows differentiation from the adjacent portal vein (*PV*) and the caudal vena cava (*CVC*).

Ductal dilation may be insufficient for detection or be hidden by bowel gas. Identification of the bile duct at the porta hepatis is a helpful window, but this area can sometimes be obscured by stomach and bowel gas.

The diameter of the common bile duct in normal dogs is less than 3 mm.[14] The common duct may be seen under optimal conditions to have parallel echogenic walls, approximately 2 to 3 mm apart ventral to the main portal vein. Usually only visible when dilated, the bile duct can be identified ventral to the portal vein in a transverse intercostal view at the dorsal aspect of the right 11th or 12th intercostal space. The normal bile duct is more consistently visualized in cats with the right intercostal or ventral oblique window.[15] The diameter of the common bile duct in normal cats has been reported to be 4 mm or less (Figure 9-52; see also Figure 9-3, K and L).[15]

In dogs, dilation of the biliary tract progresses retrogradely after complete common hepatic duct obstruction.[242-244] In dogs, one of the first indications of complete obstruction is marked gallbladder distension. This finding may be less common in cats because only 38%,[247] 62%,[248] and 43%[201] of cats with duct obstruction were reported to have gallbladder dilation. If the gallbladder is enlarged, the neck appears larger and more tortuous than is normally seen in fasted or anorectic animals (Figure 9-53). Along with gallbladder enlargement, dilation of the common duct is visualized This is followed by dilation of the extrahepatic ducts within 48 hours.

Common duct diameter measured 1 to 1.5 cm after 48 hours of complete common duct obstruction in dogs (Figure 9-54).[244] Six of seven cats with extrahepatic biliary obstruction had common duct diameters greater than 5 mm.[15] In a separate study, 97% of obstructed cats had a common bile duct diameter greater than 5 mm, and 90% had dilated extrahepatic or intrahepatic ducts.[201] However, lower percentages of common bile duct dilation have been reported in cats.[247,248] The caudate and right lateral liver lobes provide the best acoustic window to the common duct region, which otherwise may be obscured by gas in the stomach or bowel. Bile duct

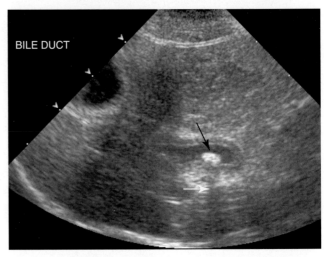

Figure 9-52 Choledocholithiasis. This calculus (*black arrow*) is located within the bile duct. A distinct acoustic shadow is easily seen (*white arrow*).

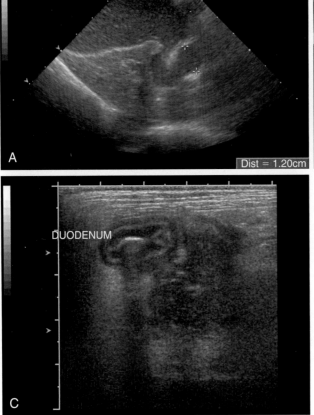

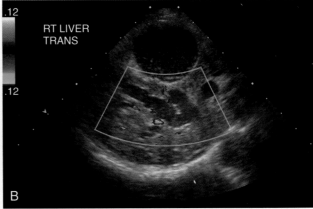

Figure 9-53 Extrahepatic bile duct obstruction secondary to pancreatitis in a dog. A, Distended gallbladder, neck, and cystic and common bile ducts (1.20 cm between electronic cursors) are the first indicators of complete obstruction, seen as early as 48 hours in dogs. **B,** Color Doppler image shows lack of flow in dilated bile duct. **C,** Transverse image of the duodenum and adjacent hypoechoic, enlarged pancreas responsible for the biliary obstruction.

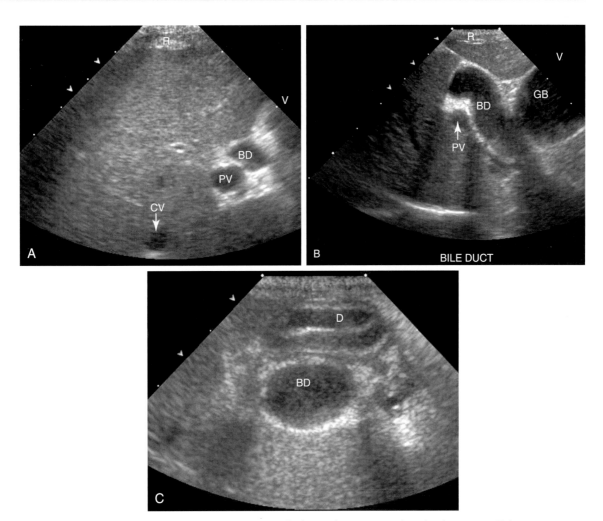

Figure 9-54 **Biliary obstruction in a dog. A,** Bile duct enlargement with early obstruction. Enlargement of the common bile duct ventral to the portal vein is another early sign of biliary obstruction. This is best seen on the lateral transverse intercostal view from the right 11th or 12th intercostal space. Note the bile duct is similar in diameter to the portal vein. **B,** The common bile duct continues to increase in size with prolonged obstruction and becomes more easily visualized on the right lateral intercostal transverse view. The bile duct can be followed from the gallbladder. The aorta and caudal vena cava are not seen on this particular scan. **C,** Common bile duct enlargement. This transverse view from the ventral abdomen shows enlargement of the bile duct as it enters the duodenal papilla in a dog with biliary obstruction. This bile duct was obstructed by a pancreatic mass (not pictured) adjacent to the duodenal papilla. *BD,* Bile duct; *CV,* caudal vena cava; *D,* duodenum; *GB,* gallbladder; *PV,* portal vein; *R,* right; *V,* ventral.

diameter is variable and cannot be used to determine chronicity of obstruction. Profound bile duct dilation can develop after 4 to 6 weeks of complete obstruction.[185]

If complete obstruction has been present for more than 48 hours in dogs, the extrahepatic ducts near the gallbladder neck become visible and may be traced to the common duct[244] (see Figures 9-53 and 9-54). The "shotgun" or "too many tubes" sign is sometimes recognized on sagittal scans of the liver after 5 to 7 days of complete obstruction. This sign refers to visualization of dilated intrahepatic ducts clustered around portal vessels. Dilated bile ducts appear similar to portal veins because they also possess echogenic walls. However, bile ducts can be differentiated from portal veins on transverse liver scans by their sudden changes in lumen caliber, irregular walls, and abrupt branching patterns. They can also be distinguished from vascular structures by Doppler ultrasonography (see

Figure 9-45, *B*). In cats with biliary obstruction, it was reported that dilation of the intrahepatic ducts occurred in 30% of the cases without extrahepatic duct dilation.[201] Therefore it seems possible that intrahepatic duct dilation, along with common duct enlargement, may be the only signs of extrahepatic biliary obstruction seen in some cats, because the gallbladder and extrahepatic ducts are not always enlarged (Figure 9-55; see also Figure 9-45).

The liver, biliary tract, pancreas, gastrointestinal tract, and lymph nodes at the porta hepatis should be evaluated to determine the cause of common duct obstruction. Surgical intervention may be indicated when extrahepatic obstruction is identified, even when the cause is not determined. When acute pancreatitis is suspected as the cause of obstruction, conservative medical therapy may be sufficient to allow spontaneous resolution once pancreatic inflammation subsides.

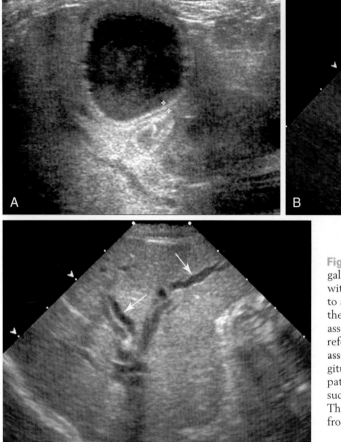

Figure 9-55 **Feline cholangitis/cholangiohepatitis. A,** The gallbladder, bile duct, and extrahepatic ducts are dilated, with thickened walls in this image. Obstruction was due to accumulation of inspissated bile. **B,** Transverse view of the liver with dilated biliary structures (*arrows*) seen in association with portal vessels. This appearance has been referred to as the "too many tubes" sign or "shotgun" sign associated with intrahepatic ductal dilation. **C,** This longitudinal view through the liver shows dilated intrahepatic bile ducts (*arrows*) with abrupt branching patterns, sudden changes in lumen caliber, and irregular walls. These features help distinguish dilated hepatic ducts from portal vessels, whose walls are also echogenic.

Cholecystocentesis has been recommended to relieve gallbladder distension in certain cases of biliary obstruction secondary to acute pancreatitis.[233]

Diagnosis of biliary obstruction may be difficult in the early stages of obstruction or if the biliary tract is dilated from previous obstruction. The biliary tract may remain dilated to some degree after prolonged or recurrent obstruction.[185] In one study, dilated intrahepatic ducts were recognized for as long as 8 to 13 days after obstruction was relieved, whereas extrahepatic biliary dilatation was still present for at least 13 weeks.[237]

Several ultrasound studies have been performed on the gallbladder in cats and dogs to determine normal volumes and emptying times after cholecystokinin administration or after ingestion of various types of meals.[8,9,11,245,249,251] In certain cases, the ultrasound measurement of gallbladder volume before and 1 hour after injection of cholecystokinin may help in the diagnosis of biliary obstruction. In dogs without obstructions, the gallbladder volume decreased by at least 40% after intravenous injection of cholecystokinin, whereas a decrease of less than 20% was noted in dogs with obstructions.[245,249] An additional method of determining gallbladder volume from linear measurements was also recently reported.[250] Normal gallbladder volume in the dog is reported to be 1.0 mL/kg or less after withholding food for 12 hours.[9] A study in cats indicated that feeding resulted in a linear decrease in gallbladder linear measurements and gallbladder volume.[251] These studies may be helpful in the identification of dogs and cats with abnormal gallbladder emptying, including those with biliary obstruction.

Neoplasia

It is generally accepted that neoplasia of the biliary tract cannot be distinguished from other types of hepatic neoplasia owing to its variable appearance.[42,43,45,46,52,83,88,89] A fine-needle liver aspiration or biopsy is required for diagnosis. Biliary cystadenomas or cystadenocarcinomas of older cats typically have a cystic appearance [62,106-108] (see Figure 9-20, *J* and *L*). Solitary or multifocal masses containing thin-walled cysts, hyperechoic masses with cystic components, or masses of mixed echogenicity with cystic components may occur. Tumors of the gallbladder, although rare, are more easily recognized if they are confined to the gallbladder wall.[186,188,252] Adenomas and adenocarcinomas of the gallbladder have been reported previously in dogs and cats.[253,254] Color flow Doppler analysis was used to help diagnose a bleeding neuroendocrine tumor in the gallbladder of a dog.[255] Figure 9-56 shows a tumor of the distal-most common bile duct in a cat.

VASCULAR ABNORMALITIES

Caudal Vena Cava and Hepatic Veins

Enlargement of the hepatic veins and caudal vena cava with passive congestion of the liver occurs most commonly from right-sided heart failure (Figure 9-57, *A* to *D*), but obstruction

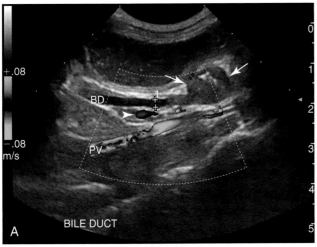

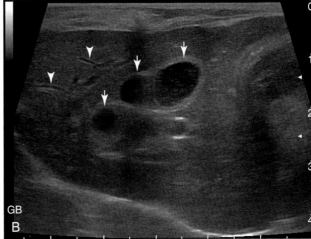

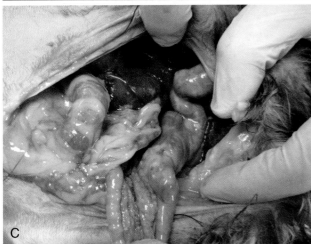

Figure 9-56 **Common bile duct obstruction. A,** Distal bile duct obstruction by solid echogenic mass (*arrows*) causing obstruction of the common bile duct (*BD*, 0.19 cm between electronic cursors +). Color Doppler image of the portal vein (*PV*) dorsal to the bile duct. The small red Doppler signal between the bile duct and the portal vein is the hepatic artery (*small arrowhead*). **B,** Dilated extrahepatic (*arrows*) and intrahepatic (*arrowheads*) bile ducts as a result of the common bile duct occlusion. **C,** Postmortem image of a dilated, tortuous common bile duct secondary to obstruction by pancreatic neoplasia in a different patient.

of the caudal vena cava by blood clots or masses near or cranial to the diaphragm is also possible. The enlarged hepatic veins are best visualized near the diaphragm where they enter the caudal vena cava.[3,4] Hepatic vein enlargement must be judged subjectively. However, finding concurrent distention of the caudal vena cava, hepatomegaly, and ascites assists with the diagnosis. Also, the heart should be assessed for pericardial effusion or other causes of right-sided heart failure. Abdominal fluid in the presence of normal-sized hepatic veins suggests the possibility of a noncardiac origin of the ascites.

Doppler Evaluation of the Caudal Vena Cava and Hepatic Veins

Dilation of the caudal vena cava and hepatic veins, hepatomegaly, and ascites may be seen secondary to right-sided heart failure in such diseases as pulmonary hypertension, pulmonic stenosis with right-sided heart failure, cor triatriatum dexter, pericardial effusion with tamponade, constrictive pericarditis, right atrial tumor, tricuspid valvular disease, caudal vena cava syndrome from heartworm disease, and myocardial disease. Increased pulsatility is noted within the hepatic veins, and the antegrade and retrograde components are more equalized. Blood flow velocities may be decreased within the caudal vena cava and hepatic veins, and especially with tricuspid insufficiency, there may be stronger than normal reversed flow during atrial systole (A wave) (Figure 9-58).[256-261] In addition, with tricuspid insufficiency the normal antegrade flow during ventricular systole (S wave) may be reversed.[19,262,263] In one

study, increases in central venous pressure could be predicted using caudal vena cava and hepatic vein diameters and v wave (on pulsed wave Doppler waveform of the hepatic vein) velocity.[264]

Thrombosis or space-occupying masses may also obstruct and dilate the caudal vena cava and hepatic veins, causing hepatomegaly and ascites. Differential diagnosis includes neoplasia, strictures, liver disease, trauma, systemic infection, and hematologic disorders. Thrombi usually produce increased intraluminal echogenicity within the vessel, although recently occurring thrombi are not always echogenic and difficult to visualize. In the case of hepatic vein thrombosis, there may be lack of flow despite the visualization of an anechoic lumen with gray-scale imaging. The intraluminal, increased echogenicity observed with a thrombus must be differentiated from slice thickness artifact, when a portion of the beam outside the vessel results in apparent intraluminal echoes. This is best accomplished by obtaining a transverse view through the vessel, which causes the artifact to disappear, whereas true echogenicity from a thrombus remains. Harmonic imaging will help to reduce this artifact. Pulsed or color Doppler analysis will indicate no flow or reduced flow with flow defects and turbulence.

In Budd-Chiari syndrome, the hepatic veins are obstructed at the point where they enter the caudal vena cava, or the caudal vena cava is obstructed cranial to the entrance of the hepatic veins.[265-270] The obstruction must occur between the heart and entry point of the hepatic veins into the caudal

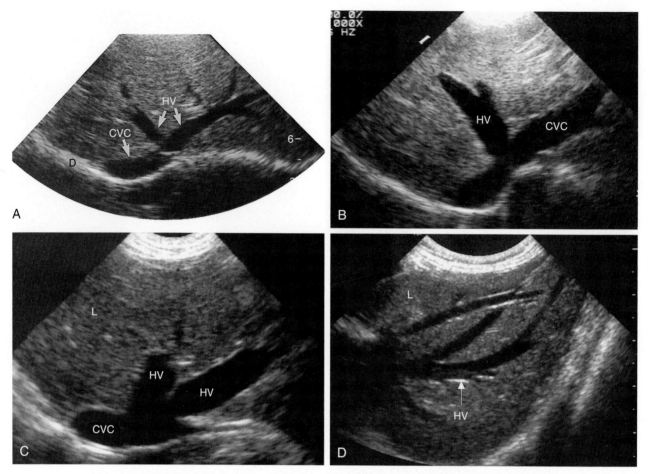

Figure 9-57 Hepatic vein distention. A, Moderately enlarged hepatic veins and caudal vena cava from right-sided heart failure. Distended hepatic veins can be traced to the caudal vena cava in this transverse view. **B** to **D,** Severely distended caudal vena cava and hepatic veins from right-sided heart failure. Sagittal (**B**) and transverse (**C**) views show markedly enlarged caudal vena cava and hepatic veins. Transverse oblique view (**D**) of the left liver lobes shows distention of the peripheral hepatic veins. *CVC,* Caudal vena cava; *D,* diaphragm; *GB,* gallbladder; *HV,* hepatic vein; *L,* liver; *PV,* portal vein.

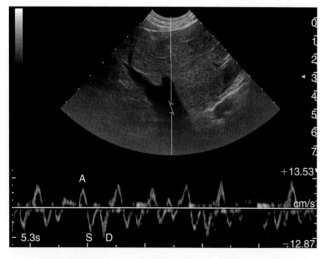

Figure 9-58 Hepatic vein pulse wave Doppler analysis in a dog with right-sided heart failure. The sample volume has been placed in a greatly distended hepatic vein, and the spectral tracing shows enlargement of the A wave. *A,* A-wave; *S,* S-wave; *D,* D-wave.

vena cava or the liver will not be affected. Doppler spectral patterns of turbulent, reduced, reversed, or absent flow may be observed within the hepatic veins and caudal vena cava, depending on the location and extent of obstruction. These changes are best seen with color flow Doppler imaging because the major hepatic vessels can easily be identified, their patency confirmed, and the direction and dynamics of flow established.

In certain types of portacaval shunts, evidence of turbulence and increased caudal vena cava diameter may be observed where the shunt vessel enters the caudal vena cava between the entrance of the right renal vein and the hepatic veins near the diaphragm or in a hepatic vein itself.[271] Turbulent flow in the caudal vena cava is best identified with color Doppler imaging.

One study addressed the possible association of Doppler waveforms in the right hepatic vein and various types of diffuse liver disease in human patients.[272] However, the results were not promising. Normal triphasic waveforms were found in a significant number of patients with diffuse liver disease such as cirrhosis, fibrosis, fatty infiltration, or metastasis. In addition, abnormal biphasic or flat waveforms were only found in only 50% or less of affected patients.

Portal Vein: Portosystemic Shunts

Portal vascular abnormalities consist of congenital or acquired portosystemic shunts and, less commonly, arteriovenous (AV) malformations. Ultrasound evaluation for portosystemic shunts may be compromised by the presence of a small liver and bowel gas and by the small size of many shunt vessels. The use of color Doppler evaluation is essential because many shunts are too small to be resolved using B-mode imaging alone. It should be emphasized that routine identification of normal portal, vena caval, and aortic blood vessels will maximize the ability to recognize abnormalities when they exist.

Ultrasound is more useful for detection of intrahepatic shunts than for many extrahepatic shunts, because the surrounding liver parenchyma makes visualization of shunt vessels easier. High speed CT angiography and available reconstruction algorithms allow much more anatomic detail that is important for surgical intervention.

An ultrasonographic diagnosis of portosystemic shunts is suspected when the liver is small, there is decreased visibility of intrahepatic portal veins, or an anomalous vessel is seen draining into the caudal vena cava, a hepatic vein, splenic vein, or the azygos vein.[271,273-278] The shunts may be congenital or acquired, single or multiple, and intrahepatic or extrahepatic.[27] Small breed dogs and cats with congenital shunts are more likely to have single extrahepatic shunts.[279] Intrahepatic shunts predominantly affect large breed dogs.[280-283] In cats, the diagnosis and treatment of congenital portosystemic shunts has also been reported.[26,275,284-288] Older dogs and cats are more likely to have multiple acquired extrahepatic shunts secondary to chronic liver disease. However, congenital shunts can be undetected for years and subsequently diagnosed in an older patient. This may be more common in dogs with portoazygos shunting.[289] The ultrasonographic diagnosis of a congenital intrahepatic portosystemic shunt may be more straightforward than that of an extrahepatic shunt because of less interference with surrounding bowel gas. The identification of an extrahepatic shunt can be difficult and time-consuming when surrounding gas and a small hepatic window are present. In one study, intrahepatic shunts were more consistently identified on ultrasound exam (sensitivity and specificity of 100%), whereas extrahepatic shunt identification had a sensitivity and specificity of 90% and 97%, respectively.[27] Thorough knowledge of vascular anatomy and various ultrasound windows that enhance shunt visualization will aid identification of both intrahepatic and extrahepatic portosystemic shunting vessels.

The use of interventional ultrasound procedures to treat congenital intrahepatic portosystemic shunts has been reported in a dog,[290] and Doppler assessment for improved portal flow after surgical treatment of portosystemic shunts is also becoming more common.

Congenital Portosystemic Shunts

Ultrasonography has assisted with the diagnosis of congenital portosystemic shunts.[26,27,271,277,278,285,288,291-293] Scintigraphic evaluation allows reliable diagnosis of the presence of a shunt, whereas CT angiography provides detailed evaluation of portal and systemic vasculature and exact shunt location. The choice of diagnostic imaging modality depends on the facilities and experience of the clinician. Ultrasonography is often the initial procedures performed because it is quick and non-invasive, and it helps to rule out coexisting abnormalities.[293] In addition to conventional ultrasound, contrast harmonic ultrasound has been used to detect solitary congenital extrahepatic shunts in dogs.[294]

The classification of congenital intrahepatic and extrahepatic portosystemic shunts in dogs and cats has been reviewed.[277,278,285] Intrahepatic shunts, which may be classified as left, central, or right divisional shunts, exhibit considerable variation in morphologic features (Figure 9-59).[285] Identification of the type of intrahepatic shunt may assist with determining prognosis and feasibility of treatment. For example, right divisional shunts involving the right medial and lateral lobes of the liver are generally more difficult to approach surgically.[285] Right divisional shunts originate from the right portal branch, running dorsolaterally and to the right, then turning medially to enter the caudal vena cava (see Figure 9-59, E and F).[277,285,295] The left portal branch is typically underdeveloped. Patent ductus venosus, considered a left divisional shunt, originates from the left portal branch. The shunting vessel runs cranioventrally and to the left, to the diaphragm, then abruptly turns dorsally to enter the caudal vena cava or left hepatic vein (see Figure 9-59, A to C).[277,285,288,295] Central divisional intrahepatic shunts can be the most difficult to identify with certainty. The anomalous vessel may be more of a "window" between the portal vein and caudal vena cava. The portal vein may appear focally enlarged and associated with a short shunt vessel connected to the caudal vena cava.[27,285,288] In some patients, only a dilated vascular segment may be seen without visualization of the actual communication between the portal and hepatic vein or caudal vena cava.[52] Color Doppler imaging may facilitate identification of a patent ductus venosus by demonstrating turbulent flow in the caudal vena cava at the site of communication with the ductus (see Figure 9-59, D).

Congenital extrahepatic shunts (Figure 9-60, A to E) can also be identified with ultrasonography (see Figure 9-20, K). A small liver, which is often present in dogs with portacaval shunts, can in some cases prevent a suitable acoustic window to the liver region. Scanning through a dorsal right lateral intercostal approach will facilitate visualization of the shunt area (see Figure 9-60, B). The liver size appears to be more normal in many cats with portosystemic shunts.[27,275] Because of reduced portal blood flow, portal vein branches within the hepatic parenchyma are often small or poorly identified. In dogs, the shunting vessel commonly arises from the main portal vein, splenic vein, or left gastric vein; in cats, it commonly arises from the left gastric vein.[296-298] The shunting vessel terminates in the caudal vena cava, cranial to the right renal vein. A right intercostal approach, or, for cats in association with the left gastric vein, a ventral approach, has been recommended.[26] Portoazygos vein shunts may be recognized through a dorsal right intercostal approach by seeing an anomalous vessel near the diaphragm, coursing close to the caudal vena cava without actually emptying into it (see Figure 9-60, B to E).[26] The azygos vein is often enlarged in these patients, and can be recognized as a large vessel running adjacent to the aorta, with flow directed cranially. In some patients, the shunt may be seen emptying directly into the azygos vein. These shunts often extend dorsally and curve around the liver.[288]

The size of the portal vein may also assist with diagnosis of certain types of portacaval shunts. The portal vein tends to be smaller in animals with extrahepatic portacaval shunts compared to those with hepatic microvascular dysplasia, intrahepatic portacaval shunts, or normal vasculature.[27] A ratio of the diameter of the portal vein to that of the aorta at the level of the porta hepatis, cranial to the entry of the gastroduodenal vein, was used to help diagnose congenital extrahepatic shunts.[27,288] A portal vein–to–aorta ratio (PV:Ao) of 0.7 to 1.25 is considered normal. All dogs and cats with a PV:Ao ratio of 0.65 or less were found to have either an extrahepatic portacaval shunt or idiopathic noncirrhotic portal hypertension (portal vein hypoplasia).[17] Dogs and cats with a PV:Ao ratio of ≥0.8 did not have an extrahepatic portacaval shunt, but may have other types of shunts or no portal venous

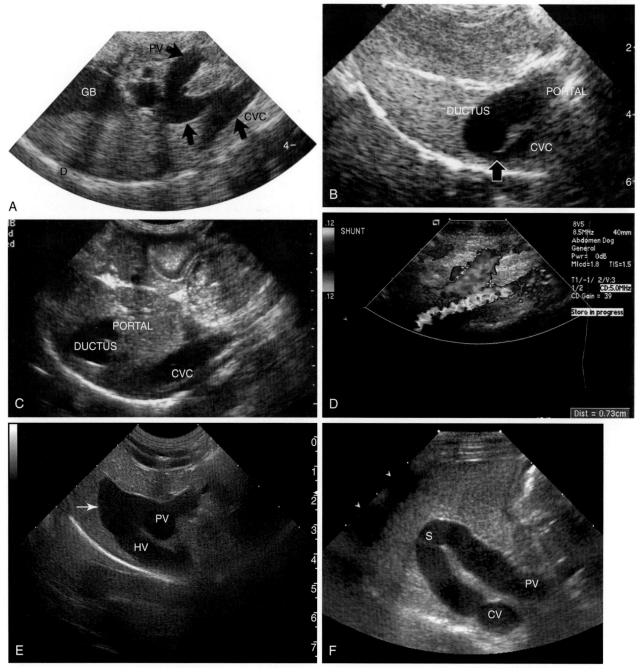

Figure 9-59 **Intrahepatic portosystemic shunts. A,** Patent ductus venosus. This congenital portosystemic shunt (*middle arrow*) was identified on a sagittal view of the liver, in which the communication between the portal vein and caudal vena cava was observed. **B and C,** Patent ductus venosus. The actual communication between the portal vein and caudal vena cava may be difficult to visualize (**B,** *arrow*) or may not be visualized (**C**). However, dilation of a vascular segment in the region of the ductus venosus can usually be identified as visualized in these examples. **D,** Color Doppler imaging may facilitate identification of the ductus (*cursors*) by demonstrating turbulent flow patterns in the caudal vena cava (seen here immediately dorsal to the ductus) near the site of communication of the ductus with the caudal vena cava. **E,** Right divisional portosystemic shunt (*arrow*) showing enlarged portal vein and hepatic vein. **F,** Right divisional intrahepatic shunt. This image was taken from a right transverse intercostal window. It shows the intrahepatic shunt vessel (*S*) extending from the right portal branch (*PV*) to the caudal vena cava (*CV*). *CVC,* caudal vena cava; *D,* diaphragm; *GB,* gallbladder; *HV,* hepatic vein; *PV,* portal vein.

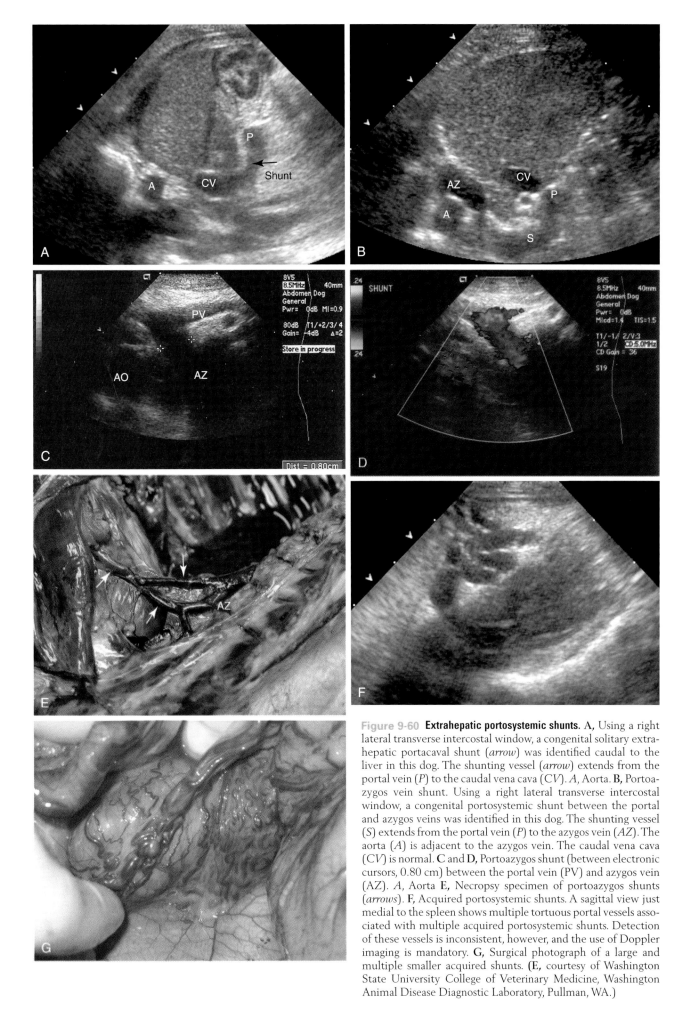

Figure 9-60 Extrahepatic portosystemic shunts. A, Using a right lateral transverse intercostal window, a congenital solitary extrahepatic portacaval shunt (*arrow*) was identified caudal to the liver in this dog. The shunting vessel (*arrow*) extends from the portal vein (*P*) to the caudal vena cava (*CV*). *A,* Aorta. **B,** Portoazygos vein shunt. Using a right lateral transverse intercostal window, a congenital portosystemic shunt between the portal and azygos veins was identified in this dog. The shunting vessel (*S*) extends from the portal vein (*P*) to the azygos vein (*AZ*). The aorta (*A*) is adjacent to the azygos vein. The caudal vena cava (*CV*) is normal. **C** and **D,** Portoazygos shunt (between electronic cursors, 0.80 cm) between the portal vein (PV) and azygos vein (AZ). *A,* Aorta **E,** Necropsy specimen of portoazygos shunts (*arrows*). **F,** Acquired portosystemic shunts. A sagittal view just medial to the spleen shows multiple tortuous portal vessels associated with multiple acquired portosystemic shunts. Detection of these vessels is inconsistent, however, and the use of Doppler imaging is mandatory. **G,** Surgical photograph of a large and multiple smaller acquired shunts. (**E,** courtesy of Washington State University College of Veterinary Medicine, Washington Animal Disease Diagnostic Laboratory, Pullman, WA.)

abnormalities. The liver of dogs with idiopathic noncirrhotic portal hypertension may appear similar to those with cirrhosis.[299-301] Multiple acquired extrahepatic shunts may be present due to portal hypertension. The PBFV is less than 10 cm/sec and the PV:Ao ratio is variable. A liver biopsy is required to make the diagnosis. It is important to make the distinction between cirrhosis and idiopathic noncirrhotic portal hypertension because dogs with the latter disease generally have a better prognosis.[301] In contrast, hepatic microvascular dysplasia (now known as hepatic portal venous hypoplasia)[278] is a disease where the portal blood is shunted through the liver bypassing the sinusoids and draining directly into the central veins of the liver.[27,278,302,303] Although portacaval shunting is present, a macroscopic shunt cannot be identified. There is no evidence of portal hypertension or multiple acquired shunts as seen with idiopathic noncirrhotic portal hypertension. PBFV is usually normal and the PV:Ao ratio is 0.65 or greater.[27,288] Obviously determinations of the PV:Ao ratio must be used with the clinical history, laboratory work, other ultrasound findings and imaging studies, and histopathology to reach a definitive diagnosis.

Positive-pressure ventilation under anesthesia can help shunt detection in some patients by displacing the liver caudally and distending venous structures.[274] Intraoperative ultrasonography can facilitate the localization and ligation of intrahepatic portacaval shunts at surgery.[273] Other methods have been reported to aid in the ultrasound diagnosis of portosystemic shunts. Ultrasound-guided transsplenic injection of agitated saline has been used to evaluate the intravascular transit of microbubbles through the portal system in normal dogs.[304] In a follow-up study, agitated saline mixed with heparinized autologous blood was injected into the splenic pulp and followed through the portal vein, caudal vena cava, and right atrium to identify the presence of both intrahepatic and extrahepatic shunts and determine the effectiveness of postoperative shunt closure.[305]

Transvenous coil embolization, surgical ligation, and placement of other external occlusion devices have been used to treat congenital intrahepatic or solitary extrahepatic portacaval shunts in dogs.[286,290,306-312] Ultrasonography has been used to diagnose the shunt, aid ligation or placement of devices, and assess outcome of treatment. After closure of the shunt vessel, the liver may return to normal size.[313,314]

Acquired Portosystemic Shunts

Portal hypertension may develop as a result of prehepatic, hepatic, or posthepatic abnormalities. This can lead to the opening of preexisting embryonic vessels that connect the portal and the systemic circulation (peripheral acquired extrahepatic portosystemic shunts).[277,315] As described previously, posthepatic causes of portal hypertension include abnormalities such as hepatic vein thrombosis (Budd-Chiari syndrome), thrombosis of the caudal vena cava cranial to the entrance of the hepatic veins, and constrictive pericarditis. Prehepatic causes of portal hypertension include portal vein thrombosis and external compression of the portal vein by masses (described later). Hepatic causes of portal hypertension are most common and occur secondary to chronic liver disease producing cirrhosis or fibrosis. In chronic liver disease, acquired extrahepatic portosystemic shunts may be diagnosed by visualizing multiple small, tortuous portal venous structures (often termed varices), primarily in the left kidney or splenic region, or a longer tortuous vessel between the splenic vein and left renal vein.[42,43,52,315] (see Figure 9-60, F and G). If Doppler imaging is available, spectral patterns typical of venous flow can be obtained. Detection of these peripheral shunt vessels is inconsistent. Doppler techniques assessing flow within the main portal vein, as described later, are becoming more useful to obtain quantitative functional information in diffuse liver diseases, such as cirrhosis, in which conventional ultrasonographic imaging has traditionally been less valuable.[16,18,28,316]

Other Portal Vein Abnormalities

Prehepatic causes of portal hypertension include portal vein stricture, thrombosis, or compression. Portal hypertension due to circumscribed fibrosis of the wall of the extrahepatic portal vein has been described in a dog.[317] Thrombosis of the portal vein has also been described in dogs in association with hepatitis, hepatic neoplasia, congenital portosystemic shunt, congenital hepatic arteriovenous fistula, cirrhosis, nonhepatic neoplasias, renal disease, pancreatitis, peritonitis, inflammatory bowel disease, hyperadrenocorticism or steroid administration, vasculitis associated with ehrlichiosis and other diseases, gastrointestinal blood loss, protein-losing nephropathy and enteropathy, immune-mediated hemolytic anemia, immune mediated thrombocytopenia, various types of infectious diseases, systemic inflammatory response syndrome, abdominal surgery or invasive procedures, and various hypercoagulable states.[318-323]

Portal vein thrombosis has also been reported in cats secondary to hepatic pathology (congenital portosystemic shunts, hepatic primary or malignant neoplasia, and acute neutrophilic cholangitis).[324,325] Thrombosis of the portal vein and obstruction of portal flow by extrinsic mass lesions near the porta hepatis are rare in the dog and cat (Figure 9-61). The thrombus may appear hyperechoic, isoechoic, or hypoechoic, and either homogeneous or heterogeneous. A hyperechoic lining around the thrombus may be present. The extent of luminal filling is variable, with some focal portal vein distention possible. Additional thrombi may be identified in splenic, mesenteric, pancreaticoduodenal veins, and caudal vena cava. Peritoneal effusion may also be present. In humans, portal vein thrombosis usually results from preexisting pathologic conditions, such as portal hypertension, or intestinal infection or inflammation (appendicitis, diverticulitis, inflammatory bowel disease).[19]

Tumors directly involving the portal vein in animals usually arise from the gastrointestinal tract.[326] Thrombosis secondary to invasion of the portal vein by a recurrent duodenal neoplasm has been described.[320] Iatrogenic portal vein thrombosis has been reported secondary to portosystemic shunt ligation.[327] Detection of thrombosis depends on identification of an intraluminal filling defect, abnormal intraluminal echoes, or evidence of abnormal swirling caused by slow blood flow. Color or duplex Doppler imaging are recommended for further evaluation.

Doppler Evaluation of the Portal Vein
Portal Vein Abnormalities with Passive Hepatic Congestion

Passive congestion of the liver can occur secondary to right-sided heart failure from diseases such as tricuspid insufficiency, pericardial effusion with tamponade, and constrictive pericarditis. This results in distention and increased pulsatility in the hepatic veins during the cardiac cycle, as previously described. In addition, Doppler waveforms showing prominent pulsatility related to the cardiac cycle can also be transmitted to the portal vein.[328-330] The minimal degree of portal vein pulsatility that would allow diagnosis of right-sided heart failure has not been established in humans, but most agree that any evidence of reversed flow in the portal vein indicates severe right-sided heart dysfunction. However, investigators have also found that portal vein pulsatility occurs in normal and cirrhotic livers without cardiac disease. Therefore it was concluded that mechanisms other than transsinusoidal

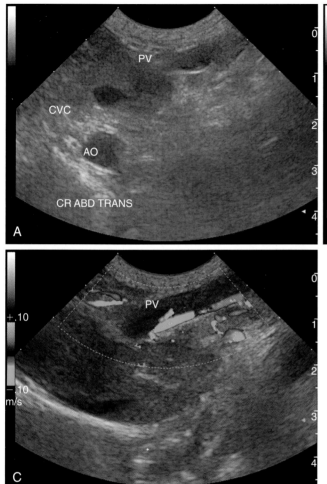

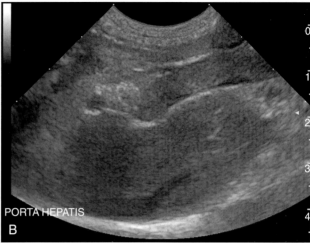

Figure 9-61 **Portal vein thrombus. A,** Transverse cranial abdominal image shows the portal vein (*PV*), caudal vena cava (*CVC*), and aorta (*AO*) in cross section. The thrombus in the portal vein cannot be identified in this image. **B,** Sagittal image shows a large thrombus in the portal vein. **C,** Color Doppler image shows near complete occlusion of the portal vein (*PV*) with only a small peripheral turbulent patency present.

transmission of atrial pulsations must also contribute to portal vein pulsatility.[331]

Doppler Abnormalities with Portacaval Shunts

The diagnosis and assessment of congenital portacaval shunts by Doppler ultrasonography has been described.[26,271,275,285,292] Preliminary experience suggests that mean portal blood flow velocity (PBFV) in normal fasted dogs is approximately 10 to 25 cm/sec.[17,18] Therefore velocities below 10 cm/sec or above 25 cm/sec are considered abnormal. Approximately 70% of dogs with congenital portosystemic shunts were reported to have increased flow velocity or abnormal variable flow patterns in the portal vein compared with normal dogs,[271] and this also appears to be true for cats.[275] This is expected for intrahepatic shunts. However, reduced or hepatofugal flow was observed with congenital extrahepatic shunts if the flow was measured between the shunt origin and the entering point of the gastroduodenal vein.[27,332] Hepatofugal flow was caused by blood flowing from the gastroduodenal vein toward the shunt. Therefore, with extrahepatic shunts, one should determine where the Doppler measurement was taken. Increased portal flow is expected if the measurement is taken caudal to the shunt, whereas reduced or reversed flow may be seen if the measurement is taken cranial to the shunt. Portal blood flow (PBF) is normally relatively uniform, and the variable flow patterns observed in the portal vein with shunts are presumably due to normal cardiac and respiratory influences transmitted from the caudal vena cava through the shunt to the portal vein.[271] Turbulence can usually be identified within

the caudal vena cava at the point where the shunt vessel enters the vena cava by color Doppler ultrasonography and a right intercostal window.[271] Increased PBF also occurs in postprandial conditions,[316] and variable flow patterns or turbulence may not always be seen in the portal vein. In addition, variable flow patterns can be transmitted to the portal vein in cases of passive hepatic congestion, as described previously.[328-330] Therefore the history, clinical findings, laboratory work, and other imaging findings should be evaluated with Doppler ultrasonography to prevent diagnostic errors.

In addition to the diagnosis of portacaval shunts, Doppler ultrasonography may be useful for evaluating PBF associated with progressive constriction of single extrahepatic portosystemic shunts after surgical banding. Devices are available that variably constrict the shunt vessel after surgical placement.[306,333-335] They provides gradual occlusion of the shunt over a prolonged period, thus reducing the possibility of acute hemodynamic effects that may occur after direct ligation. The use of Doppler ultrasound to assess the hemodynamic changes in the portal vein during surgical attenuation of congenital intrahepatic or extrahepatic portacaval shunts has also been described.[309,332,336] It is likely that similar interventional ultrasound procedures will become much more common in the future.

In dogs with acquired portosystemic shunts secondary to hepatic cirrhosis, fibrosis, or idiopathic portal hypertension, reduced mean PBFV and PBF have been described.[18,25,26,288] Ascites may be present, and in some cases, hepatofugal flow within the portal vein may be recognized.[337] Mean PBFV in 10 dogs with experimentally induced hepatic cirrhosis was markedly reduced (9.2 cm/sec versus the normal value, 18.1 cm/sec). Mean PBF was also significantly decreased compared with normal (17.2 mL/min/kg versus the normal value, 31.06 mL/min/kg), whereas portal vein diameter remained unchanged.[18] The accompanying increased portal vein diameter with hepatic cirrhosis in humans is apparently not seen in dogs, perhaps owing to the enhanced ability of dogs to develop peripheral extrahepatic shunts.[18,25] The reduced PBFV and PBF are associated with increased resistance to PBF through the liver and the development of multiple extrahepatic portosystemic shunts that move blood away from the portal system. The portal vein congestion index (CI, cm × sec), a measure of vascular resistance, may increase with hepatic cirrhosis and other liver diseases. The CI is determined by dividing the portal vein cross-sectional area (cm^2) by the average blood flow velocity (cm/sec). The mean CI for dogs with experimentally induced hepatic cirrhosis was 0.06 ± 0.018 cm × sec; that for normal, unsedated dogs is approximately 0.04 ± 0.015 cm × sec.[18] Because portal vein size does not appear to increase after hepatic fibrosis or cirrhosis,[18,25] Doppler measurement of PBFV alone is probably adequate for assessing changes in portal hemodynamics induced by chronic liver disease. Exercise and upright posture are also known to decrease portal flow and potentially cause false-positive diagnoses.[338] However, the use of standardized Doppler examination procedures will usually eliminate these possibilities.

Doppler measurements of PBFV are especially valuable because direct visualization of the shunting vessels is not required. The use of Doppler ultrasonography for evaluating various types of portosystemic shunts may be helpful, but the reliability (incidence of false-positives and false-negatives) of such measurements should be investigated in controlled studies of a large group of clinical cases, particularly those with acquired liver disease. Doppler studies may assist with evaluation of portacaval shunts and liver disease but will not substitute for proper interpretation of the history, clinical findings, laboratory work, findings of other imaging procedures, and a histologic diagnosis obtained by liver biopsy.

Doppler Abnormalities with Portal Vein Obstruction

In some cases, a portal vein thrombus may appear hypoechoic or completely anechoic, in which case color or duplex Doppler imaging is necessary for detection. The thrombus will appear as a localized flow void on color Doppler imaging (see Figure 9-61, C), or the portal vein may have dramatically reduced PBFV or complete lack of flow. However, normal PBFV has been described in some cases of portal vein thrombosis, possibly because of flow around the thrombus.[320]

In animals, tumors involving the portal vein and thus causing compression or obstruction usually arise from the gastrointestinal tract or from primary or metastatic liver tumors.[319,326] A tumor thrombus should be suspected if blood flow is detected within the thrombus with color Doppler imaging and there is expansion of the portal vein in this region. Mean PBFV in the main portal vein is usually reduced because of the obstruction and development of secondary extrahepatic portosystemic shunts.[320]

Hepatic Artery Abnormalities

Hepatic arterial flow is similar to arterial flow in other solid organs such as the kidney, with a low-resistance systolic waveform and well-maintained flow throughout diastole. A preliminary study evaluated the Doppler measurement of hepatic arterial flow in normal adult dogs and puppies, in postprandial dogs, and in dogs with AV fistulas, portal vein thrombosis, and acquired hepatic insufficiency.[17] Normal peak systolic velocity

in the hepatic artery was 1.5 ± 0.4 m/sec, and the resistive index was 0.68 ± 0.04 in 10 preprandial beagle dogs. Preliminary results indicated that hepatic arterial Doppler evaluation may be useful for dogs having arterioportal fistulas, but was not useful for dogs with portal vein thrombosis or acquired hepatic insufficiency. Two dogs with congenital arterioportal fistulas had high mean peak systolic velocities and low-normal resistive indices compared with normal dogs. The findings are compatible with markedly reduced vascular resistance associated with AV communications. However, no significant differences were detected between normal beagle dogs, three dogs with portal vein thrombosis, and two dogs with acquired hepatic insufficiency. Clearly, more investigation is needed to determine the value of hepatic arterial Doppler measurements.

Hepatic Arteriovenous Fistulas

Hepatic AV fistulas have been reported in dogs and cats.[17,325,339,340] Ultrasonography is an excellent method to detect dilated, tortuous vessels associated with hepatic AV fistulas[17,325,340-342] (Figure 9-62). The ultrasonographic findings associated with congenital hepatic AV fistulas were described in three 5-month-old dogs.[340] High fasting ammonia concentration, prolonged sulfobromophthalein dye retention, and high fasting serum bile acid concentration indicated hepatic insufficiency. Ascites was present in two of the dogs. Ultrasonography was used to detect large, tortuous, anechoic structures adjacent to or within the liver parenchyma. Doppler ultrasonography helped to identify the vascular origin of these structures with pulsatile spectral patterns typical of arterial flow. Reversal of PBF (hepatofugal) was also revealed with Doppler imaging. In addition, acquired portosystemic shunts may form as a result of a dramatic increase in hydrostatic pressure associated with portal hypertension. The Doppler findings helped differentiate the AV fistulas from conventional portosystemic shunts, in which typical venous flow patterns are expected. Celiac arteriography was used to confirm the presence of AV fistulas between the hepatic branch of the celiac artery and the portal vein, with occurrence of hepatofugal flow in two dogs and an AV fistula (unspecified site) in the

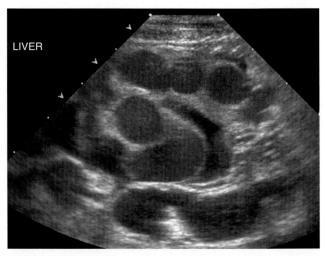

Figure 9-62 **Hepatic arteriovenous fistula.** A hepatic arteriovenous fistula was diagnosed in this dog with ascites. Multiple, round and tubular anechoic structures were identified with B-mode ultrasound. Doppler ultrasonography (not shown) revealed large, tortuous vessels with arterial flow patterns in the liver parenchyma.

third dog. Surgical resection of the affected hepatic lobes resulted in immediate improvement; however, long-term results were not known because two of the dogs were lost to follow-up and the third was evaluated for only 5 months.

The assessment of congenital hepatic AV fistulas by Doppler hepatic arterial measurements was also reported in two dogs as part of a larger study assessing the usefulness of hepatic arterial measurements in congenital or acquired liver disease.[17] Dogs with congenital arterioportal fistulas had higher mean peak systolic velocities than did normal pups (3.8 ± 1.9 m/sec versus normal 1.5 ± 0.4 m/sec) and a lower mean resistive index (0.5 ± 0.04 m/sec versus normal 0.68 ± 0.4 m/sec). Doppler evaluation of the hepatic artery may prove useful in certain cases in which the more typical signs of hepatic AV fistula are not seen.

Dual-phase CT angiography is a minimally invasive procedure that is also useful for diagnosing arterioportal fistulas in dogs.[343] The hepatic arteries, hepatic veins, and portal veins can be completely evaluated after peripheral administration of contrast medium. Hepatofugal flow and multiple acquired extrahepatic shunts caused by portal hypertension can be readily identified. For the interested reader, the surgical and interventional radiographic treatment of dogs with hepatic AV fistulas has been described in 20 dogs.[344]

REFERENCES

1. Brinckman-Ferguson EL, Biller DS. Ultrasound of the right intercostal space. *Vet Clin North Am Small Anim Pract* 2009;**39**:761–81.
2. Probst A, Kunzel W. Sonographic differentiation of liver lobes in the dog. *Wiener Tierärztliche Monatsschrift* 1993;**80**:200–7.
3. Carlisle CH, Wu JX, Heath TJ. Anatomy of the portal and hepatic veins of the dog: a basis for systematic evaluation of the liver by ultrasonography. *Vet Radiol Ultrasound* 1995;**36**:227–33.
4. Wu JX, Carlisle CH. Ultrasonographic examination of the canine liver based on recognition of hepatic and portal veins. *Vet Radiol Ultrasound* 1995;**36**:234–9.
5. Mwanza T, Miyamoto T, Okumura M, et al. Ultrasonography and angiographic examination of normal canine liver vessels. *Jpn J Vet Res* 1996;**44**:179–88.
6. Wachsberg RH, Angyal EA, Klein DM, et al. Echogenicity of hepatic versus portal vein walls revisited with histologic correlation. *J Ultrasound Med* 1997;**16**:807–10.
7. Ivancić M, Mai W. Qualitative and quantitative comparison of renal versus hepatic ultrasonographic intensity in healthy dogs. *Vet Radiol Ultrasound* 2008;**49**:368–73.
8. Rothuizen J, de Vries-Chalmers Hoynck van Papendrecht R, van den Brom WE. Post prandial and cholecystokinin-induced emptying of the gall bladder in dogs. *Vet Rec* 1990;**126**:505–7.
9. Ramstedt KL, Center SA, Randolph JF, et al. Changes in gallbladder volume in healthy dogs after food was withheld for 12 hours followed by ingestion of a meal or a meal containing erythromycin. *Am J Vet Res* 2008;**69**:647–51.
10. Bromel C, Barthez PY, Leveille R, et al. Prevalence of gallbladder sludge in dogs as assessed by ultrasonography. *Vet Radiol Ultrasound* 1998;**39**:206–10.
11. Tsukagoshi T, Ohno K, Tsukamoto A, et al. Decreased gallbladder emptying in dogs with biliary sludge or gallbladder mucocele. *Vet Radiol Ultrasound* 2012;**53**:84–91.
12. Spalding KA. Gallbladder wall thickness. *Vet Radiol Ultrasound* 1993;**34**:270–3.
13. Hittmair KM, Vielgrader HD, Loupal G. Ultrasonographic evaluation of gallbladder wall thickness in cats. *Vet Radiol Ultrasound* 2001;**42**:149–55.
14. Miller ME, Evans HE. *Miller's Anatomy of the dog*. 3rd ed. Philadelphia: Saunders; 1993.
15. Leveille R, Biller DS, Shiroma JT. Sonographic evaluation of the common bile duct in cats. *J Vet Intern Med* 1996;**10**:296–9.
16. Lamb CR, Mahoney PN. Comparison of 3 methods for calculating portal blood flow velocity in dogs using duplex-Doppler ultrasonography. *Vet Radiol Ultrasound* 1994;**35**:190–4.
17. Lamb CR, Burton CA, Carlisle CH. Doppler measurement of hepatic arterial flow in dogs: technique and preliminary findings. *Vet Radiol Ultrasound* 1999;**40**:77–81.
18. Nyland TG, Fisher PE. Evaluation of experimentally induced canine hepatic cirrhosis using duplex Doppler ultrasound. *Vet Radiol* 1990;**31**:189–94.
19. Middleton WD, Kurtz AB, Hertzberg BS. *Ultrasound: the requisites*. 2nd ed. St. Louis: Mosby; 2004.
20. Smithenson BT, Mattoon JS, Bonagura JD, et al. Pulsed-wave Doppler ultrasonographic evaluation of hepatic veins during variable hemodynamic states in healthy anesthetized dogs. *Am J Vet Res* 2004;**65**:734–40.
21. Szatmari V, Rothuizen J, Voorhout G. Standard planes for ultrasonographic examination of the portal system in dogs. *J Am Vet Med Assoc* 2004;**224**:713–16, 698-719.
22. Sartor R, Mamprim MJ, Takahira RF, et al. Hemodynamic valuation of the right portal vein in healthy dogs of different body weights. *Acta Vet Scand* 2010;**52**:36–41.
23. Lamb CR, Burton CA. Doppler ultrasonographic assessment of closure of the ductus venosus in neonatal Irish wolfhounds. *Vet Rec* 2004;**155**:699–701.
24. Lohse CL, Suter PF. Functional closure of the ductus venosus during early postnatal life in the dog. *Am J Vet Res* 1977;**38**:839–44.
25. Mwanza T, Miyamoto T, Okumura M, et al. Ultrasonographic evaluation of portal vein hemodynamics in experimentally bile duct ligated dogs. *Jpn J Vet Res* 1998;**45**:199–206.
26. Lamb CR. Ultrasonography of portosystemic shunts in dogs and cats. *Vet Clin North Am Small Anim Pract* 1998;**28**:725–53.
27. d'Anjou MA, Penninck D, Cornejo L, et al. Ultrasonographic diagnosis of portosystemic shunting in dogs and cats. *Vet Radiol Ultrasound* 2004;**45**:424–37.
28. Kantrowitz BM, Nyland TG, Fisher P. Estimation of portal blood flow using duplex real-time and pulsed Doppler ultrasound imaging in the dog. *Vet Radiol* 1989; 222–6.
29. Terry JD, Rysavy J. Peak systolic velocity and flow volume increase with blood pressure in low resistance systems. *J Ultrasound Med* 1995;**14**:199–203.
30. Mostbeck GH, Gossinger HD, Mallek R, et al. Effect of heart rate on Doppler measurements of resistive index in renal arteries. *Radiology* 1990;**175**:511–13.
31. Pierce ME, Sewell R. Identification of hepatic cirrhosis by duplex Doppler ultrasound value of the hepatic artery resistive index. *Australas Radiol* 1990;**34**:331–3.
32. Vassiliades VG, Ostrow TD, Chezmar JL, et al. Hepatic arterial resistive indices: correlation with the severity of cirrhosis. *Abdom Imaging* 1993;**18**:61–5.
33. Sacerdoti D, Merkel C, Bolognesi M, et al. Hepatic arterial resistance in cirrhosis with and without portal vein thrombosis: relationships with portal hemodynamics. *Gastroenterology* 1995;**108**:1152–8.

34. Tanaka K, Mitsui K, Morimoto M, et al. Increased hepatic arterial blood flow in acute viral hepatitis: assessment by color Doppler sonography. *Hepatology* 1993;**18**:21–7.

35. Han SH, Rice S, Cohen SM, et al. Duplex Doppler ultrasound of the hepatic artery in patients with acute alcoholic hepatitis. *J Clin Gastroenterol* 2002;**34**:573–7.

36. Platt JF, Rubin JM, Ellis JH. Hepatic artery resistance changes in portal vein thrombosis. *Radiology* 1995;**196**:95–8.

37. Stell D, Downey D, Marotta P, et al. Prospective evaluation of the role of quantitative Doppler ultrasound surveillance in liver transplantation. *Liver Transpl* 2004;**10**:1183–8.

38. Uzochukwu LN, Bluth EI, Smetherman DH, et al. Early postoperative hepatic sonography as a predictor of vascular and biliary complications in adult orthotopic liver transplant patients. *Am J Roentgenol* 2005;**185**:1558–70.

39. Chen W, Facciuto ME, Rocca JP, et al. Doppler ultrasonographic findings on hepatic arterial vasospasm early after liver transplantation. *J Ultrasound Med* 2006;**25**:631–8.

40. Loisance DY, Peronneau PA, Pellet MM, et al. Hepatic circulation after side-to-side portacaval shunt in dogs: velocity pattern and flow rate changes studied by an ultrasonic velocimeter. *Surgery* 1973;**73**:43–52.

41. Bergman JR. Nodular hyperplasia in the liver of the dog: an association with changes in the Ito cell population. *Vet Pathol* 1985;**22**:427–38.

42. Nyland TG, Hager DA. Sonography of the liver, gallbladder, and spleen. *Vet Clin North Am Small Anim Pract* 1985;**15**:1123–48.

43. Nyland TG, Hager DA, Herring DS. Sonography of the liver, gallbladder, and spleen. *Semin Vet Med Surg (Small Anim)* 1989;**4**:13–31.

44. Stowater JL, Lamb CR, Schelling SH. Ultrasonographic features of canine hepatic nodular hyperplasia. *Vet Radiol* 1990;**31**:268–72.

45. Lamb CR. Abdominal ultrasonography in small animals: examination of the liver, spleen and pancreas. *J Small Anim Pract* 1990;**31**:6–15.

46. Lamb CR. Ultrasonography of the liver and biliary tract. *Probl Vet Med* 1991;**3**:555–73.

47. Cuccovillo A, Lamb CR. Cellular features of sonographic target lesions of the liver and spleen in 21 dogs and a cat. *Vet Radiol Ultrasound* 2002;**43**:275–8.

48. Crevier FR, Wrigley RH. The Sonographic features of splenic lymphoid hyperplasia in 31 dogs: a retrospective study (1980-2000). *Vet Radiol Ultrasound* 2000;**41**:566.

49. Patnaik AK, Hurvitz AI, Lieberman PH. Canine hepatic neoplasms: a clinicopathologic study. *Vet Pathol* 1980;**17**:553–64.

50. O'Brien RT, Iani M, Matheson J, et al. Contrast harmonic ultrasound of spontaneous liver nodules in 32 dogs. *Vet Radiol Ultrasound* 2004;**45**:547–53.

51. Ochiai K, Takechi M, Matsumoto T, et al. Human focal nodular hyperplasia-like lesion in the liver of a cat. *Jpn J Vet Res* 1990;**38**:117–25.

52. Nyland TG, Park RD. Hepatic ultrasonography in the dog. *Vet Radiol* 1983;**24**:74–84.

53. Berry CR, Ackerman N, Charach M, et al. Iatrogenic biloma (biliary pseudocyst) in a cat with hepatic lipidosis. *Vet Radiol Ultrasound* 1992;**33**:145–9.

54. McKenna SC, Carpenter JL. Polycystic disease of the kidney and liver in the Cairn Terrier. *Vet Pathol* 1980;**17**:436–42.

55. McAloose D, Casal M, Patterson DF, et al. Polycystic kidney and liver disease in two related West Highland White Terrier litters. *Vet Pathol* 1998;**35**:77–81.

56. Van den Ingh TS, Rothuizen J. Congenital cystic disease of the liver in seven dogs. *J Comp Pathol* 1985;**95**:405–14.

57. Gorlinger S, Rothuizen J, Bunch S, et al. Congenital dilatation of the bile ducts (Caroli's disease) in young dogs. *J Vet Intern Med* 2003;**17**:28–32.

58. Last RD, Hill JM, Roach M, et al. Congenital dilatation of the large and segmental intrahepatic bile ducts (Caroli's disease) in two Golden retriever littermates. *J S Afr Vet Assoc* 2006;**77**:210–14.

59. Crowell WA, Hubbell JJ, Riley JC. Polycystic disease in related cats. *J Am Vet Med Assoc* 1979;**175**:286–8.

60. Stebbins KE. Polycystic disease of the kidney and liver in an adult Persian cat. *J Comp Pathol* 1989;**100**:327–30.

61. Biller DS, Chew DJ, DiBartola SP. Polycystic kidney disease in a family of Persian cats. *J Am Vet Med Assoc* 1990;**196**:1288–90.

62. Nyland TG, Koblik PD, Tellyer SE. Ultrasonographic evaluation of biliary cystadenomas in cats. *Vet Radiol Ultrasound* 1999;**40**:300–6.

63. vanSonnenberg E, Simeone JF, Mueller PR, et al. Sonographic appearance of hematoma in the liver, spleen, and kidney: a clinical, pathologic, and animal study. *Radiology* 1983;**147**:507–10.

64. Farrar ET, Washabau RJ, Saunders HM. Hepatic abscesses in dogs: 14 cases (1982-1994). *J Am Vet Med Assoc* 1996;**208**:243–7.

65. Schwarz LA, Penninck DG, Leveille-Webster C. Hepatic abscesses in 13 dogs: a review of the ultrasonographic findings, clinical data and therapeutic options. *Vet Radiol Ultrasound* 1998;**39**:357–65.

66. Grooters AM, Sherding RG, Biller DS, et al. Hepatic abscesses associated with diabetes mellitus in two dogs. *J Vet Intern Med* 1994;**8**:203–6.

67. Konde LJ, Lebel JL, Park RD, et al. Sonographic application in the diagnosis of intraabdominal abscess in the dog. *Vet Radiol* 1986;**27**:151–4.

68. Downs MO, Miller MA, Cross AR, et al. Liver lobe torsion and liver abscess in a dog. *J Am Vet Med Assoc* 1998;**212**:678–80.

69. Sergeeff JS, Armstrong PJ, Bunch SE. Hepatic abscesses in cats: 14 cases (1985-2002). *J Vet Intern Med* 2004;**18**:295–300.

70. Singh M, Krockenberger M, Martin P, et al. Hepatocellular carcinoma with secondary abscessation in a cat. *Aust Vet J* 2005;**83**:736–9.

71. Zerem E, Hadzic A. Sonographically guided percutaneous catheter drainage versus needle aspiration in the management of pyogenic liver abscess. *AJR Am J Roentgenol* 2007;**189**:W138–42.

72. Miele V, Buffa V, Stasolla A, et al. Contrast enhanced ultrasound with second generation contrast agent in traumatic liver lesions. *Radiol Med (Torino)* 2004;**108**:82–91.

73. Catalano O, Lobianco R, Raso MM, et al. Blunt hepatic trauma: evaluation with contrast-enhanced sonography: sonographic findings and clinical application. *J Ultrasound Med* 2005;**24**:299–310.

74. McGahan JP, Horton S, Gerscovich EO, et al. Appearance of solid organ injury with contrast-enhanced sonography in blunt abdominal trauma: preliminary experience. *AJR Am J Roentgenol* 2006;**187**:658–66.

75. Valentino M, Serra C, Pavlica P, et al. Contrast-enhanced ultrasound for blunt abdominal trauma. *Semin Ultrasound CT MR* 2007;**28**:130–40.

76. Tang J, Wenxiu L, Faqin L, et al. Comparison of gray-scale contrast-enhanced ultrasonography with contrast-enhanced computed tomography in different grading of blunt hepatic and splenic trauma: an animal experiment. *Ultrasound Med Biol* 2009;**35**:566–75.

77. Mihalik J, Smith R, Toevs C, et al. The use of contrast-enhanced ultrasound for the evaluation of solid abdominal organ injury in patients with blunt abdominal trauma. *J Trauma Acute Care Surg* 2012.

78. Catalano O, Cusati B, Nunziata A, et al. Active abdominal bleeding: contrast enhanced sonography. *Abdom Imaging* 2006;**31**:9–16.

79. Sato AF, Solano M. Radiographic diagnosis: liver lobe entrapment and associated emphysematous hepatitis. *Vet Radiol Ultrasound* 1998;**39**:123–4.

80. Sonnenfield JM, Armbrust LJ, Radlinsky MA, et al. Radiographic and ultrasonographic findings of liver lobe torsion in a dog. *Vet Radiol Ultrasound* 2001;**42**:344–6.

81. Schwartz SG, Mitchell SL, Keating JH, et al. Liver lobe torsion in dogs: 13 cases (1995-2004). *J Am Vet Med Assoc* 2006;**228**:242–7.

82. Swann HM, Brown DC. Hepatic lobe torsion in 3 dogs and a cat. *Vet Surg* 2001;**30**:482–6.

83. Liptak J. Hepatobiliary tumors. In: Withrow SJ, MacEwen EG, editors. *Small animal clinical oncology*. 4th ed. Philadelphia: WB Saunders; 2007. p. 484–92.

84. Strombeck DR. Clinicopathologic features of primary and metastatic neoplastic diseases of the liver in dogs. *J Am Vet Med Assoc* 1978;**173**:267.

85. Cullen JM, Popp JA. Tumors of the liver and gall bladder. In: Meuten DJ, editor. *Tumors in domestic animals*. 4th ed. Ames: Iowa State Press; 2002.

86. Thamm DH. Hepatobiliary tumors. In: Withrow SJ, MacEwen EG, editors. *Small animal clinical oncology*. 3rd ed. Philadelphia: WB Saunders; 2001.

87. Nyman HT, Kristensen AT, Flagstad A, et al. A review of the sonographic assessment of tumor metastases in liver and superficial lymph nodes. *Vet Radiol Ultrasound* 2004;**45**:438–48.

88. Feeney DA, Johnston GR, Hardy RM. Two-dimensional, gray-scale ultrasonography for assessment of hepatic and splenic neoplasia in the dog and cat. *J Am Vet Med Assoc* 1984;**184**:68–81.

89. Whiteley MB, Feeney DA, Whiteley LO, et al. Ultrasonographic appearance of primary and metastatic canine hepatic tumors. A review of 48 cases. *J Ultrasound Med* 1989;**8**:621–30.

90. Hammer AS, Sikkema DA. Hepatic neoplasia in the dog and cat. *Vet Clin North Am Small Anim Pract* 1995;**25**:419–35.

91. Eves NG. Hepatocellular adenoma in a 12-year-old crossbred German shepherd dog. *Can Vet J* 2004;**45**:326–8.

92. Murakami T, Feeney DA, Bahr KL. Analysis of clinical and ultrasonographic data by use of logistic regression models for prediction of malignant versus benign causes of ultrasonographically detected focal liver lesions in dogs. *Am J Vet Res* 2012;**73**:821–9.

93. Guillot M, d'Anjou MA, Alexander K, et al. Can sonographic findings predict the results of liver aspirates in dogs with suspected liver disease? *Vet Radiol Ultrasound* 2009;**50**:513–18.

94. Nyland TG. Ultrasonic patterns of canine hepatic lymphosarcoma. *Vet Radiol* 1984;**25**:167–72.

95. Nyland TG, Kantrowitz BM. Ultrasound in diagnosis and staging of abdominal neoplasia. *Contemp Issues Small Anim Pract* 1986;**6**:1–24.

96. Lamb CR, Hartzband LE, Tidwell AS, et al. Ultrasonographic findings in hepatic and splenic lymphosarcoma in dogs and cats. *Vet Radiol Ultrasound* 1991;**32**:117–20.

97. Crabtree AC, Spangler E, Beard D, et al. Diagnostic accuracy of gray-scale ultrasonography for the detection of hepatic and splenic lymphoma in dogs. *Vet Radiol Ultrasound* 2010;**51**:661–4.

98. Dank G, Rassnick KM, Kristal O, et al. Clinical characteristics, treatment, and outcome of dogs with presumed primary hepatic lymphoma: 18 cases (1992-2008). *J Am Vet Med Assoc* 2011;**239**:966–71.

99. Faverzani S, Chinosi S, Valenti P, et al. Comparison between ultrasonography and cytology of liver focal lesions and parenchyma in the dog and cat. *Vet Res Comm* 2006;**30**(Suppl. 1):293–6.

100. Sato AF, Solano M. Ultrasonographic findings in abdominal mast cell disease: a retrospective study of 19 patients. *Vet Radiol Ultrasound* 2004;**45**:51–7.

101. Hanson JA, Papageorges M, Girard E, et al. Ultrasonographic appearance of splenic disease in 101 cats. *Vet Radiol Ultrasound* 2001;**42**:441–5.

102. Stefanello D, Valenti P, Faverzani S. Ultrasound-guided cytology of spleen and liver: A prognostic tool in canine cutaneous mast cell tumor. *J Vet Intern Med* 2009;**23**:1051–7.

103. Book AP, Fidel J, Wills T, et al. Correlation of ultrasound findings, liver and spleen cytology, and prognosis in the clinical staging of high metastatic risk canine mast cell tumors. *Vet Radiol Ultrasound* 2011;**52**:548–54.

104. Cruz-Arambulo R, Wrigley R, Powers B. Sonographic features of histiocytic neoplasms in the canine abdomen. *Vet Radiol Ultrasound* 2004;**45**:554–8.

105. Ramirez S, Douglass JP, Robertson ID. Ultrasonographic features of canine abdominal malignant histiocytosis. *Vet Radiol Ultrasound* 2002;**43**:167–70.

106. Adler R, Wilson DW. Biliary cystadenoma of cats. *Vet Pathol* 1995;**32**:415–18.

107. Trout NJ, Berg RJ, McMillan MC, et al. Surgical treatment of hepatobiliary cystadenomas in cats: five cases (1988-1993). *J Am Vet Med Assoc* 1995;**206**:505–7.

108. Trout NJ. Surgical treatment of hepatobiliary cystadenomas in cats. *Semin Vet Med Surg (Small Anim)* 1997;**12**:51–3.

109. Warren-Smith CMR, Andrew S, Mantis P, et al. Lack of associations between ultrasonographic appearance of parenchymal lesions of the canine liver and histological diagnosis. *J Small Anim Pract* 2012;**53**:168–73.

110. Newell SM, Selcer BA, Girard E, et al. Correlations between ultrasonographic findings and specific hepatic diseases in cats: 72 cases (1985-1997). *J Am Vet Med Assoc* 1998;**213**:94–8.

111. Wang KY, Panciera DL, Al-Rukibat RK, et al. Accuracy of ultrasound-guided fine-needle aspiration of the liver and cytologic findings in dogs and cats: 97 cases (1990-2000). *J Am Vet Med Assoc* 2004;**224**:75–8.

112. Taylor KJW. Gastrointestinal Doppler ultrasound. In: Taylor KJW, Burns PN, Wells PNT, editors. *Clinical applications of Doppler ultrasound*. New York: Raven Press; 1988. p. 162–200.

113. Taylor KJ, Ramos I, Carter D, et al. Correlation of Doppler US tumor signals with neovascular morphologic features. *Radiology* 1988;**166**:57–62.

114. Bates SM, Keller MS, Ramos IM, et al. Hepatoblastoma: detection of tumor vascularity with duplex Doppler US. *Radiology* 1990;**176**:505–7.

115. Orr NM, Taylor KJW. Doppler detection of tumor vascularity. *Clin Diagn Ultrasound* 1990;**26**:149–63.

116. Cosgrove DO, Bamber JC, Davey JB, et al. Color Doppler signals from breast tumors. Work in progress. *Radiology* 1990;**176**:175–80.

117. Dock W, Grabenwoger F, Metz V, et al. Tumor vascularization: assessment with duplex sonography. *Radiology* 1991;**181**:241–4.

118. Tanaka S, Kitamura T, Fujita M, et al. Color Doppler flow imaging of liver tumors. *AJR Am J Roentgenol* 1990;**154**:509–14.

119. Numata K, Tanaka K, Mitsui K, et al. Flow characteristics of hepatic tumors at color Doppler sonography: correlation with arteriographic findings. *AJR Am J Roentgenol* 1993;**160**:515–21.

120. Murphy KJ, Rubin JM. Power Doppler: it's a good thing. *Semin Ultrasound CT MR* 1997;**18**:13–21.

121. Bartolozzi C, Lencioni R, Paolicchi A, et al. Differentiation of hepatocellular adenoma and focal nodular hyperplasia of the liver: comparison of power Doppler imaging and conventional color Doppler sonography. *Eur Radiol* 1997;**7**:1410–15.

122. Martinoli C, Pretolesi F, Crespi G, et al. Power Doppler sonography: clinical applications. *Eur J Radiol* 1998;**27**(Suppl. 2):S133–40.

123. Hosten N, Puls R, Lemke AJ, et al. Contrast-enhanced power Doppler sonography: improved detection of characteristic flow patterns in focal liver lesions. *J Clin Ultrasound* 1999;**27**:107–15.

124. Hirai T, Ohishi H, Yamada R, et al. Three-dimensional power Doppler sonography of tumor vascularity. *Radiat Med* 1998;**16**:353–7.

125. Nyman HT, Kristensen AT, Flagstad A. A review of the sonographic assessment of tumor metastases in liver and superficial lymph nodes. *Vet Radiol Ultrasound* 2004;**45**:438–48.

126. Ziegler LE, O'Brien RT, Waller KR, et al. Quantitative contrast harmonic ultrasound imaging of normal canine liver. *Vet Radiol Ultrasound* 2003;**44**:451–4.

127. Ohlerth S, O'Brien RT. Contrast ultrasound: general principles and veterinary clinical applications. *Vet J* 2007;**174**:501–12.

128. O'Brien RT, Holmes SP. Recent advances in ultrasound technology. *Clin Tech Small Anim Pract* 2007;**22**:93–103.

129. Haers H, Saunders JH. Review of clinical characteristics and applications of contrast-enhanced ultrasonography in dogs. *J Am Vet Med Assoc* 2009;**234**:460–70.

130. Kutara K, Asano K, Kito A, et al. Contrast harmonic imaging of canine hepatic tumors. *J Vet Med Sci* 2006;**68**:433–8.

131. O'Brien RT. Improved detection of metastatic hepatic hemangiosarcoma nodules with contrast ultrasound in three dogs. *Vet Radiol Ultrasound* 2007;**48**:146–8.

132. Ivančić M, Long F, Seiler G. Contrast harmonic ultrasonography of splenic masses and associated liver nodules in dogs. *J Am Vet Med Assoc* 2009;**234**:88–94.

133. Kanemoto H, Ohno K, Nakashima K, et al. Characterization of canine focal liver lesion with contrast-enhanced ultrasound using a novel contrast agent—Sonazoid. *Vet Radiol Ultrasound* 2009;**50**:188–94.

134. Nakamura K, Takagi S, Sasaki N, et al. Contrast-enhanced ultrasonography for characterization of canine focal liver lesions. *Vet Radiology Ultrasound* 2010;**51**:79–85.

135. Kanemoto H, Ohno K, Nakashima K, et al. Vascular and Kupffer imaging of canine liver and spleen using the new contrast agent Sonozoid. *J Vet Med Sci* 2008;**70**:1265–8.

136. Leinonen MR, Raekallio MR, Vainio OM, et al. Quantitative contrast-enhanced ultrasonographic analysis of perfusion in the kidneys, liver, pancreas, small intestine, and mesenteric lymph nodes in healthy cats. *Am J Vet Res* 2010;**71**:1305–11.

137. Janica JR, Serwatka W, Polakow J, et al. Evaluation of enhancement patterns of focal nodular hyperplasia in contrast-enhanced, wide-band phase-inversion harmonic power Doppler imaging of the liver. *Med Sci Monit* 2004;**10**(Suppl. 3):17–21.

138. Janica JR, Serwatka W, Polakow J, et al. Hemangiomas and focal nodular hyperplasia images in contrast-enhanced, wide-band phase-inversion harmonic power Doppler imaging. *Med Sci Monit* 2004;**10**(Suppl. 3):26–31.

139. Kim AY, Choi BI, Kim TK, et al. Hepatocellular carcinoma: power Doppler US with a contrast agent—preliminary results. *Radiology* 1998;**209**:135–40.

140. Strobel D, Kleinecke C, Hansler J, et al. Contrast-enhanced sonography for the characterisation of hepatocellular carcinomas—correlation with histological differentiation. *Ultraschall Med* 2005;**26**:270–6.

141. Genadieva-Dimitrova M, Neskovski M, Popova R, et al. Contrast-enhanced power Doppler sonography in detection and differentiation of focal liver lesions. *Prilozi* 2005;**26**:41–9.

142. Du WH, Yang WX, Xiong XQ, et al. Contrast-enhanced ultrasonographic imaging diagnosis on assessment of vascularity in liver metastatic lesions. *World J Gastroenterol* 2005;**11**:3610–13.

143. Lee JY, Choi BI, Han JK, et al. State-of-the-art ultrasonography of hepatocellular carcinoma. *Eur J Radiol* 2006;**58**:177–85.

144. Wisner ER, Ferrara KW, Short RE, et al. Sentinel node detection using contrast-enhanced power Doppler ultrasound lymphography. *Invest Radiol* 2003;**38**:358–65.

145. Salwei RM, O'Brien RT, Matheson JS. Characterization of lymphomatous lymph nodes in dogs using contrast harmonic and Power Doppler ultrasound. *Vet Radiol Ultrasound* 2005;**46**:411–16.

146. Lurie DM, Seguin B, Schneider PD, et al. Contrast-assisted ultrasound for sentinel lymph node detection in spontaneously arising canine head and neck tumors. *Invest Radiol* 2006;**41**:415–21.

147. Feeney DA, Anderson KL, Ziegler LE. Statistical relevance of ultrasonographic criteria in the assessment of diffuse liver disease in dogs and cats. *Am J Vet Res* 2008;**69**:212–21.

148. Drost WT, Henry GA, Memkoth JH, et al. Quantification of hepatic and renal cortical echogenicity in clinically normal cats. *Am J Vet Res* 2000;**61**:1016–20, 45, 52.

149. Biller DS, Kantrowitz B, Miyabayashi T. Ultrasonography of diffuse liver disease. A review. *J Vet Intern Med* 1992;**6**:71–6.

150. Wrigley RH. Radiographic and ultrasonographic diagnosis of liver diseases in dogs and cats. *Vet Clin North Am Small Anim Pract* 1985;**15**:21–38.

151. Lamb CR, Hartzband LE, Tidwell AS, et al. Ultrasonographic findings in hepatic and splenic lymphosarcoma in dogs and cats. *Vet Radiol* 1991;**32**:117–20.

152. Yeager AE, Mohammed H. Accuracy of ultrasonography in the detection of severe hepatic lipidosis in cats. *Am J Vet Res* 1992;**53**:597–9.

153. Nicoll RG, O'Brien RT, Jackson MW. Qualitative ultrasonography of the liver in obese cats. *Vet Radiol Ultrasound* 1998;**39**:47–50.

154. O'Brien RT, Zagzebski JA, Lu ZF, et al. Measurement of acoustic backscatter and attenuation in the liver of dogs

with experimentally induced steroid hepatopathy. *Am J Vet Res* 1996;**57**:1690–4.

155. Lu ZF, Zagzebski JA, O'Brien RT, et al. Ultrasound attenuation and backscatter in the liver during prednisone administration. *Ultrasound Med Biol* 1997;**23**:1–8.

156. Syakalima M, Takiguchi M, Yasuda J, et al. Comparison of attenuation and liver-kidney contrast of liver ultrasonographs with histology and biochemistry in dogs with experimentally induced steroid hepatopathy. *Vet Q* 1998;**20**:18–22.

157. Gagne JM, Armstrong PJ, Weiss DJ, et al. Clinical features of inflammatory liver disease in cats: 41 cases (1983-1993). *J Am Vet Med Assoc* 1999;**214**:513–16.

158. Nicoll RG, Jackson MW, Knipp BS, et al. Quantitative ultrasonography of the liver in cats during obesity induction and dietary restriction. *Res Vet Sci* 1998;**64**:1–6.

159. Armstrong PJ, Blanchard G. Hepatic lipidosis in cats. *Vet Clin Small Anim* 2009;**39**:599–616.

160. Penninck D, Berry C. Liver imaging in the cat. *Semin Vet Med Surg (Small Anim)* 1997;**12**:10–21.

161. Marolf AJ, Leach L, Gibbons DS, et al. Ultrasonographic findings of feline cholangitis. *J Am Anim Hosp Assoc* 2012;**48**:36–42.

162. Center SA. Diseases of the gallbladder and biliary tree. *Vet Clin Small Anim* 2009;**39**:543–98.

163. Beatty JA, Barrs VR, Martin PA, et al. Spontaneous hepatic rupture in six cats with systemic amyloidosis. *J Small Anim Pract* 2002;**43**:355–63.

164. Flatland B, Moore RR, Wolf CM, et al. Liver aspirate from a Shar Pei dog. *Vet Clin Pathol* 2007;**36**:105–8.

165. Jacobson LS, Kirberger RM, Nesbit JW. Hepatic ultrasonography and pathological findings in dogs with hepatocutaneous syndrome: new concepts. *J Vet Intern Med* 1995;**9**:399–404.

166. Nyland TG, Barthez PY, Ortega TM, et al. Hepatic ultrasonographic and pathologic findings in dogs with canine superficial necrolytic dermatitis. *Vet Radiol Ultrasound* 1996;**37**:200–4.

167. Hill PB, Auxilia ST, Munro E, et al. Resolution of skin lesions and long-term survival in a dog with superficial necrolytic dermatitis and liver cirrhosis. *J Small Anim Pract* 2000;**41**:519–23.

168. Byrne KP. Metabolic epidermal necrosis-hepatocutaneous syndrome. *Vet Clin North Am Small Anim Pract* 1999;**29**:1337–55.

169. Day MJ. Review of thymic pathology in 30 cats and 36 dogs. *J Small Anim Pract* 1997;**38**:393–403.

170. Godfrey DR, Rest JR. Suspected necrolytic migratory erythema associated with chronic hepatopathy in a cat. *J Small Anim Pract* 2000;**41**:324–8.

171. Kimmel SE, Christiansen W, Byrne KP. Clinicopathological, ultrasonographic, and histopathological findings of superficial necrolytic dermatitis with hepatopathy in a cat. *J Am Anim Hosp Assoc* 2003;**39**:23–7.

172. Bahr A, Wrigley R, Salman M. Quantitative evaluation of imagent as an abdominal ultrasound contrast medium in dogs. *Vet Radiol Ultrasound* 2000;**41**:50–5.

173. Nyman HT, Kristensen AT, Kjelgaard-Hansen M, et al. Contrast-enhanced ultrasonography in normal canine liver. Evaluation of imaging and safety parameters. *Vet Radiol Ultrasound* 2005;**46**:243–50.

174. Moentk J, Biller DS. Bilobed gallbladder in a cat: ultrasonographic appearance. *Vet Radiol Ultrasound* 1993;**34**:354–6.

175. Moores AL, Gregory SP. Duplex gall bladder associated with choledocholithiasis, cholecystitis, gall bladder rupture and septic peritonitis in a cat. *J Small Anim Pract* 2007;**48**:404–9.

176. Liptak JM, Swinney GR, Rothwell TL, et al. Aplasia of the gallbladder in a dog. *J Small Anim Pract* 2000;**41**:175–7.

177. Austin B, Tillson DM, Kuhnt LA. Gallbladder agenesis in a Maltese dog. *J Am Anim Hosp Assoc* 2006;**42**:308–11.

178. Kealy JK, McAllister H. The abdomen. In: *Diagnostic radiology & ultrasonography of the dog and cat.* 4th ed. St. Louis: Elsevier Saunders; 2005. p. 21–171.

179. Ralls PW, Quinn MF, Juttner HU, et al. Gallbladder wall thickening: patients without intrinsic gallbladder disease. *Am J Roentgenol* 1981;**137**:65–8.

180. Shlaer WJ, Leopold GR, Scheible FW. Sonography of the thickened gallbladder wall: a nonspecific finding. *Am J Roentgenol* 1981;**136**:337–9.

181. Wegener M, Borsch G, Schneider J, et al. Gallbladder wall thickening: a frequent finding in various nonbiliary disorders—a prospective ultrasonographic study. *J Clin Ultrasound* 1987;**15**:307–12.

182. Reference deleted in proof.

183. van Breda Vriesman AC, Engelbrecht MR, Smithuis RHM, et al. Diffuse gallbladder wall thickening: differential diagnosis. *AJR Am J Roentgenol* 2007;**188**:495–501.

184. Quantz JE, Miles MS, Reed AL, et al. Elevation of alanine transaminase and gallbladder wall abnormalities as biomarkers of anaphylaxis in canine hypersensitivity patients. *J Vet Emerg Crit Care* (San Antonio) 2009;**19**:536–44.

185. Center SA. Diseases of the gallbladder and biliary tree. *Vet Clin Small Anim* 2009;**39**:543–98.

186. Willard MD, Dunstan RW, Faulkner J. Neuroendocrine carcinoma of the gallbladder in a dog. *J Am Vet Med Assoc* 1988;**192**:926–8.

187. Bromel C, Smeak DD, Leveille R. Porcelain gallbladder associated with primary biliary adenocarcinoma in a dog. *J Am Vet Med Assoc* 1998;**213**:1137–9, 1131.

188. Morrell CN, Volk MV, Mankowski JL. A carcinoid tumor in the gallbladder of a dog. *Vet Pathol* 2002;**39**:756–8.

189. Pazzi P, Bamberini S, Buildrini P. Biliary sludge; the sluggish gallbladder. *Dig Liver Dis* 2003;**35**(Suppl. 3):S39–45.

190. Eich CS, Ludwig LL. The surgical treatment of cholelithiasis in cats: a study of nine cases. *J Am Anim Hosp Assoc* 2002;**38**:290–6.

191. Kirpensteijn J, Fingland RB, Ulrich T, et al. Cholelithiasis in dogs: 29 cases (1980-1990). *J Am Vet Med Assoc* 1993;**202**:1137–42.

192. Fahie MA, Martin RA. Extrahepatic biliary tract obstruction: a retrospective study of 45 cases (1983-1993). *J Am Anim Hosp Assoc* 1995;**31**:478–81.

193. Voros K, Nemeth T, Vrabely T, et al. Ultrasonography and surgery of canine biliary diseases. *Acta Vet Hung* 2001;**49**:141–54.

194. Elwood CM, White RN, Freeman K, et al. Cholelithiasis and hyperthyroidism in a cat. *J Feline Med Surg* 2001;**3**:247–52.

195. Ward R. Obstructive cholelithiasis and cholecystitis in a keeshond. *Can Vet J* 2006;**47**:1119–21.

196. Harvey AM, Holt PE, Barr FJ, et al. Treatment and long-term follow-up of extrahepatic biliary obstruction with bilirubin cholelithiasis in a Somali cat with pyruvate kinase deficiency. *J Feline Med Surg* 2007;**9**:424–31.

197. vanGeffen C, Savary-Bataille K, Chiers K, et al. Bilirubin cholelithiasis and haemosiderosis in an anaemic pyruvate kinase-deficient Somali cat. *J Small Anim Pract* 2008;**49**:479–82.

198. Smith SA, Biller DS, Kraft SL, et al. Diagnostic imaging of biliary obstruction. *Comp Cont Ed Pract Vet* 1998;**213**:94–8.

199. Kipnis RM. Cholelithiasis, gallbladder perforation, and bile peritonitis in a dog. *Canine Pract* 1986;**13**:15–27.

200. Bromel C, Leveille R, Scrivani PV, et al. Gallbladder perforation associated with cholelithiasis and cholecystitis in a dog. *J Small Anim Pract* 1998;**39**:541–4.

201. Gaillot HA, Penninck DG, Webster CR, et al. Ultrasonographic features of extrahepatic biliary obstruction in 30 cats. *Vet Radiol Ultrasound* 2007;**48**:439–47.

202. Rivers BJ, Walter PA, Johnston GR, et al. Acalculous cholecystitis in four canine cases: ultrasonographic findings and use of ultrasonographic-guided, percutaneous cholecystocentesis in diagnosis. *J Am Anim Hosp Assoc* 1997;**33**:207–14.

203. Oswald GP, Twedt DC, Steyn P. *Campylobacter jejuni* bacteremia and acute cholecystitis in two dogs. *J Am Anim Hosp Assoc* 1994;**30**:165–9.

204. Ralls PW, Halls J, Lapin SA, et al. Prospective evaluation of the sonographic Murphy sign in suspected acute cholecystitis. *J Clin Ultrasound* 1982;**10**:113–15.

205. Simeone JF, Brink JA, Mueller PR, et al. The sonographic diagnosis of acute gangrenous cholecystitis: importance of the Murphy sign. *Am J Roentgenol* 1989;**152**:289–90.

206. Lee FT Jr, DeLone DR, Bean DW, et al. Acute cholecystitis in an animal model: findings on color Doppler sonography. *AJR Am J Roentgenol* 1995;**165**:85–90.

207. Zawie DA, Garvey MS. Feline hepatic disease. *Vet Clin North Am Small Anim Pract* 1984;**14**:1201–30.

208. Callahan JE, Haddad JL, Brown DC, et al. Feline cholangitis: a necropsy study of 44 cats (1986-2008). *J Feline Med Surg* 2011;**13**:570–6.

209. Brain PH, Barrs VR, Martin P, et al. Feline cholecystitis and acute neutrophilic cholangitis: clinical findings, bacterial isolates and response to treatment in six cases. *J Feline Medicine and Surgery* 2006;**8**:91–103.

210. Neel JA, Tarigo J, Grindem CB. Gallbladder aspirate from a dog. *Vet Clin Pathol* 2006;**35**:467–70.

211. Armstrong JA, Taylor SM, Tryon KA, et al. Emphysematous cholecystitis in a Siberian Husky. *Can Vet J* 2000;**41**:60–2.

212. Lord PF, Wilkins RJ. Emphysema of the gallbladder in a diabetic dog. *J Am Vet Radiol Soc* 1972;**13**:49–52.

213. Burk RL, Johnson GF. Emphysematous cholecystitis in the nondiabetic dog: three case histories. *Vet Radiol* 1980;**21**:242–5.

214. Avgeris S, Hoskinson JJ. Emphysematous cholecystitis in a dog: a radiographic diagnosis. *J Am Anim Hosp Assoc* 1992;**28**:344–6.

215. Church EM, Matthiesen DT. Surgical treatment of 23 dogs with necrotizing cholecystitis. *J Am Anim Hosp Assoc* 1988;**24**:305–10.

216. Holt DE, Mehler SJ, Mayhew PD, et al. Canine gallbladder infarction: 12 cases (1993-2003). *Vet Pathol* 2004;**41**:416–18.

217. Jeffrey RB, Laing FC, Wong W, et al. Gangrenous cholecystitis: diagnosis by ultrasound. *Radiology* 1983;**148**:219–21.

218. Lipowitz AJ, Poffenbarger E. Gallbladder perforation in a dog. *J Am Vet Med Assoc* 1984;**184**:836–9.

219. Aguirre AL, Center SA, Randolph JF, et al. Gallbladder disease in Shetland Sheepdogs: 38 cases (1995-2005). *J Am Vet Med Assoc* 2007;**231**:79–88.

220. Mealey K, Minch J, White S, et al. An insertion mutation in ABCB4 is associated with gallbladder mucocele formation in dogs. *Comp Hepatol* 2010;**9**:1–6.

221. Kook PH, Schallenberg S, Rentsch KM, et al. Effect of twice-daily oral administration of hydrocortisone on the bile acids composition of gallbladder bile in dogs. *Am J Vet Res* 2011;**72**:1607–12.

222. Mesich ML, Mayhew PD, Pack M, et al. Gallbladder mucoceles and their association with endocrinopathies in dogs: a retrospective case-control study. *J Small Anim Pract* 2009;**50**:630–5.

223. Newell SM, Selcer BA, Mahaffey MB, et al. Gallbladder mucocele causing biliary obstruction in two dogs: ultrasonographic, scintigraphic, and pathological findings. *J Am Anim Hosp Assoc* 1995;**31**:467–72.

224. Besso JG, Wrigley RH, Gliatto JM, et al. Ultrasonographic appearance and clinical findings in 14 dogs with gallbladder mucocele. *Vet Radiol Ultrasound* 2000;**41**:261–71.

225. Pike FS, Berg J, King NW, et al. Gallbladder mucocele in dogs: 30 cases (2000-2002). *J Am Vet Med Assoc* 2004;**224**:1615–22.

226. Crews LJ, Feeney DA, Jessen CR, et al. Clinical, ultrasonographic, and laboratory findings associated with gallbladder disease and rupture in dogs: 45 cases (1997-2007). *J Am Vet Med Assoc* 2009;**234**:359–66.

227. Worley DR, Hottinger HA, Lawrence HJ. Surgical management of gallbladder mucoceles in dogs: 22 cases (1999-2003). *J Am Vet Med Assoc* 2004;**225**:1418–22.

228. Vielgrader HD. Sonographische und klinische diagnostik bei gallenblasen-und gallengangserkrankungen der katze [dissertation]. Veterinarmedizinische Universitat Wien; 1998.

229. Bennett SL, Milne M, Slocombe RF, et al. Gallbladder mucocoele and concurrent hepatic lipidosis in a cat. *Aust Vet J* 2007;**85**:397–400.

230. Walter R, Dunn ME, d'Anjou MA, et al. Nonsurgical resolution of gallbladder mucocele in two dogs. *J Am Vet Med Assoc* 2008;**232**:1688–93.

231. Voros K, Sterczer A, Manczur F, et al. Percutaneous ultrasound-guided cholecystocentesis in dogs. *Acta Vet Hung* 2002;**50**:385–93.

232. Savary-Bataille KC, Bunch SE, Spaulding KA, et al. Percutaneous ultrasound-guided cholecystocentesis in healthy cats. *J Vet Intern Med* 2003;**17**:298–303.

233. Herman BA, Brawer RS, Murtaugh RJ, et al. Therapeutic percutaneous ultrasound-guided cholecystocentesis in three dogs with extrahepatic biliary obstruction and pancreatitis. *J Am Vet Med Assoc* 2005;**227**:1782–6.

234. Ginat D, Saad WE. Cholecystostomy and transcholecystic biliary access. *Tech Vasc Interv Radiol* 2008;**11**:2–13.

235. vanSonnenberg E, D'Agostino HB, Goodacre BW, et al. Percutaneous gallbladder puncture and cholecystostomy: results, complications, and caveats for safety. *Radiology* 1992;**183**:167–70.

236. Gold JA, Zeman RK, Schwartz A. Computed tomographic cholangiography in a canine model of biliary obstruction. *Invest Radiol* 1979;**14**:498–501.

237. Raptopoulos V, Fabian TM, Silva W, et al. The effect of time and cholecystectomy on experimental biliary tree dilatation. A multi-imaging evaluation. *Invest Radiol* 1985;**20**:276–86.

238. Boothe HW, Boothe DM, Komkov A, et al. Use of hepatobiliary scintigraphy in the diagnosis of extrahepatic biliary obstruction in dogs and cats: 25 cases (1982-1989). *J Am Vet Med Assoc* 1992;**201**:134–41.

239. Head LL, Daniel GB. Correlation between hepatobiliary scintigraphy and surgery or postmortem examination findings in dogs and cats with extrahepatic biliary

obstruction, partial obstruction, or patency of the biliary system: 18 cases (1995-2004). *J Am Vet Med Assoc* 2005; **227**:1618–24.

240. Foley WD, Quiroz FA. The role of sonography in imaging of the biliary tract. *Ultrasound* Q 2007;**23**:123–35.

241. Watanabe Y, Nagayama M, Okumura A, et al. MR imaging of acute biliary disorders. *Radiographics* 2007; **27**:477–95.

242. Fried AM, Bell RM, Bivins BA. Biliary obstruction in a canine model: sequential study of the sonographic threshold. *Invest Radiol* 1981;**16**:317–19.

243. Zeman RK, Taylor KJ, Rosenfield AT, et al. Acute experimental biliary obstruction in the dog: sonographic findings and clinical implications. *AJR Am J Roentgenol* 1981;**136**:965–7.

244. Nyland TG, Gillett NA. Sonographic evaluation of experimental bile duct ligation in the dog. *Vet Radiol* 1982;**23**:252–60.

245. Finn ST, Park RD, Twedt DC, et al. Ultrasonographic assessment of sincalide-induced canine gallbladder emptying: an aid to the diagnosis of biliary obstruction. *Vet Radiol* 1991;**32**:269–76.

246. Della Santa D, Schweighauser A, Forterre F, et al. Imaging diagnosis—extrahepatic biliary tract obstruction secondary to a duodenal foreign body in a cat. *Vet Radiol Ultrasound* 2007;**48**:448–50.

247. Buote NJ, Mitchell SL, Penninck D, et al. Cholecystoenterostomy for treatment of extrahepatic biliary tract obstruction in cats: 22 cases (1994-2003). *J Am Vet Med Assoc* 2006;**228**:1376–82.

248. Mayhew PD, Holt DE, McLear RC, et al. Pathogenesis and outcome of extrahepatic biliary obstruction in cats. *J Small Anim Pract* 2002;**43**:247–53.

249. Finn-Bodner ST, Park RD, Tyler JW, et al. Ultrasonographic determination, in vitro and in vivo, of canine gallbladder volume, using four volumetric formulas and stepwise-regression models. *Am J Vet Res* 1993;**54**: 832–5.

250. Atalan G, Barr FJ, Holt PE. Estimation of the volume of the gall bladder of 32 dogs from linear ultrasonographic measurements. *Vet Rec* 2007;**160**:118–22.

251. Diana A, Guglielmini C, Specchi S, et al. Ultrasonographic evaluation of preprandial and postprandial gallbladder volume in healthy cats. *Am J Vet Res* 2012; **73**:1583–8.

252. Foley P, Miller L, Graham K, et al. Cholecystadenocarcinoma in a cat. *Can Vet J* 1998;**39**:373–4.

253. Patnaik AK, Liu S-K, Hurvitz AI, et al. Nonhematopoietic neoplasms in cats. *J Natl Cancer Inst* 1975;**54**: 855–60.

254. Patnaik AK, Hurvitz AI, Lieberman PH, et al. Canine bile duct carcinoma. *Vet Pathol* 1981;**18**:439–44.

255. Bhandal J, Head L, Francie DA, et al. Use of color flow Doppler ultrasonography to diagnose a bleeding neuroendocrine tumor in the gallbladder of a dog. *J Am Vet Med Assoc* 2009;**235**:1326–9.

256. von Bibra H, Schober K, Jenni R, et al. Diagnosis of constrictive pericarditis by pulsed Doppler echocardiography of the hepatic vein. *Am J Cardiol* 1989;**63**: 483–8.

257. Sasson Z, Gupta MK. Are hepatic pulsations in dilated cardiomyopathy with heart failure due to tricuspid regurgitation? *Am J Cardiol* 1993;**71**:355–8.

258. Jullien T, Valtier B, Hongnat JM, et al. Incidence of tricuspid regurgitation and vena caval backward flow in mechanically ventilated patients. A color Doppler and contrast echocardiographic study. *Chest* 1995;**107**: 488–93.

259. Minich LL, Tani LY, Shaddy RE, et al. Doppler systemic venous flow patterns: changes in children with mild/moderate pulmonic stenosis. *J Am Soc Echocardiogr* 1996;**9**:814–18.

260. Mehta A, Mehta M, Jain AC. Constrictive pericarditis. *Clin Cardiol* 1999;**22**:334–44.

261. Szatmari V, Sotonyi P, Fenyves B, et al. Doppler-ultrasonographic detection of retrograde pulsatile flow in the caudal vena cava of a puppy with cor triatriatum dexter. *Vet Rec* 2000;**147**:68–72.

262. Sakai K, Nakamura K, Satomi G, et al. Evaluation of tricuspid regurgitation by blood flow pattern in the hepatic vein using pulsed Doppler technique. *Am Heart J* 1984;**108**:516–23.

263. Abu-Yousef MM. Duplex Doppler sonography of the hepatic vein in tricuspid regurgitation. *AJR Am J Roentgenol* 1991;**156**:79–83.

264. Nelson NC, Drost WT, Lerch P, et al. Noninvasive estimation of central venous pressure in anesthetized dogs by measurement of hepatic venous blood flow velocity and abdominal venous diameter. *Vet Radiol Ultrasound* 2010;**51**:313–23.

265. Hosoki T, Kuroda C, Tokunaga K, et al. Hepatic venous outflow obstruction: evaluation with pulsed duplex sonography. *Radiology* 1989;**170**:733–7.

266. Cohn LA, Spaulding KA, Cullen JM, et al. Intrahepatic postsinusoidal venous obstruction in a dog. *J Vet Intern Med* 1991;**5**:317–21.

267. Cave TA, Martineau H, Dickie A, et al. Idiopathic hepatic veno-occlusive disease causing Budd-Chiari–like syndrome in a cat. *J Small Anim Pract* 2002;**43**: 411–15.

268. Fine DM, Olivier NB, Walshaw R, et al. Surgical correction of late-onset Budd-Chiari-like syndrome in a dog. *J Am Vet Med Assoc* 1998;**212**:835–7.

269. Schoeman JP, Stidworthy MF. Budd-Chiari-like syndrome associated with an adrenal phaeochromocytoma in a dog. *J Small Anim Pract* 2001;**42**:191–4.

270. Baig MA, Gemmill T, Hammond G, et al. Budd-Chiari–like syndrome caused by a congenital hiatal hernia in a shar-pei dog. *Vet Rec* 2006;**159**:322–3.

271. Lamb CR. Ultrasonographic diagnosis of congenital portosystemic shunts in dogs - results of a prospective study. *Vet Radiol Ultrasound* 1996;**37**:281–8.

272. von Herbay A, Frieling T, Haussinger D. Association between duplex Doppler sonographic flow pattern in right hepatic vein and various liver diseases. *J Clin Ultrasound* 2001;**29**:25–30.

273. Wrigley RH, Macy DW, Wykes PM. Ligation of ductus venosus in a dog, using ultrasonographic guidance. *J Am Vet Med Assoc* 1983;**183**:1461–4.

274. Wrigley RH, Konde LJ, Park RD, et al. Ultrasonographic diagnosis of portacaval shunts in young dogs. *J Am Vet Med Assoc* 1987;**191**:421–4.

275. Lamb CR, Forster-van Hijfte MA, White RN, et al. Ultrasonographic diagnosis of congenital portosystemic shunt in 14 cats. *J Small Anim Pract* 1996;**37**:205–9.

276. Santilli RA, Gerboni G. Diagnostic imaging of congenital porto-systemic shunts in dogs and cats: a review. *Vet J* 2003;**166**:7–18.

277. Szatmári V, Rothuizen J. Ultrasonographic identification and characterization of congenital portosystemic shunts and portal hypertensive disorders in dogs and cats. In: *WSAVA Standards for Clinical and Histopathological Diagnosis of Canine and Feline Liver Disease*. WSAVA. Spain: Saunders Elsevier; 2006. p. 15–39.

278. Berent AC, Tobias KM. Portosystemic Vascular Anomalies. *Vet Clin Small Anim* 2009;**39**:513–41.

279. Tivers M, Lipscomb V. Congenital portosystemic shunts in cats. Investigation, diagnosis and stabilisation. *J Feline Med Surg* 2011;**13**:173–84.

280. Martin RA. Congenital portosystemic shunts in the dog and cat. *Vet Clin North Am Small Anim Pract* 1993;**23**:609–23.

281. van den Ingh TS, Rothuizen J, Meyer HP. Circulatory disorders of the liver in dogs and cats. *Vet Q* 1995;**17**:70–6.

282. van Straten G, Leegwater PA, de Vries M, et al. Inherited congenital extrahepatic portosystemic shunts in Cairn terriers. *J Vet Intern Med* 2005;**19**:321–4.

283. van Steenbeek FG, Leegwater PAJ, van Sluijs FJ, et al. Evidence of inheritance of intrahepatic portosystemic shunts in Irish Wolfhounds. *J Vet Intern Med* 2009;**23**:950–2.

284. White RN, Forster-van Hijfte MA, Petrie G, et al. Surgical treatment of intrahepatic portosystemic shunts in six cats. *Vet Rec* 1996;**139**:314–17.

285. Lamb CR, White RN. Morphology of congenital intrahepatic portacaval shunts in dogs and cats. *Vet Rec* 1998;**142**:55–60.

286. Weisse C, Schwartz K, Stronger R, et al. Transjugular coil embolization of an intrahepatic portosystemic shunt in a cat. *J Am Vet Med Assoc* 2002;**221**:1287–91, 1266-1287.

287. Tillson DM, Winkler JT. Diagnosis and treatment of portosystemic shunts in the cat. *Vet Clin North Am Small Anim Pract* 2002;**32**:881–99, vi-vii.

288. D'Anjou MA. The sonographic search for portosystemic shunts. *Clin Tech Small Anim Pract* 2007;**22**:104–14.

289. Windsor RC, Olby NJ. Congenital portosystemic shunts in five mature dogs with neurological signs. *J Am Anim Hosp Assoc* 2007;**43**:322–31.

290. Partington BP, Partington CR, Biller DS, et al. Transvenous coil embolization for treatment of patent ductus venosus in a dog. *J Am Vet Med Assoc* 1993;**202**:281–4.

291. Moon ML. Diagnostic imaging of portosystemic shunts. *Semin Vet Med Surg (Small Anim)* 1990;**5**:120–6.

292. Holt DE, Schelling CG, Saunders HM, et al. Correlation of ultrasonographic findings with surgical, portographic, and necropsy findings in dogs and cats with portosystemic shunts: 63 cases (1987-1993). *J Am Vet Med Assoc* 1995;**207**:1190–3.

293. Tiemessen I, Rothuizen J, Voorhout G. Ultrasonography in the diagnosis of congenital portosystemic shunts in dogs. *Vet Q* 1995;**17**:50–3.

294. Salwei RM, O'Brien RT, Matheson JS. Use of contrast harmonic ultrasound for the diagnosis of congenital portosystemic shunts in three dogs. *Vet Radiol Ultrasound* 2003;**44**:301–5.

295. Szatmári V, Rothuizen J, van den Ingh TS, et al. Ultrasonographic findings in dogs with hyperammonemia: 90 cases (2000-2002). *J Am Vet Med Assoc* 2004;**224**:717–27.

296. Breznock EM, Whiting PG. Portacaval shunts and anomalies. In: Slatter DH, editor. *Textbook of small animal surgery*. Philadelphia: WB Saunders; 1985. p. 1156.

297. Scavelli TD, Hornbuckle WE, Roth L, et al. Portosystemic shunts in cats: seven cases (1976-1984). *J Am Vet Med Assoc* 1986;**189**:317–25.

298. Berger B, Whiting PG, Breznock EM, et al. Congenital feline portosystemic shunts. *J Am Vet Med Assoc* 1986;**188**:517–21.

299. Van den Ingh TS, Rothuizen J, Meyer HP. Portal hypertension associated with primary hypoplasia of the hepatic portal vein in dogs. *Vet Rec* 1995;**137**:424–7.

300. DeMarco J, Center SA, Dykes N, et al. A syndrome resembling idiopathic noncirrhotic portal hypertension in 4 young Doberman pinschers. *J Vet Intern Med* 1998;**12**:147–56.

301. Bunch SE, Johnson SE, Cullen JM. Idiopathic noncirrhotic portal hypertension in dogs: 33 cases (1982-1998). *J Am Vet Med Assoc* 2001;**218**:392–9.

302. Schermerhorn T, Center SA, Dykes NL, et al. Characterization of hepatoportal microvascular dysplasia in a kindred of cairn terriers. *J Vet Intern Med* 1996;**10**:219–30.

303. Christiansen JS, Hottinger HA, Allen L, et al. Hepatic microvascular dysplasia in dogs: a retrospective study of 24 cases (1987-1995). *J Am Anim Hosp Assoc* 2000;**36**:385–9.

304. Gómez-Ochoa P, Llabrés-Díaz F, Ruiz S, et al. Ultrasonographic appearance of the intravascular transit of agitated saline in normal dogs following ultrasound guided percutaneous splenic injection. *Vet Radiology Ultrasound* 2010;**51**:523–6.

305. Gómez-Ochoa P, Llabrés-Díaz F, Ruiz S, et al. Use of transsplenic injection of agitated saline and heparinized blood for the ultrasonographic diagnosis of macroscopic portosystemic shunts in dogs. *Vet Radiology Ultrasound* 2011;**52**:103–6.

306. Youmans KR, Hunt GB. Cellophane banding for the gradual attenuation of single extrahepatic portosystemic shunts in eleven dogs. *Aust Vet J* 1998;**76**:531–7.

307. Gonzalo-Orden JM, Altonaga JR, Costilla S, et al. Transvenous coil embolization of an intrahepatic portosystemic shunt in a dog. *Vet Radiol Ultrasound* 2000;**41**:516–18.

308. Leveille R, Pibarot P, Soulez G, et al. Transvenous coil embolization of an extrahepatic portosystemic shunt in a dog: a naturally occurring model of portosystemic malformations in humans. *Pediatr Radiol* 2000;**30**:607–9.

309. Szatmari V, van Sluijs FJ, Rothuizen J, et al. Intraoperative ultrasonography of the portal vein during attenuation of intrahepatic portocaval shunts in dogs. *J Am Vet Med Assoc* 2003;**222**:1086–92, 1077.

310. Weisse C, Mondschein JI, Itkin M, et al. Use of a percutaneous atrial septal occluder device for complete acute occlusion of an intrahepatic portosystemic shunt in a dog. *J Am Vet Med Assoc* 2005;**227**:249–52, 236.

311. Mehl ML, Kyles AE, Case JB, et al. Surgical management of left-divisional intrahepatic portosystemic shunts: outcome after partial ligation of, or ameroid ring constrictor placement on, the left hepatic vein in twenty-eight dogs (1995-2005). *Vet Surg* 2007;**36**:21–30.

312. Bussadori R, Bussadori C, Millan L, et al. Transvenous coil embolisation for the treatment of single congenital portosystemic shunts in six dogs. *Vet J* 2007.

313. Furneaux RW. Liver hemodynamics as they relate to portosystemic shunts in the dog: a review. *Res Vet Sci* 2011;**91**:175–80.

314. Kummeling A, Vrakking DJE, Rothuizen J, et al. Hepatic volume measurements in dogs with extrahepatic congenital portosysemic shunts before and after surgical attenuation. *J Vet Intern Med* 2010;**24**:114–19.

315. Bertolini G. Acquired portal collateral circulation in the dog and cat. *Vet Radiol Ultrasound* 2010;**51**:25–33.

316. Strombeck DR, Guilford WG. *Small animal gastroenterology*. 2nd ed. London: Wolfe; 1991.

317. Szatmari V, van den Ingh TS, Fenyves B, et al. Portal hypertension in a dog due to circumscribed fibrosis of the wall of the extrahepatic portal vein. *Vet Rec* 2002;**150**:602–5.

318. Willard MD, Bailey MQ, Hauptman J, et al. Obstructed portal venous flow and portal vein thrombus in a dog. *J Am Vet Med Assoc* 1989;**194**:1449–51.

319. Van Winkle TJ, Bruce E. Thrombosis of the portal vein in eleven dogs. *Vet Pathol* 1993;**30**:28–35.

320. Lamb CR, Wrigley RH, Simpson KW, et al. Ultrasonographic diagnosis of portal vein thrombosis in four dogs. *Vet Radiol Ultrasound* 1996;**37**:121–9.

321. Diaz Espineira MM, Vink-Nooteboom M, Van den Ingh TS, et al. Thrombosis of the portal vein in a miniature schnauzer. *J Small Anim Pract* 1999;**40**:540–3.

322. Bressler C, Himes LC, Moreau RE. Portal vein and aortic thromboses in a Siberian husky with ehrlichiosis and hypothyroidism. *J Small Anim Pract* 2003;**44**:408–10.

323. Respess M, O'Toole TE, Taeymans O, et al. Portal vein thrombosis in 33 dogs: 1998-2011. *J Vet Intern Med* 2012;**26**:230–7.

324. Rogers CL, O'Toole TE, Keating JH, et al. Portal vein thrombosis in cats: 6 cases (2001-2006). *J Vet Intern Med* 2008;**22**:282–7.

325. McConnell JF, Sparkes AH, Ladlow J, et al. Ultrasonographic diagnosis of unusual portal vascular abnormalities in two cats. *J Small Anim Pract* 2006;**47**:338–43.

326. Theilen GH, Madewell BR. *Veterinary cancer medicine.* 2nd ed. Philadelphia: Lea & Febiger; 1987.

327. Roy RG, Post GS, Waters DJ, et al. Portal vein thrombosis as a complication of portosystemic shunt ligation in two dogs. *J Am Anim Hosp Assoc* 1992;**28**:53–8.

328. Loperfido F, Lombardo A, Amico CM, et al. Doppler analysis of portal vein flow in tricuspid regurgitation. *J Heart Valve Dis* 1993;**2**:174–82.

329. Rengo C, Brevetti G, Sorrentino G, et al. Portal vein pulsatility ratio provides a measure of right heart function in chronic heart failure. *Ultrasound Med Biol* 1998;**24**:327–32.

330. Gorka TS, Gorka W. Doppler sonographic diagnosis of severe portal vein pulsatility in constrictive pericarditis: flow normalization after pericardiectomy. *J Clin Ultrasound* 1999;**27**:84–8.

331. Wachsberg RH, Needleman L, Wilson DJ. Portal vein pulsatility in normal and cirrhotic adults without cardiac disease. *J Clin Ultrasound* 1995;**23**:3–15.

332. Szatmari V, van Sluijs FJ, Rothuizen J, et al. Ultrasonographic assessment of hemodynamic changes in the portal vein during surgical attenuation of congenital extrahepatic portosystemic shunts in dogs. *J Am Vet Med Assoc* 2004;**224**:395–402.

333. Vogt JC, Krahwinkel DJ Jr, Bright RM, et al. Gradual occlusion of extrahepatic portosystemic shunts in dogs and cats using the ameroid constrictor. *Vet Surg* 1996;**25**:495–502.

334. Youmans KR, Hunt GB. Experimental evaluation of four methods of progressive venous attenuation in dogs. *Vet Surg* 1999;**28**:38–47.

335. Broome CJ, Walsh VP, Braddock JA. Congenital portosystemic shunts in dogs and cats. *N Z Vet J* 2004;**52**:154–62.

336. Szatmari V, Rothuizen J, van Sluijs FJ, et al. Ultrasonographic evaluation of partially attenuated congenital extrahepatic portosystemic shunts in 14 dogs. *Vet Rec* 2004;**155**:448–56.

337. McConnell JF, Sparkes AH, Ladlow J, et al. Ultrasonographic diagnosis of unusual portal vascular abnormalities in two cats. *J Small Anim Pract* 2006;**47**:338–43.

338. Ohnishi K, Saito M, Nakayama T, et al. Portal venous hemodynamics in chronic liver disease: effects of posture change and exercise. *Radiology* 1985;**155**:757–61.

339. Legendre AM, Krahwinkel DJ, Carrig CB, et al. Ascites associated with intrahepatic arteriovenous fistula in a cat. *J Am Vet Med Assoc* 1976;**168**:589–91.

340. Bailey MQ, Willard MD, McLoughlin MA, et al. Ultrasonographic findings associated with congenital hepatic arteriovenous fistula in three dogs. *J Am Vet Med Assoc* 1988;**192**:1099–101.

341. Szatmari V, Nemeth T, Kotai I, et al. Doppler ultrasonographic diagnosis and anatomy of congenital intrahepatic arterioportal fistula in a puppy. *Vet Radiol Ultrasound* 2000;**41**:284–6.

342. Koide K, Koide Y, Wada Y, et al. Congenital hepatic arteriovenous fistula with intrahepatic portosystemic shunt and aortic stenosis in a dog. *J Vet Med Sci* 2004;**66**:299–302.

343. Zwingenberger AL, McLear RC, Weisse C. Diagnosis of arterioportal fistulae in four dogs using computed tomographic angiography. *Vet Radiol Ultrasound* 2005;**46**:472–7.

344. Chanoit G, Kyles AE, Weisse C, et al. Surgical and interventional radiographic treatment of dogs with hepatic arteriovenous fistulae. *Vet Surg* 2007;**36**:199–209.

CHAPTER 10
Spleen

Thomas G. Nyland • John S. Mattoon

Ultrasonographic examination of the spleen is useful clinically to determine the size, location, and presence of parenchymal abnormalities when a pathologic condition is suspected. The main indications for examining the spleen are generalized splenomegaly, abdominal or splenic mass, trauma, and hemoperitoneum. Diseases affecting the spleen often cause enlargement, which may be detected with abdominal palpation, radiography, or ultrasonography. The primary value of ultrasonography over other imaging methods is its ability to determine whether focal or diffuse parenchymal disease is present, to differentiate cavitary from solid lesions, and to provide guidance for intralesional aspiration biopsy. Ultrasonography is particularly worthwhile in the presence of abdominal fluid. Doppler ultrasonography is also helpful in the evaluation of splenic blood flow in cases of abdominal trauma, splenic torsion, and splenic arterial or venous thrombosis; of the latter, venous thrombosis is more common.

Identifying splenic disease is easy when masses or multifocal disease are present, but ultrasound cannot be used to differentiate malignant, benign, and inflammatory/infectious disease. Many cases (the majority perhaps) of "mottled" splenic parenchyma, small nodules, and even large nodules or masses may be benign. Furthermore, splenic disease may be present even though the spleen appears to be entirely normal by ultrasound.

All figures in this chapter demonstrate confirmed disease. Categorizing figures by disease is done out of necessity; it does not imply that we can diagnose disease type by sonographic appearance; nor does normal appearance of the spleen indicate lack of disease. These two points cannot be overemphasized. Box 10-1 provides a classification guide of splenic disease. Note many of the disease processes can be diffuse or nodular, or be present without parenchymal alterations.

EXAMINATION TECHNIQUE

The spleen is located in the left cranial abdomen and usually follows the greater curvature of the stomach in the dog. The exact position of the spleen is variable, depending on the amount of gastric distention and the size of other abdominal organs. A detailed ultrasonographic-anatomic correlation and imaging protocol of the canine spleen in anesthetized dogs has been described.[1] The head (dorsal extremity) of the spleen is typically located under the border of the rib cage; the body and tail (ventral extremity) extend along the left body wall or across the ventral abdomen. The spleen lies lateral and caudal to the stomach and ventral or lateral to the left kidney. When the spleen is enlarged, it may cross the ventral midline or extend caudally to the bladder region. The left intercostal approach is used to visualize the head of the spleen at the 11th or 12th intercostal space if it cannot be seen from the ventrolateral abdomen. The remainder of the spleen is systematically scanned in sagittal and transverse planes from the ventral abdominal wall. A 7.5-MHz or higher (for dogs) or 10.0-MHz or higher (for cats) transducer may be used to provide high resolution because of the spleen's superficial location. A standoff pad is helpful to position the spleen farther from and more fully within the focal zone of the transducer if the ventral (parietal) surface is incompletely visualized in the near field.[2] However, this is usually unnecessary because of the good near-field visibility of today's blended frequency linear or curvilinear probes. See Chapter 4 for a detailed description and illustration of scanning the spleen.

NORMAL ANATOMY AND APPEARANCE

The normal spleen is a very homogenous and echogenic organ. The cat spleen is consistently small and thin (up to about 10 mm thick) because, in contrast to the dog's spleen, it is not a large blood reservoir (Figure 10-1). And though the cat spleen will slightly enlarge following sedation or general anesthesia, the effects are much less pronounced than in dogs. However, the sonographer should note that as higher frequency transducers are used, a normal spleen often appears very mildly mottled. It may be that today's most advanced transducers are able to resolve splenic lymphoid centers.

The size of the normal dog spleen is highly variable and must be assessed subjectively, similar to radiographic methods. There are no established parameters for thickness, width, or length. The usual crescent or triangular shape of the spleen seen in the near field is also variable, but the capsule is smooth and regular. The spleen has an echogenic capsule when the beam strikes it perpendicularly (Figure 10-2, *A* to *E*). This enables determination of whether an abdominal mass arises from the spleen or merely rests against it. If a mass originates from the spleen, the capsule is interrupted or deviates outward, and the splenic parenchyma is continuous with the mass. The echogenic capsule remains intact with extrasplenic masses.

The splenic parenchyma is homogeneous with a finely textured, medium- to high-level echo pattern (see Figure 10-2). This pattern contrasts with a slightly more coarse and slightly less echogenic appearance of the dog liver (the spleen and liver are often isoechoic in normal cats). Direct comparisons of the normal spleen and liver at the same depth, gain, and time-gain compensation settings can be difficult in some patients. However, when the liver or spleen is enlarged,

BOX 10-1

Splenic Diseases

FOCAL OR MULTIFOCAL DISEASE (NODULES AND/OR MASSES)

Hematoma
    Trauma, lymphoid hyperplasia, vascular tumor
Nodular hyperplasia (lymphoid hyperplasia)
Extramedullary hematopoiesis
Primary tumors
    Lymphoma
    Histiocytic sarcoma
    Hemangiosarcoma
    Hemangioma
    Fibroma
    Fibrosarcoma, osteosarcoma
    Myxosarcoma
    Myelolipoma
    Lipoma, liposarcoma
    Leiomyoma, leiomyosarcoma
Metastatic tumors
Granuloma
Abscess

INCREASE IN SIZE WITHOUT PARENCHYMAL ALTERATIONS

Anesthetic agents, tranquilizers
Lymphoid hyperplasia
Extramedullary hematopoiesis
Hemolytic anemias
Chronic anemias
Hematopoietic neoplasias
    Mast cell tumor, lymphoma, histiocytic sarcoma

DIFFUSE NODULAR DISEASE OR INHOMOGENEOUS ALTERATIONS IN PARENCHYMA

Hemangioma, hemangiosarcoma
Hematopoietic neoplasias
    Mast cell tumor, lymphoma, histiocytic sarcoma
Granulomatous disease
Histoplasmosis
Lymphoid hyperplasia
Amyloidosis

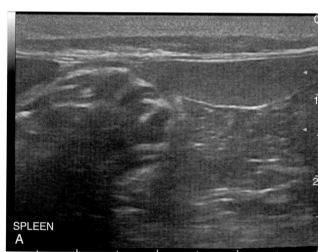

SPLEEN
A

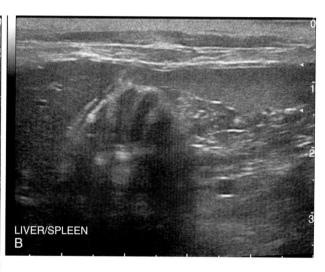

LIVER/SPLEEN
B

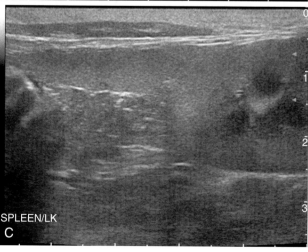

SPLEEN/LK
C

Figure 10-1 Normal spleen in an 8-year-old neutered male cat. In general, the cat splenic is nearly isoechoic to the liver and renal cortex. This is especially true when using higher frequency transducers. **A,** The spleen is present in the near field (right center), approximately 8 mm thick. The parenchyma is very homogeneous. The adjacent stomach is located in the near field, left center. **B,** Comparison of feline spleen and liver. The spleen is just slightly more echogenic and fine textured than the adjacent liver, located to the left. The stomach is located between them. **C,** Comparison of spleen and left kidney. The splenic parenchyma and renal cortex are very similar in both echogenicity and echotexture. A linear-array broadband (4-13 MHz) transducer was used, operating at the highest frequency of 13 MHz.

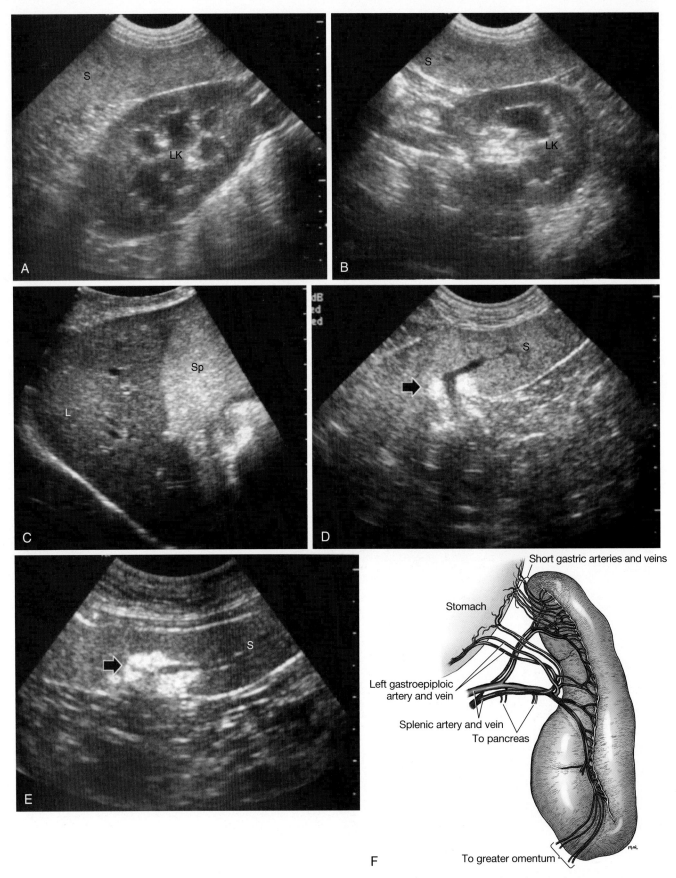

Figure 10-2 Normal dog spleen. Sagittal (**A**) and transverse (**B**) views comparing the echogenicity of the spleen (*S*) and left kidney (*LK*). The spleen is usually much more echogenic than the kidney cortex. **C,** Sagittal view of the liver and spleen in the left cranial abdomen. The echogenicity of the liver (*L*) is the same as or slightly greater than that of the kidney but less than that of the spleen (*Sp*). **D** and **E,** Splenic capsular invagination and fat surrounding the vessels at the splenic hilum produce increased echogenicity (*arrow*). This appearance should not be mistaken for an abnormality. **F,** Blood supply of the dog spleen. (From Evans H, de Lahunta A: Guide to dissection of the dog, ed. 7, St. Louis, 2009, Saunders.)

comparisons of echogenicity are much easier. For unexplained reasons, echogenicity of a seemingly normal spleen may appear similar to that of the liver. This appearance suggests an abnormality when none exists. The echogenicities of the left kidney and spleen are more easily compared in most animals. The dog spleen is normally considerably more echogenic than the cortex of the left kidney (see Figure 10-2, A and B), although this is not always the case in cats. As mentioned previously, liver parenchymal echogenicity is generally intermediate between that of the kidney and spleen. Subtle changes in the parenchymal echogenicity of the liver, spleen, and kidney are difficult to recognize clinically, and more than one organ could be abnormal. Therefore the sonographer cannot rely solely on splenic echogenicity or comparisons with other organs for a diagnosis. A recent study by Yabuki and colleagues[3] emphasizes this point. In their study, different regions of renal cortices were compared to the spleen and the liver (yielding Kid/Sp and Kid/Liv echogenicity ratios). They found that Kid/Sp using a linear-array transducer at four different settings was a reliable method for quantitative evaluation of renal echogenicity in cats. However, Kid/Sp and Kid/Liv were not consistent when using a convex transducer at different machine settings.

The splenic vasculature consists of the splenic artery (a branch of the celiac artery) and the splenic vein, which drains into the portal vein. The splenic arterial branches are difficult to see on routine splenic scans. Doppler ultrasonography can help determine their location and patency. The branches of the dog splenic vein are well visualized near the hilum of the spleen, but their course into the splenic parenchyma can be followed only for a short distance in the normal animal (see Figure 10-2, D and E). In cats, the splenic veins are less conspicuous. The splenic veins are often normally surrounded by very echogenic fat (see Figures 10-2, D and E, and 10-22, B). The size of splenic veins must be judged subjectively, similar to hepatic veins. The main splenic vein can sometimes be traced from the spleen to the main portal vein, but interference from bowel gas sometimes prevents complete visualization. The splenic veins should be assessed for thrombosis, and the splenic hilar region should be searched carefully for lymphadenopathy.

FOCAL OR MULTIFOCAL DISEASE

Focal lesions of the spleen are easily detected, but the ultrasound appearance alone usually does not allow a definitive diagnosis. Focal lesions range from small (nodules) to large (masses) and may be solitary, several, or so numerous that they represent a diffuse nodular process. Attempting to classify splenic disease in this manner can therefore become difficult at times. Complicating this is the fact that nearly all splenic parenchymal diseases can manifest as focal, multifocal, or diffuse alterations. Hyperplastic nodules, hematoma, abscess, primary or metastatic neoplasia, necrosis from vascular compromise, toxic conditions, and inflammatory disorders, can produce similar ultrasound findings.

A complete ultrasound examination is required to detect other potential abdominal abnormalities such liver nodules or peritoneal fluid. The findings must be correlated with the history, clinical information, laboratory work, and other imaging studies to arrive at a differential diagnosis or diagnoses. Cytology or histology is almost certainly necessary for a definitive diagnosis. Reviews of pathologic diagnoses from canine splenic lesions are available.[4,5] The most common diagnosis was splenic neoplasia, with hemangiosarcoma the most frequently recognized. Benign conditions such as nodular hyperplasia, hematoma, splenic congestion, hemorrhage, extramedullary hematopoiesis, and hemosiderin deposition were also seen. The remainder of the canine cases consisted of splenic infarction, with or without torsion, abscessation, and focal mast cell proliferation. A similar review is also available for a series of 455 cats.[6] Primary and metastatic neoplasia was found in 37% of splenic lesions. Mast cell tumor was the most frequently identified neoplasia in the cat, followed by lymphosarcoma, myeloproliferative disease, and hemangiosarcoma, in that order. Accessory splenic tissue from the omentum or pancreas was found in 4% of the cats (see Figure 10-43), whereas hyperplastic nodules, hematomas, or both were found in another 4%. Splenitis was found in 2% and infarction, in 1% of the affected cats. Ultrasonography is useful for guided aspiration of focal or diffuse lesions to obtain representative cytologic material. Figures 10-3 to 10-9 illustrate a variety of splenic nodules from a range of disease processes.

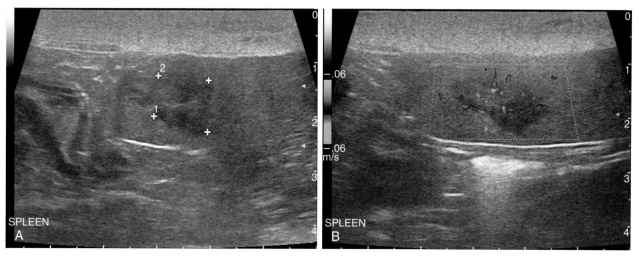

Figure 10-3 Seven-year-old Jack Russell terrier with fever. A, A poorly demarcated, solitary primarily hypoechoic nodule was present within the spleen (approximately 1.2 × 1.4 cm between electronic cursors). **B,** Color Doppler evaluation shows good blow flow within the nodule. The cytologic diagnosis was small cell lymphoma.

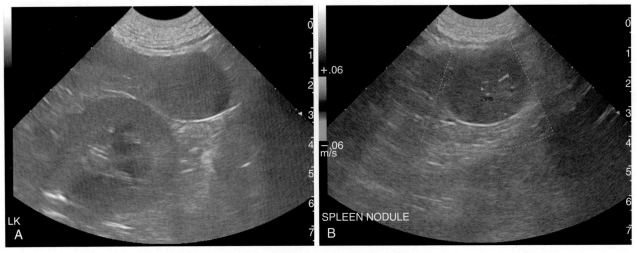

Figure 10-4 **Six-year old spayed female golden retriever in liver failure. A,** A solid, hypoechoic nodule was identified protruding from the tail of the spleen, approximately 2.5 cm in diameter. The left kidney is in the adjacent far field. **B,** Color Doppler analysis shows some blood flow within the splenic nodule. Fine-needle aspiration for cytology yielded a diagnosis of undifferentiated sarcoma.

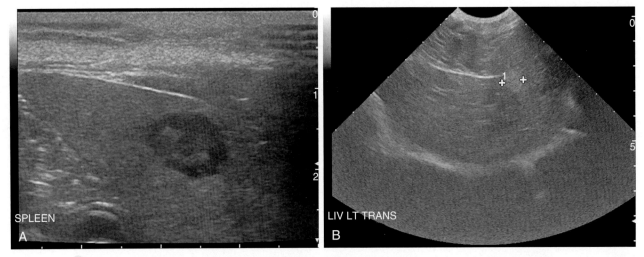

Figure 10-5 **Ten-year old German shorthaired pointer with a high-grade osteosarcoma of her mandible. A,** A small (approximately 1 cm), complex, well-demarcated nodule was identified in the spleen. On real-time examination this nodule was close to a similar nodule. **B,** A small (0.87 cm) solitary hyperechoic nodule was identified between the left lateral and medial lobes of the liver. The splenic nodule was lymphoid hyperplasia; the liver nodule was also hyperplasia.

Hematoma

Splenic hematomas usually result from abdominal trauma or clotting disorders, or they occur in association with splenic neoplasia, such as hemangiosarcoma or lymphosarcoma.[7,8] Their location varies from intraparenchymal to subcapsular, and hemorrhage may be seen adjacent to the spleen. The contour of the spleen is altered if the lesion is large or close to the surface. The ultrasonographic appearance of a hematoma is extremely variable, depending on its age, and the hematoma may appear similar to other focal inflammatory or neoplastic conditions affecting the spleen[7-11] (Figure 10-10; see also Figure 10-20). Intraparenchymal hemorrhage may

initially appear hyperechoic,[12] but larger collections of unclotted blood are initially anechoic to hypoechoic. Clotted blood within a hematoma may appear isoechoic or hyperechoic, gradually becoming hypoechoic relative to the splenic parenchyma.[13] This has been ascribed to red blood cell lysis and clot retraction.[14-15] Later, more echogenic contents appear with variable amounts of anechoic fluid as the clot organizes. A cystlike structure with posterior acoustic enhancement may eventually develop, or the echogenic contents may persist for long periods. The hematoma may also have internal septations.[7] The cystic lesion usually resolves with time, but hematomas have been suggested as one origin of acquired splenic

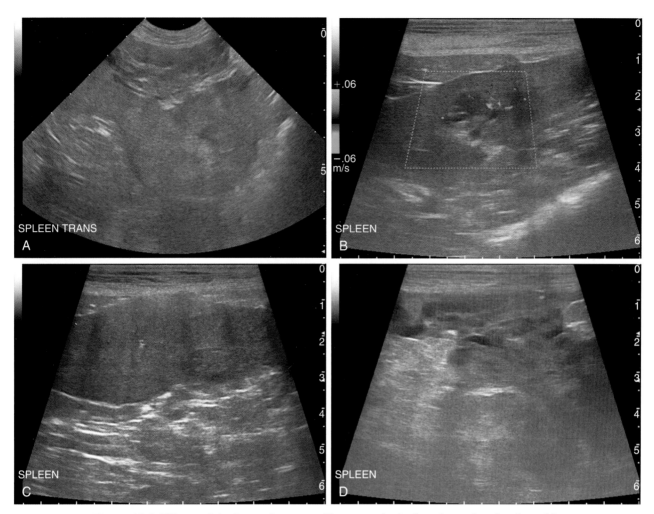

Figure 10-6 **Diffuse nodular hemangiosarcoma.** This example displays the multitude of possible appearances of splenic hemangiosarcoma. **A,** A slightly inhomogeneous 2-cm mass that appeared solid was present in the tip of the tail of the spleen. **B,** In the body of the spleen a poorly marginated, complex, and primarily hypoechoic nodule was seen. Color Doppler imaging shows the nodule to be poorly vascularized. **C,** A nearly isoechoic nodule was present in the far field of this portion of the spleen with generalized thickening of the spleen regionally. **D,** In this section, the spleen was nearly unrecognizable with marked disruption of the splenic capsule and an irregular contour. The parenchyma was very inhomogeneous.

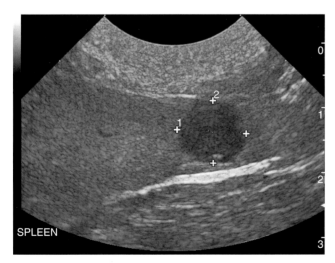

Figure 10-7 **Four-year-old Welsh corgi with a history of dietary indiscretion and possible pancreatitis.** An approximately 1-cm solitary nodule (1.08 × 0.96 cm) that was well-demarcated and homogeneous was present within the tail of the spleen. This was an incidental finding of lymphoid hyperplasia.

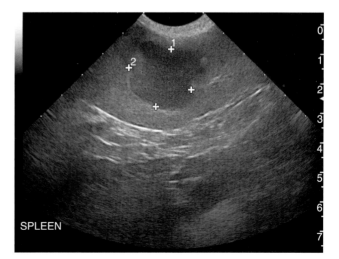

Figure 10-8 A solitary hypoechoic nodule was present within the spleen in this 10-year-old Wheaton terrier examined because of an epiglottic sarcoma (2.20 × 2.31 cm). Some of the periphery was well delineated from the surrounding parenchyma, whereas other portions were poorly demarcated. The cytologic diagnosis was lymphoid hyperplasia and extramedullary hematopoiesis.

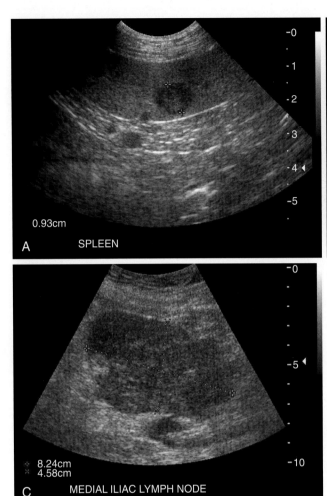

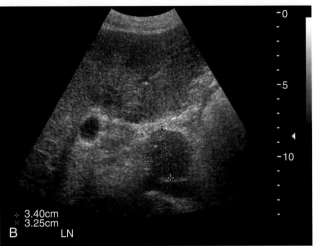

Figure 10-9 Plasma cell tumor. A, A hypoechoic nodule is present within the splenic parenchyma (0.93 cm). **B,** In another portion of the same spleen, a poorly defined mass distorting the contour of the spleen is present. The spleen is thickened and has a coarse, diffuse, hypoechoic, and slightly inhomogeneous texture. In the far field an enlarged mesenteric lymph node is identified as a round, homogeneous structure (3.40 × 3.25 cm) surrounded by echogenic mesentery. **C,** Enlarged, misshapen medial iliac lymph nodes were also present (8.24 × 4.58 cm).

cysts (pseudocysts). In one study, 57% of hematomas created in an experimental canine model resolved spontaneously within 3 months.[16] Those that persisted (43%) eventually resolved after percutaneous aspiration under ultrasound guidance. Intrasplenic hematomas in humans have been reported to take months to resorb and some may take up to a year.[13] Based on these studies, it seems that splenic hematomas may persist for extended periods. However, in our experience, benign splenic cysts are rare. Other causes of cavitary splenic lesions, such as hemangiosarcoma, occur much more frequently and therefore should always be excluded. It is generally accepted that splenic neoplasia, abscess, nodular hyperplasia, infarcts, and necrosis can appear similar to a hematoma on a single ultrasound examination.[10,11,17] A history of trauma or a bleeding disorder, age of the animal, and serial ultrasound examinations may aid diagnosis.

Contrast enhanced and three-dimensional sonography has been used for evaluation of intraabdominal hemorrhage to identify splenic hematomas in humans.[18] This technique may eventually prove useful in animals to detect active bleeding sites in the spleen. Enhancement of the normal surrounding splenic parenchyma was evident, whereas the hematomas themselves remained unenhanced. In addition, normal blood flow and extravasated blood from damaged vessels were better identified with this technique.

Fine-needle aspiration of the spleen or abdominal lymph nodes may be helpful for diagnosis of splenic lesions in certain cases, such as with hematomas associated with lymphosarcoma. However, other types of neoplasia, such as hemangiosarcoma, usually cannot be differentiated from hematomas on the basis of a fine-needle aspirate. Neoplastic cells are difficult to detect because of blood dilution. Therefore normal findings from an aspirate do not rule out neoplasia. However, other findings, such as a mass in the area of the right atrium on echocardiography or metastasis involving other sites in the abdomen or thorax, may assist with diagnosis of hemangiosarcoma. Pulmonary or abdominal metastasis suggests splenic neoplasia, although not necessarily hemangiosarcoma. In questionable cases where a suspected hematoma is identified, serial ultrasound examinations are recommended. Hematomas generally get smaller and resolve with time.

Focal Infarcts or Necrosis

Focal splenic infarcts occur secondary to embolism or thrombosis and may be associated with inflammatory diseases such as pancreatitis, endocarditis, septicemia, and neoplasia in humans.[19] Splenic infarction has also been described in dogs with bacterial endocarditis, hypercoagulable conditions secondary to liver disease, renal disease or hyperadrenocorticism, neoplasia, and thrombosis associated with cardiovascular disease.[10,20,21]

The appearance of infarcts is variable and depends on the time since the infarct occurred. Initially, infarcts appear as poorly marginated hypoechoic or complex lesions that cannot

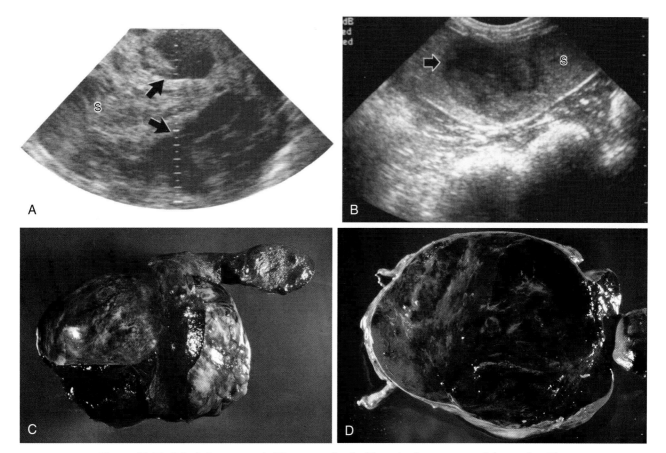

Figure 10-10 **Splenic hematoma. A,** This young dog had been hit by a car several days earlier. The spleen (*S*) was greatly enlarged with variably sized, poorly circumscribed hypoechoic areas (*arrows*) throughout the parenchyma. This was identified as a splenic hematoma at surgery when the abdomen was explored to repair a ruptured bladder. Hemangiosarcoma of the spleen could have a similar appearance ultrasonographically, so the age and history were essential to establish the most likely diagnosis. **B,** A focal lesion of mixed echogenicity (*arrow*) was identified in the spleen (*S*) of this dog. A hematoma secondary to trauma was suspected. This lesion was not identified in a follow-up examination several weeks later. **C,** Example of a large splenic hematoma. **D,** Cut surface of hematoma showing complex internal nature. (**C** and **D** courtesy of Washington State University College of Veterinary Medicine, Washington Animal Disease Diagnostic Laboratory, Pullman, WA.)

be distinguished from other focal splenic lesions on the basis of the ultrasonographic appearance alone [10,19,22,23] (Figures 10-11 and 10-12). A hypoechoic, wedge-shaped appearance with the base toward the splenic margin has been described in humans.[19] Infarcts also appear as echogenic lesions if there is postinfarctive hemorrhage.[24] Circular, hypoechoic or anechoic, irregularly delineated masses have also been described as another manifestation of splenic infarcts in dogs and humans.[10,19] The differential diagnosis must include nodular hyperplasia, abscess, hematoma undergoing clot organization or lysis, and tumor. Infarcts may or may not be infected or contain gas from gas-forming bacteria. If it is located at the periphery of the spleen, an infarct may distort the splenic capsule. The use of color or power Doppler imaging is essential in documenting lack of blood flow (see Figures 10-11, *C* and *D*, and 10-12, *B*).

Contrast-enhanced ultrasound has been used to evaluate splenic infarcts in an experimental canine model.[25] Gray-scale, color Doppler, pulsed Doppler, and power Doppler ultrasound were used to assess infarcts before and after administration of intravenous contrast material. Infarcts were more conspicuous after intravenous administration of contrast agent using color and spectral Doppler. Normally perfused tissue was markedly enhanced, whereas the ischemic areas associated with the infarct were poorly enhanced.

The diagnosis of an infarct depends on ultrasound-guided aspiration for cytology and culture to help rule out tumor or abscess. Progressive resolution of a lesion with medical therapy and abnormal results from culture and cytology strongly suggest the possibility of a splenic infarct. Infarcts also become smaller with time and sometimes scarify and appear hyperechoic after resolution. Hematomas or infarcts that become secondarily infected cannot be differentiated from abscesses.

Abscess

Abscesses produce focal or multifocal splenic lesions that cannot be differentiated from other diseases solely on the basis of their ultrasound appearance. Fortunately, they are uncommon. Their appearance varies from poorly marginated, hypoechoic lesions to complex lesions with variable cystic components and echogenic debris.[26-28] Distal acoustic enhancement is variable, depending on the viscosity of the fluid. Initially, some abscesses may appear echogenic and exhibit refractive edge shadowing, which helps determine the nature

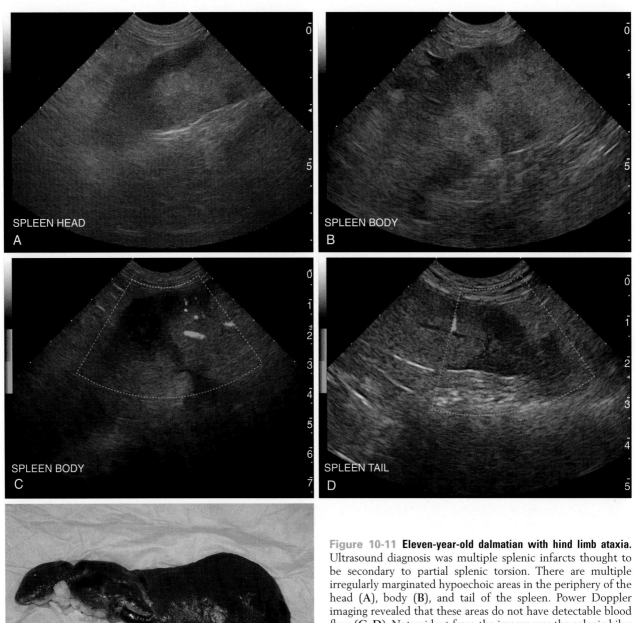

Figure 10-11 Eleven-year-old dalmatian with hind limb ataxia. Ultrasound diagnosis was multiple splenic infarcts thought to be secondary to partial splenic torsion. There are multiple irregularly marginated hypoechoic areas in the periphery of the head (**A**), body (**B**), and tail of the spleen. Power Doppler imaging revealed that these areas do not have detectable blood flow (**C, D**). Not evident from the images was the splenic hilus directed laterally toward the left abdominal wall instead of medially. Abdominal fluid was present (not shown). **E,** Surgical specimen of the spleen showing multiple dark red areas of acute infarction. Histologic diagnosis was splenic infarcts, acute, multifocal to coalescing, severe with thrombosis, consistent with torsion.

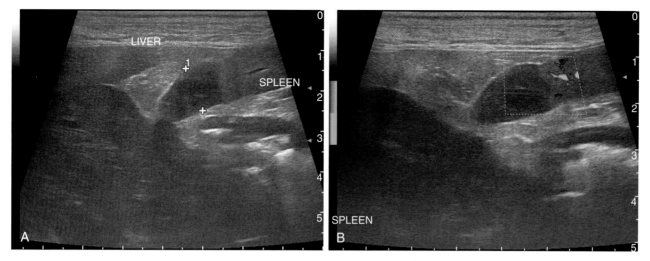

Figure 10-12 **Splenic infarct in a 9-year-old shorthaired dachshund with resolving pancreatitis, thrombocytopenia and anemia. A,** The tip of the spleen bulges and is hypoechoic compared to the adjacent normal parenchyma (1.12 cm between electronic cursors). **B,** Power Doppler evaluation shows complete absence of blood flow to this area. An enlarged, hypoechoic pancreas and peritoneal fluid was also present (not shown). Histologic diagnosis was septic splenic infarction (*Escherichia coli, Klebsiella pneumoniae*), pancreatitis, and peritonitis.

of the mass (Figure 10-13, *A*). A history consisting of fever, leukocytosis with a left shift, and peritonitis with free abdominal fluid or the presence of an extrasplenic focus of infection may assist with the diagnosis (Figure 10-13, *B*). An abscess is likely if intense areas of hyperechogenicity are present within the lesion because of gas-forming microorganisms (Figure 10-13, *C* and *D*). Shadowing from gas, if present, is "dirty" with indistinct margins, compared with the sharper borders encountered with focal parenchymal calcification. Shadowing may be indistinct or absent if gas microbubbles are present or if there is insufficient parenchymal calcification. Abdominal radiographs should be taken to assist with this determination. However, ultrasonography may be more sensitive than radiography for detecting small amounts of gas or calcification. Ultimately, the diagnosis must be confirmed by guided aspiration, cytology, and culture. Ultrasound-guided interventional treatment of splenic abscesses has been described in humans.[29] These procedures may eventually prove useful in dogs in certain cases.

Nodular Hyperplasia

Nodular (lymphoid) hyperplasia and extramedullary hematopoiesis (discussed later under Diffuse Disease) are probably the most frequently seen conditions of the spleen, encountered daily in a busy ultrasound practice. Hypoechoic to essentially isoechoic and barely perceptible nodules are typically seen; differentiation between hyperplasia and extramedullary hematopoiesis (EMH) can only be made with cytology and they are often concurrent. Although nodular hyperplasia is frequently observed in the spleen of old dogs at surgery or necropsy, the nodules are not always observed ultrasonographically. In these instances it is because the acoustic impedance of the nodules is not different from that of native spleen. In such cases, nodular hyperplasia may be suspected when the border of the spleen is smoothly irregular and no parenchymal abnormalities are detected. An isoechoic *mass* may be seen in some cases, recognized because of changes in splenic echo texture or shape (Figure 10-14, *A*). Increased echogenicity is also possible (Figure 10-14, *B* and *E*). If the hyperplastic nodule becomes congested or necrotic, complex lesions may

be observed ultrasonographically (Figure 10-14, *C* and *D*). Nodular hyperplasia can be diagnosed only by excluding other benign or neoplastic conditions of the spleen on histologic evaluation. Figures 10-15 to 10-17 show a variety of nodular hyperplasia appearances. As for the spleen, nodular hyperplasia of the *liver* may also appear as isoechoic, hypoechoic, hyperechoic target-like or complex lesions.[30-31] On the basis of our experience and one report,[32] the range of appearances in the spleen are similar. It *must* be recognized that nodular hyperplasia can present as large mass lesions (discussed later).

Neoplasia

Focal or multifocal neoplastic lesions (nodules, masses) of the spleen commonly result from sarcomas in dogs.[22,23,33,34] Hemangiosarcoma (Figures 10-18 to 10-22) and lymphosarcoma (Figures 10-23 and 10-24) are most commonly encountered; however, histiocytic sarcoma (Figures 10-25 and 10-26), malignant histiocytosis, leiomyosarcoma, fibrosarcoma, undifferentiated sarcoma (see Figure 10-4), osteosarcoma, chondrosarcoma, liposarcoma, myxosarcoma, rhabdomyosarcoma, and fibrous histiocytoma have also been reported.[5,35-43] Mast cell tumor, lymphosarcoma, myeloproliferative disease, and hemangiosarcoma, in that order, are the most common tumors in cats.[6] These tumors metastasize to the liver more often than the spleen because the liver has a dual blood supply, but carcinomas are known to involve the spleen after invading the blood stream. Retrograde involvement of the spleen from primary hepatic tumors and local invasion from tumors of adjacent abdominal structures appears to be uncommon.

The type of splenic neoplasia, or whether it is primary or metastatic, cannot be determined from its ultrasonographic appearance alone. Neoplastic lesions are commonly poorly defined, anechoic, hypoechoic, target-like, or complex in appearance, similar to those of the liver. Splenomegaly is usually present. Hemangiosarcomas of the spleen usually have variable amounts of anechoic to hyperechoic areas throughout the lesion, occasionally with weak posterior acoustic enhancement[17,44] (see Figures 10-18 to 10-23). Target lesions have

Text continued on p. 417

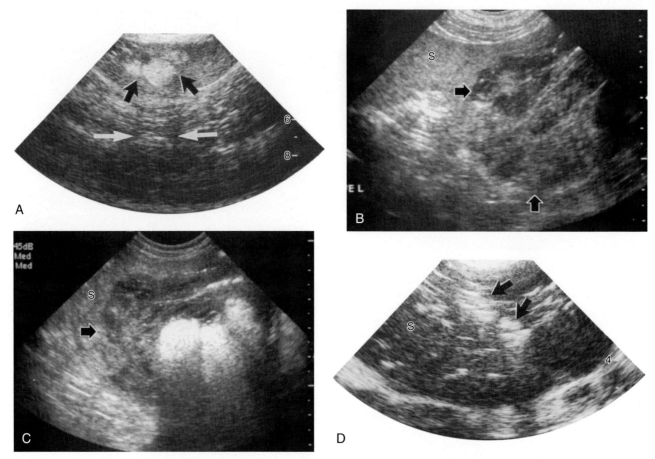

Figure 10-13 Splenic abscess, spectra of patterns. Splenic abscesses may result from bacterial septicemia, peritonitis, or diseases that produce vascular compromise, necrosis, and secondary bacterial infection. **A,** Focal splenic abscess. Multiple, hyperechoic focal lesions (*black arrows*) were identified in the spleen of a dog with bacterial septicemia. The lesions did not shadow but exhibited weak edge shadowing (*white arrows*) typical of a curved structure in which a sound velocity change has occurred. Fluid was aspirated from the lesions but culture was negative. The dog was treated with antibiotics for the septicemia, and the splenic lesions resolved. These lesions were thought to represent small abscesses, possibly hyperechoic because of centralized hemorrhage, necrosis, or bacterial gas microbubble formation. **B,** A large mass of mixed echogenicity (*arrows*) was a focal splenic abscess arising from the tail of the spleen (*S*) in this dog with bacterial septicemia. Differential diagnosis must include hematoma, focal nodular hyperplasia with necrosis, and primary or metastatic neoplasia. **C,** A splenic abscess in this dog produced a large mass (*arrow*) of mixed echogenicity with focal areas of hyperechogenicity and shadowing. The focal hyperechoic areas represented areas of bacterial gas formation within the abscess. The possibility of neoplasia with necrosis and secondary infection should also be considered. The history, clinical signs, age of the animal, laboratory work, other ultrasound and radiographic findings, and ultrasound-guided aspiration help narrow the differential diagnosis. **D,** Splenic abscess with bacterial gas formation. The spleen was markedly enlarged in this dog with a coarse, diffusely hypoechoic parenchymal pattern similar to that seen with splenic torsion, infarction, abscess formation, and necrosis. However, focal hyperechoic areas that shadowed strongly (*arrows*) were also identified within the splenic parenchyma. These represented areas of bacterial gas formation secondary to splenic abscess formation. This was confirmed on abdominal radiographs when gas was identified within the spleen. A splenic torsion was found at surgery.

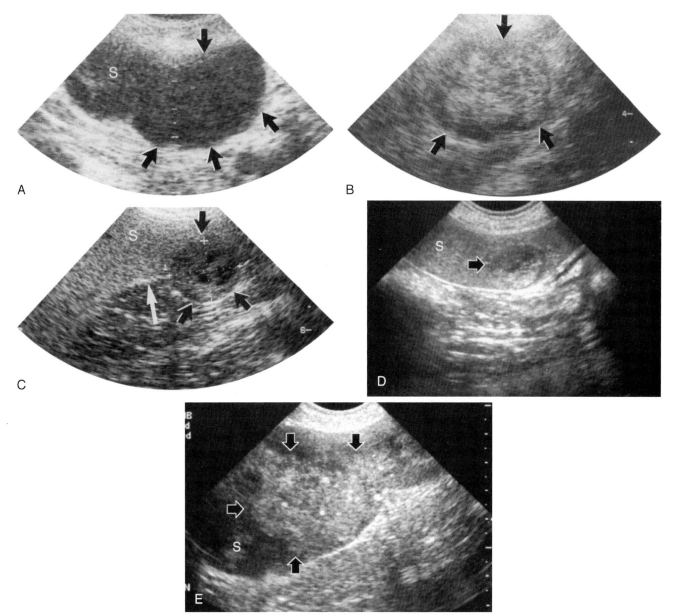

Figure 10-14 **Nodular hyperplasia, spectra of patterns. A,** A solitary mass (*arrows*), 3 to 4 cm in diameter, was identified extending from the caudal border of the spleen (*S*) in this dog. The parenchymal pattern and echogenicity of the mass were similar to the remainder of the spleen. Cytologic evaluation of an aspirate of the mass yielded normal spleen with no evidence of neoplasia. The dog underwent exploration at the owner's request, and a splenectomy was performed. The histologic diagnosis was splenic nodular hyperplasia. **B,** This irregular splenic mass (*arrows*) had a hyperechoic central region surrounded by a thin, hypoechoic rim. Cytologic evaluation of an aspirate was nondiagnostic. The animal was surgically explored. Histopathologic findings indicated nodular hyperplasia. **C,** A well-demarcated, solitary splenic mass (*black arrows*) with centralized hypoechoic areas interrupted the splenic capsule (*white arrow*) of this dog with chronic renal failure. Aspirates of the mass were not diagnostic. The dog was euthanized at the owner's request for irreversible renal disease several weeks later. The histopathologic diagnosis was nodular hyperplasia. **D,** A focal, well-demarcated mass (*arrow*) was noted in the spleen (*S*) of this older dog. Fine-needle aspirates of the mass were nondiagnostic. The appearance of the mass did not change on subsequent examinations during a 2-year period. A presumptive diagnosis of nodular hyperplasia was made. **E,** A large, hyperechoic lesion (*arrows*) within the spleen (*S*) was determined to be nodular hyperplasia after splenectomy and histopathologic evaluation.

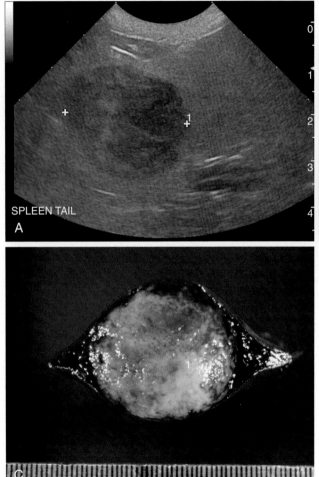

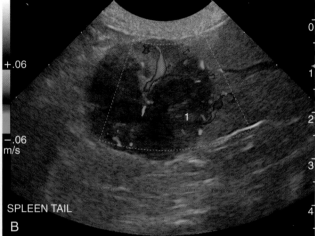

Figure 10-15 Lymphoid hyperplasia. Five-year-old spayed female miniature schnauzer presented for inappetence. **A,** A solitary 2.7-cm nodule was identified within an otherwise appearing normal spleen. The nodule was primarily hypoechoic but does contain areas that are isoechoic to hyperechoic relative to the surrounding spleen. The nodule was well demarcated from the adjacent normal splenic parenchyma and protrudes from the surface. Some would consider this a splenic mass. **B,** Color Doppler evaluation of the nodule shows the avascular nature of its hypoechoic portions but good blood flow within the more echogenic areas. The cytological diagnosis was lymphoid hyperplasia and considered incidental relative to the inappetence. **C,** Cut surface of lymphoid hyperplasia nodule. (Courtesy of Washington State University College of Veterinary Medicine, Washington Animal Disease Diagnostic Laboratory, Pullman, WA.)

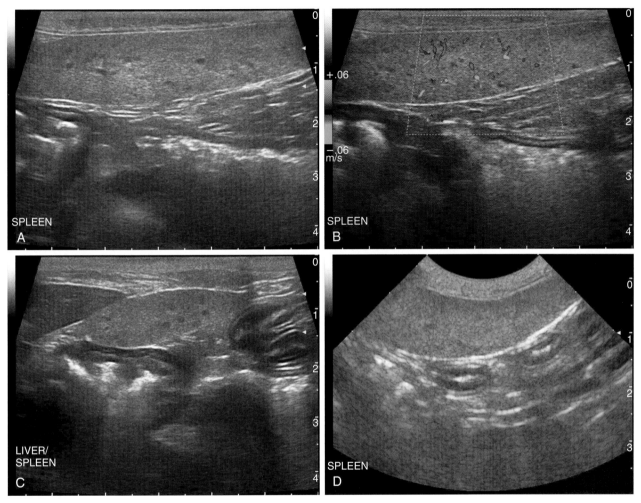

Figure 10-16 **Lymphoid hyperplasia.** Nine-year-old miniature schnauzer with renal failure. **A,** The parenchyma shows diffusely scattered, small, fairly well-demarcated hypoechoic foci. **B,** Color Doppler image showing normal splenic blood flow and the nonvascular nature of the hypoechoic foci. **C,** Multiple hypoechoic foci are present surrounded by normal-appearing and relatively hyperechoic splenic parenchyma. The caudoventral margin of the relatively hypoechoic liver can be seen in the near field to the left. The stomach and a section of small intestine are seen adjacent to the spleen. **D,** The same spleen shown in **A** to **C** but imaged using a microconvex transducer of lower frequency (9 MHz). Note that the hypoechoic foci are not nearly as readily identifiable because of a reduction in resolution compared to the 13-MHz linear array transducer used to obtain images in Figure 10-15, *A* to C.

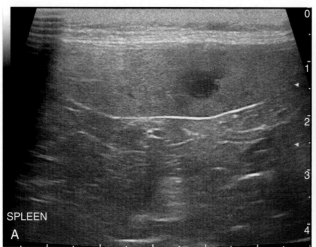

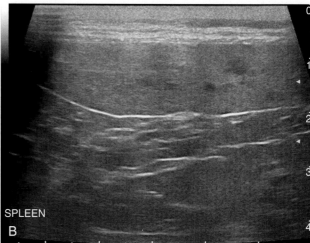

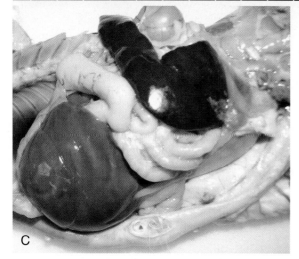

Figure 10-17 **Six-year-old neutered male cat.** Radiographs made of the abdomen because of trauma showed an enlarged spleen. **A** and **B,** The spleen is mottled, with numerous small hypoechoic nodules of various sizes present diffusely within the parenchyma. The spleen is also thicker than normal, up to 14 mm. Cytology obtained from fine-needle aspirates was diagnostic for extramedullary hematopoiesis and lymphoid hyperplasia. **C,** Gross pathology example of lymphoid hyperplasia. (Courtesy of Washington State University College of Veterinary Medicine, Washington Animal Disease Diagnostic Laboratory, Pullman, WA.)

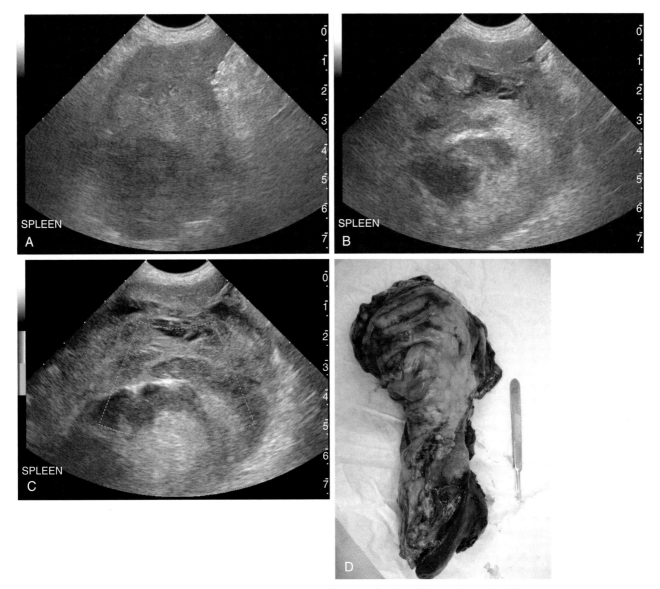

Figure 10-18 **Hemangiosarcoma in an 11-year-old neutered male golden retriever.** A, A large mass was present within the spleen. Normal splenic tissue can be seen in the near field. B, Portions of the mass had a complex internal echotexture. C, Power Doppler imaging showed an absence of blood flow within the mass. D, Splenectomized specimen. The splenic mass is to the top and covered in adhered mesentery. Normal-appearing splenic tissue is to the bottom. Histologic diagnosis was hemangiosarcoma. The majority of the mass was composed of hemorrhagic and necrotic tissue.

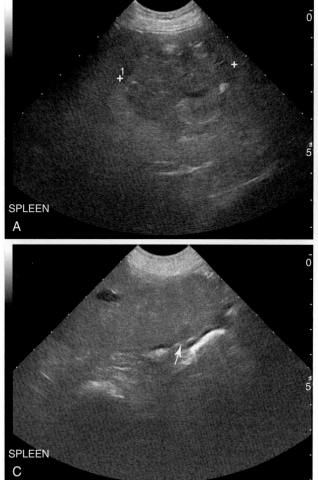

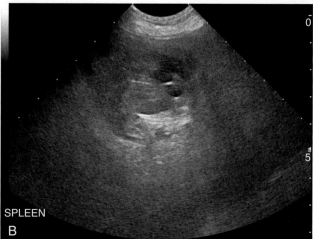

Figure 10-19 Hemangiosarcoma in an 8-year-old spayed female German shepherd with a possible abdominal mass. A, An approximately 4 cm complex mass (between electronic cursors) is present within the spleen characterized by hyperechoic, hypoechoic, and anechoic areas. **B,** It is poorly demarcated from adjacent normal appearing splenic tissue. **C,** A small nearly isoechoic nodule (arrow) is present in otherwise normal-appearing splenic tissue. At pathology, the large mass was firm and hemorrhagic. Multiple nodules were also found within the spleen, liver, pancreas, and mesentery, which were not seen during the ultrasound examination. The histologic diagnosis was disseminated hemangiosarcoma.

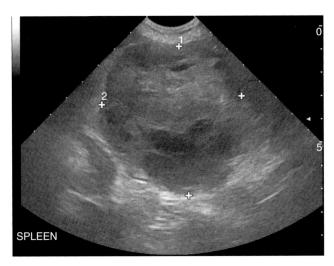

Figure 10-20 Fifteen-year-old Labrador retriever with syncope or seizure. A complex mass originating from the spleen was present, approximately 6 cm in diameter. Histologic diagnosis was hematoma secondary to hemangiosarcoma. A single hyperechoic liver nodule seen on the ultrasound examination (not shown) was determined to be a hyperplastic nodule.

also been described.[31] Hemoperitoneum often accompanies hemangiosarcoma of the spleen (see Figure 10-21, *B*). Less commonly, splenic lesions or those associated with liver metastasis of primary splenic hemangiosarcoma appear uniformly hyperechoic.

Lymphosarcoma has been reported to produce poorly marginated, anechoic to hypoechoic nodular lesions without distal acoustic enhancement.[9,44,45] However, target lesions have also been described.[31] Focal lymphomatous masses may distort the splenic contour or cavitate if they are large.[44,45] Abdominal effusion may be present.[44]

Malignant histiocytosis in dogs produces multiple well-defined, hypoechoic nodules in the spleen, some of which may distort the splenic margin.[46] The appearance is nonspecific, and an ultrasound guided aspirate is required for diagnosis. Mesenteric or medial iliac lymphadenopathy may be present. The spleen is the most common organ involved, but liver involvement is the next most common. The pancreas, kidneys, adrenal glands, ovaries and gastrointestinal tract also may be affected.[46] Thoracic abnormalities may include pulmonary nodules or consolidation, mediastinal masses, or pleural effusion. Bernese mountain dogs, golden retrievers, rottweilers, and Doberman pinschers are more commonly affected.[47] Disseminated histiocytic sarcoma has been reported in two cats, one with multiple splenic masses, the other with diffuse

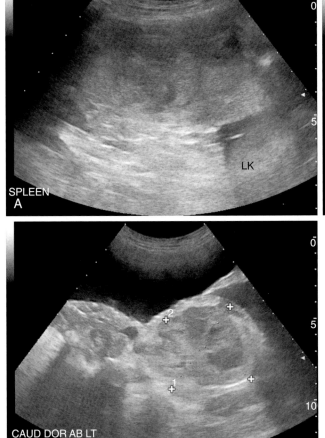

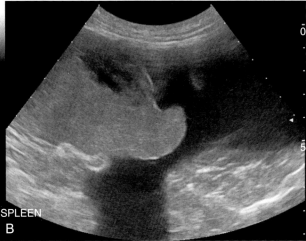

Figure 10-21 Seven-year old male Labrador retriever mix with acute hemoabdomen. A, This portion of the spleen shows a very inhomogeneous splenic parenchyma. The left kidney (*LK*) is present in the far field. **B,** A cavitary mass near the tail of the spleen is identified. The tail of the spleen is greatly distorted by the mass. A large amount of anechoic fluid (hemorrhage) is present. **C,** A complex lesion was present in the caudal retroperitoneal space (between electronic cursors). The histologic diagnosis was disseminated hemangiosarcoma. Metastatic nodules not seen on the ultrasound examination were also identified at necropsy.

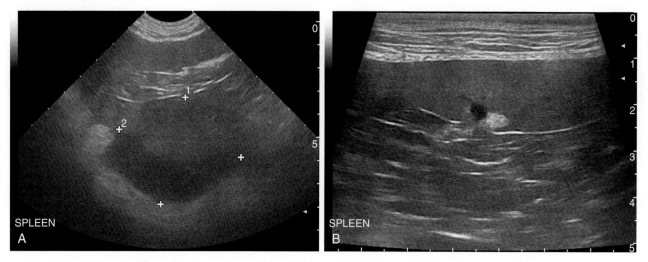

Figure 10-22 **Twelve-year-old spayed female German shepherd mix with a heart base mass found on an echocardiogram. A,** A 4.74 × 5.52 cm mass was identified arising from the head of the spleen. Half of the mass is essentially isoechoic to the normal splenic tissue, whereas the deeper portion is hypoechoic. The body of the spleen in the near field can be seen to curve to the left and dorsally, which the mass arises from. Note the very hyperechoic mesentery surrounding the mass to the left. **B,** A roughly triangular hyperechoic homogeneous focus is seen adjacent to a major splenic vein, representing an incidental finding of a myelolipoma. The histopathologic diagnosis for the mass was hemangiosarcoma.

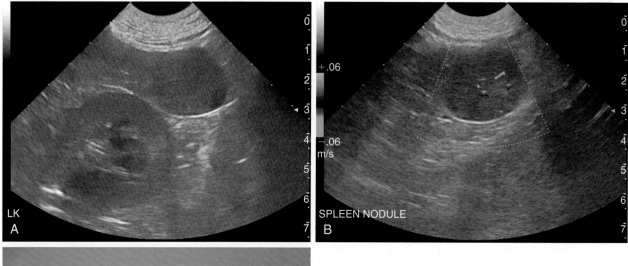

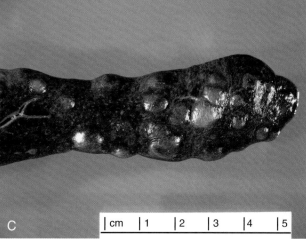

Figure 10-23 **Six-year-old spayed female golden retriever with liver failure. A,** A bulging isoechoic to slightly hypoechoic nodule protrudes from the margin of the spleen. The left kidney is in the far field. **B,** Color Doppler image of the nodule in **A** shows normal-appearing blood flow. The liver (not shown) showed an abnormally diffuse increase in echogenicity and was markedly enlarged. Cytology of the splenic nodule and the liver was diagnostic for lymphosarcoma in both organs. **C,** Gross pathology specimen of multinodular form of splenic lymphoma. (Courtesy of Washington State University College of Veterinary Medicine, Washington Animal Disease Diagnostic Laboratory, Pullman, WA.)

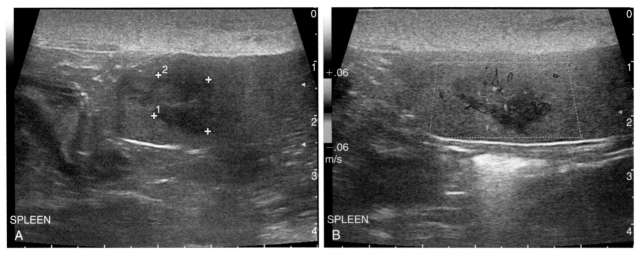

Figure 10-24 **Seven-year-old spayed female Jack Russell terrier with fever of unknown origin. A,** A small heterogeneous, primarily hypoechoic nodule was identified in the spleen (1.22 × 1.39 cm between electronic cursors). **B,** Color Doppler image of the nodule in **A** shows normal-appearing blood flow. Cytological diagnosis was small cell lymphoma.

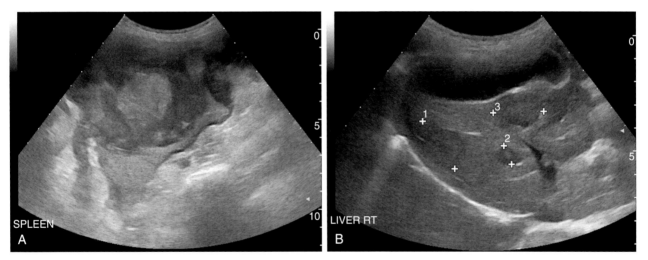

Figure 10-25 **Twelve-year-old spayed female Great Pyrenees with acute lethargy and a large abdominal mass on palpation. A,** A large and complex splenic mass was identified with very irregular margins. No normal splenic parenchyma could be identified. The surrounding mesentery is hyperechoic. **B,** Multiple hypoechoic hepatic masses were also found. Histologic diagnosis for both spleen and liver was anaplastic sarcoma (likely malignant histiocytosis or histiocytic sarcoma).

splenomegaly.[48,49] Other histiocytic tumors, such as malignant fibrous histiocytoma or histiocytic sarcoma (see Figures 10-25 and 10-26), have not been differentiated sonographically, although they may be distinguished histopathologically or with an ultrasound-guided aspirate.[50,51] Malignant histiocytosis has also been reported in cats, but it is rare and the sonographic features have not been described in detail.[52,53]

Mast cell tumors infiltrating the spleen of dogs usually cause splenomegaly with a diffuse increase in echogenicity of the spleen and one or more hypoechoic nodules (Figures 10-27 and 10-28).[54] Occasionally the spleen may be unremarkable.[54] In cats, mast cell tumors have been reported to cause splenomegaly only; a diffusely hypoechoic spleen; a mottled, irregular spleen; or a spleen containing nodules.[44,54] A hyperechoic spleen was seen less frequently, but when

found, it appears to be specific to splenic mast cell tumors in cats.[44] In some cats, only a single mass or nodule was found.[44] The nodules were usually hypoechoic, but hyperechoic nodules were also reported.[44] Hyperechoic nodules (Figure 10-29) must be differentiated from splenic myelolipomas, which are benign fatty nodules of dogs, cats, and cheetahs. Myelolipomas can also appear hyperechoic.[55-59] In questionable cases, an ultrasound-guided aspirate is indicated to determine if mast cells are present. Abdominal lymph nodes are often involved in both dogs and cats, and an ultrasound-guided aspiration of enlarged nodes is also recommended.

Metastatic melanoma produces either hypoechoic or hyperechoic lesions in humans,[60] but the appearance has not been described in dogs or cats. Metastatic carcinomas were characterized as solitary, well-defined, anechoic to hypoechoic

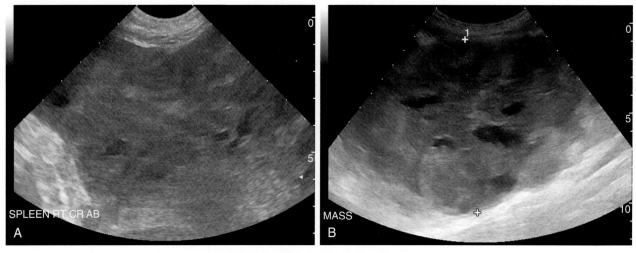

Figure 10-26 **Six-year-old Bernese mountain dog with a large abdominal mass. A,** The entire spleen is composed of abnormal inhomogeneous parenchyma. **B,** Using a convex transducer of a lower frequency allows more complete visualization of the splenic mass, with a depth of approximately 10 cm. This portion of the splenic mass contains multiple irregular anechoic areas of fluid. At pathology, the mass was friable, nodular, and greater than 35 cm in diameter, which illustrates that the limited field of view inherent to ultrasound prevents full visualization of large structures. The histologic diagnosis was histiocytic sarcoma.

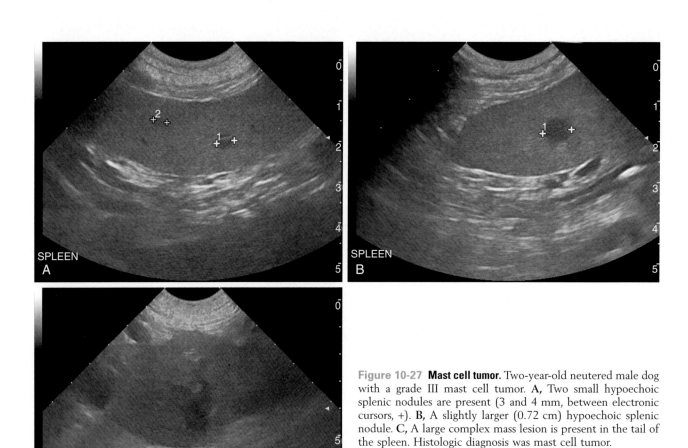

Figure 10-27 **Mast cell tumor.** Two-year-old neutered male dog with a grade III mast cell tumor. **A,** Two small hypoechoic splenic nodules are present (3 and 4 mm, between electronic cursors, +). **B,** A slightly larger (0.72 cm) hypoechoic splenic nodule. **C,** A large complex mass lesion is present in the tail of the spleen. Histologic diagnosis was mast cell tumor.

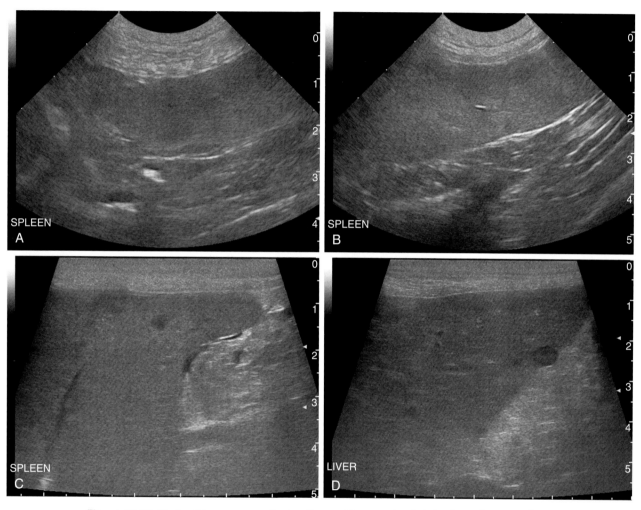

Figure 10-28 **Mast cell tumor progression in a 3-year-old neutered male Labrador retriever.** Grade III mast cell tumor removed 2 weeks prior. **A** and **B,** The spleen is mildly blotchy with large areas of hypoechoic parenchyma surrounded by more echogenic regions. Cytology of fine-needle aspirates showed few mast cells in numbers not representative of disseminated disease. **C** and **D,** Six months later the patient was presented for vomiting and disseminated peripheral lymph node enlargement. **C,** The spleen has increased in size and contains hypoechoic nodules. An abnormal liver is to the left. **D,** The liver parenchyma was mottled, less echogenic than expected, and contained multiple hypoechoic nodules, some of which protruded from the surface. Disseminated mast cell tumor was confirmed from cytology of aspirates of the spleen, liver, abdominal fluid (not shown), and peripheral lymph nodes.

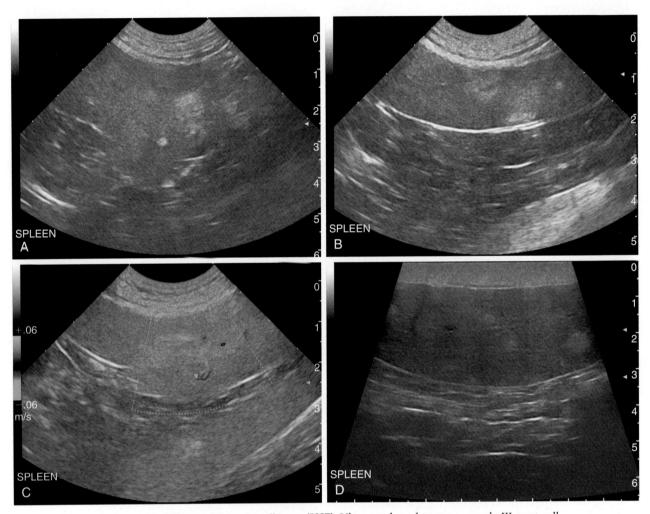

Figure 10-29 Diffuse nodular mast cell tumor (MCT). Ultrasound used to stage a grade III mast cell tumor in a 6-year-old golden retriever. **A,** The spleen is thick and distorted from bulging parenchyma. Within the splenic parenchyma are multiple poorly circumscribed hyperechoic nodules. **B,** Another section showing hyperechoic nodules without distortion of the splenic capsule. **C,** Color Doppler assessment shows blood flow similar to normal splenic parenchyma. **D,** Linear-array high frequency transducer operating in trapezoidal display mode shows more discrete hyperechoic nodules of the splenic parenchyma in addition to a more diffusely heterogeneous echogenicity. Fine-needle aspiration for cytologic analysis was diagnostic for mast cell infiltrate.

nodules in the spleens of five cats.[44] Adenocarcinomas have also been reported to produce target lesions in dogs.[31]

We have observed multifocal, hypoechoic splenic lesions with multiple myeloma in the dog. However, the spleen of a cat with multiple myeloma appeared normal, but multiple, small hyperechoic nodules were identified in the liver.[61]

When neoplasia is suspected, other abdominal organs should be evaluated for metastasis and the abdomen searched for lymphadenopathy. Ultrasonography is not reliable for detecting serosal lesions or peritoneal metastasis unless the nodules are larger than 1 to 2 cm or surrounded by peritoneal fluid. This helps differentiate the nodules from lymphadenopathy, even in the presence of considerable bowel gas. However, masses within the connecting peritoneum, visceral peritoneum, or parietal peritoneum are characteristic of abdominal carcinomatosis, and aspiration of the masses, abdominal fluid or both is recommended.[62] Thoracic and abdominal survey radiographs should also be taken to exclude additional abnormalities or metastasis to the lungs or skeletal system.

Hyperechoic Foci

Most focal splenic lesions tend to be less echogenic than the surrounding parenchyma or may be appear complex. On occasion, parenchymal hemorrhage, abscess, and primary or metastatic tumor may be hyperechoic, as described previously. However, acoustic shadowing is usually absent unless gas, fibrosis, or calcification accompanies the lesion. Gas from gas-producing organisms, foreign bodies, metastatic or dystrophic calcification, and fibrosis produce focal, hyperechoic lesions that more commonly shadow unless they are small (Figures 10-30 to 10-32). Fibrosis or calcification may occur with hematomas, old infarcts, chronic inflammation, or granulomatous disease such as histoplasmosis. Myelolipomas have also been reported in the dog, cat, and cheetah.[55-58] These are benign, hyperechoic fatty nodules of varying size that appear relatively unchanged in sequential scans (Figures 10-33 to 10-35). Myelolipomas cannot be distinguished from other poorly shadowing hyperechoic foci in the spleen, and their significance is unknown. Chronic disease or stress has been suggested as a possible cause of myelolipomas in the cheetah.[57]

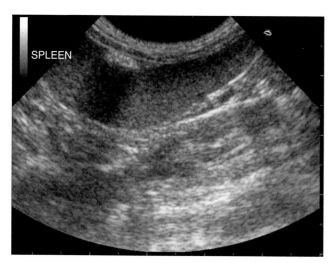

Figure 10-30 Siderocalcific plaque. A strongly hyperechoic plaque is present on the surface of this cat spleen. Note the acoustic shadow distal to the plaque, consistent with mineralization.

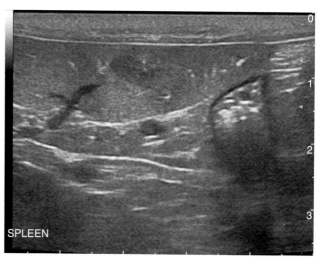

Figure 10-32 Eleven-year-old miniature schnauzer with uncontrolled diabetes. Linear and punctate mineralized foci are present within the spleen. A central hypoechoic nodule is also seen.

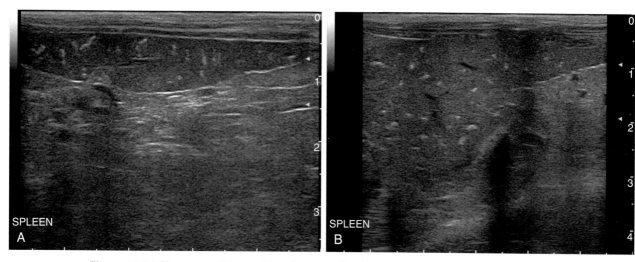

Figure 10-31 Eleven-year-old spayed female toy poodle with diabetic ketoacidosis and hyperadrenocorticism. A, Transverse image of the body of the spleen showing linear and punctuate foci of mineralization. **B,** Image of the head of the spleen showing punctate areas of mineralization.

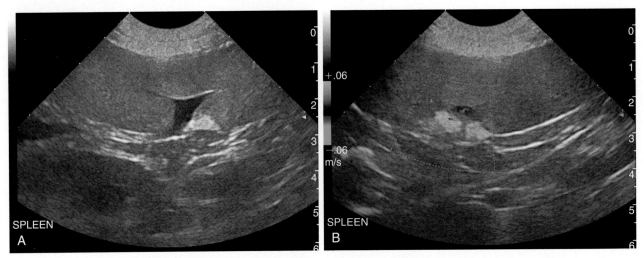

Figure 10-33 **Myelolipomas in an 11-year-old spayed female dog with dyspnea, increased appetite, and panting. A,** A triangular hyperechoic homogeneous focus is present adjacent to a major splenic vein. **B,** A different portion of the splenic hilum shows two well-demarcated irregular hyperechoic and homogeneous nodules surrounding a splenic vein (color Doppler image). This dog had a right adrenal gland mass accounting for the clinical signs (not shown).

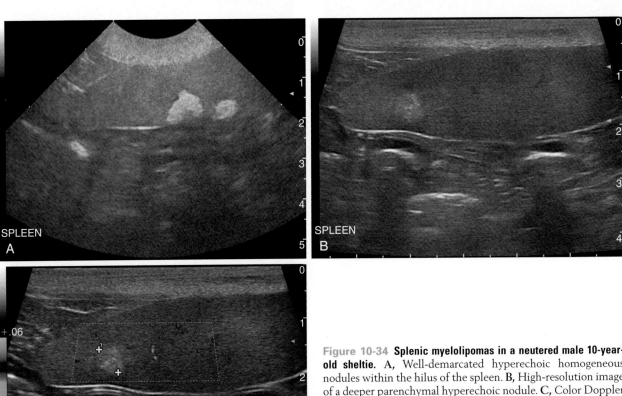

Figure 10-34 **Splenic myelolipomas in a neutered male 10-year-old sheltie. A,** Well-demarcated hyperechoic homogeneous nodules within the hilus of the spleen. **B,** High-resolution image of a deeper parenchymal hyperechoic nodule. **C,** Color Doppler evaluation shows two small blood vessels within the hyperechoic nodule.

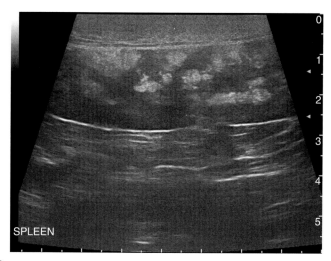

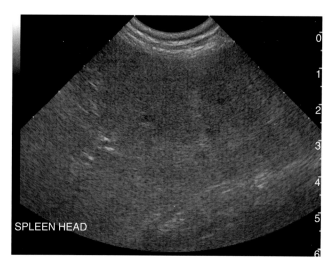

Figure 10-35 **Splenic lipomas.** The splenic parenchyma consists of multiple irregularly shaped hyperechoic foci. Histologic diagnosis was splenic lipomas.

Abdominal radiographs may provide additional information about the source of the echogenicity in the spleen, especially when gas, calcification, or foreign bodies are suspected.

DIFFUSE DISEASE

The differential diagnosis of diffuse splenomegaly is a lengthy one, and in most cases ultrasonography is not helpful in establishing its cause. Anesthetics, infection, immune-mediated disease, lymphoma, leukemias, neoplasia, vascular stasis, chronic hemolytic anemia, torsion, and parasitic infections (e.g., *Haemobartonella*, *Babesia*, or *Ehrlichia*) are known to cause diffuse enlargement of the spleen. In humans, attempts have been made to relate the splenic parenchymal echogenicity to pathologic changes in the early stages of disease. An enlarged spleen with low echogenicity has often been found with malignant diseases, such as lymphoma, plasmacytic neoplasia, and acute congestion, whereas splenomegaly caused by chronic congestion, chronic inflammatory processes, and chronic myeloproliferative disorders tends to produce a higher echogenicity than normal.[11-13] Extramedullary hematopoiesis, acute myeloproliferative disorders, and increased reticuloendothelial activity have also been reported to cause normal or reduced echogenicity of the spleen in humans.[12,13] However, there are many exceptions and inconsistencies, and splenic echogenicity may appear normal with many types of diffuse splenic disease in humans.[14] The same is true for animals. Therefore aspiration for cytology or biopsy is usually indicated unless the diagnosis is obvious from other clinical information.

Congestion
Passive congestion of the spleen occurs from disturbance of the systemic or portal circulation and with some types of hemolytic anemia or toxemic conditions. Anesthetic agents and tranquilizers are also common causes of splenic congestion.[63] Splenomegaly with normal or slightly reduced echogenicity is usually found (Figure 10-36). Venous congestion resulting from right-sided heart failure commonly produces hepatomegaly, but typically not marked splenomegaly, because the splenic vein drains into the portal vein. Obstruction of the portal vein or increased resistance to portal blood flow through the liver from inflammatory or neoplastic disease may produce diffuse splenic enlargement and congestion.

Figure 10-36 **Splenic congestion in a geriatric dog with elevated central venous pressure secondary to pericardial effusion.** The splenic parenchyma is mottled and the spleen was enlarged. The hepatic veins were markedly enlarged and peritoneal fluid was present (not shown).

Partial splenic torsion, incomplete splenic vein thrombosis, or acute splenic inflammation may initially produce passive congestion, which may later develop into more widespread thrombosis, infarction and parenchymal necrosis, or abscess formation. Marked splenomegaly with a coarse, "lacy," hypoechoic parenchymal pattern has been described as an important finding in these conditions.[10,21,64] Splenic congestion due to these causes can sometimes be differentiated from that seen with splenic torsion or severe splenic vein thrombosis by the lack of prominent parallel echogenic lines representing severely dilated intraparenchymal vessels.[64] However, Doppler ultrasonography is currently the procedure of choice for evaluating blood flow within the spleen to help distinguish passive congestion or splenic inflammation from severe vascular compromise produced by splenic torsion or thrombosis.

The splenic parenchyma may appear more echogenic than normal if chronic splenic congestion occurs from less severe causes during a longer period. The appearance cannot be differentiated from other chronic infiltrative, infectious, or inflammatory conditions. The cause of splenic congestion is frequently suspected from the clinical history, laboratory work, other ultrasound findings, or additional abdominal imaging procedures. However, differentiation from diffuse infiltrative diseases, such as lymphoma, leukemia, and extramedullary hematopoiesis, usually requires a fine-needle aspiration biopsy.

Splenic Vein Thrombosis
Thrombosis of the splenic vein is not an uncommon finding in dogs. It is often found incidentally, without clinical signs or accompanying splenic parenchymal changes. However, underlying causes of thrombosis should be investigated, such as splenic torsion, generalized vascular or clotting disorders, lymphoma, hyperadrenocorticism, mast cell disease, and other organ or systemic disease processes. Laurenson and colleagues[65] investigated concurrent diseases and conditions in dogs with splenic vein thrombosis. They found neoplasia to be the most common concurrent condition, with lymphoma the most common neoplastic process. Exogenous corticosteroid administration was the second most common condition, followed by systemic inflammatory response syndrome, disseminated intravascular coagulation, pancreatitis,

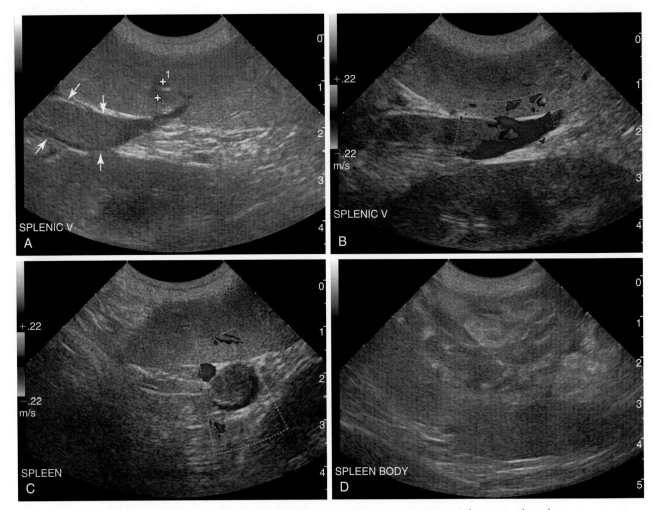

Figure 10-37 Nine-year-old spayed female dog with weight loss and lethargy. Splenic vein thrombosis was identified in addition to a large complex splenic mass. **A,** Ultrasound image of the splenic hilum showing an echogenic thrombus (*arrows*) in the lumen of the splenic vein seen in a sagittal view. Electronic cursors (+) indicate a thrombosed parenchymal splenic vein. Sagittal (**B**) and transverse (**C**) color Doppler images of the thrombosed splenic vein. **D,** Complex splenic mass.

and immune-mediated disease (immune-mediated hemolytic anemia is the most common). Protein-losing nephropathy and naturally occurring hyperadrenocorticism were uncommon associated conditions. However, splenic infarcts were present in 33% of the dogs, and portal vein thrombosis was present in 18% of the dogs. Doppler ultrasound is important for assessing splenic vein thrombosis, establishing the degree of thrombosis, and differentiating slow, turbulent flow from true thrombosis. It can also distinguish venous and arterial thromboses. Figures 10-37 and 10-38 show examples of splenic vein thrombosis. Figure 10-39 shows sluggish splenic vein blood flow, potentially mistaken for a thrombus without the use of Doppler ultrasonography.

Splenic Torsion
Splenic torsion produces a markedly enlarged spleen with diffuse anechoic areas and multiple parallel echogenic lines within the parenchyma[64] (Figure 10-40). A case report of splenic torsion in a small-breed dog, a Boston terrier, noted classic sonographic features including splenomegaly, diffuse hypoechoic parenchyma, and interspersed linear echoes.[66] The anechoic areas are thought to represent dilated sinusoids from splenic congestion, whereas the parallel echogenic lines are thought to be severely dilated vessels. The splenic veins near the hilum are also enlarged from venous outflow obstruction.

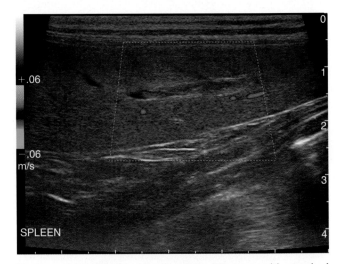

Figure 10-38 Splenic vein thrombus. Nine-year-old standard poodle examined because of an incompletely excised grade II mast cell tumor of the left cranial hind limb. An echogenic thrombus is noted incidentally in this intraparenchymal splenic vein, confirmed with lack of flow shown by color Doppler examination. Cytology of the spleen was normal.

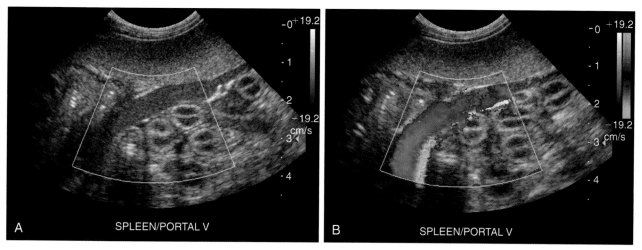

Figure 10-39 **Sluggish, echogenic blood flow in the splenic vein of a dog.** **A,** Echogenic blood is present within the splenic vein. This could be mistaken for a thrombus. **B,** Color Doppler image shows splenic vein blood flow is present.

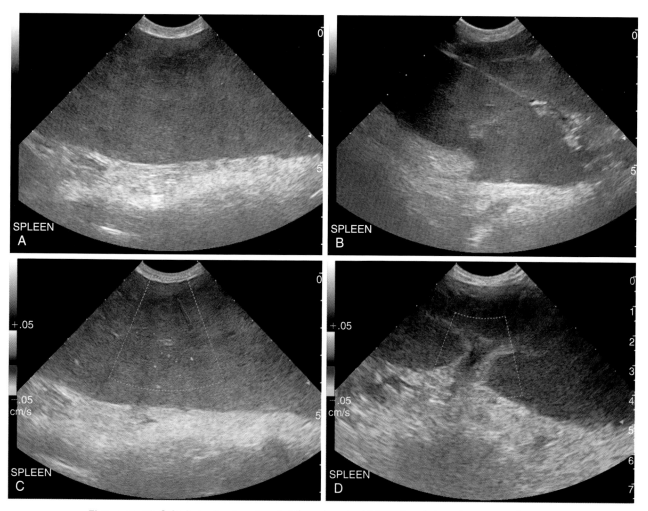

Figure 10-40 **Splenic torsion in a dog.** **A,** The spleen is thickened and the splenic parenchyma is mottled. Hyperechoic splenic hilar fat is present. **B,** This image shows the spleen folded on itself. **C,** Color Doppler image shows very little blood flow to the splenic parenchyma. **D,** Color Doppler image at the hilus of the spleen showing complete lack of blood flow.

Patterns associated with infarction, necrosis, or abscess formation may occur if vascular compromise is severe or prolonged. Gas emitted from various organisms may be identified within the spleen.[67] Free abdominal fluid may be present adjacent to the spleen. Doppler evaluation of the spleen indicates an absence of blood flow and helps to differentiate torsion from other causes of splenic congestion.

Splenic torsion and acute splenic inflammation (splenitis) produce marked splenomegaly with a similar lacy, hypoechoic parenchymal pattern. However, as described before, the presence of parallel echogenic lines (representing dilated vessels) within the splenic parenchyma and enlarged hilar veins may help distinguish torsion from at least some cases of splenic necrosis secondary to splenitis or infarction, in which the intraparenchymal veins are expected to be small. In two of three reported cases of necrosis secondary to infarction, the splenic vasculature was not identified.[10] Enlarged, slightly tortuous vessels were found in a third case of infarction, but this case also had accompanying splenic torsion.[10] In this third case, it was unclear whether vascular enlargement was limited to the hilar veins or extended to the intraparenchymal vessels, as has been described with torsion. In 16 dogs with splenic infarction due to causes other than torsion, it was reported that the parenchymal vessels appeared hyperechoic against a diffuse hypoechoic background.[21] However, there was no mention of intraparenchymal venous dilation. In another report, a *hyperechoic* triangle continuous with the mesentery around the veins at the splenic hilus was used to help diagnose splenic torsion[68] (see Figure 10-40). The hilar perivascular hyperechoic triangle was seen in 6 of 7 cases with acute splenic torsion. A diffuse enlargement of the spleen from venous flow obstruction with bulging of the parenchyma around the hilar vessels is thought to be the cause. This sonographic sign, along with the other findings mentioned previously, may help distinguish acute splenic torsion from infarction/necrosis without torsion.

Of 15 dogs with splenic torsion evaluated with conventional B-mode and Doppler ultrasonography,[69] the splenic parenchyma was mottled with hypoechoic regions in 2 dogs; in 11 others, it was diffusely hypoechoic with the typical coarse, lacy parenchymal pattern. However, the splenic parenchymal echogenicity was normal in 2 dogs. In 13 dogs, visible echogenicities were also found within the intrasplenic and mesenteric portions of the splenic veins, which is compatible with static echogenic blood or thrombi. Doppler ultrasonography failed to detect blood flow in the splenic veins of all 15 dogs, including the 2 dogs without visible thrombi. It is still unclear whether Doppler ultrasonography can reliably distinguish splenic torsion from cases with splenic vein thrombosis without torsion. However, splenectomy is usually indicated if there is severe vascular compromise or splenic necrosis, so the differential diagnosis may be largely academic.

Infectious or Inflammatory Disease

Acute systemic infectious diseases of bacterial or fungal origin may cause secondary splenomegaly with normal to reduced echogenicity (Figure 10-41). Infectious or inflammatory diseases directly involving the spleen (splenitis) usually produce

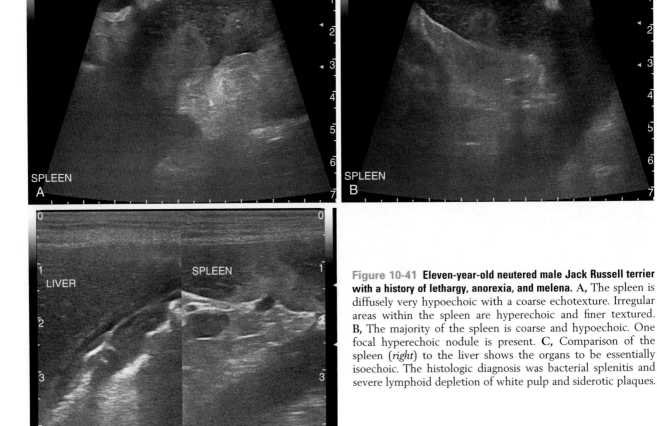

Figure 10-41 **Eleven-year-old neutered male Jack Russell terrier with a history of lethargy, anorexia, and melena. A,** The spleen is diffusely very hypoechoic with a coarse echotexture. Irregular areas within the spleen are hyperechoic and finer textured. **B,** The majority of the spleen is coarse and hypoechoic. One focal hyperechoic nodule is present. **C,** Comparison of the spleen (*right*) to the liver shows the organs to be essentially isoechoic. The histologic diagnosis was bacterial splenitis and severe lymphoid depletion of white pulp and siderotic plaques.

a similar appearance, but with more pronounced splenomegaly. A markedly hypoechoic or lacy parenchymal pattern has been described with severe, acute inflammation.[10,21] Patterns typical of thrombosis, infarction, necrosis, and abscess formation may also appear[10,21,70] (see Figure 10-12).

Chronic conditions resulting from vascular compromise, peritonitis, infection, or diffuse nonneoplastic infiltrative processes may uniformly increase splenic echogenicity. Chronic granulomatous diseases, such as histoplasmosis, can cause increased splenic echogenicity with focal areas of parenchymal calcification. However, two cats with pyogranulomatous splenitis associated with feline infectious peritonitis had abdominal effusion and splenomegaly with normal splenic echogenicity.[44] Lewis and O'Brien[71] reviewed the ultrasound findings associated with feline infectious peritonitis and found the spleen to have normal echogenicity in 14 of 16 cases; the other 2 cats had hypoechoic splenic parenchyma. Other findings included normal liver echogenicity in 11 cats, hypoechoic subcapsular rim in 5 cats, abdominal lymphadenopathy in 9 cats, peritoneal fluid in 7 cats, and retroperitoneal fluid in only 1 cat.

Diffuse Infiltrative Disease

Diffuse infiltrative diseases of the spleen usually cause generalized splenomegaly with a normal to reduced echogenicity. However, normal splenic size and echogenicity are known to occur in some cases of lymphoma and mast cell disease.[72,73] The parenchyma may have either a normal or coarse echo texture. Focal hypoechoic regions or ill-defined nodules may also be present (thus taking on a multifocal appearance). The ultrasonographic appearance is nonspecific, and differential diagnosis depends on other information. Cytologic evaluation of a fine-needle aspirate from the spleen or lymph nodes and correlation of the ultrasonographic findings with the history, physical findings, laboratory work, and other imaging procedures are essential.

Diffuse Nonneoplastic Disease

Extramedullary hematopoiesis (EMH), lymphoid hyperplasia (LH), and amyloidosis can cause diffuse changes and generalized splenomegaly. Extramedullary hematopoiesis and lymphoid hyperplasia are often diagnosed from the same spleen, in both dogs and cats. Although normal to reduced echogenicity is expected, few reports describe the ultrasonographic appearance of the spleen with these conditions (Figures 10-42 and 10-43). Approximately 40% of cats with extramedullary hematopoiesis, lymphoid hyperplasia, or both had splenomegaly with normal echogenicity (Figure 10-44).[44] Hypoechoic nodules ranging in size from 0.7 to 3.0 cm were also present in about 25% of these cats (Figure 10-45, see also Figures 10-16 and 10-17). The spleen was hypoechoic or mottled in another 25% of the cats with extramedullary hematopoiesis or lymphoid hyperplasia. Figures 10-46 to

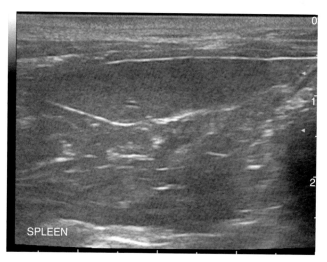

Figure 10-42 **Three-year-old male neutered cat with possible renal lymphoma.** The spleen has normal thickness (approximately 8 mm), echogenicity, and echotexture. The thin echogenic splenic capsule shows its smooth surface. Because of the clinical suspicion of lymphoma, fine-needle aspiration was performed with a cytologic diagnosis of extramedullary hematopoiesis.

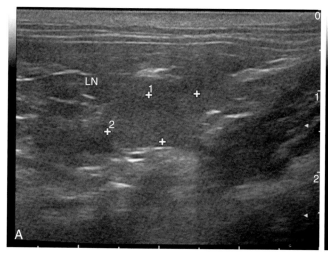

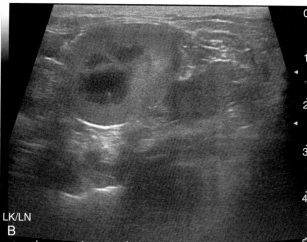

Figure 10-43 **Accessory spleen.** Eight-year-old cat investigated because of underlying bone disease suggestive of neoplasia. **A,** A small, homogeneous, solid, irregularly shaped but smoothly margined nodule (*LN,* between electronic cursors) was identified caudal and medial to the spleen. **B,** Adjacent to the left kidney. The tissue was isoechoic to splenic parenchyma. It was originally thought to represent a lymph node, and fine-needle aspiration was performed for cytologic diagnosis. Final diagnosis was splenic parenchyma with mild to moderate lymphoid hyperplasia and extramedullary hematopoiesis.

10-49 are examples of diffuse EMH and LH in dogs, showing the wide range of the potential appearances.

Diffuse Neoplastic Disease

The most common diffuse splenic neoplasia are lymphoma and mast cell disease. These along with malignant histiocytic, mastocytic, myelomatous, and leukemic infiltrations may reduce splenic echogenicity, or the parenchyma may appear *normal* (Figures 10-50 and 10-51).[72,73] The overall pattern is sometimes uneven or more coarser normal. Diffuse increased echogenicity has also been noted with lymphosarcoma and mast cell tumor in dogs. Two cats with myeloproliferative disease had splenomegaly with a diffusely hypoechoic spleen,[44] and there has since been two other case reports of histiocytic sarcoma and malignant histiocytosis in cats.[48,49]

Lymphoma of the spleen has a wide variety of appearances and may produce no abnormalities, show multiple, various size hypoechoic nodules (Figures 10-52 and 10-53), diffuse increased or decreased echogenicity with coarse texture (Figure 10-54), a honeycomb pattern (Figure 10-55), a moth-eaten appearance, or focal or multifocal hypoechoic or complex lesions[9,33,45] (see Figures 10-3, 10-23, and 10-24). Interestingly, Crabtree and co-workers[74] recommended obtaining splenic aspirates for diagnosis of lymphoma of dogs only when the spleen appears abnormal, and performing cytological analysis of the liver regardless of its sonographic appearance. The classic appearance of splenic lymphoma has been described as looking like a honeycomb or chicken wire fence. Splenic hilar or mesenteric lymphadenopathy, generalized peripheral lymphadenopathy, or involvement of other

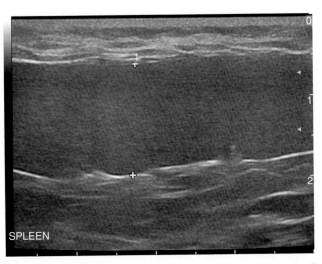

Figure 10-44 Mildly thickened spleen. Nine-year-old neutered male cat with lethargy and mild anorexia. The spleen is mildly thickened at 13.7 mm. The splenic parenchyma is homogeneous and considered normal. Fine-needle aspiration for cytologic analysis was diagnostic for extramedullary hematopoiesis.

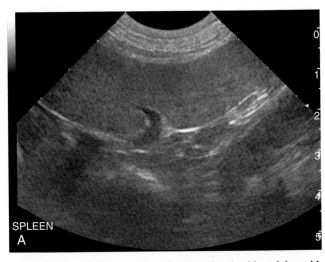

Figure 10-46 Eleven-year-old spayed female mixed breed dog with a history of a grade II mast cell tumor incompletely excised from her axilla and an enlarged axillary lymph node. The spleen was judged to be normal but fine-needle aspiration was performed because of the clinical presentation. Cytologic diagnosis of mild to moderate extramedullary hematopoiesis was made.

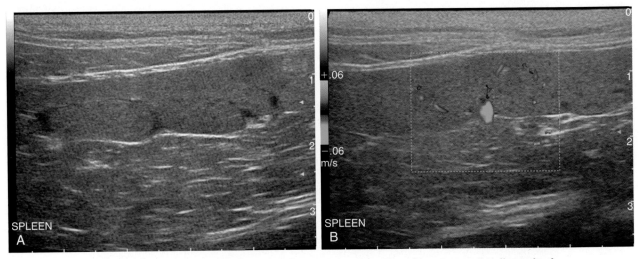

Figure 10-45 Six-year-old Siamese cat with pyrexia and anorexia, with a presumptive diagnosis of pancreatitis. A, The spleen is mildly mottled with numerous tiny hypoechoic islands evenly dispersed throughout the parenchyma. **B,** Color Doppler examination shows normal vascularity with persistence of tiny hypoechoic foci. Fine-needle aspiration was performed and a cytologic diagnosis of extramedullary hematopoiesis was made.

abdominal organs such as the liver or gastrointestinal tract may suggest the cause (see Figure 10-51, C); however, definitive diagnosis requires a fine-needle aspirate.

Splenic mast cell tumors may also appear normal, and this is often the case, requiring fine-needle aspiration for cytologic diagnosis.[72,73] The appearance of mast cell tumors in cats is similar to the patterns seen with lymphosarcoma or myeloproliferative disease and could not be distinguished from these diseases ultrasonographically (Figure 10-56; see also Figures 10-27 to 10-29).[44] However mesenteric lymphadenopathy and abdominal effusion were more likely in cats with lymphosarcoma, whereas increased splenic echogenicity (hyperechoic nodules or diffuse increase), although less common, was only

seen with mast cell tumors. In addition, the spleen of cats with mast cell tumor was more likely to have an irregular contour. It is helpful to compare the echogenicity of the spleen and left kidney to confirm the initial impressions, though this is probably not a reliable comparison in cats. Focal or multifocal hypoechoic areas or nodules may be present concurrently with these diseases as previously described for focal splenic disease. A splenic aspirate or bone marrow sample and blood work may assist with diagnosis.

DOPPLER EVALUATION, HARMONICS, AND CONTRAST ULTRASOUND

As many of the figures and references in this chapter have shown, Doppler ultrasonography is helpful to evaluate splenic blood flow. Power Doppler imaging, because of its sensitivity to low blood flow, is especially helpful for evaluating the splenic parenchyma (although more susceptible to artifact from patient motion). Doppler ultrasonography has also been used to identify lack of blood flow in the splenic veins of dogs with splenic torsion, including dogs without visible thrombi.[69] In addition, Doppler ultrasonography is helpful for diagnosing splenic vein thrombosis in abdominal inflammatory disease or other pathologic conditions predisposing to hypercoagulability. It is also the procedure of choice for distinguishing various types of splenic congestion or inflammation from severe vascular compromise produced by splenic torsion or vascular thrombosis.

Color Doppler, pulsed Doppler, and power Doppler ultrasound can also be used in combination with intravenous microbubble contrast agents. Contrast agents significantly enhance Doppler signals and have been used for a number of years for vascular studies (see Chapter 3), including confirmation of the lack of blood flow in splenic infarcts.[25] Contrast Doppler imaging has been used to identify and characterize splenic nodules and masses.

The development of new broad bandwidth transducers underlies harmonic ultrasound imaging. This procedure consists of transmitting the sound at one frequency and receiving the sound at twice or half the transmitted frequency to form

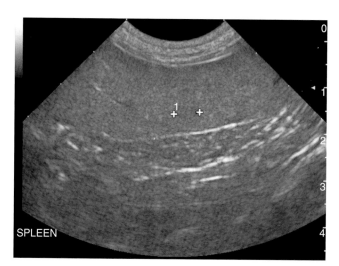

Figure 10-47 **Fourteen-year-old spayed female shih tzu mix with a cranial mediastinal mass.** Subtle small hypoechoic foci were seen throughout the parenchyma; one is identified between electronic cursors (+, 0.56 cm). The splenic foci were aspirated and yielded a cytologic diagnosis of mild extramedullary hematopoiesis and mild lymphoid hyperplasia.

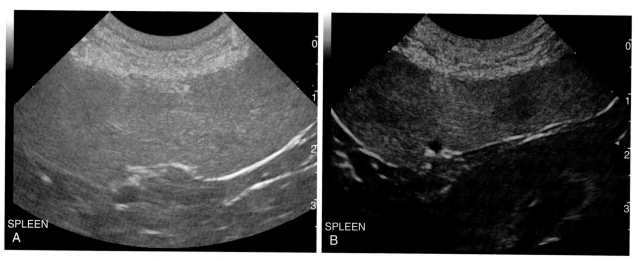

Figure 10-48 **Eleven-year-old neutered male Siberian husky with carcinoma metastasis to a regional lymph node. A,** The spleen has a barely perceptible mottled appearance. **B,** Colorized B-mode image shows better conspicuity of the mottled nature of the spleen. Multiple fine-needle aspirates were obtained for cytology and were diagnostic for extramedullary hematopoiesis and lymphoid hyperplasia.

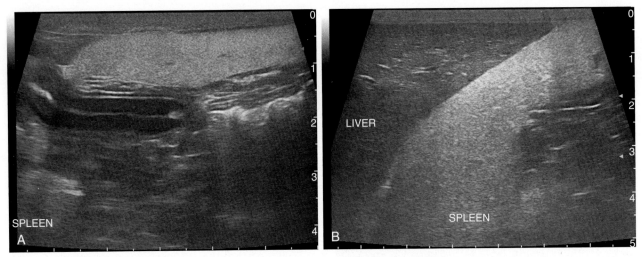

Figure 10-49 **Six-year-old spayed female miniature schnauzer with diabetes and pituitary-dependent hyperadrenocorticism. A,** The spleen is diffusely profoundly hyperechoic but not enlarged. A segment of normal small intestine is present deep to the spleen. **B,** Note the severely hyperechoic splenic parenchyma (*right*) compared to the adjacent relatively hypoechoic liver (*left*). Fine-needle aspiration for cytologic analysis was diagnostic for extramedullary hematopoiesis.

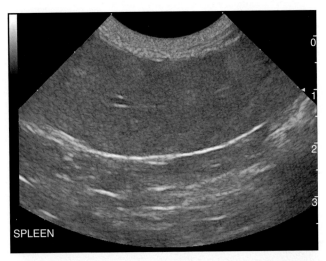

Figure 10-50 **Thirteen-year-old spayed female Australian cattle dog with a large abdominal mass.** The splenic parenchyma is subtly mottled with slightly hyperechoic and poorly defined foci throughout the spleen. The histologic diagnosis was splenic lymphoma. The abdominal mass was a large hepatocellular carcinoma (not shown).

the image. More in-depth information on the principles of harmonic ultrasound imaging can be found in Chapters 1 and 3 and in several excellent reviews.[75,76]

Two forms of harmonic ultrasound imaging have been used: (1) tissue harmonic, and (2) contrast harmonic. Tissue harmonic ultrasound relies on the tissues themselves to produce the harmonic waves, whereas contrast harmonic ultrasound requires microbubble contrast agents to generate the harmonics. With contrast harmonic ultrasound, some contrast media are taken up by the reticuloendothelial cells and others behave as blood pool media. The different properties of each contrast agent must be considered when setting the machine parameters to achieve optimal imaging. Microbubble

ultrasound contrast agents and contrast-enhanced ultrasound have been recently reviewed in humans[77] and in animals.[78]

The use of tissue harmonic ultrasound for imaging normal abdominal organs has been described in 38 cats and 48 dogs.[79] The investigators in this study concluded that the technique improved splenic image quality in dogs, but an even greater improvement was seen in cats. Currently there are no reports where tissue harmonic ultrasound has been used to evaluate animals with disease.

The preliminary use of contrast harmonic ultrasound for the evaluation of the spleen in normal dogs has been reported.[80,81] Normal perfusion values and baseline data for perfusion dynamics were obtained. Work by Ohlerth and colleagues[80] showed mean splenic parenchyma peak intensity (PI) of 6.6 dB, with mean time to peak intensity of 25.6 seconds. Although the values in dogs weighing less than 15 kg were lower than those in dogs weighing 15 kg or more, statistical differences were not found. They also found no association between hematocrit, hemoglobin concentration, red blood cell count, blood pressure, heart rate, gender, age, and perfusion variables. Nakamura and co-workers[81] found splenic parenchymal enhancement was maintained up to 30 minutes after injection in 6 healthy Beagles. Gray-scale arterial enhancement was present 5 to 22 seconds postinjection. They also showed renal perfusion could be evaluated 3.6 seconds to 3.5 minutes postinjection. Another report used contrast ultrasound to diagnose an accessory spleen, with contrast uptake similar to the parent spleen.[82]

The effect of anesthesia on contrast-enhanced ultrasound of normal cat spleens has been investigated.[83] The time to first appearance of contrast was significantly faster in awake versus anesthetized cats (3.9 ± 0.6 seconds versus 4.8 ± 1.0 seconds). Importantly, the spleen was heterogeneous for approximately 30 seconds in all cats, and a heterogeneous perfusion pattern was more pronounced in anesthetized cats than awake cats. Therefore suspected perfusion defects must be interpreted with caution.

The use of contrast harmonic imaging for evaluating splenic lesions in dogs has been investigated.[84-86] Ohlerth and colleagues[85] found moderate to extensive hypoechoic lesions clearly identified malignant splenic lesions in dogs, whereas

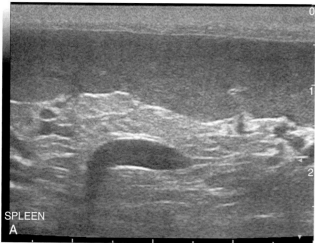

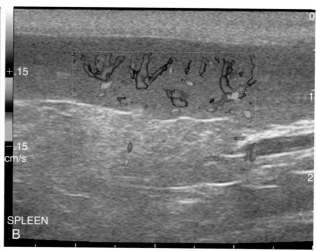

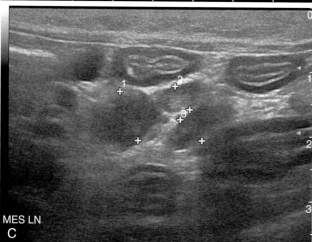

Figure 10-51 **Fifteen-year-old neutered male cat with pancytope-nia due to bone marrow arrest. A,** The spleen has an irregular contour along the mesenteric margin (far field), although maximum thickness is not increased beyond that of many normal cats (approximately 10 mm). The parenchyma is homogeneous, finely textured, and appears normal. **B,** Color Doppler evaluation of the spleen shows excellent blood flow. **C,** Mesenteric lymph nodes (between electronic cursors) are enlarged (0.81, 0.43, 0.47 cm). Note the abnormal small intestinal wall layering, with markedly disproportionate thickening of the muscularis. Lymphoma of the spleen, intestinal tract, and mesenteric lymph nodes was confirmed.

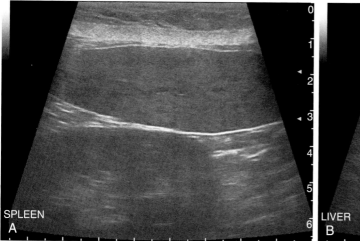

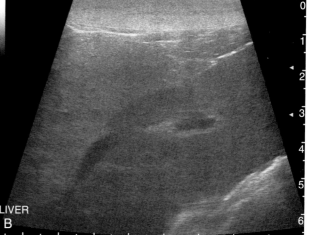

Figure 10-52 **Nine-year-old spayed female Siberian husky with generalized lymphadenopathy and confirmed lymphoma. A,** The spleen has a mottled echotexture with small, barely perceptible hypoechoic foci evenly scattered throughout the parenchyma. **B,** The spleen (*right*) is notably hypoechoic relative to the adjacent liver (*left*). Fine-needle aspirations of the spleen and liver were diagnostic for lymphoma in both organs.

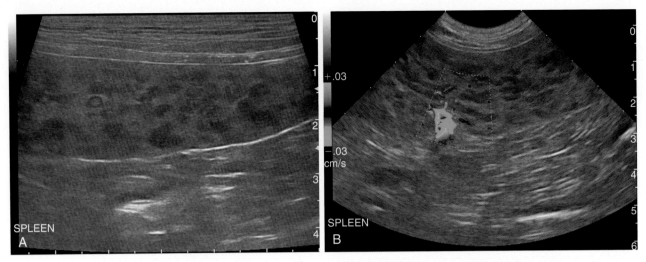

Figure 10-53 **Nine-year-old neutered male border collie mix with an enlarged abdomen and a mass effect on abdominal palpation.** A, Diffuse hypoechoic nodules of variable sizes, some of which are coalescing, are present throughout the spleen. B, Color Doppler image of the spleen. Multiple enlarged abdominal lymph nodes were also present (not shown). Lymphoma of the spleen, abdominal lymph nodes, and liver was confirmed with cytology.

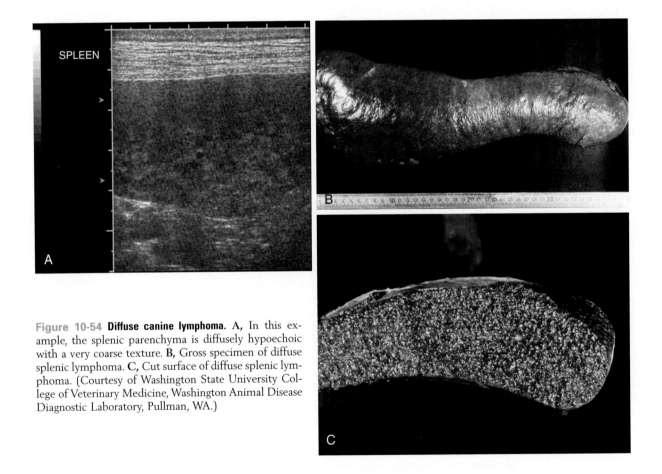

Figure 10-54 **Diffuse canine lymphoma.** A, In this example, the splenic parenchyma is diffusely hypoechoic with a very coarse texture. B, Gross specimen of diffuse splenic lymphoma. C, Cut surface of diffuse splenic lymphoma. (Courtesy of Washington State University College of Veterinary Medicine, Washington Animal Disease Diagnostic Laboratory, Pullman, WA.)

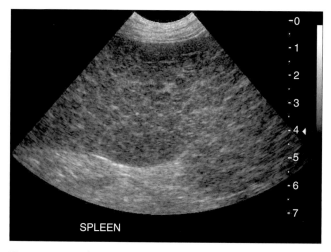

Figure 10-55 Classic appearance of the reticulated texture sometimes seen in splenic lymphosarcoma dogs.

contrast harmonic ultrasound was not useful for differentiating nodules with marked enhancement, thus necessitating histology. Rossi and associates[84] determined that malignant canine splenic lesions were all hypoechoic to surrounding splenic parenchyma 30 seconds after contrast injection. The presence of tortuous feeding vessels was also a useful criterion for malignancy. Lymphoma was shown to have a rapid time to contrast peak and a rapid wash-out phase characterized by a honeycomb appearance. Ivancic and co-workers[86] found contrast harmonic ultrasound accurate in distinguishing metastatic from benign hepatic disease in dogs with splenic hemangiosarcoma but not useful in distinguishing splenic hemangiosarcoma from hematoma.

In summary, contrast-enhanced ultrasound should improve the detection of splenic disease compared to conventional ultrasound imaging. However, definitive diagnosis will probably still require a biopsy with cytopathologic or histopathologic evaluation.

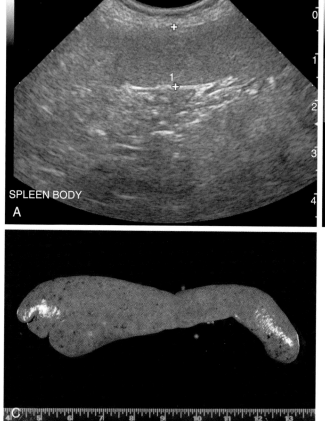

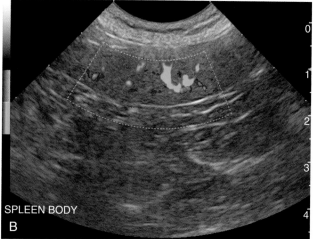

Figure 10-56 **Feline splenic mast cell tumor in a 16-year-old cat with symptoms of vomiting, anorexia, and lethargy. A,** The spleen is mildly thickened at 12.8 mm (between electronic cursors). Echogenicity is normal but there is very mild heterogeneity or coarseness to the parenchyma. **B,** Normal splenic blood flow is present using power color Doppler. Fine-needle aspiration for cytologic analysis was diagnostic for mast cell disease. **C,** Gross appearance of diffuse feline splenic mast cell disease. (Courtesy of Washington State University College of Veterinary Medicine, Washington Animal Disease Diagnostic Laboratory, Pullman, WA.)

REFERENCES

1. Wood AK, McCarthy PH, Angles JM. Ultrasonographic-anatomic correlation and imaging protocol for the spleen in anesthetized dogs. *Am J Vet Res* 1990;51:1433–8.
2. Biller DS, Myer W. Ultrasound scanning of superficial structures using an ultrasound standoff pad. *Vet Radiol* 1988;29:138–42.
3. Yabuki A, Endo Y, Sakamoto H, et al. Quantitative assessment of renal cortical echogenicity in clinically normal cats. *Anat Histol Embryol* 2008;37(5):383–6.
4. Spangler WL, Culbertson MR. Prevalence, type, and importance of splenic diseases in dogs: 1,480 cases (1985-1989). *J Am Vet Med Assoc* 1992;200:829–34.
5. Day MJ, Lucke VM, Pearson H. A review of pathological diagnoses made from 87 canine splenic biopsies. *J Small Anim Pract* 1995;36:426–33.
6. Spangler WL, Culbertson MR. Prevalence and type of splenic diseases in cats: 455 cases (1985-1991). *J Am Vet Med Assoc* 1992;201:773–6.
7. Wrigley RH, Konde LJ, Park RD, et al. Clinical features and diagnosis of splenic hematomas in dogs: 10 cases (1980-1987). *J Am Anim Hosp Assoc* 1989;25:371–5.
8. Hanson JA, Penninck DG. Ultrasonographic evaluation of a traumatic splenic hematoma and literature review. *Vet Radiol Ultrasound* 1994;35:463–6.
9. Wrigley RH, Konde LJ, Park RD, et al. Ultrasonographic features of splenic lymphosarcoma in dogs: 12 cases (1980-1986). *J Am Vet Med Assoc* 1988;193:1565–8.
10. Schelling CG, Wortman JA, Saunders HM. Ultrasonic detection of splenic necrosis in the dog: three case reports of splenic necrosis secondary to infarction. *Vet Radiol* 1988;29:227–33.
11. Lamb CR. Abdominal ultrasonography in small animals: examination of the liver, spleen and pancreas. *J Small Anim Pract* 1990;31:6–15.
12. vanSonnenberg E, Simeone JF, Mueller PR, et al. Sonographic appearance of hematoma in liver, spleen, and kidney: a clinical, pathologic, and animal study. *Radiology* 1983;147:507–10.
13. Lupien C, Sauerbrei EE. Healing in the traumatized spleen: sonographic investigation. *Radiology* 1984;151:181–5.
14. Coelho JC, Sigel B, Ryva JC, et al. B-mode sonography of blood clots. *JCU J Clin Ultrasound* 1982;10:323–7.
15. Peter DJ, Flanagan LD, Cranley JJ. Analysis of blood clot echogenicity. *JCU J Clin Ultrasound* 1986;14:111–16.
16. Sofer M, Michowitz M, Mandelbaum Y, et al. Percutaneous drainage of subcapsular splenic hematoma: an experimental model in dogs. *Am Surg* 1998;64:1212–14.
17. Wrigley RH, Park RD, Konde LJ, et al. Ultrasonographic features of splenic hemangiosarcoma in dogs: 18 cases (1980-1986). *J Am Vet Med Assoc* 1988;192:1113–17.
18. Liu JB, Merton DA, Goldberg BB, et al. Contrast-enhanced two- and three-dimensional sonography for evaluation of intra-abdominal hemorrhage. *J Ultrasound Med* 2002;21:161–9.
19. Goerg C, Schwerk WB. Splenic infarction: sonographic patterns, diagnosis, follow-up, and complications. *Radiology* 1990;174:803–7.
20. Ellison GW, King RR, Calderwood-Mays M. Medical and surgical management of multiple organ infarctions secondary to bacterial endocarditis in a dog. *J Am Vet Med Assoc* 1988;193:1289–91.
21. Hardie EM, Vaden SL, Spaulding K, et al. Splenic infarction in 16 dogs: a retrospective study. *J Vet Intern Med* 1995;9:141–8.
22. Nyland TG, Hager DA. Sonography of the liver, gallbladder, and spleen. *Vet Clin North Am Small Anim Pract* 1985;15:1123–48.
23. Nyland TG, Hager DA, Herring DS. Sonography of the liver, gallbladder, and spleen. *Semin Vet Med Surg (Small Anim)* 1989;4:13–31.
24. Shirkhoda A, Wallace S, Sokhandan M. Computed tomography and ultrasonography in splenic infarction. *J Can Assoc Radiol* 1985;36:29–33.
25. Brown JM, Quedens-Case C, Alderman JL, et al. Contrast enhanced sonography of visceral perfusion defects in dogs. *J Ultrasound Med* 1997;16:493–9.
26. Dubbins PA. Ultrasound in the diagnosis of splenic abscess. *Br J Radiol* 1980;53:488–9.
27. Konde LJ, Lebel JL, Park RD, et al. Sonographic application in the diagnosis of intraabdominal abscess in the dog. *Vet Radiol* 1986;27:151–4.
28. Ginel PJ, Lucena R, Arola J, et al. Diffuse splenomegaly caused by splenic abscessation in a dog. *Vet Rec* 2001;149:327–9.
29. Chou YH, Tiu CM, Chiou HJ, et al. Ultrasound-guided interventional procedures in splenic abscesses. *Eur J Radiol* 1998;28:167–70.
30. Stowater JL, Lamb CR, Schelling SH. Ultrasonographic features of canine hepatic nodular hyperplasia. *Vet Radiol* 1990;31:268–72.
31. Cuccovillo A, Lamb CR. Cellular features of sonographic target lesions of the liver and spleen in 21 dogs and a cat. *Vet Radiol Ultrasound* 2002;43:275–8.
32. Crevier FR, Wrigley RH. The Sonographic features of splenic lymphoid hyperplasia in 31 dogs: a retrospective study (1980-2000). *Vet Radiol Ultrasound* 2000;41:566.
33. Feeney DA, Johnston GR, Hardy RM. Two-dimensional, gray-scale ultrasonography for assessment of hepatic and splenic neoplasia in the dog and cat. *J Am Vet Med Assoc* 1984;184:68–81.
34. Nyland TG, Kantrowitz BM. Ultrasound in diagnosis and staging of abdominal neoplasia. *Contemp Issues Small Anim Pract* 1986;6:1–24.
35. Jabara AG, McLeod JB. A primary extraskeletal osteogenic sarcoma arising in the spleen of a dog. *Aust Vet J* 1989;66:27–9.
36. Schena CJ, Stickle RL, Dunstan RW, et al. Extraskeletal osteosarcoma in two dogs. *J Am Vet Med Assoc* 1989;194:1452–6.
37. Weinstein MJ, Carpenter JL, Schunk CJ. Nonangiogenic and nonlymphomatous sarcomas of the canine spleen: 57 cases (1975-1987). *J Am Vet Med Assoc* 1989;195:784–8.
38. Patnaik AK. Canine extraskeletal osteosarcoma and chondrosarcoma: a clinicopathologic study of 14 cases. *Vet Pathol* 1990;27:46–55.
39. Hendrick MJ, Brooks JJ, Bruce EH. Six cases of malignant fibrous histiocytoma of the canine spleen. *Vet Pathol* 1992;29:351–4.
40. Kapatkin AS, Mullen HS, Matthiesen DT, et al. Leiomyosarcoma in dogs: 44 cases (1983-1988). *J Am Vet Med Assoc* 1992;201:1077–9.
41. Kuntz CA, Dernell WS, Powers BE, et al. Extraskeletal osteosarcomas in dogs: 14 cases. *J Am Anim Hosp Assoc* 1998;34:26–30.
42. Langenbach A, Anderson MA, Dambach DM, et al. Extraskeletal osteosarcomas in dogs: a retrospective study of 169 cases (1986-1996). *J Am Anim Hosp Assoc* 1998;34:113–20.
43. Spangler WL, Kass PH. Pathologic and prognostic characteristics of splenomegaly in dogs due to fibrohistiocytic nodules: 98 cases. *Vet Pathol* 1998;35:488–98.

44. Hanson JA, Papageorges M, Girard E, et al. Ultrasonographic appearance of splenic disease in 101 cats. *Vet Radiol Ultrasound* 2001;**42**:441–5.

45. Lamb CR, Hartzband LE, Tidwell AS, et al. Ultrasonographic findings in hepatic and splenic lymphosarcoma in dogs and cats. *Vet Radiol* 1991;**32**:117–20.

46. Ramirez S, Douglass JP, Robertson ID. Ultrasonographic features of canine abdominal malignant histiocytosis. *Vet Radiol Ultrasound* 2002;**43**:167–70.

47. Vail DM. Histiocytic disorders. In: Stephen JW, MacEwen EG, editors. *Small Animal Clinical Oncology*. 3rd ed. Philadelphia: WB Saunders; 2001. p. 667–71.

48. Ide K, Setoguchi-Mukai A, Nakagawa T, et al. Disseminated histiocytic sarcoma with excessive hemophagocytosis in a cat. *J Vet Med Sci* 2009;**71**(6):817–20.

49. Cortese L, Paciell O, Papparella S. Morphological characterization of malignant histiocytosis in a cat. *Folia Morphol* 2008;**67**(4):299–303.

50. Cruz-Arambulo R, Wrigley R, Powers B. Sonographic features of histiocytic neoplasms in the canine abdomen. *Vet Radiol Ultrasound* 2004;**45**:554–8.

51. Dobson J, Villiers E, Roulois A, et al. Histiocytic sarcoma of the spleen in flat-coated retrievers with regenerative anaemia and hypoproteinaemia. *Vet Rec* 2006;**158**:825–9.

52. Court EA, Earnest-Koons KA, Barr SC, et al. Malignant histiocytosis in a cat. *J Am Vet Med Assoc* 1993;**203**:1300–2.

53. Kraje AC, Patton CS, Edwards DF. Malignant histiocytosis in 3 cats. *J Vet Intern Med* 2001;**15**:252–6.

54. Sato AF, Solano M. Ultrasonographic findings in abdominal mast cell disease: a retrospective study of 19 patients. *Vet Radiol Ultrasound* 2004;**45**:51–7.

55. Sandler CH, Langham RF. Myelolipomas of the spleen in a cat. *J Am Vet Med Assoc* 1972;**160**:1101–3.

56. Zimmer MA, Stair EL. Splenic myelolipomas in two dogs. *Vet Pathol* 1983;**20**:637–8.

57. Walzer C, Hittmair K, Walzer-Wagner C. Ultrasonographic identification and characterization of splenic nodular lipomatosis or myelolipomas in cheetahs (Acinonyx jubatus). *Vet Radiol Ultrasound* 1996;**37**:289–92.

58. Schwarz LA, Penninck DG, Gliatto J. Canine splenic myelolipomas. *Vet Radiol Ultrasound* 2001;**42**:347–8.

59. Al-Rukibat RK, Bani Ismail ZA. Unusual presentation of splenic myelolipoma in a dog. *Can Vet J* 2006;**47**:1112–14.

60. Murphy JF, Bernardino ME. The sonographic findings of splenic metastases. *J Clin Ultrasound* 1979;**7**:195–7.

61. Hickford FH, Stokol T, vanGessel YA, et al. Monoclonal immunoglobulin G cryoglobulinemia and multiple myeloma in a domestic shorthair cat. *J Am Vet Med Assoc* 2000;**217**:1029–33, 1007–28.

62. Monteiro CB, O'Brien RT. A retrospective study on the sonographic findings of abdominal carcinomatosis in 14 cats. *Vet Radiol Ultrasound* 2004;**45**:559–64.

63. O'Brien RT, Waller KR 3rd, Osgood TL. Sonographic features of drug-induced splenic congestion. *Vet Radiol Ultrasound* 2004;**45**:225–7.

64. Konde LJ, Wrigley RH, Lebel JL, et al. Sonographic and radiographic changes associated with splenic torsion in the dog. *Vet Radiol* 1989;**30**:41–5.

65. Laurenson MP, Hopper K, Herrera MA, et al. Concurrent diseases and conditions in dogs with splenic vein thrombosis. *J Vet Intern Med* 2010;**24**(6):1298–304.

66. Ohta H, Takagi S, Murakami M, et al. Primary splenic torsion in a Boston terrier. *J Vet Med Sci* 2009;**71**(11):1533–5.

67. Gaschen L, Kircher P, Venzin C, et al. Imaging diagnosis: the abdominal air-vasculogram in a dog with splenic torsion and clostridial infection. *Vet Radiol Ultrasound* 2003;**44**:553–5.

68. Mai W. The hilar perivenous hyperechoic triangle as a sign of acute splenic torsion in dogs. *Vet Radiol Ultrasound* 2006;**47**:487–91.

69. Saunders HM, Neath PJ, Brockman DJ. B-mode and Doppler ultrasound imaging of the spleen with canine splenic torsion: a retrospective evaluation. *Vet Radiol Ultrasound* 1998;**39**:349–53.

70. Trotta M, Carli E, Novari G, et al. Clinicopathological findings, molecular detection and characterization of Babesia gibsoni infection in a sick dog from Italy. *Vet Parasitol* 2009;**165**(3–4):318–22.

71. Lewis KM, O'Brien RT. Abdominal ultrasonographic findings associated with feline infectious peritonitis: a retrospective review of 16 cases. *J Am Anim Hops Assoc* 2010;**46**(3):152–60.

72. Stefanello D, Valenti P, Faverzani S, et al. Ultrasound-guided cytology of spleen and liver: a prognostic tool in canine cutaneous mast cell tumor. *J Vet Intern Med* 2009;**23**(5):1051–7.

73. Book AP, Fidel J, Wills T, et al. Correlation of ultrasound findings, liver and spleen cytology, and prognosis in the clinical staging of high metastatic risk canine mast cell tumors. *Vet Radiol Ultrasound* 2011;**52**(5):548–54.

74. Crabtree AC, Spangler E, Beard D, et al. Diagnostic accuracy of gray-scale ultrasonography for the detection of hepatic and splenic lymphoma in dogs. *Vet Radiol Ultrasound* 2010;**51**(6):661–4.

75. Ziegler L, O'Brien RT. Harmonic ultrasound: a review. *Vet Radiol Ultrasound* 2002;**43**:501–9.

76. Szatmari V, Harkanyi Z, Voros K. A review of nonconventional ultrasound techniques and contrast-enhanced ultrasonography of noncardiac canine disorders. *Vet Radiol Ultrasound* 2003;**44**:380–91.

77. Quaia E. Microbubble ultrasound contrast agents: an update. *Eur Radiol* 2007;**17**:1995–2008.

78. Ohlerth S, O'Brien RT. Contrast ultrasound: general principles and veterinary clinical applications. *Vet J* 2007;**174**:501–12.

79. Matheson JS, O'Brien RT, Delaney F. Tissue harmonic ultrasound for imaging normal abdominal organs in dogs and cats. *Vet Radiol Ultrasound* 2003;**44**:205–8.

80. Ohlerth S, Ruefli E, Poirier V, et al. Contrast harmonic imaging of the normal canine spleen. *Vet Radiol Ultrasound* 2007;**48**:451–6.

81. Nakamura K, Sasaki N, Yoshikawa M, et al. Quantitative contrast-enhanced ultrasonography of canine spleen. *Vet Radiol Ultrasound* 2009;**50**(1):104–8.

82. Rossi F, Rabba S, Vignoli M, et al. B-mode and contrast-enhanced sonographic assessment of accessory spleen in the dog. *Vet Radiol Ultrasound* 2010;**51**(2):173–7.

83. Leinonen MR, Raekallio MR, Vainio OM, et al. Effect of anaesthesia on contrast-enhanced ultrasound of the feline spleen. *Vet J* 2011;**190**(2):273–7.

84. Rossi F, Leone VF, Vignoli M, et al. Use of contrast-enhanced ultrasound for characterization of focal splenic lesions. *Vet Radiol Ultrasound* 2008;**49**(2):154–64.

85. Ohlerth S, Dennler M, Rüefli E, et al. Contrast harmonic imaging characterization of canine splenic lesions. *J Vet Intern Med* 2008;**22**(5):1095–102.

86. Ivancic M, Long F, Seiler GS. Contrast harmonic ultrasonography of splenic masses and associated liver nodules in dogs. *J Am Vet Med Assoc* 2009;**234**(1):88–94.

CHAPTER 11
Pancreas

Thomas G. Nyland • John S. Mattoon

INDICATIONS FOR PANCREATIC ULTRASONOGRAPHY

The pancreas is a difficult organ to evaluate by most abdominal imaging methods. In veterinary medicine, survey radiographs of the abdomen have traditionally been the initial imaging procedure of choice. Radiographic signs suggestive of pancreatic abnormalities include a soft tissue dense mass or loss of peritoneal detail in the right cranial abdomen and small amounts of duodenal gas accumulation indicative of functional ileus. An upper gastrointestinal tract series is helpful to confirm pancreatic masses that cause duodenal fixation or displacement, increased width of the cranial duodenal flexure, or thickening and deformity of the adjacent duodenum or stomach. However, the radiographic findings may be equivocal or normal in many cases of pancreatic disease.

Ultrasonography was one of the first modalities that enabled direct visualization of the pancreas in humans, and its use was quickly applied to animals. More recently, computed tomography, magnetic resonance imaging, and scintigraphy have played major roles in assessing pancreatic disease in humans. The preliminary use of these modalities to image the pancreas has also been described in animals.[1-10] Fiberoptic technology has enabled the use of endoscopic retrograde cholangiopancreatography and endoscopic ultrasonography for pancreatic evaluation in humans. The potential applications and preliminary experience with endoscopic retrograde cholangiopancreatography and endoscopic ultrasonography of the pancreas have also been described in animals.[11-17] The expense and availability of specialized equipment, as well as the need for anesthesia, have currently limited the routine use of these techniques in small animals. Ultrasonography is still the primary means for imaging the pancreas in the dog and cat because of its wider availability.

Ultrasonography complements but does not replace abdominal radiography for the work-up of the acute abdomen. Radiography is important for evaluating peritoneal detail, bowel patterns, and the displacement of viscera by large abdominal masses. Radiography is also useful for detecting gastrointestinal foreign bodies, free abdominal air, and bone abnormalities. Ultrasonography is better for evaluating pancreatic or other small abdominal masses, identifying focal fluid collections, and recognizing metastasis to adjacent organs or lymph nodes. In addition, ultrasonography is superior to radiography when there is a large amount of abdominal fluid. The discovery of a mass in the pancreatic region, with concurrent lymphadenopathy, metastasis, or other abnormalities, helps narrow the differential diagnosis and establish a prognosis for the acute abdomen. If necessary, material for cytologic analysis can be obtained from the pancreas, lymph nodes, or potential metastatic lesions by guided aspiration. Serial follow-up ultrasound examinations allow an accurate determination of treatment response.

Although there are many advantages to pancreatic ultrasonography, the technique also has significant limitations. These include poor visualization of the normal pancreas and interference from gas or barium in the gastrointestinal tract. Proper preparation of animals, judicious use of transducer pressure to displace overlying gas-filled bowel, and positional studies can usually overcome the limitations of bowel gas. Ultrasound examinations should always be performed before procedures causing aerophagia and before a barium series because of the high reflectivity of air and barium. The examination should be repeated if a diagnostic study cannot be obtained. The lack of abnormalities on an ultrasound examination of the pancreatic region does not exclude pancreatic disease, but it helps rule out significant anatomic abnormalities. In spite of these limitations, ultrasound has gained an important place in the diagnostic work-up of almost all cases of suspected pancreatic disease.

The normal canine or feline pancreas can be difficult to see as a distinct structure on ultrasound studies, but the surrounding anatomy, as described later, helps localize its position.[18-23] Fat within and surrounding the pancreas is probably responsible for the high echogenicity of this region. In some cases, the pancreas is not visualized, but newer ultrasound equipment has allowed more frequent identification of the pancreas in dogs and cats. The acoustic output and gain settings of the scanner should be kept as low as possible to decrease overall reflectivity of the region and permit the greatest chance for visualizing the pancreas.

EXAMINATION TECHNIQUE

Pancreatic ultrasound examinations may be performed in dorsal recumbency, ventral recumbency, lateral recumbency, or the standing position. The sonographer may begin the study from the ventral abdomen with the dog or cat positioned in dorsal recumbency (Figure 11-1, *A* and *B*). However, some sonographers prefer left lateral recumbency, especially with deep-chested dogs (Figure 11-1, *C*). Hair removal and imaging through the right 9th to 12th intercostal space facilitates transverse views when excessive bowel gas is present.[24,25] The ventral or lateral recumbent position is also used as needed to avoid bowel gas. An 8- to 15-MHz linear or curvilinear transducer is preferred for pancreatic examinations in small dogs and cats, but large dogs may require a 5- to 8-MHz transducer

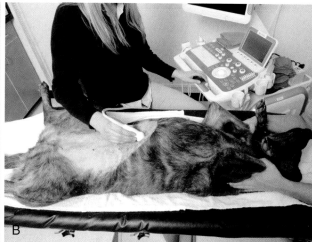

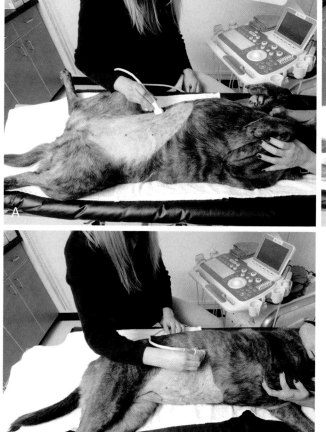

Figure 11-1 **Pancreatic imaging. A,** Dorsal recumbency. Transducer position for imaging the right lobe of the pancreas in a sagittal view. **B,** Dorsal recumbency. Transducer position for imaging the body of the pancreas in a transverse view. Moving the transducer to the animal's left across the abdomen just caudal to the stomach allows a transverse view through the left lobe of the pancreas. **C,** Left lateral recumbency for evaluating the right lobe of the pancreas (transducer positioned to view pancreas in transverse view).

to obtain better penetration. The most important advice is to position the patient so that important anatomic landmarks used to locate the pancreas can be recognized.

NORMAL ANATOMY AND ULTRASOUND APPEARANCE

The normal pancreas is usually localized by using a combination of surrounding anatomy and direct ultrasonographic visualization[18-26] (Figure 11-2). Improvements in ultrasound imaging technology provide better visualization of the pancreas than was possible a few years ago. The pancreas is more frequently seen as an isoechoic or slightly hypoechoic structure medial or dorsomedial to the descending duodenum, ventral to the portal vein, and caudal to the stomach in apparently healthy dogs and cats.

In dogs, the pancreatic body, which separates the right and left pancreatic lobes, normally lies immediately ventral to the portal vein. The right lobe is located by using the right kidney, portal vein, and descending duodenum as landmarks (see Figure 11-2). These structures are best visualized in a transverse view of the right cranial abdomen. The right kidney may be located first, followed by identification of the descending duodenum near the body wall, ventral or ventrolateral to the right kidney (Figure 11-3). The duodenum has a round, target-like appearance on cross section with hypoechoic walls and a central hyperechoic lumen. Air mixed with mucous secretions contributes to the highly echogenic appearance of the

duodenal mucosal surface. The exact location of the duodenum depends on the amount of transducer pressure exerted on the ventral abdomen. Increased pressure will displace the duodenum dorsolaterally. The right lobe of the pancreas lies medial or dorsomedial to the duodenum, to the right of the portal vein and immediately ventral to the right kidney. Cranial to the kidney, the right lobe lies ventral to the caudate lobe of the liver and caudodorsal to the cranial duodenal flexure. The pancreaticoduodenal vein, which courses through the right lobe of the pancreas parallel to the descending duodenum, may also help with localization[26,27] (see Figure 11-3). The pancreatic duct may be visible in the right pancreatic lobe in some normal dogs and can be distinguished from the pancreaticoduodenal artery and vein by Doppler ultrasonography (see Figure 11-3, C and G).[28] The descending duodenum can be differentiated from other small bowel loops by tracing it in a transverse plane from the cranial flexure to the point where the caudal duodenal flexure turns medially. Unlike other small bowel loops, the normal descending duodenum consistently maintains its target-like appearance in the transverse scanning plane because of its straight course to the caudal flexure. The descending duodenum is usually the lateral-most segment of small intestine on the right, its wall slightly thicker and diameter slightly larger than surrounding jejunum. In almost all cases, the duodenum can be identified with confidence, as can the mesoduodenum and hence the right lobe of the pancreas.

The left lobe of the pancreas is best localized by scanning the cranial abdomen in a sagittal plane. The left lobe lies

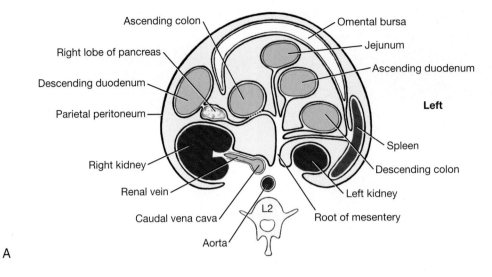

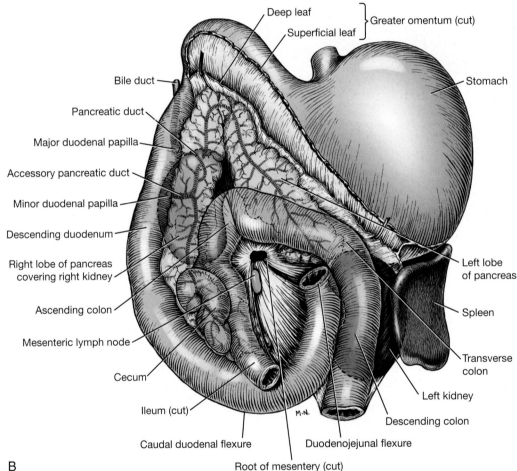

Figure 11-2 **Relationship of the pancreas to major abdominal organs. A,** Diagram of major anatomic relationships in the transverse plane through the right pancreatic lobe. Note the relationship to the descending duodenum, the right kidney, and the ascending colon. **B,** Ventral view of the pancreas and its relationship to surrounding anatomic structures. Note its relationship of the right lobe to the duodenum, the cecum and ascending colon, and the right kidney. The left lobe is bounded by the transverse colon caudally and the caudal margin of the stomach cranially. It may extend to the medial margin of the left kidney. (From Evans H, de Lahunta A: *Guide to dissection of the dog,* St. Louis, 2010, Saunders.)

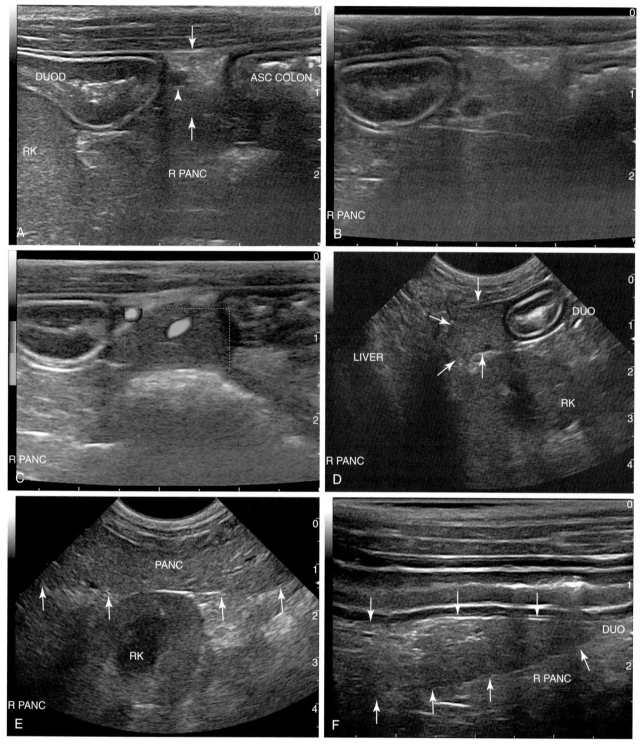

Figure 11-3 Normal dog pancreas. A, Transverse image through the right cranial abdomen showing the relationship of the right lobe of the pancreas (between arrows, *R PANC*) to surrounding organs. Transverse image of the duodenum (*DUOD*), ascending colon (*ASC COLON*) and right kidney (*RK*) are seen. The pancreaticoduodenal vein is present between the pancreas and the duodenum (*arrowhead*). **B,** Transverse image of the right lobe of the pancreas and adjacent duodenum. The pancreaticoduodenal vein is seen in cross section. **C,** Color Doppler image of the right lobe of the pancreas in showing the pancreaticoduodenal artery and vein. **D,** Transverse image through the right lobe of the pancreas (between arrows), duodenum (*DUO*), right kidney (*RK*), and liver. The pancreas is roughly rectangular to triangular in its transverse axis. The parenchyma is of medium echogenicity and normally similar to the renal cortex and liver. The leftward placement of the pancreas is due to transducer placement. **E,** Sagittal view of the right lobe of the pancreas (*PANC, arrows*). The right kidney (*RK*) is seen in the far field. **F,** Sagittal image of the right lobe of the pancreas obtained by transducer placement along the right lateral body wall with the patient in left lateral recumbency (a dorsal image plane). In this view, the descending duodenum (*DUO*) is seen in the near field with the pancreas (*R PANC*) directly adjacent in the far field (between arrows).

Continued

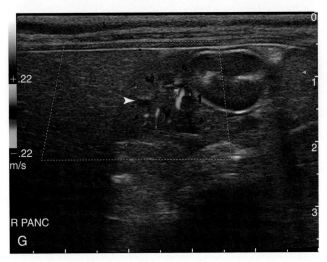

Figure 11-3, cont'd G, Color Doppler transverse image of the body/right lobe of the pancreas shows normal blood flow. The small pancreatic duct is seen in cross section (*arrowhead*). The pancreas is roughly triangular in shape and is slightly hypoechoic relative to the adjacent liver tissue to the left. The duodenum is seen to the right of the pancreas.

immediately caudal to the cranial duodenal flexure and greater curvature of the stomach as scanned leftward in a sagittal plane from the portal vein to the cranial pole of the left kidney. The antral and pyloric portions of the stomach appear as a bull's-eye near the portal vein. The region caudal and caudodorsal to the stomach is kept in view while scanning to the left from the portal vein. The splenic vein passes caudodorsal to the left pancreatic lobe and may be seen in cross section. The splenic vein can often be traced from the spleen to where it joins the cranial mesenteric vein to form the portal vein. The leftward extent of the pancreas lies near the cranial pole of the left kidney. The transverse colon lies caudal to the pancreas and often appears in cross section as a hyperechoic gas-filled bowel loop in sagittal views of the cranial abdomen. The spleen lies lateral and ventral to the left pancreatic lobe and may act as an acoustic window. The head (dorsal extremity) of the spleen can be confused with the left pancreatic lobe because both are closely associated with the cranial pole of the left kidney. However, the head of the spleen can be traced laterally where it joins the main portion of the spleen. Two separate splenic segments are occasionally present, which may simulate a pancreatic mass. The typical, finely textured appearance of splenic parenchyma and an echogenic splenic capsule usually permit the correct diagnosis. The transverse colon, when it is devoid of gas, has a target-like appearance bordering the left lobe caudodorsally.

In our experience, the thickness of the pancreas varies considerably in dogs, ranging from a minimum of 4 mm to 10 mm or more. The pancreatic duct, while not as readily identified as in cats, is now seen routinely using high frequency transducers, and using color Doppler analysis to differentiate it from pancreatic blood vessels. It is very small, from a few tenths of a millimeter up to perhaps 1 mm.

In cats, the right lobe of the pancreas is more difficult to identify than in dogs, whereas the body and left lobe are more easily seen (Figure 11-4). The normal pancreatic ducts are also much more frequently identified in the cat, particularly within the left pancreatic lobe (see Figure 11-4, *B* to *D*). The major duodenal papilla, where the common bile duct and pancreatic duct enter the duodenum, is readily seen in the cat. In dogs, the largest pancreatic duct (accessory pancreatic duct) is

infrequently seen where it enters the duodenum at the minor duodenal papilla.

Examination of the pancreas in cats should begin by localizing the portal vein in a transverse plane. The portal vein is then traced cranially to the caudal border of the stomach where the pancreatic body is seen ventral to the portal vein. Similarly, locating the portal vein in its long axis is equally effective (see Figure 11-4, *E* and *F*). The pancreatic body usually appears as an isoechoic or hypoechoic structure compared to surrounding fat with an echogenicity similar to that of the liver. The left lobe of the pancreas is caudal to the stomach and cranial to the transverse colon, closely associated with the splenic vein (see Figure 11-4, *A*). The splenic vein is caudodorsal to the pancreas. The pancreatic duct can usually be identified as an anechoic, tubular structure centrally located within the left lobe. The right pancreatic lobe is smaller and more difficult to identify than the left lobe. The right lobe can be traced caudally from the pancreatic body medial to the descending duodenum. A centrally located pancreatic duct may be visible. Normal pancreatic measurements and the diameter of the left lobe pancreatic duct have been published in cats.[20-22] Based on these studies, the approximate normal range of thickness for the body and left lobe (5 to 9 mm), thickness of the right lobe (3 to 6 mm), and diameter of the left lobe pancreatic duct (0.5 to 2.5 mm) in cats have been proposed.[23] The mean pancreatic duct diameter increases with age in normal cats.[21,22] In healthy cats less than 10 years of age the mean duct diameter is approximately 0.8 ± 0.25 mm (range 0.5 to 1.3 mm),[20] whereas the mean duct diameter in a group of cats aged 10 years and older was 1.3 ± 0.4 mm (range 0.6 to 2.4 mm).[22] Results of a recent study on secretin-induced pancreatic duct dilation in normal cats revealed that mean pancreatic duct diameter increased from 0.77 ± 0.33 to 1.42 ± 0.40 mm after secretin administration.[29] The increase in pancreatic duct diameter over baseline values was dramatic—$101.9 \pm 58.8\%$ up to 15 minutes postadministration. Secretin induces exocrine secretion of bicarbonate, causing transient pancreatic duct dilation. In people with chronic pancreatitis, pancreatic duct dilation does not occur following secretin administration, a result of periductal fibrosis. This application in veterinary medicine has yet to be investigated.

The authors routinely use color Doppler and power Doppler imaging to evaluate pancreatic blood flow, in both normal and abnormal patients. Usually, some degree of pancreatic blood flow can be detected using color and power Doppler techniques, and familiarity with normally expected pancreatic blood flow may help the sonographer in cases of pancreatic disease. In addition to identifying the pancreaticoduodenal artery and vein, and differentiating them from the pancreatic duct, Doppler imaging can be used qualitatively to assess abnormally increased pancreatic parenchymal blood flow (e.g., hyperemia in acute pancreatitis) or absence of blood flow (e.g., necrotizing pancreatitis).[5] Rademacher and colleagues[30] investigated the use of contrast-enhanced color and power Doppler analysis in to assess the pancreas in normal and diseased cats. They found significant increases in vascularization in cats with pancreatic disease (inflammation, hyperplasia, neoplasia). As expected, higher values were obtained with power Doppler than with color Doppler techniques, and with the use of contrast.

PATHOLOGY

Nodular Hyperplasia

Pancreatic nodular hyperplasia is commonly found in older dogs and does not seem to be related to the presence or

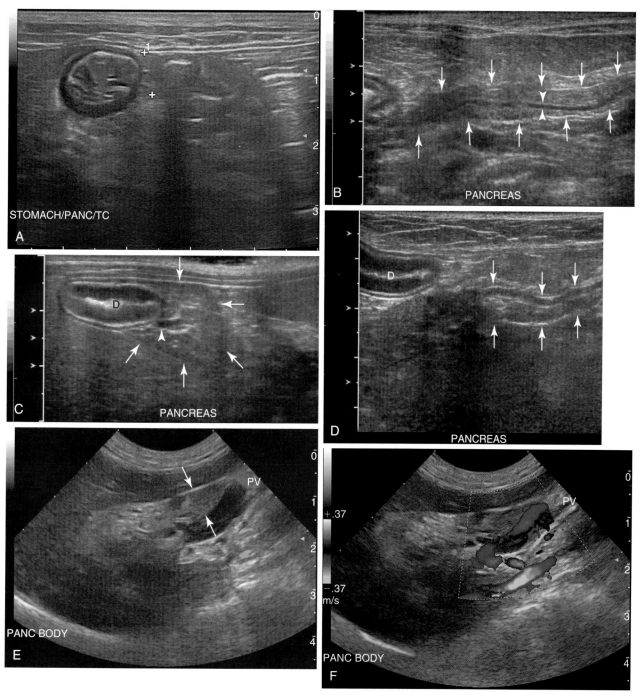

Figure 11-4 **Normal cat pancreas.** **A,** Transverse view of the left lobe of the pancreas (between electronic cursors, 0.66 cm thick; sagittal body plane). The empty stomach is to the left, the empty transverse colon to the right. **B,** Long axis view of the left lobe of the pancreas (between arrows). The pancreas is much less than 10 mm thick; the central pancreatic duct (between arrowheads) is less than 1 mm thick. Note the pancreas has echogenicity and echotexture similar to the surround mesentery and peritoneal fat (near field). **C,** Transverse view of the right lobe of the pancreas (between arrows), roughly rectangular to triangular in shape. The pancreaticoduodenal vein (*arrowhead*) is seen in cross section between the pancreas and the duodenum (*D*). **D,** Sagittal view (slightly oblique) of the right lobe of the pancreas (between arrows). A section of the duodenum (*D*) in sagittal axis is seen in the near field to the left. **E,** Sagittal body plane view showing the body of the pancreas in transverse axis (between arrows) immediately ventral to the portal vein (*PV*). **F,** Color Doppler image of E showing portal vein blood flow. The caudal vena cava is in the far field dorsal to the portal vein.

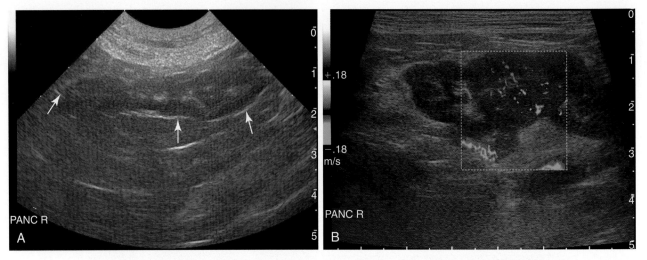

Figure 11-5 **Nodular pancreas in a 9-year-old spayed female Siberian husky in diabetic ketoacidosis.** **A,** Sagittal image of the right lobe of the pancreas (*arrows*) shows an irregular central region of hyperechogenicity surrounded by lobulated hypoechoic tissue. A microconvex transducer operating at 9 MHz was used. **B,** Color Doppler image of the right pancreatic lobe. There is good pancreatic blood flow. Note the increase in resolution of the pancreatic pathology when using a higher frequency linear-array transducer (trapezoidal mode). At necropsy the pancreas contained 3- to 9-mm firm nodules.

absence of inflammation, necrosis, or fibrosis.[31] However, the authors are unaware of any published studies on the sonographic appearance of pancreatic nodular hyperplasia in dogs; it is doubtful that benign nodular hyperplasia can be distinguished from neoplasia by ultrasound alone (Figure 11-5).

In five cats ranging in age from 10 to 16 years, multiple hypoechoic nodules less than 1 cm in size and pancreatic enlargement up to 2 cm in thickness were seen with pancreatic nodular hyperplasia.[32] Nodular hyperplasia tended to appear as smaller nodules, and pancreatic neoplasia commonly appeared as a single large lesion exceeding 2 cm in diameter. However, nodular hyperplasia and neoplasia had similar findings in many cases, making differentiation difficult.[32] Therefore cytology and histopathology are required to differentiate pancreatic nodular hyperplasia from neoplasia in cats (Figure 11-6).

Acute Pancreatitis

Pancreatitis does not always produce sufficient changes within the pancreas for detection by ultrasonography. This is especially true in cats. Therefore a normal-appearing pancreas does not rule out pancreatitis. Furthermore, diseases other than pancreatitis, such as hypoalbuminemia, portal hypertension, or overhydration, can produce pancreatic edema and be confused with pancreatitis.[33] The sensitivity of ultrasound for diagnosing acute pancreatitis in dogs was reported to be 68%.[34] Pancreatic disease is usually diagnosed by recognizing an enlarged pancreas or an ill-defined, hypoechoic to complex mass in the pancreatic region[6,18,19,28,34,35] (Figures 11-7 to 11-12). Increased echogenicity to surrounding mesentery, omentum, and variable amounts of free abdominal fluid are often present (see Figures 11-7 to 11-9; see also Figures 11-11 and 11-12). Local transducer pressure to the right cranial quadrant may cause pain. Excessive gas within the gastrointestinal tract sometimes compromises the examination and necessitates multiple positional views and judicious use of transducer pressure to displace overlying gas-filled loops. Focal peritonitis with functional small bowel ileus and pain-induced aerophagia contribute to excessive gas accumulation.

Pancreatitis cannot be differentiated from pancreatic neoplasia or focal septic peritonitis solely on ultrasound appearance.

Multifocal hypoechoic areas, cystlike lesions, hyperechoic regions, and mixed patterns of echogenicity are commonly identified with canine pancreatitis. The appearance varies with the severity and chronicity. In acute pancreatitis, the ultrasonographic appearance is due to edema, hemorrhage, or necrosis. Detail surrounding the pancreatic region may be reduced by poor visualization of normal tissue interfaces. Focal peritonitis and fat saponification result from release of pancreatic enzymes. In the subacute phase, necrosis may produce cystlike lesions that can develop into pseudocysts, as described later.[36] Localized free abdominal fluid, duodenal and stomach wall thickening (>5 mm), distortion, or displacement of the adjacent duodenum or stomach may be present in either the acute or subacute phase (see Figure 11-12, *A* and *B*). The descending duodenum is usually displaced ventrally and laterally, but medial displacement can also occur with larger masses.[19] Functional ileus or spasticity of the surrounding small bowel with fluid accumulation in the duodenum due to functional ileus may occur (see Figure 11-10, *A*). Heng and co-workers[37] reported a spontaneous intramural duodenal hematoma resulting from acute pancreatitis. Corrugated small bowel caused by spasticity has also been described in association with pancreatitis (see Figure 11-12, *E*).[38] The stomach is usually empty if the animal has been vomiting. Dilation of the pancreatic duct in association with pancreatitis has also been described in dogs[39] and cats.[40,41] (Figure 11-13). Signs of biliary obstruction with common bile duct dilation, gallbladder enlargement, and elevation of serum bilirubin may also be present with pancreatitis (see Figure 11-13, *E*).

Although the multiple causes of acute pancreatitis are well-known, a recent report on the association of peracute pancreatitis in a dog from administration of the antianxiety drug clomipramine (a selective serotonin reuptake inhibitor) is notable, and it also occurs in humans.[42]

In contrast to dogs, the clinical signs of pancreatitis in cats are often subtle (anorexia, lethargy, dehydration) and the

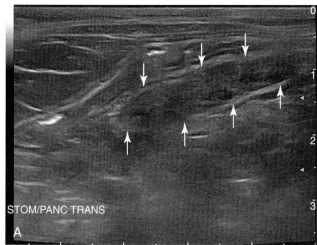

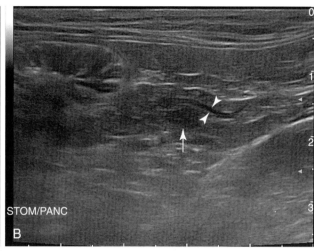

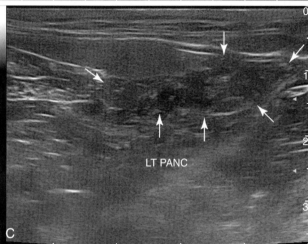

Figure 11-6 Nodular pancreas in a 15-year-old male neutered Siamese cat with presenting sign of vomiting. A, Sagittal view of the left lobe of the pancreas (*arrows*) just caudal to the stomach (transverse body plane). Multiple hypoechoic nodules are seen. The pancreas is not thickened. **B,** Oblique image through the left lobe of the pancreas shows a single hypoechoic nodule (*arrow*), the pancreatic duct (between arrowheads), and an irregular pancreatic margin. An empty stomach is present on the left side of the image. **C,** The lateral-most extent of the left lobe of the pancreas (*arrows*), abutting the spleen in the near field. Cytology was diagnostic for nodular hyperplasia and mild histiocytic inflammation. It was determined that acute renal failure was the cause of the vomiting.

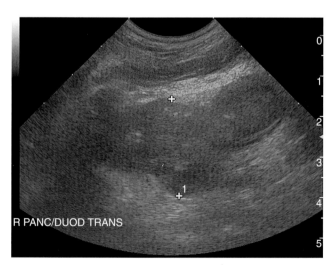

Figure 11-7 Acute pancreatitis. Ten-year-old spayed female Siberian husky with acute vomiting and a painful cranial abdomen. Transverse image of the right cranial abdomen shows a very enlarged, hypoechoic, irregularly margined right pancreatic lobe (between electronic cursors, 2.40 cm). Poor surrounding mesenteric detail is noted. The duodenum is poorly seen in transverse axis to the right of the pancreas.

pancreas may appear normal more frequently on ultrasonographic evaluation.[43] Inflammatory bowel disease or cholangiohepatitis may occur in association with feline pancreatitis.[40] Bailey and colleagues[44] found that in 23 cats with inflammatory bowel disease, 16 had elevated feline pancreatic lipase immunoreactivity (fPLI) concentrations (6.9 to >12 µg/L), and that cats with fPLI values greater than 12 µg/L had hypoalbuminemia and hypocobalaminemia. Interestingly, there was no difference in pancreatic ultrasound findings between any of the three groups of cats studied. In addition, pancreatitis was seen in 38% of cats with hepatic lipidosis.[45] The relationship of these disorders to feline pancreatitis is still unclear. If pancreatic abnormalities are identified with ultrasonography, the findings are usually similar but less extensive than those described in dogs.[43,46] The pancreas may appear hypoechoic, enlarged, or as an irregular hypoechoic mass (Figures 11-14 and 11-15). Less commonly, a complex mass is identified in the pancreatic region. Enlarged bile ducts and biliary obstruction have been reported.[3,47,48] Pancreatic duct dilatation has also been observed.[40,41] The surrounding mesentery may be hyperechoic and there may be variable amounts of free abdominal fluid. The sensitivity of ultrasound for diagnosing pancreatitis in the cat has been reported to range from 11% to 35%.[3,43,49] However, a more recent ultrasound study reported a sensitivity of 67% for diagnosing feline pancreatitis.[6] Ultrasound findings of increased pancreatic size, enhanced

Text continued on p. 451

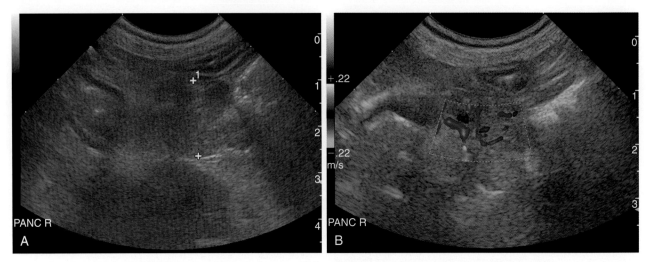

Figure 11-8 **Acute pancreatitis.** Eight-year-old female dog presented with acute vomiting. **A,** Seen in transverse axis, the right lobe of the pancreas is enlarged (between electronic cursors, 1.63 cm) and inhomogeneous. The mesoduodenum separating the pancreas from the adjacent duodenum (*left*) is inflamed with poor detail. **B,** Color Doppler image of the right pancreatic lobe shows hypervascularization thought to indicate hyperemia and acute inflammation.

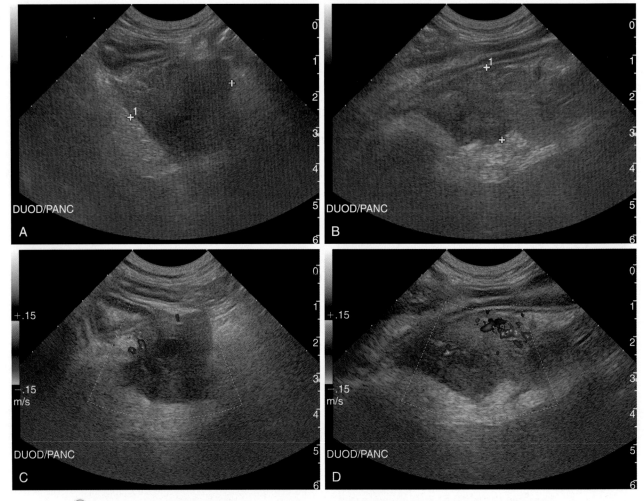

Figure 11-9 **Acute pancreatitis.** Acute vomiting in a 10-year-old neutered male dog. **A,** Transverse image of the right lobe of the pancreas that is diffusely and severely enlarged (between electronic cursors, 3.05 cm). The parenchyma is hypoechoic and fairly homogeneous. The surrounding peripancreatic tissue is hyperechoic, whereas the duodenum (*upper left*) is normal. **B,** Sagittal image of the enlarged, mildly inhomogeneous right lobe of the pancreas (between electronic cursors, 2.06 cm). The duodenum is in the near field and peripancreatic tissue is hyperechoic. **C,** Transverse color Doppler image of the right lobe of the pancreas with peripheral blood flow but poor parenchymal flow, suggesting necrosis. **D,** Sagittal color Doppler image shows increased blood flow within the inflamed parenchyma. The descending duodenum is in the near field.

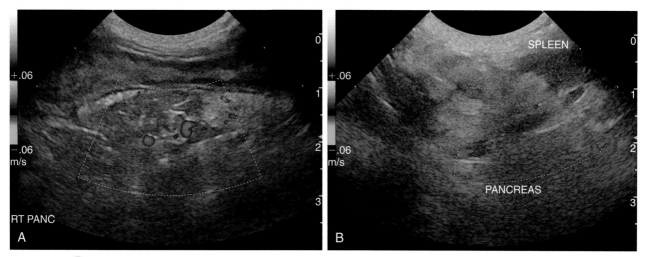

Figure 11-10 **Severe pancreatitis and peritonitis in a 14-year-old spayed female poodle with respiratory distress, vomiting, and a painful abdomen.** A, Color Doppler sagittal image of the right lobe of the pancreas shows abnormal heterogeneity with areas of good blood flow and areas of no flow. A dilated duodenum is in the near field. B, Color Doppler transverse image of the left lobe of the pancreas. The pancreas is relatively hyperechoic and avascular; only the adjacent splenic vein shows blood flow. The pathologic diagnosis was necrotic pancreatitis and peritonitis.

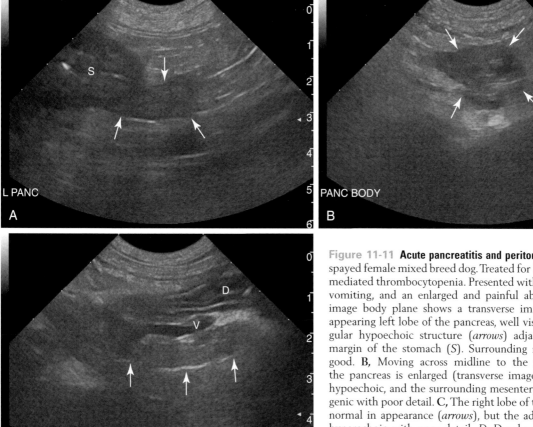

Figure 11-11 **Acute pancreatitis and peritonitis.** Seven-year-old spayed female mixed breed dog. Treated for 1 week for immune-mediated thrombocytopenia. Presented with profound lethargy, vomiting, and an enlarged and painful abdomen. A, Sagittal image body plane shows a transverse image of the normal-appearing left lobe of the pancreas, well visualized as a rectangular hypoechoic structure (*arrows*) adjacent to the caudal margin of the stomach (*S*). Surrounding mesenteric detail is good. B, Moving across midline to the right, the body of the pancreas is enlarged (transverse image, between arrows), hypoechoic, and the surrounding mesentery is now very echogenic with poor detail. C, The right lobe of the pancreas is fairly normal in appearance (*arrows*), but the adjacent mesentery is hyperechoic with poor detail. *D,* Duodenum; *V,* pancreatico-duodenal vein. Final pathologic diagnosis was suppurative acute to subacute pancreatitis and steatitis.

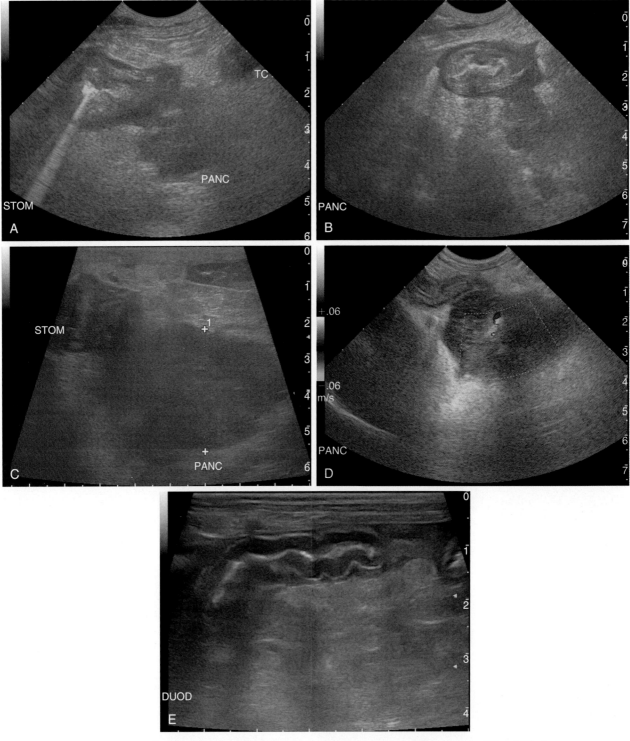

Figure 11-12 Progressive pancreatitis. Initial (**A** and **B**) and 10-day recheck images (**C** and **D**). A 5-year-old spayed female Australian terrier with vomiting of several days duration and abdominal pain. **A,** Sagittal image body plane shows the transverse image of the left lobe of the pancreas (*PANC*) is enlarged and hypoechoic with an irregular margin. The peripancreatic tissue is hyperechoic by comparison with poor detail. The caudal wall of the stomach (*STOM*) is thickened and has lost its normally layered appearance. *TC,* Transverse colon. **B,** Enlarged hypoechoic body of the pancreas. The pylorus is in the near field, with thickening of its wall adjacent to the pancreas. Note the poor regional detail. The liver is to the left. **C,** Marked progressive enlargement of the left lobe of the pancreas (between electronic cursors, 3.38 cm) in location similar to **A. D,** Color Doppler image of the body of the pancreas near the pylorus showing progressive increase in size. Poor parenchymal vascularization is present and the peripancreatic tissues are hyperechoic and have poor detail. **E,** Corrugated duodenum. The ultrasound diagnosis was severe progressive necrotizing pancreatitis. The pathologic diagnosis was necrotizing pancreatitis, chronic, multifocal to coalescent, severe.

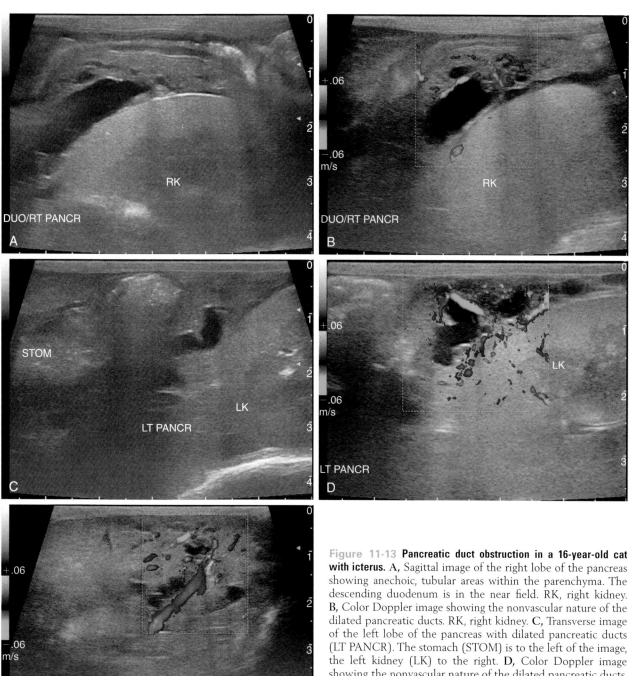

Figure 11-13 Pancreatic duct obstruction in a 16-year-old cat with icterus. A, Sagittal image of the right lobe of the pancreas showing anechoic, tubular areas within the parenchyma. The descending duodenum is in the near field. RK, right kidney. **B,** Color Doppler image showing the nonvascular nature of the dilated pancreatic ducts. RK, right kidney. **C,** Transverse image of the left lobe of the pancreas with dilated pancreatic ducts (LT PANCR). The stomach (STOM) is to the left of the image, the left kidney (LK) to the right. **D,** Color Doppler image showing the nonvascular nature of the dilated pancreatic ducts. LK, left kidney **E,** Color Doppler image of the liver showing the presence of dilated intrahepatic ducts.

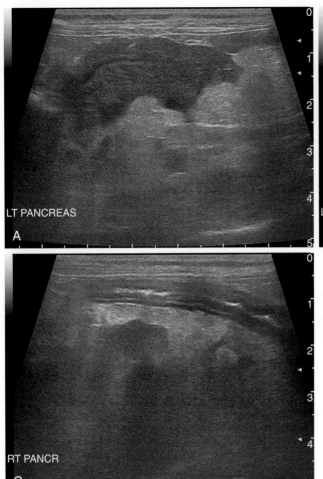

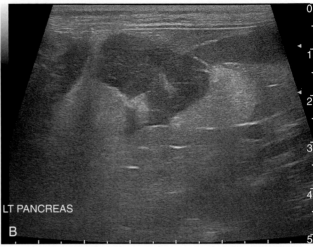

Figure 11-14 Acute pancreatitis 8-year-old neutered male cat with a 3-day history of lethargy and anorexia and prior vomiting. History of diabetes mellitus. A, A markedly enlarged, hypoechoic left pancreatic lobe was present with homogenous parenchyma and irregular margination. The pancreatic duct can be seen in the near field in this long-axis view. The peripancreatic tissue is highly hyperechoic. **B,** Transverse image of the left pancreatic lobe. Liver is to the left (cranial) and spleen is present in the near field to the right (caudal). **C,** The right lobe of the pancreas is severely enlarged, hypoechoic, and irregular in shape (central portion of image in mid to far field. The hyperechoic peripancreatic tissues are inflamed, yielding poor visualization. The duodenum in long axis is present in the near field.

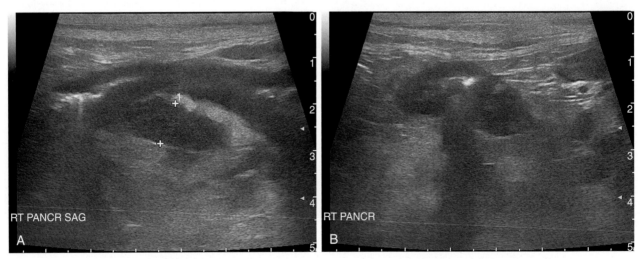

Figure 11-15 Acute pancreatitis in a 15-year-old neutered male cat with sudden anorexia. A, The right lobe of the pancreas is thick and irregular (between electronic cursors, 0.92 cm) with hypoechoic and homogeneous parenchyma in this long-axis image. The surrounding mesentery is hyperechoic and indistinct because of inflammation from the adjacent pancreas. A thickened duodenum is seen in the near field with indistinct margins and loss of normally visible wall layering. **B,** Transverse image of the right lobe of the pancreas (center of image). It is thickened, hypoechoic, and irregular in shape. The inflamed adjacent duodenum is seen in cross section to the left, with luminal gas and loss of wall layers. The tissues in the far field are indistinct because of inflammation.

visualization of the pancreatic duct or bile duct, irregular contour to the pancreas, hypoechoic parenchyma, or increased echogenicity to the surrounding mesentery, either alone or in combination, were considered consistent with feline pancreatitis.[6] Elevations in serum fPLI and pancreatic biopsy were used for confirmation. It was concluded that serum fPLI concentrations and stricter interpretation of pancreatic ultrasound findings improved the detection of pancreatitis in the cat.

On occasion, only secondary changes in the duodenum and stomach are visualized with pancreatitis. Functional ileus with fluid distention and thickening of the adjoining wall of the duodenum or stomach or free peritoneal fluid in the pancreatic region suggests pancreatitis. A corrugated small intestine associated with pancreatitis has been seen in both dogs and cats.[38] However, the final diagnosis must be confirmed in another manner because gastroenteritis, diffuse neoplastic infiltration of the stomach and bowel, septic peritonitis, and other conditions can produce secondary findings similar to pancreatitis.

Chronic Pancreatitis

Chronic pancreatitis results from recurrent episodes of pancreatitis over months or years. However, diagnosis is difficult with ultrasonography because of inconsistent pancreatic changes in both dogs and cats. A recent observational study showed an abnormal pancreas on ultrasound examination in only 56% of the patients (8 of 14).[50] Most of these dogs showed chronic low-grade gastrointestinal signs and abdominal pain; 5 dogs had exocrine pancreatic insufficiency and 5 had diabetes mellitus. Kathrani and colleagues[51] also found no difference in the ultrasound appearance of the pancreas in normal dogs and dogs with pancreatitis. It was found that canine pancreatic lipase immunoreactivity concentration in dogs with inflammatory bowel disease was associated with a negative outcome. Figure 11-16 illustrates what might be called a classic chronic pancreatitis in dogs, with mild thickening and increased echogenicity over what is normally expected. Also, note that typically the surrounding mesentery and omentum are not as echogenic and maintain clarity compared to most cases of acute pancreatitis in dogs.

In cats, it was concluded that acute necrotizing pancreatitis could not be distinguished from chronic nonsuppurative pancreatitis solely on the basis of history, physical examination findings, results of clinicopathologic testing, radiographic abnormalities, or ultrasonographic abnormalities.[46] However, findings such as decreased pancreatic size, increased or mixed echogenicity in the pancreatic region, nodularity, shadowing, or enlargement and irregularity of the pancreatic ducts may be recognized with chronic pancreatitis.[12,22,26] Healing with scarring or calcification may cause acoustic shadowing. Pancreatic duct calculi appear to be rare in small animals, and the ultrasound diagnosis has only been reported in one cat.[52] A dilated common bile duct or biliary ducts may be present if the disease has resulted in intermittent, partial, or complete common bile duct obstruction. The duodenum or stomach may be displaced because of adhesion formation. The normal symmetric, central echo complex of the duodenum or pyloric antrum may also be distorted by scarring. It is essential to use a combination of history, physical examination, laboratory data, and imaging findings to diagnose chronic pancreatitis in the dog or cat. Figure 11-17 illustrates chronic pancreatitis in a cat.

A recent report describes multisystemic mineralization of the pancreas, liver, and small intestine in a dog with *Heterobilharzia americana* infection.[53] Granulomas containing schistosome eggs were identified histologically. In a cat with a pituitary macroadenoma and enlarged adrenal glands presented for central vestibular signs, generalized toxoplasmosis was found, including tachyzoites in the pancreas, bowel, and brain.[54] Of interest, pancreatic infection was not detectable sonographically.

In conclusion, differentiating acute from chronic pancreatitis can be challenging, especially in cats. Similarly, it can be difficult to judge the clinical importance of unexpected sonographic alterations in the pancreas. Figure 11-18 demonstrates the variety of presentations that can occur with pancreatitis.

Pancreatic Cysts

Detailed ultrasonographic evaluation of pancreatic cysts has not been made in animals, although a number of case reports are available.[36,52,55-61] Differentiation of the various types of pancreatic cysts requires histologic analysis. Experience with human pancreatic cysts is presented in this section in the hope that this information may be applied to and compared with the findings in small animals.

True Cysts

In humans, simple pancreatic cysts may be unilocular or multilocular, range from microscopic to 5 cm in size, and may be associated with polycystic disease of the liver, kidney, or ovary.[62,63] The cysts do not communicate with the pancreatic duct. In contrast to inflammatory pseudocysts, true cysts are lined with a single layer of cuboidal epithelium and do not contain exudate. Little is known about the occurrence of true pancreatic cysts in small animals. However, a pedunculated, true pancreatic cyst attached to the body of the pancreas was described in a 5-year-old cat.[60] The cyst was septated, had a thickened wall, and measured approximately 4 cm in diameter. Histopathologic examination indicated that the cyst was lined with a single layer of cuboidal epithelium. In several cats and dogs, we have identified similar pancreatic cysts that did not change on serial ultrasound examinations (Figures 11-19 and 11-20). The cysts were confirmed surgically to originate from the pancreas in one cat, but the type of cyst was not determined from the biopsy. Histologic confirmation was not possible in the other cases because invasive procedures were not indicated or the animals were lost to follow-up. Most recently Branter and co-workers[61] described multiple recurrent true pancreatic cysts associated with pancreatic inflammation, atrophy, and diabetes mellitus in a cat.

Pseudocysts

In humans, pancreatic inflammatory pseudocyst formation results from acute or chronic pancreatitis.[64] It has been postulated that pseudocysts occur by continuing secretions into areas of pancreatic necrosis (Figure 11-21, *A*), with subsequent encapsulation and development of fibrotic, thickened walls[65] (Figure 11-21, *B*). The cysts contain exudate, pancreatic secretions, blood, and plasma and sometimes have posterior acoustic enhancement. The wall of the cyst is generally thicker and more irregular than the wall of true cysts, such as those found in the kidney. Solitary or multiloculated pancreatic pseudocysts have been described.[66] Biliary obstruction may occur if the common bile duct is compressed.[67] High morbidity and mortality have been associated with pseudocysts if they rupture into the peritoneal cavity before the lesion wall has matured.[68] Treatment requires anastomosis of the mature cyst to the stomach or an adjacent loop of bowel to achieve drainage and healing. Serial ultrasound examinations have shown that pseudocysts are more commonly associated with acute or chronic pancreatitis than was formerly believed, and many resolve spontaneously without complications.

Use of ultrasound in animals has enabled increased detection of similar cystlike lesions in the pancreas of the dog and cat[36,56-58] (see Figure 11-21, *B*). It remains unclear whether the

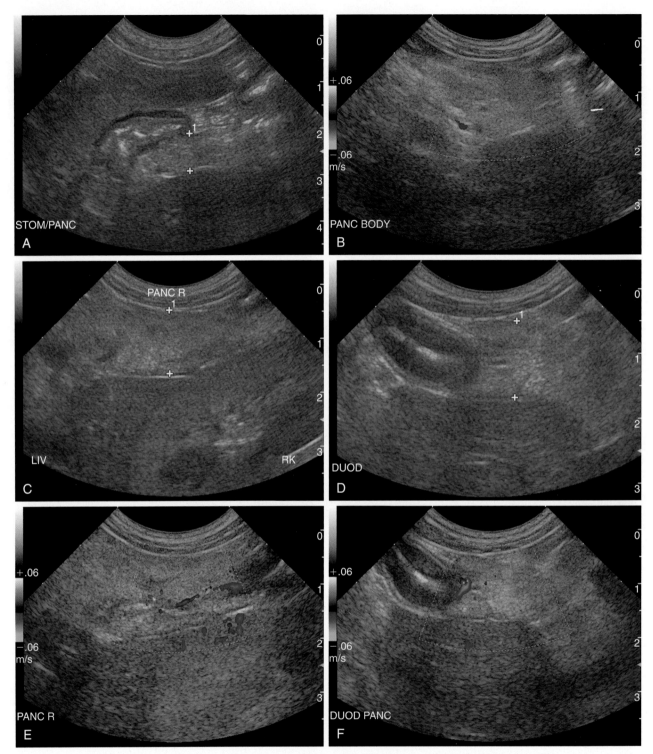

Figure 11-16 Thirteen-year-old neutered male Yorkshire terrier with chronic pancreatitis. A, In this sagittal body plane the left lobe of the pancreas is seen as a discrete hyperechoic organ in cross section (between electronic cursors, 0.81 cm). Though not considered thickened at this level, the parenchyma is abnormally hyperechoic. The stomach is to the left (cranial), and the liver is in the near field. **B,** Following the left lobe toward midline, the body of the pancreas is seen in transverse axis as an enlarged, hyperechoic and homogeneous structure. Color Doppler image shows peripheral vascularization. **C,** The right lobe of the pancreas is seen in its sagittal axis as a moderately enlarged (between electronic cursors, 1.17 cm thick) and slightly inhomogeneous structure. In the far field the liver (*left*) and right kidney (*right*) are seen. **D,** The enlarged hyperechoic right lobe of the pancreas (between electronic cursors, 1.18 cm) is seen in transverse axis with the duodenum adjacent to it (*left*). Note that there is good peripancreatic tissue detail and that the duodenal wall layers are clearly seen. **E,** Color Doppler sagittal image of the right lobe of the pancreas showing the pancreaticoduodenal vein and renal cortical blood flow. **F,** Color Doppler transverse image of the right lobe of the pancreas showing the pancreaticoduodenal vein.

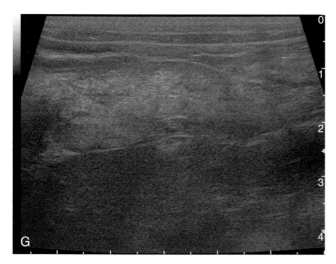

Figure 11-16, cont'd **G,** 13-MHz linear array transducer displaying in trapezoidal mode a sagittal image of the right lobe of the pancreas. The increased resolution of the higher frequency transducer clearly shows the inhomogeneous nature of the pancreatic parenchyma, which is not resolved with the lower frequency microconvex sector transducer used in images **A** to **F.** The central area of the pancreas is hyperechoic with an irregular hypoechoic periphery.

mechanism of pseudocyst formation is similar to that in humans. In most cases, the pseudocysts are associated with clinical and laboratory evidence of pancreatitis. They often disappear spontaneously within several weeks, but some may persist for extended periods and require surgical drainage. Extrahepatic biliary obstruction was reported with a pancreatic pseudocyst in a dog, but it is unclear whether the obstruction was due to recurrent pancreatitis or the pseudocyst itself.[59] Aspiration of pancreatic pseudocysts for diagnosis or treatment has been described.[57,58] The fluid was aseptic and no morbidity was associated with the aspiration procedures. Pancreatic necrosis with cavitation, pseudocysts, abscesses, and neoplasia cannot be differentiated by ultrasound evaluation alone. Pancreatic abscesses tend to be rare and must be diagnosed by positive culture results. However, pancreatic abscesses may be sterile, making their diagnosis difficult.[69] Pancreatic necrosis resolves with clinical improvement (see Figure 11-21, *A*), whereas pseudocysts tend to enlarge during this same time (see Figure 11-21, *B*). Later, pseudocysts stop enlarging and may resolve spontaneously, as previously described. Neoplasia is suspected with similar lesions that do not resolve, primarily when the animal is refractory to conservative forms of therapy (Figure 11-21, C). Figure 11-22 illustrates that pseudocysts can have a complex appearance.

Retention Cysts

Pancreatic retention cysts in humans occur from blockage of pancreatic ducts and accumulation of secretions. They tend to be smaller than either true cysts or inflammatory pseudocysts and rarely are clinically significant.[70] The contents are more likely to be anechoic with strong posterior acoustic enhancement compared with inflammatory pseudocysts. The incidence of retention cysts in small animals is unknown.

Pancreatic Bladder

Cystic dilation of the pancreatic duct, which has been called a pancreatic bladder, is a rare condition that has been described in cats.[55,71] The dilated pancreatic duct may become large enough to compress adjacent structures, such as the common

bile duct, resulting in jaundice. The cause of this condition is unknown.

Recently a case of pancreatolithiasis and pancreatic pseudobladder containing calculi was described in a cat with pancreatitis.[52] The authors preferred to use the term pancreatic pseudobladder, rather than pancreatic bladder, because the pancreas does not include a true bladder for excretory storage like the biliary or urinary system. Ultrasound examination revealed what was thought to be a bilobed or duplex gallbladder,[72,73] with one duplicate structure containing calculi. The pancreas and pancreatic duct were enlarged, and a stone was seen obstructing the pancreatic duct. At surgery a pancreatic pseudobladder containing calculi was found. The duct exiting the pseudobladder communicated with pancreatic ductal system at the point where the stone in the pancreatic duct was seen. The pseudobladder was filled with purulent material and *Escherichia coli* was cultured from its contents. Histopathology confirmed that the structure was lined by epithelial cells, ruling out a pancreatic pseudocyst. Communication with the pancreatic duct ruled out a true pancreatic cyst. Therefore the pseudobladder may have represented what has been previously termed a pancreatic bladder or an unusual complication of a pancreatic retention cyst.

Pancreatic Abscess

The sonographic appearance of pancreatic abscess in humans depends on the amount of suppurative material, the consistency of the material, and whether gas bubbles are present. The walls of an abscess are usually thick, highly echogenic, and irregular. Computed tomography is the technique of choice for diagnosis of a pancreatic abscess in humans. The presence of gas, which may interfere with ultrasound visualization, is a definitive sign of abscess on computed tomography.

Pancreatic abscess is usually a complication of pancreatitis, and definitive diagnosis requires fine-needle aspiration to obtain material for a bacterial culture and sensitivity. The clinical, radiographic, ultrasonographic, and surgical findings of pancreatic abscess in six dogs were reported.[69] In five of the six dogs, there was increased soft tissue density in the right cranial abdomen on radiography. A mass was identified in the pancreatic region in all four dogs examined with ultrasonography. Three masses were located in the proximal duodenal region, and two had hypoechoic areas consistent with fluid accumulation. The hypoechoic regions proved to be mucopurulent material at surgery. The sonographic appearance was similar to that described for intraabdominal abscesses in other locations.[74] Bacterial cultures were obtained in five dogs, and all results were negative. The investigators speculated that the abscesses may have been sterile or the culture results were affected by prior antibiotic administration.

A pericolonic mass containing chyle was described as a sequela to chronic pancreatitis in a dog.[75] The results of histopathologic evaluation after surgical removal were consistent with an abscess that had incorporated adjacent lymphatics.

These reports clearly emphasize the difficulty of differentiating pancreatic abscess (Figures 11-23 and 11-24) from acute pancreatitis, pancreatic necrosis (with or without pseudocyst formation), and pancreatic tumor. Shadowing and reverberation echoes from bacterial gas formation may assist with diagnosis. Material for cytologic or histologic analysis and bacterial culture should be obtained from ultrasound-guided aspiration or fine-needle biopsy. Surgery is indicated for diagnosis and treatment if the bacterial culture results are positive or the clinical condition does not improve quickly.

Pancreatic Neoplasia

As expected, ultrasonography is more sensitive than radiology for detecting pancreatic neoplasia.[26,32,76-79] Pancreatic

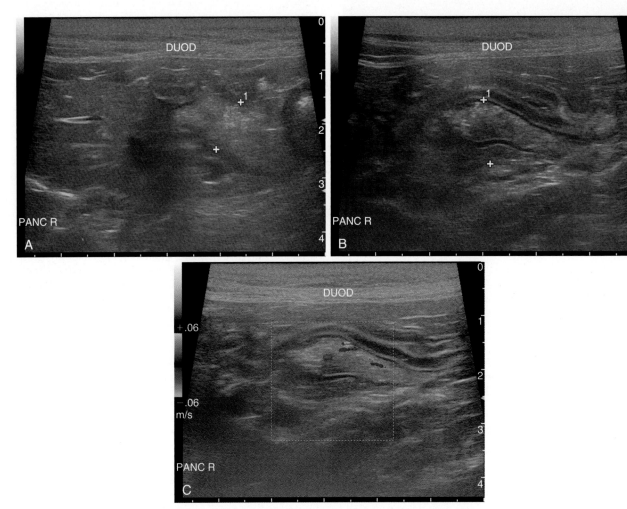

Figure 11-17 Chronic pancreatitis in a 12-year-old neutered male cat with diabetes mellitus. A, The right lobe of the pancreas is very thickened (between electronic cursors, 0.99 cm) and widened, and hyperechoic to the surrounding mesentery with a homogeneous echotexture. A thin hypoechoic rim is present. A cross section of the duodenum is central in the near field (*DUOD*); liver is present to the left, and a portion of transverse colon to the far right. The peripancreatic tissues are considered normal. **B,** Sagittal axis view of the right lobe of the pancreas (between electronic cursors, 1.19 cm). In this image plane the abnormally hyperechoic pancreatic tissue is inhomogeneous. The pancreatic duct is seen as the small, tubular, longitudinal hypoechoic structure in the central portion of the image. A sagittal section of the descending duodenum (*DUOD*) is present in the near field. **C,** Color Doppler image of the right lobe of the pancreas showing normal blood flow within the parenchyma and lack of flow in the pancreatic duct. A sagittal section of the descending duodenum (*DUOD*) is present in the near field.

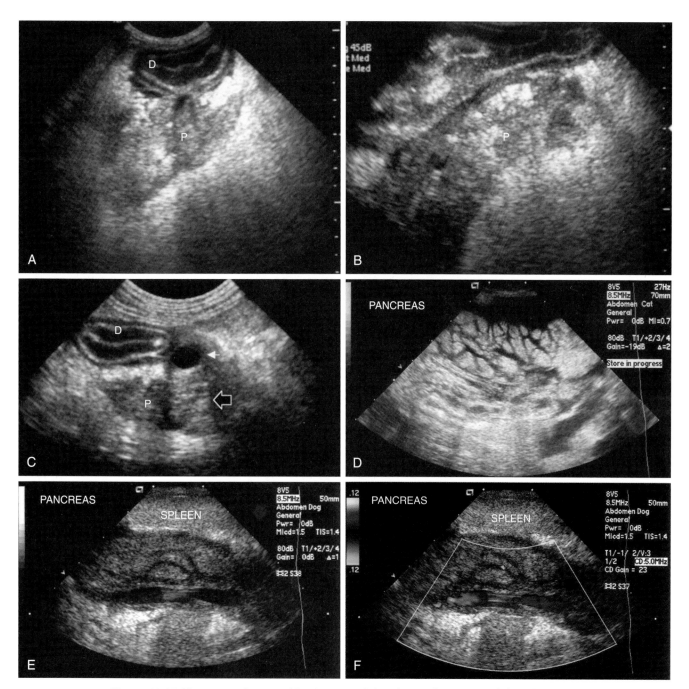

Figure 11-18 The spectra of pancreatitis. Transverse (A) and sagittal (B) views of the right cranial abdomen of a dog with pancreatitis. An enlarged, hypoechoic pancreatic mass (*P*) is seen dorsal to the duodenum (*D*). The duodenal wall is thickened, and the region around the pancreas is hyperechoic secondary to focal peritonitis. **C,** Transverse view of the right cranial abdomen of a dog with pancreatitis and icterus. An enlarged, hypoechoic pancreas (*P*) is seen dorsomedial to the duodenum (*D*). The pancreatic duct (*white arrow*) is dilated secondary to obstruction from the pancreatitis. Distal acoustic enhancement (*black arrow*) is identified dorsal to the dilated pancreatic duct. **D,** Severe pancreatic edema with ascites secondary to pancreatitis is noted in this dog. **E** and **F,** Pancreatitis with a splenic vein thrombus. **E,** A splenic vein thrombus secondary to severe, necrotizing pancreatitis is noted in this dog. The edematous pancreas is seen dorsal to the spleen with an increased echogenicity noted within the lumen of the splenic vein. **F,** On color Doppler imaging, a flow void is noted at the site of the thrombus within the vessel lumen.

Continued

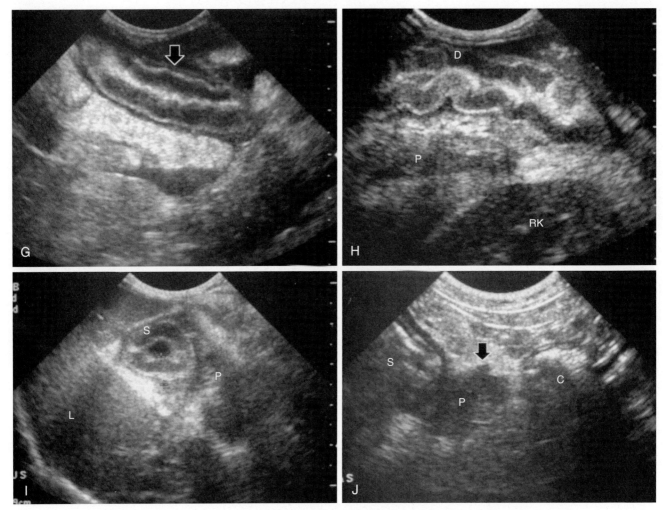

Figure 11-18, cont'd G and H, Duodenum, sagittal views, showing wall thickening and spasticity. G, The duodenal walls (*arrow*) may be thickened secondary to pancreatitis. H, The duodenum (*D*) may appear spastic and contain fluid in addition to wall thickening. In mild cases of pancreatitis, duodenal spasticity may be the only significant finding. *P,* Pancreatic mass; *RK,* right kidney. I and J, Sagittal views, mid cranial (*I*) and left cranial (*J*) abdomen of a dog with pancreatitis. I, A pancreatic mass (*P*) can be seen caudal to the stomach (*S*) in the region of the pyloric antrum. The stomach wall is thickened secondary to the inflammation. *L,* Liver. J, A pancreatic mass (*arrow*) is seen in the region of the left lobe of the pancreas (*P*). *C,* Transverse colon; *S,* stomach.

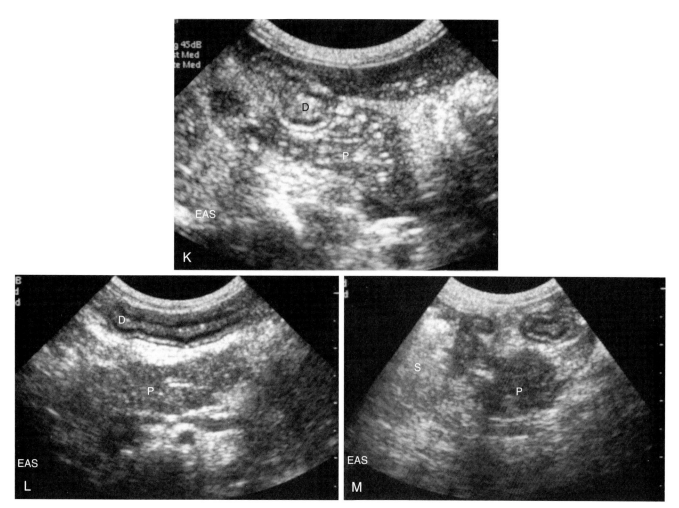

Figure 11-18, cont'd K to M, Feline pancreatitis. K and L, Transverse (K) and sagittal (L) views of the right cranial abdomen of a cat with pancreatitis. The normal feline pancreas is not easily visualized. In our experience, it is also poorly visualized in the majority of cases of feline pancreatitis. However, in this case, the right lobe of the pancreas (*P*) can be seen dorsomedial to the duodenum (*D*) in both views. M, Sagittal view, left cranial abdomen. In another cat with pancreatitis, a pancreatic mass (*P*) could be visualized in the region of the left lobe of the pancreas just caudal to the stomach (*S*). The diagnosis of feline pancreatitis remains frustrating because the majority of cases do not have easily detectable abnormalities on ultrasonography.

neoplasia usually appears as a hypoechoic nodule or mass in the pancreatic region. However, neoplasia cannot be differentiated from pancreatitis solely on the basis of the ultrasound findings, especially on a single examination. The age of the animal, history, clinical signs, and laboratory work must always be considered. Pancreatitis, when it is properly treated, tends to resolve on serial examinations, whereas neoplasia does not. Pancreatitis usually causes more localized accumulations of fluid than neoplasia does, but severe pancreatitis may produce more generalized distribution of fluid. Biliary obstruction may be present with either pancreatitis or pancreatic neoplasia. The patient should be examined for signs of lymphadenopathy and metastasis to abdominal organs or peritoneal surfaces (carcinomatosis). Pancreatic tumors are rare, which favors the diagnosis of pancreatitis. Guided fine-needle aspiration for cytologic analysis or biopsy of mass lesions may be essential in difficult cases.

Exocrine pancreatic tumors originating from acini or ductal epithelium constitute the most common tumor type; they usually affect older dogs and cats with an average age of 10 and 12 years, respectively[32,77,79,80] (Figures 11-25 to 11-28).

The Airedale terrier is said to be predisposed to pancreatic adenocarcinomas.[81] These tumors often metastasize before the appearance of clinical signs and therefore usually reach advanced stages of involvement before detection. Biliary obstruction may be present. Abdominal fluid, carcinomatosis, and metastasis to regional lymph nodes and other abdominal organs are common. Pancreatic adenomas have also been reported in cats, but no imaging findings were described.[79]

Endocrine pancreatic tumors, known as islet cell tumors, are even less common in small animals (Figures 11-29 to 11-31). Islet cell tumors include insulinomas, glucagonomas, and gastrinomas. They may be functional or nonfunctional. Islet cell tumors are often small, which makes them difficult to detect. Visualization depends on many factors including the experience of the sonographer, temperament of the animal, size of the tumor, body conformation and obesity of the patient, and the amount of bowel gas. Insulinomas are the most common of the three types of endocrine tumors in dogs.[82-85] Middle-aged, large breed dogs are more commonly affected, including Irish setters, German shepherds, golden retrievers, boxers, Labrador retrievers, and standard

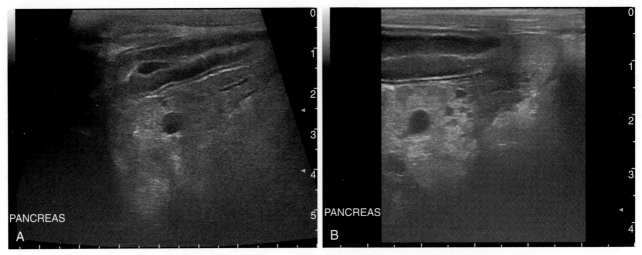

Figure 11-19 Pancreatic cysts in a 16-year-old male Yorkshire terrier with syncope and a history of hypertension and renal disease. Radiographs showed an enlarged liver, and ultrasound was requested. **A,** A cyst is present within the right lobe of the pancreas, surrounded by thickened and hyperechoic parenchyma. Normal pancreatic tissue is present to the right and the duodenum is present in the near field. A 13MHz transducer was used. **B,** Using an 18-MHz linear-array transducer, multiple cysts are now recognized within hyperechoic, thickened pancreatic tissue. The cysts were considered incidental to the presenting clinical signs and histopathology was not obtained.

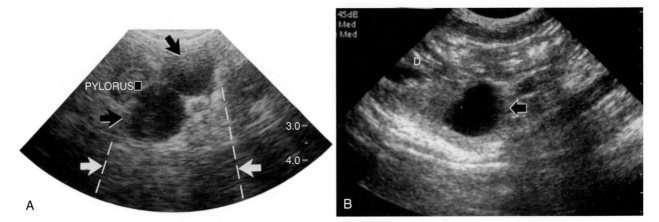

Figure 11-20 Congenital pancreatic cysts. A, This cat had cystic structures (*black arrows*) with distal acoustic enhancement (*white arrows*) in the pancreatic region caudal to the pylorus that did not change on serial ultrasound examinations during a 2-year period. They were discovered incidentally during an examination for urinary tract calculi. The cysts had all the characteristics of true pancreatic cysts, with thin and sharply demarcated walls, anechoic contents, and strong distal acoustic enhancement. This type of cyst may be congenital. Pathologic confirmation was not obtained in this case. In a similar feline case, the cysts were confirmed at surgery to arise from the pancreas, but the type of cyst (congenital versus retention) was not determined from the biopsy. Congenital cysts and retention cysts should be lined with epithelium and contain no exudate. **B,** Pancreatic cyst, transverse view, right cranial abdomen. This solitary pancreatic cyst (*arrow*) was discovered as an incidental finding in a young dog with no prior history of pancreatitis or other illness. The cyst remained unchanged on follow-up examinations during several years and was presumed to be congenital. *D,* Duodenum. These images were made using a mechanical transducer.

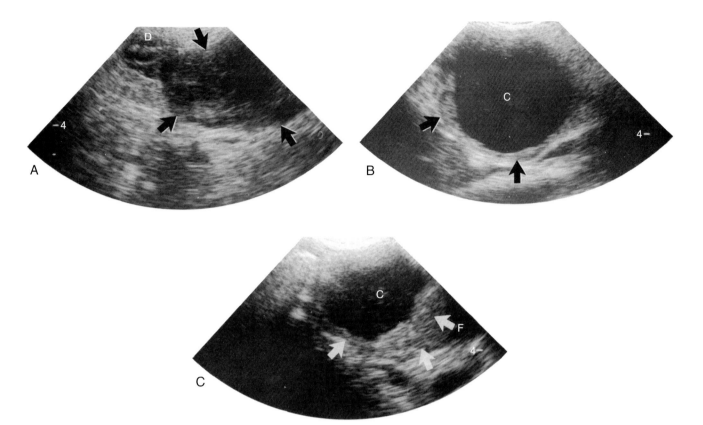

Figure 11-21 A, Pancreatic necrosis and pseudocyst formation. An irregular, cystlike lesion containing a small amount of internal debris (*arrows*) was noted in the pancreatic region of this dog with acute pancreatitis. Pancreatic necrosis and pancreatic abscess were considered in the differential diagnosis, but the dog's clinical condition improved rapidly with conservative therapy. The lesion progressively decreased in size on serial ultrasound examinations and disappeared 3 weeks later. The findings were compatible with pancreatic necrosis and resolution. *D,* Duodenum. **B,** Pancreatic pseudocyst. A cystlike lesion was noted in the pancreatic region shortly after this dog recovered from acute pancreatitis. The cyst (C) progressively enlarged and developed a thick wall (*arrows*) during the next 2 weeks. The cyst subsequently decreased in size and could not be identified 4 weeks later. The findings were compatible with a pancreatic pseudocyst and spontaneous resolution. **C,** Pancreatic adenocarcinoma. This dog had clinical signs and serum biochemistry values consistent with acute pancreatitis. However, the dog's clinical condition did not improve after 2 weeks of conservative therapy. A cystlike lesion (C) with thick walls (*arrows*), discovered in the pancreatic region on initial ultrasound examination, did not change in size during this period. Free abdominal fluid (*F*) was also present in the right cranial quadrant of the abdomen. The dog underwent surgical exploration several days later because of lack of treatment response. A pancreatic adenocarcinoma was diagnosed by biopsy. These images were made using a mechanical transducer.

poodles.[86,87] Metastasis to the regional nodes and liver was present in 60% of the reported cases in one study.[88] Insulinomas are extremely rare in cats.[89] The radiographic and sonographic findings of dogs with pancreatic neoplasia, including 13 dogs with insulinomas have been reviewed[76]; 4 of the 13 were not detected with ultrasonography and some were considered "probable pancreatic masses." When seen, insulinomas appeared hypoechoic and either spherical or lobular as described by others.[26] Hypoglycemia was present in 11 of the 13 dogs, leading to signs of weakness, ataxia, collapse, or seizures. Biliary obstruction was present in 1 dog. In another series of 14 insulinomas in 13 dogs, 5 insulinomas were correctly identified with ultrasonography.[8] Hypoglycemia was identified in all 13 dogs. Low blood glucose helps differentiate insulinomas from acute pancreatitis, in which transient hyperglycemia is commonly found. It also helps distinguish insulinomas from chronic pancreatitis, in which glucose concentration

is elevated if secondary *diabetes mellitus* develops. Biliary obstruction may be seen with either endocrine or exocrine pancreatic tumors in animals. If biliary obstruction occurs early in the course of the disease, a smaller mass will be detected. In humans, gastrinomas and glucagonomas appear as small hypoechoic, solid masses similar to islet cell tumors.[90] Gastrinomas produce excessive serum gastrin levels and Zollinger-Ellison syndrome. The abnormally high levels of gastrin result in overproduction of stomach acid with ulcers in the stomach and small intestine. A case of canine gastrinoma was reported recently where sonographic evaluation of the pancreas showed mixed echogenicity in the pancreatic region, but a discrete nodule or a mass was not identified.[91] Another report describes a canine mucinous gastric carcinoma with abdominal carcinomatosis, including a peripancreatic mass seen on ultrasound and confirmed at surgery.[92] A

Text continued on p. 465

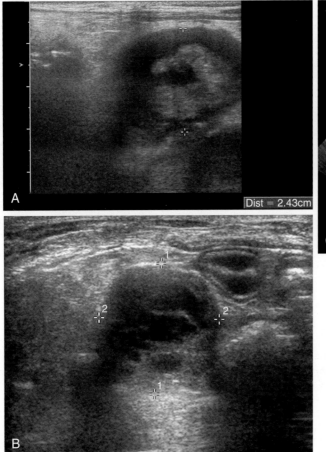

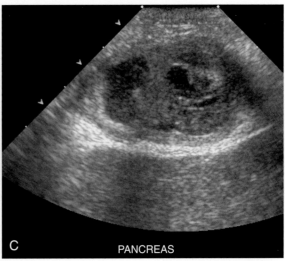

Figure 11-22 Complex pseudocysts resulting from acute pancreatitis. A, Fluid filled cystic area within the pancreas, with echogenic material centrally. The pancreas is thickened (2.43 cm between electronic cursors). **B,** Multicavitary pancreatic pseudocyst (between electronic cursors). **C,** Loculated pancreatic pseudocyst with fluid pockets peripherally and centrally. (Courtesy Dr. Marti Larson.)

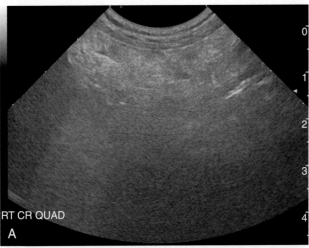

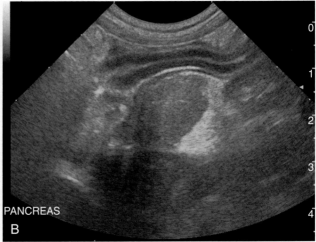

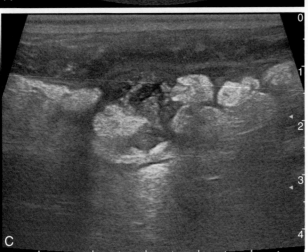

Figure 11-23 Pancreatic abscess and peritonitis in a 7-year-old neutered male Pomeranian with acute abdominal pain. A, The cranial abdomen shows extremely poor image detail. This type of image is not uncommon with severe pancreatitis and peritonitis. **B,** Displacing mesentery with transducer pressure allowed visualization of the descending duodenum and a very enlarged pancreas (center of image). **C,** Further investigation showed extremely hyperechoic islands of pancreatic tissue surrounded by hypoechoic regions with swirling motion indicative of fluid. Pathologic diagnosis was pancreatitis, necrosuppurative, hemorrhagic, severe chronic active with abscessing peritonitis.

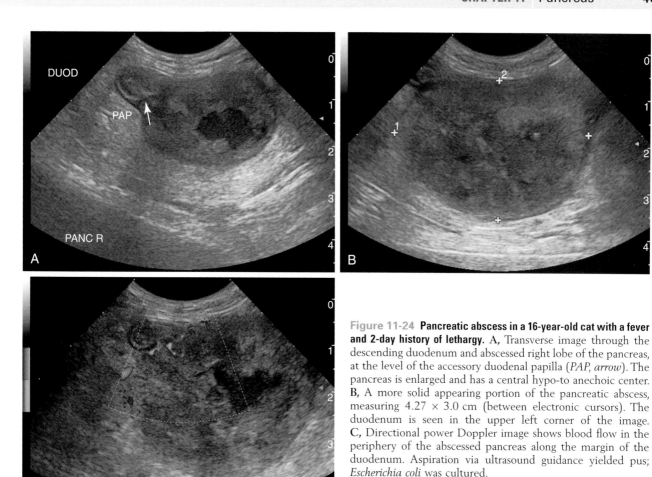

Figure 11-24 **Pancreatic abscess in a 16-year-old cat with a fever and 2-day history of lethargy. A,** Transverse image through the descending duodenum and abscessed right lobe of the pancreas, at the level of the accessory duodenal papilla (*PAP, arrow*). The pancreas is enlarged and has a central hypo-to anechoic center. **B,** A more solid appearing portion of the pancreatic abscess, measuring 4.27 × 3.0 cm (between electronic cursors). The duodenum is seen in the upper left corner of the image. **C,** Directional power Doppler image shows blood flow in the periphery of the abscessed pancreas along the margin of the duodenum. Aspiration via ultrasound guidance yielded pus; *Escherichia coli* was cultured.

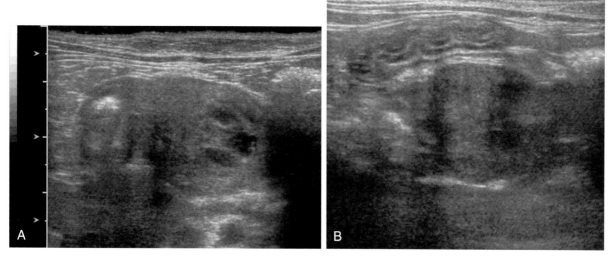

Figure 11-25 **Pancreatic adenocarcinoma.** In this example the pancreatic adenocarcinoma is nodular. **A,** Transverse image shows a small hypoechoic nodule in the right lobe of the pancreas with solid and cystic components. The duodenum is to the left. **B,** Sagittal image of the pancreatic nodule. (Courtesy Dr. Marti Larson.)

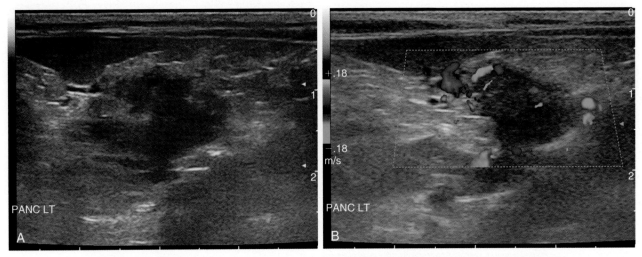

Figure 11-26 **Pancreatic adenocarcinoma in a 12-year-old neutered male cat with chronic weight loss, anorexia, and lethargy. A,** A large, lobulated mass is present within the left lobe of the pancreas. There is reduced detail to the surrounding mesentery. The spleen is present in the left near field. **B,** Color Doppler image of the pancreatic mass shows good peripancreatic blood flow but little vascularization within the mass.

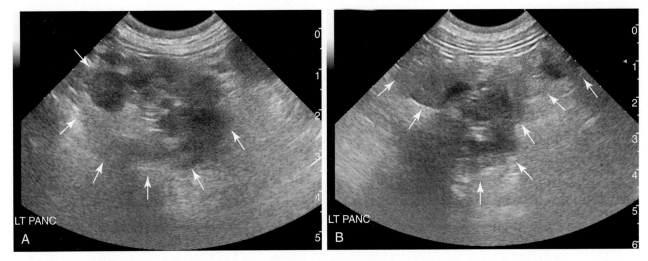

Figure 11-27 **Pancreatic carcinoma in an 11-year-old Labrador retriever mix with a month-long history of vomiting, decreased appetite, and weight loss. A,** Lobulated left pancreatic lobe mass (*arrows*) of mixed echogenicity seen in transverse-section. The surrounding tissues are poorly defined. **B,** Sagittal image of the left pancreatic lobe mass (*arrows*). There is acoustic shadowing present from part of the mass.

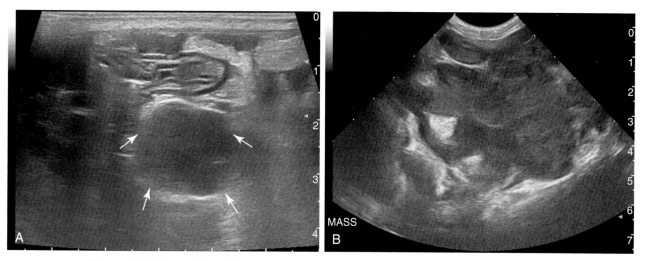

Figure 11-28 Pancreatic carcinoma is a 6-year-old standard schnauzer with a history of inappetence and undulating fever lasting longer than 1 month. A, Large hypoechoic mass seen arising from the right lobe of the pancreas. The ascending colon is in the near field, the duodenum can be seen in transverse section to the left. **B,** Further investigation using a microconvex transducer better shows the enormity of the pancreatic mass.

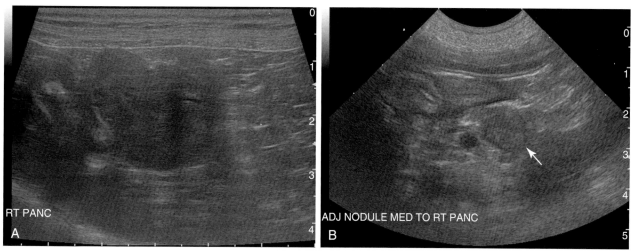

Figure 11-29 Neuroendocrine tumor (insulinoma) in a 10-year-old spayed female basset hound referred for possible insulinoma. A, A hypoechoic, homogeneous, mildly lobular nodule, approximately 2 cm in diameter, is present within the right lobe of the pancreas. The duodenum is seen in transverse axis to the left of the nodule. **B,** A small (approximately 1 cm, arrow) solid hypoechoic nodule is present in the adjacent mesentery. This was proven to be a metastatic lymph node within the mesoduodenum.

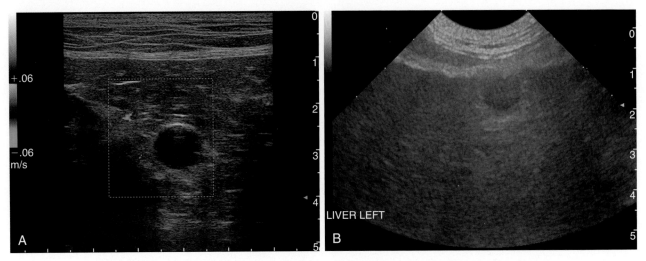

Figure 11-30 Ten-year-old neutered male German shepherd dog referred for possible insulinoma. A, An approximately 10-mm hypoechoic to anechoic nodule was identified within the left lobe of the pancreas. Color Doppler image shows no vascularization of the nodule. The left gastroepiploic artery and vein are seen in cross section to the left of the nodule, along the caudal margin of the stomach in this sagittal body image plane. B, A small hypoechoic liver nodule was identified. Fine-needle aspirates of the pancreatic nodule and the liver nodule were diagnostic for a neuroendocrine tumor.

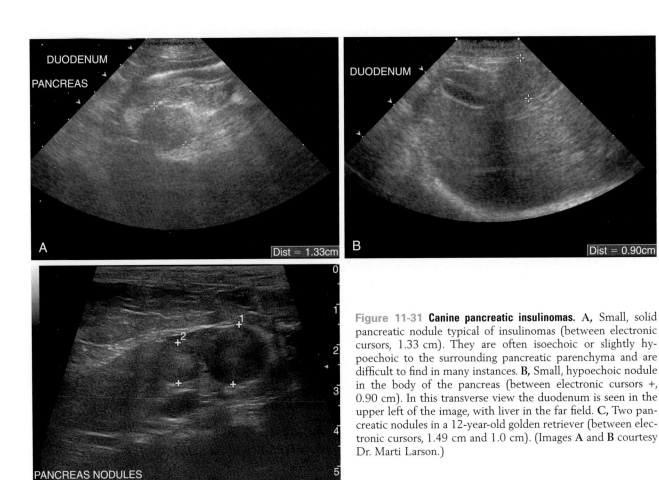

Figure 11-31 Canine pancreatic insulinomas. A, Small, solid pancreatic nodule typical of insulinomas (between electronic cursors, 1.33 cm). They are often isoechoic or slightly hypoechoic to the surrounding pancreatic parenchyma and are difficult to find in many instances. B, Small, hypoechoic nodule in the body of the pancreas (between electronic cursors +, 0.90 cm). In this transverse view the duodenum is seen in the upper left of the image, with liver in the far field. C, Two pancreatic nodules in a 12-year-old golden retriever (between electronic cursors, 1.49 cm and 1.0 cm). (Images A and B courtesy Dr. Marti Larson.)

glucagonoma is a rare pancreatic tumor secreting glucagon. Superficial necrolytic dermatitis also known as hepatocutaneous syndrome or metabolic epidermal necrosis, was reported in several dogs with glucagonomas,[83,93-95] but this syndrome has also been seen in dogs without glucagonomas.[96] A case of superficial necrolytic dermatitis in a cat was also described, but unfortunately findings related to the pancreas were not reported and plasma glucagon concentrations were not determined.[97] Cases of canine glucagonoma have been reported, but ultrasonography of the pancreas was either unremarkable or not done.[83,94,98] Endoscopic, laparoscopic, or intraoperative localization of islet cell tumors with high-frequency transducers is frequently performed in humans.[99-104] These techniques should be applicable in small animals as well.[11,13,16]

The frequency of metastasis to the pancreas in dogs and cats is unknown. In humans, pancreatic metastasis is uncommon; direct extension from the gastrointestinal tract and lymph nodes and metastasis from melanoma, breast, and lung have all been reported.[105] Direct extension from tumors of the gastrointestinal tract also occur in dogs and cats. Two dogs were reported to have secondary invasion of the pancreas by gastric carcinoma and intestinal lymphoma.[76] Squamous cell carcinoma, lymphoma, and lymphangiosarcoma were less common pancreatic tumors identified in three cats.[32] However, it was not known if these tumors were primary or secondary. A prostatic tumor metastasizing to the pancreas has also been reported in a cat.[106] Visceral hemangiosarcoma with pancreatic metastasis has also been reported.[107]

REFERENCES

1. Newell SM, Graham JP, Roberts GD, et al. Quantitative magnetic resonance imaging of the normal feline cranial abdomen. *Vet Radiol Ultrasound* 2000;**41**:27–34.
2. Probst A, Kneissl S. Computed tomographic anatomy of the canine pancreas. *Vet Radiol Ultrasound* 2001;**42**:226–30.
3. Gerhardt A, Steiner JM, Williams DA, et al. Comparison of the sensitivity of different diagnostic tests for pancreatitis in cats. *J Vet Intern Med* 2001;**15**:329–33.
4. Head LL, Daniel GB, Tobias K, et al. Evaluation of the feline pancreas using computed tomography and radiolabeled leukocytes. *Vet Radiol Ultrasound* 2003;**44**:420–8.
5. Jaeger JQ, Mattoon JS, Bateman SW, et al. Combined use of ultrasonography and contrast enhanced computed tomography to evaluate acute necrotizing pancreatitis in two dogs. *Vet Radiol Ultrasound* 2003;**44**:72–9.
6. Forman MA, Marks SL, De Cock HE, et al. Evaluation of serum feline pancreatic lipase immunoreactivity and helical computed tomography versus conventional testing for the diagnosis of feline pancreatitis. *J Vet Intern Med* 2004;**18**:807–15.
7. Head LL, Daniel GB, Becker TJ, et al. Use of computed tomography and radiolabeled leukocytes in a cat with pancreatitis. *Vet Radiol Ultrasound* 2005;**46**:263–6.
8. Robben JH, Pollak YW, Kirpensteijn J, et al. Comparison of ultrasonography, computed tomography, and single-photon emission computed tomography for the detection and localization of canine insulinoma. *J Vet Intern Med* 2005;**19**:15–22.
9. Caceres AV, Zwingenberger AL, Hardam E, et al. Helical computed tomographic angiography of the normal canine pancreas. *Vet Radiol Ultrasound* 2006;**47**:270–8.
10. Iseri T, Yamada K, Chijiwa K, et al. Dynamic computed tomography of the pancreas in normal dogs and in a dog with pancreatic insulinoma. *Vet Radiol Ultrasound* 2007;**48**:328–31.
11. Morita Y, Takiguchi M, Yasuda J, et al. Endoscopic ultrasonography of the pancreas in the dog. *Vet Radiol Ultrasound* 1998;**39**:552–6.
12. Morita Y, Takiguchi M, Yasuda J, et al. Endoscopic ultrasonographic findings of the pancreas after pancreatic duct ligation in the dog. *Vet Radiol Ultrasound* 1998;**39**:557–62.
13. Gaschen L, Kircher P, Lang J. Endoscopic ultrasound instrumentation, applications in humans, and potential veterinary applications. *Vet Radiol Ultrasound* 2003;**44**:665–80.
14. Spillmann T, Happonen I, Kahkonen T, et al. Endoscopic retrograde cholangio-pancreatography in healthy Beagles. *Vet Radiol Ultrasound* 2005;**46**:97–104.
15. Spillmann T, Schnell-Kretschmer H, Dick M, et al. Endoscopic retrograde cholangio-pancreatography in dogs with chronic gastrointestinal problems. *Vet Radiol Ultrasound* 2005;**46**:293–9.
16. Gaschen L, Kircher P, Wolfram K. Endoscopic ultrasound of the canine abdomen. *Vet Radiol Ultrasound* 2007;**48**:338–49.
17. Schweighauser A, Gaschen F, Steiner J, et al. Evaluation of endosonography as a new diagnostic tool for feline pancreatitis. *J Feline Med Surg* 2009;**11**(6):492–8.
18. Nyland TG, Mulvany MH, Strombeck DR. Ultrasonic features of experimentally induced, acute pancreatitis in the dog. *Vet Radiol* 1983;**24**:260–6.
19. Murtaugh RJ, Herring DS, Jacobs RM, et al. Pancreatic ultrasonography in dogs with experimentally induced acute pancreatitis. *Vet Radiol* 1985;**26**:27–32.
20. Etue SM, Penninck DG, Labato MA, et al. Ultrasonography of the normal feline pancreas and associated anatomic landmarks: a prospective study of 20 cats. *Vet Radiol Ultrasound* 2001;**42**:330–6.
21. Larson MM, Panciera DL, Ward DL, et al. Age-related changes in the ultrasound appearance of the normal feline pancreas. *Vet Radiol Ultrasound* 2005;**46**:238–42.
22. Hecht S, Penninck DG, Mahony OM, et al. Relationship of pancreatic duct dilation to age and clinical findings in cats. *Vet Radiol Ultrasound* 2006;**47**:287–94.
23. Hecht S, Henry G. Sonographic evaluation of the normal and abnormal pancreas. *Clin Tech Small Anim Pract* 2007;**22**:115–21.
24. Brinkman EL, Biller DS, Armbrust LJ, et al. The clinical utility of the right lateral intercostal ultrasound scan technique in dogs. *J Am Anim Hosp Assoc* 2007;**43**:179–86.
25. Brinkman-Ferguson EL, Biller DS. Ultrasound of the right lateral intercostal space. *Vet Clin N Am Small Pract* 2009;**39**(4):761–81.
26. Saunders HM. Ultrasonography of the pancreas. *Probl Vet Med* 1991;**3**:583–603.
27. Saunders HM, Pugh CR, Rhodes WH. Expanding applications of abdominal ultrasonography. *J Am Anim Hosp Assoc* 1992;**28**:369–74.
28. Lamb CR, Simpson KW. Ultrasonographic findings in cholecystokinin-induced pancreatitis in dogs. *Vet Radiol Ultrasound* 1995;**36**:139–45.
29. Baron ML, Hecht S, Matthews AR, et al. Ultrasonographic observations of secretin-induced pancreatic duct dilation in healthy cats. *Vet Radiol Ultrasound* 2010;**51**(1):86–9.
30. Rademacher N, Ohlerth S, Scharf G, et al. Contrast-enhanced power and color Doppler ultrasonography of the pancreas in healthy and diseased cats. *J Vet Intern Med* 2008;**22**(6):1310–16.

31. Newman SJ, Steiner JM, Woosley K, et al. Correlation of age and incidence of pancreatic exocrine nodular hyperplasia in the dog. *Vet Pathol* 2005;**42**:510–13.
32. Hecht S, Penninck DG, Keating JH. Imaging findings in pancreatic neoplasia and nodular hyperplasia in 19 cats. *Vet Radiol Ultrasound* 2007;**48**:45–50.
33. Lamb CR. Pancreatic edema in dogs with hypoalbuminemia or portal hypertension. *J Vet Intern Med* 1999;**13**:498–500.
34. Hess RS, Saunders HM, Van Winkle TJ, et al. Clinical, clinicopathologic, radiographic, and ultrasonographic abnormalities in dogs with fatal acute pancreatitis: 70 cases (1986-1995). *J Am Vet Med Assoc* 1998;**213**:665–70.
35. Morita Y, Takiguchi M, Yasuda J, et al. Endoscopic and transcutaneous ultrasonographic findings and grey-scale histogram analysis in dogs with caerulein-induced pancreatitis. *Vet Q* 1998;**20**:89–92.
36. Rutgers C, Herring DS, Orton EC. Pancreatic pseudocyst associated with acute pancreatitis. *J Am Anim Hosp Assoc* 1985;**21**:411–16.
37. Heng HG, Huang A, Baird DK, et al. Imaging diagnosis-spontaneous intramural canine duodenal hematoma. *Vet Radiol Ultrasound* 2010;**51**(2):178–81.
38. Moon ML, Biller DS, Armbrust LJ. Ultrasonographic appearance and etiology of corrugated small intestine. *Vet Radiol Ultrasound* 2003;**44**:199–203.
39. Lamb CR. Dilatation of the pancreatic duct: an ultrasonographic finding in acute pancreatitis. *J Small Anim Pract* 1989;**30**:410–13.
40. Weiss DJ, Gagne JM, Armstrong PJ. Relationship between inflammatory hepatic disease and inflammatory bowel disease, pancreatitis, and nephritis in cats. *J Am Vet Med Assoc* 1996;**209**:1114–16.
41. Wall M, Biller DS, Schoning P, et al. Pancreatitis in a cat demonstrating pancreatic duct dilatation ultrasonographically. *J Am Anim Hosp Assoc* 2001;**37**:49–53.
42. Kook PH, Kranjc A, Dennler M, et al. Pancreatitis associated with clomipramine administration in a dog. *J Small Anim Pract* 2009;**50**(2):95–8.
43. Saunders HM, VanWinkle TJ, Drobatz K, et al. Ultrasonographic findings in cats with clinical, gross pathologic, and histologic evidence of acute pancreatic necrosis: 20 cases (1994-2001). *J Am Vet Med Assoc* 2002;**221**:1724–30.
44. Bailey S, Benigni L, Eastwood J, et al. Comparisons between cats with normal and increased fPLI concentrations in cats diagnosed with inflammatory bowel disease. *J Small Anim Pract* 2010;**51**(9):484–9.
45. Akol KG, Washabau RJ, Saunders HM, et al. Acute pancreatitis in cats with hepatic lipidosis. *J Vet Intern Med* 1993;**7**:205–9.
46. Ferreri JA, Hardam E, Kimmel SE, et al. Clinical differentiation of acute necrotizing from chronic nonsuppurative pancreatitis in cats: 63 cases (1996-2001). *J Am Vet Med Assoc* 2003;**223**:469–74.
47. Leveille R, Biller DS, Shiroma JT. Sonographic evaluation of the common bile duct in cats. *J Vet Intern Med* 1996;**10**:296–9.
48. Mayhew PD, Holt DE, McLear RC, et al. Pathogenesis and outcome of extrahepatic biliary obstruction in cats. *J Small Anim Pract* 2002;**43**:247–53.
49. Swift NC, Marks SL, MacLachlan NJ, et al. Evaluation of serum feline trypsin-like immunoreactivity for the diagnosis of pancreatitis in cats. *J Am Vet Med Assoc* 2000;**217**:37–42.
50. Watson PJ, Archer J, Roulois AJ, et al. Observational study of 14 cases of chronic pancreatitis in dogs. *Vet Rec* 2010;**167**(25):968–76.
51. Kathrani A, Steiner JM, Suchodolski J, et al. Elevated canine pancreatic lipase immunoreactivity concentration in dogs with inflammatory bowel disease is associated with a negative outcome. *J Small Anim Pract* 2009;**50**(3):126–32.
52. Bailiff NL, Norris CR, Seguin B, et al. Pancreatolithiasis and pancreatic pseudobladder associated with pancreatitis in a cat. *J Am Anim Hosp Assoc* 2004;**40**:69–74.
53. Kvitko-White HL, Sayre RS, Corapi WV, et al. Imaging diagnosis—*Heterobilharzia americana* infection in a dog. *Vet Radiol Ultrasound* 2011;**52**(5):538–41.
54. Spada E, Proverbio D, Giudice C, et al. Pituitary-dependent hyperadrenocorticism and generalized toxoplasmosis in a cat with neurological signs. *J Feline Med Surg* 2010;**12**(8):654–8.
55. Garvey MS, Zawie DA. Feline pancreatic disease. *Vet Clin North Am Small Anim Pract* 1984;**14**:1231–46.
56. Hines BL, Salisbury SK, Jakovljevic S, et al. Pancreatic pseudocyst associated with chronic-active necrotizing pancreatitis in a cat. *J Am Anim Hosp Assoc* 1996;**32**:147–52.
57. Smith SA, Biller DS. Resolution of a pancreatic pseudocyst in a dog following percutaneous ultrasonographic-guided drainage. *J Am Anim Hosp Assoc* 1998;**34**:515–22.
58. VanEnkevort BA, O'Brien RT, Young KM. Pancreatic pseudocysts in 4 dogs and 2 cats: ultrasonographic and clinicopathologic findings. *J Vet Intern Med* 1999;**13**:309–13.
59. Marchevsky AM, Yovich JC, Wyatt KM. Pancreatic pseudocyst causing extrahepatic biliary obstruction in a dog. *Aust Vet J* 2000;**78**:99–101.
60. Coleman MG, Robson MC, Harvey C. Pancreatic cyst in a cat. *N Z Vet J* 2005;**53**:157–9.
61. Branter EM, Viviano KR. Multiple recurrent pancreatic cysts with associated pancreatic inflammation and atrophy in a cat. *J Feline Med Surg* 2010;**12**(10):822–7.
62. Cotran RS, Kumar V, Robbins SL. The pancreas. In: *Pathologic Basis of Disease*. 4th ed. Philadelphia: WB Saunders; 1989.
63. Bergin D, Ho LM, Jowell PS, et al. Simple pancreatic cysts: CT and endosonographic appearances. *AJR Am J Roentgenol* 2002;**178**:837–40.
64. Sarti DA, King W. The ultrasonic findings in inflammatory pancreatic disease. *Semin Ultrasound* 1980;**1**:178–91.
65. Lee CM, Chang-Chien CS, Lim DY, et al. Real-time ultrasonography of pancreatic pseudocyst: comparisons of infected and uninfected pseudocysts. *J Clin Ultrasound* 1988;**16**:393–7.
66. Laing FC, Gooding GAW, Brown T, et al. Atypical pseudocysts of the pancreas: an ultrasonographic evaluation. *J Clin Ultrasound* 1979;**7**:27–33.
67. Skellenger ME, Patterson D, Foley NT, et al. Cholestasis due to compression of the common bile duct by pancreatic pseudocysts. *Am J Surg* 1983;**145**:343–8.
68. Sarti DA. Rapid development and spontaneous regression of pancreatic pseudocysts documented by ultrasound. *Radiology* 1977;**125**:789–93.
69. Salisbury SK, Lantz GC, Nelson RW, et al. Pancreatic abscess in dogs: six cases (1978-1986). *J Am Vet Med Assoc* 1988;**193**:1104–8.
70. Sarti DA. Ultrasonography of the pancreas. In: Sarti DA, editor. *Diagnostic Ultrasound*. Chicago: Year Book Medical Publishers; 1987. p. 214–83.
71. Boyden EA. The problem of the pancreatic bladder. *Am J Anat* 1925;**36**:151–83.

72. Moentk J, Biller DS. Bilobed gallbladder in a cat: ultrasonographic appearance. *Vet Radiol Ultrasound* 1993;**34**: 354–6.

73. Moores AL, Gregory SP. Duplex gall bladder associated with choledocholithiasis, cholecystitis, gall bladder rupture and septic peritonitis in a cat. *J Small Anim Pract* 2007;**48**:404–9.

74. Konde LJ, Lebel JL, Park RD, et al. Sonographic application in the diagnosis of intraabdominal abscess in the dog. *Vet Radiol* 1986;**27**:151–4.

75. Barnhart MD, Smeak D. Pericolonic mass containing chyle as a presumed sequela to chronic pancreatitis in a dog. *J Am Vet Med Assoc* 1998;**212**:70–3.

76. Lamb CR, Simpson KW, Boswood A, et al. Ultrasonography of pancreatic neoplasia in the dog: a retrospective review of 16 cases. *Vet Rec* 1995;**137**:65–8.

77. Bennett PF, Hahn KA, Toal RL, et al. Ultrasonographic and cytopathological diagnosis of exocrine pancreatic carcinoma in the dog and cat. *J Am Anim Hosp Assoc* 2001;**37**:466–73.

78. Monteiro CB, O'Brien RT. A retrospective study on the sonographic findings of abdominal carcinomatosis in 14 cats. *Vet Radiol Ultrasound* 2004;**45**:559–64.

79. Seaman RL. Exocrine pancreatic neoplasia in the cat: a case series. *J Am Anim Hosp Assoc* 2004;**40**:238–45.

80. Hawks D, Peterson ME, Hawkins KL, et al. Insulinsecreting pancreatic (islet cell) carcinoma in a cat. *J Vet Intern Med* 1992;**6**:193–6.

81. Priester WA. Data from eleven United States and Canadian colleges of veterinary medicine on pancreatic carcinoma in domestic animals. *Cancer Res* 1974;**34**:1372–5.

82. Leifer CE, Peterson ME, Matus RE. Insulin-secreting tumor: diagnosis and medical and surgical management in 55 dogs. *J Am Vet Med Assoc* 1986;**188**:60–4.

83. Gross TL, O'Brien TD, Davies AP, et al. Glucagonproducing pancreatic endocrine tumors in two dogs with superficial necrolytic dermatitis. *J Am Vet Med Assoc* 1990;**197**:1619–22.

84. Simpson KW, Dykes NL. Diagnosis and treatment of gastrinoma. *Semin Vet Med Surg (Small Anim)* 1997;**12**: 274–81.

85. Fukazawa K, Kayanuma H, Kanai E, et al. Insulinoma with basal ganglion involvement detected by magnetic resonance imaging in a dog. *J Vet Med Sci* 2009;**71**(5): 689–92.

86. Priester WA. Pancreatic islet cell tumors in domestic animals. Data from 11 colleges of veterinary medicine in the United States and Canada. *J Natl Cancer Inst* 1974;**53**:227–9.

87. Caywood DD, Klausner JS, O'Leary TP, et al. Pancreatic insulin-secreting neoplasms: clinical, diagnostic and prognostic features in 73 dogs. *J Am Anim Hosp Assoc* 1988;**24**:577–84.

88. Njoku CO, Strafus AC, Dennis SM. Canine islet cell neoplasia: a review. *J Am Anim Hosp Assoc* 1972;**8**: 284–90.

89. Elie MS, Zerbe CA. Insulinoma in dogs, cats and ferrets. *Compend Contin Educ Vet* 1995;**17**:51–9.

90. Middleton WD, Kurtz AB, Hertzberg BS. *Ultrasound: the requisites.* 2nd ed. St. Louis: Mosby; 2004.

91. Fukushima R, Ichikawa K, Hirabayashi M, et al. A case of canine gastrinoma. *J Vet Med Sci* 2004;**66**:993–5.

92. de Brito Galvao JF, Pressier BM, Freeman LJ, et al. Mucinous gastric carcinoma with abdominal carcinomatosis and hypergastrinemia in a dog. *J Am Anim Hosp Assoc* 2009;**45940**:197–202.

93. Torres SM, Caywood DD, O'Brien TD, et al. Resolution of superficial necrolytic dermatitis following excision of a glucagon-secreting pancreatic neoplasm in a dog. *J Am Anim Hosp Assoc* 1997;**33**:313–19.

94. Torres S, Johnson K, McKeever P, et al. Superficial necrolytic dermatitis and a pancreatic endocrine tumour in a dog. *J Small Anim Pract* 1997;**38**:246–50.

95. Allenspach K, Arnold P, Glaus T, et al. Glucagonproducing neuroendocrine tumour associated with hypoaminoacidaemia and skin lesions. *J Small Anim Pract* 2000;**41**:402–6.

96. Nyland TG, Barthez PY, Ortega TM, et al. Hepatic ultrasonographic and pathologic findings in dogs with canine superficial necrolytic dermatitis. *Vet Radiol Ultrasound* 1996;**37**:200–4.

97. Kimmel SE, Christiansen W, Byrne KP. Clinicopathological, ultrasonographic, and histopathological findings of superficial necrolytic dermatitis with hepatopathy in a cat. *J Am Anim Hosp Assoc* 2003;**39**:23–7.

98. Bond R, McNeil PE, Evans H, et al. Metabolic epidermal necrosis in two dogs with different underlying diseases. *Vet Rec* 1995;**136**:466–71.

99. Gouya H, Vignaux O, Augui J, et al. CT, endoscopic sonography, and a combined protocol for preoperative evaluation of pancreatic insulinomas. *AJR Am J Roentgenol* 2003;**181**:987–92.

100. Jaroszewski DE, Schlinkert RT, Thompson GB, et al. Laparoscopic localization and resection of insulinomas. *Arch Surg* 2004;**139**:270–4.

101. Kaczirek K, Ba-Ssalamah A, Schima W, et al. The importance of preoperative localisation procedures in organic hyperinsulinism—experience in 67 patients. *Wien Klin Wochenschr* 2004;**116**:373–8.

102. Chung JC, Choi SH, Jo SH, et al. Localization and surgical treatment of the pancreatic insulinomas. *ANZ J Surg* 2006;**76**:1051–5.

103. Kang CM, Park SH, Kim KS, et al. Surgical experiences of functioning neuroendocrine neoplasm of the pancreas. *Yonsei Med J* 2006;**47**:833–9.

104. Sweet MP, Izumisato Y, Way LW, et al. Laparoscopic enucleation of insulinomas. *Arch Surg* 2007;**142**:1202–4, discussion 1205.

105. Hagen-Ansert SL. *Textbook of diagnostic ultrasonography.* 6th ed. St. Louis: Mosby Elsevier; 2006.

106. Hubbard BS, Vulgamott JC, Liska WD. Prostatic adenocarcinoma in a cat. *J Am Vet Med Assoc* 1990;**197**: 1493–4.

107. Culp WT, Drobatz KJ, Glassman MM, et al. Feline visceral hemangiosarcoma. *J Vet Intern Med* 2008;**22**(1): 148–52.

CHAPTER 12
Gastrointestinal Tract

Thomas G. Nyland • Dana A. Neelis • John S. Mattoon

Ultrasound examination of the gastrointestinal tract can provide important diagnostic information despite the potential limitations imposed by bowel gas. Although ultrasonography may be performed as the initial imaging procedure in cases of suspected gastrointestinal disease, obtaining survey radiographs before the ultrasound study is recommended to assess the amount, location, and pattern of intestinal gas and fluid. Survey radiographs help guide the ultrasound study and assist in further investigations of any radiographic abnormalities detected, such as gastric distention or bowel dilation. Ultrasound and radiography provide complementary information. As a result, the clinician may then decide to perform additional diagnostic procedures such as a gastrointestinal contrast study, endoscopy, or an exploratory laparotomy. Ultrasonography may not always provide a definitive diagnosis or reliably distinguish between neoplastic and nonneoplastic conditions. However, ultrasound-guided aspirations and biopsies are easily performed and will help establish a cytologic or histologic diagnosis.

EXAMINATION TECHNIQUE

If possible, the patient should fast for 6 to 12 hours before the ultrasound examination to reduce the amount of food and gas in the gastrointestinal tract. However, this may not be possible in busy clinical situations. Sedation is usually not required. If sedation is necessary, drugs that do not alter gastrointestinal motility, such as acepromazine, should be used. The ventral abdominal hair is clipped and acoustic gel is applied to the skin before the ultrasonographic procedure. A 7.5-MHz transducer can be used for the majority of the examination in dogs, but a 10-MHz or higher transducer is preferred for cats. The latter is also used to evaluate bowel wall layers in both species. In some larger dogs, a 5-MHz transducer may be required to penetrate to the area of interest.

Animals are routinely scanned in dorsal recumbency, although left and right lateral recumbency and other positions are also used as needed to shift gas and fluid in the gastrointestinal tract. For example, the pyloric region of the stomach may be imaged better in right lateral recumbency because gastric fluid accumulates in the pyloric region, whereas gas migrates to the nondependent portions of the stomach. The standing position may also facilitate visualization of the ventral pylorus and body of the stomach. A flexible approach is required depending on the conformation of the animal and the nature of the gastric contents.

Systematic transverse and longitudinal views of the gastrointestinal tract are needed for a complete examination. The axis of the view is defined by the luminal axis of the segment. Thus, a transverse view of the stomach would actually be taken in a sagittal or parasagittal plane through the cranial abdomen. A longitudinal view of the stomach would be taken in a transverse plane through the cranial abdomen. A longitudinal view of the bowel would be parallel to the lumen, and a transverse view would be obtained at right angles to the lumen.

The stomach is initially scanned in a transverse view (transverse axis of stomach, sagittal body plane). It is easily recognized by its location just caudal to the liver and presence of rugae (depending on degree of distension), and peristaltic contractions (Figure 12-1; see also Figure 4-20). The transducer is moved from the fundic portion of the stomach in the left cranial abdomen to the pyloric portion on the right, while including as much of the stomach as possible in the field of view. The fundus on the left is the lateral-most portion of the stomach (Figure 12-1, *A*), whereas the gastric body is more medial (Figure 12-1, *B* and *C*). The greater and less curvatures of the stomach and ventral stomach wall are readily seen. The left lobe of the pancreas lies dorsocaudal to the stomach in this region. The antrum (Figure 12-1, *D*) and pyloric portions of the stomach are seen by moving the transducer to the right of midline. The transducer must be rotated clockwise and moved cranially to follow and maintain a transverse view of the antrum and pylorus. The pyloric sphincter is recognized by its thick, muscular wall and narrow lumen. Gastric fluid can be moved to the pyloric region by tilting the sternum to the right to obtain a better view of the pylorus. In some cases, a right intercostal approach may be required to visualize the pylorus and proximal duodenum in deep-chested dogs. Longitudinal views of the fundus, body, antrum, and pylorus may be taken as needed to complete the study. In the cat, the stomach crosses the abdomen more obliquely, and the pylorus lies closer to midline than in the dog (Figure 12-2; see also Figure 4-19). Therefore a true longitudinal view of the stomach in a cat requires the transducer to be oriented more obliquely than in the dog.

The progression from pylorus to duodenum is seen as a transition from the muscular pylorus to the layered wall appearance of the duodenum. The transducer must now be rotated counterclockwise compared with transverse views of the stomach to maintain a transverse view through the proximal descending duodenum (see Figure 4-21 and accompanying video). The duodenum is followed caudally along the right body wall, ventral or ventrolateral to the right kidney. The right lobe of the pancreas is medial or dorsomedial to the descending duodenum. The exact position of the duodenum and pancreas relative to the right kidney depends on transducer pressure. In the cat, the pylorus and descending duodenum are closer to midline, as described previously.

The remainder of the small bowel is evaluated by slow, systematic sweeps through the abdomen in transverse and

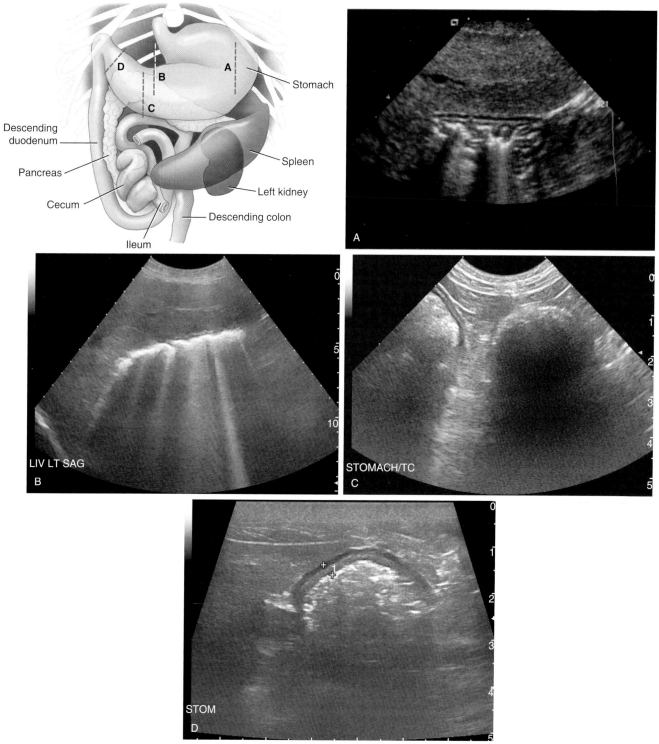

Figure 12-1 **Illustration of dog stomach and its relationship to surrounding organs.** The labels *A, B, C,* and *D* in this illustration correspond to the locations where ultrasound images in parts **A** to **D** were obtained. **A,** Transverse view through the fundus of the stomach. The near field wall is denoted by the electronic cursors (0.29 cm). A portion of the liver is seen to the left (cranial) in the image. A large amount of very echogenic reverberation artifact is present from intraluminal gas. Intraluminal gas inhibits visualization of the gastric lumen, potentially hiding gastric wall disease or intraluminal foreign bodies. **B,** Transverse view through the body of the stomach. The liver is seen ventral and cranial to the stomach. Strong reverberation artifact and comet tails from stomach gas prevents visualization of the gastric lumen. The wall is poorly defined in this example. **C,** Transverse images through the body of the stomach and transverse colon. This is a good starting point to attempt visualization of the left lobe of the pancreas, located dorsal to and between the greater curvature of the stomach and the transverse colon. In cases where the stomach and transverse colon contact each other, the left pancreatic lobe cannot be seen. **D** Transverse image through the pyloric antrum. The liver is in the near field.

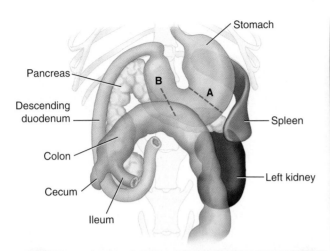

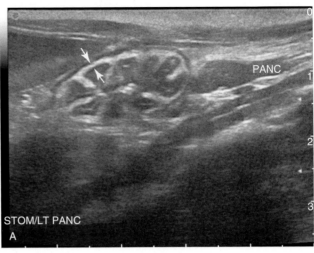

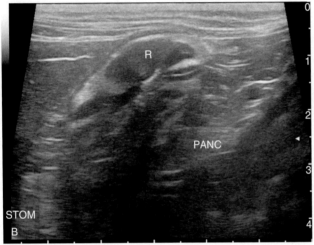

Figure 12-2 **Illustration of cat stomach and its relationship to surrounding organs.** The labels *A* and *B* on the stomach correspond to the locations where ultrasound images in parts **A** and **B** were obtained. **A,** Ultrasound beam transversely oriented to the body of an empty stomach. Note the thick hyperechoic submucosa layer commonly seen because of fat deposition (between arrows), which differs from dogs. Hypoechoic mucosal folds represent rugae. A portion of the left lobe of the pancreas is seen to the right of the stomach (*PANC*). **B,** A more longitudinal view through the body of the stomach shows an elongated rugal fold (*R*) with the appearance of gastric wall thickening. A small portion of the pancreas can be seen (*PANC*).

sagittal planes. A good method is to scan the abdomen from cranial to caudal in the transverse body plane in three successive sweeps. The first sweep is down the midline, whereas the other two sweeps overlap the first sweep to the right and left of midline. Successive overlapping sweeps in the sagittal body plane are then taken from right to left in the cranial abdomen, mid abdomen, and caudal abdomen. Variable transducer pressure should be applied throughout the sweeps to visualize the entire bowel and mesentery.

The colon is identified by its consistent location and the presence of shadowing and reverberation artifacts caused by intraluminal fecal material and gas. It is easiest for beginning sonographers to trace the colon from caudal to cranial. The distinctive crescent shaped colonic gas shadow is first located dorsal to the bladder in the transverse view. The transducer is then moved cranially to follow the descending colon to the level of the transverse colon in the left abdomen. The transducer is then rotated 90 degrees to follow the transverse colon across midline in a transverse view. Finally, the transducer is again rotated 90 degrees to obtain a transverse view of the ascending colon and trace it caudally to the cecum. The more experienced sonographer can identify the different portions of the colon without the need to trace its entire length.

Endoscopic ultrasonography has been introduced to veterinary medicine, and the potential uses of endosonography in veterinary medicine have been reviewed.[1] High-frequency transducers can be placed in the bowel lumen to better delineate mucosal abnormalities and bowel wall layers, and to

increase visibility of surrounding structures adjacent to the bowel, such as regional lymph nodes. This technique has been used to image the stomach wall, cranial duodenal flexure, and structures immediately adjacent to the stomach in normal dogs.[2] Better visualization of the gastric wall layers has the potential to provide increased accuracy for staging neoplastic lesions.[3] Endosonography has also been used to evaluate alimentary lymphoma in a dog[4] and to image the pancreas of normal dogs and dogs with experimentally induced pancreatic duct obstruction.[5,6] Endoscopic ultrasonography of the pancreas may prove useful to evaluate pancreatitis, pancreatic cysts, pancreatic abscesses, and small pancreatic tumors such as insulinomas and gastrinomas.

In humans, endoscopic ultrasonography of the colon has been used to evaluate colorectal cancer, inflammatory bowel disease, ulcerative colitis, and Crohn disease.[7-12] Endorectal sonography and endovaginal sonography have been used to stage rectal carcinoma, and anal endosonography has been used to assess fecal incontinence and perianal inflammatory disease.[13]

NORMAL ULTRASOUND APPEARANCE

Stomach

The size of a normal stomach can vary significantly depending on its contents. Peristaltic contractions average about five per minute.[14,15] Normal gastric wall thickness in the dog is approximately 3 to 5 mm depending on degree of distention (Figure 12-3),[15] with a slightly smaller thickness of 2.2 to 3.7 mm reported in beagle puppies up to 12 weeks of age.[16] The rugal folds of the stomach are commonly visualized, especially when the stomach is empty. The rugal folds of the cat are often very prominent and increased in echogenicity, associated with the layer of fat found in the submucosa (see Figure 12-2).[17] In the cat, interrugal thickness has been reported as approximately 2 mm,[18,19] and rugal fold thickness as 4.4 mm.[18] Gastric wall thickness is measured from the hyperechoic mucosal surface to the outer hyperechoic serosal layer of the stomach. Wall thickness measurements should always be interpreted in the context of stomach distention. We have been fooled on multiple occasions by an apparently thickened stomach wall only to recheck it later in the day and determine that it is completely normal.

Small Intestine and Colon

The intestinal tract should be assessed for uniformity in diameter, wall thickness, discrete wall layers, luminal contents, and peristalsis. The small intestine normally averages one to three peristaltic contractions per minute.[15]

Duodenal thickness can measure up to 5 mm in the dog, which is greater than the remainder of the canine small bowel[16,20] (Figures 12-4 and 12-5). The duodenal papilla can sometimes be identified with a high-resolution transducer (see Figure 12-5). In the cat, duodenal thickness is also greater than the rest of the bowel, measuring approximately 2 to 4 mm (see Figure 12-7, C).[18,19,21] The duodenal papilla in the cat varies from 2.9 to 5.5 mm in width and has a maximum thickness of 4 mm on the transverse view.[21] Occasionally mucosal indentations corresponding to Peyer patches are also seen on the antimesenteric border of the descending duodenum.

The intestinal wall is 2 to 3 mm thick in both the dog and cat.[15,16,18,19]

The ileum of cats is slightly thicker than the rest of the feline intestinal tract (see Figure 12-6). It ranges from 2.5 to 3.2 mm in thickness and has a distinctive "wagon wheel" appearance in transverse view.[19] A mucosal surface is not usually seen in the feline ileum, perhaps because its narrow,

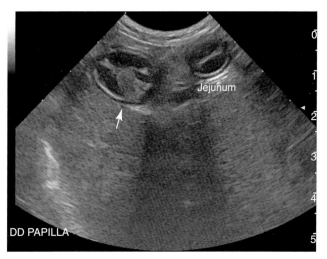

Figure 12-5 **Normal dog duodenal papilla.** The duodenal papilla is seen as a hyperechoic area within the proximal duodenal mucosa (*arrow*) is this transverse image. Note that the adjacent segment of jejunum (*Jejunum*) is smaller in diameter than the duodenum. This is very consistent and easily observable in dogs, helpful in differentiating duodenum from jejunum. Though also true for cats, the differences in thickness are less pronounced and therefore less noticeable.

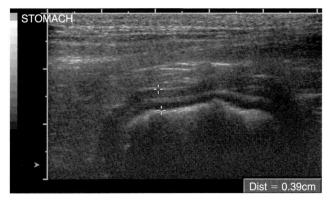

Figure 12-3 **Normal dog stomach wall.** Normal layering of the stomach wall is easily seen in this example. The layers visible are the same as those for the small intestine (see Figure 12-8). The stomach wall is 0.39 cm thick (between electronic cursors).

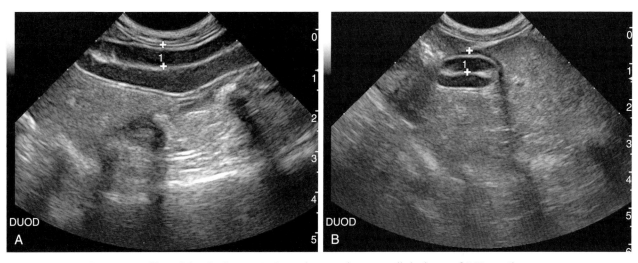

Figure 12-4 **Normal dog duodenum. A,** Sagittal image shows a wall thickness of 0.53 cm (between electronic cursors). **B,** Transverse image of the same dog shows the wall thickness of 0.60 cm (between electronic cursors).

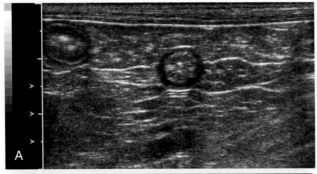

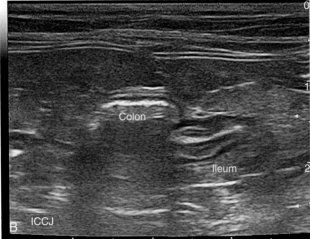

Figure 12-6 **Ileum. A,** Transverse image showing normal segment of jejunum (*far left*) compared to the stellate or "wagon wheel" appearance of the ileum (*center*) in a dog. **B,** Longitudinal image of the ileum as it enters the ileocecocolic junction in a cat.

sphincter-like lumen may limit the accumulation of mucus and gas.[19] Figure 12-6 shows examples of the dog and cat ileum.

The colonic wall is usually not as thick as it is in the small intestine, and peristaltic contractions are not normally detected (Figure 12-7). Colonic wall thickness is 1 to 2 mm in dogs and ranges from 1.5 to 2.0 mm in cats.[16,18,19] The thinner wall of the colon helps distinguish it from the small intestine in some instances.

Normal Wall Layers
The walls of the gastrointestinal tract have a five-layered appearance with alternating hyperechoic and hypoechoic layers from the lumen outwards (Figure 12-8). These layers correspond to the mucosal surface, mucosa, submucosa, muscularis, and serosa.[15,22] The mucosal and muscular layers are hypoechoic, whereas the other layers are hyperechoic. A high-resolution 7.5- to 10.0-MHz transducer is best for visualizing the wall layers clearly. When assessing wall thickness, the near wall is usually measured to avoid interference from luminal gas.

ABNORMALITIES OF THE STOMACH

Dilation
An enlarged, fluid- or gas-filled stomach is found with dilation. Fluid dilation of the stomach can be caused by a recent meal, gastric atony, or pyloric outflow obstruction. A gas-dilated stomach may occur secondary to aerophagia, gastric dilatation,

or gastric volvulus. If gastric volvulus is suspected, ultrasonography is not indicated and emergency procedures to decompress the stomach are recommended. The relevance of gastric dilation must be considered in light of the history, clinical findings, laboratory work, and other imaging procedures. Positional studies may be useful to shift fluid and gas so that all regions of the stomach can be evaluated.

Fluid dilation of the stomach is recognized by a large fluid-filled stomach (Figure 12-9). The fluid contents may be anechoic or somewhat hyperechoic depending on the mixture of fluid, ingesta, and gas. Foreign material may be noted within the gastric lumen. The stomach wall may appear thinner than normal and gastric rugal folds will be less prominent or absent because the stomach is distended.

A gas-dilated stomach is recognized by a large hyperechoic interface in the near field with gas reverberation artifacts (Figure 12-10). Only the near field stomach wall can be evaluated, and positional studies are of limited value because of the large amount of intraluminal gas.

The presence of gastric dilation requires a search for the etiology. Primary or secondary gastric dysfunction should be suspected if gastric contractions are reduced in number or intensity. For example, reduced motility may occur secondary to sedation or other medications, neuromuscular disorders, gastric or duodenal ulceration, pancreatitis, or peritonitis. Reduced motility of the stomach also may be observed in cases of chronic pyloric outflow obstruction. Gastric fluid should be used as a window to search for foreign bodies and wall thickening. The pylorus should be observed for passage of gastric contents into the duodenum. In most cases survey radiographs are also indicated, followed by an upper gastrointestinal contrast study or endoscopy to confirm the ultrasound findings.

Pyloric Obstruction
Pyloric stenosis, foreign bodies, inflammatory disease, and neoplasia may cause gastric outflow obstruction. Chronic vomiting is a consistent clinical finding. A large, fluid-filled stomach is identified unless there is a partial obstruction or the animal has recently vomited. Normal to increased peristaltic contractions are usually evident, but reduced motility may be observed with prolonged obstruction.

Congenital hypertrophic pyloric stenosis (HPS) is more common in dogs than in cats and is usually diagnosed by radiographic contrast studies. However, circumferential thickening of the pylorus, especially the muscular layer, and lack of passage of gastric contents through the pyloric canal, may be observed ultrasonographically (Figure 12-11). There are no reports describing the ultrasonographic diagnosis of HPS based on specific ultrasound criteria, but gastric wall thickness greater than 6 to 7 mm and a muscular layer thickness greater than 4 mm is generally considered pathologic.[15]

Chronic hypertrophic pyloric gastropathy (CHPG) is another disorder that has been reported to cause muscular or mucosal hypertrophy of the pylorus and may appear similar to HPS[23-26] (Figure 12-12). CHPG tends to occur in middle-aged to older small purebred dogs; twice as many males as females are affected.[23,24] Pyloric obstruction is a consistent finding with this disease. In six dogs with CHPG evaluated ultrasonographically, pyloric wall thickness ranged from 9.0 to 15.3 mm, and the thickness of the muscular layer ranged from 3.0 to 5.4 mm.[26]

Pyloric outflow obstruction may also occur from inflammatory or neoplastic mass lesions. The appearance of these disorders varies with duration and extent of the pathologic process, but wall thickening is a characteristic feature. These conditions will be discussed later with diseases that cause wall thickening.

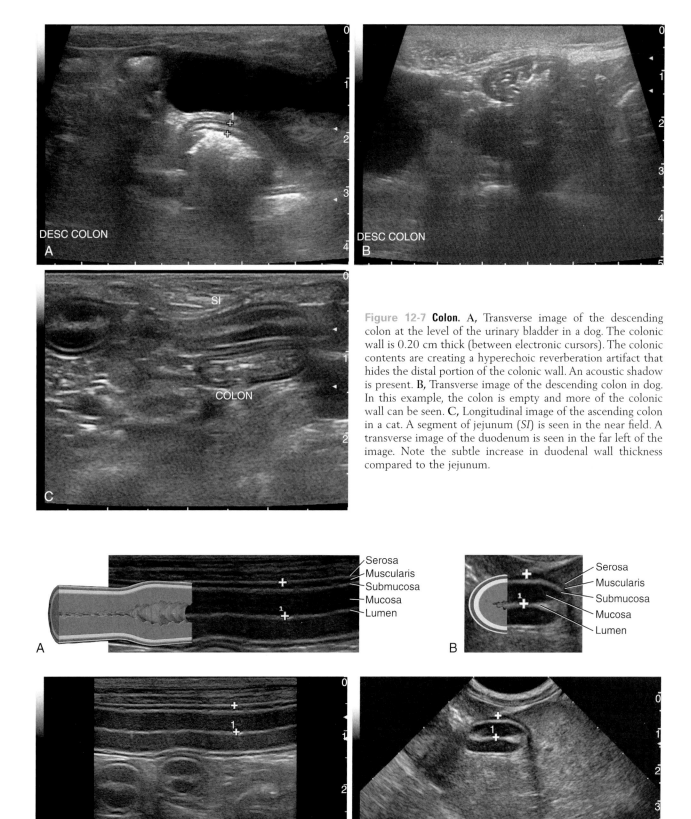

Figure 12-7 Colon. A, Transverse image of the descending colon at the level of the urinary bladder in a dog. The colonic wall is 0.20 cm thick (between electronic cursors). The colonic contents are creating a hyperechoic reverberation artifact that hides the distal portion of the colonic wall. An acoustic shadow is present. **B,** Transverse image of the descending colon in dog. In this example, the colon is empty and more of the colonic wall can be seen. **C,** Longitudinal image of the ascending colon in a cat. A segment of jejunum (*SI*) is seen in the near field. A transverse image of the duodenum is seen in the far left of the image. Note the subtle increase in duodenal wall thickness compared to the jejunum.

Figure 12-8 Intestinal layers. A, Illustration showing the layers of the small intestine in sagittal section. **B,** Illustration showing the layers of the small intestine in transverse section. **C,** Ultrasound image showing the layers of the small intestine (sagittal duodenum, 0.49 cm between electronic cursors). Two transverse sections of small intestine are seen deep to the duodenum. **D,** Transverse ultrasound image of the duodenum (between electronic cursors, 0.60 cm).

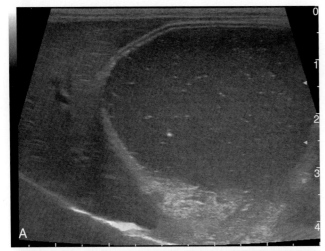

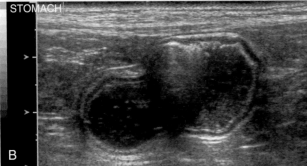

Figure 12-9 Gastric dilation. A, Severe gastric dilation in a cat with alimentary lymphoma (small intestine) and a linear duodenal foreign body. The stomach contents are echogenic but are allowing through transmission. Note the thin gastric wall. More echogenic gastric content has settled into the dependent portion of the stomach. **B,** Less severe gastric distension in a cat with nearly anechoic fluid.

Gastric Foreign Bodies

Gastric foreign bodies are usually diagnosed on survey radiographs or upper gastrointestinal contrast studies. Vomiting will occur if gastric outflow obstruction is present. Foreign bodies may also be seen with ultrasonography if they have a hyperechoic interface or intense shadowing; they may also be outlined by gastric fluid.[22,27,28] If there is partial or complete pyloric obstruction, gastric fluid will help outline the foreign body. Balls or ball fragments, rocks, string, cloth, plastic toys, hairballs, fruit pits, and corncobs have been identified. The specific pattern observed depends on the nature of the foreign body. Corncobs may be recognized by their characteristic

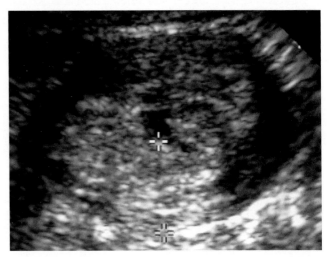

Figure 12-11 Transverse ultrasound image of a thickened pyloric canal in a 10-week-old bull terrier with persistent vomiting. There is evidence of circumferential thickening of the wall, with a thickness of 0.83 cm (between electronic cursors). This dog had congenital hypertrophic pyloric stenosis confirmed surgically.

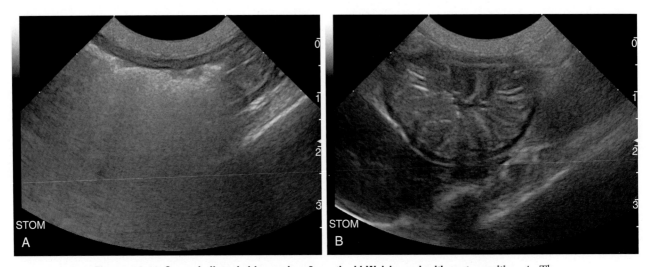

Figure 12-10 Stomach distended by gas in a 3-month-old Welsh corgi with acute vomiting. A, The stomach is distended by gas, with reverberation artifact obscuring the view of the majority of the gastric wall and the entire lumen. **B,** Reevaluation after a vomiting episode now shows an empty stomach.

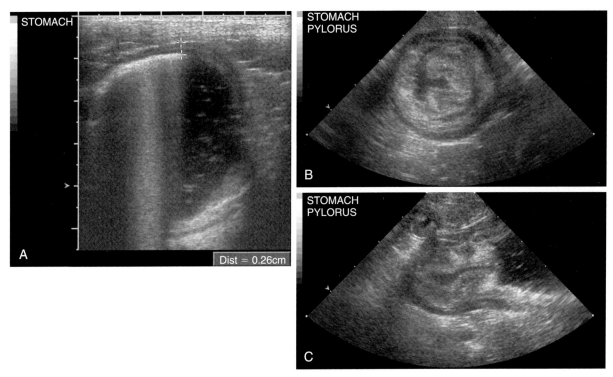

Figure 12-12 Chronic hypertrophic pyloric gastropathy in a dog with chronic vomiting. A, Distended stomach is a clue to search for an underlying anatomic cause of vomiting. Gas is seen in a portion of the stomach, creating reverberation artifact, whereas adjacent fluid allows the stomach lumen to be seen. The gastric wall has a normal appearance and thickness (0.26 cm between electronic cursors). **B,** Transverse image of the thickened, hyperechoic pylorus. **C,** Sagittal image of the thickened pylorus with a fluid-filled pyloric antrum seen to the right.

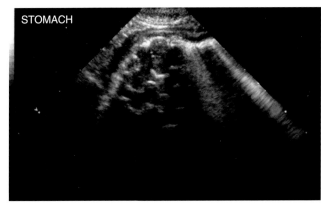

Figure 12-13 Corncob gastric foreign body. The multicavitary nature created by the corn kernel cavities is evident as small curved hyperechoic gas pockets. The corncob moved freely within the stomach as the patient's position was changed.

appearance (Figure 12-13). Dense balls, rocks, or fruit pits tend to produce hyperechoic curvilinear lines with strong acoustic shadowing (Figure 12-14A and 12-15). With soft rubber balls, the sound may penetrate and the entire ball may be seen (see Figure 12-14, B). An anechoic center may be seen if a hollow ball is punctured during ingestion or the ball has a fluid-filled center that transmits sound. Fragments of balls or plastic toys tend to produce irregular echogenic borders with shadowing. Sticks or metallic sewing needles produce straight hyperechoic lines that shadow.[27,29] Perforation of the stomach with evidence of peritonitis may occur.[29] Cloth

foreign bodies or string may produce an echogenic line within the stomach that extends into the duodenum and small intestine.[28,30] Plication of the bowel may also be seen with linear foreign bodies.[30] Hairballs are most common in cats, but also may be found in dogs. They usually produce masses of mixed echogenicity with variable shadowing depending on the hairball's density and size. The hairball may be cylindrical or occupy the entire gastric lumen, simulating a gastric mass. Fortunately many foreign bodies are radiopaque and can be confirmed on survey radiographs. Radiolucent foreign bodies may require an upper gastrointestinal contrast study to make a definitive diagnosis.

Gastric Wall Thickening

Gastric wall thickening is commonly found with inflammatory disease or neoplasia. The distribution, symmetry, and extent of wall thickening and the appearance of wall layers can help differentiate nonmalignant diseases from neoplasia. Nonmalignant disease tends to produce diffuse, mild to moderate wall thickening with preservation of the wall layers. Neoplastic lesions characteristically cause extensive focal thickening or mass lesions with disruption or loss of the wall layers.[28,31,32] However, significant overlap exists between inflammatory and neoplastic disease,[33] and the history, clinical signs, and laboratory work must be considered to formulate a differential diagnosis. An ultrasound-guided aspiration or biopsy is almost always required to make a final diagnosis.

Diffuse Wall Thickening

The differential diagnosis for gastric disease is extensive.[34] As mentioned previously, nonmalignant disease typically produces diffuse, uniform wall thickening with preservation of

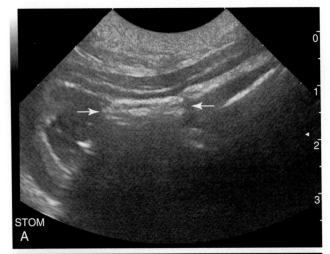

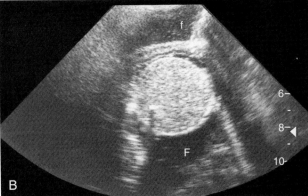

the wall layers. Generalized enlargement of the rugal folds may be seen. Various types of gastritis commonly produce these findings.

In severe cases of nonmalignant disease or with long-standing involvement, there may be greater wall thickening with disruption or loss of the wall layers. Motility of the stomach may be impaired. If gastric ulcers are present, ulcer craters and more localized wall thickening may be seen at the site of the ulcer (Figure 12-16). A defect in the mucosal layer may be visible and the ulcer crater may appear hyperechoic because of the accumulation of microbubbles and blood clots[35] (Figure 12-17; see also Figure 12-16). There may be reduced gastric motility and the accumulation of fluid within the stomach.[35] Perforating gastric ulcers and concurrent peritonitis can produce a mass effect involving the stomach wall and adjacent mesentery (Figure 12-18). There may be evidence of a hyperechoic mesentery, peritoneal fluid, and free abdominal air following perforation.[32,36,37] Linear echogenicities representing gas dissection within the wall of

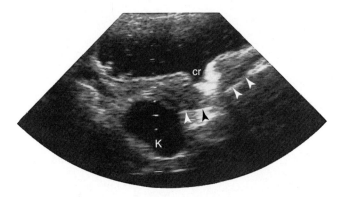

Figure 12-14 Gastric foreign bodies. A, Gastric foreign body (*arrows*) in a dog showing characteristic hyperechoic interface and strong acoustic shadowing. **B,** Gastric foreign body (ball) surrounded by gastric fluid (*F*). The ball has been punctured and contains echogenic fluid with through transmission. Note the free peritoneal fluid (*f*). (B. From Penninck DP, Nyland TG, Kerr LY, et al: Ultrasonographic evaluation of gastrointestinal diseases in small animals. *Vet Radiol* 1990;31:134-141.)

Figure 12-16 Transverse ultrasound image of the pylorus. Localized thickening of the gastric wall (*arrowheads*) with irregular ulceration (*cr*) is seen. Incidental finding of hepatic cyst (*K*) is noted. (From Penninck DP, Nyland TG, Kerr LY, et al: Ultrasonographic evaluation of gastrointestinal diseases in small animals. *Vet Radiol* 1990;31:134-141.)

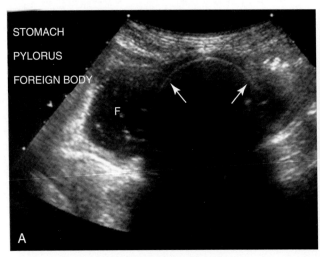

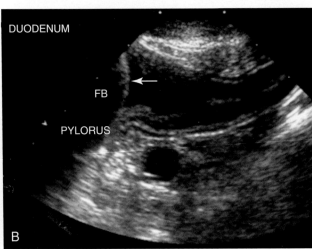

Figure 12-15 Ball gastric foreign body. A, A highly reflective, curved interface is present in the stomach lumen (*arrows*), with very strong acoustic shadowing, representing a racquetball. Fluid (*F*) surrounds a portion of the ball. **B,** The ball foreign body (FB) is seen wedged in the pylorus/proximal duodenum (*arrow*). The descending duodenum is present in long axis to the right.

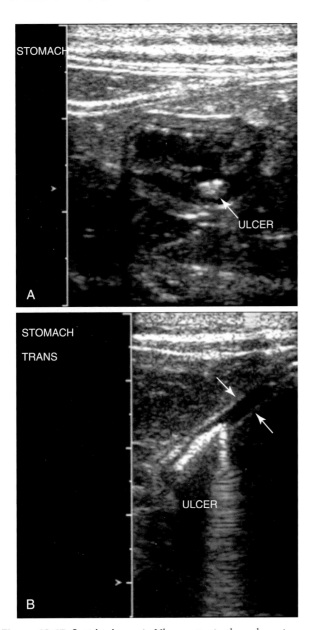

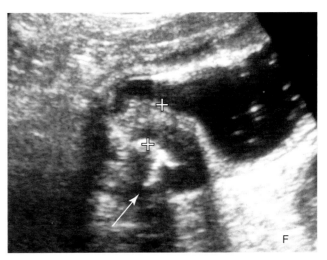

Figure 12-18 Longitudinal ultrasound image of the pyloric region of a dog with symptoms of intermittent vomiting and recent weakness. The stomach was moderately fluid filled. A focal thickening associated with a deep crater was noted (between electronic cursors). An irregularly linear hyperechoic tract (*arrow*) was seen crossing the ulcerated area toward the mesentery. A marked increased echogenicity of the adjacent fat (*F*) suggested localized peritonitis, possibly resulting from a perforated ulcer. The ulceration was confirmed at surgery. The suspected cause of this perforated ulcer was a foreign body.

Figure 12-17 **Gastric ulcers.** A, Ulcer crater in the pylorus is seen as a small focal hyperechoic depression in the gastric wall. The adjacent wall is slightly thicker and less echogenic than the near-field wall. **B,** Large, flat, hyperechoic depression in the stomach wall is present. The adjacent stomach wall (between arrows) is not thickened.

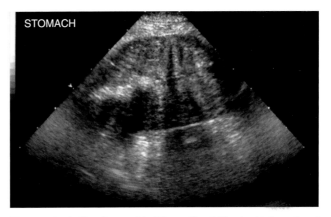

Figure 12-19 **Uremic gastritis.** The wall is diffusely thickened and more echogenic than expected. Layering has been lost. The empty status of this stomach suggests caution when interpreting its appearance.

the stomach have also been observed with gastric ulcers or severe necrosis.[38]

Uremic gastropathy due to chronic renal disease produces a thickened gastric wall, thickened rugal folds, mucosal ulceration, and a hyperechoic line representing mineralization of the gastric mucosa at the mucosal-luminal interface[39] (Figure 12-19). Gastric wall thickness was reported to range from 9.0 to 14 mm with poor definition of the wall layers in the majority of cases.[39]

Zollinger-Ellison syndrome is caused by a non–beta islet cell tumor of the pancreas that secretes gastrin and causes gastric and duodenal wall thickening with ulceration.[40-42] The findings are caused by hypersecretion of gastric acid. This syndrome should be considered in the differential diagnosis

when unexplained ulcers are found in the stomach and duodenum. Gastrinomas are usually small and difficult to detect with ultrasonography before surgery, and the diagnosis is usually made by documentation of hypergastrinemia. However, intraoperative ultrasound may be useful for localizing gastrinomas and other pancreatic islet cell tumors at surgery. Extrapancreatic gastrinomas are rare, but a duodenal gastrinoma has been reported in a dog with extrahepatic biliary obstruction.[43]

Certain neoplastic diseases can also diffusely thicken the stomach wall. Lymphoma is the best example.[44,45] Gastric lymphoma can appear as a focal mass or diffuse infiltrative lesion with loss of wall layers (Figures 12-20 to 12-22). Ulceration or perforation of the stomach wall has been reported with lymphoma.[36,44,46]

Mast cell tumors can cause gastric and duodenal ulceration, sometimes with perforation, secondary to high circulating levels of histamine.[47,48] The authors are not aware of any reports describing the sonographic appearance of mast cell disease directly involving the stomach, although the features of small intestinal, ileocolic, and colonic mast cell disease have been described in the cat.[49,50]

In one report of a dog, malignant histiocytosis was found to diffusely thicken the gastric wall and increase echogenicity while preserving the wall layers.[31] However, in another report, a single focal hypoechoic mass effacing the wall layers was described.[51]

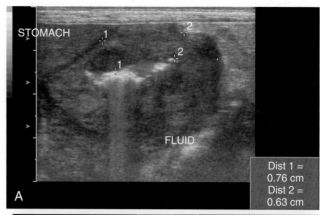

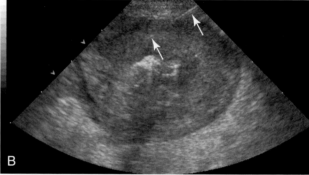

Figure 12-22 Gastric lymphoma in a dog. A, The wall is thickened (0.76 cm and 0.63 cm between electronic cursors) and heterogeneous in echotexture and echogenicity. **B,** Fine-needle aspiration (*arrows*) was used for a cytologic diagnosis.

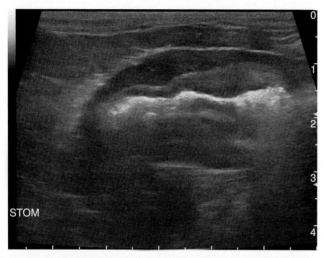

Figure 12-20 Diffuse gastric lymphoma in a 16-year-old dog. The stomach wall is thickened and normal layering has been lost.

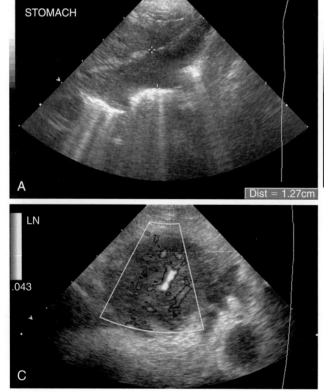

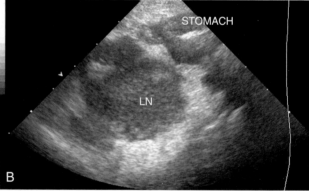

Figure 12-21 Diffuse gastric lymphoma in a dog. A, The gastric wall is markedly thickened (1.27 cm, between electronic cursors) and normal wall layering has been lost. **B,** Severe regional lymph node (*LN*) enlargement is present. A portion of the thickened stomach is seen in the near field. **C,** Power Doppler image shows a very vascular lymph node. Cytology from the stomach wall and lymph node was diagnostic for lymphoma.

Lesions in the liver, spleen, and intestinal tract, and the presence of lymphadenopathy may help distinguish malignant from nonmalignant disease. Lymphadenopathy is usually more pronounced with neoplasia. Aspirates from the stomach wall, adjacent lymph nodes, and other abdominal organs, such as the liver and spleen, will help provide a definitive diagnosis.

Focal Wall Thickening or Mass Lesions

Focal wall thickening or mass lesions usually indicate neoplasia. In most cases, the amount of wall thickening is greater than that seen with nonmalignant disease, and obliteration of the wall layers may also be observed.[31,32,52] Tumor-associated gastric ulcers may be evident, wall motility in the affected area may be absent, and perforation of the stomach wall may occur with diffuse wall thickening, as described previously. Regional lymph nodes are often involved. Tumors may appear hypoechoic, hyperechoic, or of mixed echogenicity, and the type of tumor usually cannot be determined strictly from its ultrasound appearance (Figures 12-23 to 12-26).[31,53]

Carcinoma is the most common gastric neoplasm in the dog.[31,54] Most carcinomas are located in the lesser curvature and pylorus, and they often involve the body of the stomach (see Figure 12-23).[54] The ultrasonographic features of gastric carcinoma have been described in a number of reports.[52-56] A pseudolayered pattern was described as a characteristic feature of gastric carcinoma.[55] This pattern consists of a poorly echogenic lining to the innermost, outermost, or both portions of the gastric wall separated by a more echogenic central zone.

Other canine gastric tumors include leiomyosarcoma and lymphoma. Leiomyosarcoma tends to produce focal mass lesions[22,53,57] (see Figure 12-24). Gastric lymphoma can appear as a focal mass or diffuse infiltrative lesion (see Figure 12-25).[46,53] Malignant histiocytosis with loss of wall layers has also been reported in a dog.[51]

Benign tumors are rare and consist of adenomas and leiomyomas. Adenomas can appear flat or polypoid.[54] Leiomyomas can be single or multiple and appear as a sessile, round polyps protruding into the gastric lumen.[22,58] Leiomyomas are usually covered by normal mucosa.[54,58] Figure 12-26 shows metastatic pyloric carcinoma from regional pancreatic carcinoma.

Lymphoma is the most common gastric neoplasm in the cat.[54] Focal or diffuse thickening of the gastric wall was reported to range from 5.0 to 22 mm, and a tumor-associated ulcer was noted in one case.[44] Gastric adenocarcinomas occur in cats but are extremely rare.[54]

Focal wall thickening can also be seen with nonmalignant disease. Solitary or multiple polyps from 0.5 to 1.0 cm have been found in the antral mucosa of old dogs.[54,59] Chronic hypertrophic gastritis may result from either mucosal gland hypertrophy or gastric gland hyperplasia. Asymmetrical thickening of the gastric wall and focal polypoid lesions resembling gastric tumors are sometimes seen. Eosinophilic sclerosing fibroplasia has been reported to cause focal mass lesions at the pyloric antrum in cats.[60] Pythiosis is a chronic pyogranulomatous infection caused by the water mold, *Pythium insidiosum*.[61,62] Focal thickening of the stomach wall with partial or complete obliteration of the wall layers has been reported. Additionally, focal thickening with alteration of normal wall layers has been reported postoperatively following gastropexy procedures.[63]

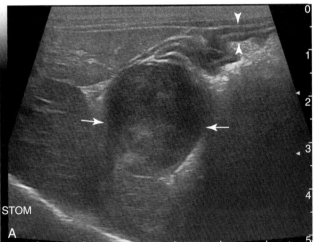

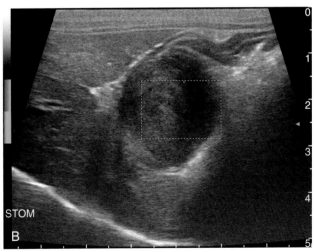

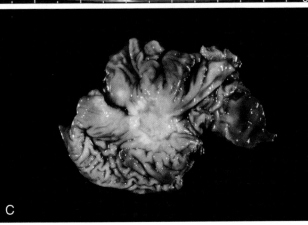

Figure 12-23 Gastric adenocarcinoma in a 14-year-old dog. A, Large, homogeneous, well demarcated mass (between arrows) extends from the lesser curvature of the stomach. Portions of normal stomach wall are seen to the right in the image (between arrowheads). **B,** Power Doppler image shows very little detectable blood flow within the mass. **C,** Gastric carcinoma. (Courtesy of Washington State University College of Veterinary Medicine, Washington Animal Disease Diagnostic Laboratory, Pullman, WA.)

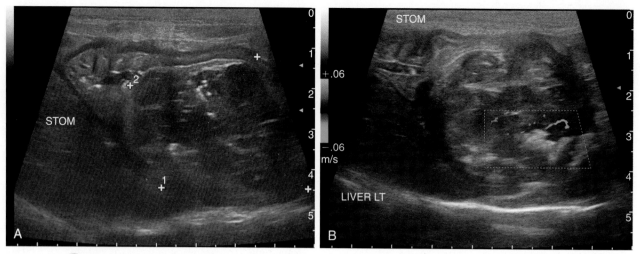

Figure 12-24 **Gastric leiomyosarcoma in a dog. A,** Large, complex mass arising from the stomach wall (4.04 × 5.16 cm between electronic cursors) is present. **B,** Color Doppler analysis shows some blood flow within the mass.

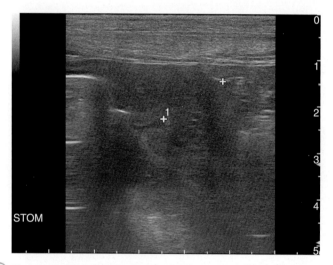

Figure 12-25 **Gastric lymphoma in a dog.** Regional, homogeneous gastric wall thickening is present (1.54 cm between electronic cursors), with loss of layering.

ABNORMALITIES OF THE SMALL INTESTINE

Corrugated Bowel Pattern

An abnormal corrugated small bowel pattern has been described in the duodenum or jejunum of dogs and cats. This pattern has been defined as an undulating or rippled wall, best visualized by noting the undulating hyperechoic line of the mucosa/lumen interface, the submucosa, or both.[28,64] The bowel wall is sometimes thickened as well as corrugated. This pattern was originally described with pancreatitis (Figure 12-27, *A*),[65] intestinal lymphangiectasia,[66] and intestinal lymphoma.[67] Other etiologies of so-called corrugated bowel include enteritis, peritonitis (Figure 12-27, *B*), neoplasia, and bowel wall ischemia.[64,68] Although abnormal, this pattern is a nonspecific finding that could be caused by any of the previously listed conditions. Therefore the specific cause of bowel wall corrugation should be identified.

Dilation

Dilation of the small intestine may be due to a functional disorder or a mechanical obstruction. A functional disorder is one in which paralysis of the intestinal musculature (paralytic ileus) impedes progression of bowel contents. Functional disorders can produce either localized or generalized dilation of the small bowel (Figure 12-28). Peristalsis may be markedly reduced or absent. Pancreatitis is an example of a disease that may cause localized functional dilation of the stomach, duodenum, and proximal small bowel caused by focal peritonitis. Generalized functional bowel dilation may be seen with severe gastroenteritis (e.g., salmon poisoning disease,[69] parvoviral infection[70]), generalized peritonitis, postoperative abdomen, pain, drugs, or electrolyte imbalances. In most generalized functional disorders, uniform dilation of the bowel is present.

Mechanical bowel obstruction also can result in either localized or generalized small bowel dilation (Figure 12-29). A mechanical obstruction is a physical impediment to the progression of bowel contents. The amount of dilation depends on the location, duration, and completeness of the obstruction. A mechanical obstruction is more likely to be characterized by dilated, fluid-filled bowel loops that are unequal in size compared to functional disorders, where the dilated loops are more uniform in size. A high small bowel obstruction usually results in localized dilation of only a small number of proximal small bowel loops, whereas a lower small bowel obstruction results in more generalized bowel distention. The diameter of affected loops is smaller with high small bowel obstructions than with lower bowel obstructions because the animal usually vomits more frequently. Partial obstructions also cause less dilation than complete obstructions. Additionally, the duration of an obstruction affects the amount of dilation, with longer-standing obstructions of the middle and lower bowel causing greater dilation.

Ultrasonography has good sensitivity for diagnosing small intestinal obstructions, especially when performed by experienced sonographers; however, obstructions can be missed with when ultrasonography is the only diagnostic tool used.[71-74] Therefore abdominal radiographs should always be taken in cases of suspected small bowel obstruction to better delineate the pattern of fluid and gas distention. In some cases, upper gastrointestinal contrast series may be required to rule out

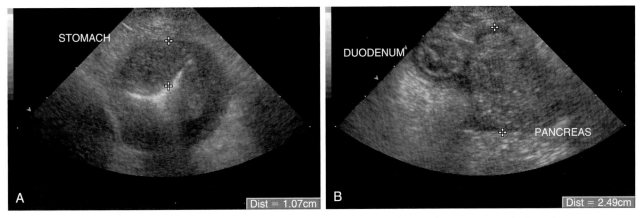

Figure 12-26 **Pancreatic carcinoma with metastasis to the stomach. A,** Pyloric antrum is thickened (1.07 cm between electronic cursors) and normal wall layering has been lost. **B,** Transverse image of the pancreatic mass (2.49 cm between electronic cursors) with adjacent descending duodenum.

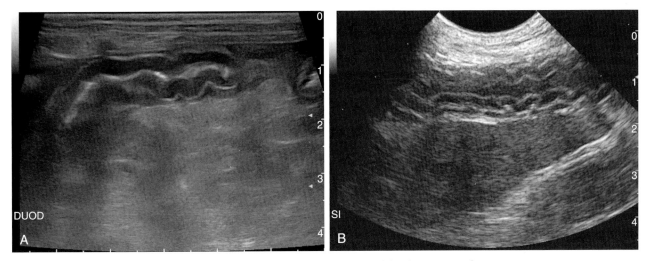

Figure 12-27 **Corrugated small intestine. A,** Mildly corrugated duodenum secondary to pancreatitis. **B,** Corrugated small intestine in a dog with peritonitis.

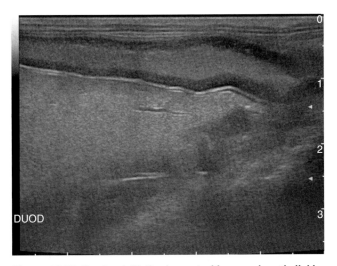

Figure 12-28 **Duodenal dilation in a cat with severe hepatic lipidosis.** The duodenum is dilated (near field), with echogenic yet sonolucent luminal content. Note the extremely hyperechoic and finely textured liver parenchyma in the far field. Much of the small intestine was dilated, in this case secondary to physiologic (functional) abnormalities rather than mechanical obstruction.

obstruction, depending on the survey radiographic and ultrasound findings.

Obstruction

Partial or complete small intestinal obstruction may be caused by a foreign body, stricture, granuloma, abscess, intussusception, or tumor. Other conditions such as strangulation of bowel in an abdominal hernia or mesenteric tear, or mesenteric root torsion are more rare.

Differentiation of mechanical obstructive versus functional bowel dilation is possible when both dilated and normal small bowel loops are seen or the cause of the obstruction is identified. Dilation of the bowel occurs proximal to a mechanical obstruction but not distal to it. Hyperperistalsis is also noted proximal to a mechanical obstruction as the bowel attempts to pass the contents distally. However, in chronic mechanical obstructions, the bowel may become exhausted and reduced peristaltic activity may be observed instead.

If localized bowel dilation is present with normal bowel proximal and distal to the dilation, the cause is likely a localized, functional disorder. However, a partial mechanical obstruction at this site cannot be ruled out, and a search for the cause of a partial obstruction should be undertaken. If normal small bowel loops cannot be identified, then either a

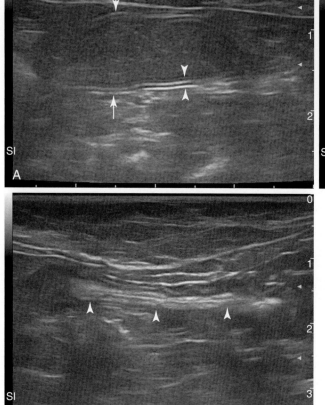

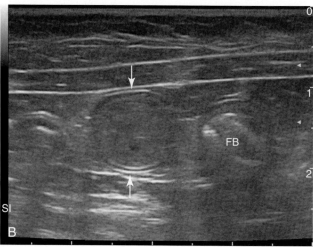

Figure 12-29 **Small intestinal dilation secondary to linear foreign body obstruction in a cat.** **A,** A dilated segment of small intestine (between arrows) contains echogenic but sonolucent fluid. The bowel wall is very thin (between arrowheads), with preservation of layers. **B,** Transverse image shows the dilated segment of small intestine (between arrows). To the left is the segment of intestine containing the linear foreign body (*FB*). **C,** The linear foreign body is seen as a highly echogenic luminal structure in this sagittal image of small intestine (*arrowheads*).

lower small bowel mechanical obstruction or a generalized functional disorder of the bowel may be present. Finding the cause of a mechanical obstruction, if present, will help differentiate these two conditions. Also with mechanical obstruction, the dilated bowel loops tend to be unequal in size. Generalized functional disorders usually have uniformly dilated bowel loops.

As stated previously, increased peristaltic contractions are frequently seen in dilated small bowel proximal to an acute mechanical obstruction. However, reduced peristaltic activity cannot always differentiate functional from mechanical obstruction. If dilated loops with reduced peristaltic contractions are seen, either a functional disorder or a chronic lower small bowel mechanical obstruction could be present. Prolonged mechanical obstruction may lead to bowel exhaustion, electrolyte imbalances, or other changes resulting in decreased motility.

Foreign Bodies

Intestinal foreign bodies may be difficult to detect unless they partially or completely obstruct the small bowel. The bowel is usually dilated proximal to the obstruction and normal distal to the obstruction. The foreign body may be partially outlined by luminal fluid. A distinct hyperechoic interface with strong acoustic shadowing is usually seen with larger foreign bodies (Figures 12-30 and 12-31).[22,27,28,71,75] The hyperechoic interface may be curvilinear with foreign bodies such as a ball, bone, or fruit pit. Trichobezoar foreign bodies

have been reported to cause intestinal obstruction, most commonly in cats.[37] There may be bowel wall thickening, hemorrhage, and perforation of the wall in the region of intestinal foreign bodies.[37] Hyperechoic mesentery, peritoneal fluid, or free abdominal air may be seen.

Linear foreign bodies such as string, fishing line, or linear cloth fragments have a distinctive appearance because they cause plication of the small bowel[27,30] (Figure 12-32; see also Figure 12-31). Fluid accumulates within the plicated loops, and in many cases a thin hyperechoic line representing the string or fishing line can be seen.[28,30] With linear cloth fragments or pieces of rug, a larger elongated shadowing structure can be identified within the bowel lumen (Figure 12-33). The stomach should also be checked carefully for foreign bodies, because many linear foreign bodies extend from the stomach distally.

Intussusception

An intussusception occurs when a bowel segment invaginates within itself. Most intussusceptions are found in young animals and usually occur secondary to primary intestinal disease such as bacterial, viral, or parasitic enteritis.[76] However, they may also occur with foreign bodies, mesenteric cysts, or intestinal neoplasia.[77,78] Intussusceptions are named according to the segment of bowel involved. Enteroenteric, ileocolic, and cecocolic intussusceptions are the most common, but gastroduodenal, pylorogastric, and colocolic intussusceptions have also been reported.[77,79,80]

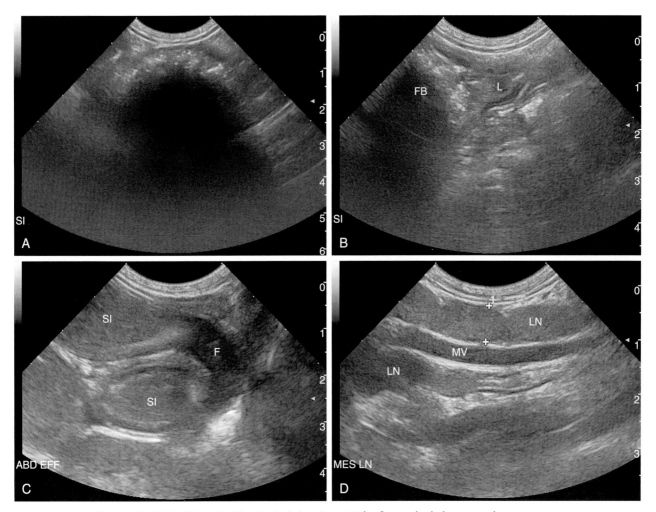

Figure 12-30 Small intestinal foreign body in a dog. A, The foreign body has created a very strong acoustic shadow. **B,** The foreign body (*FB*) is seen within the small intestinal lumen (*L*), with transition to nondistended bowel distal to the foreign body seen to the right. **C,** Markedly dilated segment of small intestine (*SI*) proximal to the obstruction. Peritoneal fluid is present (*F*). **D,** Mesenteric lymph node (*LN*) enlargement is present (0.67 cm, between electronic cursors). *MV,* Mesenteric vein. This dog had a small rupture of his bowel and resultant peritonitis.

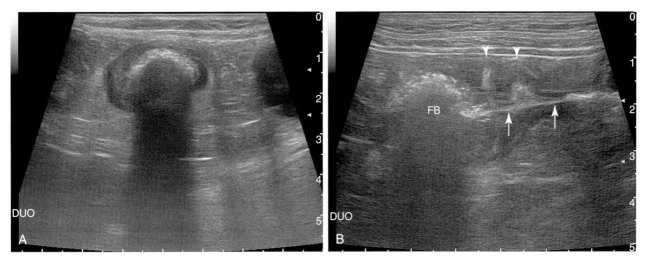

Figure 12-31 Duodenal foreign body. A, Transverse image shows a dilated duodenum with a hyperechoic foreign body, with strong acoustic shadowing. **B,** Long axis view shows a portion of the linear foreign body (*FB, arrows*) and has caused plication (*arrowheads*) of the bowel.

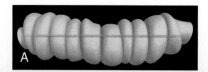

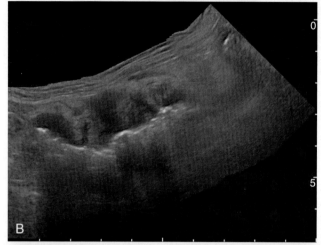

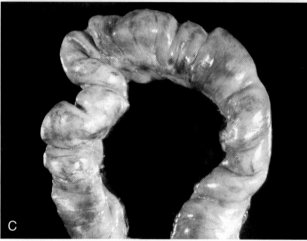

Figure 12-32 **Linear foreign body. A,** Illustration of bowel plication from a linear foreign body. **B,** Panoramic view of a chronic linear foreign body in a dog. The bowel is plicated, and the central luminal content is very hyperechoic. Surrounding mesentery shows poor detail, compatible with peritonitis. The foreign body was cloth. **C,** Pathology specimen of a small intestinal linear foreign body shows plication and bunching. (Courtesy of Washington State University College of Veterinary Medicine, Washington Animal Disease Diagnostic Laboratory, Pullman, WA.)

An intussusception appears as a multilayered structure in the longitudinal view and as multiple concentric rings (target lesion) in the transverse view[22,28,71,77,78,81] (Figures 12-34 and 12-35). The appearance is due to the multiple wall layers making up the intussusception. Hyperechoic mesentery may also be incorporated within the intussusception. A variable amount of bowel dilation is seen proximal to the intussusception, depending on whether a partial or complete bowel obstruction is present. Intussusceptions can spontaneously reduce, so reexamination is recommended immediately after anesthesia but before surgery.[82] Occasionally, the layered appearance of an intussusception is obscured by inflammation and edema of the wall layers. In these cases, the symmetrically increased diameter of the intussuscepted bowel segment may help make the diagnosis.

Healthy intestine, enteritis associated with a foreign body, and a postpartum uterus have been reported to simulate a small intestinal intussusception by producing a target-like lesion in some imaging planes.[83] Linear foreign bodies can sometimes mimic an intussusception if there is extensive plication of the bowel.[27] However, the wall layers do not form a complete concentric ring. To prevent misdiagnosis, the sonographer should view the suspected lesion in multiple imaging planes and verify that the concentric rings are complete. If they are not complete, the target-like lesion may not be an intussusception, and the differential diagnosis should be widened. Clear visualization of the inner bowel loop (intussusceptum) within the outer bowel loop (intussuscipiens) separated by mesenteric fat also helps confirm the diagnosis of an intussusception.

Intestinal Wall Thickening

As in the stomach, intestinal wall thickening is commonly found with inflammatory disease or neoplasia. Diffuse edema causing thickening of the bowel wall may also be seen with a variety of conditions such as hypoproteinemia, congestive heart failure, or vascular abnormalities. The distribution, symmetry, and extent of wall thickening and the appearance of wall layers can help differentiate nonmalignant diseases from neoplasia. Nonmalignant disease tends to induce diffuse, mild to moderate wall thickening with preservation of the wall layers. Neoplastic lesions characteristically produce more extensive focal thickening or mass lesions with disruption or loss of the wall layers.[22,84] The exception is lymphosarcoma, which can either diffusely infiltrate the bowel or produce mass lesions. In either case, there is loss or alteration of the wall layers, which may help differentiate lymphosarcoma from other nonneoplastic conditions. Lymphadenopathy is usually more extensive with neoplasia, which can also help differentiate benign from malignant disease. In addition, recognition of metastasis to other abdominal organs helps confirm the diagnosis of neoplasia. The history, clinical signs, and laboratory work should be considered to formulate a differential diagnosis. However, ultrasound-guided aspirations or biopsies of the bowel, lymph nodes, and suspected metastatic lesions are usually required for final diagnosis.

Diffuse Wall Thickening

Diffuse thickening of the wall of the small intestine is seen with various types of generalized enteritis (e.g., bacterial, viral, lymphocytic-plasmacytic, eosinophilic, uremic) and lymphosarcoma. Enteritis generally produces diffuse, concentric wall thickening, which often is only 1 to 2 mm thicker than normal. However, normal findings during an ultrasound examination do not completely rule out disease because some dogs with confirmed bowel inflammation have no detectable bowel thickening on ultrasound.[85] The degree of wall thickening may not be the same throughout the bowel, with some segments affected more than others. In some cases of enteritis, wall thickening may be limited to only one segment of bowel. Duodenitis secondary to pancreatitis, for example, may produce diffuse thickening of only the duodenum.

In most cases of enteritis, the wall layers will be preserved, although they may be altered (Figure 12-36). Altering of the wall layers may consist of poor definition, thickening, or echogenicity changes. In one study, mucosal echogenicity was used in dogs in an attempt to differentiate types of chronic enteropathies, which were categorized by response to treatment.[86] Hyperechoic striations were most common in cases of protein-losing enteropathy, whereas no changes in mucosal echogenicity were identified in patients responsive to a change in diet. Hyperechoic speckles within the mucosa were identified in cases of inflammatory bowel disease, but were not specific

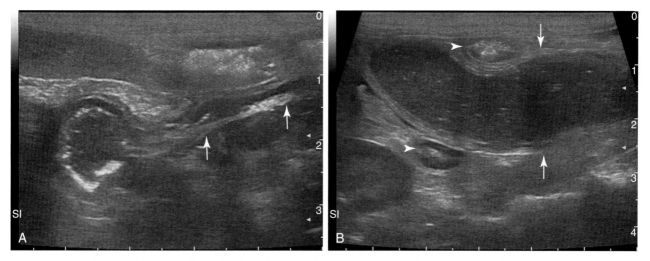

Figure 12-33 **Linear foreign body. A,** A hyperechoic linear foreign body (*arrows*) is identified within a segment of small intestine. The portion of bowel to the left is dilated. **B,** Markedly distended segment of small intestine (between arrows) proximal to the obstruction. Note the two segments of nondistended small intestine postobstruction (*arrowheads*).

for type or severity of the disease. Hyperechoic speckles have also been identified in cases of parvoviral infection, possibly caused by mucus, cellular debris, and protein accumulation.[70] In a recent retrospective report of cats with intestinal mucosal fibrosis, all 11 cats had a hyperechoic linear band within the mucosal layer of the bowel identified with ultrasound. This hyperechoic band was parallel to the submucosa, corresponded to linear mucosal fibrosis on histopathology, and was most frequently identified in the jejunum.[87] However, this hyperechoic band has also been identified in animals without gastrointestinal disease.[88]

In severe cases of enteritis or with long-standing involvement, there may be greater wall thickening and disruption or loss of the wall layers. In one report, 4 of 61 dogs (6.5%) with enteritis had intestinal wall thickness equal to or exceeding 1 cm.[84] All dogs had severe hemorrhagic, necrotizing, and/or suppurative enteritis. Ultrasound-guided fine-needle aspirations of the bowel are usually not very rewarding in enteritis cases,[84,89] although lymph node aspirates may help differentiate inflammatory from neoplastic conditions. Lymphangiectasia in dogs was reported to produce generalized intestinal wall thickening and indistinct wall layering in approximately 50% of the cases.[66] Abdominal fluid was present in about 60% of the cases (Figure 12-37). Other less common abnormal findings included hyperechogenicity of the intestinal mucosal layer, hyperechoic mesentery, hypermotility, and corrugation of the small intestine. The authors reported that the changes were not specific enough to differentiate this disease from other gastrointestinal disorders. Lymphangiectasia presenting as circumferential, more localized intestinal thickening with loss of wall layering has also been described in one dog.[90] In other reports, lymphangiectasia with protein-losing enteropathy was associated with mild wall thickening, preservation of wall layering, and hyperechoic mucosal striations in dogs (see Figure 12-37, C and D).[86,91] Although wall layering was preserved, the mucosal layer was more hyperechoic than normal. The hyperechoic mucosal striations were associated with lacteal dilation on histopathology. Hypoalbuminemia, hypoproteinemia, and abdominal effusion consistent with a protein-losing enteropathy were present in nearly all dogs in both reports, and concurrent inflammation was a consistent feature of the lacteal dilation on histopathology. In the earlier report,

one dog had disseminated villus histiocytic sarcoma, and the authors state that it was impossible to determine whether primary inflammatory disease, primary lymphangiectasia, or villus histiocytic sarcoma were possible causes of the protein-losing enteropathy.[91]

Mild to moderate thickening of a specific layer of the intestinal wall with preservation of the other wall layers has also been reported. Lymphocytic-plasmacytic enteritis may affect specific wall layers in the early stages. A prominent mucosa with an irregular increase in echogenicity and an unevenly thickened submucosa has been described.[20] (Figure 12-36). Changes specific to the submucosal layer of the bowel have also been reported in certain diseases, such as canine schistosomiasis. A thickened submucosal layer, with or without mineralization, has been associated with edema, granulomatous inflammation, and fragmented schistosome eggs in multiple cases of *Heterobilharzia americana* infection.[92,93]

Thickening of the muscularis layer in the small bowel, equal to or thicker than the mucosal layer, has been frequently reported in cats. In one study, four cats had moderate thickening of the bowel wall measuring 7 to 8 mm, primarily caused by thickening of only the muscular layer.[94] The muscular layer measured approximately 5 mm in thickness, whereas the other wall layers were normal. Two of these cats had chronic enteritis. The other two cats had muscular layer thickening proximal to a stenosis caused by lymphosarcoma and an intestinal foreign body. The cause of the muscular thickening in these cases may have been secondary to inflammatory infiltrates or hypertrophy as a compensatory response, as suggested by the two cases with bowel obstruction. Multiple additional cases of cats with inflammatory bowel disease have also reported a thickened muscularis layer on ultrasound, which could be caused by the lymphocytic and/or eosinophilic infiltrates within the lamina propria identified on histopathology (see Figure 12-36).[20,95,96] A solitary case of muscularis thickening in a cat with disseminated histoplasmosis has also been reported.[18,97] Neoplasms, such as lymphoma and mast cell tumors, have also been found to cause muscularis thickening in the small intestine of cats.[49,96,98] In a more recent retrospective study, cats with thickening of the muscularis layer identified with ultrasound were more likely to have lymphoma, specifically T-cell lymphoma, when compared

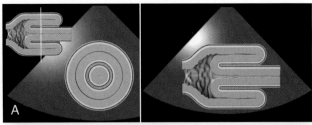

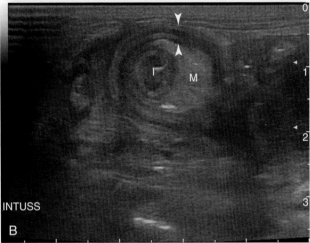

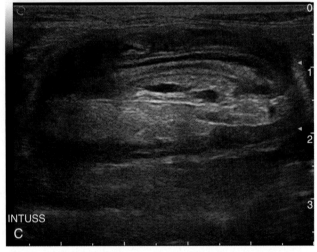

Figure 12-34 **Intussusception.** A, Illustration of transverse and long-axis intussusception. B, Transverse image of an intussusception. The inner small intestinal loop (*I*, intussusceptum) is easily identified within the outer bowel loop (between arrowheads, intussuscipiens), surrounded by echogenic mesenteric fat (*M*). C, Long-axis view of the intussusception.

with normal cats or those diagnosed with inflammatory bowel disease.[98] In this study, cats with lymphoma were 18 times more likely to have a thickened muscularis than cats with inflammatory bowel disease. The authors hypothesize that the discrepancy between the current study and earlier studies may be associated with the difficulty in distinguishing the two diseases on routine histopathology.

A thicker, hypoechoic wall (5.0 to 20.0 mm or more) with loss of the wall layers is also commonly seen in cases of lymphosarcoma (Figure 12-39; see also Figure 12-38).[44,45,67,99] Bowel hypomotility may be evident in the affected segments. Lymphosarcoma can also present as a bowel mass and with diffuse thickening of the wall.[44,99] Regional lymphadenopathy is generally more pronounced with lymphosarcoma than with

enteritis, which assists with diagnosis. Other abdominal organs, such as the liver and spleen, may also be involved with lymphosarcoma. Ultrasound-guided aspiration of the bowel, lymph nodes, or other organs will help establish the correct diagnosis.

Focal Wall Thickening or Mass Lesions

Focal wall thickening with loss of wall layers or intestinal mass lesions are commonly seen with neoplasia.[22,32,84,100] Leiomyosarcoma, lymphosarcoma, and adenocarcinoma are the most common intestinal tumors in dogs.[46,57,67,101-104] A single case report of a benign hemangioma, described as a well-defined cavitary mass, has been reported in the ileum of a dog.[105] In cats, lymphosarcoma and adenocarcinoma are most common, but mast cell tumors and hemangiosarcoma have also been reported in the small bowel, at the ileocolic junction or in the colon.[44,45,49,50,106-109] Adenomatous polyps have been described in the duodenum of cats,[110] but these have not been documented ultrasonographically.

Lymphoma can either diffusely infiltrate the bowel and break down wall layers (see Figures 12-38 and 12-39) or induce mass lesions (Figure 12-40).[44,45,99] Wall thickening may be circumferential. The lesion usually appears distinctly hypoechoic, ulceration may be present, and regional lymphadenopathy is common. Adenocarcinomas tend to cause circumferential thickening of the bowel with loss of wall layering and partial or complete intestinal obstruction[108,111] (Figures 12-41 and 12-42). Carcinomas of the bowel are usually solitary masses but can spread throughout the peritoneal cavity (carcinomatosis).[88,111] Their echogenicity is usually hypoechoic to mixed, and the intestinal lumen appears irregular.

Leiomyomas are more commonly found in the stomach of older dogs, but those in the bowel are usually small (<3 cm) and have smooth contours (Figure 12-43).[104] However, a large jejunal leiomyoma measuring 10 × 17 cm has also been described.[100]

Leiomyosarcomas are generally large, eccentric masses[104] (Figure 12-44). The echogenicity is usually heterogeneous with single or multiple hypoechoic or anechoic areas associated with larger tumors. The appearance may result from centralized necrosis as the tumor outstrips its blood supply.

Mast cell disease can produce diffuse wall thickening or a focal mass in the duodenum, jejunum, ileocecocolic junction, or colon of cats.[49,50] Mast cell tumors have been reported in the small intestine of dogs; however, the sonographic characteristics of these abnormalities have not been widely reported. One case report of mast cell disease in an adult Boxer dog describes two masses, one in the duodenum and one in the jejunum, of mixed echogenicity.[112] Another retrospective description of visceral mast cell tumors, which involved the duodenum, jejunum, ileum, and colon, state that of the six dogs that underwent ultrasonography, solid tumors were identified in five.[113] However, no additional details on sonographic description were included. Additionally, gastric and duodenal ulceration can result from high histamine levels with mast cell tumors located elsewhere.[47,48] Although in one case series of dogs with abdominal mast cell disease, which included mast cell disease in the liver, spleen, kidney, and abdominal lymph nodes, no abnormalities were identified in the gastrointestinal tract of any of the dogs.[50] Nonneoplastic lesions can also cause focal wall thickening with indistinct wall layering, although this is less common. Infarction of the bowel has been reported in a cat with focal thickening of the bowel and progressive loss of wall layering.[114] Masses associated with the bowel have been seen with pyogranulomas secondary to foreign bodies,[115] hematomas, feline eosinophilic sclerosing fibroplasia,[60] fungal infection (histoplasmosis),[97] chronic granulomatous enteritis

Text continued on p. 491

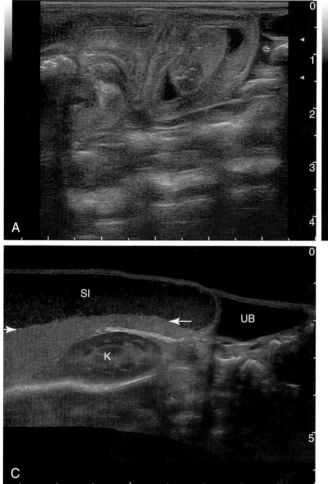

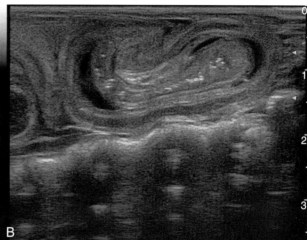

Figure 12-35 Intussusception. A, Transverse image of an intussusception. B, Long-axis image of the intussusception. C, Extended field of view image shows a very large segment of distended small intestine (*SI*) proximal to the intussusception. The bowel loop contains dependent sediment (*arrows*), creating a layered appearance to the fluid-filled intestine. The urinary bladder (*UB*) and a kidney (*K*) are also visible.

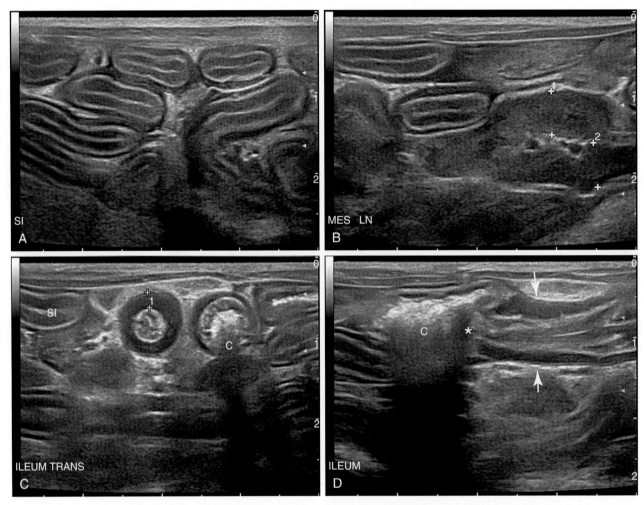

Figure 12-36 Diffuse inflammatory bowel disease in a cat. A, Although not thickened overall, the muscularis layer is disproportionately thickened in all of the small intestine. **B,** Mesenteric lymph nodes are very prominent in this patient (between electronic cursors, 0.54cm and 0.55 cm). **C,** The ileum is seen in transverse section, recognizable by a thicker muscle layer (0.19 cm between electronic cursors) than the jejunum. C, Colon; *SI,* small intestine. **D,** Long axis image of the ileum (between arrows) entering the cecocolic junction (*). C, Cecum/colon.

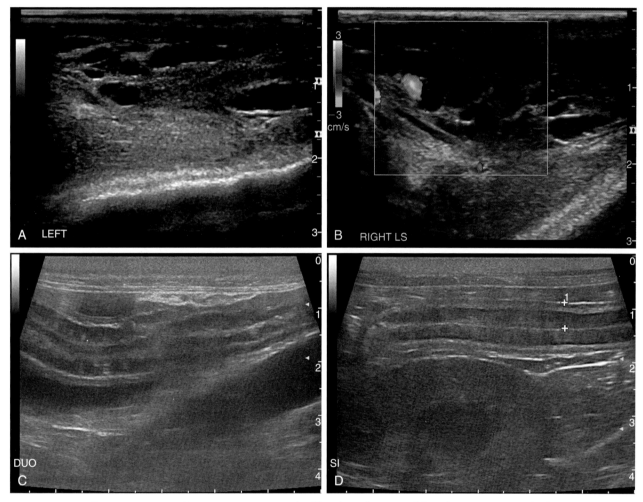

Figure 12-37 **Lymphangiectasia. A,** Severely dilated small intestinal lymphatics seen as multiple fluid-filled areas within the mucosa. **B,** Color Doppler image of **A. C,** Much less severe lymphangiectasia ultrasonographically in a patient with severe hypoalbuminemia and ascites. The mucosa has hyperechoic striations that are perpendicular to the lumen. The mucosa is also thicker than expected. **D,** Echogenic mucosa (bowel thickness is 0.48 cm between electronic cursors). (**A** and **B** courtesy Dr. Fraser McConnell, University of Liverpool, England.)

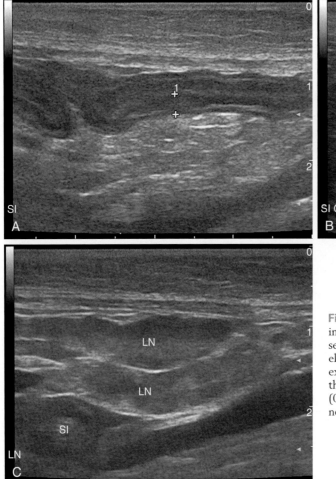

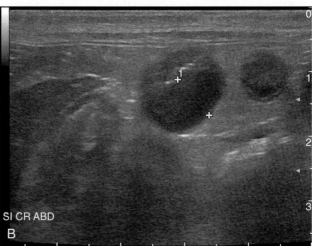

Figure 12-38 Alimentary lymphoma in a cat. A, Diffuse increase in echogenicity of this segment of small intestine, with preserved layering and normal wall thickness (0.25 cm between electronic cursors). The submucosal layer is thicker than expected. **B,** Transverse image through an area of small intestine that is eccentrically thickened and has lost wall layering (0.74 cm between electronic cursors). **C,** Mesenteric lymph node (*LN*) enlargement. *SI,* Small intestine.

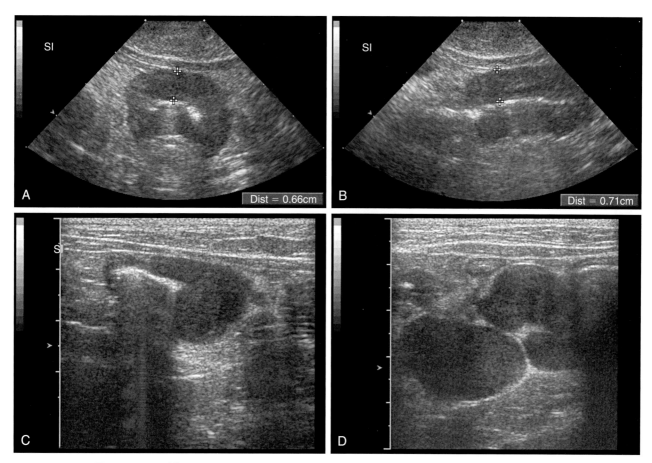

Figure 12-39 **Alimentary lymphoma in a cat. A,** Transverse image of thickened small intestine (0.66 cm between electronic cursors) and complete loss of intestinal layering. **B,** Longitudinal image of small intestine shows thickening and loss of layering (0.71 cm between electronic cursors). **C,** Eccentric thickening is seen in this section of small intestine, also with complete loss of wall layers. **D,** Very enlarged, rounded, hypoechoic mesenteric lymph nodes.

(pythiosis), or ganglioneuromatosis. Pythiosis is a chronic pyogranulomatous infection caused by the water mold, *P. insidiosum*.[61] Focal thickening of the gastric and/or intestinal walls with partial or complete obliteration of the wall layers has been reported. Ganglioneuromatosis is a rare proliferation of the intestinal ganglia, with lesions ranging from well-demarcated solitary or multifocal masses to diffuse abnormalities of an entire bowel segment. In the only case report of ganglioneuromatosis in the small bowel of a dog, the lesion was characterized by marked thickening of the distal jejunal and ileal wall with loss of normal wall layering on ultrasound.[116] Differentiation of nonmalignant lesions, such as pythiosis or ganglioneuromatosis, from neoplasia usually requires histopathology.

Additionally, focal thickening of the bowel can be found with ultrasound postoperatively. In one prospective study evaluating enterotomy and enterectomy sites in dogs, the majority of the patients had wall thickening and absent wall layering at the surgical site for the duration of the project, with the final ultrasound performed 20 days postoperatively (Figures 12-45 and 12-46).[117] In another study assessing enterotomy sites from 6 months to 7 years after surgery, mild focal intestinal wall thickening and altered to absent wall layering was still visualized with ultrasound in most of the dogs.[118]

Doppler Ultrasonography

Intestinal peristalsis has been quantitatively assessed using pulsed Doppler ultrasound in normal dogs.[119] Peristalsis in dogs after fasting was compared to dogs after feeding and to dogs sedated with xylazine hydrochloride, ketamine hydrochloride, or acepromazine. A peristaltic wave was described as a ring of constriction that moves aborally over a short segment of the intestine. Peristaltic contractions were differentiated from nonperistaltic segmental or mixing waves by pulsed Doppler technique. Peristaltic waves occurred at a rate of approximately 0.1/min (1 every 10 min) in fasted dogs. This increased to approximately 1.7/min immediately after feeding and gradually decreased over a 24-hour period. In dogs sedated with xylazine, the number of peristaltic contractions was significantly reduced. There was no change in the rate of peristaltic contractions in the dogs sedated with ketamine or acepromazine. This study provides baseline information on the use of pulsed Doppler ultrasound to differentiate peristaltic waves from nonperistaltic waves and may prove useful to quantitate bowel motility under abnormal physiologic conditions.

Color Doppler ultrasonography has also been used to help predict the whether a given intussusception could be reduced.[120] Presence of blood flow in the mesentery along the entire length of the intussuscepted bowel segment was

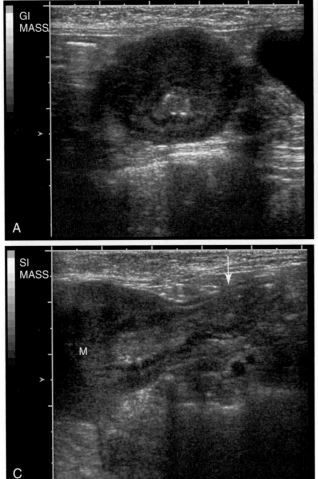

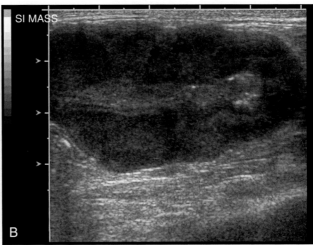

Figure 12-40 Lymphosarcoma in a cat. In this example, the lymphoma only involved a portion of small intestine. **A,** Transverse image through the intestinal mass. The wall is markedly thickened and normal layering has been lost. **B,** Long-axis image of the mass in the small intestine. **C,** Transition of intestinal mass (*M*) into normal-appearing small intestine (*arrow*).

considered a positive sign. Reduction of the intussusception was achieved at surgery in 9 of 12 dogs that had mesenteric blood flow (75%), but it was not achieved in any of the 3 dogs without blood flow. In the 3 dogs with mesenteric flow that could not be reduced, adhesions at the apex of the intussusception prevented complete reduction, although most of the intussuscepted segment could be reduced. If internal vascularization was detected within an intussusception, bowel wall necrosis was less likely to occur.

In humans, neoplasia and inflammatory disease have been reported to show increased bowel wall vascularization on color Doppler analysis when compared to normal, but ischemic and edematous bowel tend to be hypovascular.[13] Color Doppler ultrasonography has also been used to differentiate inflammatory from ischemic bowel wall thickening.[121] Absent or barely visible color Doppler flow and the absence of arterial signals suggests ischemia. Readily visible Doppler flow and a stratified echotexture suggests inflammation. A resistive index (RI) less than 0.60 was also considered consistent with inflammation, compared to an RI of 0.71 ± 03, which was considered normal. The authors concluded that vasodilation secondary to inflammation leads to increased diastolic flow and a decreased RI.

Chronic enteropathies have also been evaluated with Doppler ultrasound.[122-124] Mild thickening of the bowel wall with preservation of wall layering is common to many types of inflammatory bowel disease and food allergies. However, Doppler techniques have the potential to provide additional information about the hemodynamics of blood flow during the digestion of food. Analysis of the RI and pulsatility index (PI) in the celiac and cranial mesenteric arteries can be used to assess capillary bed resistance downstream. An RI of approximately 0.80 in the cranial mesenteric artery is considered normal in fasted dogs.[125] Measurements are made in both vessels after a 12-hour fast and at 20, 40, 60, and 90 minutes following ingestion of a meal. Normally, RI and PI values decrease until 40 to 60 minutes following a meal, after which they increase to nearly normal at 90 minutes.[125] Dogs with inflammatory bowel disease show lower RI and PI values during digestion than normal dogs.[123] Dogs with food hypersensitivities also show lower RI and PI values during digestion than normal.[122] The lowered RI and PI values in dogs with inflammatory bowel disease may be due to the lack of response of the vascular bed to feeding, because the mean postprandial increase in diastolic blood flow velocity was below that of normal dogs.[123] In the case of food hypersensitivity, a local inflammatory response with increased and prolonged vasodilation may be responsible for the lowered RI and PI values.[124] The RI, PI, and other Doppler waveform patterns in response to feeding may eventually allow differentiation of specific chronic enteropathies.

Ultrasonographic contrast media have also been used to assess vascularization of various abdominal organs in small animals. Recently, the enhancement pattern of normal jejunum has been described intraoperatively, with the transducer placed directly on a loop of jejunum.[126] This technique may be useful in the future for assessing intestinal viability; however, further research is needed.

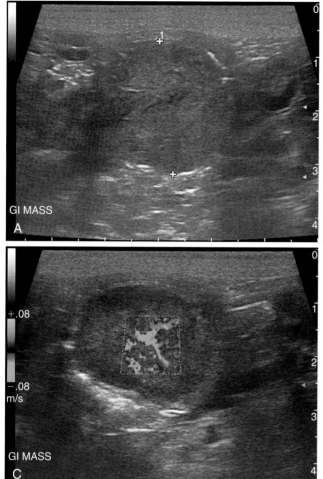

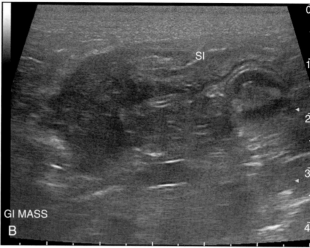

Figure 12-41 **Adenocarcinoma of the small intestine in a dog.** A, Transverse image through the intestinal mass (2.49 cm between electronic cursors) shows a very solid appearance. B, In long axis the mass has a more complex composition. C, Color Doppler evaluation shows the mass to be very well vascularized.

ABNORMALITIES OF THE CECUM AND COLON

Many diseases of the cecum and colon appear similar to those of the small intestine. However, interference from gas and feces makes it much more difficult to evaluate the colon ultrasonographically. In addition, the terminal colon and rectum are hidden from view by the bony pelvis. Survey radiographs, radiographic contrast studies, and endoscopy are usually employed instead. However, the cecum and colon should always be evaluated as part of a complete ultrasonographic examination. If there is a stricture of the colon due to scarring or neoplasia, it may not be possible to evaluate the proximal colon with radiographic contrast studies or endoscopy. Ultrasound is most useful for diagnosing intussusceptions or identifying wall thickening. However, congenital abnormalities such as colonic duplication may be recognized occasionally.[127] A colonic foreign body may also be discovered if the history is compatible and the colon is filled with fluid or there is adjacent wall thickening.[75] The ultrasonographic findings with cecal or colonic wall thickening are usually nonspecific, but a combination of the ultrasound findings and clinical information may suggest a differential diagnosis. Fine-needle aspirations or biopsies of the colon or regional lymph nodes under ultrasound guidance will help determine the final diagnosis.

Intussusception

Intussusceptions involving the cecum or colon appear similar to those described earlier for the small bowel. Multiple concentric rings are seen on the transverse view, and a multilayered structure is seen on the longitudinal view. There is a variable amount of fluid accumulation proximal to the intussusception depending on the degree of obstruction. Ileocolic, cecocolic, and colocolic intussusceptions are the three types associated with the colon. An ileocolic intussusception is seen within the ascending and transverse colon, but it also may extend distally into the descending colon. A cecocolic intussusception is rather short and localized to the area of the cecum and proximal ascending colon. Colocolic intussusceptions involve the colon only. Intussusceptions are rather easy to diagnose despite the limitations of bowel gas and feces.

Wall Thickening

Inflammation, infection, ischemia, edema, hemorrhage, and neoplasia can produce colonic wall thickening. Ulceration or perforation can occur and the ultrasonographic findings are similar to those described previously for with small bowel lesions.[37]

Diffuse Wall Thickening

Inflammation generally produces mild, diffuse wall thickening similar to the small bowel (Figure 12-47). The wall layers are

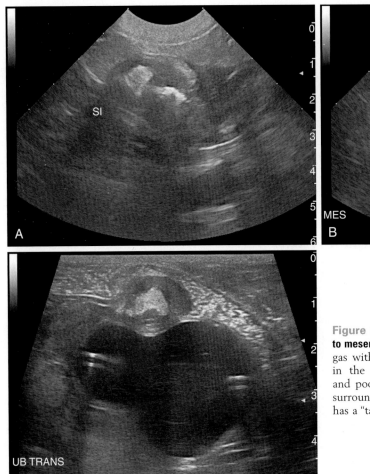

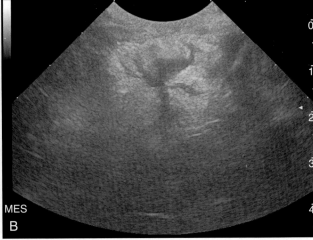

Figure 12-42 Adenocarcinoma of small intestine with metastasis to mesentery. **A,** Mass in small intestine. Note the hyperechoic gas within the lumen of the mass. Also note the poor detail in the surrounding peritoneum. **B,** Extremely hyperechoic and poor detail of the central abdomen. **C,** Multiple masses surround the urinary bladder. The mass in the central near field has a "target" appearance, with a hyperechoic central area.

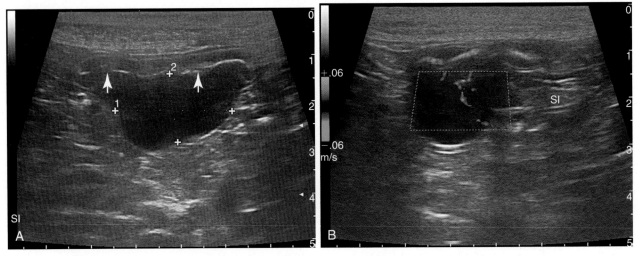

Figure 12-43 Leiomyoma of the small intestine in a 7-year-old dog. **A,** Hypoechoic, nearly anechoic eccentric mass in the small intestine is identified (2.61 × 1.50 cm between electronic cursors). The intestinal lumen is identified with arrows. **B,** Color Doppler image shows moderate blood flow within the mass. *SI,* Small intestine.

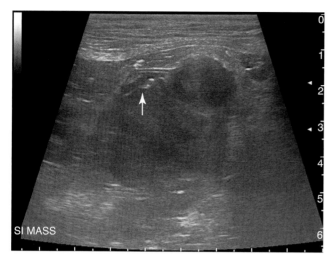

Figure 12-44 **Leiomyosarcoma of the small intestine in a 6-year-old dog.** The mass has a smooth but uneven margin, is somewhat lobulated, and is eccentric relative to the lumen. A tiny amount of intraluminal bowel gas is seen (*arrow*), and remnants of bowel wall layers are noted adjacent to the gas. Identification of intraluminal gas and the ability to follow the mass into normal intestine allows determination of bowel origin.

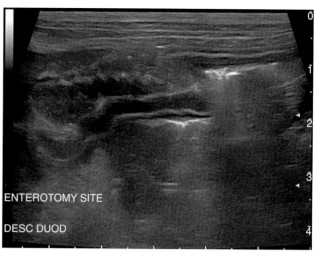

Figure 12-45 **Enterotomy site.** The near field duodenal wall is thickened and irregular secondary to an enterotomy 2 days prior. Corrugated appearance is a result of sutures.

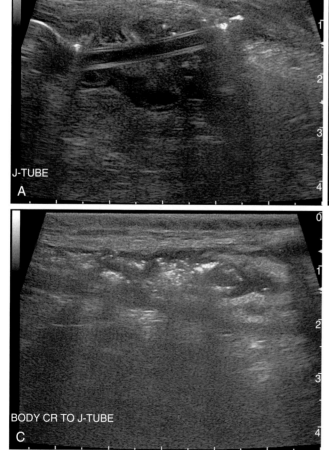

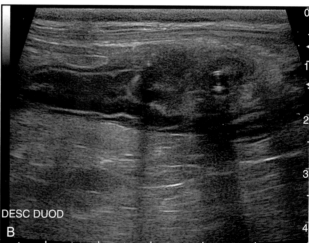

Figure 12-46 **Duodenal enterotomy J-tube placement shows focal thickening and loss of layering of the intestine. A,** The enterotomy tube can be seen as an anechoic tube with thin parallel walls, surrounded by focally thickened intestine. **B,** Same area as A, but with the tube now seen in cross section. **C,** Regional body wall and peritoneal inflammation from a J-tube enterotomy leakage.

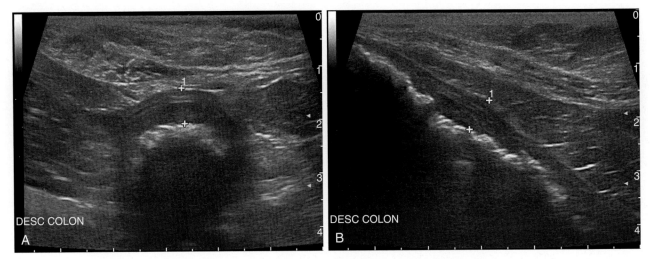

Figure 12-47 **Diffuse thickening in wall of descending colon in a 12-year-old dog. A,** Transverse image shows thickening of the near-field colonic wall (0.67 cm between electronic cursors). **B,** Sagittal image of wall thickening in the descending colon (0.66 cm between electronic cursors).

usually preserved, but may be altered or lost in severe cases. High-frequency endoscopic ultrasonography is the best way to evaluate colonic wall layers, because they are more difficult to identify than in the small intestine. Infectious, parasitic, ulcerative, granulomatous, lymphocytic-plasmacytic-eosinophilic disorders involving the cecum and colon have been described in the literature, but there are few reports detailing the ultrasonographic features of inflammatory diseases of the colon.[128]

Neoplasia can also produce diffuse, symmetric wall thickening in the cecum or colon. Lymphoma is the most likely tumor to cause this abnormality.

Focal Wall Thickening

Eccentric wall thickening or thickening associated with focal masses generally indicates neoplasia. The wall layers are usually lost and the appearance is similar to neoplasia in the small bowel. Carcinoma and lymphoma are commonly encountered tumors of the cecum and colon[44,111,129] (Figures 12-48 and 12-49). Carcinomas often cause annular thickening with obstruction of the colon similar to that in the small bowel.[130] Obstruction of the small bowel or colon were not mentioned as features of lymphosarcoma in two reports.[44,45] Other tumors such as leiomyosarcoma or leiomyoma of the cecum or colon also occur, but have lower incidence.[56,103] The features are likely similar to leiomyosarcomas and leiomyomas found in the small bowel, but no reports describing their sonographic appearance in the colon are available. Malignant histiocytosis with circumferential, asymmetric wall thickening has also been reported in the colon of a dog.[131] Mast cell tumors have been described at the ileocolic junction or colon in cats.[49,50] Additionally, hemangiosarcoma has been identified at the ileocolic junction, colon and rectum in cats, often causing luminal narrowing.[106,109]

Nonmalignant diseases such as histiocytic, granulomatous, and fungal colitis can also cause focal wall thickening or masses. Eosinophilic fibrosing fibroplasia has been reported in the cat at the ileocecocolic junction and in the colon.[60] Pythiosis, found in subtropical regions, is a water mold that causes multifocal pyogranulomatous infections of the stomach, small intestine, and colon.[61] In the colon, it most commonly induces focal wall thickening with loss of wall layers, although an eccentric colonic mural mass was identified in one dog.[61]

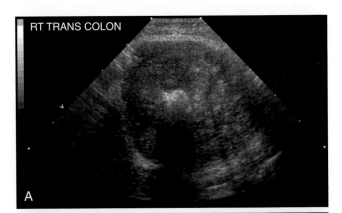

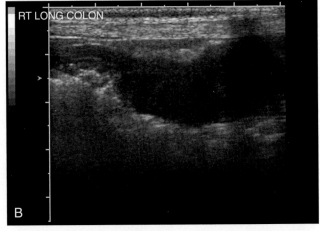

Figure 12-48 **Colonic mass in a dog. A,** Transverse image shows an extremely thickened colonic wall. The hyperechoic center represents the lumen. **B,** Sagittal image shows transition from mild thickening of the colon with preservation of wall layering on the left to marked hypoechoic thickening with complete loss of layering.

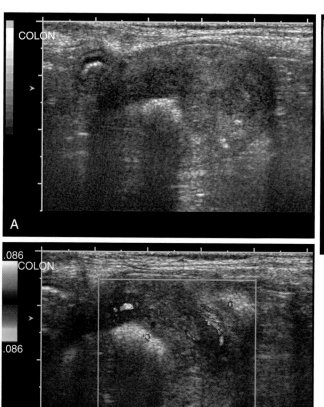

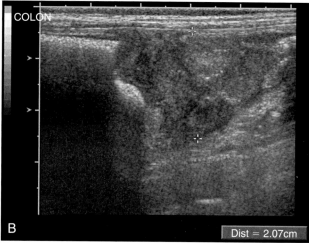

Figure 12-49 **Colonic mass in a dog. A,** Transverse image shows a markedly thickened colonic wall. A small intestinal loop is seen to the left of the image. **B,** Sagittal image shows abrupt transition from normal colon to markedly thickened colon (2.07 cm between electronic cursors), with loss of layering. **C,** Color Doppler image shows the colonic mass has a good blood supply.

REFERENCES

1. Gaschen L, Kircher P, Lang J. Endoscopic ultrasound instrumentation, applications in humans, and potential veterinary applications. *Vet Radiol Ultrasound* 2003;**44**:665–80.
2. Gaschen L, Kircher P, Wolfram K. Endoscopic ultrasound of the canine abdomen. *Vet Radiol Ultrasound* 2007;**48**:338–49.
3. Zerbey AL III, Lee MJ, Brugge WR, et al. Endoscopic sonography of the upper gastrointestinal tract and pancreas. *AJR Am J Roentgenol* 1996;**166**:45–50.
4. Miura T, Maruyama H, Sakai M, et al. Endoscopic findings on alimentary lymphoma in 7 dogs. *J Vet Med Sci* 2004;**66**:577–80.
5. Morita Y, Takiguchi M, Yasuda J, et al. Endoscopic ultrasonography of the pancreas in the dog. *Vet Radiol Ultrasound* 1998;**39**:552–6.
6. Morita Y, Takiguchi M, Yasuda J, et al. Endoscopic ultrasonographic findings of the pancreas after pancreatic duct ligation in the dog. *Vet Radiol Ultrasound* 1998;**39**:557–62.
7. Cho E, Nakajima M, Yasuda K, et al. Endoscopic ultrasonography in the diagnosis of colorectal cancer invasion. *Gastrointest Endosc* 1993;**39**:521–7.
8. Cho E, Mochizuki N, Ashihara T, et al. Endoscopic ultrasonography in the evaluation of inflammatory bowel disease. *Endoscopy* 1998;**30**(Suppl. 1):A94–6.
9. Nakazawa S. Recent advances in endoscopic ultrasonography. *J Gastroenterol* 2000;**35**:257–60.
10. Mallery S, Van Dam J. Current status of diagnostic and therapeutic endoscopic ultrasonography. *Radiol Clin North Am* 2001;**39**:449–63.
11. Frascio F, Giacosa A. Role of endoscopy in staging colorectal cancer. *Semin Surg Oncol* 2001;**20**:82–5.
12. Irisawa A, Bhutani MS. Cystic lymphangioma of the colon: endosonographic diagnosis with through-the-scope catheter miniprobe and determination of further management. Report of a case. *Dis Colon Rectum* 2001;**44**:1040–2.
13. Wilson SR. The gastrointestinal tract. In: Rumack CM, Wilson SR, Charboneau JW, editors. *Diagnostic ultrasound.* 3rd ed. St. Louis: Elsevier Mosby; 2005. p. 269–320.
14. O'Brien TR. Stomach. In: O'Brien TR, editor. *Radiographic Diagnosis of Abdominal Disorders of the Dog and Cat.* Philadelphia: WB Saunders; 1978. p. 204–78.
15. Penninck DG, Nyland TG, Fisher PE, et al. Ultrasonography of the normal canine gastrointestinal tract. *Vet Radiol Ultrasound* 1989;**30**:272–6.
16. Stander N, Wagner WM, Goddard A, et al. Normal canine pediatric gastrointestinal ultrasonography. *Vet Radiol Ultrasound* 2010;**51**:75–8.
17. Heng HG, Wrigley RH, Kraft SL, et al. Fat is responsible for an intramural radiolucency band in the feline stomach wall. *Vet Rad Ultrasound* 2005;**46**:54-6.

18. Newell SM, Graham JP, Roberts GD, et al. Sonography of the normal feline gastrointestinal tract. *Vet Radiol Ultrasound* 1999;**40**:40–3.

19. Goggin JM, Biller DS, Debey BM, et al. Ultrasonographic measurement of gastrointestinal wall thickness and the ultrasonographic appearance of the ileocolic region in healthy cats. *J Am Anim Hosp Assoc* 2000;**36**:224–8.

20. Penninck DG. Gastrointestinal tract. In: Nyland TG, Mattoon JS, editors. *Small animal diagnostic ultrasound*. 2nd ed. Philadelphia: WB Saunders; 2002. p. 207–30.

21. Etue SM, Penninck DG, Labato MA, et al. Ultrasonography of the normal feline pancreas and associated anatomic landmarks: a prospective study of 20 cats. *Vet Radiol Ultrasound* 2001;**42**:330–6.

22. Penninck DG, Nyland TG, Kerr LY, et al. Ultrasonographic evaluation of gastrointestinal diseases in small animals. *Vet Radiol Ultrasound* 1990;**31**:134–41.

23. Walter MC, Goldschmidt MH, Stone EA, et al. Chronic hypertrophic pyloric gastropathy as a cause of pyloric obstruction in the dog. *J Am Vet Med Assoc* 1985;**186**:157–61.

24. Sikes RI, Birchard S, Patnaik A, et al. Chronic hypertrophic pyloric gastropathy: a review of 16 cases. *Vet Radiol Ultrasound* 1986;**22**:99–104.

25. Bellenger CR, Maddison JE, MacPherson GC, et al. Chronic hypertrophic pyloric gastropathy in 14 dogs. *Aust Vet J* 1990;**67**:317–20.

26. Biller DS, Partington BP, Miyabayashi T, et al. Ultrasonographic appearance of chronic hypertrophic pyloric gastropathy in the dog. *Vet Radiol Ultrasound* 1994;**30**:30–3.

27. Tidwell AS, Penninck DG. Ultrasonography of gastrointestinal foreign bodies. *Vet Radiol Ultrasound* 1992;**33**:160–9.

28. Larson MM, Biller DS. Ultrasound of the gastrointestinal tract. *Vet Clin Small Anim* 2009;**39**:747–59.

29. Penninck D, Mitchell SL. Ultrasonographic detection of ingested and perforating wooden foreign bodies in four dogs. *J Am Vet Med Assoc* 2003;**223**:206–9, 196.

30. Hoffmann KL. Sonographic signs of gastroduodenal linear foreign body in 3 dogs. *Vet Radiol Ultrasound* 2003;**44**:466–9.

31. Kaser-Hotz B, Hauser B, Arnold P. Ultrasonographic findings in canine gastric neoplasia in 13 patients. *Vet Radiol Ultrasound* 1996;**37**:51–6.

32. Manczur F, Vörös K. Gastrointestinal ultrasonography of the dog: a review of 265 cases (1996-1998). *Acta Vet Hung* 2000;**48**:9–21.

33. Easton S. A retrospective study into the effects of operator experience on the accuracy of ultrasound in the diagnosis of gastric neoplasia in dogs. *Vet Radiol Ultrasound* 2001;**42**:47–50.

34. Webb C, Twedt DC. Canine gastritis. *Vet Clin North Am Small Anim Pract* 2003;**33**:969–85.

35. Penninck D, Matz M, Tidwell A. Ultrasonography of gastric ulceration in the dog. *Vet Radiol Ultrasound* 1997;**38**:308–12.

36. Mellanby RJ, Baines EA, Herrtage ME. Spontaneous pneumoperitoneum in two cats. *J Small Anim Pract* 2002;**43**:543–6.

37. Boysen SR, Tidwell AS, Penninck DG. Ultrasonographic findings in dogs and cats with gastrointestinal perforation. *Vet Radiol Ultrasound* 2003;**44**:556–64.

38. Lang LG, Greatting HH, Spaulding KA. Imaging diagnosis—gastric pneumatosis in a cat. *Vet Radiol Ultrasound* 2011;**52**:658–60.

39. Grooters AM, Miyabayashi T, Biller DS, et al. Sonographic appearance of uremic gastropathy in four dogs. *Vet Radiol Ultrasound* 1994;**35**:35–40.

40. Green RA, Gartrell CL. Gastrinoma: a retrospective study of four cases (1985-1995). *J Am Anim Hosp Assoc* 1997;**33**:524–7.

41. Lurye JC, Behrend EN. Endocrine tumors. *Vet Clin North Am Small Anim Pract* 2001;**31**:1083–110.

42. Fukushima R, Ichikawa K, Hirabayashi M, et al. A case of canine gastrinoma. *J Vet Med Sci* 2004;**66**:993–5.

43. Vergine M, Pozzo S, Pogliani E, et al. Common bile duct obstruction due to a duodenal gastrinoma in a dog. *Vet J* 2005;**170**:141–3.

44. Grooters AM, Biller DS, Ward H, et al. Ultrasonographic appearance of feline alimentary lymphoma. *Vet Radiol Ultrasound* 1994;**35**:468–72.

45. Penninck DG, Moore AS, Tidwell AS, et al. Ultrasonography of alimentary lymphosarcoma in the cat. *Vet Radiol Ultrasound* 1994;**35**:299–304.

46. Couto CG, Rutgers HC, Sherding RG, et al. Gastrointestinal lymphoma in 20 dogs: a retrospective study. *J Vet Intern Med* 1989;**3**:73–8.

47. Howard EB, Sawa TR, Nielsen SW, et al. Mastocytoma and gastroduodenal ulceration. Gastric and duodenal ulcers in dogs with mastocytoma. *Pathol Vet* 1969;**6**:146–58.

48. Allan GS, Watson AD, Duff BC, et al. Disseminated mastocytoma and mastocytemia in a dog. *J Am Vet Med Assoc* 1974;**165**:346–9.

49. Laurenson MP, Skorupski KA, Moore PF. Ultrasonography of intestinal mast cell tumors in the cat. *Vet Radiol Ultrasound* 2011;**52**:330–4.

50. Sato AF, Solano M. Ultrasonographic findings in abdominal mast cell disease: a retrospective study of 19 patients. *Vet Radiol Ultrasound* 2004;**45**:51–7.

51. Cruz-Arambulo R, Wrigley R, Powers B. Sonographic features of histiocytic neoplasms in the canine abdomen. *Vet Radiol Ultrasound* 2004;**45**:554–8.

52. Rivers BJ, Walter PA, Johnston GR, et al. Canine gastric neoplasia: utility of ultrasonography in diagnosis. *J Am Anim Hosp Assoc* 1997;**33**:144–55.

53. Lamb CR, Grierson J. Ultrasonographic appearance of primary gastric neoplasia in 21 dogs. *J Small Anim Pract* 1999;**40**:211–15.

54. Gualtieri M, Monzeglio MG, Scanziani E. Gastric neoplasia. *Vet Clin North Am Small Anim Pract* 1999;**29**:415–40.

55. Penninck DG, Moore AS, Gliatto J. Ultrasonography of canine gastric epithelial neoplasia. *Vet Radiol Ultrasound* 1998;**39**:342–8.

56. Beck C, Slocombe RF, O'Neill T, et al. The use of ultrasound in the investigation of gastric carcinoma in a dog. *Aust Vet J* 2001;**79**:332–4.

57. Kapatkin AS, Mullen HS, Matthiesen DT, et al. Leiomyosarcoma in dogs: 44 cases (1983-1988). *J Am Vet Med Assoc* 1992;**201**:1077–9.

58. Beck JA, Simpson DS. Surgical treatment of gastric leiomyoma in a dog. *Aust Vet J* 1999;**77**:161–3.

59. Diana A, Penninck DG, Keating JH. Ultrasonographic appearance of canine gastric polyps. *Vet Radiol Ultrasound* 2009;**50**:201–4.

60. Craig LE, Hardam EE, Hertzke DM, et al. Feline gastrointestinal eosinophilic sclerosing fibroplasia. *Vet Pathol* 2009;**46**:63–9.

61. Graham JP, Newell SM, Roberts GD, et al. Ultrasonographic features of canine gastrointestinal pythiosis. *Vet Radiol Ultrasound* 2000;**41**:273–7.

62. Leblanc CJ, Echandi RL, Moore RR, et al. Hypercalcemia associated with gastric pythiosis in a dog. *Vet Clin Pathol* 2008;**37**:115–20.

63. Wacker CA, Weber UT, Tanno F, et al. Ultrasonographic evaluation of adhesions induced by incisional gastropexy in 16 dogs. *J Small Anim Pract* 1998;**39**:379–84.

64. Moon ML, Biller DS, Armbrust LJ. Ultrasonographic appearance and etiology of corrugated small intestine. *Vet Radiol Ultrasound* 2003;**44**:199–203.

65. Saunders HM. Ultrasonography of the pancreas. *Probl Vet Med* 1991;**3**:583–603.

66. Kull PA, Hess RS, Craig LE, et al. Clinical, clinicopathologic, radiographic, and ultrasonographic characteristics of intestinal lymphangiectasia in dogs: 17 cases (1996-1998). *J Am Vet Med Assoc* 2001;**219**:197–202.

67. Yam PS, Johnson VS, Martineau HM, et al. Multicentric lymphoma with intestinal involvement in a dog. *Vet Radiol Ultrasound* 2002;**43**:138–43.

68. Swift I. Ultrasonographic features of intestinal entrapment in dogs. *Vet Radiol Ultrasound* 2009;**50**:205–7.

69. Sykes JE, Marks SL, Mapes S. Salmon poisoning disease in dogs: 29 cases. *J Vet Intern Med* 2010;**24**:504–13.

70. Stander N, Wagner WM, Goddard A, et al. Ultrasonographic appearance of canine parvoviral enteritis in puppies. *Vet Rad Ultrasound* 2010;**51**:69–74.

71. Garcia DA, Froes TR, Vilani RG, et al. Ultrasonography of small intestinal obstructions: a contemporary approach. *J Small Anim Prac* 2011;**52**:484–90.

72. Maczur F, Vörös K, Vrabély T, et al. Sonographic diagnosis of intestinal obstruction in the dog. *Acta Vet Hung* 1998;**46**:35–45.

73. Pastore GE, Lamb CR, Lipscomb V. Comparison of the results of abdominal ultrasonography and exploratory laparotomy in the dog and cat. *J Am Anim Hosp Assoc* 2007;**43**:264–9.

74. Sharma A, Thompson MS, Scrivani PV, et al. Comparison of radiography and ultrasonography for diagnosing small-intestinal mechanical obstruction in vomiting dogs. *Vet Radiol Ultrasound* 2011;**52**:248–55.

75. Tyrrell D, Beck C. Survey of the use of radiography vs. ultrasonography in the investigation of gastrointestinal foreign bodies in small animals. *Vet Radiol Ultrasound* 2006;**47**:404–8.

76. Rallis TS, Papazoglou LG, Adamama-Moraitou KK, et al. Acute enteritis or gastroenteritis in young dogs as a predisposing factor for intestinal intussusception: a retrospective study. *J Vet Med A Physiol Pathol Clin Med* 2000;**47**:507–11.

77. Lamb CR, Mantis P. Ultrasonographic features of intestinal intussusception in 10 dogs. *J Small Anim Pract* 1998;**39**:437–41.

78. Patsikas MN, Papazoglou LG, Papaioannou NG, et al. Ultrasonographic findings of intestinal intussusception in seven cats. *J Feline Med Surg* 2003;**5**:335–43.

79. Watson PJ. Gastroduodenal intussusception in a young dog. *J Small Anim Pract* 1997;**38**:163–7.

80. Lee H, Yeon S, Lee H, et al. Ultrasonographic diagnosis—pylorogastric intussusception in a dog. *Vet Radiol Ultrasound* 2005;**46**:317–18.

81. Patsikas MN, Jakovljevic S, Moustardas N, et al. Ultrasonographic signs of intestinal intussusception associated with acute enteritis or gastroenteritis in 19 young dogs. *J Am Anim Hosp Assoc* 2003;**39**:57–66.

82. Patsikas MN, Papazoglou LG, Adamama-Moraitou KK. Spontaneous reduction of intestinal intussusception in five young dogs. *J Am Anim Hosp Assoc* 2008;**44**:41–7.

83. Patsikas MN, Papazoglou LG, Papaioannou NG, et al. Normal and abnormal ultrasonographic findings that mimic small intestinal intussusception in the dog. *J Am Anim Hosp Assoc* 2004;**40**:147–51.

84. Penninck D, Smyers B, Webster CR, et al. Diagnostic value of ultrasonography in differentiating enteritis from intestinal neoplasia in dogs. *Vet Radiol Ultrasound* 2003;**44**:570–5.

85. Rudorf H, van Schaik G, O'Brien RT, et al. Ultrasonographic evaluation of the thickness of the small intestinal wall in dogs with inflammatory bowel disease. *J Small Anim Pract* 2005;**46**:322–6.

86. Gaschen L, Kirscher P, Stüssi A, et al. Comparison of ultrasonographic findings with clinical activity index (CIBDAI) and diagnosis in dogs with chronic enteropathies. *Vet Radiol Ultrasound* 2008;**49**:56–64.

87. Penninck DG, Webster CR, Keating JH. The sonographic appearance of intestinal mucosal fibrosis in cats. *Vet Rad Ultrasound* 2010;**51**:458–61.

88. Gaschen L. Ultrasonography of small intestinal inflammatory and neoplastic disease in dogs and cats. *Vet Clin Small Anim* 2011;**41**:329–44.

89. Crystal MA, Penninck DG, Matz ME, et al. Use of ultrasound-guided fine-needle aspiration biopsy and automated core biopsy for the diagnosis of gastrointestinal diseases in small animals. *Vet Radiol Ultrasound* 1993;**34**:438–44.

90. Louvet A, Denis B. Ultrasonographic diagnosis—small bowel lymphangiectasia in a dog. *Vet Radiol Ultrasound* 2004;**45**:565–7.

91. Sutherland-Smith J, Penninck DG, Keating JH, et al. Ultrasonographic intestinal hyperechoic mucosal striations in dogs are associated with lacteal dilation. *Vet Radiol Ultrasound* 2007;**48**:51–7.

92. Fabrick C, Bugbee A, Fosgate G. Clinical features and outcome of *Heterobilharzia americana* infection in dogs. *J Vet Intern Med* 2010;**24**:140–4.

93. Kvitko-White HL, Sayre RS, Corapi WV, et al. Imaging diagnosis—*Heterobilharzia americana* infection in a dog. *Vet Radiol Ultrasound* 2011;**52**:538–41.

94. Diana A, Pietra M, Guglielmini C, et al. Ultrasonographic and pathologic features of intestinal smooth muscle hypertrophy in four cats. *Vet Radiol Ultrasound* 2003;**44**:566–9.

95. Baez JL, Hendrick MJ, Walker LM, et al. Radiographic, ultrasonographic, and endoscopic findings in cats with inflammatory bowel disease of the stomach and small intestine: 33 cases (1990-1997). *J Am Vet Med Assoc* 1999;**215**:349–54.

96. Evans SE, Bonczynski JJ, Broussard JD, et al. Comparison of endoscopic and full-thickness biopsy specimens for diagnosis of inflammatory bowel disease and alimentary tract lymphoma in cats. *J Am Vet Med Assoc* 2006;**229**:1447–50.

97. Mavropoulou A, Grandi G, Calvi L, et al. Disseminated histoplasmosis in a cat in Europe. *J Small Anim Pract* 2010;**51**:176–80.

98. Zwingenberger AL, Marks SL, Baker TW, et al. Ultrasonographic evaluation of the muscularis propria in cats with diffuse small intestinal lymphoma or inflammatory bowel disease. *J Vet Intern Med* 2010;**24**:289–92.

99. Geiger T. Alimentary lymphoma in cats and dogs. *Vet Clin Small Anim* 2011;**41**:419–32.

100. Penninck DG. Characterization of gastrointestinal tumors. *Vet Clin North Am Small Anim Pract* 1998;**28**:777–97.

101. Patnaik AK, Hurvitz AI, Johnson GF. Canine gastrointestinal neoplasms. *Vet Pathol* 1977;**14**:547–55.

102. Birchard SJ, Couto CG, Johnson S. Nonlymphoid intestinal neoplasia in 32 dogs and 14 cats. *J Am Anim Hosp Assoc* 1986;**22**:533–7.

103. Gibbs C, Pearson H. Localized tumors of the canine small intestine: a report of twenty cases. *J Small Anim Pract* 1986;**27**:507–19.

104. Myers NC, Penninck DG. Ultrasonographic diagnosis of gastrointestinal smooth muscle tumors in the dog. *Vet Radiol Ultrasound* 1994;**35**:391–7.

105. Aita N, Iso H, Uchida K. Hemangioma of the ileum in a dog. *J Vet Med Sci* 2010;**72**:1071–3.

106. Culp WTN, Drobatz KH, Glassman MM, et al. Feline visceral hemangiosarcoma. *J Vet Intern Med* 2008;**22**:148–52.

107. Monteiro CB, O'Brien RT. A retrospective study on the sonographic findings of abdominal carcinomatosis in 14 cats. *Vet Rad Ultrasound* 2004;**45**:559–64.

108. Rivers BJ, Walter PA, Feeney DA, et al. Ultrasonographic features of intestinal adenocarcinoma in five cats. *Vet Radiol Ultrasound* 1997;**38**:300–6.

109. Sharpe A, Canon MJ, Lucke VM, et al. Intestinal haemangiosarcoma in the cat: clinical and pathological features of four cases. *J Small Anim Pract* 2000;**41**:411–15.

110. MacDonald J, Mullen H, Moroff S. Adenomatous polyps of the duodenum in cats: 18 cases (1985-1990). *J Am Vet Med Assoc* 1993;**202**:647–51.

111. Paoloni MC, Penninck DG, Moore AS. Ultrasonographic and clinicopathologic findings in 21 dogs with intestinal adenocarcinoma. *Vet Radiol Ultrasound* 2002;**43**:562–7.

112. Baldi A, Colloca E. Spugnini EP. Lomustine for the treatment of gastrointestinal mast cell tumour in a dog. *J Small Anim Pract* 2006;**47**:465–7.

113. Takahashi T, Kadosawa T, Nagase M, et al. Visceral mast cell tumors in dogs: 10 cases (1982-1997). *J Am Vet Med Assoc* 2000;**216**:222–6.

114. Wallack ST, Hornof WJ, Herrgesell EJ. Ultrasonographic diagnosis – small bowel infarction in a cat. *Vet Rad Ultrasound* 2003;**44**:81–5.

115. Papazoglou LG, Tontis D, Loukopoulos P, et al. Foreign body-associated intestinal pyogranuloma resulting in intestinal obstruction in four dogs. *Vet Rec* 2010;**166**:494–7.

116. Hazell KLA, Reeves MP, Swift IM. Small intestinal ganglioneuromatosis in a dog. *Aust Vet J* 2011;**89**:15–18.

117. Matthews AR, Penninck DG, Webster CRL. Postoperative ultrasonographic appearance of uncomplicated enterotomy or enterectomy sites in dogs. *Vet Radiol Ultrasound* 2008;**49**:477–83.

118. Mareschal A, Penninck D, Webster CRL. Ultrasonographic assessment of long-term enterectomy sites in dogs. *Vet Radiol Ultrasound* 2010;**51**:652–5.

119. An YJ, Lee H, Chang D, et al. Application of pulsed Doppler ultrasound for the evaluation of small intestinal motility in dogs. *J Vet Sci* 2001;**2**:71–4.

120. Patsikas MN, Papazoglou LG, Jakovljevic S, et al. Color Doppler ultrasonography in prediction of the reducibility of intussuscepted bowel in 15 young dogs. *Vet Radiol Ultrasound* 2005;**46**:313–16.

121. Teefey SA, Roarke MC, Brink JA, et al. Bowel wall thickening: differentiation of inflammation from ischemia with color Doppler and duplex US. *Radiology* 1996;**198**:547–51.

122. Kircher PR, Spaulding KA, Vaden S, et al. Doppler ultrasonographic evaluation of gastrointestinal hemodynamics in food hypersensitivities: a canine model. *J Vet Intern Med* 2004;**18**:605–11.

123. Gaschen L, Kircher P, Lang J, et al. Pattern recognition and feature extraction of canine celiac and cranial mesenteric arterial waveforms: normal versus chronic enteropathy—a pilot study. *Vet J* 2005;**169**:242–50.

124. Gaschen L, Kircher P. Two-dimensional grayscale ultrasound and spectral Doppler waveform evaluation of dogs with chronic enteropathies. *Clin Tech Small Anim Pract* 2007;**22**:122–7.

125. Kircher P, Lang J, Blum J, et al. Influence of food composition on splanchnic blood flow during digestion in unsedated normal dogs: a Doppler study. *Vet J* 2003;**166**:265–72.

126. Jimenez DA, O'Brien RT, Wallace JD, et al. Intraoperative contrast-enhanced ultrasonography of normal canine jejunum. *Vet Radiol Ultrasound* 2011;**52**:196–200.

127. Arthur EG, Fox DB, Essman SC, et al. Surgical treatment of noncommunicating duplication of the colon in a dog. *J Am Vet Med Assoc* 2003;**223**:210–14, 196.

128. Brellou GD, Kleinschmidt S, Meneses F, et al. Eosinophilic granulomatous gastroenterocolitis and hepatitis in a 1-year-old male Siberian Husky. *Vet Pathol* 2006;**43**:1022–5.

129. Slawienski MJ, Mauldin GE, Mauldin GN, et al. Malignant colonic neoplasia in cats: 46 cases (1990-1996). *J Am Vet Med Assoc* 1997;**211**:878–81.

130. Hume DZ, Solomon JA, Weisse CW. Palliative use of a stent for colonic obstruction caused by adenocarcinoma in two cats. *J Am Vet Med Assoc* 2006;**228**:392–6.

131. Ramirez S, Douglass JP, Robertson ID. Ultrasonographic features of canine abdominal malignant histiocytosis. *Vet Radiol Ultrasound* 2002;**43**:167–70.

CHAPTER 13

Peritoneal Fluid, Lymph Nodes, Masses, Peritoneal Cavity, Great Vessel Thrombosis, and Focused Examinations

William R. Widmer • John S. Mattoon • Thomas G. Nyland

This chapter describes the ultrasonographic appearance of peritoneal fluid, lymphadenopathy, masses not originating from specific organs, abnormal mesentery, free peritoneal air, and thrombosis of the peritoneal aorta and caudal vena cava. Focused sonographic examinations of the abdomen are also described. Pathologic changes of specific organs and associated vascular structures are covered in dedicated chapters.

SCANNING TECHNIQUE

The majority of peritoneal sonograms are performed with the patient in dorsal recumbency. The ventral peritoneal hair coat should be clipped to allow good contact of the transducer with the skin when it is coupled with acoustic gel. Patients may also be scanned in right or left lateral recumbency as well as in the standing position (see Chapter 4). The highest frequency transducer allowing sufficient field-of-view depth is used to maximize image resolution. A 7.5-MHz or higher frequency transducer is preferred for cats and small to medium-sized dogs. A 5.0-MHz or lower frequency transducer may be required for larger patients. Transducers with a small footprint such as those with a curved array scan head are recommended to minimize effects of intestinal gas on the incident ultrasound beam.

PERITONEAL FLUID

Intraperitoneal (free peritoneal) fluid is detected by the presence of anechoic areas separating the various intraperitoneal structures. Ultrasonography is more sensitive than survey radiography in detecting free peritoneal fluid,[1] and as little as 2 mL of free fluid per pound of body weight can be identified. Dorsal or sternal recumbency with the head and body elevated are the most helpful positions for detecting a small amount of peritoneal fluid, which is appears as an angular anechoic or hypoechoic region near the vertex of the urinary bladder (Figure 13-1) or dorsal (far field) to it (Figure 13-2). Small amounts of free fluid can also be detected between the hepatic lobes, between the diaphragm and liver, between the stomach and liver, and between the body wall and spleen (Figure 13-3). Peritoneal fluid can also be found between the gallbladder and the liver, where it can mimic gallbladder wall thickening (Figures 13-4 and 13-5). Small amounts of peritoneal fluid are best identified with high quality ultrasound equipment featuring high frequency transducers and high contrast resolution.

Moderate to severe accumulation of peritoneal fluid is easily recognized by the appearance of intraperitoneal organs separated by large anechoic spaces (Figures 13-6 to 13-12). The presence of peritoneal fluid, especially large amounts, greatly enhances the visualization of various abdominal organs. Intraabdominal organs become easier to identify and assess because they are surrounded by fluid rather than mesenteric fat. In particular, the serosal surfaces become readily visible. However, with large fluid accumulations, increased depth is required to visualize organs because the abdominal cavity has an increased cross-sectional area caused by fluid distention (see Figure 13-9). The small intestine will appear to be floating because it is suspended within fluid (see Figure 13-12). The pancreas, ovaries, uterus, and lymph nodes can be easily visualized, as can other structures normally difficult to identify. The omentum and mesentery are readily apparent as echogenic tissues surrounding the intestines and may also appear to be floating within the fluid (Figure 13-13). Vascular structures are also easily detected. Whenever there is a large amount of free fluid, the intraabdominal organs appear more echoic than they would without the presence of fluid. This is due to nonattenuation of the ultrasound beam as it passes through the fluid (through transmission, distal acoustic enhancement). Thus the sonographer must use caution when ascribing a perceived increase in echogenicity to a particular organ when it is surrounded by fluid.

Although the typical presentation of ascites is generalized fluid accumulation within the abdomen, focal areas of fluid collection may be detected when regional disease is present. An example of this is peritoneal fluid within the right cranial quadrant secondary to pancreatitis (see Figure 13-36). In this instance, fluid may be seen surrounding the duodenum, separating the right kidney from the caudate liver lobe or pancreas and adjacent mesenteric fat, or it may be found between the stomach and the liver. Other examples of regional peritoneal effusion include cholecystitis and acute nephrosis.

Ultrasound can give the sonographer some indication of the physical characteristics of the peritoneal fluid, but *it is not a reliable test to differentiate types of effusion* (Figure 13-14). In addition to variations and similarities in appearance between classifications of peritoneal fluid (transudate, modified transudate, exudate, hemorrhage), ultrasound machine control settings can greatly alter the appearance of fluid (Figure 13-15).

A transudate or a modified transudate usually appears anechoic, without any evidence of suspended echogenicities. Intraperitoneal hemorrhage may appear echogenic, with multiple echoes from red blood cells within the fluid. Such echoes often have a swirling movement. Chronic inflammatory transudates and neoplastic transudates (including carcinomatosis) can have multifocal echogenicities from cells and fibrin. Evaluation of the serosal surfaces of the intraabdominal organs and the peritoneum may provide clues as to the cause of the fluid. Patients with carcinomatosis or chronic peritonitis may show

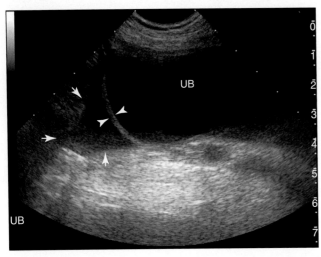

Figure 13-1 A small amount of nearly anechoic peritoneal fluid (between arrows) is present cranial to the urinary bladder (*UB*). Note the normal, thin appearance of the echogenic bladder wall (between arrowheads).

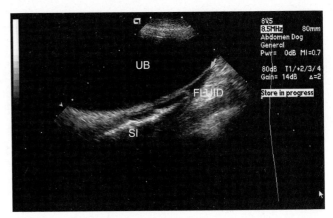

Figure 13-2 Small amount of peritoneal fluid accumulation in a dog. A small amount of fluid (*arrow*) is seen as a thin triangular anechoic area adjacent to the dorsal surface of the urinary bladder (*UB*) and a small intestinal loop (*SI*). The fluid was a transudate.

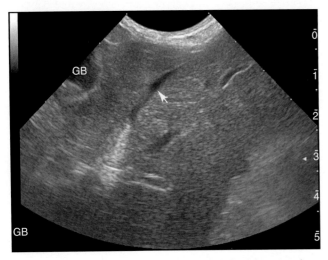

Figure 13-3 A small amount of peritoneal fluid between liver lobes is present (*arrow*). *GB*, Gallbladder. The fluid was a transudate.

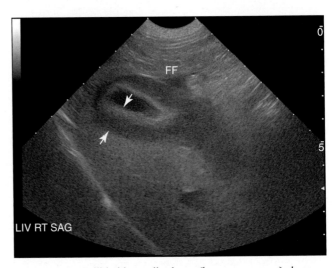

Figure 13-4 Gallbladder wall edema (between arrows) that can mimic perigallbladder peritoneal fluid. A hyperechoic inner surface of the gallbladder is surrounded by a thickened hypoechoic wall. The small amount of bile present is anechoic. Peritoneal fluid (*FF*) is seen as a small triangular anechoic area adjacent to the gallbladder in the near field.

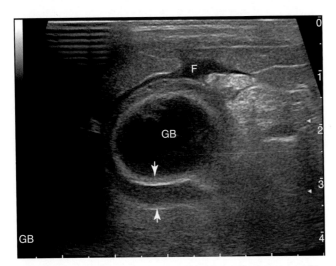

Figure 13-5 Peritoneal fluid and gallbladder wall edema caused by fluid overload in a dog An area of anechoic peritoneal fluid (*F*) is present, with a thin rim adjacent to the gallbladder wall. The gallbladder (*GB*) wall (between arrows) is very thick, with a hyperechoic mucosal surface and a hypoechoic outer wall.

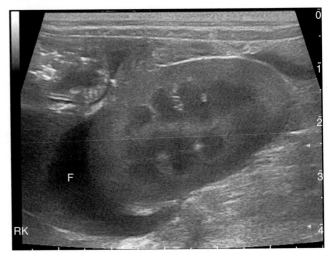

Figure 13-6 Anechoic peritoneal fluid (*F*) separating the right kidney from the liver. The fluid was an exudate from a ruptured duodenal ulcer.

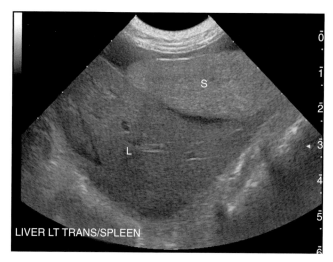

Figure 13-7 Anechoic exudate is seen in the near field and between the liver (*L*) and spleen (*S*) in this dog with septic peritonitis.

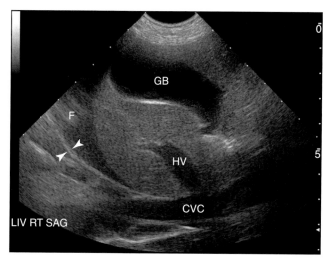

Figure 13-8 Peritoneal fluid is present cranial to the liver in this dog with right-sided heart failure. The diaphragm is seen as a thin echogenic curvilinear structure (between arrowheads). A distended hepatic vein (*HV*) is seen entering the caudal vena cava (*CVC*). *F*, Peritoneal fluid; *GB*, gallbladder. There is also pleural fluid present cranial to the diaphragm.

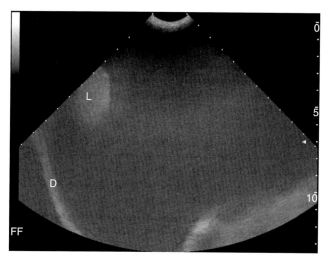

Figure 13-9 Massive peritoneal fluid accumulation in a dog with lymphangiectasia. The character of the fluid is difficult to determine. It appears to be composed of tiny echogenic specks, but this must be differentiated from artifact and is very dependent on gain settings. *L*, Liver. Pleural fluid is also present to the left of the diaphragm (*D*).

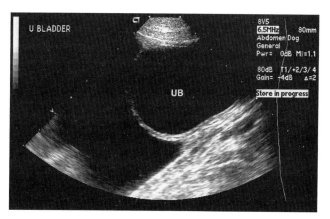

Figure 13-10 Severe peritoneal fluid accumulation in a dog. Anechoic transudate surrounds the urinary bladder (*UB*) secondary to an aortic thrombus. The thin, layered echogenic bladder wall is easily seen because of fluid surrounding the serosal surface and anechoic urine within this normal, moderately distended urinary bladder.

roughened, irregular serosal surfaces. Nodular lesions can be seen along peritoneal surfaces with carcinomatosis (Figure 13-16). With chronic peritoneal disease, fibrinous tags can often be seen floating within the fluid because of the mechanical effects of chronic effusion (see Figure 13-13). Although the previous discussion implies ultrasonographic interpretation may provide some insight regarding classification of peritoneal effusion, abdominocentesis and fluid analysis are mandatory for accurate evaluation of peritoneal fluid. Some transudates appear echogenic, whereas some exudates and hemorrhage may appear anechoic (see Figure 13-14; see also Chapter 7, Figure 7-14).

Retroperitoneal fluid can be easily detected with ultrasound examination and is typified by focal, crescent-shaped anechoic areas surrounding the kidneys. Perinephric cysts are a classic example this type of fluid accumulation. Retroperitoneal fluid may be seen secondary to renal or ureteral trauma

or other disease processes involving the retroperitoneal space, such as abscess formation or hemorrhage (Figures 13-17 and 13-18). Retroperitoneal fluid and peritoneal fluid are often present in cases of ethylene glycol toxicity. In some instances retroperitoneal fluid may be difficult to distinguish from peritoneal fluid. Evaluation of the abdomen from various scan planes for the signs of free peritoneal fluid may be helpful, because peritoneal fluid moves to different areas whereas retroperitoneal fluid will not.

The presence of peritoneal fluid should prompt the sonographer to carefully examine the peritoneal organs for a potential cause of the fluid. Common causes of hemorrhagic effusions are splenic and liver tumors. However, the sonographer should be aware that bleeding from parenchymal tumors is due to leakage with a low flow rate that will not be seen with Doppler interrogation. Transudates may be secondary to elevated central venous pressure and right-sided heart failure,

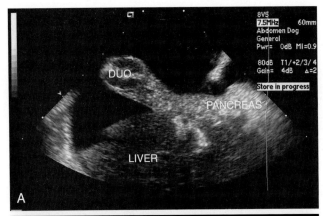

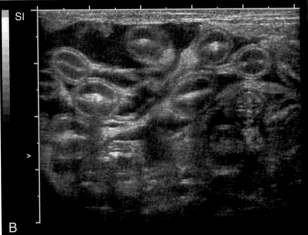

Figure 13-11 Severe peritoneal fluid accumulation. A, Anechoic fluid surrounds the duodenum (*DUO*), seen in transverse section. The right lobe of the pancreas is seen as a homogeneous, coarsely echogenic structure in the mesoduodenum. The dorsal portion of the liver is in the far field. **B,** Multiple segments of small intestine are seen in cross section surrounded by anechoic fluid.

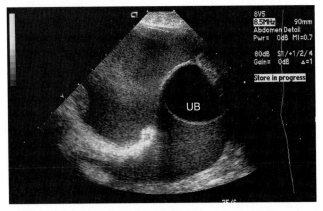

Figure 13-12 Massive peritoneal fluid in a dog. Echogenic fluid contrasts nicely with the anechoic urine within the bladder (*UB*). The serosal surface of the ventral urinary bladder wall is irregular and echogenic. A markedly echogenic small intestinal loop and mesentery are present in the far field. Note the acoustic shadow edge (refraction) artifact created by the apex of the urinary bladder.

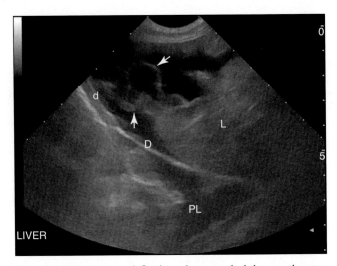

Figure 13-13 Peritoneal fluid in the cranial abdomen showing the presence of wavy, linear structures, felt to omentum or fibrin strands (*arrows*). Their presence makes the anechoic fluid appear loculated. This image shows both the tendinous (*D*) and muscular portion (*d*) of the diaphragm. Pleural fluid (*PL*) is also present. *L*, Liver.

in which case an enlarged caudal vena cava and distended hepatic veins may be recognized (see Figure 13-8). Liver disease may also cause a transudate or modified transudate when hypoproteinemia, portal hypertension, or intraparenchymal lesions are present. As stated previously, a definitive diagnosis of the type of fluid requires aspiration for analysis.

INTRAPERITONEAL LYMPHADENOPATHY

Accurate evaluation of the intraabdominal lymph nodes requires a good understanding of the location of the various abdominal lymphocenters and their normal size, shape, and variations in echotexture.[2-4] Abdominal lymph nodes can be classified by location along the lumbar spine as parietal, including lumbar, aortic, medial iliac, hypogastric, sacral, and deep inguinal; and visceral, which serve specific organs. The reader is referred to Chapter 4 for a description of normal appearance and scanning technique. Lymphadenopathy is characterized by enlarged lymph nodes that are usually homogeneous, hypoechoic, and smoothly marginated.[5] Multiple nodes are frequently affected (Figures 13-19 to 13-21), and a thin hyperechoic capsule is often present. With nodal enlargement acoustic enhancement is commonly encountered, which is an unusual finding in solid organs (Figure 13-22). Because lymph nodes can be hypoechoic to nearly anechoic, they must be differentiated from cystic or fluid-filled structures (Figure 13-23). Sometimes lymph nodes can become cystic (Figure 13-24). As the lymph nodes become larger, they may become distorted, have irregular margins, and develop a heterogeneous echotexture (Figure 13-25). In addition, lymph nodes can occasionally have a "target" lesion or bull's-eye appearance. The hyperechoic central area of the gland is surrounded by a hypoechoic margin (Figure 13-26).

Ultrasonic differentiation between benign and neoplastic lymph nodes is problematic because criteria such as size, echotexture, and shape may be similar.[6-8] In addition, the appearance of abdominal lymph nodes varies considerably in asymptomatic dogs and cats. For instance, normal canine jejunal lymph nodes are the largest of the intraabdominal nodes and have age-related variable echotexture and size. In

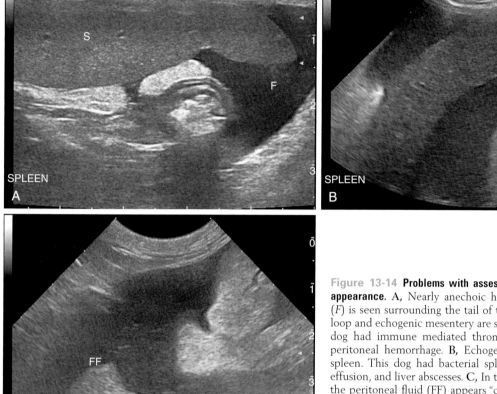

Figure 13-14 **Problems with assessing fluid type by ultrasound appearance. A,** Nearly anechoic hemorrhagic peritoneal fluid (*F*) is seen surrounding the tail of the spleen (*S*). An intestinal loop and echogenic mesentery are seen deep to the spleen. This dog had immune mediated thrombocytopenia and resultant peritoneal hemorrhage. **B,** Echogenic exudate surrounds the spleen. This dog had bacterial splenitis, exudative peritoneal effusion, and liver abscesses. **C,** In this example of a transudate, the peritoneal fluid (FF) appears "cellular."

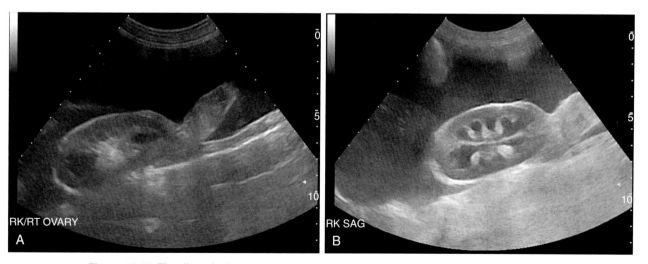

Figure 13-15 **The effect of gain settings on the appearance of peritoneal fluid. A,** The peritoneal fluid has an anechoic appearance, seen surrounding the right kidney and right ovary. **B,** The gain has been increased in this example, and the peritoneal fluid has become more echogenic. Note the thick, irregular surface of the right kidney in each view. This was a chronic transudate from right-sided heart failure.

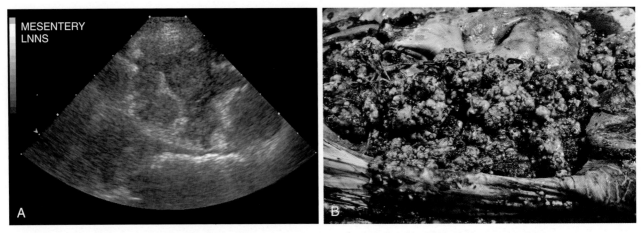

Figure 13-16 Carcinomatosis. A, Nodules are seen throughout the abdominal cavity. **B,** Gross specimen of carcinomatosis. (Courtesy of Washington State University College of Veterinary Medicine, Washington Animal Disease Diagnostic Laboratory, Pullman, WA.)

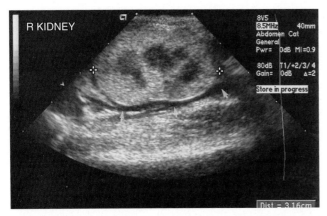

Figure 13-17 A thin rim of anechoic retroperitoneal fluid (*arrows*) surrounds the right kidney in a cat. The kidney in this older cat is smaller than expected (3.16 cm between electronic cursors), but creatinine and blood urea nitrogen concentrations were normal.

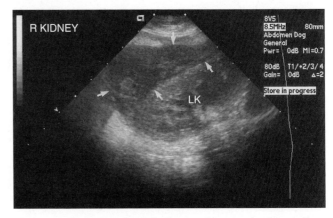

Figure 13-18 Retroperitoneal abscess. A triangular hypoechoic, slightly heterogeneous area of abscess formation (*arrows*) surrounds an abnormal left kidney (*LK*).

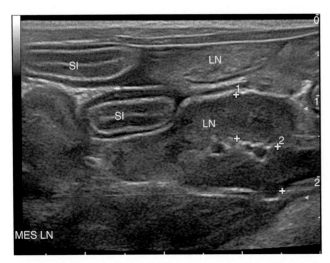

Figure 13-19 Mesenteric lymph nodes in a 15-year-old cat with a 5-week history of small bowel diarrhea. The mesenteric lymph nodes (*LN*) are seen as homogeneous, elongated structures within the mesentery. Small intestines (*SI*) are seen immediately adjacent to the lymph nodes. Though striking in appearance and readily identified in this thin cat, fine needle aspirates yielded only lymph node hyperplasia. Electronic cursors indicate their small size (0.54 and 0.55 cm in thickness).

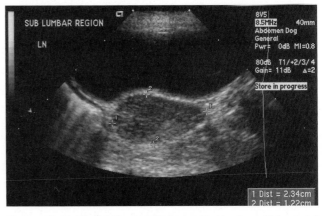

Figure 13-20 Medial iliac lymphadenopathy in a dog with bacterial prostatitis. The node is moderately enlarged (between electronic cursors) and is misshapen and swollen.

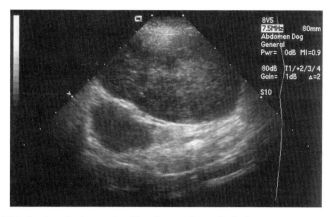

Figure 13-21 Massive lymphadenopathy. Two hypoechoic, fairly homogeneous peritoneal lymph nodes in a dog with malignant histiocytosis.

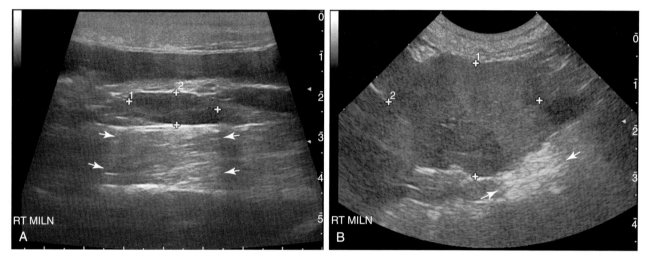

Figure 13-22 Acoustic enhancement with lymph node enlargement. A, This mildly enlarged, homogeneous, and hypoechoic medial iliac lymph node (*RT MILN;* between electronic cursors, 2.24 × 0.80 cm) displays distal acoustic enhancement (between arrows). This dog had multicentric lymphoma including this medial iliac lymph node. **B,** This very enlarged, fairly homogenous, and mildly irregularly shaped right medial iliac lymph node (*RT MILN;* between electronic cursors, 2.25 × 3.45 cm) displays acoustic enhancement (between arrows). This lymph node enlargement was secondary to metastasis from an anal gland carcinoma.

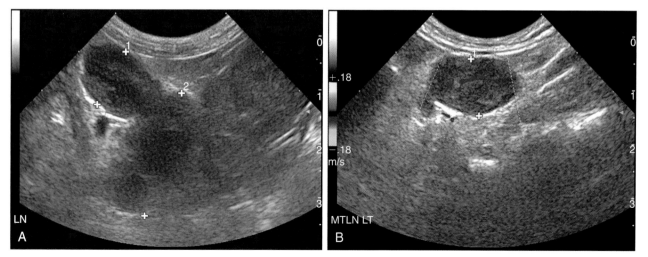

Figure 13-23 Hypoechoic lymph nodes can be distinguished from cystic structures using Doppler analysis. A, Collection of enlarged, hypoechoic, lobulated mesenteric lymph nodes (between electronic cursors, 1.12 × 2.38 cm). **B,** Color Doppler image of an adjacent lymph node (1.07 cm between electronic cursors) shows central blood flow. This patient had multicentric lymphoma.

57 asymptomatic dogs, median maximum diameter (width) was 7.5 mm (range, 2.6 to 14.7 mm), and dogs younger than 6 years had larger lymph nodes that were more heterogeneous and less uniform than nodes of dogs older than 6 years.[3] Features of benign and neoplastic nodes were compared in a study of 31 dogs.[9] Deep (2 intrathoracic and 29 intraabdominal) nodes were subjected to ultrasonic examination with follow-up cytologic or histopathologic evaluation. Maximal short- (diameter) and long-axis measures and short axis–to–long axis ratio were significantly increased for neoplastic versus benign nodes of the same anatomic group. However, all nodes were hypoechoic to the expected norm, whether benign or malignant. Other features including shape, contour, presence of cavitation, and Doppler evaluation were not useful in determining benign versus neoplastic nodes. Heterogeneity is an additional feature that has been associated with malignancy in canine and feline intraabdominal lymph nodes. In a case-control study, 91% of heterogeneous lymph nodes in dogs were malignant, and 63% of heterogeneous nodes in cats were malignant.[8]

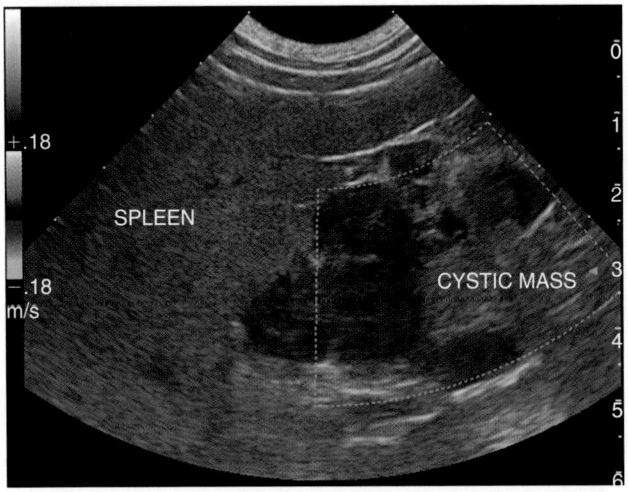

Abdominal lymph node enlargement is commonly seen with lymphosarcoma and other types of abdominal neoplasia in the dog and cat. Enlargement can occur with inflammatory and infectious diseases of the gastrointestinal tract, which cause reactivity of regional nodes. Reactive lymphadenopathy is usually typified by less enlargement and shape change than with neoplastic invasion. Cats with lymphosarcoma often develop a large midabdominal mass that is not associated with a specific intraabdominal organ. This mass frequently originates from mesenteric nodes and may also involve adjacent small intestine. Ultrasonographic abnormalities of the ileocecocolic area have been documented in a study of 29 cats without neoplasia.[10] Most of the cats (28 of 29) had gastrointestinal signs, and common findings included lymphadenopathy, increased cecal wall thickness, and hyperechoic fat. The authors concluded that ultrasonic abnormalities of the ileocecocolic junction are significant and are usually associated with underlying gastrointestinal disease; in some instances, abnormalities occur with disease in other abdominal organs such as the liver and pancreas.

Evaluation of the lumbar, medial iliac, hypogastric, and sacral lymph nodes is important in assessing abnormalities of the prostate, urinary bladder, and anorectal area. The medial iliac nodes are easily detected ultrasonographically because of their consistent relationship to the terminal aorta and external iliac arteries (Figure 13-27; see also Chapter 4, Figure 4-31, E). They are routinely measured and assessed for echotexture by sonographers; however, the hypogastric and sacral nodes are smaller and are rarely observed, even though they are included in the sublumbar group. In normal dogs, medial iliac nodes are fusiform, isoechoic or hypoechoic to surrounding tissues, with either a distinct corticomedullary demarcation or a homogeneous appearance. Medial iliac nodes should be evaluated cautiously for enlargement, because their dimensions vary with body size and weight.[4] Mean width of left and right nodes was, respectively, 0.43 and 0.45 cm in small dogs; 0.64 and 0.63 in medium-sized dogs; and 0.7 and 0.75 in large dogs.[4] Although these nodes are routinely evaluated for signs of regional metastasis, one should also direct the transducer caudally and examine for the presence of enlarged hypogastric

Figure 13-24 Lobulated multicystic lymph node (*CYSTIC MASS*). The color Doppler image shows minimal blood flow. Aspiration yielded fluid. The cytologic analysis showed intermediate lymphocytes suggesting a reactive lymphoid population without evidence of neoplasia.

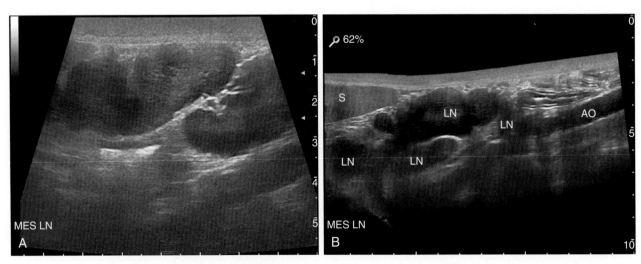

Figure 13-25 Severely enlarged mesenteric lymph nodes in a dog with lymphoma. A, Very large, hypoechoic, mildly irregular jejunal lymph nodes (mesenteric lymph nodes). **B,** Extended field of view showing multiple enlarged lymph nodes (*LN*). *AO,* Aorta; *S,* spleen.

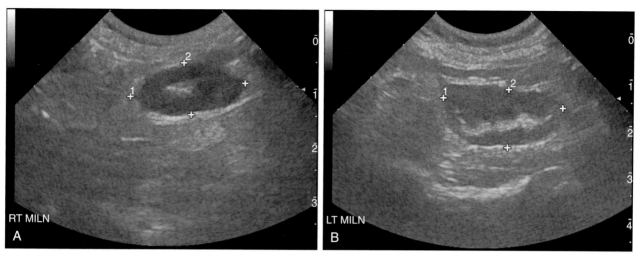

Figure 13-26 Target lesion or bull's-eye appearance of an enlarged medial iliac lymph nodes in a dog with multicentric lymphoma. A, Transverse image through an enlarged, misshapen right medial iliac lymph node (*RT MILN;* 2.17 × 0.97 cm, between electronic cursors). The lymph node contains a central hyperechoic area surrounded by homogeneous hypoechoic tissue. **B,** Long axis image of the contralateral left medial iliac lymph node shows that the node has lost its fusiform shape and become much more rounded, increasing the width-to-length ratio (2.66 × 1.25 cm, between electronic cursors).

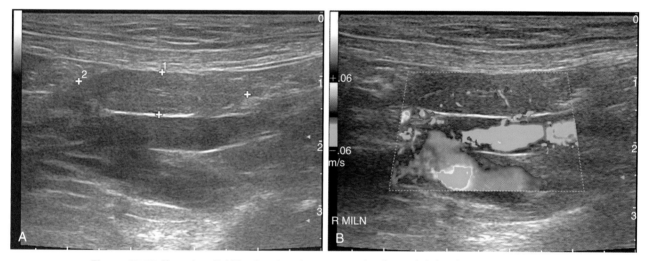

Figure 13-27 Normal medial iliac lymph node. A, Normal right medial iliac lymph node in a dog is homogeneous and slightly hypoechoic to the surrounding soft tissues, yet slightly hyperechoic to the adjacent great blood vessels. The medial iliac lymph nodes is 2.66 cm long and 0.66 cm wide, between the electronic cursors. **B,** Color Doppler assessment showing blood flow within the node and surrounding great vessels.

or sacral nodes. The detection of enlarged lymph nodes in the sublumbar regions is a strong indicator of neoplasia, although severe inflammatory disease (e.g., bacterial prostatitis, abscessation) can result in lymphadenopathy.

MASSES

In addition to lymphadenopathy, other types of intraabdominal masses not associated with specific organs occur. These include abscesses, granulomas, hematomas, lipomas, and mesotheliomas. Abscesses have a variable ultrasonographic appearance (Figures 13-28 to 13-30).[11] They classically are thick, have irregular walls, and vary in size. The center of the mass usually contains semisolid or fluid material and echoic debris.

When fluid content is present, agitation of the mass may produce swirling or wavelike motions that can be seen during real-time examination. Distal acoustic enhancement may also be present if significant fluid has accumulated. Other components of an abscess may be more solid or contain echogenic gas. The internal architecture of abscesses may be complex (see Figure 13-29). Lipomas are occasionally found in the abdominal cavity and typically are well-marginated masses of variable echotexture. In a study of deep and superficial canine lipomas, reliable sonographic characteristics included sharp edge definition, a thin hyperechoic capsule, and a striated appearance.[12]

Retained surgical sponges can cause a mass effect. In a postsurgical study of eight dogs with retained sponges, ultrasound examination revealed sonolucent masses with irregular echogenic centers in all eight dogs.[13] Onset of clinical signs with retained sponges may be delayed for several years and can produce tissue reactions that can be confused with neoplasia.[14] Sublumbar or retroperitoneal granulomas and abscesses can occur, frequently as a sequela of grass awn (foxtail) migration. Neoplasias of the retroperitoneal space and pelvic inlet occasionally are encountered (Figures 13-31 and 13-32).

Hematomas have a wide spectrum of sonographic appearances, depending on duration. They usually have low echogenicity and a solid appearance. They may have a homogeneous parenchymal texture or be more heterogeneous (Figure 13-33). Doppler evaluation determines that they are nonvascular and differentiates them from other types of masses. They may be detected after known acute trauma (such as an automobile accident), be secondary to cystocentesis (see Chapter 1, Figure 1-37, B and C), occur with bleeding disorders, or have no known cause. Thus hematomas are always considered in the differential diagnosis of intraabdominal masses without an obvious organ of origin. A duodenal hematoma was reported in a dog with pancreatitis.[15] Sonographic findings were typified by a heterogeneous intramural mass in the tunica muscularis of the descending duodenum. Although duodenal hematomas are rare in dogs, the authors concluded that they should be included along with neoplasia in differential diagnosis of intramural masses.

Lipomas are typically characterized by homogeneous, echoic mass lesions, often with distinct margination. They usually have uniform echogenicity with a coarse internal echotexture, but they may appear relatively hypoechoic or have a heterogeneous, mixed internal echo pattern (Figure 13-34). The definitive diagnosis of intraperitoneal masses requires a fine-needle aspiration or biopsy, which can be performed safely under ultrasonographic guidance.

MESENTERY

Normal mesentery and omentum are echogenic with a coarse architecture but, unlike parenchymal organs such as the liver and kidney, they do not have a distinguishing echotexture. The mesentery normally appears as a "background" echogenicity because it contains fatty tissue. Obese patients usually have decreased image detail because of increased scattering of the ultrasound beam by adipose tissue. This is opposite to abdominal radiography, where increased intraperitoneal fat increases contrast of peritoneal organs and is desirable. In obese human patients, harmonic ultrasound techniques have been used to overcome poor image quality. Harmonic imaging is commonly available on newer ultrasound equipment and can improve image detail and contrast with obese animals. In patients with peritonitis, inflamed mesentery is hyperechoic (to normal), homogeneous, and solid (Figures 13-35 to 13-37), but it may also have a coarse architecture (Figure 13-38). The mesentery can become more echogenic in cases of abdominal trauma, reducing image detail (Figure 13-39).

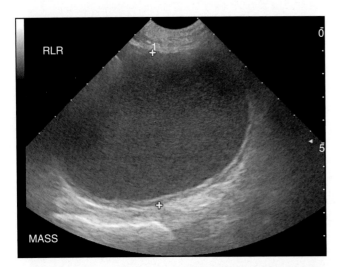

Figure 13-28 Omental abscess in a 4-year-old dog with thrombocytopenia. A thin but discernible wall surrounds echogenic central contents that were swirling during examination (between electronic cursors, 6.60 cm). Pus was obtained via fine-needle aspiration and surgery revealed a large omental abscess. *RLR*, right lateral recumbency.

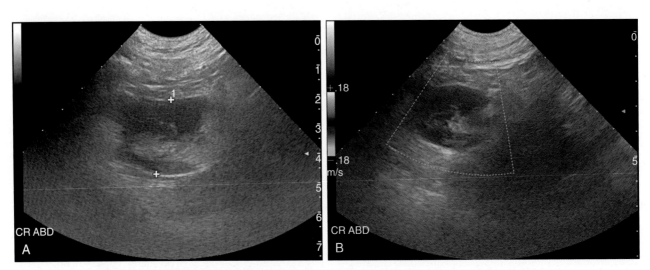

Figure 13-29 Mesenteric abscess in a dog. A, A small, thin-walled structure with heterogeneous, movable contents was identified and was unassociated with any organ (2.58 cm between electronic cursors). **B,** Color Doppler image showed an absence of blood flow. Surgery revealed a mesenteric abscess. Note the poor detail of the tissue surrounding the abscess.

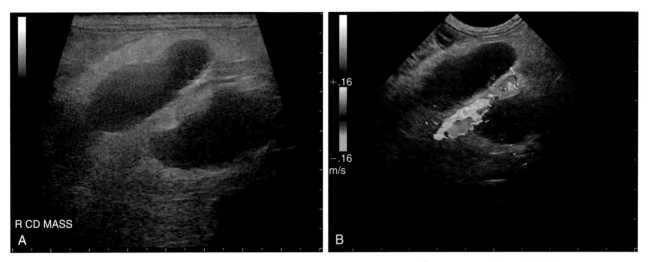

Figure 13-30 Mesenteric abscess in a dog. A, Bicavitary appearance of a mesenteric abscess. Thick, hyperechoic and irregular walls surround two large pockets of nearly anechoic fluid. Aspiration yield thick pus. **B,** Color Doppler image shows blood flow within the central portion of the abscess, which was thought to be a jejunal vein and a jejunal artery.

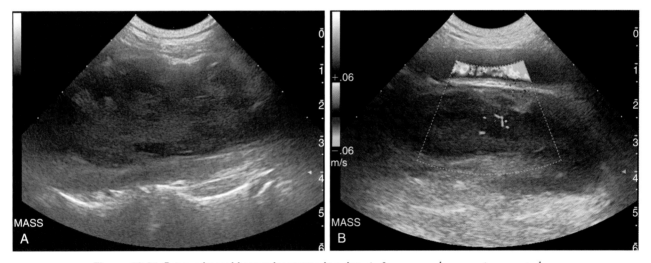

Figure 13-31 Retroperitoneal hemangiosarcoma in a dog. A, Large complex mass is present along the lumbar spine. **B,** Color Doppler image shows a portion of the abdominal aorta in the near field and very little blood flow within the mass.

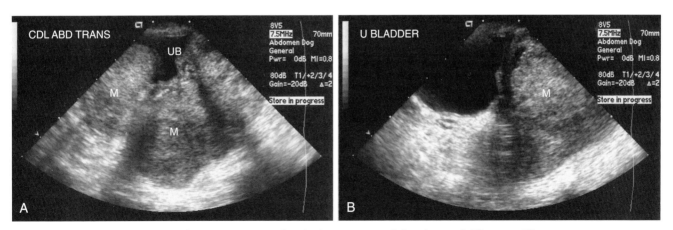

Figure 13-32 Pelvic carcinoma in a female dog, transverse **(A)** and sagittal **(B)** images. The mass (*M*) is large, solid, slightly heterogeneous, and irregularly marginated; it distorts the neck of the urinary bladder (*UB*).

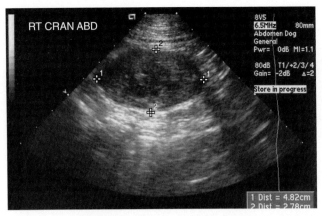

Figure 13-33 Hematoma. This hypoechoic discrete structure had islands of anechoic foci within it. Its appearance mimicked an abnormal kidney. Doppler examination indicated absence of blood flow, differentiating it from a lymph node and a kidney. Fine-needle aspiration was inconclusive; the diagnosis was made at surgery.

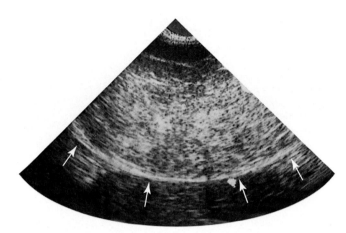

Figure 13-34 Intraabdominal lipoma (*arrows*), characterized by a coarse echotexture.

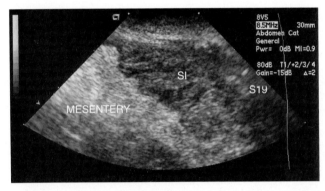

Figure 13-35 Peritonitis. The mesentery is hyperechoic. Stacked loops of relatively hypoechoic small intestine (*SI*) are poorly demarcated because of inflammation. Small irregular anechoic pockets of free peritoneal fluid are noted between the small intestinal segments.

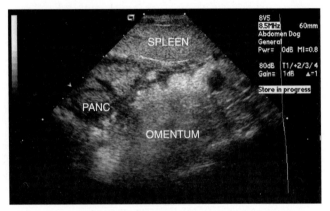

Figure 13-36 Peritonitis secondary to pancreatitis. Hyperechoic mesentery (*OMENTUM*) obscures normal anatomic detail centrally. The pancreas (*PANC*) is severely inflamed. Central area is abnormally echogenic; periphery is hypoechoic to anechoic. A small amount of regional peritoneal fluid is also noted. The spleen is in the near field.

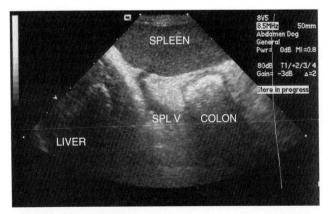

Figure 13-37 Peritonitis. The mesentery is hyperechoic. The mesentery surrounds the anechoic splenic vein (*SPL V*) and colon in transverse section.

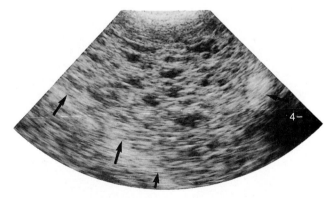

Figure 13-38 Peritonitis in which the mesentery (*arrows*) is inflamed. A coarse, echoic, "lacy" appearance is noted. *Mesocestoides* was found.

FREE PERITONEAL AIR

Free peritoneal air creates a poor ultrasound imaging environment. Imaging of the abdomen can be extremely difficult when free peritoneal air is present because air reflects the ultrasound beam, creating various artifacts and decreasing image quality (Figure 13-40; see also Chapter 1, Reverberation, Ring-down and Comet Tail Artifacts). Quality can be improved by using firm transducer pressure or scanning the patient from the dependent side. If free peritoneal air is suspected, radiography, including horizontal beam techniques, should be used for confirmation. Free peritoneal air is considered a surgical emergency; it often indicates the rupture of a hollow viscus or, rarely, an abdominal abscess. At times, the sonographer is also asked to evaluate a postoperative abdomen for the presence of hemorrhage, bowel obstruction, or other surgical complications. This often requires positional studies

to redistribute the air so that a satisfactory acoustic window can be obtained. The sonographer must be careful to distinguish between free intraperitoneal air (gas) and gas within the lumen of the intestines (see Figure 13-40, B). This can usually be accomplished by examining the patient with the transducer positioned nondependently and using a short depth setting. Free peritoneal gas lies next to the body wall, adjacent to the margin of the parietal peritoneum, and causes an intense specular echo and reverberation, or in some instances, a comet-tail artifact. With intraluminal intestinal gas, the same specular echo and artifacts are present, but in the near field, the intestinal wall lies between the specular echo and the body wall and parietal peritoneal surface. The intestinal wall will not be seen in the near field with peritoneal gas.

THROMBOSIS OF THE ABDOMINAL AORTA AND CAUDAL VENA CAVA

Thrombus formation within the peritoneal aorta and caudal vena cava is not uncommon and can be diagnosed on a B-mode ultrasound examination (Figures 13-41 to 13-43). Thrombi may be associated with cardiac disease, systemic disorders, or localized pathologic processes. They may be hypoechoic to near anechoic in their formative phase and difficult to identify. Increasing the gain setting may be helpful for distinguishing immature thrombi from anechoic flowing blood. Doppler evaluation is particularly helpful in many of these cases for more thorough assessment of vascular compromise. Figure 13-44 shows the presence of heartworms within the caudal vena cava.

FOCUSED SONOGRAPHIC EXAMINATIONS

Most veterinary radiologists and other specialists providing ultrasound examinations advocate a complete abdominal ultrasound exam, because it often yields additional information that would have been undetected during a focused exam. However, focused or targeted exams based on presenting

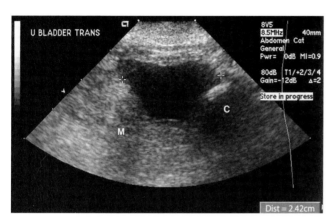

Figure 13-39 **Traumatized mesentery.** This cat was hit by a car 2 days earlier. The mesentery (*M*) is diffusely hyperechoic, reducing image detail within the abdomen. A transverse image of a small urinary bladder is present between the electronic cursors. *C,* Colon.

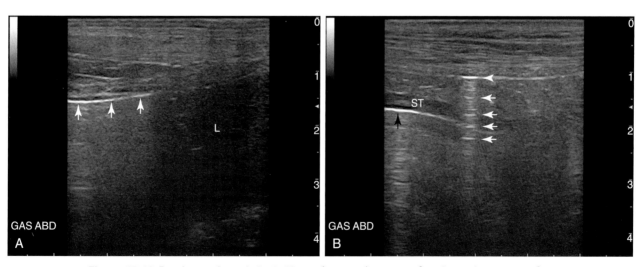

Figure 13-40 **Free intraperitoneal air. A,** Very echogenic, linear interface (*arrows*) represents free peritoneal air. The air masks the underlying liver (*L*), which can be seen to the right, where free air is not present. **B,** Small pocket of free air (*white arrowhead*) is present in the near field. Reverberation artifact is present (*white arrows*), and a comet-tail type of reverberation artifact has resulted. An identical artifact is seen in the left of the image from gas reverberating (*black arrow*) from the stomach. *ST,* Stomach wall.

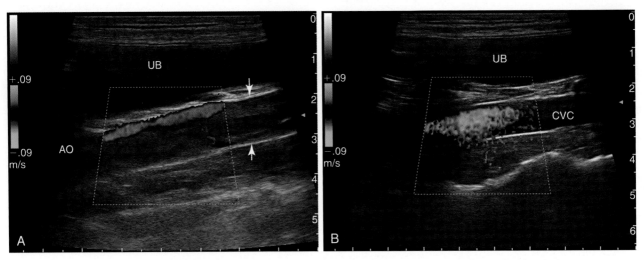

Figure 13-41 **Aortic thrombus. A,** A large, echogenic thrombus is present in the terminal aorta (*AO,* between arrows). Color Doppler image shows a small peripheral area of maintained blood flow. The urinary bladder (*UB*) is in the near field. **B,** Color Doppler image of the adjacent caudal vena cava (*CVC*) at the same level showing normal blood flow. *UB,* Urinary bladder.

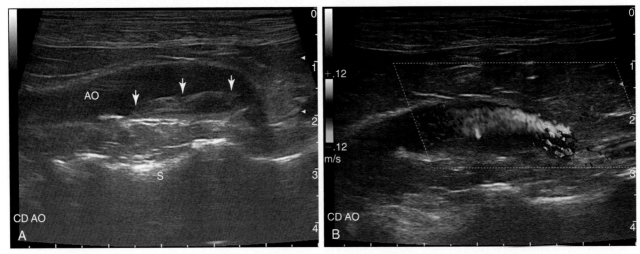

Figure 13-42 **Aortic thrombus. A,** An echogenic thrombus (*arrows*) is present in the lumen of the terminal aorta (*AO*). *S,* Spine. **B,** Color Doppler image shows good blood flow around the thrombus.

clinical signs are a reasonable approach for general practitioners, provided inherent limitations are fully understood.

Focused ultrasound examinations of the abdominal cavity include organ- and system-specific studies (e.g., hepatobiliary and urinary tracts), and examination for peritoneal fluid and parenchymal trauma. The latter has been termed focused assessment with sonography in trauma (FAST) and is commonly used with humans treated in emergency departments.[16,17] Peritoneal fluid in unstable patients can be readily detected with FAST and triaged to surgery without other more complicated, expensive tests. Patients who are stable or have negative findings on sonographic examinations may need CT or other examinations. In humans, ultrasound exam is based on detection of peritoneal fluid; but according to recent studies, sonography has a sensitivity rate of approximately 40% in direct detection of solid organ injuries. Use of FAST in humans has been shown to significantly alter patient man-

agement, reducing the incidence of needless laparotomy, peritoneal lavage, and CT examinations in trauma patients.[17]

Applications of FAST in veterinary patients with trauma are similar to those of human patients, and both abdominal FAST (AFAST) and thoracic FAST (TFAST) examinations have been reported.[18-21] The first study described using a quadrant approach for the detection of fluid.[18] Figure 13-45 illustrates the basic windows for rapid detection of abdominal fluid as described by Boysen and co-workers[18] Basic search patterns for fluid accumulation are the same as described for peritoneal effusion.

In a more recent study, an abdominal fluid scoring (AFS) system was evaluated in dogs sustaining motor vehicle trauma.[20] Using a 4-point scale (0, no abdominal fluid; 4, fluid detected in all four quadrants), it was found that dogs with an AFS of 3 or 4 had lower packed cell volume (PCV) and total plasma protein, had higher alanine aminotransferase, and

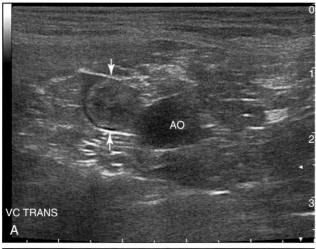

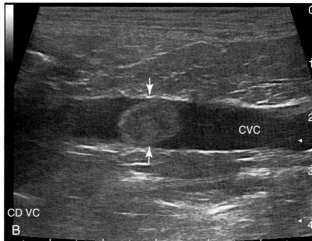

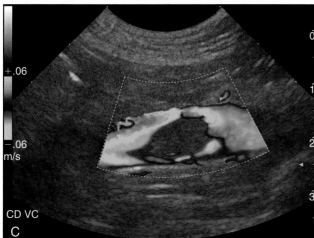

Figure 13-43 **Caudal vena cava thrombus. A,** Transverse image of the caudal vena cava with an echogenic thrombus (*arrows*). To the right in the image is the abdominal aorta (*AO*). **B,** Sagittal image of the caudal vena cava (*CVC*) and thrombus (*arrows*). **C,** Color Doppler image shows vessel patency.

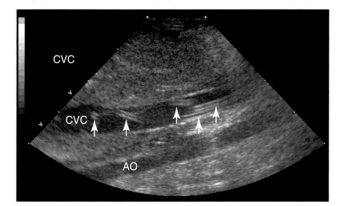

Figure 13-44 **Heartworms within the caudal vena cava.** Multiple, linear echogenic heartworms (*arrows*) are present within the caudal vena cava (*CVC*). *AO,* Aorta.

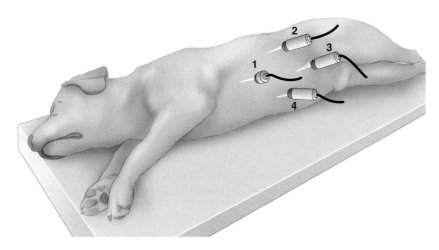

Figure 13-45 Illustration depicting areas for rapid assessment of possible peritoneal fluid. Position 1 has the transducer positioned on midline just caudal to the xiphoid process of the sternum. This has been termed the Diaphragmatic-Hepatic (DH) view. Position 2 is termed the Splenic-Renal (SR) view, with the transducer placed on the left side of the patient's mid-abdomen. Position 3, termed the Cysto-Colic (CC) view, places the transducer on midline in the caudal abdomen. Position 4 places the transducer on the right (recumbent) side of the mid-abdomen, termed the Hepato-Renal (HR) view. (Adapted from Boysen SR, Rozanski EA, Tidwell AS, et al. Evaluation of a focused assessment with sonography for trauma protocol to detect free abdominal fluid in dogs involved in motor vehicle accidents. *J Am Vet Med Assoc* 2004; 225(8):1198-1204.)

needed more blood transfusions than dogs with lower scores. Serial exams also showed that some dogs changed scores, usually worsening. The conclusion was that initial and serial AFAST combined with ASF was a reliable semiquantitative process to measure peritoneal fluid, and it effectively guided clinical management.

As in human emergency and critical care medicine, FAST techniques in veterinary medicine serve as an extension of the physical examination, expediting diagnosis and potentially lifesaving intervention while guiding patient management.[21]

REFERENCES

1. Henley RK, Hager DA, Ackerman N. A comparison of two-dimensional ultrasonography and radiography for the detection of small amounts of free peritoneal fluid in the dog. *Vet Radiol* 1989;**30**:121–4.
2. Schreurs E, Vermote K, Barberet V, et al. Ultrasonographic anatomy of abdominal lymph nodes in the normal cat. *Vet Radiol Ultrasound* 2008;**49**(1):68–72.
3. Agthe P, Caine AR, Posch B, et al. Ultrasonographic appearance of jejunal lymph nodes in dogs without clinical signs of gastrointestinal disease. *Vet Radiol Ultrasound* 2009;**50**(2):195–200.
4. Mayer MN, Lawson JA, Silver TI. Sonographic characteristics of presumptively normal canine medial iliac and superficial inguinal lymph nodes. *Vet Radiol Ultrasound* 2010;**51**(6):638–41.
5. Pugh CR. Ultrasonographic examination of abdominal lymph nodes in the dog. *Vet Radiol Ultrasound* 1994;**35**:110–15.
6. Nyman HT, Kristensen AT, Skovgaard IM, et al. Characterization of normal and abnormal canine superficial lymph nodes using gray-scale B-mode, color flow mapping, power, and spectral Doppler ultrasonography: a multivariate study. *Vet Radiol Ultrasound* 2005;**46**:404–10.
7. Nyman HT, Lee MH, McEvoy FJ, et al. Comparison of B-mode and Doppler ultrasonographic findings with histologic features of benign and malignant superficial lymph nodes in dogs. *Am J Vet Res* 2006;**67**:978–84.
8. Kinns J, Mai W. Association between malignancy and sonographic heterogeneity in canine and feline abdominal lymph nodes. *Vet Radiol Ultrasound* 2007;**48**:565–9.
9. De Swarte M, Alexander K, Rannou B, et al. Comparison of sonographic features of benign and neoplastic deep lymph nodes in dogs. *Vet Radiol Ultrasound* 2011;**52**:451–6.
10. Taeymens O, Holt N, Penninck DG, et al. Ultrasonographic characterization of feline ileocecocolic abnormalities. *Vet Radiol Ultrasound* 2011;**52**:302–5.
11. Konde LJ, Lebel JL, Park RD, et al. Sonographic application in the diagnosis of intraabdominal abscess in the dog. *Vet Radiol* 1986;**27**:151–4.
12. Volta A, Bonazzi M, Gnudi G, et al. Ultrasonographic features of canine lipomas. *Vet Radiol Ultrasound* 2006;**47**:589–91.
13. Merlo M, Lamb CR. Radiographic and ultrasonographic features of retained surgical sponge in eight dogs. *Vet Radiol Ultrasound* 2000;**41**:279–83.
14. Deschamps JY, Roux FA. Extravesical textiloma (gossypiboma) mimicking a bladder tumor in a dog. *J Am Anim Hosp Assoc* 2009;**45**:89–92.
15. Heng HG, Huang A, Baird DK, et al. Imaging diagnosis—spontaneous intramural canine duodenal hematoma. *Vet Radiol Ultrasound* 2010;**51**:178–81.
16. Blackbourne LH, Soffer D, McKenney M, et al. Secondary ultrasound examination increases the sensitivity of the FAST exam in blunt trauma. *J Trauma* 2004;**57**(5):934–8.
17. Ollerton JE, Sugrue M, Balogh Z, et al. Prospective study to evaluate the influence of FAST on trauma patient management. *J Trauma* 2006;**60**(4):785–91.
18. Boysen SR, Rozanski EA, Tidwell AS, et al. Evaluation of a focused assessment with sonography for trauma protocol to detect free abdominal fluid in dogs involved in motor vehicle accidents. *J Am Vet Med Assoc* 2004;**225**(8):1198–204.
19. Lisciandro GR, Lagutchik MS, Mann KA, et al. Evaluation of a thoracic focused assessment with sonography for trauma (TFAST) protocol to detect pneumothorax and concurrent thoracic injury in 145 traumatized dogs. *J Vet Emerg Crit Care* 2008;**18**(3):258–69.
20. Lisciandro GR, Lagutchik MS, Mann KA, et al. Evaluation of an abdominal fluid scoring system determined using abdominal focused assessment with sonography for trauma (AFAST) in 101 dogs with motor vehicle trauma. *J Vet Emerg Crit Care* 2009;**19**(5):426–37.
21. Lisciandro GR. Focused abdominal (AFAST) and thoracic (TFAST) focused assessment with sonography for trauma, triage and monitoring in small animals. *J Vet Emerg Crit Care* 2011;**20**(2):104–22.

CHAPTER 14

Musculoskeletal System

Allison Zwingenberger • Livia Benigni • Christopher R. Lamb

Ultrasonography is a relatively versatile, convenient, and cost-effective method that is complementary to radiography for examining musculoskeletal structures. In instances when radiography does not elucidate the diagnosis, ultrasonography should be considered before more expensive imaging modalities, such as computed tomography and magnetic resonance imaging. As for any body part, ultrasonography of musculoskeletal structures requires knowledge of the relevant anatomy and careful attention to scanning technique. Musculoskeletal ultrasonography is particularly demanding because many important structures are small, which necessitates use of high-frequency transducers and accurate placement of transducers to obtain optimal images.

EXAMINATION TECHNIQUE

The area to be examined is first clipped, and then a wetting agent such as isopropyl alcohol is applied to the skin, followed by coupling gel. In general, the highest frequency transducer available is used to examine musculoskeletal structures. Linear transducers are preferred because of their wide superficial field of view and uniform angle of insonation. In contrast, a sector or curvilinear transducer is not optimal for examination of straight tendons because the variable angle of insonation makes tendon appear falsely hypoechoic toward the edges of longitudinal images.[1-3] Modern linear transducers also provide satisfactory image quality close to the transducer face, so a standoff pad[4-6] is not usually necessary, although it may aid coupling between a flat transducer face and a curved skin surface. In the absence of a flexible standoff pad, fitting a linear transducer to a curved protuberance requires abundant coupling gel and firm transducer pressure. Harmonic and compound imaging decrease artifacts and increase signal-to-noise ratio, and they are beneficial for ultrasonography of musculoskeletal structures.[7,8] Doppler ultrasonography is routinely used when attempting to identify blood vessels, distinguish blood vessels from nerves, and assess the vascularity of tissue.[9]

Many musculoskeletal ultrasound studies can be completed without anesthesia or sedation, although a still, relaxed patient facilitates a detailed and thorough examination, which includes scanning structures during passive movement. Comparison scanning of contralateral structures may be necessary when a suitable anatomic reference is lacking. For patients that also require radiography, and patients with lesions that are painful or may need ultrasound-guided fine-needle aspiration or biopsy, performing the entire examination during one session with general anesthesia may be most efficient. Ultrasonography of bones of clinical patients is best preceded by radiography in order to assess the nature and extent of lesions, and to guide the ultrasonographer.

Skin, Subcutaneous Tissues, and Muscle
Normal Findings

Normal skin is 2 to 3 mm thick with a laminar hyperechoic appearance. The subcutaneous tissues directly beneath the skin are composed primarily of connective tissue and fat and are less echogenic than skin. The depth of subcutaneous tissues depends on location and the amount of subcutaneous fat deposition. Subcutaneous fat appears moderately hypoechoic, with uniform but coarse hyperechoic speckling (Figure 14-1). The echogenicity of fat is somewhat variable and depends on its heterogeneity.[9a] A light touch with a high-frequency linear transducer is recommended for scanning superficial structures, which can be obscured by excessive transducer pressure.

Muscle appears as a relatively hypoechoic structure with fine, oblique, echogenic striations visible when scanning parallel to the long axis of the muscle belly.[10] The fine striations represent connective tissue between the muscle fascicles. In the transverse plane, these appear as multiple echogenic foci (Figure 14-2). Muscles are delineated by thin hyperechoic lines corresponding to their epimysium and surrounding fascia. In addition to using 2-D, gray-scale ultrasonography for diagnosis of muscle injuries, 3-D ultrasonography may be used to determine volume of muscles in live animals.[11]

Abnormal Findings

Cellulitis and Edema. In the early stages of cellulitis, affected tissues appear hyperechoic and thickened. Later, tissues may have distorted architecture and appear marbled with fusiform or linear anechoic to hypoechoic areas dispersed randomly in a hyperechoic background (Figure 14-3). Defined cavities containing fluid are usually not present.[12] A similar appearance to that associated with cellulitis may also be observed in patients with subcutaneous edema (Figure 14-4). Doppler evidence of increased blood flow to the affected tissues can help to distinguish these conditions.[13]

Cavitary Lesions: Seroma, Abscess, and Hematoma. Seromas are frequently observed at surgical sites.[14] They may be single or multiple, usually have well-defined, regular margins and anechoic contents, sometimes with thin linear septa (Figure 14-5). A seroma may contain a horizontal fluid-fluid level as red blood cells sediment on the dependent aspect, leaving serum above.

Abscesses may be found in subcutaneous sites or deeper structures.[13,15] Abscesses may be rounded, tubular, or complex; they usually have a well-defined hyperechoic capsule that may have a regular or irregular inner margin, and heterogeneous, isoechoic, hypoechoic, or anechoic contents (Figure 14-6). As with seromas, abscesses may contain sedimentary echogenic debris. Hyperechoic foci within an abscess may represent gas bubbles, occurring either as a result of anaerobic bacteria or

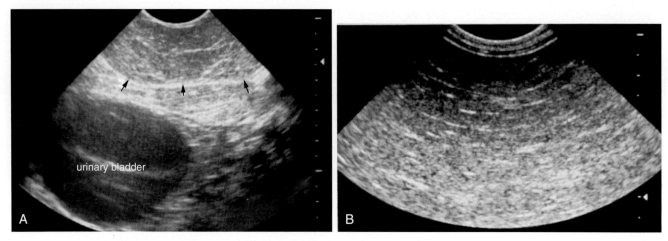

Figure 14-1 Lipoma. A, Fat is characteristically hypoechoic in appearance with hyperechoic speckling as seen in this example of a subcutaneous lipoma ventral to the caudal abdominal body wall (*arrows*). **B,** Near field image of the lipoma shown in **A.**

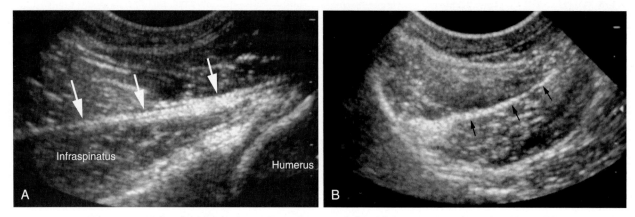

Figure 14-2 Infraspinatus muscle. A, Sagittal image of the infraspinatus muscle with its hyperechoic central tendinous band (*arrows*). **B,** Transverse image through the infraspinatus muscle. The hyperechoic band running through the muscle (*arrows*) represents the infraspinatus tendon.

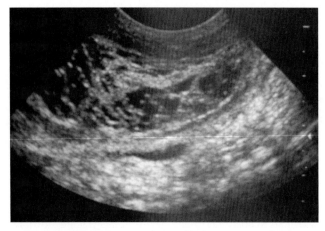

Figure 14-3 Cellulitis. Note the marbled appearance characteristic of an inflammatory process, with anechoic areas dispersed randomly in a hyperechoic background.

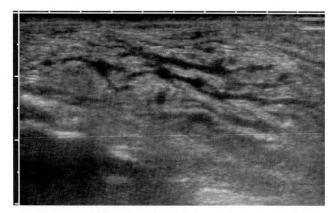

Figure 14-4 Edema. A striped appearance affecting thickened subcutaneous tissues on the ventral abdominal wall of a dog with hypoproteinemia.

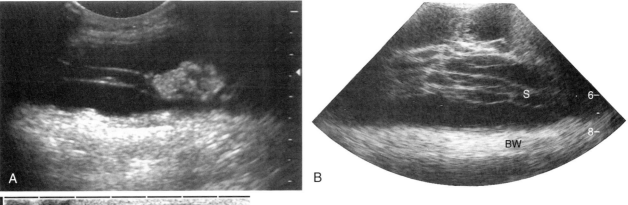

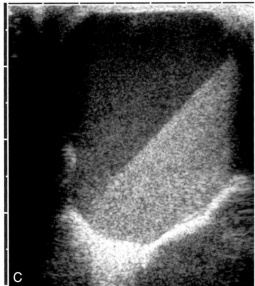

Figure 14-5 **Seromas. A,** Anechoic pocket of fluid beneath the skin. Note the echogenic fibrin clot and strands of fibrin within the fluid pocket. **B,** A large body wall seroma that followed abdominal surgery. The seroma (*S*) is characterized by anechoic regions of fluid separated by hyperechoic septum-like structures. The underlying body wall (*BW*), although thickened, is intact. **C,** Seroma containing a fluid-fluid level from sedimentation of red cells.

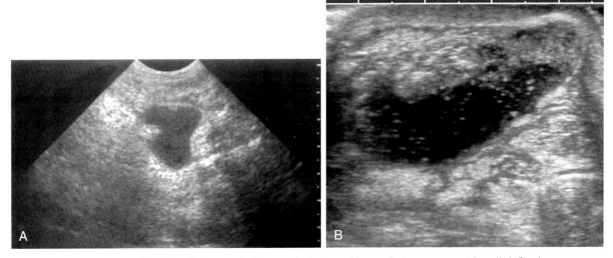

Figure 14-6 **Examples of abscess. A,** An irregularly shaped hypoechoic structure with well-defined wall. **B,** Abscess with heterogeneous contents, including numerous tiny echoes representing gas bubbles. In each case, the tissues surrounding the abscess appear hyperechoic and disorganized secondary to inflammation.

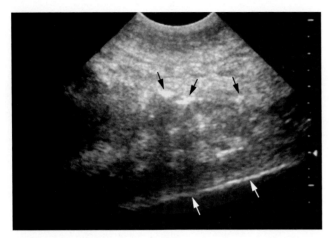

Figure 14-7 **Gas foci within soft tissues secondary to a bite wound.** Note the hyperechoic speckles (*black arrows*) with acoustic shadowing artifacts. The smooth, linear hyperechoic line in the far field (*white arrows*) represents the normal-appearing cortical surface of an adjacent bone.

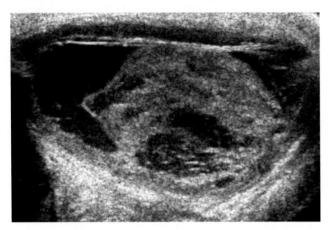

Figure 14-8 **Hematoma.** Subcutaneous cavitary mass with complex appearance including anechoic, hyperechoic, and strandlike components. Hematoma and seroma may appear similar ultrasonographically.

communication with the skin surface (Figure 14-7). Distal acoustic enhancement may be observed with a cyst, seroma, or abscess. Aspiration of the contents may be necessary for diagnosis.

Hematomas are variable in appearance, depending on their age and the coagulation status of the patient. A hematoma may initially appear as a homogeneous or heterogeneous mass lesion (Figure 14-8), depending on the proportion of liquid and clotted blood.[16] Application of transducer pressure causes movement of the internal echoes, which helps distinguish hematoma from a more solid mass; however, an organizing hematoma may be difficult to distinguish from a hemorrhagic or necrotic neoplasm without biopsy.

Hematomas associated with partial muscle tears or blunt trauma are hypoechoic relative to surrounding tissues[17-22] (Figure 14-9). Normal muscle architecture is usually lost, but with time, normal structures generally return with healing. With complete muscle rupture, the muscle contracts, and the severed ends on either side of the hematoma appear blunted and thickened with loss of normal architecture and increased heterogeneous echogenicity. After several days, clots begin to break down, producing complex cystic and solid areas within

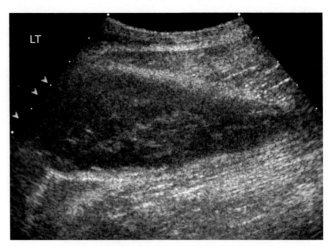

Figure 14-9 **Muscle hematoma.** Well demarcated hypoechoic lesion dividing the fibers of a thigh muscle in a Doberman pinscher with von Willebrand coagulopathy.

the hematoma. After several weeks, the area will be fluid filled.[22] Chronic hematomas are gradually resorbed and the tissues remodel. Residual scarring may be visible as hyperechoic patches. Discrete, hyperechoic foci, sometimes with distinct distal shadowing, may represent calcification of a chronic hematoma.

Pseudoaneurysm is a blood-filled cavity adjacent to an artery following disruption of the arterial wall as a result of iatrogenic or traumatic puncture.[23] This condition may be differentiated ultrasonographically from a hematoma by the presence of a persistent patent channel between the artery lumen and the cavity, which allows blood to continually flow into the pseudoaneurysm, causing the blood to swirl within the cavity (Figure 14-10).

Draining Sinus. Ultrasonography is an alternative to contrast radiography for examination of a draining sinus. Using the cutaneous sinus as a starting point, it may be possible to follow the tract to a foreign body (Figure 14-11). Tracts may appear hypoechoic or hyperechoic, depending on whether they contain fluid or gas.[15] In dogs with a draining sinus in the flank, the tissues ventral to the lumbar spine should be examined for signs of abscess (Figure 14-12).

Mass Lesions: Lipoma, Other Neoplasms, and Granulation Tissue. Lipomas are frequently seen in the subcutaneous tissues of older dogs and appear as thinly encapsulated accumulations of fat (see Figure 14-1). Although they usually have a relatively hyperechoic echotexture, lipomas have been reported to have isoechoic, hyperechoic, or hypoechoic appearances.[24] Infiltrative lipomas or liposarcomas tend to have less well-defined margins than superficial lipomas, and they can be difficult to delineate because fat and muscle may appear similar ultrasonographically. Liposarcomas tend to be slightly more echogenic and less homogeneous than lipomas, with multiple septa and nodules, but ultrasonography is not accurate for distinguishing lipomas from liposarcomas.[25] Histopathology is necessary for definitive diagnosis.

Most other neoplasms arising from musculoskeletal soft tissues generally have a heterogeneous echotexture, often with central hypoechoic regions that represent areas of necrosis (Figure 14-13). In general, neoplasia is highly variable in appearance, and ultrasound findings alone are nonspecific. The principal role of ultrasonography in diagnosis of soft tissue masses is to guide biopsy.

Granulation tissue must be distinguished from neoplasia. It tends to be hypoechoic, and Doppler examination may

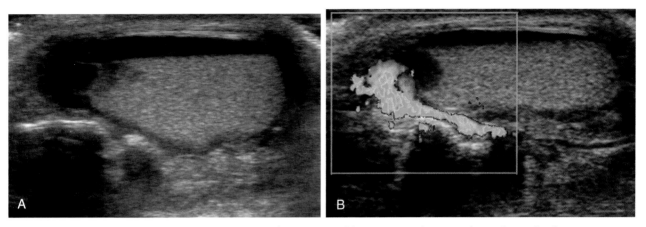

Figure 14-10 **Pseudoaneurysm.** A, Subcutaneous, oblong cavitary lesion with regular wall of uniform thickness and sedimentation of contents. B, Corresponding color-flow Doppler image showing flow from the radial artery swirling into the distal aspect of the cavity.

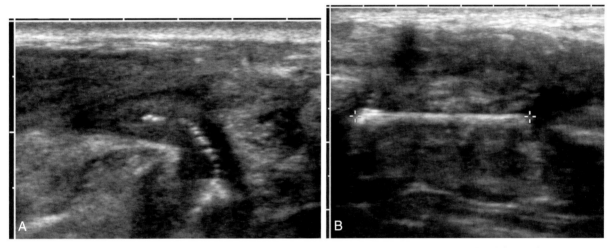

Figure 14-11 **Draining tract.** A, Thickened, heterogeneous subcutaneous tissues on the abdominal wall contain numerous small echoes within a curvilinear structure compatible with a draining tract. B, 2.7-cm linear echogenic structure found in the depths of the tract was a fragment of wood.

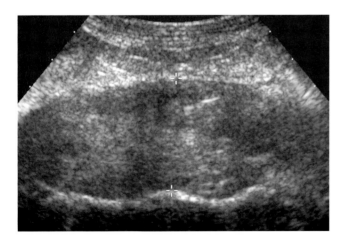

Figure 14-12 **Sublumbar abscess.** Hypoechoic mass on the ventral aspects of the midlumbar vertebrae. Although a cavity is not evident ultrasonographically, aspiration produces exudates compatible with abscess. Migrating foreign body was suspected as the underlying cause and the lesion was resected.

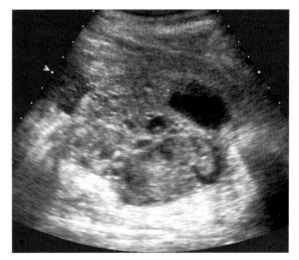

Figure 14-13 **Soft tissue neoplasm.** Hemangiosarcoma appearing as a complex mass affecting the iliopsoas muscle.

demonstrate that it is uniformly vascularized, which is not a feature associated with soft tissue neoplasms, except possibly lymphoma.[26]

Nerves

Nerves can be recognized in animals as hypoechoic structures surrounded by a thin hyperechoic rim and containing discontinuous hyperechoic bands.[27] Peripheral nerve routes are usually closely associated with the arteries and veins supplying the limbs. If necessary, Doppler can be used to differentiate these structures. The peripheral nerves travel in the soft tissue as a single nerve unit or as a group of multiple units close together.[27,28]

Ultrasonographic anatomy of the brachial plexus and major nerves of the canine thoracic limb has been described.[28] The brachial plexus is seen lateral to the first rib with the scapula pulled caudally and in the axillary region as a net of multiple nerves (Figure 14-14). The musculocutaneous, ulnar, and median nerves are seen on the medial aspect at midhumerus and are formed by a single nerve component. The radial nerve, formed by multiple small components, is seen on the mediocaudal aspect of the humerus.[28]

Ultrasonographic anatomy of the canine[27] and feline[27a] sciatic nerves has been described. The caudal part of the lumbosacral trunk and the origin of the sciatic nerve are visible through the greater ischiatic foramen[27] (Figure 14-15). The sciatic nerve is made of two units that will give rise to the common peroneal and the tibial nerves. These two components are distinctly visible and can be followed as they travel together distally until they diverge on the distal third of the femur. The common peroneal component has the smaller diameter and is located cranial to the tibial component.[27] The sciatic nerve is an example of a nerve that is not closely associated with an artery or a vein.

The canine femoral nerve is formed by multiple small nerves bundled together, and is difficult to distinguish from the surrounding tissue.[29] The femoral artery at the level of the inguinal crease is the landmark used to identify the femoral nerve, which can be seen in cross section as a slightly hyperechoic triangular area located cranial to the femoral artery.

Ultrasound-guided nerve blocks using local anesthetic injections around the brachial plexus or sciatic nerve may help optimize anesthesia in patients undergoing surgery for painful limb conditions.[30]

Abnormal Findings

Ultrasonography has been used to examine various lesions affecting the peripheral nerves in humans.[31-33] In small animals, reports have emphasized the use of ultrasound in diagnosis of peripheral nerve sheath tumors.[34-40] These tumors generally appear as hypoechoic or heterogeneous fusiform swellings of the nerve (Figure 14-16). The most common location of peripheral nerve sheath tumors in dogs is the brachial plexus, followed by the lumbosacral trunk and the sciatic nerve. A mass in the axillary region could only be palpated in roughly 30% of the cases reported with a peripheral brachial plexus tumor. Approximately half of the tumors are located in the area of the plexus or distal to it and therefore can be easily visualized ultrasonographically.[37-39] Following the nerves more proximally and visualizing the ventral branches of the spinal nerves by ultrasound can be quite challenging. Computed tomography (CT) and magnetic resonance imaging (MRI) enable visualization of the most proximal part of the plexus and may be used to complete the imaging investigation in patients in which spinal cord involvement is suspected. Preliminary diagnosis of peripheral nerve sheath tumor can be achieved by ultrasound-guided fine-needle aspiration of the lesion.[36]

Bone

Normal Findings

Sound waves are predominantly reflected by the intact cortical surface of bone, producing a high amplitude specular echo[41] (Figure 14-17). Reverberation artifact may be observed deep to the cortical surface because of repeated reflection of sound between the bone and the skin or transducer.[41] Scanning with the image plane parallel to the long axis of the bone may aid orientation and recognition of landmarks; however, examination of a long bone may also be achieved efficiently by sweeping the transducer along the bone with the image plane transverse to its long axis. Suitable ultrasound windows include cranial for the proximal humerus, lateral for the distal humerus, craniolateral for the radius and ulna, medial for the femur, and craniolateral for the tibia.[42]

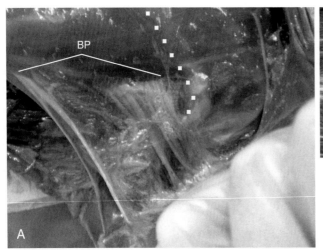

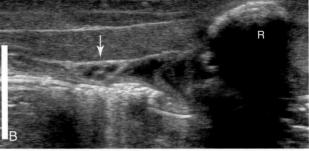

Figure 14-14 **The brachial plexus. A,** Photograph of the brachial plexus in a cadaver; image obtained by removing the scapula. Note the position of the brachial plexus (*BP*) relative to the first rib (dotted line at cranial edge). **B,** Ultrasound image transverse to the first rib (*R*) showing multiple neural components (*arrow*) of the C8 spinal nerve. White bar is 1 cm. (From Guilherme S, Benigni L. Ultrasonographic anatomy of the brachial plexus and major nerves of the canine thoracic limb. *Vet Radiol Ultrasound* 2008;49:577–83.)

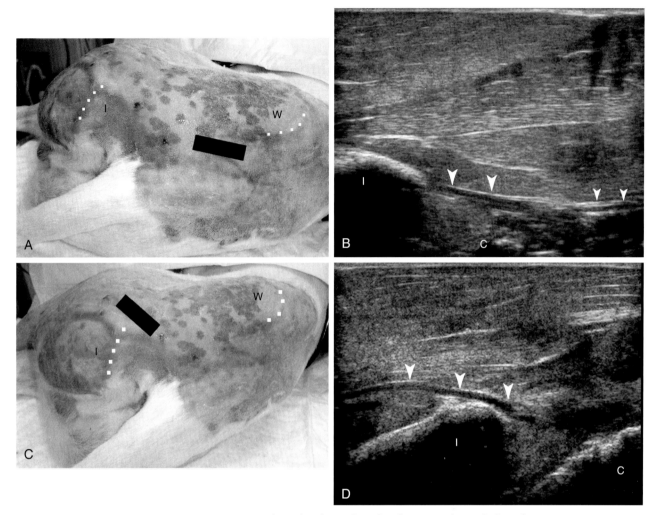

Figure 14-15 **Sciatic nerve. A,** Greyhound cadaver, shaved and positioned in right lateral recumbency. The wing of the ilium (*W*) and the sciatic tuberosity (*I*) are outlined by white dots. The transducer (footprint indicated by black rectangle) is positioned on the dorsal aspect, caudal to the sacroiliac joint and nearly parallel to the shaft of the ilium. **B,** Corresponding longitudinal ultrasound image of the left lumbosacral trunk (*small arrowheads*) and the origin of the sciatic nerve (*large arrowheads*) visible lateral to the colon (C) and cranial to the ischium (*I*). **C,** The wing of the ilium (*W*) and the ischiatic tuberosity (*I*) of a cadaver are outlined by white dots. The transducer (footprint indicated by black rectangle) is positioned caudal to the greater trochanter, cranial to the ischiatic tuberosity (*I*), and parallel to the femoral neck. **D,** Corresponding ultrasound image of the sciatic nerve (*arrowheads*) as it passes over the ischium (*I*). C, colon. (From Benigni L, Corr SA, Lamb CR. Ultrasonographic assessment of the canine sciatic nerve. *Vet Radiol Ultrasound* 2007;**48:**428–33.)

Abnormal Findings

Ultrasonographic evaluation of intact bone is limited to the cortical surface. Lesions affecting the cortical surface may be evident as loss of the normal specular echo, either as a result of roughening or discontinuity of the cortex.[41]

Fractures. Radiography is the principal modality used when fracture is suspected, but fractures may be detected ultrasonographically when there is a gap or step in the cortical surface of a bone. Ultrasonography has been investigated as a means of evaluating fracture healing more than as method for detecting fractures[42-44] because, although radiography is a practical method for fracture diagnosis, radiography is insensitive for fibrous callus formation in the early stages of healing. With ultrasound imaging, evaluation of fracture healing from post-trauma hematoma formation through fibrous callus to ossified callus formation is possible. The ultrasonographic appearance of the stages of fracture healing have been described in dogs.[43,44] In dogs with long bone fractures, signs of healing may be detected earlier with ultrasound than with radiographs.[44] In the first week after fracture, hypoechoic hematoma fills the fracture, becoming more heterogeneous as it is resorbed in the second week. By 2 to 4 weeks after fracture, the bone edges become blunted and irregular as callus forms; any remaining hematoma is isoechoic to hyperechoic (Figure 14-18). Callus becomes smoother in outline and more echogenic as healing progresses until the laminar hyperechoic interface at the bone cortex is restored. Power Doppler signals at the fracture site decreases as healing progresses. In dogs with fractures surgically repaired using plates, Doppler signals were visible along the length of the plate after Doppler signals at the fracture site had diminished and the fractures were healed.[45] This may indicate persistent inflammation associated with the implants.

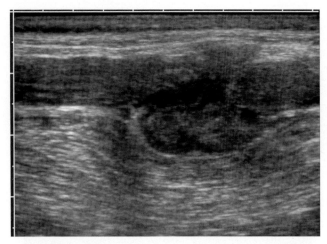

Figure 14-16 Nerve tumor. Longitudinal image of the sciatic nerve, which is diffusely thickened and hypoechoic as a result of a malignant peripheral nerve sheath tumor. The tumor breaks through the perineurium into the surrounding tissues.

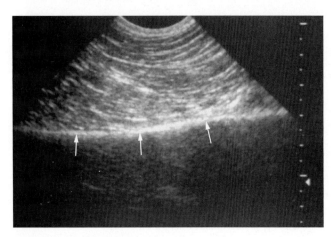

Figure 14-17 Normal bone. The echogenic line across the image (*arrows*) represents the cortical surface of normal bone. Note the lack of image detail deep to the cortical surface because of acoustic impedance.

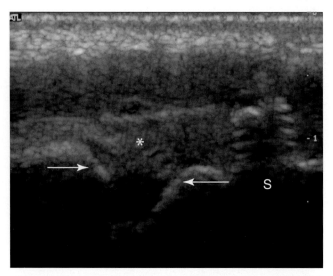

Figure 14-18 Healing fracture. Sagittal image of the tibia 1 month postosteotomy. The tibial fracture has a visible fracture gap, and the ends of the bone fragments are rounded (*white arrows*). The hyperechoic tissue in the fracture gap represents organizing callus (*). The tip of a screw is visible in the distal fracture fragment (*S*).

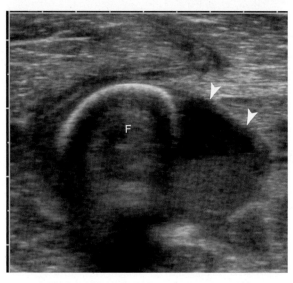

Figure 14-19 Subperiosteal abscess in a puppy with necrotizing fasciitis. The periosteum (*arrowheads*) is elevated from the femur (*F*) by a fluid collection that has a faint fluid-fluid level. Culture of aspirates grew *Streptococcus canis*.

Osteomyelitis. Ultrasonography enables detection of acute bone infections before they are visible on radiographs. Subperiosteal abscesses were identified in 24 children with clinically suspected acute hematogenous osteomyelitis 4 to 14 days after onset.[46,47] In another report of 25 children, abscesses were identified 4 to 7 days after the onset of illness.[48] The earliest changes are isoechoic thickening of the soft tissues adjacent to bone and periosteal thickening. Increased power Doppler signal affecting the periosteal tissues may be observed, and may be the only abnormality in the acute stages of infection.[48] As the infection progresses, hypoechoic subperiosteal fluid collections and cortical irregularity[47] may appear (Figure 14-19). Radiographic signs of osteomyelitis are not usually evident until at least 10 to 14 days after infection. Ultrasonography offers the potential for earlier diagnosis and treatment.

In chronic osteomyelitis, cortical disruption is likely to be more marked and any fluid collections more echoic than in acute cases.[49,50,50a] Cloaca and sinus tracts may be identified. Hyperechoic foci with distal shadowing representing sequestra or foreign bodies may also be visualized (Figure 14-20). Ultrasonography is an excellent tool for guiding fine-needle aspiration or drainage of fluid collections in patients with suspected osteomyelitis.[50,50a]

Neoplasia. Ultrasonography can be used to assess the osseous and extraosseous components of bone neoplasms or soft tissue neoplasms invading bone. Periosteal reaction, cortical destruction, pathologic fracture, matrix mineralization, fluid levels, and involvement of the neurovascular bundle and regional soft tissues may be identified.[51] The affected periosteum appears hyperechoic and irregular, and the cortical margin loses its normal smooth crisp appearance (Figure 14-21). For bone tumors with a predominantly osseous proliferative component, such as multilobular osteosarcoma, ultrasonographic evaluation is fairly unrewarding owing to the inability of sound to penetrate the bone interface. In patients with more lytic neoplasms, the cortex may appear porous, and

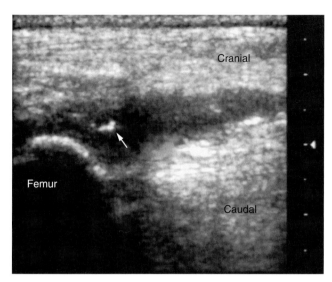

Figure 14-20 Osteomyelitis with sequestration. A large, hypoechoic triangle-shaped area is noted adjacent to the caudomedial aspect of a femur imaged in a transverse plane. Note the hyperechoic focus within the hypoechoic region (*arrow*). This represents a sequestered fragment of bone within an abscessed tissue pocket adjacent to the irregular femoral cortical surface.

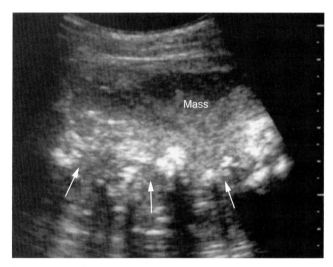

Figure 14-21 Bone neoplasia with complete disruption of the cortical surface. A homogeneous-appearing hypoechoic mass can be seen in the near field adjacent to the fragmented cortical surface (*arrows*).

discontinuity secondary to neoplastic infiltration or pathologic fracture may be evident. Pronounced bone thinning or bone loss may enable visualization of the medullary cavity in long bones or underlying structures through flat bones.

There is no significant advantage in the use of ultrasonography over radiography for the diagnosis or staging of osseous neoplasia. Ultrasonography may sometimes be a more convenient method than radiography for guiding percutaneous needle biopsy of bone lesions.[52,53]

Joints

Normal Findings

Radiographs of suspected joint conditions should be obtained before considering ultrasonography. In selected cases, ultrasonography may provide supplementary information about joints but is technically challenging, primarily because of the difficulty obtaining suitable acoustic windows for examination of articular surfaces. Several approaches at varying angles are required for thorough investigation of a joint, and even then, certain regions will remain inaccessible. Because of the tightly curved skin around many joints, obtaining optimal transducer-skin coupling is difficult. For this reason, there may be an advantage to using a transducer with a small footprint; however, sector (or vector) transducers, which have small footprints, are not well suited to imaging convex surfaces. Sector transducers also produce more artifacts associated with anisotropism of tendons[3] or ligaments adjacent to joints. For these reasons, a linear transducer may be preferred even though it does not fit the skin surface well. Careful skin preparation, abundant coupling gel, and firm transducer pressure will help maximize image quality under these circumstances.

Passive joint motion during scanning can help identify anatomic landmarks and may also reveal dynamic lesions. Examination of the contralateral joint is essential when the anatomy is unfamiliar or when bilateral lesions are suspected.

Normal hyaline articular cartilage is hypoechoic because of its homogeneous texture and high water content.[54] In contrast, fibrocartilage, such as in the menisci of the stifle and the annulus fibrosus of intervertebral disks, is heterogeneous and hyperechoic.[55,56] Small amounts of anechoic joint fluid may be seen in normal joints. The joint capsule is seldom visualized in normal patients because it is thin and blends with the echoes of overlying soft tissues; however, in the presence of joint effusion, it can more easily be distinguished from the surrounding soft tissue.

Shoulder. Techniques and the normal ultrasonographic appearance of the shoulder joint have been described in dogs and horses.[57,58] Structures that may be visualized ultrasonographically include the biceps brachii tendon and its bursa, the supraspinatus and infraspinatus muscles and tendons, and the superficial muscles of the shoulder and the underlying humerus and scapula (Figure 14-22). The patient is normally positioned in lateral recumbency with the affected side up. The joint may be extended or flexed during the examination, which aids recognition of anatomic landmarks.

Elbow. The elbow joint is amenable to ultrasound imaging because of its small size and superficial location. Many soft tissue and osseous structures can be seen, including the lateral and medial epicondyles, the collateral ligaments, the medial coronoid process of the ulna, the anconeal process of the ulna, the humeroradial and humeroulnar joint spaces, and the tendons of the supinator, biceps, and triceps muscles.[59]

Coxofemoral Joint. The coxofemoral joint can be superficially evaluated by ultrasonography from a dorsolateral approach.[60] The concave acetabular shelf and convex femoral surface can be imaged just craniomedial to the palpable greater trochanter (Figure 14-23). This window has proved suitable for guiding joint aspirations.

Stifle Joint. Ultrasonographic evaluation of the equine[61,62] and canine[55,56,63] stifle joint has been described. In the dog, normal anatomic structures consistently seen are the patellar tendon, patellar fat pad, medial and lateral menisci, cranial and caudal cruciate ligaments, and femoral condylar cartilage. The caudal cruciate ligament is less consistently seen than the cranial cruciate ligament. The tendon of the long digital extensor muscle can be seen crossing the joint on the lateral aspect. The collateral, meniscal, and intermeniscal ligaments are not typically identified because they are thin and close to bone.

The joint is best examined in sagittal and transverse planes from five separate windows: cranial, craniomedial, craniolateral, caudomedial, and caudolateral. The cranial cruciate

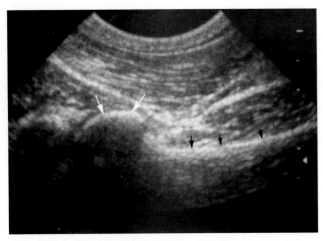

Figure 14-22 Normal caudal humeral head. The convex surface of the caudal humeral head (*white arrows*) and caudal surface of the proximal humerus (*black arrows*) are clearly visualized.

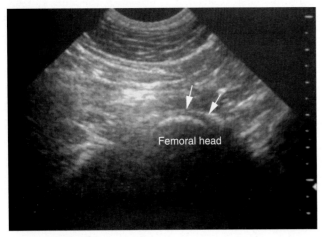

Figure 14-23 Normal coxofemoral joint. The parallel curvilinear surfaces of the dorsal acetabular rim (*arrows*) and femoral head can be imaged just craniomedial to the palpable greater trochanter.

ligament and cranial menisci are best imaged in a sagittal plane from a cranial approach with the joint in full flexion. The patellar ligament is best imaged in extension. Both the cranial cruciate and meniscal ligaments are more hypoechoic than the patellar ligament. In large dogs, the caudal cruciate ligament can be seen by positioning the stifle in extension with the transducer 15 degrees medial to the sagittal plane. In medium-size dogs, the caudal cruciate ligament is seen in the same image as the cranial cruciate ligament with the joint in full flexion.[63] The infrapatellar fat pad is visualized as a hyperechoic zone between the patellar and cruciate ligaments.

Tarsus. The trochlear ridges of the talus are predilection sites for developmental joint disease. The normal ultrasonographic appearance of the distal tibia and trochlear ridges of the talus has been described, in which the joint is imaged dorsally in extension with a linear transducer, and from the plantar aspect with the joint flexed using either a linear or microconvex transducer. Approximately 75% of the trochlear ridges can be seen using these approaches.[64]

Abnormal Findings
Osteochondrosis. Articular cartilage defects of the caudal aspect of the humeral head (and femoral condyle) may be detected ultrasonographically, depending on the size and position of the defect.[65,66] The caudal humeral head is imaged with the transducer in a craniocaudal orientation, and the shoulder is rotated medially to expose the articular cartilage. The subchondral bone defects appear as an irregular concavity in the normally smooth convex curve of the caudal humerus. Cartilage flaps and mineralized cartilage flaps can appear as a hyperechoic line proximal to the subchondral defect. An echogenic, shadowing intracapsular fragment (joint mouse) may be identified adherent to a portion of thickened synovium on the caudal aspect of the joint[63] or in the bicipital tendon sheath.[65] Concurrent joint effusion and bicipital tendon sheath distension are often present in dogs with humeral osteochondrosis.

Elbow Dysplasia. Ultrasonographic identification of a fragmented medial coronoid process has been described.[67] Independent movement of the fragment in relation to the rest of the bone could be seen during passive movement of the joint. Ununited anconeal process may also be identified, and, again, separation of the process from the ulna is best seen on flexion of the joint.

Hip Dysplasia. Ultrasonography of the coxofemoral joint during manipulation is a promising method for revealing excessive joint laxity in puppies with dysplasia.[68,69] Additional studies are focused on the possible use of ultrasonography to identify onset of femoral head mineralization as a sign of hip dysplasia.[68] Although hip dysplasia has been associated with decreased blood flow to the femoral head in humans, abnormal pulsatility index and mean flow velocity were not evident in dogs with hip joint laxity and degenerative joint disease.[70]

Avascular Necrosis of the Femoral Head. Ultrasonography typically reveals an irregular contour of the femoral head and adjacent acetabulum in humans with avascular necrosis of the femoral head.[71,71a] The joint capsule is often thickened, and periarticular tissues have increased echogenicity because of inflammation. Joint effusion may or may not be present, depending on the chronicity of the disease.

Osteoarthrosis. Radiographs are more informative than ultrasound imaging for staging the severity of osteoarthrosis; however, ultrasonography may help distinguish synovial thickening from effusion and can guide arthrocentesis. Ultrasonography at 25 MHz has been used experimentally to assess cartilage thickness in vitro and subsurface characteristics in normal and arthritic joints.[54]

Joint Effusions. Both septic and aseptic joint effusions can readily be identified with ultrasound imaging. The echogenicity of these effusions is similar to that of effusions previously described in other locations (Figure 14-24).

Neoplasia. Although various neoplasms may affect joints,[72] the neoplasm that most frequently arises in joints is synovial cell sarcoma (Figure 14-25). Ultrasound may be helpful in guiding diagnostic aspiration of proliferative synovium or destructive osseous lesions (Figure 14-26).

Tendons and Ligaments
Normal Findings
Ultrasonography of tendons and ligaments is a well established and common practice of equine patients, but similar analyses in small animal patients have a shorter history. Many of the tendons and ligaments in the distal limbs of small animal patients are too small for detailed examination, hence studies have concentrated on larger tendons and ligaments around the shoulder, elbow, stifle, and hock.

The ultrasonographic appearance of tendons is similar across species.[1,3,73] Linear transducers are preferred because of their wide superficial field of view and uniform angle of insonation, which renders a uniform echogenicity for a straight tendon.[1-3] Longitudinally, tendons exhibit a moderately echogenic echotexture composed of multiple parallel lines (Figure 14-27). In transverse section, tendons are round to oval with multiple small internal echoes. The peritenon is thin and hyperechoic. A slight amount of anechoic fluid may be identified within the sheathed portions of tendons. The tendon sheath appears thin and hyperechoic at the peritenon–superficial soft tissue interface. Excessive pressure applied with the transducer over a superficial tendon will compress the tendon sheath and displace fluid such that it is not visible.

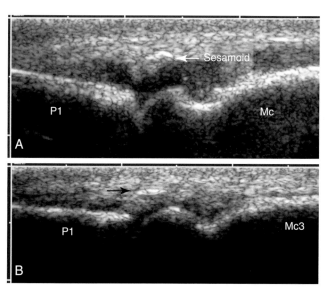

Figure 14-24 Joint effusion. A, Sagittal image of the metacarpophalangeal joint in a dog with a painful swelling of the joint. The dorsal sesamoid (*arrow*) is displaced dorsally by an anechoic effusion. *P1,* first phalanx. *Mc* third metacarpal bone. **B,** Comparison image made 6 weeks later after treatment shows normal appearance. *P1,* first phalanx. *Mc3,* third metacarpal bone.

Abnormal Findings

Tendon Sheath Effusion. Tenosynovitis is the most common cause of tendon sheath effusion in small animal patients. The tendon sheath contents are typically anechoic to hypoechoic (Figure 14-28). More chronic effusions may contain echogenic debris representative of fibrin, and the sheath may become thicker with a more irregular internal surface. Similarly, in patients with septic or acute hemorrhagic effusions, the fluid within the tendon sheath is usually echogenic and the tendon sheath is thickened and irregular.

MUSCLE, TENDON, AND LIGAMENT TRAUMA

Muscle

Muscle trauma can be categorized as external, resulting in hematomas, and internal, which usually causes strains and

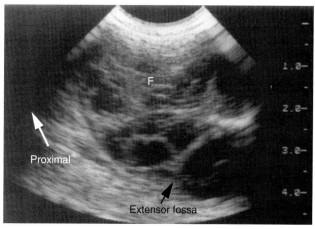

Figure 14-25 Lateral parasagittal image of a femoral condyle (*F*) in a dog with highly invasive synovial cell sarcoma of the stifle joint. The cortex and articular condyle are "paper thin," allowing the intraosseous tissues to be imaged in this region. Note the many cystic and lytic areas within the condyle compatible with a neoplastic infiltrate.

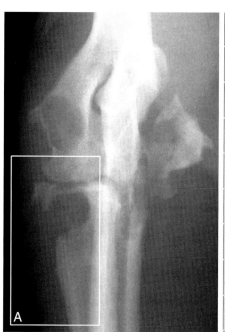
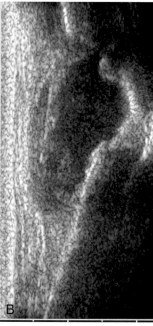

Figure 14-26 Synovial sarcoma. A, Craniocaudal radiograph of the elbow of a dog with multiple lytic bone lesions as a result of synovial cell sarcoma. There is a pathologic fracture of the medial aspect of the humeral condyle. **B,** Ultrasound image corresponding to the white rectangle in **A** shows hypoechoic mass occupying an osseous defect. Ultrasound-guided biopsy was performed of this lesion.

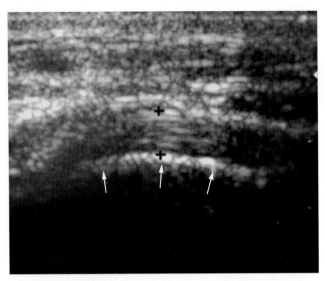

Figure 14-27 **Normal appearance of the biceps tendon imaged in a sagittal plane (+).** Note the linear echogenic fiber pattern. The curvilinear echogenic structure deep to the tendon represents the proximal humeral cortical surface (*arrows*).

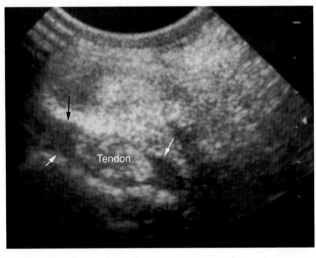

Figure 14-28 Biceps tendon in transverse plane as it passes within the bicipital groove of the proximal humerus. Note the hypoechoic areas on either side of the tendon representing flocculent fluid accumulation within the tendon sheath (*arrows*).

ruptures.[18,74] Muscle trauma may also result in compartmental syndromes, rhabdomyolysis, fibrotic myopathies, and myositis ossificans. Injuries can also be characterized as acute or chronic.

Acute strains from overstretching muscle may result in stiffness and soreness but no macroscopic lesion, hence ultrasonography does not usually demonstrate any abnormalities. Acute partial ruptures result in discontinuity of muscle fibers and the presence of a hematoma. The hematoma is usually contained within the compartment of origin and may cause focal or diffuse muscle enlargement. Examination during contracture of the muscle may facilitate visualization of a partial tear. In a complete rupture, the retracted muscle ends may be visible and surrounded by a hematoma (Figure 14-29). The ultrasonographic appearance of muscle contusions and hematomas varies significantly with the age of the hematoma. Hemorrhage initially appears as a diffuse, increased echogenicity

within the muscle. A hematoma of a few days' duration is usually hypoechoic or anechoic. Subsequent clot reorganization produces internal echoes and septations. Finally, the hematoma liquefies and is eventually resorbed. Hematomas that result in increased pressure within a fascial compartment can compromise venous return and lead to irreversible ischemia, necrosis, and nerve damage (compartment syndrome). A decompressive fasciotomy or drainage of the hematoma may be necessary to prevent such a complication. With rhabdomyolysis, the smooth architecture of the muscle is replaced with heterogeneous areas of mixed echogenicity. These areas may later appear more hypoechoic and can become fluid-filled collections.[22,23,75]

In the chronic stages, a partial muscle tear may heal without ultrasonographic sequelae or may heal with a focal, small, echogenic scar within the muscle belly. The muscle belly may contract, resulting in an abnormal gait and conformation of the limb. A chronic, complete rupture will result in a thick, ropelike scar between the two torn fragments.[18-20,75] Significant hemorrhage from direct muscle trauma can result in myositis ossificans, the formation of heterotopic, nonneoplastic bone in or adjacent to the injured muscle. This is most commonly seen within the semitendinosus, semimembranosus, supraspinatus, and quadriceps muscles in dogs.[18] In the early stages of myositis ossificans, ultrasonography may reveal lamellar sheets of echogenic material. In more chronic cases, the lesion appears as coarse, echogenic foci with distal shadowing, usually aligned parallel with the diaphysis of the bone.

Tendon and Ligament

The ultrasonographic appearance of normal and traumatized tendons and ligaments is universal throughout the body, and their response to injury is similar; therefore the description of tendon injury that follows also applies to ligaments. Damage to tendons is a continuum from fiber slippage (which is microscopic) to complete rupture. Tendon injuries have a variable ultrasonographic appearance depending on the severity of the injury and the stage of healing. In the acute stage, a partial tear is characterized by focal replacement of the normal striated echotexture with hemorrhage and edema, which thickens the tendon and produces a heterogeneous, hypoechoic echotexture (Figure 14-30). Fluid may also be present in the peritendinous tissues or tendon sheath. Reexamination after a period of rest may reveal a more homogeneous appearance. With chronic injuries, the tendon remains thickened and heterogeneous, sometimes with small echogenic, shadowing foci that represent intratendinous calcification. Chronic tears may also appear hypoechoic compared to surrounding tendon because of immature collagen formation. It can be difficult to age a lesion on the basis of its ultrasonographic appearance if the results of a previous examination are not available for comparison. It can also be difficult to differentiate a partial tendon tear from a degenerative tendinopathy because the two may coexist. Complete tendon rupture is associated with focal replacement of the normal striated echotexture by a hypoechoic defect between the hyperechoic, retracted ends of the tendon. Dynamic examinations, in which the tendon is scanned while the limb is manipulated to apply tension to the tendon, can facilitate identification of complete tendon rupture.

In general, the criteria for characterizing a tendon injury are (1) cross-sectional area of the tendon and the lesion; (2) percentage of fibers that appear disrupted within the lesion; (3) echogenicity and echotexture; (4) pattern: homogeneous, heterogeneous, focal, or diffuse; and (5) changes in appearance over time. Assessment of tendon and ligament size and echogenicity are facilitated by comparison with corresponding

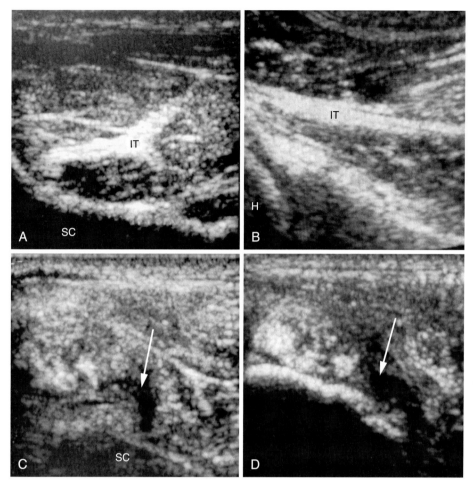

Figure 14-29 Transverse (**A**) and sagittal (**B**) images of a normal canine infraspinatus muscle. The central hyperechoic regions represent the proximal extent of the infraspinatus tendon (*IT*). The humerus (*H*) and scapula (*SC*) are visible as the reflective surfaces underlying the muscle. Transverse (**C**) and sagittal (**D**) images of the infraspinatus muscle from a dog with acute onset of non–weight-bearing lameness. The normal pattern of muscle is disrupted, and there is a hematoma (*arrows*) between separated sections of tendon. *SC*, Scapula.

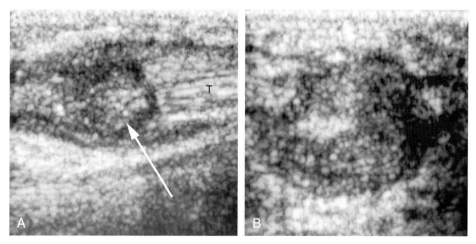

Figure 14-30 Sagittal (**A**) and transverse (**B**) images of a torn calcaneal tendon (*T*) showing a large area of edema and hemorrhage (*arrow*) that has developed within the region of the tear.

structures in the contralateral limb. Care should be taken to evaluate tendons in two planes to ensure that suspected lesions are within the tendon and not artifacts resulting from variable angle of insonation or partial volume effects.

As healing of a tendon injury progresses, hemorrhage, edema, and immature collagen are replaced by mature collagen fibers, fibrous scar tissue, or both, and the echogenicity of lesions increases. Although the healing period is extremely variable, it frequently takes 3 to 5 months for the fiber pattern to return to a damaged area. In all but the mildest lesions, some degree of fiber pattern disruption remains in the "healed" tendon, making the endpoint of the healing process difficult to determine. Even if there is ultrasonographic evidence of healing, the tendon will remain weak and susceptible to reinjury if the animal is allowed to return to exercise too soon. Significant reorganization of the tendon fibers occurs with the increased loading associated with exercise, but this change is not usually visible ultrasonographically.[76]

Individual Tendon Examinations

Ultrasound of the shoulder has been recently evaluated in diagnosing disorders of tendons, ligaments, synovium, and cartilage. In one study, ultrasonography had a sensitivity of 86% and specificity of 91% for diagnosis of a range of disorders (not including instability of the joint).[77]

Biceps Brachii

The biceps tendon originates on the supraglenoid tubercle of the scapula, crosses the cranial aspect of the shoulder joint, and passes within the bicipital groove where it is held in place by a small transverse ligament. An invagination of the shoulder joint forms the bicipital bursa. Distal to the bicipital groove, the tendon blends into the spindle-shaped biceps brachii muscle.[78]

The biceps tendon is easily palpable within the bicipital groove, just medial to the prominent greater tubercle at the cranial aspect of the shoulder. The overlying skin must be depressed with slight pressure from the transducer to orient the transducer perpendicular to the tendon fibers. The brachiocephalic and pectoral muscles are superficial to the biceps tendon. The tendon is best located with the probe initially in the longitudinal plane. The biceps tendon has a dense, linear, homogeneous hyperechoic fiber pattern (Figure 14-31; see also Figure 14-28). At the musculotendinous junction, the compact, hyperechoic appearance of the biceps tendon is rapidly replaced by the coarse, hypoechoic biceps muscle

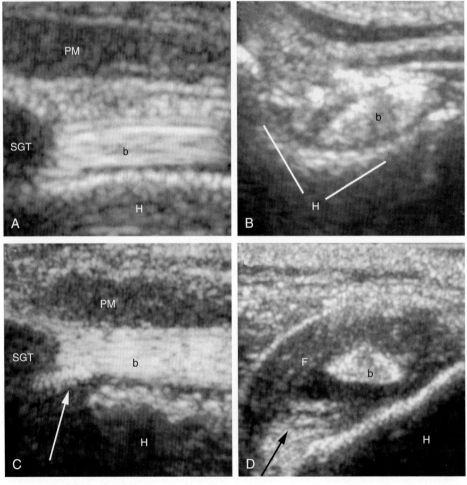

Figure 14-31 Sagittal (**A**) and transverse (**B**) images of a normal canine biceps tendon (*b*) near its origin on the scapula. Similar sagittal (**C**) and transverse (**D**) images from a dog with clinical signs compatible with bicipital tenosynovitis. A focus of mineralization (*white arrow*) is present within the bicipital bursa under the biceps tendon (**C**). The transverse image shows a large volume of fluid (*F*) surrounding the biceps tendon and proliferative synovium within the bicipital bursa (*black arrow*). *H,* Humerus; *PM,* pectoral muscle; *SGT,* supraglenoid tubercle of the scapula.

fibers. Evaluation of the tendon is easiest if the shoulder joint is marginally flexed with the humerus slightly supinated, which places tension on the biceps tendon. The probe has to be moved distally in a curvilinear fashion during the examination to maintain a perpendicular angle of insonation to the curved tendon. In transverse section, the tendon shape typically changes from circular near its origin to oblong distally, but the cross-sectional area remains fairly constant. In the normal dog, the biceps bursa is visible as a small accumulation of anechoic fluid in a pouch medial to the tendon, near its junction with the muscle. A small amount of joint fluid is also typically seen under the tendon at its origin on the supraglenoid tubercle. The underlying surface of the intertubercular groove is smooth and uniformly echogenic.

Injuries to the biceps tendon of origin are well recognized in middle-aged, medium to large dogs.[79] Injuries affecting the biceps tendon of insertion have also been described.[80] Signs of bicipital tenosynovitis include an anechoic zone around the biceps tendon from excess fluid in the tendon sheath, enlarged and hypoechoic tendon, altered echotexture from fiber pattern disruption, partial or complete rupture, an irregular or proliferative synovial lining, and in chronic cases, an irregular surface of the bicipital groove[57,81] (see Figure 14-31). Free osseous bodies and proliferative synovium may also be seen in the bicipital bursa.[81] Fluid within the bursa is a nonspecific finding because it may also occur secondary to inflammation of the scapulohumeral joint (see Figure 14-31). Nonvisualization of the biceps tendon indicates a complete tear or medial luxation associated with rupture of the transverse intertubercular ligament. Medial displacement of the tendon may be seen during

dynamic examination.[81] Small avulsion fragments from the supraglenoid tubercle may be observed in patients with rupture of the biceps brachii tendon.[81]

In addition to diagnosis of biceps tendon injuries, ultrasonography has been used to guide biceps tenotomy.[82,83]

Supraspinatus Tendon

The supraspinatus tendon fills the supraspinous fossa of the scapula. Distally, the muscle curves around the neck of the scapula and has a short, strong tendon that inserts on the greater tubercle of the humerus. Like the biceps tendon, this tendon is easier to examine if the shoulder joint is flexed and the limb adducted. The supraspinatus tendon should be evaluated along its entire insertion on the greater tubercle. The longitudinal fiber pattern of the tendon can be seen on the lateral and cranial aspects of the tubercle with the transducer in an oblique position parallel with the spine of the scapula. The tendon is short, but dense fibers can be followed far proximally within the less echogenic, heterogeneous pattern of the large supraspinatus muscle (Figures 14-32 and 14-33). A portion of the supraspinatus tendon inserts on the medial aspect of the tubercle near the biceps bursa. Dystrophic calcification may form in this region.[57,77,81]

Calcifying tendinopathy of the supraspinatus tendon has been reported as a cause of lameness and as an incidental finding in dogs, particularly large breeds such as the Rottweiler. Calcification is more likely to be associated with lameness if it affects the supraspinatus tendon near the biceps bursa, potentially resulting in a synovitis.[57] Ultrasonography can help differentiate supraspinatus calcification from sclerosis of the

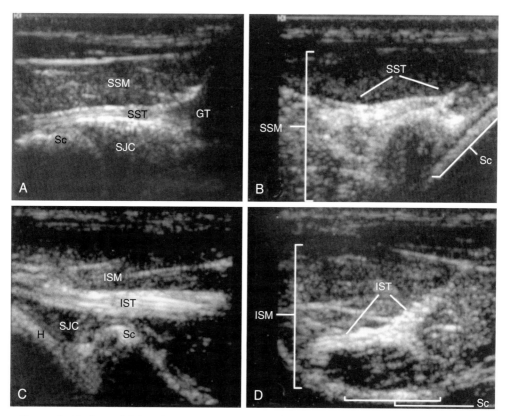

Figure 14-32 Sagittal (**A**) and transverse (**B**) images of the supraspinatus tendon (*SST*) and muscle (*SSM*) near insertion on the greater tubercle of the humerus (*GT*). Sagittal (**C**) and transverse (**D**) images of the infraspinatus tendon (*IST*) and muscle (*ISM*) near insertion on the proximal humerus (*H*). The rim of the glenoid fossa (*Sc*) and shoulder joint capsule (*SJC*) are visible under the tendons.

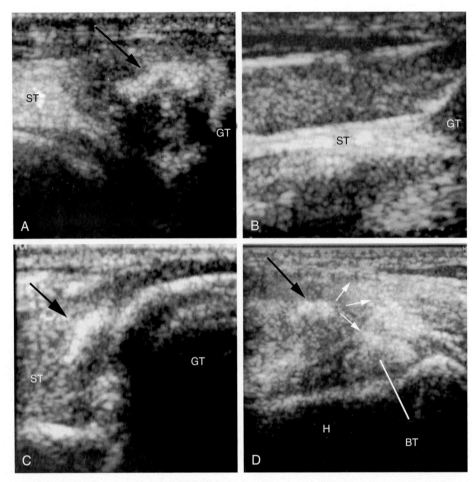

Figure 14-33 Sagittal images (**A** and **C**) and a transverse image (**D**) of an injured (**D**) and comparative normal (**B**) canine supraspinatus tendon (*ST*). In **A** and **C**, the normal hyperechoic fiber pattern of the tendon has been disrupted, and there are foci of mineralization (*black arrows*) near the insertion on the greater tubercle of the humerus (*GT*). Transverse image (**D**) of the biceps tendon (*BT*) and bursa shows the medial aspect of the injured supraspinatus tendon (*white arrows*) close to the biceps bursa. Mineralization within the supraspinatus tendon is noted (*black arrow*). Fluid in the biceps tendon indicates an associated biceps bursitis. *H*, Humerus.

bicipital groove, calcifying tendinopathy of the biceps tendon, and entrapped joint mice within the bicipital bursa, all of which can appear similar radiographically. Ultrasonography may reveal a disrupted fiber pattern of the supraspinatus tendon, and dystrophic mineralization can be recognized as discrete, hyperechoic foci with distal acoustic shadowing[57,77] (see Figure 14-33). Acoustically mixed lesions with sonolucent and echogenic areas can be seen with trauma of the supraspinatus muscle.[21]

Infraspinatus and Teres Minor Tendons
The infraspinatus muscle lies in the infraspinous fossa at the caudolateral aspect of the scapula. The muscle has a strong, long tendon that crosses the lateral aspect of the shoulder joint to insert on the lateral aspect of the greater tubercle of the humerus (see Figure 14-32). The belly of the infraspinatus muscle can be visualized deep to the scapular head of the deltoid muscle by positioning the probe on the caudal aspect of the scapular spine. The tendon fibers begin to form in the central part of the muscle belly.[78]

The teres minor tendon, which looks like the infraspinatus tendon but is smaller, lies just caudal to it and also inserts at

the proximolateral aspect of the humerus. The lateral aspect of the shoulder joint capsule lies under the infraspinatus and teres minor tendons but does not normally have identifiable characteristics. Ultrasonography may be used to look for signs of contracture or strain of the infraspinatus muscle,[21] calcification,[77] and teres minor myopathy.[84] The ultrasonographic characteristics of these lesions are variable, depending on the chronicity of the lesion, but they follow the usual patterns of tendon and muscle trauma (Figure 14-34).

Carpal Canal. The ultrasonographic anatomy of the canine carpal canal has been described recently.[85]

Calcaneal Tendon
The canine calcaneal tendon (Achilles tendon) is formed by three closely associated tendons: the tendons of insertion of the gastrocnemius and superficial digital flexor muscles, and a conjoined tendon formed by tendons from the biceps femoris, semitendinosus, and gracilis muscles (Figure 14-35).[86] The calcaneal bursa lies between the superficial digital flexor tendon (SDFT) and the gastrocnemius tendon and distally between the SDFT and the plantar ligament, but it is not visible ultrasonographically.[86]

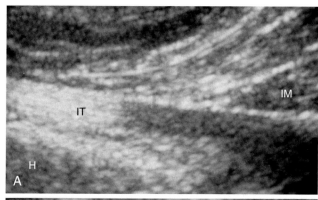

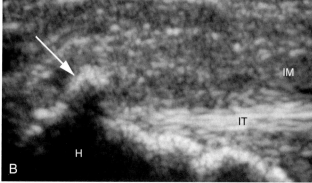

Figure 14-34 Sagittal images of a normal (**A**) and avulsed (**B**) canine infraspinatus tendon (*IT*) near its insertion on the proximal humerus (*H*). An avulsed fragment of the humerus is seen in **B** (*white arrow*). *IM*, Infraspinatus muscle.

Ultrasonography of the normal canine calcaneal tendon has been described in some detail.[86] In the proximal portion of the tendon in the sagittal plane, the SDFT or the gastrocnemius is in the near field, depending on the location of the transducer. The conjoined tendon is the structure closest to the tibia. Near the insertion on the calcaneus, the SDFT is in the near field, and the gastrocnemius tendon is between it and the conjoined tendon. Transverse images are the most useful for identifying the tendons of the superficial digital flexor and gastrocnemius muscles, which are difficult to distinguish in longitudinal images. For the majority of the length of the calcaneal tendon, the component tendons are rounded in transverse section. Each of these tendons becomes slightly wider and flatter as they approach the tuber calcis, with the SDFT sliding over the gastrocnemius tendon into a more superficial position and the conjoined tendon becoming deeper. Each of these tendons has a fairly uniform thickness, although the gastrocnemius tendon and SDFT became thinner immediately proximal to the tuber calcis.

Injuries affecting the calcaneal tendon in dogs are usually the result of direct trauma.[70,87,88] There is evidence that certain breeds, such as the Doberman pinscher, are predisposed to calcaneal tendon injuries.[89,90] In many dogs, calcaneal injuries are relatively severe, involving rupture of one or more components.[70,87,88] In these cases, ultrasonography may add little information to that obtained by physical examination; however, in dogs with less severe injuries, it is possible to differentiate patients with tendon edema or tendon sheath swelling from those with tendon displacement, partial ruptures, or associated muscle tears.[89-91] (Figure 14-36). Partial calcaneal tendon ruptures can also be classified as deep or superficial ruptures, or muscle tears.[90] This is an important distinction

clinically because surgery is indicated for large transverse or complete tears, but conservative therapy is used for tenosynovitis. Partial superficial tears near the calcaneus often have associated bone fragments.[90] Partially or completely ruptured tendons are associated with hematomas that are initially hypoechoic, then inhomogeneous with hyperechoic areas in the first 1 to 2 weeks. Healing tendons are initially enlarged and heterogeneous, then decrease in size and regain some normal fiber pattern over a period of 10 to 12 weeks.[90]

Cruciate Ligaments and Menisci. The cranial cruciate ligament is difficult to visualize clearly by ultrasonography. Although recent studies have had greater success than those performed previously,[92-95] it is easy to miss partial or complete ligament tears. Stifles with cranial cruciate ligament rupture may have irregular, hyperechoic tissue between the tibial eminences that represents fibrous tissue, or they may have hypoechoic tissue that represents hematoma.[92] A ruptured cranial cruciate ligament may be visible as a short, echogenic band attached to the intercondylar area of the tibia and surrounded by the infrapatellar fat pad. The peripheral portions of the lateral and medial menisci are also visible with ultrasound. In one study, bucket handle tears and complex tears of the menisci were identified with a sensitivity of 90% and a specificity of 93%.[95]

Patellar Ligament and Quadriceps Tendon
The patellar ligament is an extension of the extensor mechanism of the stifle below the apex of the patella and inserts distally on the tibial tuberosity. The quadriceps tendon represents the common tendon insertion of the rectus femoris, vastus lateralis, vastus medialis, and vastus intermedius muscles. Both of these structures are relatively large and superficial and are amenable to sonographic examination (Figure 14-37). Thickening of the patellar ligament occurs in some dogs following tibial plateau leveling osteotomy,[96] however the clinical significance of this observation is unknown.

Tarsal Soft Tissues. Ultrasonographic anatomy of the soft tissues around the tarsal joints has been described recently.[97]

Iliopsoas Muscle and Tendon
The iliopsoas originates from the ventral aspect of the lumbar vertebrae and descends caudally as one of the sublumbar, hypaxial group of muscles. The muscle belly lies between the quadratus lumborum muscle dorsolaterally and the psoas minor muscle ventromedially.[78] It inserts on the lesser trochanter of the femur and is susceptible to hyperextension injury.[22] The iliopsoas muscle is identified ultrasonographically by examination through the abdomen; it is between the lumbar vertebrae and the sublumbar retroperitoneal fat.[10] The origin of the muscle from the third lumbar vertebra can be seen consistently. In the transverse plane, the muscle is a round, well-defined structure between the transverse processes and vertebral bodies of the lumbar vertebrae (Figure 14-38, *A*). The insertion of the short tendon can be seen on the lesser trochanter of the femur (see Figure 14-38, *B*). In one study, ultrasonographically detectable injuries to the iliopsoas muscle and tendon were considered to be the cause of lameness in three dogs.[22]

Abdominal Wall Trauma
The body wall typically appears as several echoic and anechoic layers, representing the skin, subcutaneous tissues, muscle layers, and parietal peritoneum. The abdominal wall may be assessed ultrasonographically in animals with suspected hernia (e.g., umbilical) or traumatic abdominal wall rupture. Lack of continuity of the abdominal wall layers may be observed, along with bowel loops or other viscera in the subcutaneous tissues (Figure 14-39).

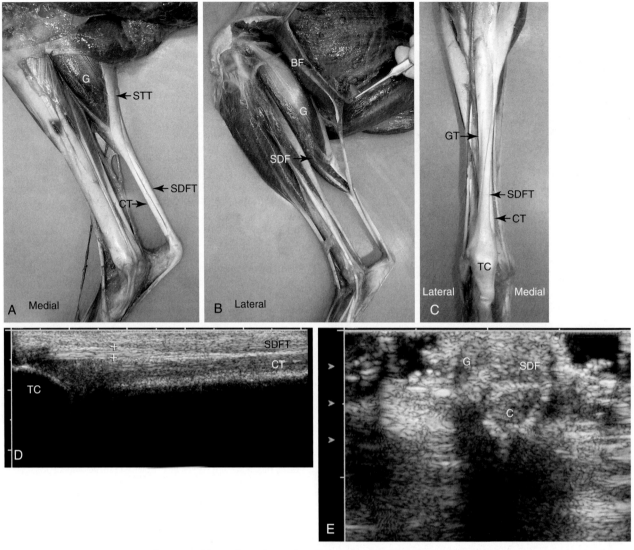

Figure 14-35 **Anatomy of the canine calcaneal tendon. A,** Medial aspect. **B,** Lateral aspect. **C,** Caudal aspect. *BF,* Biceps femoris muscle belly (reflected); *CT,* conjoined tendon; *G,* gastrocnemius muscle; *GT,* gastrocnemius tendon; *SDF,* superficial digital flexor muscle; *SDFT,* superficial digital flexor tendon; *STT,* semitendinosus tendon; *TC,* tuber calcis. **D,** In longitudinal images of the distal part of the tendon, the gastrocnemius tendon (between electronic cursors) lies between the superficial digital flexor tendon (*SDFT*) and the conjoined tendon (*CT*). **E,** In transverse images, the components of the calcaneal tendon are more easily distinguished. C, Conjoined tendon; G, gastrocnemius muscle; *SDF,* superficial digital flexor muscle. (From: Lamb CR, Duvernois A. Ultrasonographic anatomy of the normal canine calcaneal tendon. *Vet Radiol Ultrasound* 2005;**46**:326–30.)

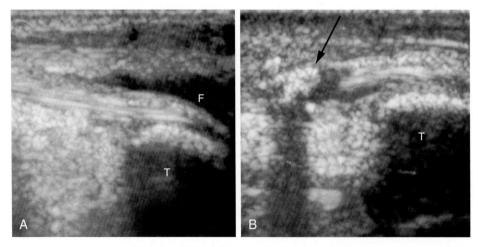

Figure 14-36 **A,** Calcaneal bursitis with fluid (*F*) within the bursa. **B,** Chronic calcaneal tendinitis with dystrophic mineralization within the gastrocnemius tendon (*arrow*) and resultant acoustic shadowing. *T,* Tuber calcaneus.

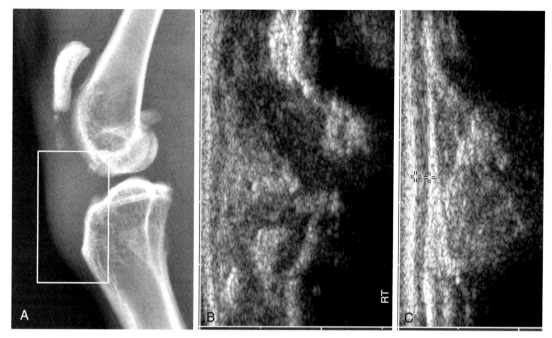

Figure 14-37 **Chronic patellar desmopathy in a cat. A,** Lateral radiograph of the stifle of a cat with firm swelling on its cranial aspect. There are two calcified bodies distal to the patella, probably representing dystrophic calcification. **B,** Sagittal ultrasound image corresponding to the white rectangle in **A** shows heterogeneous tissue replacing the normal anatomy. The patellar ligament is not visible. **C,** Ultrasound image of the contralateral stifle shows a normal feline patellar ligament (measures less than 2 mm between electronic cursors).

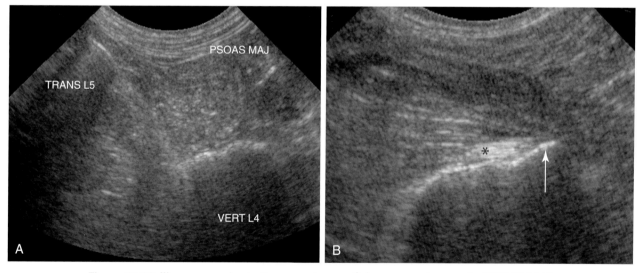

Figure 14-38 **Iliopsoas muscle. A,** Transverse image of the psoas major muscle (*PSOAS MAJ*) between the transverse process of the fifth lumbar vertebra (*TRANS L5*) and the body of the fourth lumbar vertebra (*VERT L4*). **B,** Insertion of the iliopsoas tendon (*) on the lesser trochanter of the femur (*arrow*).

ULTRASOUND-GUIDED PROCEDURES BASED ON NEEDLE INSERTION INTO MUSCULOSKELETAL STRUCTURES

Ultrasonography represents a convenient method for guiding needle insertions into musculoskeletal lesions or normal structures to sample tissue, drain fluid, or inject drugs, local anesthetics, or radiographic contrast media.[98]

Technical Considerations

A thorough ultrasonographic examination of the area of interest is performed before any interventional procedure to characterize the lesion and its relationship with surrounding structures, to obtain the clearest image of the target, and to select a safe path for the needle. The lesion should be evaluated in multiple planes so the shortest path for the needle can be found that avoids critical structures, such as recognizable

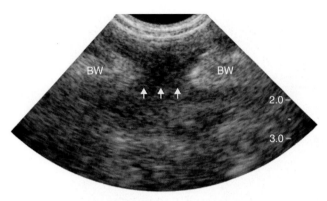

Figure 14-39 Body wall hernia secondary to bite wound. The defect in the body wall (*arrows*) is easily seen as a hypoechoic region separating the hyperechoic body wall (*BW*). The body wall is thickened and has lost the layered appearance of normal body wall.

vascular structures or nerves. Doppler examination can help identify vessels that should be avoided during the procedure and avascular areas that may represent necrotic tissue or fluid collections.

Most ultrasound-guided needle insertions can be performed under local anesthesia or with sedation. The skin and transducer are sterilized with alcohol or chlorhexidine gluconate; adjacent nonsterile parts of the body may be draped. Sterile gel may be used on the skin, or a no-touch technique may be employed, in which the sterile area of skin is not touched by the transducer or gel but only by a sterile needle or other instrument. Passage of the needle through the soft tissues must be controlled by observing the ultrasound image continuously during the procedure. It is helpful to visualize the needle tip immediately after insertion—while it is still subcutaneous—so that its direction can be adjusted precisely before inserting it more deeply. The needle tip appears as a small echogenic focus, but the shaft of the needle is not clearly visible unless it is inserted shallow enough to be perpendicular to the ultrasound beam. Oscillating the needle slightly facilitates visualization of the tip in echogenic tissue.

Percutaneous Tissue Sampling
Biopsy is essential for diagnosis of many musculoskeletal lesions, particularly neoplasms. The decision to perform the biopsy is based on clinical findings and results of the imaging studies. Percutaneous tissue sampling is quicker and less expensive than surgical biopsy and may also have decreased morbidity in some circumstances. These advantages are balanced by the small size of biopsies obtained, which limit diagnostic quality and accuracy.

Percutaneous tissue sampling includes tissue-core biopsy for histology and fine-needle aspiration for cytology. Tissue-core biopsy is performed with 14- to 18-gauge needles of various types, such as the Craig, Turkel, Ackerman, Franseen, and Tru-Cut needles. Use of automated biopsy guns improves the reliability of the procedure and the quality of samples obtained. Needles with a diameter less than 1 mm (21 to 27 gauge) are used for fine-needle aspiration and yield a small amount of nonsolid material suitable for cytology and microbial culture. Ordinary hypodermic or spinal needles are most commonly used. Evidence suggests that more tissue is collected with large-bore needles than small-bore needles.[98]

Percutaneous tissue sampling is indicated when neoplasia must be differentiated from lesions caused by inflammation or other processes. There are no absolute contraindications for percutaneous biopsy of the musculoskeletal structures. In animals with possible coagulopathy, clotting tests should be considered before tissue-core biopsy. More specific information about percutaneous biopsy technique is provided in Chapter 2.

Tissue-core biopsies of soft tissue masses can be performed quickly and safely under ultrasound guidance. The potential for spreading malignant cells along the biopsy needle tract should be considered when selecting the needle puncture site.[81] The needle tract should be resected along with the mass if the lesion is found to be neoplastic. For smaller lesions, aspiration biopsy with end-cutting 20- or 22-gauge spinal needles is usually sufficient for cytologic examination. For large masses, an 18-gauge core biopsy side-cutting needle can be used manually or with a biopsy gun. These techniques are excellent for obtaining diagnostic samples of soft tissue masses.[99]

Biopsy of Bone Lesions
Although bone is known to be a barrier to ultrasound, a lytic lesion that has destroyed bone cortex can easily be identified as a break in the normal smooth echogenic line of the cortex. A mass will often be seen extending from the lytic areas. The defect within the cortex acts as a window through which a needle can be inserted under ultrasound guidance. An aspiration biopsy with a 22-gauge needle usually yields enough tissue for cytologic examination. Studies of small animal bone lesions have demonstrated the feasibility of this method.[52,53] A similar approach can be used to aspirate subperiosteal fluid in cases of osteomyelitis.[98]

Fluid Collection
Ultrasound-guided percutaneous drainage of fluid collections can be diagnostic and/or therapeutic; ultrasound can also allow serial monitoring for recurrence. Assessment of the character of aspirated fluid can complement gray-scale ultrasonographic criteria of lesion type and enable diagnosis of cyst, abscess, hematoma, hygroma ,or abnormal synovial cavity.

Ultrasound-Guided Arthrocentesis
Synovial fluid analysis is indicated in a variety of infectious and inflammatory conditions. When unguided attempts to collect fluid fail, ultrasonography may be useful in identifying small pockets of fluid that can be successfully aspirated. Ultrasound guidance can also confirm the correct placement of a needle within the joint capsule before deposition of contrast media, local anesthetic, or drugs such as corticosteroids. In most joints, a small amount of synovial fluid can be visualized and used as the target for needle insertion. If little fluid is present, saline may be injected into the joint and aspirated for analysis.[98] Also, joint distention with saline or contrast media can enhance visualization of synovial structures and articular cartilage.

The shoulder joint is usually accessed through a lateral approach. The needle can be directed into the lateral joint pouch immediately distal to the acromion of the scapula; or it can be inserted into the pocket at the distal aspect of the biceps bursa, which normally contains a small amount of fluid.[57] Synovial fluid is most frequently found at the craniodorsal aspect of the elbow joint. Aspiration of the coxofemoral joint can be achieved from a craniodorsal approach with the transducer probe oriented parallel to the femoral neck. There is usually a small pocket of fluid in this aspect of the joint. Indications for coxofemoral arthrocentesis include septic arthritis, painful hip prosthesis, and lytic lesions involving the joint. Fluid within the stifle joint can usually be obtained from a cranial approach on either side of the patella.

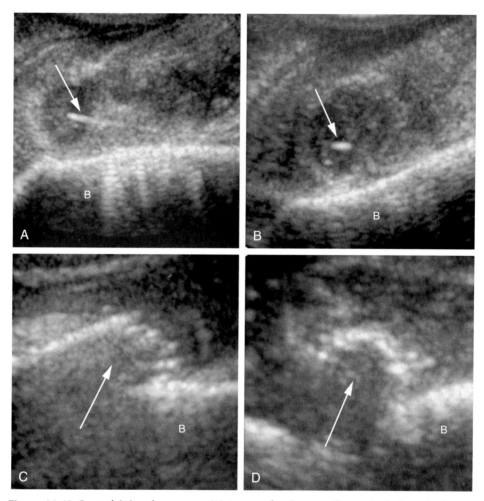

Figure 14-40 Sagittal (**A**) and transverse (**B**) images of a plant awn foreign body (*arrow*) adjacent to the ulna (*B*) of a dog. Note the surrounding hypoechoic region of abscessation. Sagittal (**C**) and transverse (**D**) images of a stick (*arrows*) that impaled the periorbital region of a dog. The lack of fluid pocketing in the surrounding temporal musculature reflects the acute nature of the injury. *B*, Calvaria.

Tendon Sheath and Bursae

Inflammation within synovial structures results in fluid distention and improved visualization with ultrasound examination. Inflammation may result from trauma, infection, arthritis, systemic diseases, and polyarthritis. The fluid distention is often accompanied by synovial proliferation in chronic cases. Aspiration of fluid may be needed for synovial fluid analysis, steroid injection, or decompression. When synovial fluid cannot be aspirated, lavage of the bursa or tendon sheath can be performed by injecting physiologic saline, which is then re-aspirated.

Foreign Body Retrieval

Foreign bodies within soft tissues are a common problem in veterinary practice. Opaque foreign bodies, such as metal, stone, and some types of glass, are visible radiographically, although accurate localization using orthogonal and oblique radiographs can be difficult. Nonopaque foreign bodies, such as wood, plant, or plastic items may not be visible radiographically unless they trap gas. Ultrasound is worth considering as a method for searching for nonopaque foreign bodies and may enable more accurate localization than radiography, depending on the affected structures.[15] Ultrasonography can be used for preoperative or intraoperative localization of a foreign body. A needle inserted adjacent to the foreign body under ultrasound guidance facilitates localization by a surgeon.

The typical ultrasonographic appearance of a foreign body is a hyperechoic structure with distal acoustic shadowing.[15,100,101] Metallic foreign bodies may have a reverberating comet-tail artifact within the distal shadow. Plant awn foreign bodies produce distal acoustic shadowing, and may have a double or triple spindle shape[102,103] (Figure 14-40). There is often a hypoechoic area around the foreign body that represents inflammation, but this may not be present in the acute stages. One study reported a sensitivity and specificity of 86.7% and 96.7%, respectively, for 2.5-mm wooden foreign bodies, and 93.3% and 92.3%, respectively, for 5-mm wooden foreign bodies in humans.[104]

Other structures that are liable to be erroneously identified as foreign material include scar tissue, calcification, ossified cartilage, normal bone structures (e.g., sesamoids), and air introduced from lacerations. In one study, gas in soft tissue did not hinder detection of foreign bodies by ultrasonography, but did reduce ability to distinguish between bone, metal, and glass.[105] If a drainage tract is present, a foreign body can often be localized and retrieved percutaneously with forceps under ultrasound guidance, thus avoiding open surgery.[106]

REFERENCES

1. Miles CA, Fursey GA, Birch HL, et al. Factors affecting the ultrasonic properties of equine digital flexor tendons. *Ultrasound Med Biol* 1996;**22**:907–15.
2. Connolly DJ, Berman L, McNally EG. The use of beam angulation to overcome anisotropy when viewing human tendon with high frequency linear array ultrasound. *Br J Radiol* 2001;**74**:183–5.
3. Garcia T, Hornof WJ, Insana MF. On the ultrasonic properties of tendon. *Ultrasound Med Biol* 2003;**29**:1787–97.
4. Bianchi S, Martinoli C. *Ultrasound of the Musculoskeletal System*. Berlin: Springer; 2007.
5. Chhem RK, Kaplan PA, Dussault RG. Ultrasonography of the musculoskeletal system. *Radiol Clin North Am* 1994;**32**:275–89.
6. Kramer M, Gerwing M, Hach V, et al. Sonography of the musculoskeletal system in dogs and cats. *Vet Radiol Ultrasound* 1997;**38**:139–49.
7. Ziegler L, O'Brien RT. Harmonic ultrasound: a review. *Vet Radiol Ultrasound* 2002;**43**:501–9.
8. Whatmough C, Guitian J, Baines E, et al. Ultrasound image compounding: effect on perceived image quality. *Vet Radiol Ultrasound* 2007;**48**:141–5.
9. Teh J. Applications of Doppler imaging in the musculoskeletal system. *Curr Probl Diagn Radiol* 2006;**35**:22–34.
9a. Sanders RC. Sonography of fat. In: Sanders RC, Hill M, editors. *Ultrasound annual*. New York: Raven; 1984. p. 71–95.
10. Cannon MS, Puchalski SM. Ultrasonographic evaluation of normal canine iliopsoas muscle. *Vet Radiol Ultrasound* 2008;**49**(4):378–82.
11. Weller R, Pfau T, Ferrari M, et al. The determination of muscle volume with a freehand 3D ultrasonography system. *Ultrasound Med Biol* 2007;**33**:402–7.
12. Chao HC, Lin SJ, Huang YC, et al. Sonographic evaluation of cellulitis in children. *J Ultrasound Med* 2000;**19**:743–9.
13. Chau CL, Griffith JF. Musculoskeletal infections: ultrasound appearances. *Clin Radiol* 2005;**60**:149–59.
14. Trout NJ, Penninck DG, Boudrieau RJ, et al. Early postoperative ultrasonographic evaluation of incisional sites in dogs: 15 cases (1990-1992). *J Am Vet Med Assoc* 1994;**205**:1565–8.
15. Armbrust LJ, et al. Ultrasonographic diagnosis of foreign bodies associated with chronic draining tracts and abscesses in dogs. *Vet Radiol Ultrasound* 2003;**44**(1):66–70.
16. Davison BD, Polak JF. Arterial injuries: a sonographic approach. *Radiol Clin North Am* 2004;**42**:383–96.
17. Hall J, Lee K, Priestnall S, et al. Radial artery pseudoaneurysm in a Maine Coon cat. *Vet Surg* submitted.
18. Fitch RB, Jaffe MH, Montgomery RD. Muscle injuries in dogs. *Compend Contin Educ Pract Vet* 1997;**19**:947–57.
19. Steiss JE. Muscle disorders and rehabilitation in canine athletes. *Vet Clin North Am Small Anim Pract* 2002;**32**(1):267–85.
20. Lewis DD, Shelton GD, Piras A, et al. Gracilis or semitendinosus myopathy in 18 dogs. *J Am Anim Hosp Assoc* 1997;**33**:177–88.
21. Siems JJ, Breur GJ, Blevins WE, et al. Use of two-dimensional real-time ultrasonography for diagnosing contracture and strain of the infraspinatus muscle in a dog. *J Am Vet Med Assoc* 1998;**212**:77–80.
22. Breur GJ, Blevins WE. Traumatic injury of the iliopsoas muscle in three dogs. *J Am Vet Med Assoc* 1997;**210**:1631–4.
23. Fukuda T, Sakamoto I, Kohzaki S, et al. Spontaneous rectus sheath hematomas: clinical and radiological features. *Abdom Imaging* 1996;**21**:58–61.
24. Inampudi P, Jacobson JA, Fessell DP, et al. Soft-tissue lipomas: accuracy of sonography in diagnosis with pathologic correlation. *Radiology* 2004;**233**:763–7.
25. Murphey MD, Arcara LK, Fanburg-Smith J. From the archives of the AFIP: imaging of musculoskeletal liposarcoma with radiologic-pathologic correlation. *Radiographics* 2005;**25**:1371–95.
26. Belli P, Costantini M, Mirk P, et al. Role of color Doppler sonography in the assessment of musculoskeletal soft tissue masses. *J Ultrasound Med* 2000;**19**:823–30.
27. Benigni L, Corr SA, Lamb CR. Ultrasonographic assessment of the canine sciatic nerve. *Vet Radiol Ultrasound* 2007;**48**:428–33.
27a. Haro P, Gil F, Laredo F, et al. Ultrasonographic study of the feline sciatic nerve. *J Feline Med Surg* 2011;**13**:259–65.
28. Guilherme S, Benigni L. Ultrasonographic anatomy of the brachial plexus and major nerves of the canine thoracic limb. *Vet Radiol Ultrasound* 2008;**49**:577–83.
29. Echeverry DF, Gil F, Laredo F, et al. Ultrasound-guided block of the sciatic and femoral nerves in dogs: a descriptive study. *Vet J* 2010;**186**:210–15.
30. Campoy L, Bezuidenhout AJ, Gleed RD, et al. Ultrasound-guided approach for axillary brachial plexus, femoral nerve, and sciatic nerve blocks in dogs. *Vet Anaesth Analg* 2010;**37**:144–53.
31. Reynolds DL Jr, Jacobson JA, Inampudi P, et al. Sonographic characteristics of peripheral nerve sheath tumors. *Am J Roentgenol* 2004;**182**:741–4.
32. Gruber H, Glodny B, Bendix N, et al. High-resolution ultrasound of peripheral neurogenic tumors. *Eur Radiol* 2007;**17**:2880–8.
33. Tagliafico A, Altafini L, Garrello I, et al. Traumatic neuropathies: spectrum of imaging findings and postoperative assessment. *Semin Musculoskeletal Radiol* 2010;**14**(5):512–22.
34. Platt SR, Graham J, Chrisman CL, et al. Magnetic resonance imaging and ultrasonography in the diagnosis of a malignant peripheral nerve sheath tumor in a dog. *Vet Radiol Ultrasound* 1999;**40**:367–71.
35. Montoliu P, Pumarola M, Zamora À, et al. Femoral mononeuropathy caused by a malignant sarcoma: two case reports. *Veterinary Journal* 2008;**178**(2):298–301.
36. Da Costa RC, Parent JM, Dobson H, et al. Ultrasound-guided fine needle aspiration in the diagnosis of peripheral nerve sheath tumors in 4 dogs. *Can Vet J* 2008;**49**:77–81.
37. Rose S, Long C, Knipe M, et al. Ultrasonographic evaluation of brachial plexus tumors in five dogs. *Vet Radiol Ultrasound* 2005;**46**(6):514–17.
38. Bradley RL, Withrow SJ, Snyder SP. Nerve sheath tumors in the dog. *J Am Anim Hosp Assoc* 1982;**18**:915–21.
39. Brehm DM, Vite CH, Steinberg HS, et al. A retrospective evaluation of 51 cases of peripheral nerve sheath tumors in the dog. *J Am Anim Hosp Assoc* 1995;**31**:349–59.
40. Targett MP, Dyce J, Houlton JEF. Tumors involving the nerve sheaths of the forelimb in dogs. *J Small Anim Pract* 1993;**34**:221–5.
41. Cho KH, Lee YH, Lee SM, et al. Sonography of bone and bone-related diseases of the extremities. *J Clin Ultrasound* 2004;**32**:511–21.
42. Risselada M, Kramer M, van Bree H. Approaches for ultrasonographic evaluation of long bones in the dog. *Vet Radiol Ultrasound* 2003;**44**:214–20.

43. Risselada M, Van Bree H, Kramer M, et al. Ultrasonographic assessment of fracture healing after plate osteosynthesis. *Vet Radiol Ultrasound* 2007;**48**:368–72.
44. Risselada M, Kramer M, de Rooster H, et al. Ultrasonographic and radiographic assessment of uncomplicated secondary fracture healing of long bones in dogs and cats. *Vet Surg* 2005;**34**:99–107.
45. Maffulli N, Thornton A. Ultrasonographic appearance of external callus in long-bone fractures. *Injury* 1995;**26**:5–12.
46. Kang B, Zhu TB, Du JY, et al. Sonographic diagnosis of acute hematogenous osteomyelitis in the early stage. *J Tongji Med Univ* 1994;**14**:61–4.
47. Taneja K, Mittal SK, Marya SK, et al. Acute osteomyelitis: early diagnosis by ultrasonography. *Australas Radiol* 1992;**36**:77–9.
48. Collado P, Naredo E, Calvo C, et al. Role of power Doppler sonography in early diagnosis of osteomyelitis in children. *J Clin Ultrasound* 2008;**36**:251–3.
49. Cleveland TJ, Peck RJ. Case report: chronic osteomyelitis demonstrated by high resolution ultrasonography. *Clin Radiol* 1994;**49**:429–31.
50. Pineda C, Vargas A, Rodriguez AV. Imaging of osteomyelitis: current concepts. *Infect Dis Clin North Am* 2006;**20**:789–825.
50a. Kulendra E, Corr S. Necrotizing fasciitis with subperiosteal *Streptococcus canis* infection in two puppies. *Vet Comp Orthop Traumatol* 2008;**21**:474–7.
51. Saifuddin A, Burnett SJ, Mitchell R. Pictorial review: ultrasonography of primary bone tumours. *Clin Radiol* 1998;**53**:239–46.
52. Samii VF, Nyland TG, Werner LL, et al. Ultrasound-guided fine-needle aspiration biopsy of bone lesions: a preliminary report. *Vet Radiol Ultrasound* 1999;**40**:82–6.
53. Britt T, Clifford C, Barger A, et al. Diagnosing appendicular osteosarcoma with ultrasound-guided fine-needle aspiration: 36 cases. *J Small Anim Pract* 2007;**48**:145–50.
54. Myers SL, Dines K, Brandt DA, et al. Experimental assessment by high frequency ultrasound of articular cartilage thickness and osteoarthritic changes. *J Rheumatol* 1995;**22**:109–16.
55. Reed AL, Payne JT, Constantinescu GM. Ultrasonographic anatomy of the normal canine stifle. *Vet Radiol Ultrasound* 1995;**36**:315–21.
56. Kramer M, Stengel H, Gerwing M, et al. Sonography of the canine stifle. *Vet Radiol Ultrasound* 1999;**40**:282–93.
57. Long CD, Nyland TG. Ultrasonographic evaluation of the canine shoulder. *Vet Radiol Ultrasound* 1999;**40**:372–9.
58. Tnibar MA, Auer JA, Bakkali S. Ultrasonography of the equine shoulder: technique and normal appearance. *Vet Radiol Ultrasound* 1999;**40**:44–57.
59. Lamb CR, Wong K. Ultrasonographic anatomy of the canine elbow. *Vet Radiol Ultrasound* 2005;**46**:319–25.
60. Greshake RJ, Ackerman N. Ultrasound evaluation of the coxofemoral joints of the canine neonate. *Vet Radiol Ultrasound* 1993;**34**:99–104.
61. Penninck DG, Nyland TG, O'Brien TR, et al. Ultrasonography of the equine stifle. *Vet Radiol* 1990;**31**:293–8.
62. Cauvin ER, Munroe GA, Boyd JS, et al. Ultrasonographic examination of the femorotibial articulation in horses: imaging of the cranial and caudal aspects. *Equine Vet J* 1996;**28**:285–96.
63. Soler M, Murciano J, Latorre R, et al. Ultrasonographic, computed tomographic and magnetic resonance imaging anatomy of the normal canine stifle joint. *Vet J* 2007;**174**:351–61.
64. Liuti T, Saunders JH, Gielen I, et al. Ultrasound approach to the canine distal tibia and trochlear ridges of the talus. *Vet Radiol Ultrasound* 2007;**48**:361–7.
65. Vandevelde B, Van Ryssen B, Saunders JH, et al. Comparison of the ultrasonographic appearance of osteochondrosis lesions in the canine shoulder with radiography, arthrography, and arthroscopy. *Vet Radiol Ultrasound* 2006;**47**:174–84.
66. Piorek A, Adamiak Z. Ultrasonography of the canine shoulder joint and its pathological changes. *Pol J Vet Sci* 2010;**13**(1):193–200.
67. Seyrek-Intas D, Michele U, Tacke S, et al. Accuracy of ultrasonography in detecting fragmentation of the medial coronoid process in dogs. *J Am Vet Med Assoc* 2009;**234**(4):480–5.
68. Lonsdale R, Todhunter R, Yeager A, et al. Ultrasound assessment of femoral head epiphyseal mineralization and subluxation in Labrador retrievers. *Vet Radiol Ultrasound* 1998;**39**:595.
69. O'Brien RT, Dueland RT, Adams WC, et al. Dynamic ultrasonographic measurement of passive coxofemoral joint laxity in puppies. *J Am Anim Hosp Assoc* 1997;**33**:275–81.
70. Rademacher N, Ohlerth S, Doherr MG, et al. Doppler sonography of the medial arterial blood supply to the coxofemoral joints of 36 medium to large breed dogs and its relationship with radiographic signs of joint disease. *Vet Rec* 2005;**156**:305–9.
71. Suzuki S, Awaya G, Okada Y, et al. Examination by ultrasound of Legg-Calve-Perthes disease. *Clin Orthop Relat Res* 1987 Jul;**220**:130–6.
71a. Eckerwall G, Hochbergs P, Wingstrand H, et al. Sonography and intracapsular pressure in Perthes' disease. 39 children examined 2-36 months after onset. *Acta Orthop Scand* 1994;**65**(6):575–80.
72. Whitelock RG, Dyce J, Houlton JEF, et al. A review of 30 tumours affecting joints. *Vet Comp Orthop Traumatol* 1997;**10**:146–52.
73. Martinoli C, Derchi LE, Pastorino C, et al. Analysis of echotexture of tendons with US. *Radiology* 1993;**186**:839–43.
74. Vaughan LC. Muscle and tendon injuries in dogs. *J Small Anim Pract* 1979;**20**:711–36.
75. Jacobson JA, van Holsbeeck MT. Musculoskeletal ultrasonography. *Orthop Clin North Am* 1998;**29**:135–67.
76. Crass JR, Genovese RL, Render JA, et al. Magnetic resonance, ultrasound and histopathologic correlation of acute and healing equine tendon injuries. *Vet Radiol Ultrasound* 1992;**33**:206–16.
77. Cogar SM, Cook CR, Curry SL, et al. Prospective evaluation of techniques for differentiating shoulder pathology as a source of forelimb lameness in medium and large breed dogs. *Vet Surg* 2008;**37**:132–41.
78. Evans HE. *Miller's Anatomy of the Dog*. Philadelphia: WB Saunders; 1993.
79. Bruce WJ, Burbidge HM, Bray JP, et al. Bicipital tendinitis and tenosynovitis in the dog: a study of 15 cases. *N Z Vet J* 2000;**48**:44–52.
80. Schaaf OR, Eaton-Wells R, Mitchell RAS. Biceps brachii and brachialis tendon of insertion injuries in eleven racing Greyhounds. *Vet Surg* 2009;**38**(7):825–33.
81. Kramer M, Gerwing M, Sheppard C, et al. Ultrasonography for the diagnosis of diseases of the tendon and

tendon sheath of the biceps brachii muscle. *Vet Surg* 2001;**30**:64–71.

82. Esterline ML, Armbrust L, Roush JK. A comparison of palpation guided and ultrasound guided percutaneous biceps brachii tenotomy in dogs. *Vet Comp Orthop Traumatol* 2005;**18**(3):135–9.

83. Peppler C, Kramer M, Gerwing M. Ultrasound guided percutaneous tenotomy of the biceps tendon in five dogs with tendovaginitis—preliminary results. *Tieraerztliche Praxis Ausgabe Kleintiere Heimtiere* 2009;**37**(3):167–72.

84. Bruce WJ, Spence S, Miller A. Teres minor myopathy as a cause of lameness in a dog. *J Small Anim Pract* 1997;**38**:74–7.

85. Turan E, Ozsunar Y, Yildirim IG. Ultrasonographic examination of the carpal canal in dogs. *J Vet Sci* 2009;**10**(1):77–80.

86. Lamb CR, Duvernois A. Ultrasonographic anatomy of the normal canine calcaneal tendon. *Vet Radiol Ultrasound* 2005;**46**:326–30.

87. Reinke JD, Kus SP. Calcaneal mechanism injury in the dog. *Compend Contin Educ Pract Vet* 1982;**4**:639–45.

88. Meutstege FJ. The classification of canine Achilles' tendon lesions. *Vet Comp Orthop Traumatol* 1993;**6**: 53–5.

89. Reinke JD, Mughannam AJ, Owens JM. Avulsion of the gastrocnemius tendon in 11 dogs. *J Am Anim Hosp Assoc* 1993;**29**:410–18.

90. Kramer M, Gerwing M, Michele U, et al. Ultrasonographic examination of injuries to the Achilles tendon in dogs and cats. *J Small Anim Pract* 2001;**42**:531–5.

91. Rivers BJ, Walter PA, Kramek B, et al. Sonographic findings in canine common calcaneal tendon injury. *Vet Comp Orthop Traumatol* 1997;**10**:45–53.

92. Gnudi G, Bertoni G. Echographic examination of the stifle joint affected by cranial cruciate ligament rupture in the dog. *Vet Radiol Ultrasound* 2001;**42**:266–70.

93. Seong Y, Eom K, Lee H, et al. Ultrasonographic evaluation of cranial cruciate ligament rupture via dynamic intra-articular saline injection. *Vet Radiol Ultrasound* 2005;**46**:80–2.

94. Arnault F, Cauvin E, Viguier E, et al. Diagnostic value of ultrasonography to assess stifle lesions in dogs after cranial cruciate ligament rupture: 13 cases. *Vet Comp Orthop Traumatol* 2009;**22**(6):479–85.

95. Mahn MM, Cook JL, Cook CR, et al. Arthroscopic verification of ultrasonographic diagnosis of meniscal pathology in dogs. *Vet Surg* 2005;**34**:318–23.

96. Mattern KL, Berry CR, Peck JN, et al. Radiographic and ultrasonographic evaluation of the patellar ligament following tibial plateau leveling osteotomy. *Vet Radiol Ultrasound* 2006;**47**:185–91.

97. Caine A, Agthe P, Posch B, et al. Sonography of the soft tissue structures of the canine tarsus. *Vet Radiol Ultrasound* 2009;**50**(3):304–8.

98. Cardinal E, Chhem RK, Beauregard CG. Ultrasound-guided interventional procedures in the musculoskeletal system. *Radiol Clin North Am* 1998;**36**:597–604.

99. Soudack M, Nachtigal A, Vladovski E, et al. Sonographically guided percutaneous needle biopsy of soft tissue masses with histopathologic correlation. *J Ultrasound Med* 2006;**25**:1271–7, quiz 1278–79.

100. Shah ZR, Crass JR, Oravec DC, et al. Ultrasonographic detection of foreign bodies in soft tissues using turkey muscle as a model. *Vet Radiol Ultrasound* 1992;**33**: 94–100.

101. Matteucci ML, Spaulding K, Dassler C, et al. Ultrasound diagnosis: intra-abdominal wood foreign body. *Vet Radiol Ultrasound* 1999;**40**:513–16.

102. Gnudi G, Volta A, Bonazzi M, et al. Ultrasonographic features of grass awn migration in the dog. *Vet Radiol Ultrasound* 2005;**46**:423–6.

103. Frendin J, Funkquist B, Hansson K, et al. Diagnostic imaging of foreign body reactions in dogs with diffuse back pain. *J Small Anim Pract* 1999;**40**:278–85.

104. Jacobson JA, Powell A, Craig JG, et al. Wooden foreign bodies in soft tissue: detection at US. *Radiology* 1998;**206**:45–8.

105. Lyon M, Brannam L, Johnson D, et al. Detection of soft tissue foreign bodies in the presence of soft tissue gas. *J Ultrasound Med* 2004;**23**:677–81.

106. Shiels WE 2nd, Babcock DS, Wilson JL, et al. Localization and guided removal of soft-tissue foreign bodies with sonography. *Am J Roentgenol* 1990;**155**:1277–81.

CHAPTER 15
Adrenal Glands

Thomas G. Nyland • Dana A. Neelis • John S. Mattoon

Computed tomography (CT) and magnetic resonance imaging (MRI) are the preferred methods of adrenal gland imaging in humans. These modalities have also been used to image the adrenal glands in small animals.[1-17] CT and MRI are advantageous because they can be used to evaluate the pituitary gland concurrently. However, these modalities may not be readily available to all veterinarians, and their use generally requires anesthesia. Improved resolution of newer ultrasound equipment has enabled consistent visualization of the adrenal glands in the dog and cat. This has greatly facilitated the detection of adrenal gland enlargement and masses. Invasion of surrounding structures and identification of distant metastasis by adrenal tumors can also be assessed. Therefore ultrasonography is currently the initial imaging procedure of choice for evaluating suspected adrenal gland abnormalities in small animals.

EXAMINATION TECHNIQUE

The adrenal glands are usually evaluated with either a 5- or 7.5-MHz transducer, or higher frequency, depending on the animal's body size. The highest frequency that will penetrate to the adrenal region should be used, and a 10- to 18-MHz transducer can often be used on small dogs and cats. It is not uncommon to use a lower frequency convex or microconvex transducer to initially locate the adrenal gland, and then use a higher frequency linear-array transducer for further examination. Transverse, sagittal, and dorsal scans, like those used for the kidney, are made from the ventral or lateral abdomen with the animal restrained in dorsal, left, or right lateral recumbency (see Chapter 4, Figure 4-24). Hair must be removed from the lateral aspects of the abdomen to obtain optimal visualization of the adrenal glands in most cases. A combination of views and positions may be required to avoid bowel gas. In lateral recumbency, the uppermost adrenal can be imaged. However, one or both adrenal glands may not be visualized in every animal. The small size of the adrenals, deep-chested conformation, large body size, obesity, overlying gas-filled viscera, or lack of the patient's compliance may contribute to nonvisualization.

The left adrenal gland is best seen from the left lateral abdomen or, less commonly, the left 12th intercostal space in deep-chested animals. The right adrenal gland is best evaluated from the right craniolateral abdomen or through the 11th or 12th intercostal space, depending on body conformation.

The right adrenal gland is more difficult to visualize than the left because of its deeper, more cranial location under the ribs. In one early investigation of 10 dogs, the normal left and right adrenal glands were visualized in 70% and 50% of the dogs, respectively.[2] Later studies with 50 dogs and another with 100 canine patients of varying size, found that an experienced sonographer could visualize the left and right adrenal glands in 91% to 100% and 83% to 86% of cases, respectively.[18] Obesity, deep-chested conformation, and bowel gas were cited as the most common reasons for nonvisualization. The increased resolution of newer ultrasound equipment, better familiarity with normal adrenal gland location, and improved skills of sonographers have contributed to the improved success of adrenal gland visualization.

NORMAL ANATOMY AND ULTRASOUND APPEARANCE

The adrenal glands are flattened, bilobed organs located craniomedial to the kidneys (Figures 15-1 to 15-3). In dogs the left adrenal gland is usually larger than the right.[15,19-21] The size and shape of the adrenals may vary with body weight, age, or breed.[19,22] In dogs, the left adrenal gland is often constricted to a greater degree centrally, with widened, well-defined poles (see Figure 15-2, *A* to *E*), whereas the right adrenal gland may be comma shaped (see Figure 15-3, *H* to *J*). In cats the adrenal glands are generally more oval or cylindrical than in the dog and are more uniform in both size and shape (Figure 15-4). The adrenal glands are usually uniformly hypoechoic on ultrasound scans, and they are sometimes difficult to distinguish from vascular structures in the region without Doppler ultrasonography. Identifying the right adrenal gland is particularly problematic (see Figures 15-3, *D* to *F*). The phrenicoabdominal artery passes dorsal to and the phrenicoabdominal vein ventral to each adrenal gland (see Figures 15-2, *C*, *E*, and *G*). On occasion, a distinct layering may be seen in normal dogs (often referred to as the corticomedullary junction, which may not be histologically accurate); it is even less common in cats (see Figures 15-2, *A* to *C*; 15-3, *A* and *G*; and 15-4, *E* to *H*). Layering has been seen in normal animals and in patients with adrenal disease. The adrenal glands appear oval or round in cross section (see Figures 15-3, *B*, and 15-4, *B* and *D*). Mineralization of the adrenal glands, sometimes visible radiographically, is an incidental finding in older cats (Figure 15-5; see also Figure 15-4, *A* to *D*).[23-26] This finding has more significance in dogs, in which mineralization associated with adrenal gland enlargement suggests an adrenocortical tumor.[27] It is not unusual for the size and shape of the adrenal glands to vary from this general description. In some cases, the adrenal glands may appear nearly round in all planes.

Recently, the enhancement pattern of normal canine adrenal glands has been described following intravenous

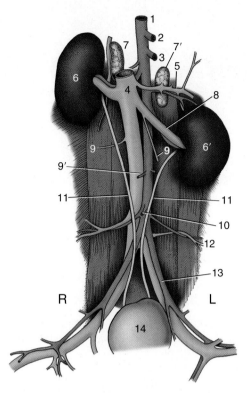

Figure 15-1 Illustration showing the adrenal glands and adjacent anatomic structures. It is the surrounding anatomy that allows localization of the adrenal glands when they are difficult to identify. (From Dyce K, Sack W, Wensing CJG. *Textbook of veterinary anatomy.* 4th ed. St. Louis: Saunders; 2010.)

administration of a microbubble contrast agent.[28] The enhancement pattern in these cases was uniform, quick to peak, and centrifugal from medulla to cortex. Contrast enhancement has been helpful in human medicine for distinguishing adenomatous nodules from neoplasia,[29] however further studies are needed before the usefulness of this procedure can be determined in veterinary patients.

Left Adrenal Gland
The left adrenal gland is medial and cranial to the cranial pole of the left kidney. It is ventrolateral to the aorta between the origin of the cranial mesenteric and left renal arteries[2,30-32] (see Figure 15-2). Therefore the aorta, the cranial pole of the left kidney, and the left renal artery serve as the primary landmarks for localization. However, these structures may not be seen in the scan plane when optimal visualization of the adrenal gland is eventually obtained.

There are a number of techniques for locating the left adrenal with the dog in either lateral or dorsal recumbency, as previously described. We prefer to scan in a dorsal plane from the left lateral abdomen with the dog in dorsal recumbency. This allows gas to migrate upward, away from the kidneys and adrenal glands. Considerable transducer pressure must be applied to reduce the distance to the adrenal gland, to displace overlying bowel gas, and to clearly visualize the pertinent anatomy. The ultrasound beam is first aligned parallel to the aorta at the level of the cranial pole of the left kidney. The beam is then swept slowly upward (ventrally) until the left adrenal gland is located cranial to the left renal artery. In the dog, it often appears as a bilobed or peanut-shaped hypoechoic structure in long axis relative to the surrounding

hyperechoic fat (see Figure 15-2, *A*). In the cat, the adrenal gland is more oval, and a distinct waist is not usually identified (see Figure 15-4). The long axis of the adrenal gland is frequently not parallel to either the kidney or aorta, and the transducer must be rotated clockwise or counterclockwise to maximize length. The short-axis view is obtained by rotating the transducer 90 degrees from the long-axis view. The adrenal gland appears oval in this view. The left kidney can be displaced by transducer pressure; therefore, if the left adrenal gland is not found within a reasonable time, the transducer should be removed from the abdomen to allow the left kidney to return to its normal position before re-attempting visualization.

Right Adrenal Gland
The right adrenal gland lies between the medial aspect of the cranial pole of the right kidney and the caudal vena cava (CVC). It is deeper and more cranial than the left adrenal gland, where overlying ribs and bowel gas can compromise visualization. It is found craniomedial to the renal hilus, lateral or dorsolateral to the CVC, and cranial to the right renal artery and vein.[30-32]

The right adrenal gland is best imaged from the ventral or right lateral abdomen just caudal to the last rib or through the right 11th or 12th intercostal space in deep-chested dogs. If scanning is done from the right lateral abdomen, the CVC is first located in a dorsal plane near the cranial pole of the right kidney, and the beam is then swept slightly upward (ventrally) or downward (dorsally) until the adrenal gland is identified (see Figure 15-3, *C*, *E*, *F*, and *J*). If scanning is done from the ventral abdomen, the CVC is first located in a long-axis view, and the beam is then moved slightly to the animal's right. With either method, the right adrenal gland appears as a hypoechoic structure surrounded by hyperechoic fat (see Figure 15-3). Neither the CVC nor the right kidney may be visible when adrenal gland visualization is optimized, depending on the exact scan plane (see Figure 15-3, *A*, *G* to *I*). The transducer must usually be rotated clockwise or counterclockwise slightly to maximize adrenal length. However, at times, it is still difficult to incorporate the entire length of the right adrenal gland in a single long-axis view because of its comma shape. The short-axis view is obtained by rotating the transducer 90 degrees from the long-axis view. The adrenal gland generally appears oval in this view.

Normal Adrenal Gland Size
The maximal diameter of the adrenal gland has been found to be the most reliable indicator of its size.[18,20,30,33,34] Unfortunately, there is an overlap in size between normal dogs and those with adrenal gland or other endocrine abnormalities. A maximal diameter of 7.4 mm (in either width or thickness) has been proposed as the upper limit of adrenal gland diameter in normal dogs.[20] However, it was found that 23% of dogs with pituitary-dependent hyperadrenocorticism (PDH) did not have adrenal gland enlargement,[31] whereas 20% of dogs without evidence of endocrine disease[20] and, in another study, 9% without evidence of adrenal disease[21] had adrenal enlargement on the basis of the upper limit of 7.4 mm in diameter. Consequently, preliminary findings indicate a sensitivity and specificity of approximately 77% and 80% to 90%, respectively, for diagnosis of PDH based on the upper limit of 7.4 mm in diameter. A more recent retrospective study of small breed dogs (body weight <10 kg), found an adrenal gland diameter greater than 6 mm to be 75% sensitive and 94% specific for identification of PDH.[35]

The diameter of the adrenal glands in 10 normal adult cats was reported to be 4.3 ± 0.3 mm.[36] In another report, the normal upper limit of width was reported as 5.3 mm in 20

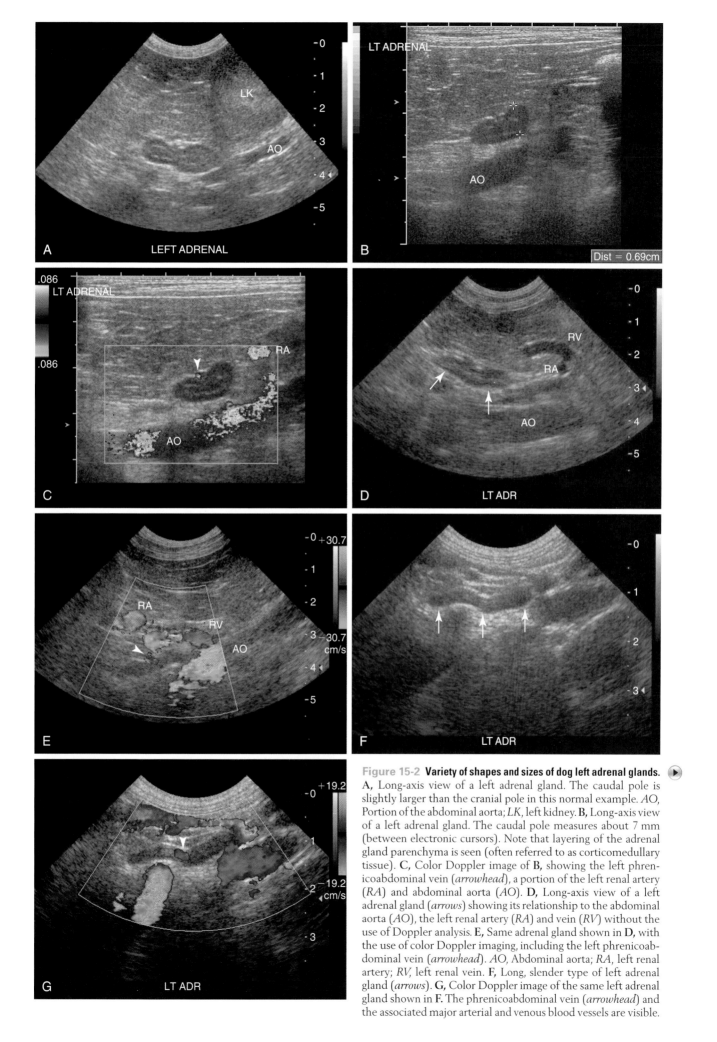

Figure 15-2 **Variety of shapes and sizes of dog left adrenal glands.**
A, Long-axis view of a left adrenal gland. The caudal pole is
slightly larger than the cranial pole in this normal example. *AO,*
Portion of the abdominal aorta; *LK,* left kidney. **B,** Long-axis view
of a left adrenal gland. The caudal pole measures about 7 mm
(between electronic cursors). Note that layering of the adrenal
gland parenchyma is seen (often referred to as corticomedullary
tissue). **C,** Color Doppler image of **B,** showing the left phrenicoabdominal vein (*arrowhead*), a portion of the left renal artery
(*RA*) and abdominal aorta (*AO*). **D,** Long-axis view of a left
adrenal gland (*arrows*) showing its relationship to the abdominal
aorta (*AO*), the left renal artery (*RA*) and vein (*RV*) without the
use of Doppler analysis. **E,** Same adrenal gland shown in **D,** with
the use of color Doppler imaging, including the left phrenicoabdominal vein (*arrowhead*). *AO,* Abdominal aorta; *RA,* left renal
artery; *RV,* left renal vein. **F,** Long, slender type of left adrenal
gland (*arrows*). **G,** Color Doppler image of the same left adrenal
gland shown in **F.** The phrenicoabdominal vein (*arrowhead*) and
the associated major arterial and venous blood vessels are visible.

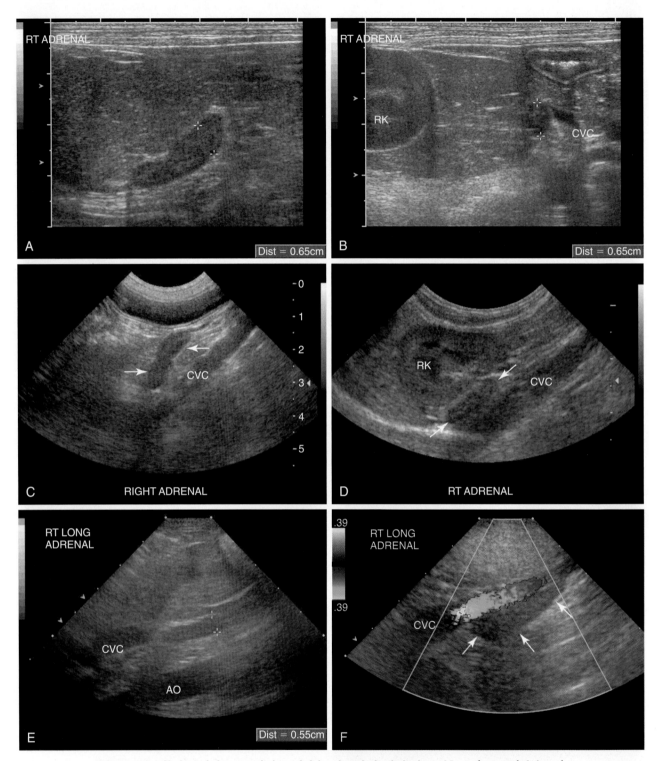

Figure 15-3 Variety of shapes and sizes of right adrenal glands in dogs. Normal sagittal (**A**) and transverse (**B**) images of the right adrenal gland (0.65 cm between electronic cursors). In **B**, the caudal vena cava (*CVC*) is partially compressed by transducer pressure, distorting its lumen. *RK,* Right kidney. **C,** Dorsal image plane showing a long-axis view of the right adrenal gland (*arrows*) and the caudal vena cava (*CVC*). **D,** In this dorsal image plane the right kidney (*RK*) is noted to be distorted by transducer pressure with the right adrenal gland (*arrows*) between it and the caudal vena cava (*CVC*). **E,** Right adrenal gland (0.55 cm) seen between the caudal vena cava (*CVC*) and the abdominal aorta (*AO*). **F,** Right adrenal gland in long axis (*arrows*) with color Doppler imaging depicting blood flow in the adjacent caudal vena cava (*CVC*).

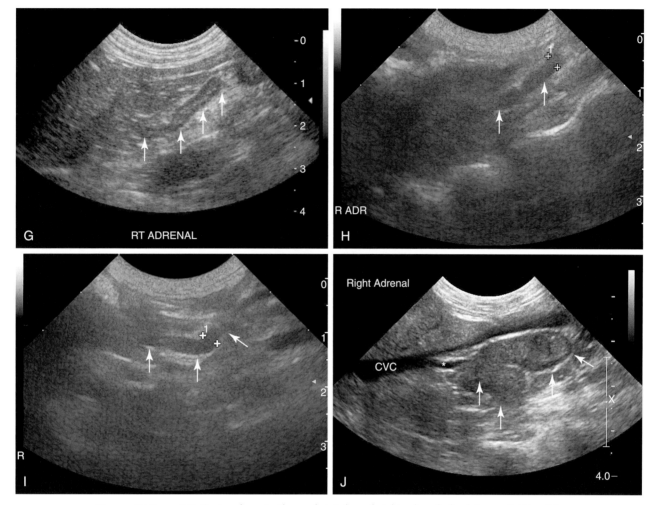

Figure 15-3, cont'd **G,** An elongate "lawn chair" shaped right adrenal gland (*arrows*). **H** and **I,** The V shape of some right adrenal glands (*arrows*) may not be appreciated (**H**) unless the transducer is properly positioned (**I**). **J,** V-shaped right adrenal gland (*arrows*). The caudal vena cava (*CVC*) is partially collapsed secondary to transducer pressure. The phrenicoabdominal vein (*) is seen branching off the CVC.

healthy cats.[37] The interpretation of ultrasound measurements should always be made in the context of the clinical findings and laboratory work in animals with suspected adrenal disease.

There are a number of pitfalls associated with measuring adrenal glands. Ideally, adrenal gland measurements should be done in both dorsal and sagittal planes whenever possible and the results of diameter measurements compared. Failure to maximize either the length or the diameter of the adrenal gland in the long-axis view may underestimate measurements. This may result from poor technique or, in the case of length, the inability to image the entire adrenal gland in one scan plane. Short-axis views may overestimate diameter if there is scan obliquity. Therefore, for greatest accuracy, adrenal gland diameter should always be maximized in long-axis views or minimized in short-axis views before measurement.

Subjective criteria may also help identify abnormal adrenal glands when diameter measurements do not indicate enlargement. Abnormal adrenal glands may lose their flattened shape and become rounded or more irregular in outline. Clinical experience indicates that consideration of both the size and the shape of the adrenal gland is useful to reach a tentative diagnosis.

ADRENAL GLAND ENLARGEMENT AND MASSES

PDH is identified in approximately 80% of the cases of hyperadrenocorticism in dogs; adrenal tumors account for about 20%.[38] Bilateral symmetrical adrenal gland enlargement is most common with PDH (Figures 15-6 and 15-7), but unilateral or bilateral unequal adrenal gland enlargement has also been reported[20,22,39-41] (Figure 15-8). Adrenal nodules (Figures 15-9 and 15-10) and less commonly adrenal nodules or masses associated with PDH have been reported.[40] It is also clear from preliminary investigations and clinical experience that the adrenal gland may be normal in size in dogs with PDH[20,22] or enlarged in dogs without adrenal gland disease.[20,21] Whereas mild to moderate bilateral enlargement suggests PDH, moderate unilateral enlargement makes differentiation of PDH from primary adrenal gland tumors or secondary metastasis to the adrenal glands potentially difficult. PDH may be more common in poodles, dachshunds, beagles, boxers, Boston terriers, and German shepherds, which may assist with diagnosis.[38]

Canine adrenal tumors primarily include adrenocortical adenoma and carcinoma, pheochromocytoma, and tumors

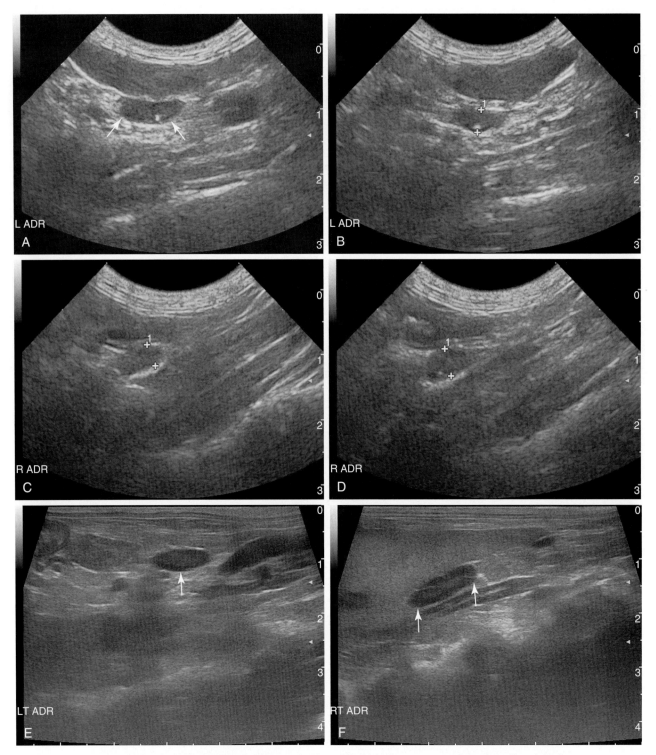

Figure 15-4 Normal cat adrenal glands. Left adrenal gland is shown in A and B. The right adrenal gland is shown in C and D. A, Sagittal image of the left adrenal gland (*arrows*) shows a hypoechoic, homogeneous parenchyma, with the exception of a solitary tiny hyperechoic focus that could represent mineralization. B, Transverse image of the left adrenal gland in A (0.35 cm between electronic cursors). The tiny focus of mineralization is noted. C, Sagittal image of the right adrenal gland (between electronic cursors 0.35 cm). D, Transverse image of C (between electronic cursors, 0.43 cm). E, Left adrenal gland in long axis (*arrow*) using a linear-array transducer. Note a faint hypoechoic periphery with a more echogenic central area. A portion of the aorta is seen to the right. F, Right adrenal gland in long axis (*arrows*). Hypoechoic periphery surrounds a more echogenic central area. An enlarged, hyperechoic liver is present in the near field in this cat with hepatic lipidosis.

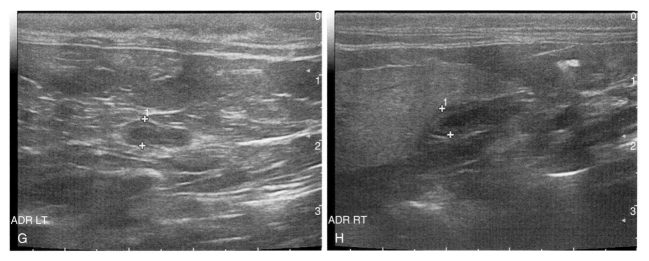

Figure 15-4, cont'd **G,** Sagittal image of the left adrenal gland (0.41 cm between electronic cursors). In this example, the periphery is hyperechoic to the central region. **H,** Sagittal image of the right adrenal gland (0.42 cm between electronic cursors), also showing a hyperechoic periphery surrounding hypoechoic central parenchyma.

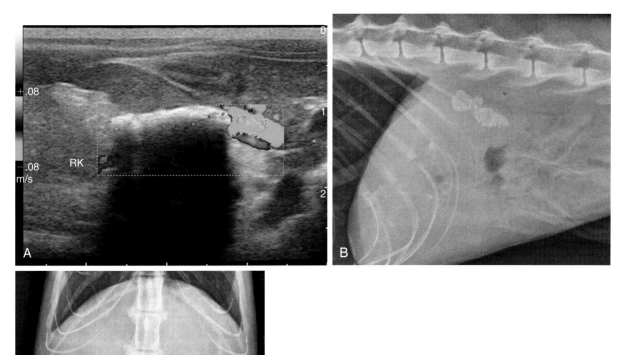

Figure 15-5 **Mineralization of cat adrenal glands. A,** Sagittal image of the hyperechoic interface of the mineralized right adrenal gland, casting a strong acoustic shadow. Color Doppler image shows the adjacent caudal vena cava. *RK,* right kidney. **B,** Close-up lateral radiograph showing bilateral adrenal gland mineralization. **C,** Close-up ventrodorsal radiograph showing bilateral adrenal gland mineralization (*arrows*).

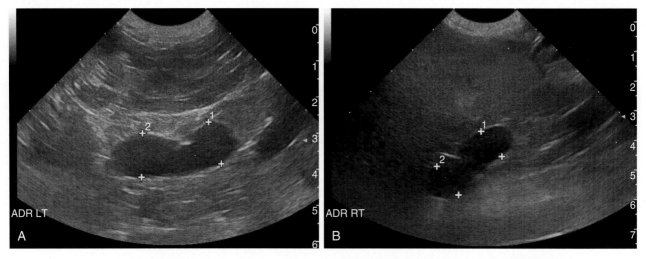

Figure 15-6 **Bilateral symmetrical adrenal gland enlargement secondary to pituitary dependent hyperadrenocorticism in a 7-year-old husky dog.** A, Sagittal image of the left adrenal gland, measuring 1.21 cm in height at the caudal pole, 1.22 cm at the cranial pole. Note the indentation (waist) of the central portion of the gland and its homogeneous hypoechoic parenchyma. **B,** Sagittal image of the right adrenal gland shows its size, shape, and homogeneous hypoechoic parenchyma to be nearly identical to the left (1.22 cm caudal pole, 1.22 cm cranial pole). Note the enlarged, hyperechoic and slightly heterogeneous liver in the near field.

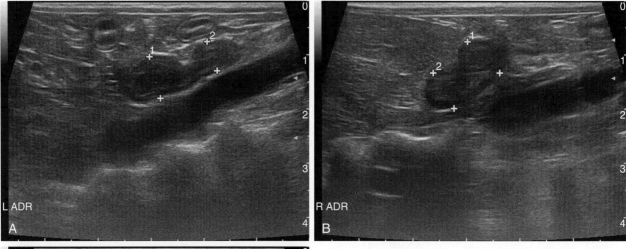

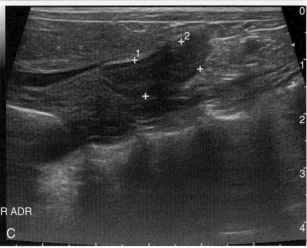

Figure 15-7 **Mild bilateral adrenal gland enlargement in a 13-year-old Yorkshire terrier with pituitary-dependent hyperadrenocorticism.** A, Dorsal image plane of the left adrenal gland, measuring 0.79 cm at the cranial pole, 0.57 cm at the caudal pole. There is layering of the parenchyma. The abdominal aorta and the hyperechoic surfaces of the lumbar vertebrae are seen in the far field; cross sections of small intestine are present in the near field. **B,** Dorsal image of the right adrenal gland (0.76 cm cranial pole, 0.83 cm caudal pole), also showing a layered parenchyma. The caudal vena cava and hyperechoic surfaces of the lumbar vertebrae are noted in the far field. **C,** Sagittal image of the right adrenal gland in **B,** showing a difference in shape and size (0.70 cm cranial pole, 0.62 cm caudal pole). This illustrates that determining the true size and shape of the right adrenal gland in dogs is more difficult than it is for the left adrenal. The compressed caudal vena cava is noted in the near field, vertebral bodies in the far field.

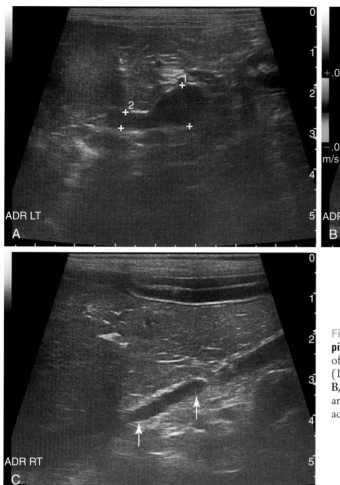

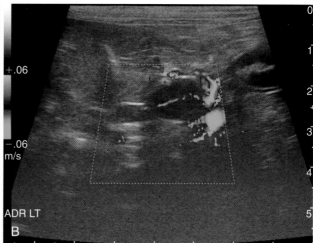

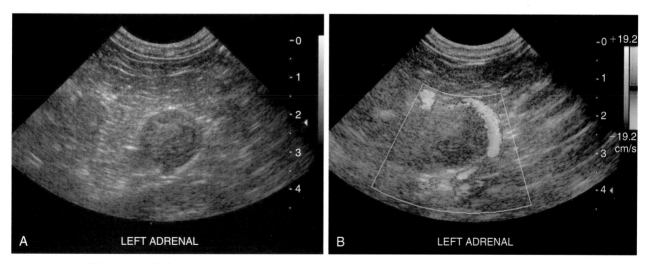

Figure 15-8 **Asymmetric adrenal gland enlargement in a dog with pituitary-dependent hyperadrenocorticism (PDH).** A, Sagittal image of the left adrenal gland shows enlargement of the caudal pole (1.03 cm), whereas the cranial pole appears normal (0.41 cm). B, Color Doppler image shows renal vasculature coursing around the enlarged caudal pole. C, Sagittal image of the right adrenal gland (*arrows*) shows a normal, slender shape.

Figure 15-9 **Left adrenal gland nodular enlargement secondary to pituitary-dependent hyperadrenocorticism (PDH) in a dog.** A, Solid, homogeneous nodular enlargement of the left adrenal gland. B, Color Doppler image shows adjacent renal vasculature.

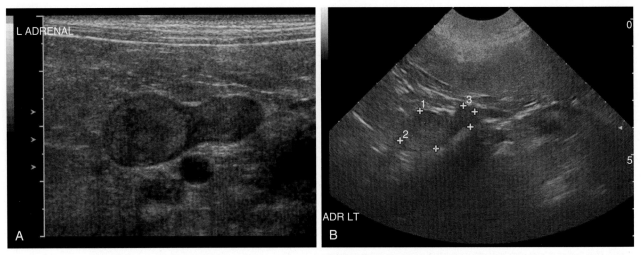

Figure 15-10 **Dog adrenal gland nodules. A,** Large cranial pole nodule in the left adrenal gland of a dog. **B,** The cranial pole nodule of the left adrenal gland (1.51 cm between electronic cursors) was an unexpected finding in this dog being examined for a cutaneous mast cell tumor.

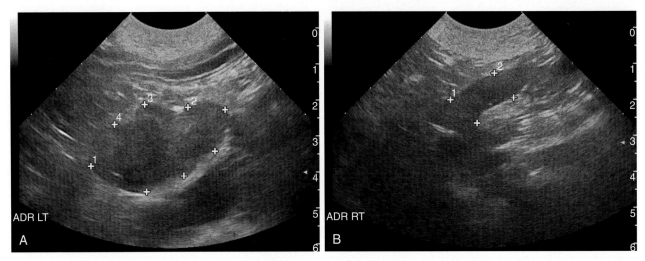

Figure 15-11 **Large left adrenal gland mass in a geriatric dog with symmetric enlargement of the right adrenal gland. A,** Sagittal image of the enlarged, irregularly shaped left adrenal gland mass (between cursors). **B,** Long-axis view of symmetric enlargement of the right adrenal gland (0.99 cm cranial pole, 0.87 cm caudal pole).

that metastasize to the adrenal gland (Figures 15-11 to 15-13). However, other types of tumors also occur.[14,42,43] Adrenocortical tumors have been reported more frequently in females and in larger breeds, which may help facilitate diagnosis.[38] A nodule or mass causing unilateral enlargement of the adrenal gland is usually identified (see Figures 15-9 and 15-10). If the tumor is hormonally active, the contralateral adrenal gland may be difficult to identify because of atrophy. One study suggested that adrenal dependent hyperadrenocorticism (HAC) is more likely if the adrenal glands are asymmetric and the maximal thickness of the smaller gland is less than 5 mm.[44] However, other studies have found that the contralateral adrenal has a normal size.[45,46] Adrenal tumors are sometimes nonfunctional,[47,48] cortisol secreting,[49] or destructive, leading to hypoadrenocorticism,[50] which contributes to the difficulty in diagnosing them. They may be discovered incidentally on routine abdominal ultrasonography (adrenal incidentaloma;

see Figures 15-9 and 15-10), or the clinical signs may relate to local tumor invasion or metastasis rather than secondary hormone effects.

The type of adrenal tumor cannot be determined from its ultrasonographic appearance, and a variety of sonographic appearances from solid to complex have been reported.[45,51,52] Adrenocortical tumors and pheochromocytomas have also been found in the same gland on histopathologic evaluation, which may contribute to the variable ultrasound appearance.[53] Although considerable size overlap exists, clinical experience and several reports indicate that an adrenal tumor is more likely than PDH if the diameter of the gland exceeds 2 cm.[45,52] However, exceptions occur as reported in several cases of PDH in which the adrenal gland measured 2 cm or more in diameter.[39,45] If there is unilateral adrenal gland enlargement with a diameter of 1 to 2 cm, either PDH or a tumor may be present. Further complicating differentiation of PDH from

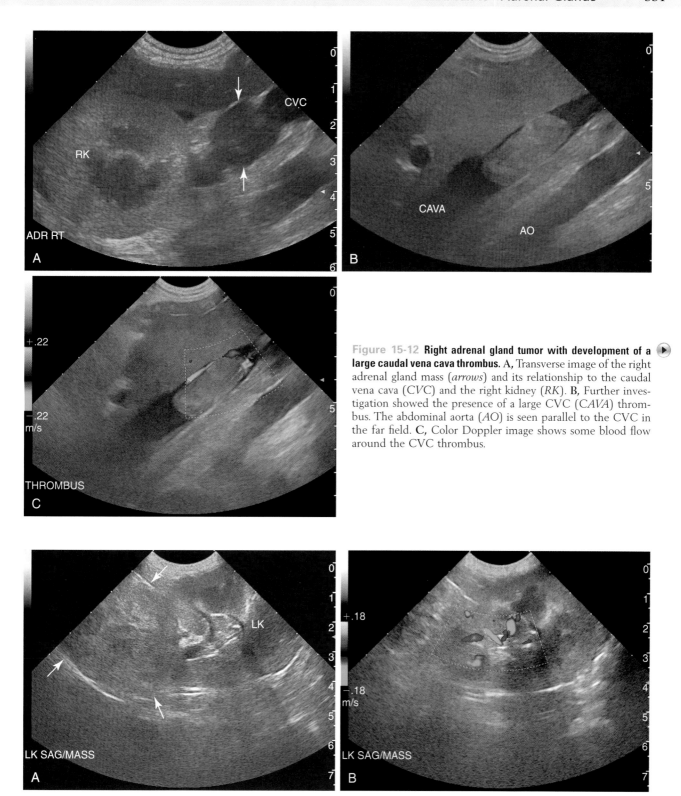

Figure 15-12 **Right adrenal gland tumor with development of a large caudal vena cava thrombus.** A, Transverse image of the right adrenal gland mass (*arrows*) and its relationship to the caudal vena cava (*CVC*) and the right kidney (*RK*). B, Further investigation showed the presence of a large CVC (*CAVA*) thrombus. The abdominal aorta (*AO*) is seen parallel to the CVC in the far field. C, Color Doppler image shows some blood flow around the CVC thrombus.

Figure 15-13 **Left adrenal gland mass in a dog.** A, A large, complex left adrenal gland mass (*arrows*) is distorting the adjacent left kidney (*LK*). B, Color Doppler image of A.

adrenal tumor, bilateral adrenal tumors[45,46,54-57] or a combination of PDH and adrenal tumors (unilateral or bilateral) may exist in the same animal.[53,56,58]

Hyperechoic foci or acoustic shadowing (from mineralization) within an enlarged canine adrenal gland suggests an adrenocortical tumor.[27,45,57] Mineralization is less common with pheochromocytomas but may occur in approximately 10% of the cases.[47,48] However, mineralization has also been reported in some cases of PDH.[22,45] All adrenal gland tumors are known to locally invade the kidney, renal artery, renal vein, aorta, or CVC and to metastasize to distant sites.[45,47,48,53] If a mass is seen in the CVC adjacent to an adrenal mass, invasion

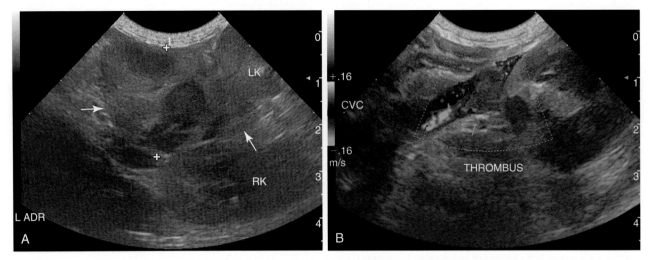

Figure 15-14 Left adrenal gland tumor in a cat. A, Large, complex mass (between electronic cursors; *arrows*) identified cranial to the left kidney (*LK*). The right kidney (*RK*) is seen in the far field. **B,** Color Doppler examination shows the presence of a thrombus and/or invasion of the caudal vena cava by the mass.

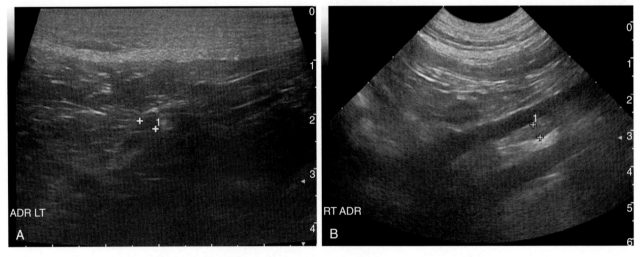

Figure 15-15 Hypoadrenocorticism in a middle-aged dog. A, Long-axis image of the left adrenal gland, only 0.34 cm thick. **B,** Right adrenal gland seen between the caudal vena cava and aorta, 0.4 cm thick. Adrenal glands this small are quite difficult to locate and surrounding anatomic landmarks need to be used as guides in most cases.

of the CVC and tumor thrombosis are likely[7,59-62] (Figure 15-14; see also Figure 15-12). However, CVC thrombosis in the absence of an adrenal tumor must also be considered because of the hypercoagulable state that accompanies hyperadrenocorticism.[45]

Adrenocortical carcinomas or pheochromocytomas can spontaneously rupture, resulting in hematomas or extensive hemorrhage into the retroperitoneal space or peritoneal cavity.[7,45,48,63,64] A careful search of adjacent structures, other abdominal organs, and thoracic radiographs to rule out metastasis is recommended when an adrenal tumor is suspected.

Percutaneous biopsy of adrenal gland masses is routinely performed in humans with a low complication rate.[65] However, biopsy of pheochromocytomas is not recommended because a hypertensive crisis may result.[66] Biopsy or aspiration of adrenal gland masses under ultrasound guidance has also been reported in small animals.[7,45,67,68] Hemorrhage, fatal hypertensive crisis, or arrhythmic episodes associated

with percutaneous biopsy of unsuspected pheochromocytomas are potential complications.[69] However, ultrasound-guided aspiration or biopsy of pheochromocytomas was reported in one cat[67] and three dogs[7] without apparent adverse effects.

REDUCED ADRENAL GLAND SIZE

Few studies have been performed to describe the size and appearance of the adrenal glands in dogs with hypoadrenocorticism.[70,71] These investigators reported decreased adrenal gland size (length and thickness) in dogs with hypoadrenocorticism compared with normal dogs. In the more recent study, a left adrenal gland diameter of less than 3.2 mm was strongly suggestive of hypoadrenocorticism when compared to healthy dogs.[71] Figure 15-15 shows the appearance of bilateral small adrenal glands in a dog with hypoadrenocorticism.

ADRENAL GLAND PATHOLOGY IN THE CAT

Hyperadrenocorticism is less common in cats than in dogs. However, both PDH and adrenal tumors (adrenocortical adenomas and carcinomas) have been described, and the findings are similar to those of dogs[72-75] (see Figure 15-14). PDH accounts for about 80% of the cases, whereas adrenal tumors are identified in about 20% of the cases.[75,76] Approximately 50% of the adrenal tumors are adenomas and 50% are carcinomas.[77] The size of the adrenal glands in cats with PDH has not been reported, although bilateral enlargement has been described.[25,72-75] A unilateral adrenal mass is usually found in cats with an adrenocortical tumor,[75] although bilateral adrenal tumors are possible.[78] Diabetes mellitus is a concurrent finding in approximately 80% of cats with hyperadrenocorticism.[75,79]

Feline hyperaldosteronism may also occur secondary to a unilateral aldosterone-secreting adrenal tumor or bilateral adrenal hyperplasia.[9,68,80-87] A polymyopathy due to hypokalemia and systemic hypertension has been observed with this disorder.

Adrenal tumors producing sex hormones have also been reported. Progesterone-secreting adrenocortical tumors produce clinical signs identical to those of hyperadrenocorticism and may also result in diabetes mellitus.[82,88,89] Androgen-secreting tumors can result in behavior changes in affected individuals.[90]

Pheochromocytomas are apparently rare in cats; only three cases have been described in the literature, one of which was an extraadrenal tumor arising from the periadrenal tissue.[67,91,92] Clinical signs of polyuria and polydipsia were observed, but hypertension was reported in only one cat.[92]

OTHER ADRENAL LESIONS

Nonneoplastic masses of the adrenal gland, such as hematomas, granulomas, cysts, and abscesses, have been described in humans.[93] Infectious diseases, such as tuberculosis, histoplasmosis, and blastomycosis, are also known to affect the adrenal glands.[93] The ultrasonographic appearance is variable, depending on the stage of the disease.

Toxoplasmosis, cryptococcosis, coccidioidomycosis, and histoplasmosis are known to involve the adrenal glands of small animals.[94] Acute intoxications and systemic bacterial infections are also known to produce inflammatory edema, necrosis, or hemorrhage of the adrenal glands.[94] However, there are no reports describing the ultrasonographic findings in these disorders. It is hoped that the descriptions will be forthcoming with more frequent evaluation of the adrenal glands of animals with these diseases.

When mitotane is used to treat PDH, we have observed sonographic changes consistent with adrenal gland necrosis on follow-up studies. Anechoic to hypoechoic areas were noted within the adrenal glands bilaterally that subsequently disappeared after several weeks. Additionally, the size of the adrenal glands has been reported to decrease following mitotane therapy.[95] In contrast, ultrasound examinations performed after trilostane therapy found an increase in adrenal size and better definition between the cortex and medulla in two different studies.[96,97] However, similar to those treated with mitotane, necrosis of the adrenal glands has been identified histopathologically in a small number of patients taking trilostane, which may explain why some adrenal glands appear heterogeneous or irregularly margined on posttreatment examinations.[98,99,100]

A variety of well-known laboratory tests are used to differentiate pituitary and adrenal cortical tumors and to document persistent hypertension with pheochromocytomas. Therefore the diagnosis of adrenal gland disorders cannot be made exclusively from the ultrasound findings. In practice, ultrasonography is used to determine whether there is adrenal gland enlargement, whether the enlargement is unilateral or bilateral, and whether there is metastasis or local invasion of adrenal tumor. These findings, in conjunction with laboratory test results, help establish a tentative diagnosis. If available, CT or MRI studies of the pituitary or adrenal region may add additional important information to help establish the diagnosis.

REFERENCES

1. Voorhout G, Stolp R, Lubberink AA, et al. Computed tomography in the diagnosis of canine hyperadrenocorticism not suppressible by dexamethasone. *J Am Vet Med Assoc* 1988;**192**:641–6.
2. Voorhout G. X-ray-computed tomography, nephrotomography, and ultrasonography of the adrenal glands of healthy dogs. *Am J Vet Res* 1990;**51**:625–31.
3. Voorhout G, Stolp R, Rijnberk A, et al. Assessment of survey radiography and comparison with x-ray computed tomography for detection of hyperfunctioning adrenocortical tumors in dogs. *J Am Vet Med Assoc* 1990;**196**:1799–803.
4. Guptill L, Scott-Moncrieff JC, Widmer WR. Diagnosis of canine hyperadrenocorticism. *Vet Clin North Am Small Anim Pract* 1997;**27**:215–35.
5. Galac S, Kooistra HS, Teske E, et al. Urinary corticoid/creatinine ratios in the differentiation between pituitary-dependent hyperadrenocorticism and hyperadrenocorticism due to adrenocortical tumour in the dog. *Vet Q* 1997;**19**:17–20.
6. Tidwell AS, Penninck DG, Besso JG. Imaging of adrenal gland disorders. *Vet Clin North Am Small Anim Pract* 1997;**27**:237–54.
7. Rosenstein DS. Diagnostic imaging in canine pheochromocytoma. *Vet Radiol Ultrasound* 2000;**41**:499–506.
8. Behrend EN, Kemppainen RJ. Diagnosis of canine hyperadrenocorticism. *Vet Clin North Am Small Anim Pract* 2001;**31**:985–1003, viii.
9. Rijnberk A, Voorhout G, Kooistra HS, et al. Hyperaldosteronism in a cat with metastasised adrenocortical tumour. *Vet Q* 2001;**23**:38–43.
10. Llabres-Diaz FJ, Dennis R. Magnetic resonance imaging of the presumed normal canine adrenal glands. *Vet Radiol Ultrasound* 2003;**44**:5–19.
11. Behrend EN, Weigand CM, Whitley EM, et al. Corticosterone- and aldosterone-secreting adrenocortical tumor in a dog. *J Am Vet Med Assoc* 2005;**226**:1662–6, 1659.
12. Javadi S, Djajadiningrat-Laanen SC, Kooistra HS, et al. Primary hyperaldosteronism, a mediator of progressive renal disease in cats. *Domest Anim Endocrinol* 2005;**28**:85–104.
13. Bertolini G, Furlanello T, De Lorenzi D, et al. Computed tomographic quantification of canine adrenal gland volume and attenuation. *Vet Radiol Ultrasound* 2006;**47**:444–8.
14. Morandi F, Mays JL, Newman SJ, et al. Imaging diagnosis—bilateral adrenal adenomas and myelolipomas in a dog. *Vet Radiol Ultrasound* 2007;**48**:246–9.
15. Bertolini G, Furlanello T, Drigo M, et al. Computed tomographic adrenal gland quantification in canine adrenocorticotroph hormone-dependent hyperadrenocorticism. *Vet Radiol Ultrasound* 2008;**49**(5):449–53.

16. Massari F, Nicoli S, Romanelli G, et al. Adrenalectomy in dogs with adrenal gland tumors: 52 cases (2002-2008). *J Am Vet Med Assoc* 2011;15(2):216–21.

17. Rodriguez Pineiro MI, De Fornel-Thibaud P, Benchekroun G, et al. Use of computed tomography adrenal gland measurement for differentiating ACTH dependence from ACTH independence in 64 dogs with hyperadrenocorticism. *J Vet Intern Med* 2011;25:1066–74.

18. Grooters AM, Biller DS, Miyabiashi T, et al. Evaluation of routine abdominal ultrasonography as a technique for imaging the canine adrenal glands. *J Am Anim Hosp Assoc* 1994;30:457–62.

19. Miller ME, Evans HE. *Miller's anatomy of the dog*. 3rd ed. Philadelphia: Saunders; 1993.

20. Grooters AM, Biller DS, Theisen SK, et al. Ultrasonographic characteristics of the adrenal glands in dogs with pituitary-dependent hyperadrenocorticism: comparison with normal dogs. *J Vet Intern Med* 1996;10: 110–15.

21. Ross MA, Gainer JH, Innes JRM. Dystrophic calcification in the adrenal glands of monkeys, cats, and dogs. *Arch Pathol* 1955;60:655.

22. Howell JM, Pickering CM. Calcium deposits in the adrenal glands of dogs and cats. *J Comp Pathol* 1964;74: 280.

23. Widmer WR, Guptill L. Imaging techniques for facilitating diagnosis of hyperadrenocorticism in dogs and cats. *J Am Vet Med Assoc* 1995;206:1857–64.

24. Burk RL, Feeney DA. *The abdomen. Small animal radiography and ultrasonography*. 3rd ed. Philadelphia: WB Saunders; 2003. p. 456.

25. Penninck DG, Feldman EC, Nyland TG. Radiographic features of canine hyperadrenocorticism caused by autonomously functioning adrenocortical tumors: 23 cases (1978-1986). *J Am Vet Med Assoc* 1988;192: 1604–8.

26. Pey P, Vignoli M, Haers H, et al. Contrast-enhanced ultrasonography of the normal canine adrenal gland. *Vet Radiol Ultrasound* 2011;52(5):560–7.

27. Friedrich-Rust M, Schneider G, Bohle RM, et al. Contrast-enhanced sonography of adrenal masses: differentiation of adenomas and nonadenomatous lesions. *Am J Roentgenol* 2008;191:1852–60.

28. Grooters AM, Biller DS, Merryman J. Ultrasonographic parameters of normal canine adrenal glands: comparison to necropsy findings. *Vet Radiol Ultrasound* 1995;36: 126–30.

29. Spaulding KA. A review of sonographic identification of abdominal blood vessels and juxtavascular organs. *Vet Radiol Ultrasound* 1997;38:4–23.

30. Barthez PY, Nyland TG, Feldman EC. Ultrasonography of the adrenal glands in the dog, cat, and ferret. *Vet Clin North Am Small Anim Pract* 1998;28:869–85.

31. Barthez PY, Nyland TG, Feldman EC. Ultrasonographic evaluation of the adrenal glands in dogs. *J Am Vet Med Assoc* 1995;207:1180–3.

32. Barberet V, Pey P, Duchateau L, et al. Intra- and interobserver variability of ultrasonographic measurements of the adrenal glands in healthy beagles. *Vet Radiol Ultrasound* 2010;51(6):656–60.

33. Mogicato G, Layssol-Lamour C, Conchou F, et al. Ultrasonographic evaluation of the adrenal glands in healthy dogs: repeatability, reproducibility, observer-dependent variability, and the effect of bodyweight, age and sex. *Vet Rec* 2011;168(5):130.

34. Douglass JP, Berry CR, James S. Ultrasonographic adrenal gland measurements in dogs without evidence of adrenal disease. *Vet Radiol Ultrasound* 1997;38:124–30.

35. Choi J, Hyunwook K, Yoon J. Ultrasonographic adrenal gland measurements in clinically normal small breed dogs and comparison with pituitary-dependent hyperadrenocorticism. *J Vet Med Sci* 2011;73(8):985–9.

36. Cartee RL, Finn-Bodner ST, Gray BW. Ultrasonography of the normal feline adrenal gland. *J Diagn Med Sonogr* 1993;9:327–30.

37. Zimmer C, Horauf A, Reusch C. Ultrasonographic examination of the adrenal gland and evaluation of the hypophyseal-adrenal axis in 20 cats. *J Small Anim Pract* 2000;41:156–60.

38. Feldman EC, Nelson RW. Canine hyperadrenocorticism. In: Feldman EC, Nelson RW, editors. *Canine and feline endocrinology and reproduction*. 3rd ed. Philadelphia: WB Saunders; 2004. p. 252–357.

39. Kantrowitz BM, Nyland TG, Feldman EC. Adrenal ultrasonography in the dog: detection of tumors and hyperplasia in hyperadrenocorticism. *Vet Radiol* 1986;27: 91–6.

40. Besso JG, Wrigley RH, Gliatto JM, et al. Ultrasonographic appearance and clinical findings in 14 dogs with gallbladder mucocele. *Vet Radiol Ultrasound* 2000;41: 261–71.

41. Gould SM, Baines EA, Mannion PA, et al. Use of endogenous ACTH concentration and adrenal ultrasonography to distinguish the cause of canine hyperadrenocorticism. *J Small Anim Pract* 2001;42:113–21.

42. Marcotte L, McConkey SE, Hanna P, et al. Malignant adrenal neuroblastoma in a young dog. *Can Vet J* 2004; 45:773–6.

43. Castro LCG, Infantozzi CM, Kamikawa L, et al. Adrenal neuroblastoma in an adult dog - case report. In: *Proceedings of the World Small Animal Veterinary Association World Congress*. 2009.

44. Benchekroun G, De Fornel-Thibaud P, Rodriguez Pineiro MI, et al. Ultrasonography criteria for differentiating ACTH dependency from ACTH independency in 47 dogs with hyperadrenocorticism and equivocal adrenal asymmetry. *J Vet Intern Med* 2010;24:1077–85.

45. Besso JG, Penninck DG, Gliatto JM. Retrospective ultrasonographic evaluation of adrenal lesions in 26 dogs. *Vet Radiol Ultrasound* 1997;38:448–55.

46. Hoerauf A, Reusch C. Ultrasonographic characteristics of both adrenal glands in 15 dogs with functional adrenocortical tumors. *J Am Anim Hosp Assoc* 1999;35: 193–9.

47. Gilson SD, Withrow SJ, Wheeler SL, et al. Pheochromocytoma in 50 dogs. *J Vet Intern Med* 1994;8:228–32.

48. Barthez PY, Marks SL, Woo J, et al. Pheochromocytoma in dogs: 61 cases (1984-1995). *J Vet Intern Med* 1997;11:272–8.

49. Machida T, Uchida E, Matsuda K, et al. Aldosterone-, corticosterone- and cortisol-secreting adrenocortical carcinoma in a dog: case report. *J Vet Med Sci* 2008; 70(3):317–20.

50. Kook PH, Grest P, Raute-Kreinsen U, et al. Addison's disease due to bilateral adrenal malignancy in a dog. *J Small Anim Pract* 2010;51:333–6.

51. Poffenbarger EM, Feeney DA, Hayden DW. Gray-scale ultrasonography in the diagnosis of adrenal neoplasia in dogs: six cases (1981-1986). *J Am Vet Med Assoc* 1988; 192:228–32.

52. Voorhout G, Rijnberk A, Sjollema BE, et al. Nephrotomography and ultrasonography for the localization of hyperfunctioning adrenocortical tumors in dogs. *Am J Vet Res* 1990;51:1280–5.

53. van Sluijs FJ, Sjollema BE, Voorhout G, et al. Results of adrenalectomy in 36 dogs with hyperadrenocorticism

caused by adrenocortical tumour. *Vet Q* 1995;**17**: 113–16.

54. Ford SL, Feldman EC, Nelson RW. Hyperadrenocorticism caused by bilateral adrenocortical neoplasia in dogs: four cases (1983-1988). *J Am Vet Med Assoc* 1993;**202**: 789–92.

55. Thuroczy J, van Sluijs FJ, Kooistra HS, et al. Multiple endocrine neoplasias in a dog: corticotrophic tumour, bilateral adrenocortical tumours, and pheochromocytoma. *Vet Q* 1998;**20**:56–61.

56. Greco DS, Peterson ME, Davidson AP, et al. Concurrent pituitary and adrenal tumors in dogs with hyperadrenocorticism: 17 cases (1978-1995). *J Am Vet Med Assoc* 1999;**214**:1349–53.

57. Reusch CE, Feldman EC. Canine hyperadrenocorticism due to adrenocortical neoplasia. *J Vet Intern Med* 1991;**5**:3–10.

58. von Dehn BJ, Nelson RW, Feldman EC, et al. Pheochromocytoma and hyperadrenocorticism in dogs: six cases (1982-1992). *J Am Vet Med Assoc* 1995;**207**: 322–4.

59. Schoeman JP, Stidworthy MF. Budd-Chiari-like syndrome associated with an adrenal phaeochromocytoma in a dog. *J Small Anim Pract* 2001;**42**:191–4.

60. Kyles AE, Feldman EC, De Cock HE, et al. Surgical management of adrenal gland tumors with and without associated tumor thrombi in dogs: 40 cases (1994-2001). *J Am Vet Med Assoc* 2003;**223**:654–62.

61. Louvet A, Lazard P, Denis B. Phaeochromocytoma treated by en bloc resection including the suprarenal caudal vena cava in a dog. *J Small Anim Pract* 2005;**46**: 591–6.

62. Schultz RM, Wisner ER, Johnson EG, et al. Contrast-enhanced computed tomography as a preoperative indicator of vascular invasion from adrenal masses in dogs. *Vet Radiol Ultrasound* 2009;**50**(6):625–9.

63. Whittemore JC, Preston CA, Kyles AE, et al. Nontraumatic rupture of an adrenal gland tumor causing intra-abdominal or retroperitoneal hemorrhage in four dogs. *J Am Vet Med Assoc* 2001;**219**:329–33, 324.

64. Lang JM, Schertel E, Kennedy S, et al. Elective and emergency surgical management of adrenal gland tumors: 60 cases (1999-2006). *J Am Anim Hosp Assoc* 2011;**47**:428–35.

65. Welch TJ, Sheedy PF 2nd, Stephens DH, et al. Percutaneous adrenal biopsy: review of a 10-year experience. *Radiology* 1994;**193**:341–4.

66. Casola G, Nicolet V, vanSonnenberg E, et al. Unsuspected pheochromocytoma: risk of blood-pressure alterations during percutaneous adrenal biopsy. *Radiology* 1986;**159**:733–5.

67. Chun R, Jakovljevic S, Morrison WB, et al. Apocrine gland adenocarcinoma and pheochromocytoma in a cat. *J Am Anim Hosp Assoc* 1997;**33**:33–6.

68. Moore LE, Biller DS, Smith TA. Use of abdominal ultrasonography in the diagnosis of primary hyperaldosteronism in a cat. *J Am Vet Med Assoc* 2000;**217**:213–15, 197.

69. Bouayad H, Feeney DA, Caywood DD, et al. Pheochromocytoma in dogs: 13 cases (1980-1985). *J Am Vet Med Assoc* 1987;**191**:1610–15.

70. Hoerauf A, Reusch C. Ultrasonographic evaluation of the adrenal glands in six dogs with hypoadrenocorticism. *J Am Anim Hosp Assoc* 1999;**35**:214–18.

71. Wenger M, Mueller C, Kook PH, et al. Ultrasonographic evaluation of adrenal glands in dogs with primary hypoadrenocorticism or mimicking diseases. *Vet Rec* 2010;**167**: 207–10.

72. Nelson RW, Feldman EC, Smith MC. Hyperadrenocorticism in cats: seven cases (1978-1987). *J Am Vet Med Assoc* 1988;**193**:245–50.

73. Immink WF, van Toor AJ, Vos JH, et al. Hyperadrenocorticism in four cats. *Vet Q* 1992;**14**:81–5.

74. Duesberg CA, Nelson RW, Feldman EC, et al. Adrenalectomy for treatment of hyperadrenocorticism in cats: 10 cases (1988-1992). *J Am Vet Med Assoc* 1995;**207**: 1066–70.

75. Duesberg C, Peterson ME. Adrenal disorders in cats. *Vet Clin North Am Small Anim Pract* 1997;**27**:321–47.

76. Feldman EC, Nelson RW. Hyperadrenocorticism in cats (Cushing's syndrome). In: Feldman EC, Nelson RW, editors. *Canine and feline endocrinology and reproduction*. 3rd ed. Philadelphia: WB Saunders; 2004. p. 358–93.

77. Watson PJ, Herrtage ME. Hyperadrenocorticism in six cats. *J Small Anim Pract* 1998;**39**:175–84.

78. Calsyn JDR, Green RA, Davis GJ, et al. Adrenal pheochromocytoma with contralateral adrenocortical adenoma in a cat. *J Am Anim Hosp Assoc* 2010;**46**: 36–42.

79. Nichols R. Complications and concurrent disease associated with diabetes mellitus. *Semin Vet Med Surg (Small Anim)* 1997;**12**:263–7.

80. Ahn A. Hyperaldosteronism in cats. *Semin Vet Med Surg (Small Anim)* 1994;**9**:153–7.

81. MacKay AD, Holt PE, Sparkes AH. Successful surgical treatment of a cat with primary aldosteronism. *J Feline Med Surg* 1999;**1**:117–22.

82. DeClue AE, Breshears LA, Pardo ID, et al. Hyperaldosteronism and hyperprogesteronism in a cat with an adrenal cortical carcinoma. *J Vet Intern Med* 2005;**19**: 355–8.

83. Gunn-Moore D. Feline endocrinopathies. *Vet Clin North Am Small Anim Pract* 2005;**35**:171–210, vii.

84. Ash RA, Harvey AM, Tasker S. Primary hyperaldosteronism in the cat: a series of 13 cases. *J Feline Med Surg* 2005;**7**:173–82.

85. Rose SA, Kyles AE, Labelle P, et al. Adrenalectomy and caval thrombectomy in a cat with primary hyperaldosteronism. *J Am Anim Hosp Assoc* 2007;**43**:209–14.

86. Chiaramonte D, Greco DS. Feline adrenal disorders. *Clin Tech Small Anim Pract* 2007;**22**:26–31.

87. Schulman RL. Feline primary hyperaldosteronism. *Vet Clinics Small Anim* 2010;**40**:353–9.

88. Boord M, Griffin C. Progesterone secreting adrenal mass in a cat with clinical signs of hyperadrenocorticism. *J Am Vet Med Assoc* 1999;**214**:666–9.

89. Rossmeisl JH Jr, Scott-Moncrieff JC, Siems J, et al. Hyperadrenocorticism and hyperprogesteronemia in a cat with an adrenocortical adenocarcinoma. *J Am Anim Hosp Assoc* 2000;**36**:512–17.

90. Millard RP, Pickens EH, Wells KL. Excessive production of sex hormones in a cat with an adrenocortical tumor. *J Am Vet Med Assoc* 2009;**234**:505–8.

91. Patnaik AK, Erlandson RA, Lieberman PH, et al. Extra-adrenal pheochromocytoma (paraganglioma) in a cat. *J Am Vet Med Assoc* 1990;**197**:104–6.

92. Henry CJ, Brewer WG Jr, Montgomery RD, et al. Clinical vignette. Adrenal pheochromocytoma. *J Vet Intern Med* 1993;**7**:199–201.

93. Thurston W, Wilson SR. The adrenal glands. In: Rumack CM, Wilson SR, Charboneau JW, editors. *Diagnostic ultrasound*. St. Louis: Mosby; 2005. p. 425–42.

94. Jubb KVF, Kennedy PF. The endocrine glands. In: Jubb KVF, Kennedy PF, editors. *Pathology of domestic animals*. New York: Academic Press; 1970. p. 407–42.

95. Horauf A, Reusch C. Effects of mitotane therapy in dogs with pituitary dependent Cushing syndrome on the adrenal gland size—an ultrasonographic study. *Schweiz Arch Tierheilkd* 1999;**141**:239–45.

96. Mantis P, Lamb CR, Witt AL. Changes in ultrasonographic appearance of adrenal glands in dogs with pituitary-dependent hyperadrenocorticism treated with trilostane. *Vet Rad Ultrasound* 2003;**44**(6):682–5.

97. Ruckstuhl NS, Nett CS, Reusch CE. Results of clinical examinations, laboratory tests, and ultrasonography in dogs with pituitary-dependent hyperadrenocorticism treated with trilostane. *Am J Vet Res* 2002;**63**:506–12.

98. Chapman PS, Kelly DF, Archer J, et al. Adrenal necrosis in a dog received trilostane for the treatment of hyperadrenocorticism. *J Small Anim Pract* 2004;**45**:307–10.

99. Ramsey IK, Richardson J, Lenard Z. Persistent isolated hypocortisolism following brief treatment with trilostane. *Aust Vet J* 2008;**86**:491–5.

100. Reusch CE, Sieber-Ruckstuhl N, Wenger M, et al. Histological evaluation of the adrenal glands of seven dogs with hyperadrenocorticism treated with trilostane. *Vet Rec* 2007;**160**:219–24.

CHAPTER 16
Urinary Tract

Thomas G. Nyland • William R. Widmer • John S. Mattoon

Ultrasonographic evaluation of the urinary tract has become a routine procedure in veterinary medicine. Ultrasound imaging is usually one of the first studies performed to assess the kidneys because important anatomic information concerning the size, shape, and internal architecture can be obtained even in the presence of impaired renal function or abdominal fluid. Advantages over conventional radiology are well known and include the ability to visualize the kidneys in emaciated animals and those with retroperitoneal fluid. Subcapsular fluid, localized perirenal fluid, small renal or perirenal masses, and pelvic or ureteral dilation are also easily detected compared with conventional radiographic imaging. Percutaneous ultrasound-guided kidney aspirations and biopsies are now favored over more invasive, less selective biopsy methods. Ultrasound-guided interventional procedures such as percutaneous nephropyelocentesis and antegrade pyelography can be performed for diagnostic or therapeutic purposes. Doppler ultrasound imaging also permits functional assessment of renal blood flow. Although the normal ureters are not easily identified with ultrasonography, abnormalities causing ureteral dilation are easily detected.

Ultrasonography is superior to conventional radiography in many cases, but there are also limitations. These include the inability to completely visualize the kidneys in some large or obese dogs and in those with excessive bowel gas. Radiopaque calculi, especially if they are ureteral, may be easier to localize with conventional radiography. Excretory urography is superior for qualitative assessment of renal function, visualization of nondilated ureters, identification of subtle pelvic or ureteral dilation, and localization of the site of trauma-induced urine leakage.

KIDNEYS AND PROXIMAL URETERS

Examination Technique

A 5- to 8-MHz transducer is adequate for most dogs; an 8- to 15-MHz transducer is optimal for cats. The abdomen is prepared by clipping the hair and applying acoustic coupling gel to the skin. The kidneys are initially examined from the ventral abdomen with the animal in dorsal recumbency (see Chapter 4, Figure 4-23). It is easiest for beginners to locate the kidneys in the transverse plane. The sagittal plane is then readily obtained to complete the examination. It is important that firm transducer pressure be applied to displace overlying bowel loops and to scan through the kidney slowly in each plane. The left kidney is easier to visualize because of its more caudal position and because of the acoustic window sometimes provided by the spleen. The cranial position of the dog's right kidney within the rib cage and its location dorsal to gas-filled bowel make it difficult to visualize. Feline kidneys are

much easier to examine because of the smaller body size of the cat and the more caudal location of the kidneys.

Supplemental views in dorsal recumbency may be needed to fully evaluate the kidneys. These views require removal of the hair from the lateral aspects of the abdomen. Views of the kidney from the lateral abdomen in a dorsal (frontal) plane and lateral transverse plane are less affected by bowel gas. High-quality images of the right kidney may require evaluation through the right 11th to 12th intercostal space. If necessary, the animal may be placed in left or right lateral recumbency. The uppermost kidney may be evaluated if bowel gas does not compromise visualization. However, it is also possible to scan the dependent kidney through a hole cut in a Plexiglas table. In addition, the kidneys can be examined from the dorsal paralumbar region with the animal in sternal recumbency or in a standing position. This view is particularly useful in animals with marked ascites or large masses because it reduces the distance to the kidneys.

Mistakes in interpretation can result from failure to completely visualize the kidneys. Therefore the sonographer must be patient, use multiple views, and if necessary repeat the examination at a later time to ensure a high-quality study.

Normal Anatomy

The cranial pole of the left kidney contacts the greater curvature of the stomach and dorsomedial aspect of the spleen laterally. The spleen is often ventral to the kidney, providing an ideal acoustic window. The left kidney contacts the left limb of the pancreas cranially and the left adrenal gland more medially. The left adrenal gland is positioned ventrolateral to the aorta. The cranial pole of the right kidney is located in the renal fossa of the caudate liver lobe. The caudal vena cava is closely associated with the right kidney's medial border. The right adrenal gland lies lateral or dorsolateral to the caudal vena cava at this location. The descending duodenum and right pancreatic limb lie immediately ventral to the right kidney.

The renal arteries in the dog originate from the lateral aspect of the aorta and measure 3 to 4 mm in diameter.[1] They often divide into a dorsal and ventral branch before reaching the kidneys. In 20% of dogs, the renal arteries may be double, particularly the left renal artery. The right renal artery arises about 4 cm caudal to the cranial mesenteric artery and travels dorsal to the caudal vena cava about 4 to 5 cm to the right kidney. The left renal artery originates about 2 cm caudal to the right renal artery and measures approximately 3 cm in length. The renal veins are immediately ventral to their corresponding arteries, with the left renal vein being longer than the right.

In a sagittal sonogram of the kidney, three distinct regions can clearly be recognized (Figures 16-1, *A*, and 16-2, *A*).

557

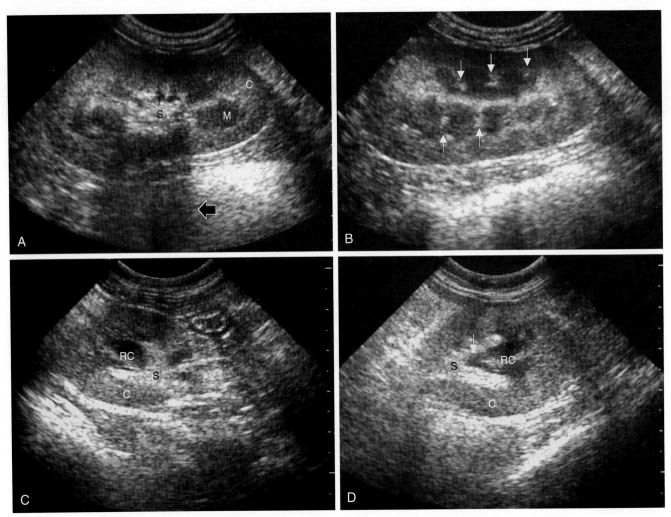

Figure 16-1 Normal dog kidney. A and **B,** Kidney, sagittal view. **A,** Three distinct regions of the kidney consisting of the renal sinus (*S*), renal medulla (*M*), and renal cortex (*C*) can be identified. The renal medulla is the least echogenic region. The renal cortex is more echogenic than the medulla but less echogenic than the renal sinus with its peripelvic fat. Some shadowing may be identified distal to the renal sinus (*arrow*). **B,** In a scanning plane lateral to **A,** echogenicities corresponding to the dorsal and ventral sets of diverticula and interlobar vessels can be seen (*arrows*). **C** and **D,** Midtransverse view. **C,** Right kidney. The renal sinus (*S*), renal crest (*RC*), and renal cortex (*C*) are identified. Urine is not identified within the renal pelvis or ureter in most normal dogs. **D,** Left kidney. An anechoic region at the tip of the renal crest (*arrow*) corresponds to urine in the renal pelvis of this normal dog. Slight pelvic dilation is sometimes seen in normal dogs undergoing diuresis from fluid therapy or diuretics.

These regions consist of a bright central echo complex, corresponding to the renal sinus and peripelvic fat; a hypoechoic region surrounding the pelvis, representing renal medulla; and an outer zone of intermediate echogenicity, the renal cortex.[2-4] The medial border of the kidney is indented by an oval opening called the hilum, which opens into the renal sinus. On scanning from medial to lateral in the sagittal plane, the bright central echo representing the renal sinus disappears, and a central hypoechoic region bordered by two parallel linear echogenicities appears. The central hypoechoic region represents the renal crest (also termed the renal pyramid or renal papilla); the linear echogenicities are the dorsal and ventral sets of pelvic diverticula (recesses) accompanied by interlobar arteries and veins. The diverticula and vessels can be recognized as short, evenly spaced linear echogenic structures traversing the medullary region toward the cortex as

they are being followed farther peripherally in the kidney (see Figure 16-1, *B*). The hypoechoic medulla is separated into multiple sections by the diverticula and interlobar vessels. The kidney of the dog is unipyramidal with no calyces, so these sections represent separations of the same renal pyramid.[5] The diverticula and vessels are cut transversely in the sagittal plane so that only a short length may be visualized in any one section. The arcuate and intralobar arteries are sometimes recognized as discrete echogenicities at the corticomedullary junction and within the cortex, respectively, of the kidneys.[4]

Imaging the kidney in a dorsal (frontal) plane from the lateral body wall or in a transverse plane results in visualization of a greater length of the diverticula and vessels because the plane passes through the long axis of these structures. In a middorsal plane, however, the beam passes between the dorsal and ventral sets of diverticula so that neither is visible.

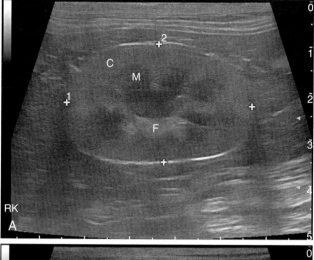

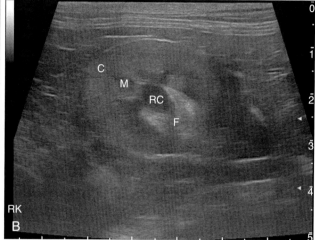

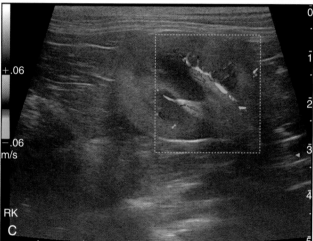

Figure 16-2 **Normal kidney from an older cat. A,** Sagittal image of the right kidney (4.09 cm in length by 2.56 cm in height, between electronic cursors). **B,** Transverse image of the right kidney. Renal sinus fat (*F*) is readily seen as hyperechoic V-shaped tissue, adjacent to the hypoechoic renal crest (*RC*). **C,** Transverse color Doppler image shows normal perfusion of the right kidney. C, Renal cortex; *M*, renal medulla.

Therefore a plane parallel to the dorsal or ventral set of diverticula is more properly termed a dorsal oblique plane.

The renal pelvis and peripelvic fat, proximal ureter, diverticula, medulla, and cortex can be identified on transverse kidney scans from the ventral or lateral abdomen with high-resolution equipment (see Figures 16-1, C and D, and 16-2, B). Linear echogenicities representing the dorsal and ventral sets of pelvic diverticula and interlobar vessels can be seen radiating to the cortex from the central pelvic region. The medullary region appears to be separated into sections by the diverticula and vessels as one scans from cranial to caudal through the kidney in a transverse plane. The solitary renal crest, flanked by the two sets of diverticula, is easily identified in midtransverse scans. In normal dogs and cats, urine is not normally identified within the pelvis or diverticula, nor is urine seen in the ureter, unless there is accompanying diuresis.

Kidney Echogenicity

The normal relationship of the echogenicity of the dog kidney to that of the liver and spleen is important for recognizing major abnormalities.[5,6] The renal medulla is the least echogenic, followed by the renal cortex. Echogenicity of the renal cortex is similar to or slightly less than that of normal liver parenchyma and quite a bit less than that of splenic parenchyma using a 5-MHz transducer at approximately the same depth (Figure 16-3, A). In a study of healthy dogs[6a] using an 8-MHz transducer and both qualitative and quantitative analysis, the normal renal cortex was *hyperechoic* with respect to the liver (see Figure 16-3, B). Perirenal fat surrounding the kidney has an echogenicity similar to or greater than the prominent central echo complex of the renal sinus. A marked change in these relationships suggests possible pathologic changes in one or more of these organs. There is evidence, however, that organ echogenicity may vary with the frequency and type of the transducer used.[7] In addition, fat vacuoles in the cortical tubular epithelium may increase cortical echogenicity of normal cats[8] (Figure 16-4). In cats, it is not unusual for the renal cortical tissue to be isoechoic or hyperechoic to the adjacent liver parenchyma. It is not often hypoechoic relative to the liver tissue (Figure 16-4B). Therefore the diagnosis of subtle abnormalities requires familiarity with the normal echogenicity of organs at a particular frequency and imaging depth on the sonographer's own equipment.

Kidney and Ureteral Size

To date, there is no widely accepted method for determining normal kidney size by ultrasonographic measurements in the dog. Kidney size is still judged primarily by subjective evaluation. Several studies attempting to correlate linear kidney measurements or kidney volume with body weight or surface area have met with limited success. Although there is a positive correlation of kidney length or volume with body weight, the standard deviation is large.[9-12] There is also a marked variation of kidney length and volume among normal dogs of similar body weights.[11] Recently a ratio of kidney length to

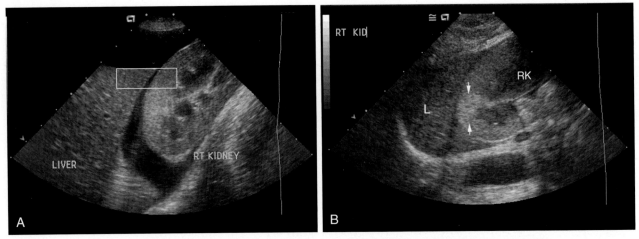

Figure 16-3 Renal cortical echogenicity relative to liver parenchyma in normal dogs. A, Right renal cortex is isoechoic to the adjacent liver parenchyma. Comparing echogenicity of two structures should be made at the same depth. In this example, the liver and kidney are isoechoic within the box. Anechoic peritoneal fluid is present. **B,** The right renal cortex is hyperechoic relative to the liver parenchyma. Note the even more hyperechoic cranial pole renal cortex (*white arrows*), because the renal tubules and vessels are perpendicular to the ultrasound beam at this level. (Courtesy Dr. Ben Young, Texas A&M University.)

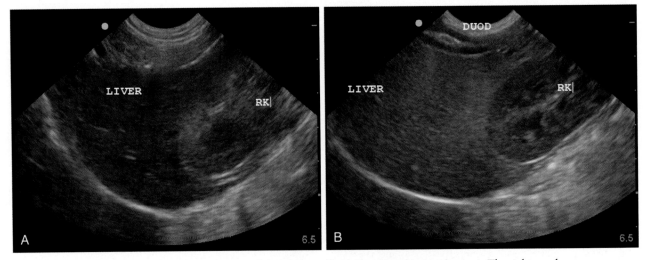

Figure 16-4 Renal cortical echogenicity relative to liver parenchyma in normal cats. A, The right renal cortex is hyperechoic relative to the liver parenchyma. **B,** The right renal cortex is hypoechoic relative to the liver parenchyma. The duodenum (DUOD) is present in the near field.

aortic diameter was investigated as a means of estimating normal kidney size in the dog.[13] The investigators concluded that a ratio of kidney length to aorta diameter of 5.5 to 9.1 was normal. A ratio of less than 5.5 indicates the kidneys are small, whereas a ratio greater than 9.1 indicates that they are enlarged. However, the ratio's interval is rather broad, and the usefulness has yet to be established in dogs with various types of renal disease.

In the cat, linear, volume, or area measurements of the kidney are more useful because there is less variation in body size. One investigation of 10 normal young cats reported that kidney length was approximately 3.2 to 4.1 cm, kidney width was 2.2 to 2.8 cm, and kidney height was 1.9 to 2.5 cm.[14] Kidney length has also been reported to range from 3.8 to 4.4 cm; kidney width, from 2.7 to 3.1 cm; and kidney height,

from 2.0 to 2.5 cm by direct anatomic measurement.[15] Based on these reports, kidney length is commonly used to estimate kidney size; a range of approximately 3.0 to 4.5 cm is considered normal. Renal cross-sectional area or volume can also be used to estimate kidney size. Normal renal cross-sectional area, measured in a transverse plane at the renal crest, ranged from approximately 4.0 to 6.0 cm^2 in 14 normal young adult cats.[16] Normal renal volume was 11.9 to 17.7 cm^3 using the prolate ellipsoid method of measurement (volume = length × width × height × 0.523) in a group of 5 normal female cats.[17]

Renal enlargement with a smooth contour has been seen with compensatory hypertrophy, acute renal failure, ethylene glycol poisoning, hydronephrosis, acute nephritis, early amyloidosis, portosystemic shunts, diffuse infiltrative diseases, and diffuse neoplasia. Enlarged kidneys with an irregular contour are most often seen with granulomas, abscesses, cysts, polycystic renal disease, and primary or metastatic neoplasia. A regular or irregular kidney contour has been seen with lymphoma or feline infectious peritonitis depending on whether there is focal, multifocal, or diffuse involvement. Small kidneys are found with congenital renal hypoplasia or dysplasia[18-21] and with chronic end-stage renal disease.

By administering furosemide and intravenous contrast agents to dogs, the renal medulla was shown to increase in size during diuresis, owing to increased fluid flow through the kidney.[2] This results in an increase in kidney size, although the appearance of the renal cortex, pelvis, and diverticula is unchanged. Water-soluble iodinated contrast agents do not interfere with ultrasonographic evaluation of the kidneys. The effect of excretory urography alone on the ultrasonographic appearance of the kidney has not been reported in the dog, but a slight increase in linear dimensions without a change in appearance was reported in the cat.[3] The same result is anticipated for dogs because a combination of intravenous contrast medium and furosemide reportedly did not produce visible pelvic dilation.[2] However, these observations should be confirmed with newer high-resolution ultrasound equipment, which can detect even subtle pelvic dilation.

The upper limit of proximal ureteral diameter in normal adult dogs not undergoing diuresis has been reported to be 1.8 mm.[22] We have observed mild renal pelvic dilation resulting from intravenous fluid administration in some dogs with apparently normal renal function, and this has also been described by others.[23] In one study, mild renal pelvic dilation was observed in 16 of 23 dogs (70%) without renal disease after the administration of intravenous saline to induce diuresis (2.7 to 18.8 mL/kg/hr).[24] In 11 of these 16 dogs (69%) with pelvic dilation, the dilation was unilateral. Neither proximal ureteral dilation nor a change in kidney dimensions was observed during saline diuresis. It is clear that the improved resolution of newer ultrasound equipment makes it possible to detect even minimal renal pelvic dilation. Poorer resolution of older equipment may partly explain the lack of pelvic dilation observed with furosemide diuresis in an earlier study.[2] The effect of furosemide and other diuretics on pelvic dilation should be reevaluated with newer high-resolution equipment.

In summary, diuresis associated with the administration of furosemide produces a transient increase in kidney size due to medullary enlargement in normal dogs.[2] Diuresis associated with hypertonic contrast agents during urography causes lesser degrees of transient kidney enlargement.[3] Saline diuresis produces no kidney size changes in dogs.[24] Mild renal pelvic dilation (pyelectasia), sometimes unilateral, has been reported with saline diuresis in dogs.[23,24] Ureteral dilation distal to the ureteropelvic junction has not been reported with diuresis in normal dogs or cats. Therefore a renal pelvis or proximal ureter transverse diameter of more than 3 to 4 mm warrants further investigation to rule out pyelonephritis or early ureteral obstruction. Figure 16-5 shows pyelectasia in a cat after administration of intravenous fluids.

Absent or Ectopic Kidneys

Absence of a kidney may result from agenesis[25,26] or previous nephrectomy. Failure to visualize one kidney on an excretory urogram indicates that the kidney is either absent or nonfunctional because of disease. Ultrasonography can easily answer that question. If both kidneys have severely impaired function, an excretory urogram may fail to opacify either kidney. Ultrasonography is useful in determining whether both kidneys are present and whether their appearance is normal. Compensatory hypertrophy of the remaining kidney in unilateral renal agenesis can occur. The kidney is enlarged but retains normal

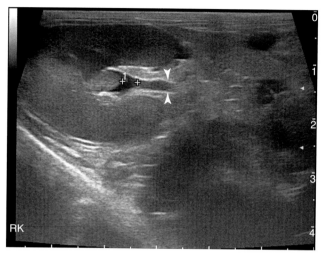

Figure 16-5 **Mild pyelectasia in a cat administered intravenous fluids.** Transverse image of the right kidney shows mild pelvic and proximal ureter dilation. The electronic cursors have been placed between the renal crest and the origin of the ureter (0.29 cm). The ureter is approximately 2 mm in diameter (between white arrowheads). Note the near-field Time gain compensation (TGC) is improperly adjusted, creating the dark (hypoechoic) band across the near field.

internal architecture. Ectopic kidneys may require a search for kidneys that are not in a normal location.[27] Fusion of the kidneys may rarely occur.[28]

Focal Abnormalities of the Renal Parenchyma

Distortion of the renal contour by intrinsic masses is easily demonstrated by ultrasound examination. However, the sonographic appearance and internal characteristics of the mass usually do not permit a definitive diagnosis except in renal cysts and some focal kidney masses produced by lymphosarcoma. Therefore a fine-needle aspiration or biopsy of the mass is often required for diagnosis. On occasion, when a mass in the kidney region is exceptionally large, it may be difficult to determine whether the mass arises from the kidney or has instead displaced the kidney from its normal position. The correct diagnosis requires a thorough search of the abdomen to locate both kidneys when survey radiographs or excretory urography is not available.

Renal Cysts

Renal cysts may be solitary or multiple, sometimes involving both kidneys and may be inherited or acquired[29-33] (Figures 16-6 and 16-7). The sonographic features of simple cysts include a round to ovoid contour, echo-free contents, smooth and sharply demarcated thin walls with a distinct far-wall border, and strong distal echo enhancement. Unlike similar-appearing solid masses, cysts remain anechoic despite an increase of the scanner's gain settings. Cysts also have strong distal acoustic enhancement, whereas in similar-appearing solid masses, enhancement is weak or absent. The near wall of the cyst may not appear smooth because of overlying reverberation artifacts. Near the edge of the cyst, the anechoic contents may appear to contain echoes, but this is a slice thickness artifact resulting from echoes originating outside the cyst. Cysts are thin walled, although this may be difficult to determine if normal renal tissue surrounds the cyst. Cysts may deform the kidney outline if they are large or if polycystic disease is present. Displacement, distortion, and dilation of the collecting system from partial obstruction may occur.[34] A zone

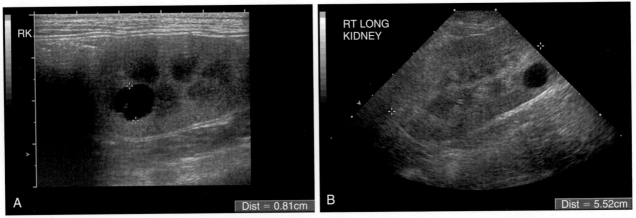

Figure 16-6 Solitary renal cortical cysts. A, Solitary cyst in the cranial pole of the right kidney in a cat (0.81 cm between electronic cursors). **B,** Solitary cyst in the caudal pole of the right kidney of a dachshund.

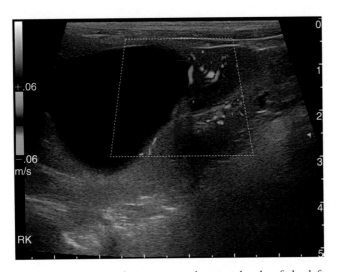

Figure 16-7 Large solitary cyst in the cranial pole of the left kidney. Color Doppler image shows normal blood flow in the remaining kidney.

of reduced echo intensity may be seen extending distally from the lateral margins of the cyst. This appearance, termed edge shadowing, results from refraction of the sound beam as it passes through the cyst. Simple cysts are usually incidental findings without clinical signs. Solitary renal cysts have been successfully ablated with ultrasound-guided ethanol injection.[35]

Small 1- to 3-mm cystlike lesions are frequently seen in end-stage kidney disease and might be part of the degenerative processes affecting these kidneys. In a study of familial juvenile glomerulonephropathy in French mastiff (Bordeaux) dogs, pertinent ultrasound findings include hyperechoic/thickened renal cortices, poor corticomedullary demarcation, and small cortical cysts.[36] Histopathologic analysis revealed numerous areas of cystic glomerular atrophy that may correspond to the ultrasonographic findings.

Other disorders, such as complicated cysts, hematoma, abscess, and tumor, must be included in the differential diagnosis if the cyst walls are thick or irregular, internal septations are present, or the contents of the cyst are not completely anechoic (Figure 16-8). In humans and cats, a large number of very small cysts produce a hyperechoic or complex sonographic lesion because of multiple reflecting interfaces.[32,37] This pattern may be confused with other hyperechoic or complex kidney lesions.

Inherited polycystic renal disease has been reported mostly in Persian or Persian-cross cats, cairn terriers, and bull terriers, but can occur in other breeds, including Chartreux cats.[17,38-51] Polycystic renal disease an autosomal dominant mutation, is the most common inherited renal disease of cats and prevalence in Persians is 37% to 49%. Multiple parenchymal cystic areas are present at birth enlarge with maturity and may cause significant loss of renal function, depending on the number and volume of cystic change.[50-53] In a study evaluating repeatability and progression, of ultrasound scanning for feline polycystic disease, repeatability was 100% and signs of progression were seen during a 1-year period.[54] While an accurate genetic test is available for the autosomal dominant genome, it cannot predict severity or progression of polycystic disease over time. Figure 16-9 shows several examples of polycystic kidney disease.

In congenital renal cystic disorders of humans, the liver and pancreas may also contain cysts. Cystic changes of the biliary tree accompanying renal polycystic disease have been reported in dogs.[39,55-57] Two cats with renal polycystic disease were also reported to have concurrent hepatic cysts, but their locations were not discussed.[32] Acquired cysts may occur from various types of chronic nephropathies. Histopathologic examination of the kidney is required for a definitive diagnosis.

Uniform blood clots, unclotted blood, hematomas, abscesses without debris, lymphomatous masses, and necrosis associated with tumors or cystadenocarcinomas of the kidney may occasionally have many of the characteristics of cysts. However, most of these lesions lack one or more of the criteria of simple cysts listed earlier. Lymphomatous masses, for example, although appearing anechoic, have weaker and less distinct far-wall echoes and distal enhancement than true cysts. Increasing instrument gain may increase internal echoes in lymphomatous masses, but not in true renal cysts. Cysts associated with cystadenocarcinomas of the kidney may have irregular contours, thicker walls, and internal debris. The diagnosis can usually be reached with the aid of the history, physical findings, or laboratory work. For example, cystadenocarcinomas of the kidney have commonly been associated with female German shepherds and accompany a nodular dermatofibrosis skin disorder.[58,59] If other information is not helpful, further diagnostic procedures, such as aspiration or biopsy, can be performed.

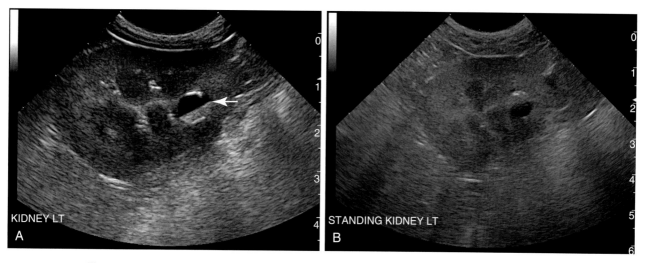

Figure 16-8 **Solitary renal cyst in a dog. A,** A small cortical cyst (approximately 8 mm) is present, containing echogenic, layering sediment (*arrow*). This was an incidental, nonclinical finding in a dog with severe pancreatitis. **B,** With the patient standing, the contents of the cyst are seen to shift to the new gravity-dependent position. Note that the depth of field was 47 mm in **A** and increased to 61 mm in **B,** accounting for the change in relative size of the kidney between the two images.

Solid Masses

Solid renal masses are commonly neoplastic and may appear hypoechoic, isoechoic, or hyperechoic, or have a mixed pattern[29-32,60-62] (Figures 16-10 to 16-12). In dogs, the most common primary malignant neoplasm is renal carcinoma, which is more common in males.[63] The most common benign primary renal tumor in dogs is hemangioma.[64-66] In cats, primary renal lymphoma has been recognized most commonly.[67] The pattern is not characteristic of the tumor type, although uniformly hypoechoic masses have often been associated with lymphoma. The internal echoes of a solid mass increase as the gain settings of the instrument are increased, and they possess much weaker distal wall echoes and acoustic enhancement than fluid-filled or complex masses. This usually helps differentiate uniform solid, anechoic to hypoechoic masses, such as those produced by lymphoma, from true cysts. Solid masses can contain small areas of hemorrhage, necrosis, or calcification, but the majority of the mass has a solid pattern (see Figure 16-12, *A*). Isoechoic masses may not be recognized unless a border, change in echo texture, distortion of internal architecture, or change in renal contour is also identified (see Figure 16-11). In contrast to small cysts, small solid renal masses are difficult to recognize without meticulous scanning technique. Hyperechoic masses have been reported with primary chondrosarcoma, metastatic hemangiosarcoma (see Figure 16-10, *B*), and metastatic thyroid adenocarcinoma in the dog.[30,31,54] We have also observed a solid, hyperechoic mass with renal hemangioma, hemangiosarcoma, and osteosarcoma.

Nonneoplastic renal masses with a solid pattern may also be recognized occasionally. Granulomas, although rare, fit this category. Calcification within a hematoma, abscess, or cyst wall may prevent sufficient sound transmission to properly characterize the far wall. This may lead to an erroneous diagnosis of a solid mass. Radiographic evaluation should enable a correct interpretation, provided that the calcification is sufficient to be recognized radiographically. An acute renal infarct may initially appear as an isoechoic or hypoechoic lesion.[68,69] A hematoma or abscess containing homogeneous, viscous internal debris may occasionally also simulate a solid mass. A fine-needle aspiration should be performed in questionable cases before tissue-core biopsy. However, renal abscesses are rare, particularly with a solid pattern, and much less common than primary or metastatic neoplasia.

Complex Masses

Many renal masses have a complex sonographic appearance; that is, they may contain a variable mixture of anechoic, hypoechoic, and hyperechoic components (Figure 16-13). The anechoic and hypoechoic regions represent areas of hemorrhage or necrosis that sonographers sometimes refer to as cystic areas despite the fact that their appearance does not resemble true cysts. The majority of the mass contains these cystic components. The solid portions represent a smaller percentage of the mass and usually appear isoechoic or hyperechoic compared with normal renal tissue. Hyperechoic areas with dirty shadowing may also occur if gas-producing organisms are present. Distal acoustic enhancement may be seen with some complex masses, but the enhancement is not as prominent as with true cysts.

Complex masses may be produced by hematomas,[30] granulomas, abscesses,[30,70,71] acute infarcts, and primary or metastatic neoplasia.[29-31,33,61,72] However, infarcts or neoplasia may also have a solid pattern as described previously. The diagnosis of hematomas and abscesses requires a compatible history and laboratory work. For example, a hematoma is more probable in a young animal with a clotting disorder or recent trauma, whereas an abscess is more likely if fever and leukocytosis are present. A hematoma or abscess may have a variable pattern depending on age. Therefore aspiration for cytologic analysis and bacterial culture may be required for a diagnosis. In an older animal without such signs, a primary renal neoplasm or metastasis to the kidney should be suspected. Evidence of tumor in the opposite kidney, lymphadenopathy, metastasis to other abdominal organs, or discovery of a primary tumor elsewhere in the abdomen may help confirm the diagnosis. There may be accompanying ureteral obstruction or invasion of the renal artery, caudal vena cava, or aorta. If the lesion is solitary, fine-needle aspiration for fluid analysis, cytologic evaluation, or bacterial culture or a tissue-core biopsy is recommended for diagnosis. When a hematoma is suspected, progressive resolution should occur on serial ultrasound

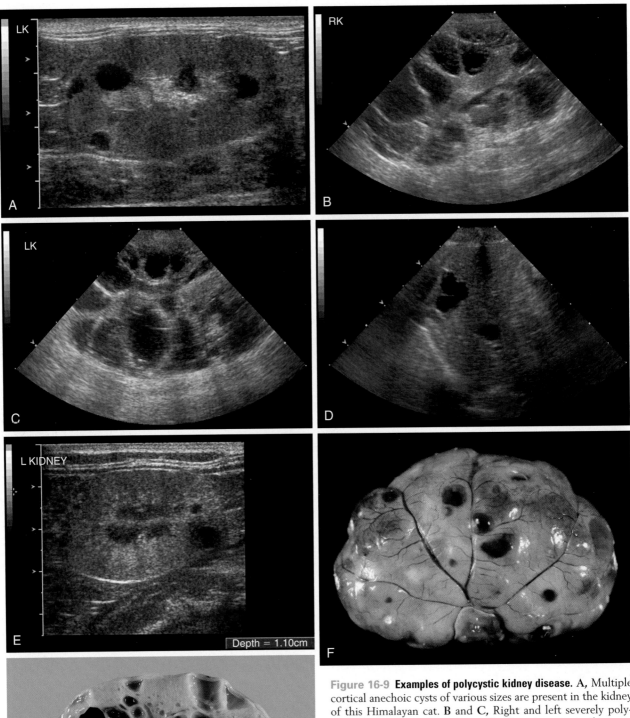

Figure 16-9 **Examples of polycystic kidney disease. A,** Multiple cortical anechoic cysts of various sizes are present in the kidney of this Himalayan cat. **B** and **C,** Right and left severely polycystic kidneys in a Persian cat. **D,** Hepatic cysts in the same Persian cat used for images in **B** and **C. E,** One large and one small caudal pole cortical cyst are present in this domestic shorthair cat. The very hyperechoic renal cortex is a result of hundreds of tiny cysts, too small to be resolved, that are collectively creating acoustic enhancement. **F,** Gross image of the external appearance of a kidney from a cat with polycystic kidney disease (capsule removed). The external contour of the kidney is distorted by the disease. **G,** Sectioned polycystic kidney. (*F, G* Courtesy of Washington State University College of Veterinary Medicine, Washington Animal Disease Diagnostic Laboratory, Pullman, WA.)

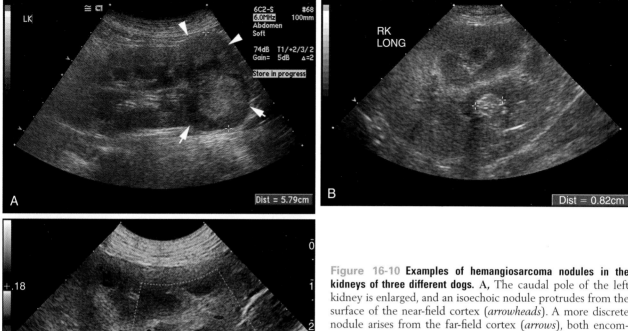

Figure 16-10 Examples of hemangiosarcoma nodules in the kidneys of three different dogs. A, The caudal pole of the left kidney is enlarged, and an isoechoic nodule protrudes from the surface of the near-field cortex (*arrowheads*). A more discrete nodule arises from the far-field cortex (*arrows*), both encompassed by the electronic cursors (5.79 cm). The latter nodule has a hypoechoic rim surrounding slightly hyperechoic internal tissue. **B,** A solitary hyperechoic nodule (0.82 cm between electronic cursors). **C,** Multiple hypoechoic nodules are present within the left kidney, which is distorted and enlarged, with only a portion of it fitting within the field of view.

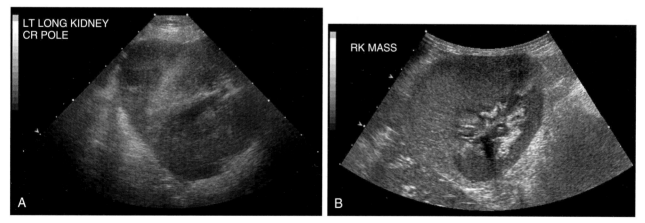

Figure 16-11 Renal lymphoma in two dogs. A, Isoechoic lymphoma nodules bulging from the cranial pole of the left kidney. **B,** Large, convex bulging from the near-field cortex of the right kidney.

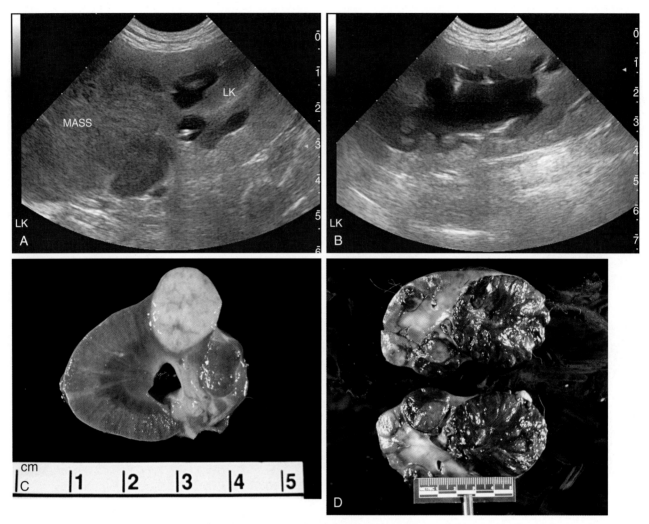

Figure 16-12 Renal neoplasia in a dog. A, A large mass is seen originating from the cranial pole of the left kidney. **B,** The origin of the mass from the left kidney is determined by identification of its dilated pelvis (moderate to severe hydronephrosis). The diagnosis was malignant histiocytosis, involving the liver, abdominal lymph nodes, and the left kidney. **C,** Metastatic carcinoma, seen as a large solitary nodule. **D,** Metastatic melanoma shows extensive tumor within the kidney. (C, D, Courtesy of Washington State University College of Veterinary Medicine, Washington Animal Disease Diagnostic Laboratory, Pullman, WA.)

examinations. Infected, hemorrhagic, or multilocular cysts and renal infarcts are also capable of producing complex masses in humans. It is reasonable to assume that such diseases could produce similar findings in animals.

Focal Hyperechoic Areas in the Renal Cortex

In addition to hyperechoic neoplastic nodules and masses mentioned previously, other causes of hyperechoic areas or lesions in the renal cortex are infection, calcification, fibrosis, gas, and older renal infarcts. Infection may cause patchy areas of hyperechogenicity.[22] Focal parenchymal calcification may occasionally simulate calculi. Fibrosis or gas in the parenchyma or collecting system may produce a similar appearance.[73] Older infarcts may have a wedge-shaped, hyperechoic appearance with a broader base at the surface of the kidney that narrows toward the corticomedullary junction (Figure 16-14).[74] There is often a corresponding defect in the renal contour and thinning of the cortex at this location. Theoretically, an infarct can be differentiated from scarring due to pyelonephritis by the lack of pelvic and diverticular

abnormalities. However, survey radiographs and excretory urography are required for a definitive diagnosis. Gas associated with an abscess or within the renal collecting system and calcific densities are usually visible on survey radiographs, although there still may be difficulty localizing them to the kidney. Calculi produce luminal filling defects on the pyelographic phase of the excretory urogram, whereas parenchymal fibrosis and calcification do not. Fibrosis or calcification may be accompanied by distortion of the collecting system or renal contour. Nonshadowing lesions observed in the pelvis on ultrasonography or filling defects seen on urography may be blood clots, inflammatory debris, or masses of inflammatory or neoplastic origin.

Diffuse Abnormalities of the Renal Parenchyma

There are no specific ultrasound findings that can be used to distinguish most diffuse renal diseases. In fact, the kidneys may appear normal in many cases, even in the face of renal failure. The history and clinical findings may suggest the diagnosis, but a renal aspiration or biopsy is usually needed for

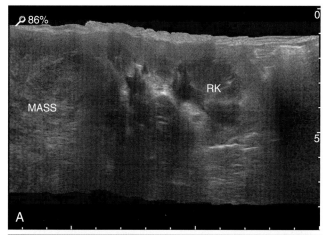

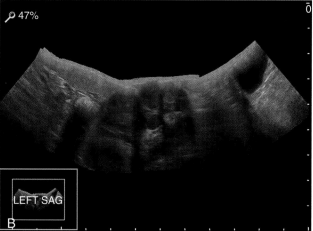

Figure 16-13 **Bilateral renal neoplasia in a dog. A,** Barely recognizable right kidney (*RK*) mass. This extended field of view does not encompass the entire mass. **B,** Extended field of view shows a panoramic image of the left side of the abdomen with the relatively large left renal mass (*center*) in relation to the spleen and transverse colon (to the left) and urinary bladder (to the right).

confirmation. However, ethylene glycol toxicity is one exception where a dramatic increase in renal cortical echogenicity is apparent (Figure 16-15).

In dogs, increased cortical echogenicity can be found with glomerular or interstitial nephritis, pyelonephritis, leptospirosis, acute tubular necrosis, ethylene glycol toxicosis, end-stage renal disease, and parenchymal calcification (nephrocalcinosis).[22,31,33,75-78] (Figure 16-16, *A* to *C*, *F* to *H*; see also Figure 16-25, *A* and *B*). In dogs with hypercalcemic nephropathy, a hyperechoic medullary band (referred to as a medullary rim sign; or, if a hypoechoic gap exists between the medullary rim sign and the corticomedullary junction, it is called a halo sign) has been observed at the corticomedullary junction during ultrasonography[79] (Figure 16-17, *A*). This appearance was associated with calcification of the basement membrane of Bowman capsule and tubular epithelium of the adjacent cortex and medulla. The prognosis is poor because of the presence of severe renal damage from hypercalcemia. In three cases, two were associated with lymphosarcoma and one with multiple myeloma. However, a similar hyperechoic medullary band has also been reported with acute tubular necrosis (ethylene glycol toxicity and idiopathic), pyogranulomatous vasculitis due to feline infectious peritonitis, chronic

interstitial nephritis, and leptospirosis, and in normal dogs and cats[8,75-77,80,81] (see Figure 16-17, *B* to *E*). This hyperechoic band is associated with deposition of minerals in the tubular epithelium of the outer zone of the medulla in some cases, but infiltrates that cause an increase in the size and number of acoustic interfaces may also account for this finding in other instances.[77] The presence of a hyperechoic medullary band suggests the possibility of a renal abnormality, but is also found in clinically normal dogs and cats.[8,81] In one report, 72% of dogs having a medullary rim sign as the only renal abnormality did not have renal dysfunction.[81] However, 78% of dogs with a medullary rim sign and other renal abnormalities (e.g., decreased kidney size, increased medullary echogenicity, or pyelectasia) had renal disease. In some animals, the dense vascular network within the outer portion of the medullary tissue may be responsible for the rim of increased echogenicity. Therefore the significance of the medullary rim sign must be interpreted cautiously in light of other renal findings.

In the cat, increased renal cortical echogenicity has been reported with glomerular and interstitial nephritis (see Figure 16-16, *D*, and 16-24, *A* and *B*), ethylene glycol toxicity, diffuse renal lymphosarcoma (see Figure 16-16, *E*), metastatic squamous cell carcinoma, and feline infectious peritonitis (see Figure 16-16, *I*).[32,76,82] Figure 16-16, *J*, is an example of renal amyloidosis. In normal cats, it was also noted that increased cortical echogenicity can be produced by fat vacuoles in the proximal convoluted tubular epithelium of the renal cortex.[8] This was especially evident in older castrated males and in one pregnant female. Therefore a perceived increase in relative echogenicity of the renal cortex may be normal or abnormal in the cat. Definitive diagnosis requires a renal biopsy. Loss of corticomedullary definition with increased cortical echogenicity was also noted in one cat with multiple small renal cysts less than 1 cm in diameter.[32] Increased cortical echogenicity must be judged subjectively and by comparison with the echogenicity of the liver and spleen. As noted previously, a medullary hyperechoic band extending parallel to the corticomedullary junction has been observed in many clinically normal cats.[8] This band was associated with mineral deposits in the medullary tubular lumen.

Overall increased renal echogenicity and reduced corticomedullary definition have been described with congenital renal dysplasia, juvenile nephropathy, chronic inflammatory diseases, and end-stage kidney disease from a variety of causes in dogs and cats[18-21,31,32,83] (see Figure 16-16, *G* and *H*). In end-stage renal disease, kidneys are typically small, irregular, and diffusely echogenic with poor visualization of the corticomedullary junction and internal renal architecture. In cairn terriers with renal dysplasia and no clinical evidence of renal dysfunction, ultrasound changes included poor corticomedullary definition and multifocal hyperechoic foci in the renal medulla, and a diffusely hyperechoic medulla. The degree of ultrasonographic changes was related to the severity of histopathologic glomerular lesions.[84] Figure 16-16, *K* and *L* show the very hyperechoic nature, distortion of shape and internal architecture, and small size of chronic amyloidosis in a Shar Pei dog.

Reduced cortical echogenicity, multifocal hypoechoic areas, hypoechoic nodules, or hypoechoic masses may be seen with lymphosarcoma of the kidneys in the dog and cat (see also Figure 16-11).[30-32] As noted earlier, lymphosarcoma in cats may also produce a diffuse increase in cortical echogenicity, which is probably the most common presentation (Figure 16-18, *A* to *E*).[32] It is clear that lymphosarcoma of the kidneys can have a variety of ultrasonographic appearances, and kidney aspiration or biopsy is recommended for diagnosis.

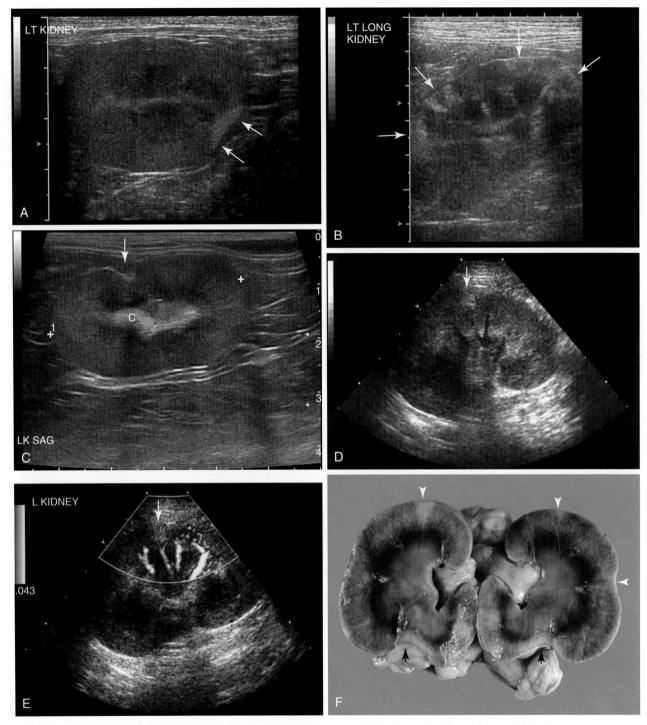

Figure 16-14 **Renal infarcts. A,** Focal depression surrounded by hyperechoic cortical tissue (*arrows*) is present in the caudal pole of the left kidney of this cat, representing an infarct. **B,** Hyperechoic, wedge-shaped cortical pathology (*arrows*) represent cortical artifacts. **C,** A focal depression of the near-field cortex is present in the left kidney of this dog, representing an infarct (*arrow*). A renal pelvic calculus (C) is present, with some acoustic shadowing. **D,** Dorsal image plane of a cat kidney with a hyperechoic cortical infarct (*arrow*). **E,** Power Doppler image of **D** showing lack of blood flow to the hyperechoic cortical infarct (*arrow*). Also note the truncation of the arcuate vessels to the left and lack of cortical blood flow. **F,** Necropsy specimen of renal infarcts. Large depressed area is a chronic infarct (*black arrows*). This would be easily recognized sonographically as an alteration of renal contour. Smaller cortical infarcts are also seen (*white arrowheads*). (F, Courtesy of Washington State University College of Veterinary Medicine, Washington Animal Disease Diagnostic Laboratory, Pullman, WA.)

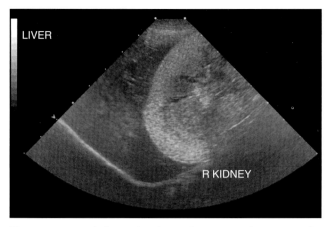

Figure 16-15 Ethylene glycol (antifreeze) renal toxicity. The renal cortex is extremely hyperechoic, with striking contrast to the hypoechoic adjacent liver tissue.

Abnormalities of the Renal Pelvis and Proximal Ureter

Pelvic and Ureteral Dilatation

In the normal animal, urine is not usually visualized within the renal pelvis, and the ureter is not seen between the kidney and bladder. However, current high-resolution ultrasound equipment allows visualization of mild pelvic dilation during diuresis in normal animals (pyelectasia). Diuresis may produce no detectable pelvic dilation, mild symmetric dilation, or mild asymmetric dilation.[2,14,23,24,73,85] Mild, unilateral pelvic dilation has been observed with saline diuresis or secondary to increased urine flow when the contralateral kidney was badly diseased or missing. The ureter usually cannot be traced to the bladder in animals undergoing diuresis. Recent work has shown that normal dogs and cats not receiving IV fluids may have renal pelvic dilation with a width up to 3 mm (Figure 16-19; see also Figures 16-5 and 16-18, B to E).[85]

The differential diagnosis for renal pelvic dilation includes congenital disease, pyelonephritis, obstruction to urine flow,

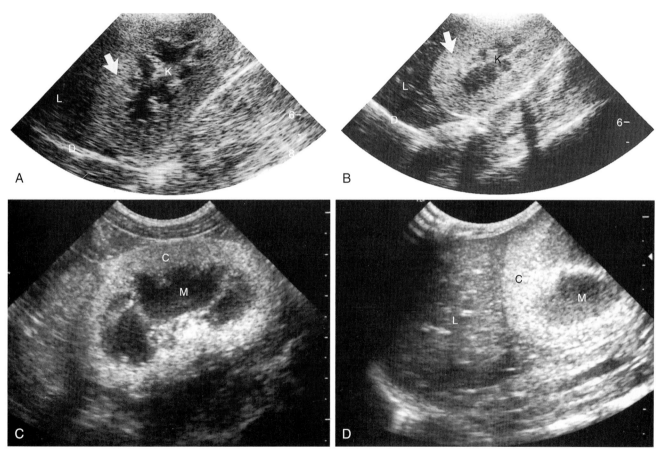

Figure 16-16 **Increased renal cortical echogenicity. A,** Chronic glomerulonephritis. The renal cortex (*arrow*) appears more echogenic than the liver (*L*) in this dog with glomerulonephritis confirmed by biopsy. *D,* Diaphragm; *K,* kidney. **B,** Chronic interstitial nephritis. The renal cortex (*arrow*) is much more echogenic than the liver (*L*) in this dog with interstitial nephritis confirmed by biopsy. *D,* Diaphragm; *K,* kidney. **C,** Chronic nephritis. The renal cortex (*C*) is much more echogenic than expected compared with the echogenicity of the renal medulla (*M*) in this dog with long-standing chronic nephritis. **D,** Chronic nephritis. The renal cortex (*C*) is more echogenic than expected for this cat. Cats normally have more echogenic renal cortices than dogs do, but the echogenicity of the renal cortex in this case is more than expected compared with that of the renal medulla (*M*) and liver (*L*).   *Continued*

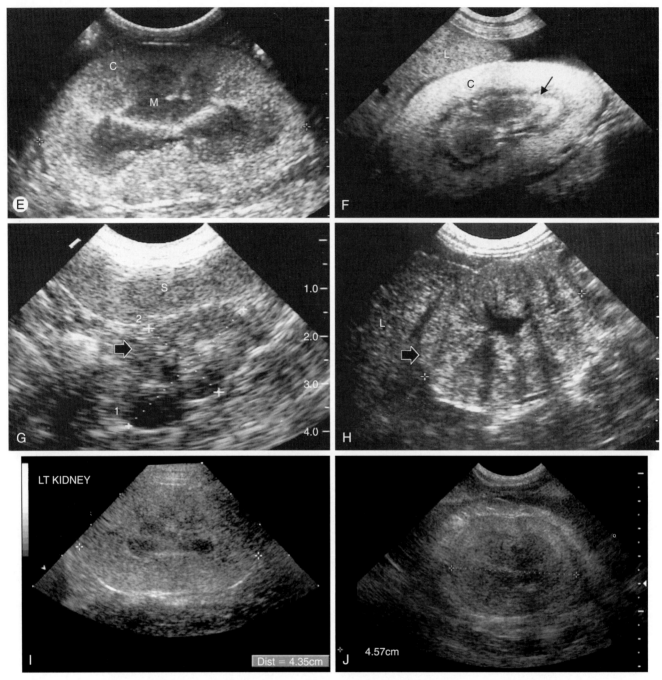

Figure 16-16, cont'd **E,** Lymphosarcoma. This kidney is enlarged and there is increased echogenicity of the renal cortex (*C*) in this cat with renal lymphosarcoma. *M,* Renal medulla. **F,** Ethylene glycol poisoning. Ingestion of ethylene glycol produces highly echogenic kidneys, particularly the renal cortex (*C*). The kidney was much more echogenic than the liver (*L*) or spleen. An echogenic band (*arrow*), termed a medullary rim, is frequently noted in the outer zone of the medulla. The medullary rim sign is a nonspecific finding seen with other diseases and may also be found in animals with no current evidence of disease. **G and H,** Small kidneys from congenital or acquired disease. End-stage or congenital kidney diseases may produce small, irregular, echogenic kidneys (*arrows*) with loss of corticomedullary definition. *L,* Liver; *S,* spleen. Decreased cortical echogenicity. **I,** Left kidney (4.35 cm between electronic cursors) in a cat with feline infectious peritonitis (FIP). There is poor corticomedullary distinction and the cortical tissue appears thicker than expected. This cannot be differentiated from lymphoma and other diffuse diseases of the kidney. **J,** Renal amyloidosis in a cat. The kidney is seen between electronic cursors (4.57 cm) and is surrounded by thick, hyperechoic tissue. There is poor corticomedullary definition and the kidney is barely recognizable.

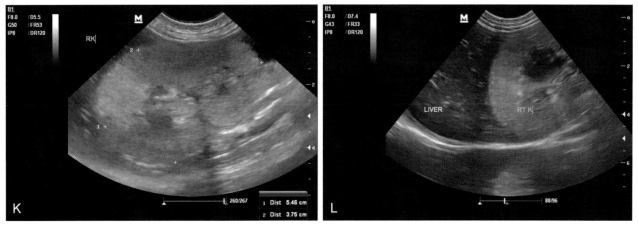

Figure 16-16, cont'd K, Renal amyloidosis in a shar-pei dog. The renal parenchyma is extremely hyperechoic with little distinction between cortical and medullary tissue. The kidney is misshapen and smaller than expected (5.46 x 3.75 cm between electronic cursors). **L,** Extremely hyperechoic right kidney (RT K) adjacent to relatively hypoechoic liver in a shar-pei with renal amyloidosis. (K, L Courtesy of Dr. Robert Williams, Labrador, Queensland, Australia)

and diuresis.[73] If the dilation is more than 3 to 4 mm, diuresis is considered less likely and further investigation is warranted to rule out disease. Dilation of the renal pelvis is recognized by separation of the normal, uniformly hyperechoic central renal sinus echoes by an anechoic space (Figure 16-20, *A* and *B*). This is best recognized in the transverse view, on which an anechoic space can be seen around the renal crest. In cases of minimal pelvic distention, it may be difficult to determine whether this appearance is produced by normal renal vasculature. The correct diagnosis can readily be obtained by following the vessel to the aorta or vena cava or by using Doppler ultrasonography. Otherwise, excretory urography is required. With careful examination of the kidney in the transverse plane, however, the dilated pelvis can usually be seen surrounding the renal crest.

The absence of dilation does not necessarily rule out disease, particularly with pyelonephritis. However, a dilated ureter may be traced medially and caudally for a short distance from the pelvis in either the transverse or sagittal plane. It should be traced as far distally as possible in an attempt to determine whether ureteral dilation involves only the proximal ureter or extends to the bladder. It may be helpful to look for a dilated ureter near the bladder to make this determination. In more advanced stages of pelvic dilation, the diagnosis is readily apparent with ultrasonography, because the dilated pelvic diverticula and proximal ureter are easily visualized.[29,33]

The differential diagnosis of a dilated ureter includes infection, obstruction, ruptured ureter, ureterocele, and ectopic ureter. These conditions will be described later in this chapter. We have also observed ureteral dilation in young animals without any known cause. This may be due to a congenital or idiopathic condition.

In some cases in which conventional ultrasonography, urography, and urethrocystography are unsuccessful in determining the cause of renal pelvic or ureteral dilation, ultrasound-guided nephropyelocentesis may be useful to obtain urine for culture, perform contrast studies, administer therapeutic agents, or provide temporary relief of obstruction.[86-88]

Pyelonephritis
Pyelonephritis may occur unilaterally or bilaterally and usually results from ascending urinary infection. In mild cases there

may be no sonographic abnormalities.[89] However, mild renal enlargement and mild to moderate pelvic and ureteral dilation is usually present (Figures 16-21 and 16-22; see also Figure 16-20, *A* and *B*).[73] This may occur secondary to bacterial endotoxins interfering with ureteral peristalsis. A hyperechoic mucosal margin line has been seen parallel to the wall of the pelvis and proximal ureter in the transverse view with experimentally induced acute pyelonephritis in the dog.[22] An echogenic medullary band may also be seen at the corticomedullary junction.[22,77,90] Focal hyperechoic areas have been noted in the renal medulla as well as patchy, focal hypoechoic or hyperechoic areas in the renal cortex.[22,33] Occasionally, hyperechoic areas with dirty shadowing may be seen in the renal parenchyma if gas-producing organisms are present. This should not be confused with gas in the renal pelvis that may have resulted from vesicoureteral reflux during a recent double-contrast cystogram procedure. Occasionally, pyelonephritis leading to retroperitoneal abscess and regional cellulitis may occur.[91] Successful ultrasound-guided percutaneous drainage and lavage has also been reported in cases of severe pyonephrosis with ureteral obstruction.[88]

In chronic pyelonephritis, dilation and distortion of the collecting system, reduced renal size, increased renal echogenicity, poor corticomedullary definition, and irregular renal contour have been noted. Ureteral dilation is also present in most cases, and if sufficient dilation is present, the ureter may be traced to the bladder or recognized near its insertion into the bladder.

Hydronephrosis
Hydronephrosis is defined as dilation of the renal collecting system secondary to obstruction. Obstruction of the ureter produces a much greater degree of ureteral and pelvic dilation than diuresis or infection.[60,73,92] It is of great diagnostic and prognostic significance to determine whether there is bilateral involvement, whether the collecting system is displaced or distorted, and the distal extent of ureteral dilation. The appearance of the kidney parenchyma and the degree of pelvic dilation vary with the completeness and duration of obstruction. After several months of complete obstruction, only a thin rim of renal tissue remains around the grossly dilated pelvis. Several echogenic linear bands extending from the hilum toward the capsule are characteristically found.

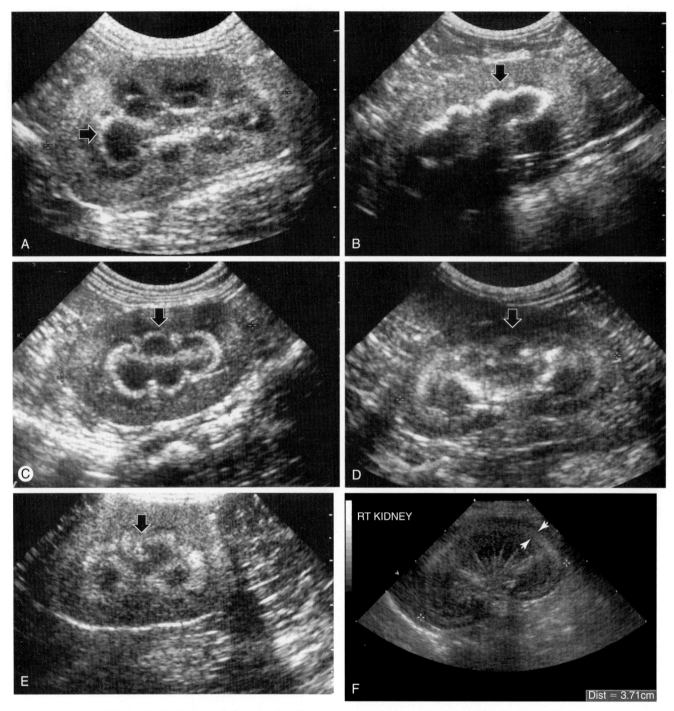

Figure 16-17 Corticomedullary rim sign. The appearance of a hyperechoic band (*black arrows*) that parallels the corticomedullary junction is a nonspecific finding. More specifically, it may be located within the outer zone of the medulla. It has been seen in normal animals (**A**), in animals with hypercalcemic nephropathy (**B**), and in animals with ethylene glycol toxicity. The band appears discrete in some cases (**C**) and ill-defined in other cases (**D** and **E**). **F,** A wide rim of hyperechogenicity is present (*white arrows*) in the outer medulla or cortex of this kidney in a dog with a portosystemic shunt. Also present are radiating linear hyperechoic striations. Though not proven, the hyperechoic structures in this kidney may represent abnormal urate deposition. The urinary bladder also contained echogenic, gravity-dependent sediment.

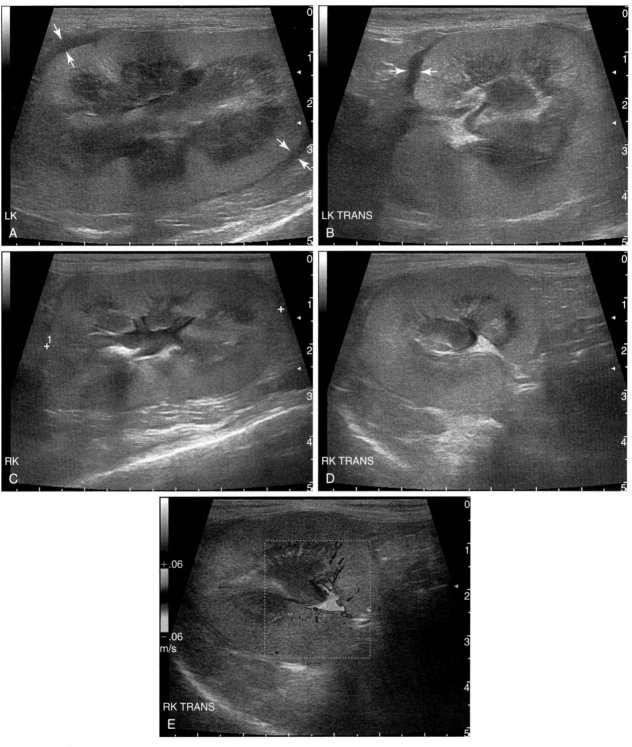

Figure 16-18 **Renal lymphoma in a cat. A,** Sagittal image of the left kidney. The kidney is enlarged, and only part of the organ is visible in this 5-cm field of view. The renal cortex is extremely hyperechoic and fine textured. The medulla is also more echogenic than normal and contains fine hyperechoic strands. There is a lumpy contour to the kidney (best seen in the near-field cortex). A thin hypoechoic to anechoic rim surrounds the poles of the kidney (*arrows*). **B,** Transverse image shows the same hypoechoic to anechoic perinephric rim (*arrows*). The renal pelvis is seen as an anechoic slit of fluid separating the renal pyramid from the Y-shaped renal sinus fat. The perinephric rim likely represents a layer of abnormal lymphocytes, known to occur with renal lymphoma. Sonographically, this cannot be differentiated from perinephric fluid from other disease processes (e.g., ethylene glycol, acute nephritis, feline infectious peritonitis, chronic kidney failure, and many others). Regardless of etiology, a perinephric rim sign indicates renal (or retroperitoneal) pathology. **C,** Sagittal image of the right kidney shows a lumpy contour and a mildly dilated renal pelvis. **D,** Transverse image of the right kidney shows mild renal pelvic dilation. A thin hypoechoic perinephric rim is seen. **E,** Transverse color Doppler image of the right kidney.

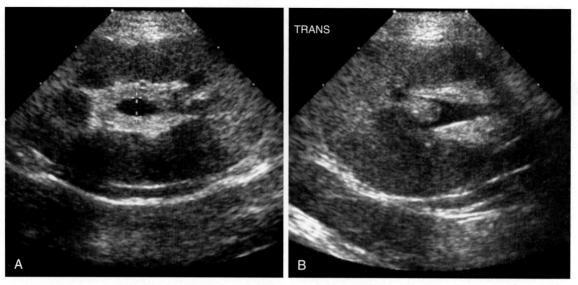

Figure 16-19 **Mild pelvic dilation (pyelectasia) in a cat undergoing fluid therapy. A,** Sagittal image of the right kidney at the level of the renal pelvis (between electronic cursors, 3 mm). The mild dilation of the pelvis is seen surrounded by highly echogenic renal sinus fat. **B,** Transverse image of the same kidney shows mild renal pelvic dilation surrounded by renal sinus fat.

Hydronephrosis may progress to pyonephrosis, caused by urinary stasis and subsequent infection.[93] Pyonephrosis is a collection of sloughed uroepithelium Ultrasonographic features include hyperechoic content of the collecting system, retroperitoneal effusion, and peritoneal effusion. Pyonephrosis should be differentiated from hydronephrosis because of risk of complications from infection.

Whenever hydronephrosis is diagnosed, a search for an accompanying dilated ureter should be undertaken from the kidney region to the bladder. In most cases, a bladder, urethral, or prostatic tumor involving the trigone is responsible for ureteral obstruction.[29,30,92,94-96] Obstruction due to ureteral inflammation, blood clots, fibroepithelial polyps, calculi, extrinsic masses, ureteral fibrosis, or strictures is less common[97-103] (see Figures 16-20, C to I, and 16-25). Ureteral tumors are rare, but leiomyoma, leiomyosarcoma, fibropapilloma, and transitional cell carcinoma have been reported.[104-108] In cats, clinical experience indicates that obstruction of the ureter from a ureteral calculus is more common than other causes.[100,102,109] Hydroureter and ureteral obstruction were associated with infarction of retroperitoneal fat in a mature cat.[110] A urinoma (paraureteral pseudocyst) has also been reported to cause obstruction by extravasation and encapsulation of urine around a ruptured ureter.[111,112] The flow of urine into the bladder can be observed as ureteral jets with gray-scale imaging.[113,114] Color Doppler imaging makes these ureteral jets even easier to see. If complete obstruction is present, ureteral jets will be absent on the affected side. The jets will still be visible if nonobstructive renal pelvic dilation exists. On occasion, symmetric pelvic dilation without ureteral enlargement occurs from pelviureteral junction obstruction due to inflammation, tumor, or congenital conditions. Smaller isoechoic masses or those less than 1 cm and strictures in this region may be difficult to detect, and excretory urography may aid in diagnosis if the obstruction is not complete. Ultrasound-guided antegrade pyelography may also be useful to obtain better visualization of the ureter and confirm obstruction.[87,98,115]

Asymmetric pelvic dilation and distortion of the renal collecting system unilaterally or bilaterally may occur from partial obstruction by a renal mass lesion such as cyst or tumor.

These lesions are usually large and therefore easily detected with ultrasonography. The ureter may be involved but is usually not completely obstructed.

New sonographers may potentially confuse renal cysts with a dilated renal collecting system or even the normal hypoechoic medulla with hydronephrosis (Figure 16-23). With experience, this is not a diagnostic problem because cysts are usually round and eccentrically located, and the bright renal sinus echoes remain. On the other hand, a dilated renal pelvis gradually replaces the normally hyperechoic renal sinus with a central, symmetric anechoic region that extends into the diverticula. Asymmetric pelvic dilation can be differentiated from renal cysts because of the noncircular, sometimes branching shape. A dilated ureter may also be seen. As stated previously, an excretory urogram should always be compared with the ultrasound findings. If renal function is still adequate, a dilated collecting system will opacify, sometimes on a delayed basis, whereas cysts usually do not. Urography is not helpful in long-standing obstruction because of poor renal function.

Congenital or Idiopathic Disorders
The most common congenital condition producing a dilated ureter and renal pelvis is unilateral or bilateral ectopic ureter.[113,114,116,117] The ectopic ureters may be dilated owing to concurrent infection or partial obstruction at the point where they enter the urethra or another location. Ectopic ureters are more common in female dogs. A ureterocele is a congenital dilation of the distal ureter that is sometimes accompanied by an ectopic ureter or obstruction.[30,73,114,118] These conditions are described in more detail later in this chapter.

Little is known about the various other types of congenital or idiopathic conditions causing dilation of the urinary tract. In most cases, the diagnosis of this type of disorder is made by ruling out other causes of pelvic and ureteral dilation, such as diuresis, infection, ectopic ureter, or obstruction.[119] There may be concurrent urinary tract infection, which makes the diagnosis difficult. However, if no cause of the dilation is identified on imaging studies and the results of urine bacterial culture are negative, a congenital or idiopathic condition is suspected.

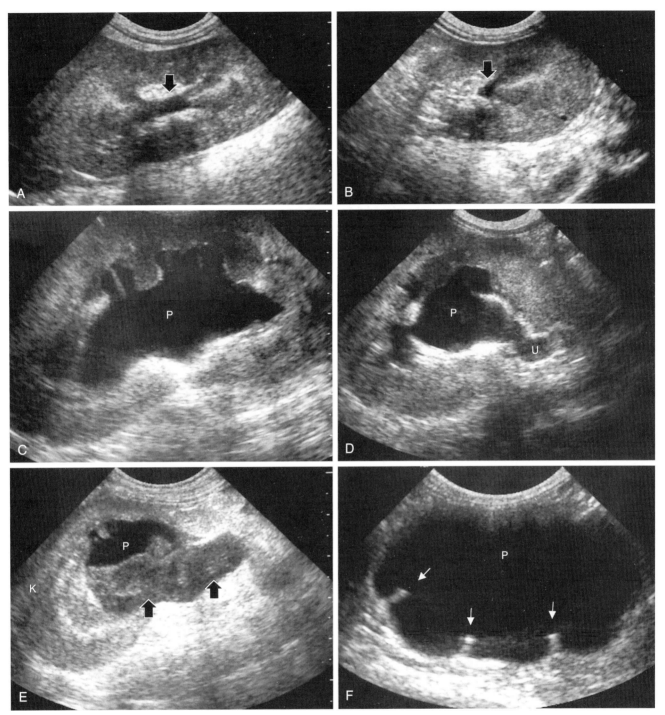

Figure 16-20 **Renal pelvic dilation.** Pyelonephritis, sagittal (A) and transverse (B) views through the kidney. Mild to moderate renal pelvic dilation (*arrows*) is seen with acute pyelonephritis. The amount of dilation is usually not as extensive as that seen with hydronephrosis. C to F, Hydronephrosis, sagittal (C and F) and transverse (D and E) views. C and D, Extensive renal pelvic (*P*) and ureteral dilation (*U*) is evident in this dog with obstruction of the right ureter due to bladder tumor. E, A large blood clot (*arrows*) obstructed the proximal ureter of this dog, resulting in pelvic dilation (*P*). *K*, Kidney. F, Severe hydronephrosis from a ureteral obstruction produced extreme pelvic dilation (P) and atrophy of renal tissue in this dog. Only a thin rim of functional renal tissue remains. Echogenic bands extending toward the hilum (*arrows*) help identify this large, cystic structure as a hydronephrotic kidney. *Continued*

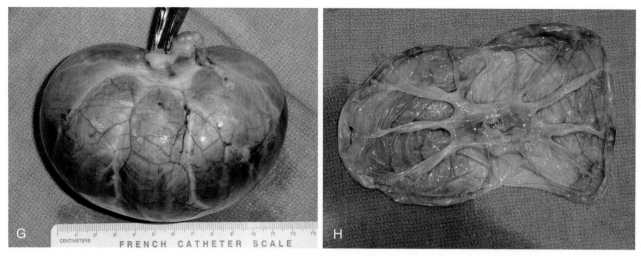

Figure 16-20, cont'd G and **H,** Images of gross specimens showing severe hydronephrosis that corresponds to kidney shown in **F. G,** Intact specimen. **H,** Opened specimen.

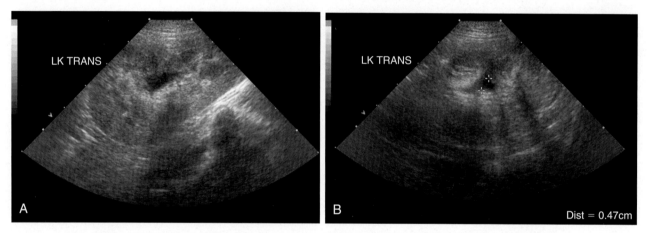

Figure 16-21 **Pyelonephritis in a puppy. A,** Sagittal image of the left kidney shows abnormal hyperechoic cortical and medullary tissue, with lack of distinction between them. The renal tissue is inhomogeneous. An irregular dilated renal pelvis is seen centrally. **B,** Transverse image shows the kidney is barely recognizable. The dilated renal pelvis is surrounded by very echogenic tissue.

Calculi and Blood Clots

Renal or ureteral calculi usually produce intense hyperechoic foci with strong acoustic shadowing on images of the kidney or ureter[29,33,60,73,99,100,102,103,120,121] (Figure 16-24). However, visualization may be obscured by overlying bowel gas. Most calculi are sufficiently radiopaque for their presence to be confirmed on survey radiographs. Therefore radiography is usually done in conjunction with ultrasonography. Although ultrasonography is accurate for urolith identification, survey radiographs provide additional information, including shape and opacity, which help determine mineral composition.[122] However, radiolucent calculi are not detected on survey radiographs but exhibit some degree of shadowing on ultrasonography. Recent work has shown that the absence of acoustic shadowing may not exclude the presence of a nephrolith in dogs and cats. The authors suggest that optimal diagnosis of nephroliths requires paired radiography and sonography.[123] This feature helps differentiate them from blood clots (see Figure 16-20, *E*). For maximal shadowing to be obtained, it is important to use the highest frequency transducer possible, to direct the beam perpendicular to the suspected calculus, and to locate the calculus within the focal zone of the transducer.

Pelvic or ureteral dilation makes visualization of calculi much easier. Smaller calculi or renal parenchymal calcification may be difficult to distinguish from the slight shadowing normally seen from the walls of the renal collecting system. Color Doppler imaging can sometimes help identify questionable calculi if a "twinkling artifact" can be seen[124] (see Chapter 1, Figure 1-78). This is a sort of color artifact, similar to a ringdown artifact that occurs distal to some calculi. Nephroliths may be located in the pelvic recesses or the renal pelvis. Caution should be exercised when evaluating the area of the pelvic recesses in a sagittal or dorsal plane because the arcuate arteries and adjacent fat often cause small specular echoes that resemble calculus in the recess, and either may cause acoustic shadowing. Scanning in a transverse plane, using Doppler interrogation to identify the arcuate arteries is helpful for determining if calculi are actually present in the pelvic recesses.

Gas in the renal pelvis or ureter may also produce hyperechoic foci with shadowing. The gas is usually present in the renal pelvis because of vesicoureteral reflux accompanying double-contrast cystography. However, gas-producing organisms are occasionally responsible. Gas usually causes dirty shadowing because of the presence of multiple reverberation

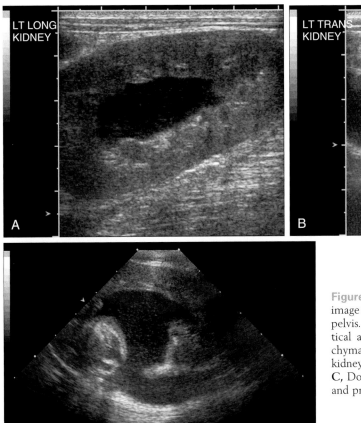

Figure 16-22 Pyelonephritis in a dog. A, Sagittal image shows a moderate dilation of the left renal pelvis. There is no longer distinction between cortical and medullary tissue, and the renal parenchyma is mottled. **B,** Transverse image of the left kidney shows pelvic and proximal ureter dilation. **C,** Dorsal image of the right kidney shows pelvic and proximal ureter dilation.

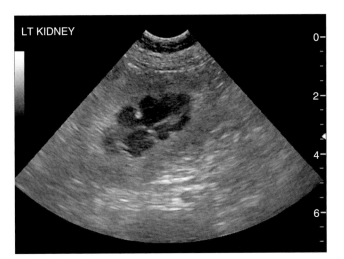

Figure 16-23 Nearly anechoic normal medullary tissue of a sagittal view of the left kidney could be mistaken for hydronephrosis.

artifacts within the shadow, whereas calculi produce "cleaner" shadowing. However, abdominal radiography and excretory urography are recommended for definitive diagnosis in doubtful cases.

Calculi obstructing the ureter may be difficult to detect ultrasonographically because of bowel gas, although a dilated ureter can usually be traced to the point where the dilation ends and an echogenic focus with shadowing is seen. The lack

of shadowing or a mass in this region suggests obstruction by a stricture[121,125] or blood clot,[87] although small calculi may shadow poorly. Retrograde movement of calculi within the ureter or back into the renal pelvis has also been described in dogs and cats, so the position of the calculi should be confirmed immediately before surgery.[103] Abdominal radiographs and an intravenous urogram are recommended in questionable cases or when visualization of the ureteral region is incomplete. Ultrasound-guided antegrade pyelography may also be useful to better visualize the ureter and confirm obstruction in certain cases.[87,115] Figure 16-25 is an example of hydronephrosis secondary to a ureteral calculus.

Ruptured Ureter and Retroperitoneal Disease
Retroperitoneal perinephric or paraureteral accumulations of fluid can occur from trauma, acute renal failure (nephrotoxicity, leptospirosis, ureteral obstruction, interstitial nephritis),[121] urine leakage,[111,112,126] hemorrhage or hematomas,[127,128] perinephric abscesses,[120,129,130] and neoplasia[131-133] (Figure 16-26, D). The ultrasound appearance may not be distinctive so that the history, clinical findings, laboratory work, other imaging procedures, and guided aspiration for fluid analysis may be required for diagnosis.

Urine collections from a ruptured ureter are usually anechoic and may be large if the retroperitoneum remains intact or if the fluid is otherwise encapsulated in a urinoma.[111,112] If the ureter is ruptured by trauma, it is common to see dilation of the proximal ureter and renal pelvis on the same side. However, the actual site of ureteral rupture is difficult to determine with sonography, and usually an excretory urogram is required to make a definitive diagnosis. If a urinoma develops from encapsulation of the extravasated urine, obstruction

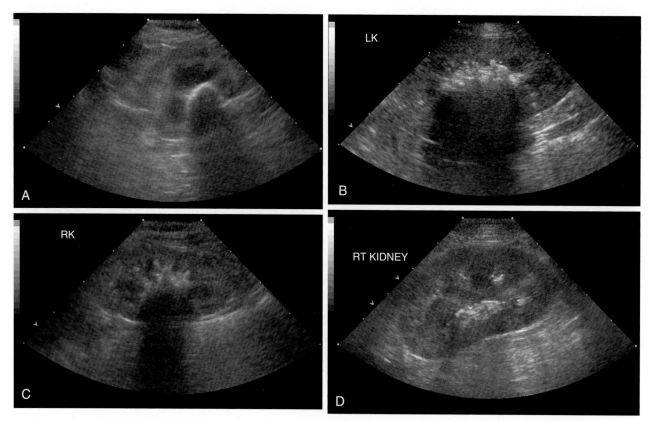

Figure 16-24 **Renal calculi. A,** Single large calculus in the renal pelvis in this dog creates a smooth, hyperechoic interface and casts a strong acoustic shadow. **B,** Multiple calculi in the renal pelvis create an irregular, very hyperechoic surface with acoustic shadowing. This could be mistaken for a single calculus. **C,** Large calculus in the renal pelvis with smaller calculi within the renal diverticula. **D,** Small calculi in the renal pelvis and diverticula are seen as hyperechoic foci but are small enough that they do not create much of an acoustic shadow.

of the ureter and hydronephrosis may result.[111,112] Urine leakage initiates a fibroblastic reaction encapsulating the urine in the retroperitoneal tissues, which may obstruct the ureter.[111]

Sublumbar hemorrhage or hematomas vary in appearance with age and the stage of clot formation; hematomas may have irregular walls and contain clumps of particulate material representing clots. Retroperitoneal hemorrhage may occur from trauma, coagulopathies, renal and adrenal gland tumors, retroperitoneal foreign bodies or tumors, and vascular anomalies.[127,128,131]

Retroperitoneal abscesses are usually complex masses that have thickened, irregular walls; they often present as anechoic to hypoechoic masses, with or without septa and particulate internal debris.[91,130] On occasion, abscesses may appear solid because of the nature of the internal contents. Migrating plant awns are a common cause of sublumbar abscesses in certain regions of the country. Ultrasound-guided aspiration of fluid for cytologic analysis, bacterial culture, and chemical tests are helpful to establish the diagnosis. Excretory urography is indicated if a ruptured ureter is suspected.

Retroperitoneal masses, in addition to those described, may occur secondary to granulomas, neoplasia, or enlarged sublumbar lymph nodes. Neoplasia produces solid or complex patterns, depending on the presence of hemorrhage or necrosis. The location of the mass is important to establish a differential diagnosis. A retroperitoneal mass may cause ureteral obstruction if it incorporates the ureter. Ureteral tumors are rare, but leiomyoma, leiomyosarcoma, fibropapilloma, and transitional cell carcinoma have been reported.[104-108] Sublumbar lymphadenopathy is recognized by the presence of a hypoechoic mass or multiple masses dorsal to the bladder and ventral to the aorta and caudal vena cava. A mass craniomedial to the kidney may arise from the adrenal gland, whereas one caudal to the kidney may arise from peritoneal structures such as an ovary, an ovarian stump, or a retained testicle. Retroperitoneal versus peritoneal origin cannot be determined with certainty in all cases. This explains why a small ovarian mass, which is actually peritoneal, appears to originate retroperitoneally on ultrasonography. The relationship of the mass to a known retroperitoneal or peritoneal structure usually permits the correct diagnosis. Localization may be confirmed with abdominal radiographs, if necessary. Ultrasound-guided aspiration or tissue-core biopsies may be indicated to help establish the diagnosis and determine a prognosis for treatment.

Subcapsular Fluid or Thickening and Perirenal Fluid

Subcapsular or perirenal fluid may occur from urine, blood, transudates, or exudates. With smaller amounts of fluid, it may be difficult to determine if the fluid is subcapsular or perirenal and therefore they are considered together here. Subcapsular or perirenal fluid may result from urine leakage,[121] hemorrhage,[128] abscess,[71,91,117,120,129,130,134] acute renal failure,[121] ureteral obstruction,[121] toxicity[76,121] (e.g., ethylene glycol), leptospirosis,[77,121] transplant rejection,[135] or renal neoplasia (Figure 16-26, *A*). The amount of fluid is usually much less than that seen with perinephric pseudocysts or conditions

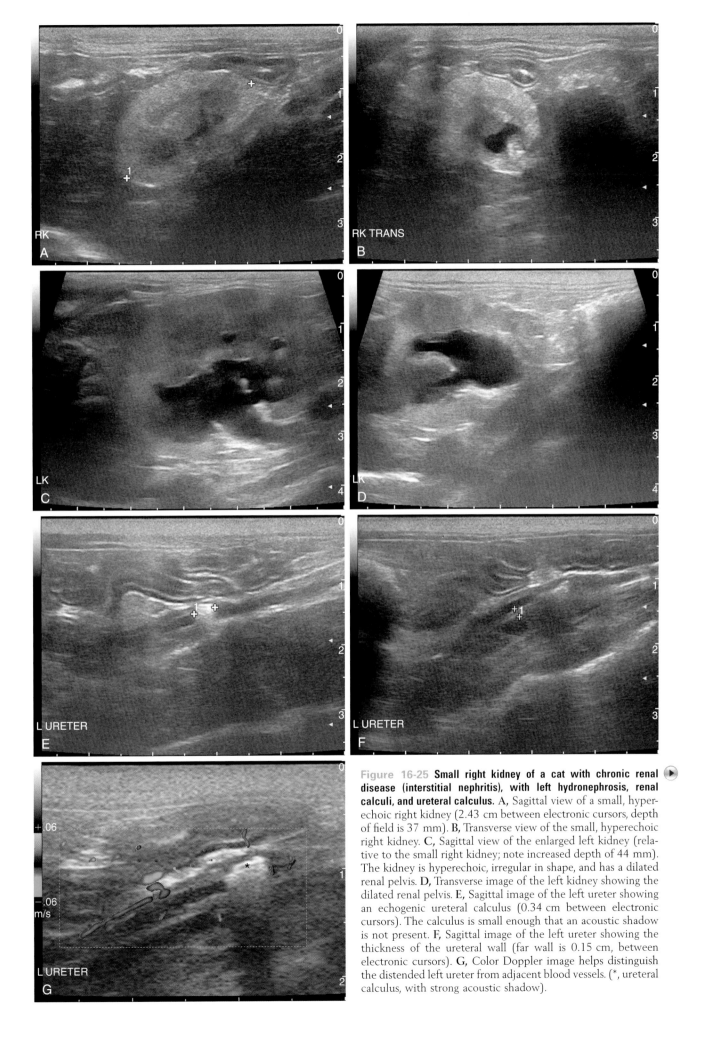

Figure 16-25 Small right kidney of a cat with chronic renal disease (interstitial nephritis), with left hydronephrosis, renal calculi, and ureteral calculus. A, Sagittal view of a small, hyperechoic right kidney (2.43 cm between electronic cursors, depth of field is 37 mm). B, Transverse view of the small, hyperechoic right kidney. C, Sagittal view of the enlarged left kidney (relative to the small right kidney; note increased depth of 44 mm). The kidney is hyperechoic, irregular in shape, and has a dilated renal pelvis. D, Transverse image of the left kidney showing the dilated renal pelvis. E, Sagittal image of the left ureter showing an echogenic ureteral calculus (0.34 cm between electronic cursors). The calculus is small enough that an acoustic shadow is not present. F, Sagittal image of the left ureter showing the thickness of the ureteral wall (far wall is 0.15 cm, between electronic cursors). G, Color Doppler image helps distinguish the distended left ureter from adjacent blood vessels. (*, ureteral calculus, with strong acoustic shadow).

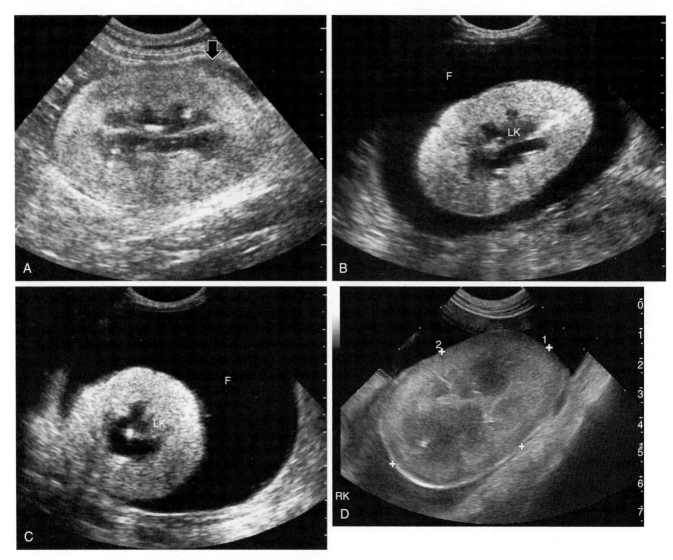

Figure 16-26 Perirenal fluid and perinephric pseudocysts. A, Perirenal fluid. A small amount of perirenal fluid or collection of lymphocytes (*arrow*) can be identified in this cat with lymphosarcoma. **B** and **C,** Perinephric pseudocyst, sagittal (**B**) and transverse (**C**) views through the left kidney. A large amount of anechoic fluid (*F*) surrounds the kidney (*LK*) in this cat with a perinephric pseudocyst. **D,** Retroperitoneal fluid.

causing generalized retroperitoneal fluid accumulation. Hypoechoic subcapsular thickening mimicking subcapsular fluid has also been described in cats with renal lymphosarcoma.[136] Blood flow was identified with color Doppler analysis in the subcapsular region in these cats, indicating that the sonographic appearance was not due to fluid. Subcapsular thickening was primarily seen in cats with renal lymphosarcoma, but also seen in cats with undifferentiated malignant neoplasia, renal anaplastic carcinoma, chronic active nephritis, and feline infectious peritonitis.[136] It is possible that some of the previous reports of subcapsular fluid with these conditions actually represented hypoechoic subcapsular thickening. Renal parenchymal, perirenal, and other abdominal abnormalities may suggest the origin of the subcapsular fluid or thickening and perirenal fluid. Aspiration to obtain samples for cytologic and fluid analysis and bacterial culture is easily accomplished with ultrasound guidance. Hypoechoic subcapsular fluid and capsular thickening secondary to renal abscessation were indentified in a cat with pyelonephritis. Excretory urography and histopathologic evaluation confirmed leakage of suppurative fluid from the renal parenchyma into the subcapsular space.[134]

Perinephric Pseudocysts
Accumulation of large amounts of fluid around one or both kidneys in a subcapsular or extracapsular location has been observed in cats and one dog[137-142] (see Figure 16-26, *B* and C). These cysts are termed pseudocysts because they are not lined by epithelium. Nearly all pseudocysts are subcapsular with the fluid accumulating between the kidney and capsule.[142] However, two extracapsular pseudocysts have been reported.[137,143] The cysts are usually palpated in the kidney region during a physical examination in cats. The entire kidney is usually found to be completely surrounded by a large amount of encapsulated, anechoic fluid on the ultrasound examination. However, fluid did not surround the entire kidney in the one dog[138] or in all the cats.[137] Analysis of aspirated fluid is usually consistent with a transudate. The cause of feline perinephric pseudocysts is unknown. They have been associated with renal diseases of various types including

interstitial nephritis, hydronephrosis, polycystic renal disease, and neoplasia.[142] Treatment requires surgical removal of pseudocysts because percutaneous drainage has met with limited success.[142] Fluid usually re-forms over time if the pseudocysts are drained percutaneously. Surgery is preferred so that the wall of the cyst can be removed and biopsy of the kidney performed. An omentalization procedure has also been used to facilitate drainage after pseudocyst removal.[140]

Doppler Evaluation of the Kidneys

Doppler ultrasound equipment has become affordable and therefore more widely available to veterinary practices. Potential uses of Doppler ultrasonography for evaluation of the kidney in animals have emerged from human studies. The technique has been used in humans to provide additional functional information in patients with acute renal failure, urinary tract obstruction, renal artery or vein thrombosis, renal infarcts, renal transplants, and renal neoplasia. Reduced renal artery diastolic flow indicates a generalized increase in renal vascular resistance. This finding is nonspecific and has been associated with a variety of disorders, including acute renal disease, acute tubular necrosis, and renal obstruction. Renal vascular resistance is determined by calculating a unitless resistive index (RI) with use of Doppler ultrasonography. Signals from the arteries near the renal hilum (segmental or interlobar) and corticomedullary junction (arcuate) are evaluated. The RI is calculated by subtracting the end-diastolic frequency shift (or end-diastolic velocity) from the peak systolic frequency shift (or peak systolic velocity) and dividing the result by the peak systolic frequency shift (or peak systolic velocity) (Figure 16-27). Because the Doppler angle to these small vessels cannot be measured, the frequency shift is typically used to provide a relative assessment of blood flow in systole and diastole. However, if the angle to the vessel can be measured then velocity measurements can be used. An RI of less than 0.70 is considered normal in the dog and cat. Increased vascular resistance reduces diastolic flow in greater proportion to systolic flow, thereby increasing RI.

Normal Doppler velocimetry values were reported in a study of 50 clinically normal Persian cats.[144] The renal and intralobar arteries were successfully interrogated, obtaining adequate waveform for analysis; however the arcuate arteries could not be successfully mapped because of their small size and respiratory motion. Mean RI for the renal arteries was 0.54 ± 0.07 and the mean RI for the interlobar arteries was 0.52 ± 0.06 cm/s. Because decreased renal blood flow may occur before RI is affected, its documentation may be helpful in early identification of renal disease. Therefore the authors reported peak systolic velocities in the same Persian cats. Mean peak systolic velocities for the renal and interlobar arteries were 41.17 ± 9.40 cm/sec and 32.16 ± 9.33 cm/sec, respectively.

Sedation will affect the RI determination. A decreased RI was observed in dogs sedated with a combination of atropine, acepromazine maleate, diazepam, and ketamine hydrochloride in comparison with unsedated dogs.[145] The authors suggested that these lower values were presumably due to the positive chronotropic effect of ketamine hydrochloride. In contrast, the RI was significantly increased in dogs sedated with midazolam and butorphanol administered intramuscularly compared to unsedated dogs.[146] The authors noted a significant decrease in blood pressure and diastolic velocity compared to unsedated dogs. An RI less than 0.79 was considered normal in these sedated dogs.

Renal Vein Occlusion or Thrombosis

In humans, renal vein occlusion occurs with trauma, dehydration, coagulopathies, nephropathies, and vena cava thrombosis.[89] The cause of renal vein occlusion in animals is likely similar. The sonographic findings in humans or animals are variable, depending on the duration and completeness of the occlusion. A clot of low or high echogenicity may be visible within the renal vein that sometimes extends to the vena cava and forward to the heart. Enlarged kidneys with increased or decreased cortical echogenicity are noted acutely, probably from hemorrhage and edema, and there may be a collection of perinephric fluid.[147] Later, anechoic areas within the cortex may be seen because of infarction. Increased cortical echogenicity from cellular infiltrate may follow after 10 days, but corticomedullary distinctness is usually maintained. If venous collaterals develop, the appearance gradually returns to normal. Otherwise, parenchymal echogenicity continues to increase with loss of corticomedullary definition and decreased kidney size. Figure 16-28 has video clips of a large renal vein thrombus.

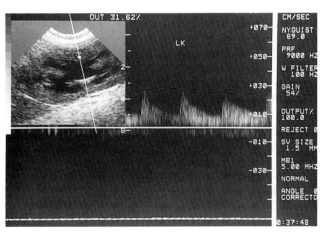

Figure 16-27 **Doppler evaluation of the kidney.** Unilateral ureteral obstruction. This dog's symptoms included sudden onset of pain in the flank region and reluctance to move. Unilateral left renal pelvic dilation and proximal ureteral dilation were found on ultrasonography. However, there was no evidence of obstructing lesions in the visible portion of the left ureter or in the bladder. Pulse wave Doppler evaluation of the left kidney revealed an elevated resistive index of 0.75 compared with a normal 0.65 in the right kidney. Tentative diagnosis of ureteral obstruction was later confirmed on survey radiographs and an intravenous urogram when a calculus was found in the distal left ureter.

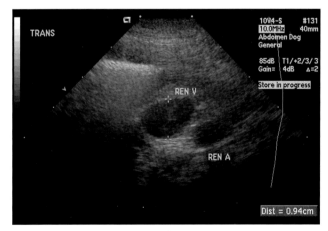

Figure 16-28 **Renal vein thrombus in a dog.** Transverse image of the renal vein (REN V) and artery REN A). The renal vein (0.94 cm between electronic cursors) contains a large thrombus.

On Doppler ultrasonography, renal vein thrombosis is characterized by reduced or absent venous flow and decreased arterial inflow. There is often a characteristic Doppler arterial pattern consisting of a narrow systolic peak and a sharp reversal of diastolic flow, often with a biphasic reversed M pattern.[148,149] However, collateral venous pathways are established rapidly in humans, so this Doppler pattern may not be so characteristic or may be nearly normal. It is not known whether this finding is similar in animals.

Renal Artery Occlusion and Infarcts

Thrombosis of the renal artery in humans has been described as a narrowed arterial lumen containing low-intensity echoes.[150] These sonographic findings were best visualized in a transverse plane parallel to the renal artery. Subsequent kidney infarction may be focal or diffuse and characterized by scattered areas of parenchymal hypoechogenicity or hyperechogenicity similar to renal vein thrombosis. Later, scarring with an irregular renal contour may be evident. If duplex Doppler ultrasonography is available, signals from the renal artery and the interlobar and arcuate artery regions can be compared with those of the contralateral kidney, if that kidney is normal. These principles may be useful in cats that have thrombosis of the renal arteries secondary to cardiomyopathy.

The sonographic findings of experimental acute renal artery occlusion in autologously transplanted kidneys in dogs have been described.[68] In segmental occlusion, a focal hypoechoic renal mass was identified at 24 hours and remained unchanged for 5 to 7 days. There was an increase in echogenicity of the mass after 7 days and a gradual progression to a depressed, echogenic focus by day 17. The investigators found that acute, total renal artery occlusion caused only a slight increase in kidney size and minimal parenchymal changes during a 100-day period. The results of this study may not reflect findings in dogs with an intact collateral blood supply.

Acute renal infarcts have a variable appearance, depending on the size, number, and duration. There may be focal or multifocal areas of hypoechogenicity or hyperechogenicity due to hemorrhage and edema.[151] They may show reduced or absent flow in an arterial segment or low systolic and low diastolic flow in a few vessels. However, it has been noted that a normal finding on Doppler study does not exclude the diagnosis.[151]

As mentioned previously, older infarcts may have a wedge-shaped, hyperechoic appearance, with a broader base at the surface of the kidney that narrows toward the corticomedullary junction.[74] There is often a corresponding defect in the renal contour and thinning of the cortex at this location. Theoretically an infarct can be differentiated from scarring due to pyelonephritis by the lack of pelvic and diverticular abnormalities. However, survey radiographs and excretory urography are required for a definitive diagnosis.

Acute Renal Failure

In certain types of acute renal failure in children, it has been shown that there may be an absence of renal blood flow in late diastole or throughout the diastolic phase.[152] This may result from increased resistance to blood flow caused by swelling or enlargement of the interstitium. These observations had significant diagnostic and prognostic value because surviving children had less depression of diastolic flow and their flow gradually returned to normal with recovery. A similar technique has proved useful in animals as a noninvasive means of assessing severity and potential for recovery in acute renal disease.[153] Serial evaluation may be especially helpful if the Doppler findings predate renal function changes.

Acute tubular necrosis is a specific type of acute renal failure that is usually considered separately from other causes of acute renal failure. There is reduced renal artery diastolic flow and elevation of the RI in severe cases of acute tubular necrosis.[154,155] Doppler evaluation is most helpful to distinguish acute tubular necrosis from prerenal failure. In some cases of acute tubular necrosis, such as that produced by aminoglycoside toxicity in dogs, the RI may not be elevated.[156]

Obstructive versus Nonobstructive Pelvic Dilation

Dilation of the renal pelvis in the dog and cat may occur with infection, congenital conditions, or obstruction. In humans it was initially reported that obstruction causes a rise in renal vascular resistance that disappears with release of the obstruction.[157] An RI exceeding 0.70 was measured in obstructed kidneys, whereas the RI in all nonobstructed kidneys was less than this value. In addition, a comparison of the RI between kidneys was found to increase sensitivity of detecting unilateral obstruction. A difference of 0.1 in RI between the two sides was significant and assisted with diagnosis. However, in subsequent human studies, the use of RI to diagnose obstruction has proven less reliable and is now considered somewhat controversial.[89]

RI determinations may still have application in small animals if used early in acute obstruction (see Figure 16-27). Elevated RI has been reported in the first 24 hours of acute unilateral obstruction in dogs, but high false-positive and false-negative rates limited Doppler RI assessment thereafter.[158,159] The conclusion in another study was that RI was not significantly elevated (RI > 0.70) until 3 to 4 hours after obstruction. An RI difference greater than 0.15 between kidneys was found at 3, 4, and 5 hours in 83%, 100%, and 100% of the dogs studied.[160] In a subsequent investigation, RI was reportedly elevated in the obstructed kidney for 5 days following unilateral obstruction.[161] In this study, an RI of 0.73 was used as an upper limit of normal,[155] and a 76% true-positive and 26% false-negative rate for obstruction was obtained. The false-negative rate was decreased to 12% by comparing the RI difference between the obstructed and nonobstructed kidneys in the same dog, with a difference greater than 0.1 indicating obstruction. Therefore finding an elevated RI and an RI difference of more than 0.1 between kidneys may help detect acute unilateral obstruction in dogs.

In humans, diuretics have been used to increase the RI difference between normal and obstructed kidneys to increase the sensitivity of detecting unilateral obstruction.[162] In dogs, an infusion of furosemide and normal saline was found to increase the RI in the obstructed kidney and decrease the RI of the nonobstructed kidney with experimentally created unilateral, partial ureteral obstruction.[163,164] Recently, the use of a mannitol infusion (0.5 g/kg administered as a 20% solution over 10 minutes) was also described as an aid for detecting unilateral renal obstruction in dogs.[161] It was determined that the mannitol administration did not affect the RI values of normal dogs. However, after unilateral obstruction, the mean RI difference between obstructed and nonobstructed kidneys increased significantly at 30 minutes after mannitol infusion. The difference was primarily attributed to a decrease in RI of the unobstructed kidney. Thus the administration of diuretics may help confirm acute unilateral renal obstruction by increasing the RI difference between kidneys.

Renal Masses

The vascularity of renal masses can be assessed with Doppler ultrasonography for evidence of signals that suggest a tumor. Increased diastolic flow suggests neovascularity and the possibility of a tumor. In humans, an RI value below 0.4 has been reported to suggest malignancy in adnexal masses.[165] However, this value was proven unreliable in subsequent studies.[166,167] The RI of benign and malignant small renal masses was also not significantly different and therefore considered unreliable for diagnostic purposes.[168]

In humans, kidney "tumor signals" have been described as those arising from the margins of masses with Doppler-shifted frequencies exceeding those of the ipsilateral main renal artery (higher than 2.5 kHz at 3.0-MHz insonating frequency). In one study, tumor signals were obtained in 77% (20 of 26 cases) of malignant renal tumors, whereas no signals were obtained in 23 benign masses and one case of lymphoma.[169] Renal carcinomas exhibited tumor signals 83% of the time (15 of 18 cases), Wilms tumors 75% of the time (3 of 4 cases), and metastases 100% of the time (2 of 2 cases) in these 20 cases. This technique may also prove useful in selected small animal cases to help differentiate benign from malignant renal masses.

In humans, power Doppler imaging and contrast-enhanced color Doppler imaging using microbubble contrast agents has improved the detection and characterization of small renal tumors.[168,170] Quantitative gray-scale contrast enhancement of the spleen and kidney was studied in normal dogs. Renal perfusion could be evaluated 3.5 minutes after injection of a microbubble contrast agent and it persisted for 6 minutes before returning to baseline. The authors concluded that this technique may prove useful for identifying renal parenchymal lesions not otherwise visualized with unenhanced gray-scale imaging. These techniques can also be used with animals when the ultrasound equipment and contrast agents become more affordable to veterinarians.

Other Potential Uses of Renal Resistive Index

An elevated renal RI was noted in a dog with Addison disease.[171] It was postulated that renal vasoconstriction from increased activity of the renin-angiotensin system may be responsible for the abnormal blood flow observed. The authors suggest that this technique may be a quick, noninvasive method of managing certain cases Addison disease. However, there have been no additional reports verifying these findings or describing the potential usefulness of this procedure.

Renal Transplants

Renal transplants in cats are becoming increasingly more common at veterinary institutions across the country. Ultrasound is primarily used to evaluate renal size and to detect hydronephrosis or perinephric fluid collections.

Ideally, the potential allograft should be scanned and an intravenous pyelogram performed before removal from the donor to detect any abnormalities. This should be followed by a baseline scan within 24 to 48 hours after the transplantation surgery. The size, shape, echo characteristics, and cross-sectional area or volume of the kidney should be determined. Renal cross-sectional area measurements are obtained from a transverse image of the kidney at the level of the renal pelvis. A sufficiently accurate estimate of renal volume (V) can be made by using the prolate ellipsoid method (V = length × height × width × 0.523).

Feline renal autografts and allografts have been studied to better understand what should be expected with renal transplants. Autografts are kidneys transplanted into the same animal; allografts are kidneys received from another animal. Autografts eliminate the possibility of rejection, and the effects of the transplantation procedure itself can be evaluated. In two studies of renal autografts, the mean increase in kidney cross-sectional area was reported to be 63%[16] and 81%[172] of preoperative values one day following surgery. Also, a mean increase of 30% in cross-sectional area between preoperative values and a 2-week postoperative period following

transplantation was found in a study of feline allografts with immunosuppressive therapy (cyclosporine and prednisolone).[173] Immunosuppressive therapy may affect the magnitude of allograft enlargement in the postoperative period. The variability of results in these studies could reflect a combination of factors, such as use of autografts versus allografts, transplant procedures, kidney ischemia time, fluid therapy, immunosuppressive therapy, or other medications.[16,172,173] A standard protocol would be required to more accurately assess the expected postoperative changes in renal transplant size. However, initial enlargement of the graft is a consistent finding.[16,172,173] Graft enlargement in the immediate postoperative period likely results from transient ischemia, acute tubular necrosis, interstitial edema, or other changes associated with the transplant procedure.[16,172,173] Acute tubular necrosis in the early posttransplant period is the result of ischemia before revascularization. Compensatory hypertrophy or redistribution of blood flow may also play a role in renal enlargement if the transplanted kidney is essentially the sole functioning kidney. If the kidney fails to enlarge, this may indicate an impaired vascular supply. Kidney size may decline slightly as the initial acute effects of the transplantation procedure resolve.[16] After 7 to 10 days, graft size should remain relatively constant.[173] The initial appearance of a renal transplant without complications should be similar to a untransplanted kidney, except that the transplanted kidney is larger. However, the renal pelvis may be slightly dilated and a small amount of perinephric fluid is possible. A transient increase in medullary echogenicity that disappears in 7 to 10 days has also been reported.[173]

After 1 week, any increase in renal size that occurs over a short period of time warrants further investigation to rule out rejection. In an experimental allograft study where immunosuppressive therapy was discontinued, the cross-sectional area of the rejecting allograft increased by at least 10% and averaged 34% at 7 days following the cessation of immunosuppression. However, it should be remembered that increased graft size is not specific for rejection. In humans, other conditions such as acute tubular necrosis, cyclosporine nephrotoxicity, ureteral obstruction, or infection have also been reported to cause acute graft dysfunction.[174-178] Unfortunately, sonography cannot be used to reliably distinguish these various conditions. A renal biopsy is often required for definitive diagnosis. In a recent retrospective study of feline allografts, significantly greater graft volume was seen with ureteral obstruction and rejection compared to clinically normal transplants.[179] Cross-sectional area was also significantly greater in grafts with obstruction and rejection than those with delayed graft function. Delayed graft function was defined as a serum creatinine level higher than 3 mg/dL at 3 days after transplantation with no potential causes (cyclosporine toxicity, uroabdomen, ureteral obstruction, or vascular thrombosis). In humans, a rapid increase in serum creatinine of 25% or greater in the period of 1 to 3 weeks following transplantation suggests acute rejection.[176,180-182]

As mentioned previously, acute renal failure in renal transplants may occur secondary to acute tubular necrosis, acute rejection, cyclosporine nephrotoxicity, or vascular thrombosis. In dogs, acute tubular necrosis was reported to cause little change in kidney echogenicity.[183] Acute rejection may lead to increased renal size, reduced echogenicity, and reduced corticomedullary definition.[184] Cellular infiltration may decrease or increase cortical echogenicity, but increased echogenicity is more common in the later stages of rejection. Infarction and necrosis may produce focal hypoechoic areas in severe cases. In chronic rejection, the kidney is enlarged, with poor definition between the cortex, medulla, and renal sinus because of an overall increase in echogenicity. Later, with end-stage renal disease, the kidney will have a small, highly echogenic, irregular contour.

Cyclosporine nephrotoxity induces acute renal vasoconstriction and interstitial fibrosis in chronic cases. Cyclosporine nephrotoxity may be diagnosed by a renal biopsy or by response to altered drug levels.[175,176]

In total renal artery thrombosis, the gross anatomy may remain unaltered initially, but color Doppler studies reflect reduced or absent flow throughout the kidney.[68] If complete renal artery thrombosis occurs in the postoperative period, normal posttransplant renal enlargement will not occur. Focal areas of decreased perfusion may be seen if branches of the renal artery are occluded. In humans, power Doppler ultrasonography has been recommended for assessing cortical perfusion because of its sensitivity to low-velocity flow. The normal transplant should have visible flow extending all the way to the renal cortex.[185,186]

Renal vein thrombosis may cause edema and kidney enlargement. The main renal vein is usually enlarged and a thrombus may be visible within its lumen. On color Doppler examination with complete venous obstruction, no flow can be detected within the renal vein and there may be reversal of diastolic flow in the renal artery.[187-190]

In humans, perinephric fluid collections consisting of hematomas, lymphoceles, urinomas, or abscesses are seen occasionally with renal transplants and must be differentiated by clinical signs, ultrasonographic appearance, and fine-needle aspiration.[191,192] Hematomas, abscesses, and urinomas tend to occur early in the postsurgical period, whereas lymphoceles are usually discovered as an incidental finding 2 weeks to 6 months after transplantation. Urine leakage may also occur in the early postoperative period, most commonly at the site of ureterovesical anastomosis.

Ureteral obstruction may complicate transplantation. Renal pelvic dilation is recognized by a progressive increase in separation of the renal sinus echoes on serial examinations. If there is a question whether renal pelvic dilation represents obstruction, a furosemide challenge test may be helpful, as previously described. In obstruction, the degree of pelvic dilation increases with furosemide-induced diuresis but remains unchanged if there is no obstruction.

Doppler RI determinations were originally considered to have high potential for evaluating human renal transplants and detecting rejection. However, subsequent clinical and laboratory studies have been less encouraging. There is still disagreement about the value of RI measurements for diagnosis of rejection, but most clinicians consider them too nonspecific unless severe rejection is present. The kidney becomes edematous and swollen in acute rejection, but RI elevation is usually not observed until the later, more severe stages of acute rejection. Therefore RI determinations are not considered useful for detection of mild to moderate rejection, and a renal biopsy remains a necessity.[154,193-195]

A number studies have also reported the Doppler findings with renal transplants in dogs and cats.[16,154,172,173,179,196,197] In a preliminary study in dogs, an elevated RI was reported immediately after surgery in the normal group and those with acute tubular necrosis, but it returned to baseline within 10 days.[154] No changes in RI occurred with cyclosporine nephrotoxicity. The RI was also decreased in the early acute rejection stage but rapidly increased as rejection progressed.

In two studies of feline autografts, no significant change in mean RI from presurgical values was noted during the posttransplant period.[16,172] A study of feline allografts also found no significant changes in mean RI during the 2 weeks following renal transplantation. Also, the RI values did not significantly change in this study after immunosuppression was discontinued and the kidneys underwent acute rejection. In a

retrospective study of feline allografts, RI was only increased with graft thrombosis or possibly cyclosporine toxicity, but was not useful for differentiating delayed graft function, ureteral obstruction, uroabdomen, or acute rejection.[179] Therefore RI does not appear to be a sensitive indicator of acute allograft rejection in cats.

Renal biopsy is currently considered the gold standard for determining allograft rejection, and no single biochemical or imaging study is able to differentiate rejection from acute tubular necrosis, cyclosporine nephrotoxity, pyelonephritis, or vessel thrombosis. Consequently a combination of biochemical tests, ultrasonography, scintigraphy, and renal biopsy may be needed to accurately determine the status of allografts. In an individual animal, it would be very difficult to rely on the ultrasound findings alone for management decisions. However, serial ultrasound examinations may indicate the need for further workup and a renal biopsy.

DISTAL URETERS, URINARY BLADDER, AND URETHRA

The bladder is readily examined when it is distended with urine (see Chapter 4, Figure 4-28) and can serve as a useful acoustic window for visualizing adjacent structures, such as the colon, uterus, and iliac lymph nodes. Bladder wall thickness, mass lesions, foreign bodies, calculi, blood clots, diverticula, ectopic ureters, and ureteroceles are easily evaluated.[92,116,198] An attempt should always be made to visualize the distal ureters while evaluating the bladder.[113,117,198] Although the distal ureters are not seen in the normal animal, a small convex protuberance (ureteral papilla, or tubercle) can often be seen in the dorsal bladder wall near the cranial aspect of the trigone where the intramural portion of the ureter enters the bladder[199] (Figure 16-29, A). Echogenic ureteral jets are occasionally seen swirling within the bladder lumen because of ureteral peristalsis (see Figure 16-29, B).[113,114] In cases of incontinence, ectopic ureters may sometimes be diagnosed by lack of a ureteral jet or the ability to trace a dilated ureter distally to the urethra.[113,116,117] A dilated ureter may also be seen if there is urinary tract infection or ureteral obstruction.[92,198] Examination of the proximal urethra in the male or female is helpful for detecting tumors or calculi. The distal urethra in the male can also be evaluated, but urethrography should be performed first to localize the area to be evaluated.

As with other regions of the body, full assessment of the distal ureters, bladder, or urethra requires that ultrasonography be used in combination with appropriate radiographic procedures. In many cases, radiographic studies are the only ones needed to define the location and extent of disease. Ultrasonography is sometimes done before radiography because it is quicker, it can be used to evaluate other parts of the abdomen as well as the urinary tract, and it aids selection of the most appropriate radiographic contrast procedure. However, when ultrasonography follows radiographic studies, it is also valuable to answer any specific questions raised by study results.

Examination Technique
A 7.5- or 10-MHz transducer is usually suitable for examination of the lower urinary tract. On occasion, a 5-MHz transducer may be required to evaluate adjacent structures in large dogs. A standoff pad may assist with visualization of the ventral bladder wall by reducing reverberation artifacts and positioning this portion of the bladder within the focal zone of the transducer. A low dose of injectable diuretic or bladder catheterization with the addition of sterile saline may be used

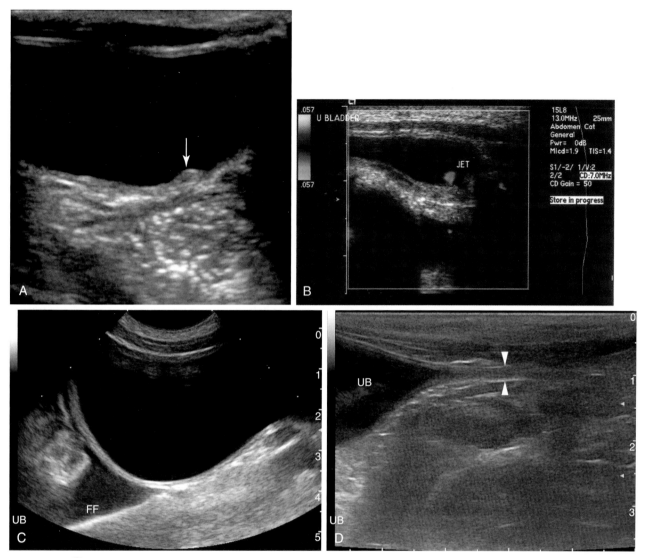

Figure 16-29 **Ureteral papilla and ureteral jet.** A, Sagittal image of the urinary bladder shows a small protuberance (*arrow*) representing the one of the two ureteral papillae. B, Sagittal color Doppler image shows a ureteral jet caused by emptying of the ureter. C, Visualization of the normal layered appearance of the urinary bladder wall is enhanced by the presence of peritoneal fluid (*FF*). D, High resolution image of the neck of a cat urinary bladder (*UB*) as it transitions into the urethra (*arrowheads*).

to distend the bladder if an insufficient amount of urine is present. However, a baseline examination should be done first.

The bladder should be scanned in two planes from the ventral abdomen (Figure 16-30; see also Chapter 4, Figures 4-27 and 4-28). If wall thickening or mass lesions are suspected, the transducer should be oriented so that the sound beam passes through the wall perpendicular to the region of interest to obtain accurate measurements. This may require placement of the transducer on the lateral aspect of the caudal abdomen. Side lobe artifacts are often identified when evaluating the urinary bladder (Figure 16-31). This type of artifact is not simply a benign annoyance; they may lead to a misdiagnosis of urinary sediment or bladder wall thickening. Side lobe artifacts are minimized by keeping the gain low; altering the transducer frequency, the focal zone, or both; and using harmonic imaging. Slice thickness or reverberation artifacts can also simulate intraluminal or mural abnormalities. Slice

thickness artifacts result from placing the beam near the bladder's edge. The beam's width causes echoes that have originated outside the lumen to appear within the bladder. Reverberation echoes from the transducer, skin, or adjacent gas-filled bowel may also cause confusing echogenicities within the bladder. These artifacts can usually be eliminated, or at least recognized, by changing the transducer's position and imaging the bladder in multiple planes.

A variable portion of urethra can be imaged from the ventral abdomen in males and females (see Chapter 4, Figure 4-28, C). However, in the male, the portion caudal to the prostate is not usually seen because of the overlying pubis or ischium. On occasion, the urethra can be visualized in its long axis from the perineal region or by use of a small linear-array transducer through a transrectal window. The membranous and penile urethra can be imaged, with use of a standoff pad if necessary, after removing the overlying hair.

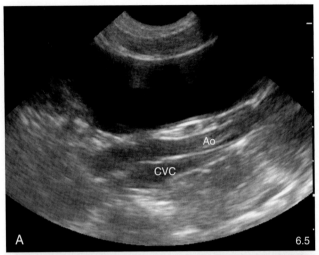

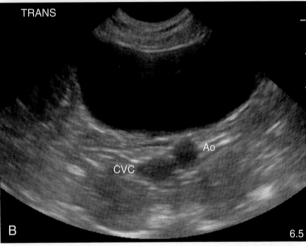

Figure 16-30 **Normal urinary bladder. A,** Longitudinal image of a normal anechoic urinary bladder. The abdominal aorta (*Ao*) and caudal vena cava (*CVC*) are seen in the far field. Note the caudal vena cava is partially collapsed, compressed by moderate transducer pressure. **B,** Transverse image. The great vessels are seen in cross section. *Ao,* Aorta; *CVC,* caudal vena cava.

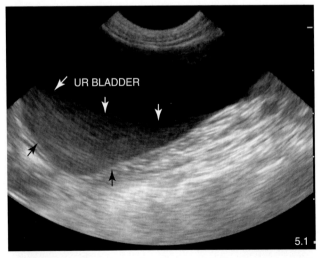

Figure 16-31 Side lobe artifact (between black and white arrows) creating a haze of echoes overlying the urinary bladder. This is most commonly mistaken for urinary sediment or sludge and can be reduced or eliminated by reducing gain.

Special sector or radial endoluminal transducers, designed to image the human prostate or vagina, can also be used to evaluate the bladder or urethra if the transducer is small enough for animals. Sonoendoscopic probes are also becoming available, which may allow transurethral evaluation of the bladder.

Normal Anatomy

The bladder wall consists of an outer hyperechoic serosa, three smooth muscle layers that are hypoechoic, and a hyperechoic lamina propria submucosa that parallels the inner hypoechoic mucosa. The bladder wall appears as two thin hyperechoic lines separated in the middle by a thin hypoechoic line in most animals with the bladder distended (Figure 16-32, *A*).[200] These three lines are appreciated only with use of high-frequency transducers directed perpendicular to the bladder wall. A hypoechoic mucosal layer may be seen in less distended bladders, but the mucosa blends with the hyperechoic submucosal layer with increased bladder distention.[200] The inner and outer layers of muscle are longitudinally oriented, whereas the middle layer is circular and thicker. The mucosa is made up of transitional epithelium. A loose submucosa is present between the mucosal and muscular layers. The serosal surface is lined with visceral peritoneum.

Bladder wall thickness varies with the degree of bladder distention. Mean bladder wall thickness is 2.3 mm in minimally distended canine bladders (see Figure 16-32, *B*); it measures approximately 1.4 mm in moderately distended bladders.[201] In addition, mean bladder wall thickness increases with body weight; the heaviest dogs have a bladder wall that is approximately 1 mm thicker than it is in the lightest dogs.[201] Bladder wall thickness varies from 1.3 to 1.7 mm in normal cats.[200]

The bladder trigone region and entrance of the ureters are not easily recognized ultrasonographically unless ureteral dilation is present. However, small protuberances representing ureteric orifices may be seen in the dorsal trigone region and should not be mistaken for an abnormality[113,114,199] (see Figure 16-29, *A*). Periodic streaming of bright, specular echoes has been noted within the anechoic urine at the trigone. This flow effect may be caused by turbulence or cavitation produced by intermittent emptying of the ureters or a difference in specific gravity between ureteral and bladder urine.[113,114,202-204] In humans, the phenomenon has been termed the ureteral jet effect and can be seen on conventional real-time imaging or on color Doppler imaging (see Figure 16-29, *B* to *D*). The bladder sphincter and ligaments are not recognized as distinct structures.

The cervix and uterine body lie immediately dorsal to the bladder in the female, whereas the descending colon occupies this position in the male. The prostate gland surrounds the proximal urethra and bladder neck in the male. The bladder is bounded cranially by small intestine. The bladder region is surrounded by hyperechoic fat that greatly contrasts with its anechoic luminal contents.

The female urethra has three smooth muscle layers similar to those of the bladder. The male urethra consists of an inner longitudinal smooth muscle layer and an outer layer of transverse skeletal muscle. The corpus cavernosum urethrae immediately surrounds the skeletal muscle layer of the penile urethra in the male. The mucosa of the urethra is transitional epithelium in both sexes, except near the external orifice where it changes to stratified squamous epithelium.

The layers of the bladder and urethra are not clearly demarcated unless high-frequency or specialized sonoendoscopic transducers are used. The presence of peritoneal fluid does allow excellent visualization of the bladder wall (see Figure 16-29, *C*). As newer probes become available to

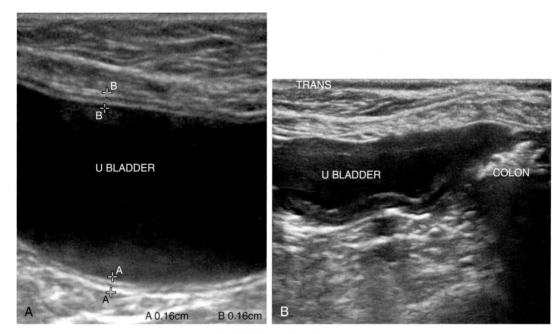

Figure 16-32 **Normal bladder. A,** The bladder wall is thin (0.16 cm between electronic cursors), and normal layering can be seen in this moderately distended bladder. **B,** The bladder wall appears thick, but is within normal limits (approximately 2 mm) in this example of a nondistended bladder. As the bladder distends, the hypoechoic muscular layer becomes progressively thinner.

veterinarians, familiarity with the normal appearance of these wall layers may help to stage neoplasia.

Distal Ureters
Although the distal ureters are not technically part of the bladder, they are included in this section because they are usually evaluated at the time of bladder examination. The distal ureters can be detected with ultrasonography only if they are dilated from ectopia, ureteritis, obstruction, or other congenital conditions.[114] Ureteral jets are often seen in the region of the bladder trigone and are helpful to confirm passage of urine into the bladder.

Antegrade Pyelography for Evaluating the Distal Ureters
In certain cases, percutaneous ultrasound-guided antegrade pyelography may help diagnose a ureteral abnormality that is not demonstrated by conventional urography or ultrasonography.[86,87,115] A needle is placed percutaneously into the dilated renal pelvis under ultrasound guidance, and water-soluble contrast material is administered to achieve optimal opacification of the ureter. This procedure may help identify the cause and location of ureteral obstruction, detect congenital or acquired ureteral abnormalities, or provide better visualization of ureteral abnormalities that were poorly seen with conventional urography.

Vesicoureteral Reflux
Vesicoureteral reflux is the retrograde passage of urine from the bladder into the ureter because of an incompetent vesicoureteral junction. It can predispose the upper urinary tract to infection. Reflux may occur in younger dogs less than 6 months of age without underlying pathology. However, in older animals it has been associated with cystitis, urethral obstruction, neurogenic bladder disease, and congenital anomalies at the ureterovesical junction. In humans, bladder infusion with agitated saline or contrast-enhanced ultrasound has been used to evaluate vesicoureteral reflux in children where it is desirable to limit radiation exposure normally received with voiding cystourethrography.[205,206] With contrast enhanced ultrasound, a galactose based echo-enhancing agent and sterile saline are instilled into the bladder via a urethral catheter until the bladder is full. The kidneys and bladder are scanned before filling, during filling, and while voiding to observe for vesicoureteral reflux. This technique may be applicable in animals with certain types of abnormalities, but its usefulness remains to be investigated.

Acquired Ureterovaginal Fistula
Ureterovaginal fistulas may develop from penetrating trauma or inadvertent ligation of the ureter during ovariohysterectomy.[86,207-209] A fistula between the affected ureter and vagina likely develops because of necrosis of tissue. Urinary incontinence is present and a dilated ureter and renal pelvis may occur from ascending infection and pyelonephritis. Sonographic diagnosis depends on a compatible history, finding a dilated ureter and renal pelvis, and the identification of an abnormally located terminal ureter. A vaginourethrogram, vaginoscopy, or computed tomographic (CT) urography may be helpful to confirm the diagnosis. Ultrasound-guided antegrade pyelography has also been described to better visualize the distal ureter.[86]

Ectopic Ureter
An ectopic ureter is a congenital condition where the ureters do not empty into the trigone region of the bladder and incontinence may result. Ectopic ureters may be unilateral or bilateral and occur most often in female dogs,[210] but they have also been reported in cats.[211-214] Incontinence is not always present,[212] especially in males.[215] Dilation of the affected ureter and renal pelvis from ureteritis and pyelonephritis can occur secondary to ascending bacterial infection.

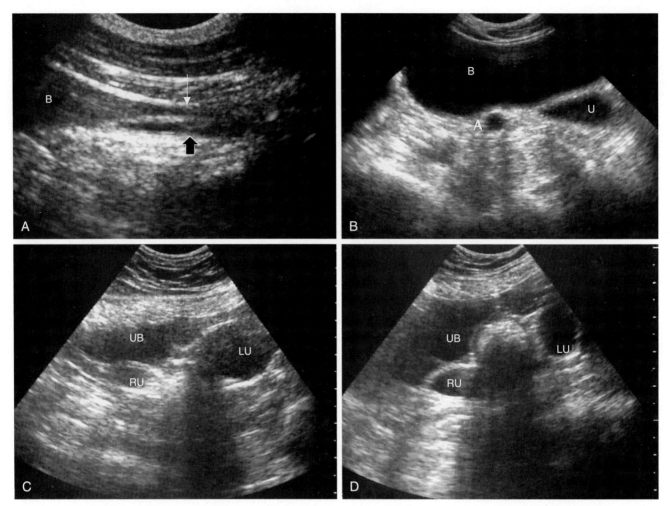

Figure 16-33 Ectopic ureter, sagittal (**A**) and transverse (**B** to **D**) views near the bladder neck. **A,** A dilated ectopic ureter (*black arrow*) can be seen near the bladder neck (*white arrow*), running parallel to the urethra. *B,* Bladder. **B,** Transverse view of the bladder (*B*) showing a dilated, left ectopic ureter (*U*). *A,* Aorta. **C** and **D,** Bilateral dilated ectopic ureters can be seen dorsal to the bladder. *LU,* Left ureter; *RU,* right ureter; *UB,* urinary bladder.

The radiographic and ultrasonographic diagnoses of ectopic ureter were compared in a series of 14 dogs[117]; the ectopic ureters were unilateral in 5 dogs and bilateral in 9 dogs. It was concluded that there was no difference in detection rate (91%) between radiography and ultrasonography by an experienced sonographer. However, the radiographic studies (intravenous pyelography, vaginourethrography [females], urethrography [males]) were conducted just before the ultrasound examination, and all studies were performed with anesthesia. Before the ultrasonographic study, the bladder was also moderately distended with saline. Termination of the five normal ureters in this investigation was considered normal when the vesicoureteral junction or a normal ureteral jet was observed. Two ectopic ureters of the 14 dogs were not detected with either radiography or ultrasonography. The renal pelvis or ureter was dilated in 10 (43%) ectopic ureters, which helped with diagnosis. Other ultrasonographic findings that helped confirm an ectopic ureter included absence of a ureteral jet, visualization of the ectopic ureter passing caudal to the bladder trigone, visualization of the ectopic ureter opening into the urethra close to the bladder neck (5 instances), and visualization of the ectopic ureter opening into the prostatic

urethra (2 cases). Figure 16-33 illustrates a case of bilateral ectopic ureter in a dog.

It has been reported that normal ureteral jets are better visualized with either conventional or color Doppler ultrasonography if the specific gravity of the urine in the bladder is different from that in the ureter.[113,203,204] Therefore filling the bladder with saline of lower specific gravity than ureteral urine will enhance visualization of normal ureteral jets. An alternative approach is to empty the bladder, withhold water for several hours to concentrate bladder urine, and then allow access to water or administer a diuretic to produce dilute ureteral urine. Failure to observe normal ureteral jets under these circumstances suggests the possibility of an ectopic ureter, whereas visualization of normal ureteral jets helps confirm normalcy.

There are also several limitations to the ultrasonographic identification of ectopic ureters. It may be difficult to detect ectopic ureters when there is an intrapelvic bladder neck due to the interference of overlying bone.[216] In addition, a normal ureteral jet may not be observed in all normal dogs or in dogs with ureteral infection or obstruction. Ectopic ureters may not be visualized on ultrasonographic studies for a variety of

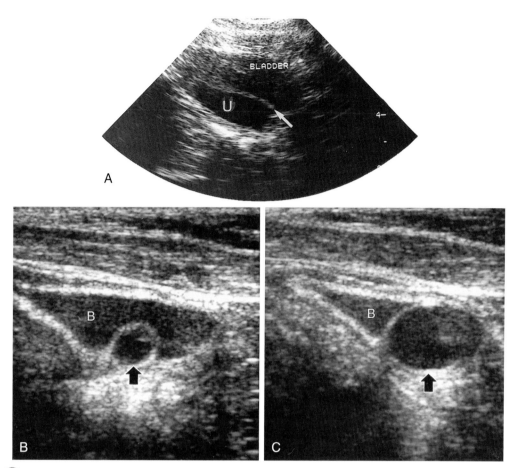

Figure 16-34 **Ureterocele. A,** Ureterocele, sagittal plane through the bladder. This young female dog developed urinary incontinence. A thin, linear echogenicity resembling a thin membrane (*arrow*) was noted dorsally within the bladder lumen near the neck. A ureterocele (*U*) with associated dilated ectopic ureter was suspected and later confirmed at surgery. **B** and **C,** Cystic structures (*arrows*) within the bladder (*B*) represent additional examples of ureteroceles.

reasons. Therefore standard urography, urethrography, or vaginourethrography are often required for diagnosis. However, not all ectopic ureters are seen even on these studies. Digital fluoroscopic urography, contrast-enhanced CT and transurethral cystoscopy can be used when other methods fail.[217,218] However, these techniques may not be available to all veterinary practitioners. Therefore one must carefully consider the clinical information, laboratory data, and the findings on available imaging procedures to reach the correct diagnosis.

Ruptured Ureter
A ruptured distal ureter is best detected on excretory urography as described previously when discussing the proximal ureter. On ultrasonography, a dilated ureter and renal pelvis may be identified on the affected side with urine accumulating retroperitoneally or collecting in the caudal abdomen around the bladder. However, excretory urography, positive-contrast cystography, and urethrography are required to identify leakage and the site of rupture (kidney, ureter, bladder, or urethra).

Ureteral Obstruction
Calculi and intrinsic or extrinsic masses can obstruct the distal ureter as described previously for the proximal ureter. Obstruction due to ureteral inflammation, blood clots, fibroepithelial polyps, calculi, extrinsic masses, ureteral fibrosis, or

strictures may occur.[97-103] Ureteral tumors are rare, but leiomyoma, leiomyosarcoma, fibropapilloma, and transitional cell carcinoma have been reported.[104-108] In the cat, distal ureteral obstruction is more commonly caused by calculi than by other conditions.[100,102,109] In the dog, primary neoplasia of the bladder, urethra, or prostate more commonly obstructs the distal ureter by involving the trigone region.[29,30,92-96]

Ureteroceles
Ureteroceles are congenital dilations of the terminal ureter. They may be unilateral or bilateral and usually appear as smooth, thin-walled cystic structures that project into the bladder lumen or occur within the bladder wall in the trigone region[114,118,219] (Figure 16-34). The affected ureter may be orthotopic (i.e., inserting in its normal position) or ectopic, and hydroureter with renal pelvic dilation due to infection or obstruction may be present. Ectopic ureteroceles usually present with incontinence.[220] In some cases, a ureterocele may also cause a partial urine outflow obstruction at the bladder neck.[221]

Bladder Pathology
Bladder Neck Position
A comparison of stress incontinence in women and sphincter mechanism incontinence in female dogs was reported.[222] It has been noted that both women and female dogs have a

shorter functional urethra and lower maximal urethral pressures with these conditions. Ultrasonography has been used to measure bladder neck positional changes in continent dogs and dogs with urinary incontinence attributable to sphincter mechanism incontinence.[223] This type of incontinence occurs mainly when the animal is recumbent or relaxed. It was found that incontinent dogs had a greater degree of caudal bladder movement under anesthesia as measured with ultrasonography. The reasons are not yet known but may be attributable to deficient vesicourethral support mechanisms in the incontinent dogs. The bladder may also have an abnormal shape and not taper normally at its junction with the urethra. It is possible that ultrasonography may not only rule out the obvious causes of incontinence, such as ectopic ureter, but may also assist with diagnosis of sphincter mechanism incontinence by assessing dynamic changes in bladder neck position. However, the usefulness of these procedures remains to be investigated. A caudally displaced bladder may make it nearly impossible to rule out other causes of incontinence, such as ectopic ureters, because of poor visualization of the trigone region.

Bladder Volume

Formulas have been devised for measurement of urine volume and postvoid residual volume in humans by ultrasonography.[224] This technique has been used to evaluate bladder contractility, neurogenic bladder, and bladder outlet obstruction, and the formula for a prolate ellipsoid is commonly employed (volume = length × width × height × 0.523).[225]

Bladder volume determinations also have the potential to characterize bladder dysfunction and assess improvement in bladder emptying after medical or surgical therapy in animals. Methods for calculating bladder volume in normal dogs by ultrasonography have been reported.[226-229] In a study where six formulas were compared, one formula was found to be the most accurate for determining bladder volume in dogs (volume = length × width × mean height × 0.625).[226] Mean height is the average of bladder height measured on the longitudinal and transverse scans. Sonographic estimates of residual urine volume have been used to evaluate dysuric dogs and the progress of dogs undergoing treatment for thoracolumbar disk disease.[230,231]

Urachal Abnormalities and Acquired Diverticuli

The location and extent of congenital or acquired bladder diverticula or fistulas are best evaluated with positive-contrast cystography. Few reports describe the diagnosis of these types of abnormalities with ultrasonography.[232] However, urachal abnormalities, diverticula, or fistulas may be suspected during ultrasonography initially if the ultrasound study is the first imaging procedure done.

On ultrasonographic evaluation, a diverticulum appears as a fluid-filled structure extending from the bladder lumen. Urachal abnormalities are located in the cranioventral bladder wall or between the bladder and umbilicus, whereas acquired diverticula may originate at any bladder location.

The urachus forms a communication between the bladder and allantoic sac in the fetus that atrophies to a fibrous structure before birth. If the urachus remains patent after birth, the diagnosis is obvious because urine exits at the umbilicus. The patent urachus may be evident ultrasonographically between the cranioventral bladder wall and umbilicus, or the bladder vertex may have an unusually pointed appearance. If the communication is incomplete, a urachal diverticulum may be seen extending from the bladder cranioventrally as a convex outpouching of the lumen. The bladder wall is often thickened in this area. Urachal diverticula may predispose the bladder to recurrent infections unless they are surgically excised.

Urachal cysts form when secretions continue in an isolated section of urachal epithelium while the remainder of the urachus undergoes fibrosis. A typical urachal cyst appears as a thin-walled, anechoic structure cranial to the bladder on an ultrasound examination. It sometimes becomes infected in later life and takes on the appearance of an abscess. A nonpatent urachal ligament has also been reported to prevent adequate bladder emptying in cats by causing elongation of the bladder with a pointed vertex.

An acquired diverticulum may result from trauma or infection. Herniation of intact mucosa through a tear in the muscular layers of the bladder wall has been identified with trauma. Acquired diverticula or fistulas between the bladder and other organs may form as a result of inflammation in the bladder wall or adjacent organs. Persistent deformity of the lumen with masses or adhesions may be noted with ultrasonography, but the diagnosis must be confirmed with contrast cystography.

Ultrasonography was used to diagnose eversion of the bladder in a female domestic shorthair cat with persistent stranguria, hematuria, and inappropriate urination. A multilayered mass, consistent with a full-thickness evagination, was detected near the apex of the bladder, and surgical correction was performed. Ultrasound examination was helpful in limiting diagnostic choices because it was noninvasive and allowed identification of all four layers of the bladder.[233]

Ruptured Bladder

A ruptured bladder is best diagnosed by positive-contrast cystography. Discontinuity of the wall may be falsely suspected because of echo dropout from the curved bladder wall (edge or refraction artifact) (see Chapter 1, Figure 1-48). In addition, small mural defects may not be seen and other parts of the urinary tract may be involved. In most trauma cases, the integrity of the entire urinary tract should be evaluated with excretory urography, positive-contrast cystography, and urethrography if urine leakage is detected on abdominocentesis.

Cystitis

Chronic cystitis causes wall thickening that is usually most pronounced cranioventrally, but it can become generalized in severe cases[234] (Figure 16-35). Normal wall thickness in a fully distended bladder is approximately 1 to 2 mm. In a nondistended bladder, subjective evaluation of wall thickness is required according to the amount of distention. In many cases of cystitis, the urinary bladder wall is normal. This may be true even in the presence of sediment or calculi.

In polypoid cystitis, wall thickening is accompanied by multiple small masses that project into the bladder lumen (Figure 16-36).[235,236] In most cases the polyps are located cranioventrally within the bladder, but they can also occur craniodorsally. Large polyps with a pedunculated base of attachment may occasionally be seen. If the base of attachment is sessile or there is a single mass, neoplasia is more likely. Because neoplasia is much more common than polyps, the diagnosis of a polyp must be confirmed with a biopsy. Cytologic or histologic evaluation is mandatory as wall thickening or masses become more conspicuous, particularly when there has been little response to treatment.

Emphysematous cystitis is a unique form of cystitis in which gas produced by certain organisms accumulates within the bladder wall, the bladder lumen, and sometimes in the bladder ligaments (Figure 16-37).[232,237-240] This is most commonly seen with diabetes mellitus and is produced by glucose-fermenting bacteria such as *Escherichia coli*.[237] However, it can also occur with *Aerobacter* or *Proteus* infections[240] and in conditions where the bladder wall becomes

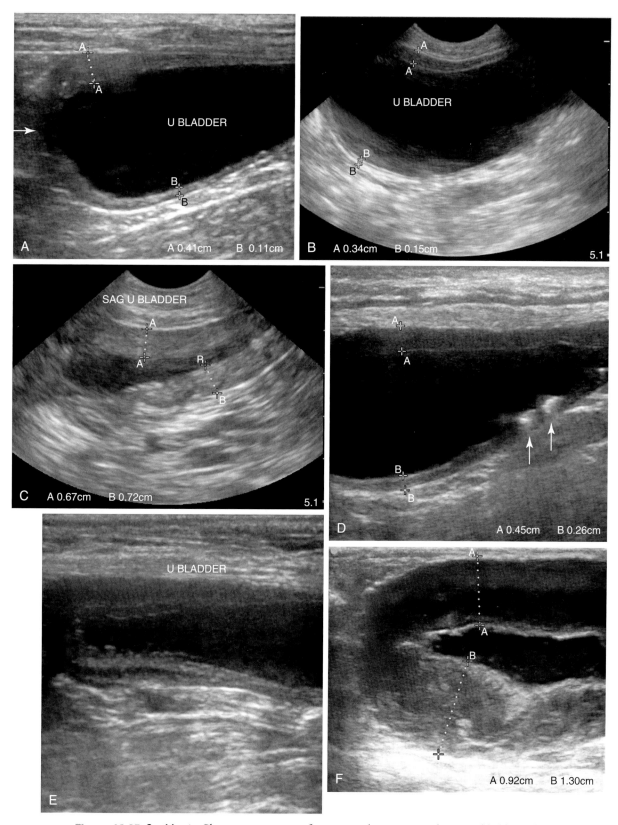

Figure 16-35 Cystitis. A, Classic presentation of cystitis with cranioventral urinary bladder wall thickening. The cranioventral wall measures 0.41 cm, whereas the thickness of the dorsal wall is normal (0.11 cm). Refraction (edge) artifact accounts for the "drop-out" of urinary bladder wall at the apex (*arrow*). **B,** Ventral bladder wall thickening (0.34 cm between electronic cursors) is present, whereas the thickness of the dorsal bladder wall is normal (0.15 cm between electronic cursors). Echogenic side lobe artifact overlays the craniodorsal portion of the bladder lumen and makes visualization of the far field (dorsal) wall more difficult (pseudosludge); it is could be misdiagnosed as sediment. **C,** Diffusely thickened urinary bladder wall in this case of cystitis. The bladder wall is much thicker than expected, even when taking into account the non-distended state of the bladder. **D,** Cystitis in the presence of cystic calculi (arrows). The ventral bladder wall is thicker than the dorsal wall. **E,** Diffuse cystitis with wall thickening and mucosal irregularity. **F,** Severe cystitis with marked diffuse bladder wall thickening (0.92 cm ventrally, 1.30 cm dorsally).

Continued

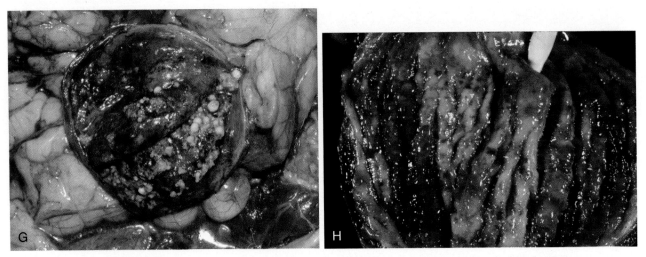

Figure 16-35, cont'd G, Specimen of thickened, erythematous urinary bladder secondary to chronic infection and the presence of multiple cystic calculi. **H,** Close-up view of thickened, erythematous and hemorrhagic urinary bladder mucosa with severe cystitis. (G, H, Courtesy of Washington State University College of Veterinary Medicine, Washington Animal Disease Diagnostic Laboratory, Pullman, WA.)

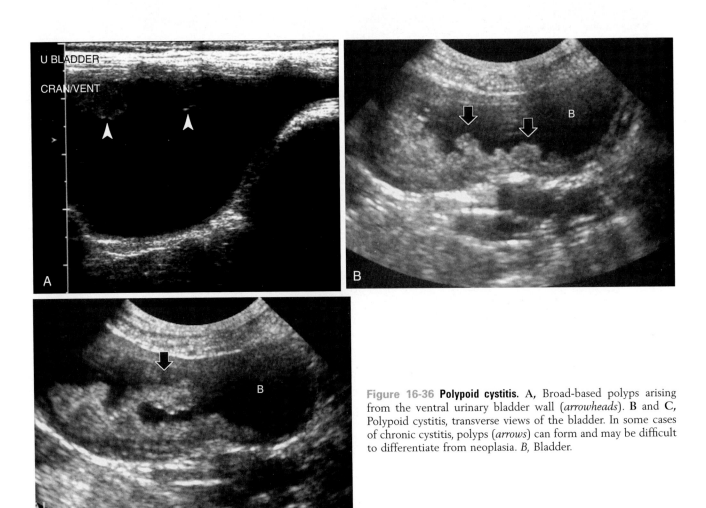

Figure 16-36 Polypoid cystitis. A, Broad-based polyps arising from the ventral urinary bladder wall (*arrowheads*). **B** and **C,** Polypoid cystitis, transverse views of the bladder. In some cases of chronic cystitis, polyps (*arrows*) can form and may be difficult to differentiate from neoplasia. *B,* Bladder.

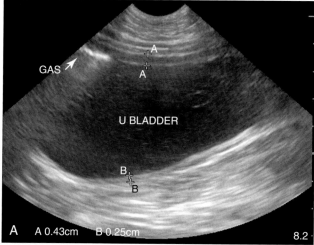

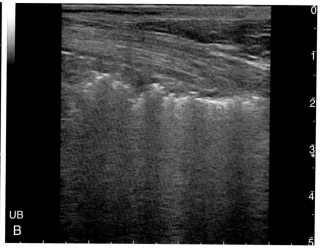

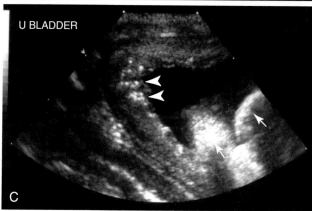

Figure 16-37 Emphysematous cystitis. A, Echogenic gas (*GAS, arrow*) is seen in the nondependent portion of the urinary bladder. **B,** Severe intraluminal gas accumulation is present in this bladder, completely shadowing the deeper portion of the bladder. The uneven gas interface indicates mucosal irregularity. **C,** Tiny pockets of gas (*arrowheads*) are identified embedded in folds of very inflamed bladder wall in this dog with *Escherichia coli* cystitis secondary to diabetes. Two large cystic calculi are also present (*arrows*).

hypoxic and infection with *Clostridium* species occurs.[238,239] The ultrasonographic appearance is one of a hyperechoic bladder wall with irregular, dirty shadowing produced by the gas. This appearance can be distinguished from gas within the bladder lumen because it is localized within the wall, follows the wall contour closely, and maintains a fixed location with positional changes. The condition can be confirmed by visualizing lucencies associated with the bladder wall on abdominal radiographs.

Pseudomembranous cystitis occurs in humans and has been presumptively diagnosed in four cats with azotemia, renal failure, and outflow obstruction.[241] Ultrasonography revealed bladder wall thickening, suspended echogenic debris, and unusual hyperechoic septa dividing the lumen into compartments.

Blood Clots and Hematomas
Blood clots may occur secondary to trauma, bleeding disorders, infection, or neoplasia. Blood clots are usually anticipated at the time of the ultrasound study on the basis of the history or clinical signs. Clots are commonly hyperechoic, nonshadowing echogenicities with an irregular shape that settle to the dependent portion of the bladder lumen on positional studies[198,242] (Figure 16-38). If the clots are large or adherent to the wall, the appearance may be more hypoechoic with less mobility and could be mistaken for a mural mass (see Figure 16-38, C). Doppler evaluation can be used to differentiate between masses and blood clots or hematomas, the former of which should demonstrate some vascularity. Quick

back-and-forth agitation of the transducer temporarily resuspends smaller clots and sediment if adequate urine is present. This is not seen with mural masses or larger calculi.

Hematoma of the bladder wall due to contusion is occasionally produced by trauma. This may appear as a hypoechoic mass associated with a thickened bladder wall. Lack of blood flow within the hematoma on Doppler analysis helps differentiate it from a tumor. Adherent blood clots extending into the bladder lumen or free fluid representing hemorrhage around the outer wall of the bladder may be seen. A history of trauma or other evidence of trauma on the physical examination, ultrasound study, or radiographic examination is required to make the diagnosis. The hematoma gradually resolves with time unless there is bladder wall necrosis and leakage of urine into the peritoneal cavity.

Cystic Calculi
Radiopaque or radiolucent calculi are detected as hyperechoic focal echogenicities that shadow in the dependent portion of the bladder[60,116,198,234,242,243] (Figure 16-39). The amount of shadowing varies with the composition and compactness of the calculus, its location with respect to the focal zone of the transducer, and the ultrasound frequency used. More pronounced shadowing is noted at higher frequencies within the focal zone. Very small calculi, smaller than the width of the ultrasound beam in the x-axis or z-axis, will not show acoustic shadowing. Calculi usually migrate to the dependent portion of the bladder but may adhere to the wall with severe inflammation. Color Doppler imaging can sometimes help identify

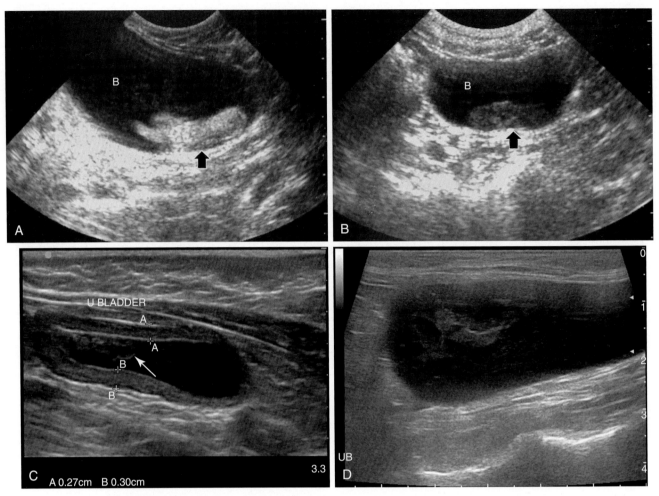

Figure 16-38 Blood clots, transverse views (**A** and **B**) of the bladder. Blood clots form amorphous echogenicities (*arrows*) within the urinary bladder that do not shadow and are located in the dependent portion of the bladder (*B*). The presence of hemorrhage or clots in the voided urine helps with the differential diagnosis. **C,** Adherent blood clot (*arrow*) in a cat with cystitis. **D,** Amorphous clotted blood in a cat with renal lymphoma.

questionable calculi if a twinkling artifact can be seen.[124] This is a short color artifact, similar to a ring-down artifact that occurs distal to some calculi.

Shadowing sediment, which layers in the dependent portion of the bladder, is also identified (Figure 16-40). The sediment suspends easily with bladder agitation, and no discrete echogenic foci the size of calculi are seen (Figure 16-41). The appearance of calculi or sediment contrasts with intraluminal gas bubbles, which also shadow but rise to the top of the bladder on positional views. This appearance must be differentiated from near-field reverberation artifacts. Fibrosis or calcification of the bladder wall may cause mural hyperechogenicity and shadowing. In most cases, repositioning the animal or imaging the bladder in multiple planes, or both, will distinguish fibrosis or calcification from calculi, blood clots, sediment, or gas bubbles.

Nonshadowing, dependent sediment indicates the presence of nonmineral substances such as cellular debris with cystitis, or small amounts of minerals such as crystalluria.

Foreign Bodies
Retained catheters, BBs, plant awns, and suture material are foreign bodies that may be found occasionally within the urinary bladder. Catheters appear as parallel echogenic lines when the sound beam is perpendicular to the wall. These parallel lines represent the walls of the catheter. A BB or other metallic foreign body may shadow (depending on size) and has a unique reverberation artifact within the shadow distally. Plant awns have a variable appearance, but may be seen as hyperechoic structures without shadowing.[244]

Bladder Neoplasia
Female dogs and male cats are more likely to develop bladder cancer.[245-248] The dog is affected more often than the cat.[246,249] The most common bladder neoplasm is transitional cell carcinoma. Transitional cell carcinomas are generally characterized by focal wall thickening with an irregular, sessile mass extending into the bladder lumen.[92,198] (Figures 16-42 and 16-43). It is clear that very small masses can be detected if the bladder is sufficiently distended with urine. Masses can easily be overlooked in a collapsed bladder. The bladder should be catheterized and distended with sterile saline, if needed. On occasion, the bladder wall may be diffusely involved by tumor with no focal mass, and the appearance may resemble the more uniform thickening seen with severe, chronic cystitis.[92] Transabdominal

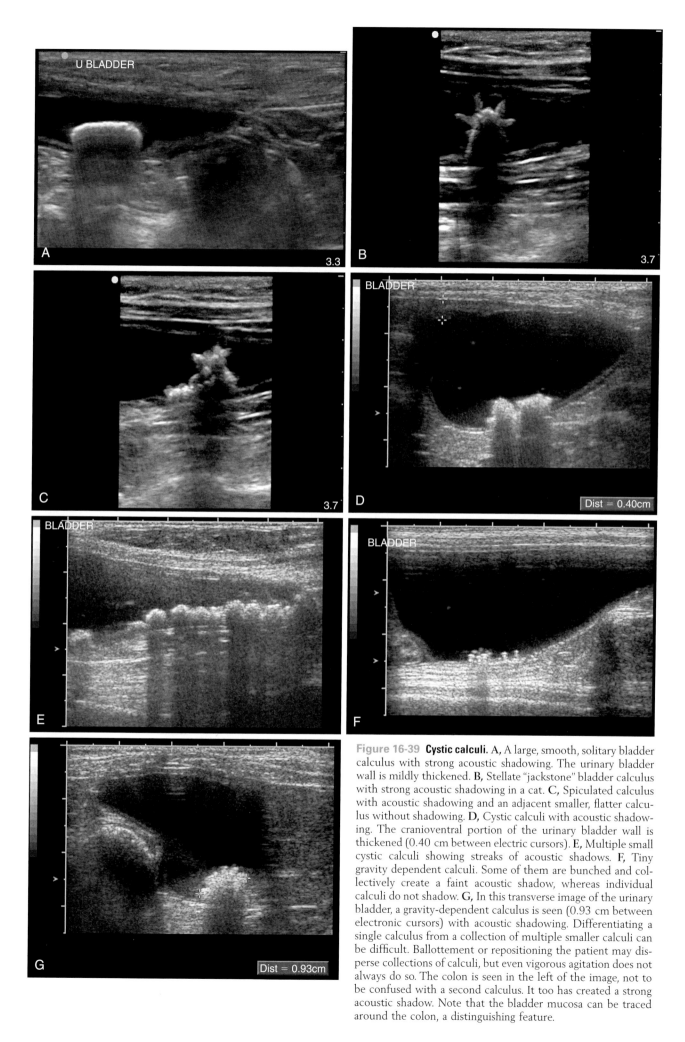

Figure 16-39 Cystic calculi. A, A large, smooth, solitary bladder calculus with strong acoustic shadowing. The urinary bladder wall is mildly thickened. **B,** Stellate "jackstone" bladder calculus with strong acoustic shadowing in a cat. **C,** Spiculated calculus with acoustic shadowing and an adjacent smaller, flatter calculus without shadowing. **D,** Cystic calculi with acoustic shadowing. The cranioventral portion of the urinary bladder wall is thickened (0.40 cm between electric cursors). **E,** Multiple small cystic calculi showing streaks of acoustic shadows. **F,** Tiny gravity dependent calculi. Some of them are bunched and collectively create a faint acoustic shadow, whereas individual calculi do not shadow. **G,** In this transverse image of the urinary bladder, a gravity-dependent calculus is seen (0.93 cm between electronic cursors) with acoustic shadowing. Differentiating a single calculus from a collection of multiple smaller calculi can be difficult. Ballottement or repositioning the patient may disperse collections of calculi, but even vigorous agitation does not always do so. The colon is seen in the left of the image, not to be confused with a second calculus. It too has created a strong acoustic shadow. Note that the bladder mucosa can be traced around the colon, a distinguishing feature.

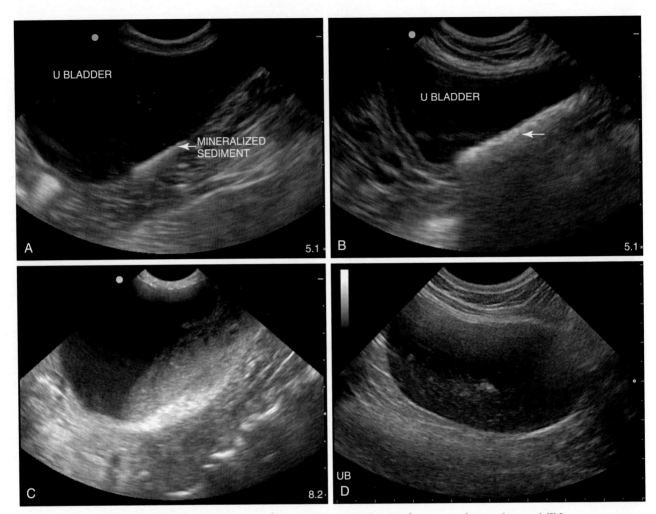

Figure 16-40 Urinary bladder sediment. A, small accumulation of urinary sediment (*arrow; MIN-ERALIZED SEDIMENT*) is seen in the dependent portion of the urinary bladder (*U BLADDER*). **B,** Large layer of gravity dependent sediment (*arrow*) has completely settled, creating an acoustic shadow. The bladder wall is mildly thickened. **C,** Settling sediment. A very echogenic, thick layer has settled while some sediment is still suspended. **D,** Echogenic, non–gravity dependent material is suspended in this cat's urine. Usually nonsettling echoes such as this are normal, usually droplets of fat. Note the urinary bladder wall is very thin.

ultrasonography has been used for endoscopically-guided laser ablation of transitional cell carcinomas affecting the cystourethral junction of dogs.[250] Ultrasonography was important for ensuring correct placement of the endoscope and the laser fiber. Figure 16-44 illustrates a case of focal cystitis secondary to surgery for removal of cystic calculi several months prior. This lesion could easily mimic bladder wall neoplasia, illustrating the importance of accurate clinical history.

Other epithelial (squamous cell carcinoma, adenocarcinoma) and mesenchymal (leiomyoma, leiomyosarcoma, fibromas, fibrosarcoma, osteosarcoma, lymphoma, rhabdomyosarcoma, hemangioma, hemangiosarcoma, myxoma, and chemodectoma) tumors have also been described in the bladder. The tumor type probably cannot be determined by its ultrasound appearance alone. However, epithelial tumors are known to have an irregular luminal surface compared with mesenchymal tumors. A tumor can be differentiated from a blood clot by its immobility and the presence of blood flow within the mass.

Percutaneous aspiration of suspected bladder tumors under ultrasound guidance is somewhat controversial because there is the potential for seeding tumor along the needle track (see Figure 16-42, G).[251,252] This is minimized by use of a small-gauge needle, but the spread of transitional cell carcinoma to the ventral abdominal wall has been observed.[251,252] Therefore an ultrasound-guided catheter biopsy is preferred.[253] A catheter is inserted into the bladder and the lesion is displaced toward the catheter by transducer pressure. Saline may be infused to distend the bladder if the tumor is poorly visualized. Suction is then applied to the catheter to obtain material from the mass for cytologic analysis.

The sublumbar (iliac) lymph nodes should also be evaluated for metastasis, and ureteral obstruction should be ruled out by examining the ureter and renal pelvis for dilation secondary to ureteral obstruction. The sonographer should remember that urethral or prostatic tumors can extend into the bladder, simulating a bladder tumor. Thoracic and abdominal radiographs should be taken to rule out metastasis to the lung, iliac lymph nodes, pelvis, and lumbar spine.

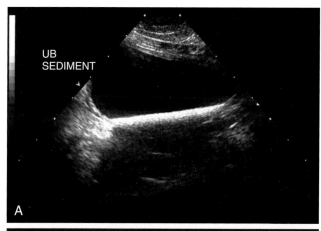

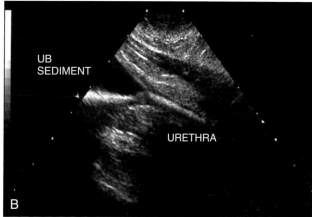

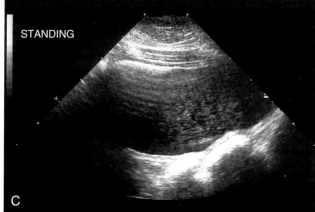

Figure 16-41 **Urinary sediment ("sand") in a cat. A,** Sagittal image of the urinary bladder shows a smooth, flat hyperechoic layer of gravity-dependent crystals, creating a very strong acoustic shadow. **B,** Sagittal image showing sediment in the neck of the urinary bladder and urethra. **C,** Standing sagittal image shows resuspension of the sediment, with early hyperechoic collection along the near field ventral wall. The colon is seen in the far field.

Accurate staging or grading of bladder cancer according to the extent of bladder wall layer invasion has been used to establish the prognosis and appropriate treatment.[245,254] The World Health Organization clinical staging system classifies T1 as a superficial papillary tumor, T2 as a tumor invading the bladder wall with induration, and T3 as a tumor invading adjacent organs (prostate, uterus, vagina, pelvic canal).[255] Staging also considers regional lymph node involvement and distant metastasis. Abdominal ultrasound is useful to assess tumor size, degree of bladder wall invasion, and abdominal metastasis. Doppler ultrasonography should be used to determine if there is blood flow within the mass to distinguish a tumor from a blood clot or sludge. In humans, the current opinion is that the extent of invasion of the bladder wall cannot be accurately assessed by transabdominal ultrasound.[256,257] However, if the tumor has spread beyond the bladder wall or involves the perivesical or retroperitoneal lymph nodes, transabdominal ultrasound can be used to stage these lesions accurately.[258] Ultrasonography was reported to be as accurate as CT for staging bladder tumors when transurethral ultrasonography of the bladder was employed.[259] Currently, CT urography and MRI are preferred for diagnosing and staging bladder tumors.[257] Some investigators consider MRI to be superior to CT because of its intrinsic high soft-tissue contrast and direct multiplanar imaging capability.[260,261]

Urethral Pathology

Ultrasonographic evaluation of the urethra is limited in the dog and cat. It is most useful for evaluating the proximal urethra in females and the prostatic urethra in males. However, with the endoluminal capability of specialized high-frequency ultrasound equipment, the entire urethra can be examined. Detection of urethral tumors, evaluation of metastasis to adjacent lymph nodes, or localization of calculi can certainly be of direct benefit. Larger calculi cause shadowing and may displace the walls of the urethra outward, but many urethral calculi are small and do not shadow (Figure 16-45). Urethrovaginal and urethrorectal fistulae have been reported but are rare and best diagnosed with positive-contrast urethrography or vaginourethrography. Ultrasound examination aided detection of urethral obstruction from a fibroblastic ischemic response in a female shih tzu. The ischemia was thought to be induced from previous torsion of a gravid uterus.[262] Urethral tumors may appear as masses projecting into the urethral lumen or diffuse thickening of the urethra[94,263,264] (Figure 16-46). Transitional cell carcinoma and squamous cell carcinoma are the common histologic types. They may invade the bladder neck and obstruct the ureters. Older female dogs are most commonly affected.[265] Tumors of the prostate may also involve the urethra and extend to the bladder neck. Retrograde positive-contrast urethrography or vaginourethrography, often combined with double-contrast cystography, remain the best methods for characterizing the location and extent of urethral tumors. However, these procedures may not be possible if the urethra is obstructed. Thoracic and abdominal radiographs should be taken to rule out metastasis to the lungs, iliac lymph nodes, pelvis, and lumbar spine. Positive-contrast urethrography is also preferred for evaluating urethral rupture, urethral diverticuli, or partial obstruction caused by calculi, strictures, and congenital conditions, especially when abnormalities are suspected in the distal urethra.

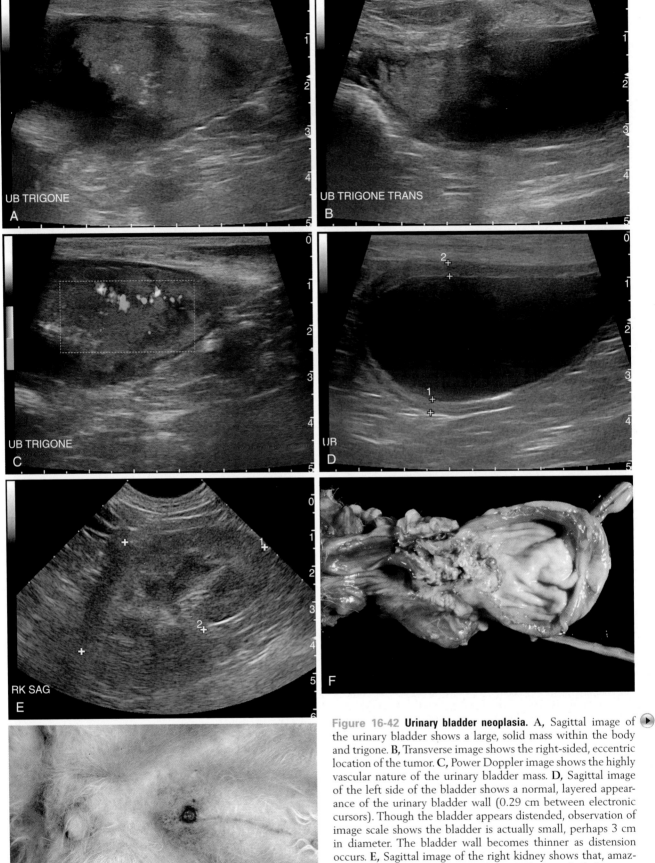

Figure 16-42 Urinary bladder neoplasia. A, Sagittal image of the urinary bladder shows a large, solid mass within the body and trigone. **B,** Transverse image shows the right-sided, eccentric location of the tumor. **C,** Power Doppler image shows the highly vascular nature of the urinary bladder mass. **D,** Sagittal image of the left side of the bladder shows a normal, layered appearance of the urinary bladder wall (0.29 cm between electronic cursors). Though the bladder appears distended, observation of image scale shows the bladder is actually small, perhaps 3 cm in diameter. The bladder wall becomes thinner as distension occurs. **E,** Sagittal image of the right kidney shows that, amazingly, the right ureter was not obstructed; the right kidney was not hydronephrotic. **F,** Specimen of a transitional cell carcinoma of the bladder trigone/neck. **G,** Needle tract spread of bladder transitional cell carcinoma in a dog. (F, Courtesy of Washington State University College of Veterinary Medicine, Washington Animal Disease Diagnostic Laboratory, Pullman, WA.)

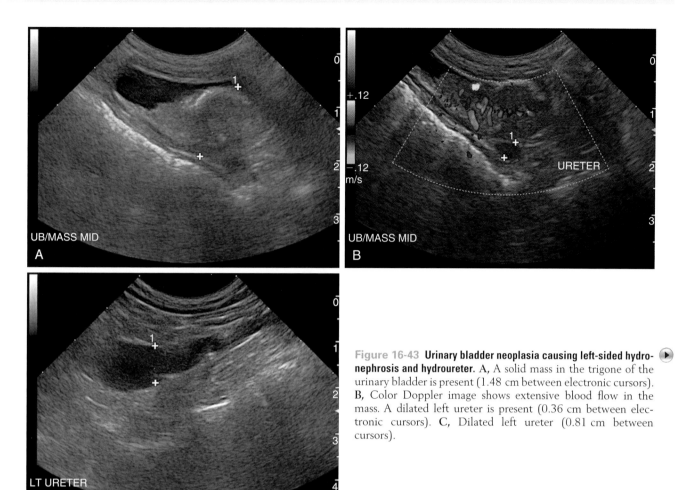

Figure 16-43 **Urinary bladder neoplasia causing left-sided hydronephrosis and hydroureter. A,** A solid mass in the trigone of the urinary bladder is present (1.48 cm between electronic cursors). **B,** Color Doppler image shows extensive blood flow in the mass. A dilated left ureter is present (0.36 cm between electronic cursors). **C,** Dilated left ureter (0.81 cm between cursors).

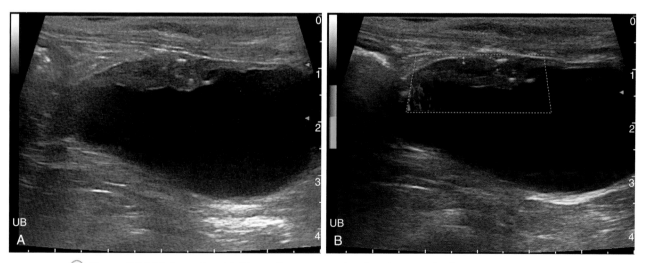

Figure 16-44 **Inflammatory bladder wall mass secondary to suture reaction from recent cystotomy. A,** Sagittal image shows focal area of heterogeneous ventral bladder wall thickening. **B,** Power Doppler shows good vascularization of the lesion.

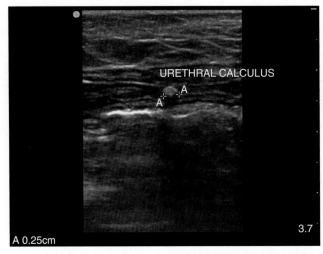

Figure 16-45 Urethral calculus. A small calculus (0.25 cm between electronic cursors) is identified in the proximal urethra, with only minimal acoustic shadowing.

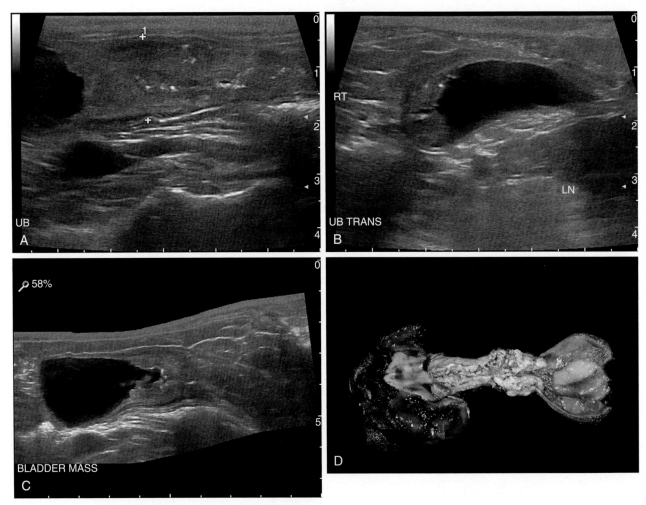

Figure 16-46 Urinary bladder and urethral tumor. A, Sagittal image of the caudal portion of the urinary bladder with extension into the urethra. The mass (1.56 cm in height between electronic cursors) has small, multifocal areas of mineralization. **B,** Transverse image of the caudal urinary bladder shows the mass is eccentric and on the right side of the bladder. An enlarged medial iliac lymph node is seen in the far field (*LN*). **C,** Extended field of view image in sagittal plane shows the extent of the trigonal and urethral mass. **D,** Specimen of urethra neoplasia in a female dog. (D, Courtesy of Washington State University College of Veterinary Medicine, Washington Animal Disease Diagnostic Laboratory, Pullman, WA.)

REFERENCES

1. Miller ME, Evans HE. *Miller's anatomy of the dog.* 3rd ed. Philadelphia: Saunders; 1993.
2. Konde LJ, Wrigley RH, Park RD, et al. Ultrasonographic anatomy of the normal canine kidney. *Vet Radiol* 1984;**25**:173–8.
3. Walter PA, Johnston GR, Feeney DA, et al. Renal ultrasonography in healthy cats. *Am J Vet Res* 1987;**48**:600–7.
4. Wood AK, McCarthy PH. Ultrasonographic-anatomic correlation and an imaging protocol of the normal canine kidney. *Am J Vet Res* 1990;**51**:103–8.
5. Nyland TG, Hager DA. Sonography of the liver, gallbladder, and spleen. *Vet Clin North Am Small Anim Pract* 1985;**15**:1123–48.
6. Nyland TG, Hager DA, Herring DS. Sonography of the liver, gallbladder, and spleen. *Semin Vet Med Surg (Small Anim)* 1989;**4**:13–31.
6a. Ivančić M, Mai W. Qualitative and quantitative comparison of renal versus hepatic ultrasonographic intensity in healthy dogs. *Vet Radiol Ultrasound* 2008;**49**:368–73.
7. Platt JF, Rubin JM, Bowerman RA, et al. The inability to detect kidney disease on the basis of echogenicity. *Am J Roentgenol* 1988;**151**:317–19.
8. Yeager AE, Anderson WI. Study of association between histologic features and echogenicity of architecturally normal cat kidneys. *Am J Vet Res* 1989;**50**:860–3.
9. Nyland TG, Kantrowitz BM, Fisher P, et al. Ultrasonic determination of kidney volume in the dog. *Vet Radiol* 1989;**30**:174–80.
10. Barr FJ. Evaluation of ultrasound as a method for assessing renal size in the dog. *J Small Anim Pract* 1990;**31**:174–9.
11. Barr FJ, Holt PE, Gibbs C. Ultrasonographic measurement of normal renal parameters. *J Small Anim Pract* 1990;**31**:180–4.
12. Felkai CS, Voros K, Vrabely T, et al. Ultrasonographic determination of renal volume in the dog. *Vet Radiol Ultrasound* 1992;**33**:292–6.
13. Mareschal A, d'Anjou MA, Moreau M, et al. Ultrasonographic measurement of kidney-to-aorta ratio as a method of estimating renal size in dogs. *Vet Radiol Ultrasound* 2007;**48**:434–8.
14. Walter PA, Feeney DA, Johnston GR, et al. Feline renal ultrasonography: quantitative analyses of imaged anatomy. *Am J Vet Res* 1987;**48**:596–9.
15. Nickel R, Schummer A, Seiferle E, et al. *Urogenital system.* The viscera of domestic mammals. Berlin: Verlag Paul Parey; 1973. p. 291–3.
16. Pollard R, Nyland TG, Bernsteen L, et al. Ultrasonographic evaluation of renal autografts in normal cats. *Vet Radiol Ultrasound* 1999;**40**:380–5.
17. Reichle JK, DiBartola SP, Leveille R. Renal ultrasonographic and computed tomographic appearance, volume, and function of cats with autosomal dominant polycystic kidney disease. *Vet Radiol Ultrasound* 2002;**43**:368–73.
18. Lobetti RG, Pearson J, Jimenez M. Renal dysplasia in a Rhodesian ridgeback dog. *J Small Anim Pract* 1996;**37**:552–5.
19. Felkai C, Voros K, Vrabely T, et al. Ultrasonographic findings of renal dysplasia in cocker spaniels: eight cases. *Acta Vet Hung* 1997;**45**:397–408.
20. Miyamoto T, Wakizaka S, Matsuyama S, et al. A control of a golden retriever with renal dysplasia. *J Vet Med Sci* 1997;**59**:939–42.
21. Abraham LA, Beck C, Slocombe RF. Renal dysplasia and urinary tract infection in a Bull Mastiff puppy. *Aust Vet J* 2003;**81**:336–9.
22. Neuwirth L, Mahaffey M, Crowell W, et al. Comparison of excretory urography and ultrasonography for detection of experimentally induced pyelonephritis in dogs. *Am J Vet Res* 1993;**54**:660–9.
23. Pugh CR, Schelling CG, Moreau RE, et al. Ultrasound corner. Iatrogenic renal pyelectasia in the dog. *Vet Radiol Ultrasound* 1994;**35**:50–1.
24. Jakovljevic S, Rivers WJ, Chun R, et al. Results of renal ultrasonography performed before and during administration of saline (0.9% NaCl) solution to induce diuresis in dogs without evidence of renal disease. *Am J Vet Res* 1999;**60**:405–9.
25. Diez-Prieto I, Garcia-Rodriguez MB, Rios-Granja MA, et al. Diagnosis of renal agenesis in a beagle. *J Small Anim Pract* 2001;**42**:599–602.
26. Agut A, Fernandez del Palacio MJ, Laredo FG, et al. Unilateral renal agenesis associated with additional congenital abnormalities of the urinary tract in a Pekingese bitch. *J Small Anim Pract* 2002;**43**:32–5.
27. Hecht S, McCarthy RJ, Tidwell AS. What is your diagnosis? Ectopic left kidney. *J Am Vet Med Assoc* 2005;**227**:223–4.
28. Allworth MS, Hoffmann KL. Crossed renal ectopia with fusion in a cat. *Vet Radiol Ultrasound* 1999;**40**:357–60.
29. Konde LJ. Sonography of the kidney. *Vet Clin North Am Small Anim Pract* 1985;**15**:1149–58.
30. Konde LJ, Park RD, Wrigley RH, et al. Comparison of radiography and ultrasonography in the evaluation of renal lesions in the dog. *J Am Vet Med Assoc* 1986;**188**:1420–5.
31. Walter PA, Feeney DA, Johnston GR, et al. Ultrasonographic evaluation of renal parenchymal diseases in dogs: 32 cases (1981-1986). *J Am Vet Med Assoc* 1987;**191**:999–1007.
32. Walter PA, Johnston GR, Feeney DA, et al. Applications of ultrasonography in the diagnosis of parenchymal kidney disease in cats: 24 cases (1981-1986). *J Am Vet Med Assoc* 1988;**192**:92–8.
33. Konde LJ. Renal sonography. *Semin Vet Med Surg (Small Anim)* 1989;**4**:32–43.
34. Zatelli A, Bonfanti U, D'Ippolito P. Obstructive renal cyst in a dog: ultrasonography-guided treatment using puncture aspiration and injection with 95% ethanol. *J Vet Intern Med* 2005;**19**:252–4.
35. Agut A, Soler M, Laredo FG, et al. Imaging diagnosis-ultrasound-guided ethanol sclerotherapy for a simple real cyst. *Vet Radiol Ultrasound* 2008;**49**:65–7.
36. Lavoue R, van der Lugt JJ, Day MJ, et al. Progressive juvenile glomerulonephropathy in 16 related French Mastiff (Bordeaux) dogs. *J Vet Intern Med* 2010;**24**:314–22.
37. Boal DK, Teele RL. Sonography of infantile polycystic disease. *AJR* 1980;**135**:575–80.
38. Crowell WA, Hubbell JJ, Riley JC. Polycystic disease in related cats. *J Am Vet Med Assoc* 1979;**175**:286–8.
39. McKenna SC, Carpenter JL. Polycystic disease of the kidney and liver in the Cairn Terrier. *Vet Pathol* 1980;**17**:436–42.
40. Biller DS, Chew DJ, DiBartola SP. Polycystic kidney disease in a family of Persian cats. *J Am Vet Med Assoc* 1990;**196**:1288–90.
41. Biller DS, DiBartola SP, Eaton KA, et al. Inheritance of polycystic kidney disease in Persian cats. *J Hered* 1996;**87**:1–5.

42. O'Leary CA, Mackay BM, Malik R, et al. Polycystic kidney disease in bull terriers: an autosomal dominant inherited disorder. *Aust Vet J* 1999;**77**:361–6.

43. Barrs VR, Gunew M, Foster SF, et al. Prevalence of autosomal dominant polycystic kidney disease in Persian cats and related-breeds in Sydney and Brisbane. *Aust Vet J* 2001;**79**:257–9.

44. Beck C, Lavelle RB. Feline polycystic kidney disease in Persian and other cats: a prospective study using ultrasonography. *Aust Vet J* 2001;**79**:181–4.

45. Cannon MJ, MacKay AD, Barr FJ, et al. Prevalence of polycystic kidney disease in Persian cats in the United Kingdom. *Vet Rec* 2001;**149**:409–11.

46. Barthez PY, Rivier P, Begon D. Prevalence of polycystic kidney disease in Persian and Persian related cats in France. *J Feline Med Surg* 2003;**5**:345–7.

47. O'Leary CA, Turner S. Chronic renal failure in an English bull terrier with polycystic kidney disease. *J Small Anim Pract* 2004;**45**:563–7.

48. Domanjko-Petric A, Cernec D, Cotman M. Polycystic kidney disease: a review and occurrence in Slovenia with comparison between ultrasound and genetic testing. *J Feline Med Surg* 2008;**10**:115–19.

49. Bonazzi M, Volta A, Gnudi G, et al. Prevalence of the polycystic kidney disease and renal and urinary bladder ultrasonographic abnormalities in Persian and Exotic Shorthair cats in Italy. *J Feline Med Surg* 2007;**9**:387–91.

50. Lee Y, Chen HY, Hsu WL, et al. Diagnosis of feline polycystic kidney disease by a combination of ultrasonographic examination and *PKD1* gene analysis. *Vet Rec* 2010;**167**:614–18.

51. Volta A, Manfredi S, Gnudi G, et al. Polycystic kidney disease in a Chartreux cat. *J Feline Med Surg* 2010;**12**:138–40.

52. Beck C, Lavelle RB. Feline polycystic kidney disease in Persian and other cats: a prospective study using ultrasonography. *Aust Vet J* 2001;**79**:181–4.

53. Bonazzi M, Onazzi M, Volta A, et al. Comparison between ultrasound and genetic testing for the early diagnosis of polycystic kidney disease in Persian and Exotic Shorthair cats. *J Feline Med Surg* 2009;**11**:430–4.

54. Wills SJ, Barrett EL, Barr FJ, et al. Evaluation of the repeatability of ultrasound scanning for detection of feline polycystic kidney disease. *J Feline Med Surg* 2009;**11**:993–6.

55. McAloose D, Casal M, Patterson DF, et al. Polycystic kidney and liver disease in two related West Highland White Terrier litters. *Vet Pathol* 1998;**35**:77–81.

56. Gorlinger S, Rothuizen J, Bunch S, et al. Congenital dilatation of the bile ducts (Caroli's disease) in young dogs. *J Vet Intern Med* 2003;**17**:28–32.

57. Last RD, Hill JM, Roach M, et al. Congenital dilatation of the large and segmental intrahepatic bile ducts (Caroli's disease) in two Golden retriever littermates. *J S Afr Vet Assoc* 2006;**77**:210–14.

58. Lium B, Moe L. Hereditary multifocal renal cystadenocarcinomas and nodular dermatofibrosis in the German Shepherd Dog: macroscopic and histopathologic changes. *Vet Pathol* 1985;**17**:447–55.

59. Atlee BA, DeBoer DJ, Irke PJ, et al. Nodular dermatofibrosis in German Shepherd Dogs as a marker for renal cystadenocarcinoma. *J Am Anim Hosp Assoc* 1991;**27**:481–7.

60. Cartee RE, Selcer BA, Patton CS. Ultrasonographic diagnosis of renal disease in small animals. *J Am Vet Med Assoc* 1980;**176**:426–30.

61. Konde LJ, Wrigley RH, Park RD, et al. Sonographic appearance of renal neoplasia in the dog. *Vet Radiol* 1985;**26**:74–81.

62. Bennett F. Unilateral renal cell carcinoma in a Labrador retriever. *Can Vet J* 2004;**45**:860–2.

63. Klein MK, Cockerell GL, Harris CK, et al. Canine primary renal neoplasms: a retrospective review of 54 cases. *J Am Anim Hosp Assoc* 1988;**24**:443–52.

64. Widmer WR, Carlton WW. Persistent hematuria in a dog with renal hemangioma. *J Am Vet Med Assoc* 1990;**197**:237–9.

65. Mott JC, McAnulty JF, Darien DL, et al. Nephron sparing by partial median nephrectomy for treatment of renal hemangioma in a dog. *J Am Vet Med Assoc* 1996;**208**:1274–6.

66. Eddlestone S, Taboada J, Senior D, et al. Renal haemangioma in a dog. *J Small Anim Pract* 1999;**40**:132–5.

67. Weller RE, Stann SE. Renal lymphosarcoma in the cat. *J Am Hosp Assoc* 1983;**19**:363–7.

68. Spies JB, Hricak H, Slemmer TM, et al. Sonographic evaluation of experimental acute renal arterial occlusion in dogs. *AJR Am J Roentgenol* 1984;**142**:341–6.

69. Brown JM, Quedens-Case C, Alderman JL, et al. Contrast enhanced sonography of visceral perfusion defects in dogs. *J Ultrasound Med* 1997;**16**:493–9.

70. Konde LJ, Lebel JL, Park RD, et al. Sonographic application in the diagnosis of intraabdominal abscess in the dog. *Vet Radiol* 1986;**27**:151–4.

71. Hess RS, Ilan I. Renal abscess in a dog with transient diabetes mellitus. *J Small Anim Pract* 2003;**44**:13–16.

72. Nyland TG, Park RD, Lattimer JC, et al. Gray-scale ultrasonography of the canine abdomen. *Vet Radiol* 1981;**22**:220–7.

73. Felkai C, Voros K, Fenyves B. Lesions of the renal pelvis and proximal ureter in various nephro-urological conditions: an ultrasonographic study. *Vet Radiol Ultrasound* 1995;**36**:397–401.

74. Biller DS, Schenkman DI, Bortnowski H. Ultrasonic appearance of renal infarcts in a dog. *J Am Anim Hosp Assoc* 1991;**27**:370–2.

75. Adams WH, Toal RL, Walker MA, et al. Early renal ultrasonographic findings in dogs with experimentally induced ethylene glycol nephrosis. *Am J Vet Res* 1989;**50**:1370–6.

76. Adams WH, Toal RL, Breider MA. Ultrasonographic findings in dogs and cats with oxalate nephrosis attributed to ethylene glycol intoxication: 15 cases (1984-1988). *J Am Vet Med Assoc* 1991;**199**:492–6.

77. Forrest LJ, O'Brien RT, Tremelling MS, et al. Sonographic renal findings in 20 dogs with leptospirosis. *Vet Radiol Ultrasound* 1998;**39**:337–40.

78. Adin CA, Cowgill LD. Treatment and outcome of dogs with leptospirosis: 36 cases (1990-1998). *J Am Vet Med Assoc* 2000;**216**:371–5.

79. Barr FJ, Patteson MW, Lucke VM, et al. Hypercalcemic nephropathy in 3 dogs: sonographic appearance. *Vet Radiol* 1989;**30**:169–73.

80. Biller DS, Bradley GA, Partington BP. Renal medullary rim sign: ultrasonographic evidence of renal disease. *Vet Radiol Ultrasound* 1992;**33**:286–90.

81. Mantis P, Lamb CR. Most dogs with medullary rim sign on ultrasonography have no demonstrable renal dysfunction. *Vet Radiol Ultrasound* 2000;**41**:164–6.

82. Adams WH, Toal RL, Breider MA. Ultrasonographic findings in ethylene glycol (antifreeze) poisoning in a pregnant queen and 4 fetal kittens. *Vet Radiol* 1991;**32**:60–2.

83. Chandler ML, Elwood C, Murphy KF, et al. Juvenile nephropathy in 37 boxer dogs. *J Small Anim Pract* 2007;**48**:690–4.

84. Seiler GS, Rhodes J, Cianciolo R, et al. Ultrasonographic findings in Cairn terriers with preclinical renal dysplasia. *Vet Radiol Ultrasound* 2010;**51**:453–7.

85. D'Anjou MA, Bedard A, Dunn ME. Clinical significance of renal pelvic dilation in dogs and cats. *Vet Radiol Ultrasound* 2001;**52**:88–94.

86. Lamb CR. Acquired ureterovaginal fistula secondary to ovariohysterectomy in a dog: diagnosis using ultrasound-guided nephropyelocentesis and antegrade ureterography. *Vet Radiol Ultrasound* 1994;**35**:201–3.

87. Rivers BJ, Walter PA, Polzin DJ. Ultrasonographic-guided, percutaneous antegrade pyelography: technique and clinical application in the dog and cat. *J Am Anim Hosp Assoc* 1997;**33**:61–8.

88. Szatmari V, Osi Z, Manczur F. Ultrasound-guided percutaneous drainage for treatment of pyonephrosis in two dogs. *J Am Vet Med Assoc* 2001;**218**:1796–9, 1778–99.

89. Middleton WD, Kurtz AB, Hertzberg BS. *Kidney*. Ultrasound: the requisites. 2nd ed. St. Louis: Mosby; 2004. p. 103–51.

90. Neuwirth L, Kuperus JH, Calderwoodmays M, et al. Comparative study of indium-111 leukocytes and nephrosonography for detection of experimental pyelonephritis in dogs. *Vet Radiol Ultrasound* 1995;**36**:253–8.

91. Hylands R. Veterinary diagnostic imaging. Retroperitoneal abscess and regional cellulitis secondary to a pyelonephritis within the left kidney. *Can Vet J* 2006;**47**:1033–5.

92. Leveille R, Biller DS, Partington BP, et al. Sonographic investigation of transitional cell carcinoma of the urinary bladder in small animals. *Vet Radiol Ultrasound* 1992;**33**:103–7.

93. Choi J, Jang J, Choi H, et al. Ultrasound features of pyonephrosis in dogs. *Vet Radiol Ultrasound* 2010;**51**:548–53.

94. Hanson JA, Tidwell AS. Ultrasonographic appearance of urethral transitional cell carcinoma in ten dogs. *Vet Radiol Ultrasound* 1996;**37**:293–9.

95. Winter MD, Locke JE, Penninck DG. Imaging diagnosis—urinary obstruction secondary to prostatic lymphoma in a young dog. *Vet Radiol Ultrasound* 2006;**47**:597–601.

96. Benigni L, Lamb CR, Corzo-Menendez N, et al. Lymphoma affecting the urinary bladder in three dogs and a cat. *Vet Radiol Ultrasound* 2006;**47**:592–6.

97. Leib MS, Allen TA, Konde LJ, et al. Bilateral hydronephrosis attributable to bilateral ureteral fibrosis in a cat. *J Am Vet Med Assoc* 1988;**192**:795–7.

98. Fox LE, Ackerman N, Buergelt CD. Urinary obstruction secondary to a retroperitoneal carcinoma in a dog. *Vet Radiol Ultrasound* 1993;**34**:181–4.

99. Armbrust L, Kraft SL, Cowan LA, et al. Radiographic diagnosis: canine ureteral calculus. *Vet Radiol Ultrasound* 1997;**38**:360–2.

100. Moon ML, Dallman MA. Calcium oxalate ureterolith in a cat. *Vet Radiol* 1991;**32**:261–3.

101. Reichle JK, Peterson RA 2nd, Mahaffey MB, et al. Ureteral fibroepithelial polyps in four dogs. *Vet Radiol Ultrasound* 2003;**44**:433–7.

102. Kyles AE, Hardie EM, Wooden BG, et al. Clinical, clinicopathologic, radiographic, and ultrasonographic abnormalities in cats with ureteral calculi: 163 cases (1984-2002). *J Am Vet Med Assoc* 2005;**226**:932–6.

103. Dalby AM, Adams LG, Salisbury SK, et al. Spontaneous retrograde movement of ureteroliths in two dogs and five cats. *J Am Vet Med Assoc* 2006;**229**:1118–21.

104. Liska WD, Patnaik AK. Leiomyoma of the ureter of the dog. *J Am Anim Hosp Assoc* 1977;**13**:83–4.

105. Berzon JL. Primary leiomyosarcoma of the ureter in a dog: clinical reports. *J Am Vet Med Assoc* 1979;**175**:374–6.

106. Hanika C, Rebar AH. Ureteral transitional cell carcinoma in a dog. *Vet Pathol* 1980;**17**:643–6.

107. Hattel AL, Diters RW, Snavely DA. Ureteral fibropapilloma in a dog. *J Am Vet Med Assoc* 1986;**188**:873.

108. Deschamps JY, Roux FA, Fantinato M, et al. Ureteral sarcoma in a dog. *J Small Anim Pract* 2007;**48**:699–701.

109. Ragone JM, Allen HS. What is your diagnosis? Ureteral calculus. *J Am Vet Med Assoc* 2005;**226**:35–6.

110. Ragni RA, Fews D. Ureteral obstruction and hydronephrosis in a cat associated with retroperitoneal infarction. *J Feline Med Surg* 2008;**10**:259–63.

111. Tidwell AS, Ullman SL, Schelling SH. Urinoma (para-ureteral pseudocyst) in a dog. *Vet Radiol* 1990;**31**:203–6.

112. Moores AP, Bell AM, Costello M. Urinoma (para-ureteral pseudocyst) as a consequence of trauma in a cat. *J Small Anim Pract* 2002;**43**:213–16.

113. Lamb CR, Gregory SP. Ultrasonography of the ureterovesicular junction in the dog: a preliminary report. *Vet Rec* 1994;**134**:36–8.

114. Lamb CR. Ultrasonography of the ureters. *Vet Clin North Am Small Anim Pract* 1998;**28**:823–48.

115. Adin CA, Herrgesell EJ, Nyland TG, et al. Antegrade pyelography for suspected ureteral obstruction in cats: 11 cases (1995-2001). *J Am Vet Med Assoc* 2003;**222**:1576–81.

116. Biller DS, Kantrowitz B, Partington BP, et al. Diagnostic ultrasound of the urinary bladder. *J Am Anim Hosp Assoc* 1990;**26**:397–402.

117. Lamb CR, Gregory SP. Ultrasonographic findings in 14 dogs with ectopic ureter. *Vet Radiol Ultrasound* 1998;**39**:218–23.

118. Stiffler KS, Stevenson MA, Mahaffey MB, et al. Intravesical ureterocele with concurrent renal dysfunction in a dog: a case report and proposed classification system. *J Am Anim Hosp Assoc* 2002;**38**:33–9.

119. Ruiz de Gopegui R, Espada Y, Majo N. Bilateral hydroureter and hydronephrosis in a nine-year-old female German shepherd dog. *J Small Anim Pract* 1999;**40**:224–6.

120. Agut A, Laredo FG, Belda E, et al. Left perinephric abscess associated with nephrolithiasis and bladder calculi in a bitch. *Vet Rec* 2004;**154**:562–5.

121. Holloway A, O'Brien R. Perirenal effusion in dogs and cats with acute renal failure. *Vet Radiol Ultrasound* 2007;**48**:574–9.

122. Lulich J, Osborne CA. Changing paradigms in the diagnosis of urolithiasis. *Vet Clin North Am Small Anim Pract* 2009;**39**:79–91.

123. Heng HG, Rohleder JJ, Pressler BM. Comparative sonographic appearance of nephroliths and associated acoustic shadowing artifacts in conventional vs. spatial compound imaging. *Vet Radiol Ultrasound* 2012;**53**:217–20.

124. Louvet A. Twinkling artifact in small animal color-Doppler sonography. *Vet Radiol Ultrasound* 2006;**47**:384–90.

125. Zotti A, Poser H, Chiavegato D. Asymptomatic double ureteral stricture in an 8-month-old Maine Coon cat: an

imaging-based case report. *J Feline Med Surg* 2004;**6**: 371–5.

126. Weisse C, Aronson LR, Drobatz K. Traumatic rupture of the ureter: 10 cases. *J Am Anim Hosp Assoc* 2002;**38**: 188–92.

127. Vandenbergh AG, Voorhout G, van Sluijs FJ, et al. Haemorrhage from a canine adrenocortical tumour: a clinical emergency. *Vet Rec* 1992;**131**:539–40.

128. Whittemore JC, Preston CA, Kyles AE, et al. Nontraumatic rupture of an adrenal gland tumor causing intraabdominal or retroperitoneal hemorrhage in four dogs. *J Am Vet Med Assoc* 2001;**219**:329–33, 324.

129. Lucy RJ. What is your diagnosis? Perirenal abscess and pyelonephritis. *J Small Anim Pract* 2003;**44**(55):90.

130. Zatelli A, D'Ippolito P. Bilateral perirenal abscesses in a domestic neutered shorthair cat. *J Vet Intern Med* 2004;**18**:902–3.

131. Liptak JM, Dernell WS, Ehrhart EJ, et al. Retroperitoneal sarcomas in dogs: 14 cases (1992-2002). *J Am Vet Med Assoc* 2004;**224**:1471–7.

132. Jones JC, Rossmeisl JH, Waldron DR, et al. Retroperitoneal hemangiosarcoma causing chronic hindlimb lameness in a dog. *Vet Comp Orthop Traumatol* 2007;**20**: 335–9.

133. Bae IH, Kim Y, Pakhrin B, et al. Genitourinary rhabdomyosarcoma with systemic metastasis in a young dog. *Vet Pathol* 2007;**44**:518–20.

134. HyeYeon L, JinHwa C, JooHyun J, et al. Unilateral renal subcapsular abscess associated with pyelonephritis in a cat. *J Vet Clin* 2010;**27**:79–82.

135. Nyland TG, Fisher PE, Gregory CR, et al. Ultrasonographic evaluation of renal size in dogs with acute allograft rejection. *Vet Radiol Ultrasound* 1997;**38**: 55–61.

136. Valdes-Martinez A, Cianciolo R, Mai W. Association between renal hypoechoic subcapsular thickening and lymphosarcoma in cats. *Vet Radiol Ultrasound* 2007;**48**: 357–60.

137. Abinoor DJ. Perinephric pseudocysts in a cat. *J Am Anim Hosp Assoc* 1980;**16**:763–7.

138. Miles KG, Jergens AE. Unilateral perinephric pseudocyst of undetermined origin in a dog. *Vet Radiol Ultrasound* 1992;**33**:277–81.

139. Ochoa VB, DiBartola SP, Chew DJ, et al. Perinephric pseudocysts in the cat: a retrospective study and review of the literature. *J Vet Intern Med* 1999;**13**:47–55.

140. Hill TP, Odesnik BJ. Omentalisation of perinephric pseudocysts in a cat. *J Small Anim Pract* 2000;**41**:115–18.

141. Essman SC, Drost WT, Hoover JP, et al. Imaging of a cat with perirenal pseudocysts. *Vet Radiol Ultrasound* 2000;**41**:329–34.

142. Beck JA, Bellenger CR, Lamb WA, et al. Perirenal pseudocysts in 26 cats. *Aust Vet J* 2000;**78**:166–71.

143. Rishniw M, Weidman J, Hornof WJ. Hydrothorax secondary to a perinephric pseudocyst in a cat. *Vet Radiol Ultrasound* 1998;**39**:193–6.

144. Carvalho CF, Chammas MC. Normal Doppler velocimetry of renal vasculature in Persian cats. *J Feline Med Surg* 2011;**13**:399–404.

145. Rivers BJ, Walter PA, Letourneau JG, et al. Duplex Doppler estimation of resistive index in arcuate arteries of sedated, normal female dogs: implications for use in the diagnosis of renal failure. *J Am Anim Hosp Assoc* 1997;**33**:69–76.

146. Novellas R, Ruiz de Gopegui R, Espada Y. Effects of sedation with midazolam and butorphanol on resistive and pulsatility indices in healthy dogs. *Vet Radiol Ultrasound* 2007;**48**:276–80.

147. Hricak H, Sandler MA, Madrazo BL, et al. Sonographic manifestations of acute renal vein thrombosis: an experimental study. *Invest Radiol* 1981;**16**:30–5.

148. Platt JF, Ellis JH, Rubin JM, et al. Intrarenal arterial Doppler sonography in patients with nonobstructive renal disease: correlation of resistive index with biopsy findings. *AJR Am J Roentgenol* 1990;**154**:1223–7.

149. Parvey HR, Eisenberg RL. Image-directed Doppler sonography of the intrarenal arteries in acute renal vein thrombosis. *J Clin Ultrasound* 1990;**18**:512–16.

150. Barber-Riley P, Patel AS. Ultrasonic demonstration of renal artery thrombosis. *Br J Radiol* 1981;**54**:351–2.

151. Erwin BC, Carroll BA, Walter JF, et al. Renal infarction appearing as an echogenic mass. *AJR Am J Roentgenol* 1982;**138**:759–61.

152. Wong SN, Lo RN, Yu EC. Renal blood flow pattern by noninvasive Doppler ultrasound in normal children and acute renal failure patients. *J Ultrasound Med* 1989;**8**: 135–41.

153. Morrow KL, Salman MD, Lappin MR, et al. Comparison of the resistive index to clinical parameters in dogs with renal disease. *Vet Radiol Ultrasound* 1996;**37**: 193–9.

154. Pozniak MA, Kelcz F, D'Alessandro A, et al. Sonography of renal transplants in dogs: the effect of acute tubular necrosis, cyclosporine nephrotoxicity, and acute rejection on resistive index and renal length. *AJR Am J Roentgenol* 1992;**158**:791–7.

155. Rivers BJ, Walter PA, Polzin DJ, et al. Duplex doppler estimation of intrarenal pourcelot resistive index in dogs and cats with renal disease. *J Vet Intern Med* 1997;**11**: 250–60.

156. Rivers BJ, Walter PA, Letourneau JG, et al. Estimation of arcuate artery resistive index as a diagnostic tool for aminoglycoside-induced acute renal failure in dogs. *Am J Vet Res* 1996;**57**:1536–44.

157. Platt JF, Rubin JM, Ellis JH, et al. Duplex Doppler US of the kidney: differentiation of obstructive from nonobstructive dilatation. *Radiology* 1989;**171**:515–17.

158. Dodd GD 3rd, Kaufman PN, Bracken RB. Renal arterial duplex Doppler ultrasound in dogs with urinary obstruction. *J Urol* 1991;**145**:644–6.

159. Nyland TG, Fisher PE, Doverspike M, et al. Diagnosis of urinary tract obstruction in dogs using duplex doppler ultrasonography. *Vet Radiol Ultrasound* 1993;**34**: 348–52.

160. Ulrich JC, York JP, Koff SA. The renal vascular response to acutely elevated intrapelvic pressure: resistive index measurements in experimental urinary obstruction. *J Urol* 1995;**154**:1202–4.

161. Choi H, Won S, Chung W, et al. Effect of intravenous mannitol upon the resistive index in complete unilateral renal obstruction in dogs. *J Vet Intern Med* 2003;**17**: 158–62.

162. Bude RO, DiPietro MA, Platt JF, et al. Effect of furosemide and intravenous normal saline fluid load upon the renal resistive index in nonobstructed kidneys in children. *J Urol* 1994;**151**:438–41.

163. Shokeir AA, Nijman RJ, el Azab M, et al. Partial ureteral obstruction: effect of intravenous normal saline and furosemide upon the renal resistive index. *J Urol* 1997; **157**:1074–7.

164. Yokoyama H, Tsuji Y. Diuretic Doppler ultrasonography in chronic unilateral partial ureteric obstruction in dogs. *BJU Int* 2002;**90**:100–4.

165. Kurjak A, Zalud I, Alfirevic Z. Evaluation of adnexal masses with transvaginal color ultrasound. *J Ultrasound Med* 1991;**10**:295–7.

166. Angeid-Backman E, Coleman BG, Arger PH, et al. Comparison of resistive index versus pulsatility index in assessing the benign etiology of adnexal masses. *Clin Imaging* 1998;**22**:284–91.
167. Ueland FR, DePriest PD, Pavlik EJ, et al. Preoperative differentiation of malignant from benign ovarian tumors: the efficacy of morphology indexing and Doppler flow sonography. *Gynecol Oncol* 2003;**91**:46–50.
168. Pallwein L, Mitterberger M, Aigner F, et al. Small renal masses: the value of contrast-enhanced colour Doppler imaging. *BJU Int* 2007;**99**:579–85.
169. Ramos IM, Taylor KJ, Kier R, et al. Tumor vascular signals in renal masses: detection with Doppler US. *Radiology* 1988;**168**:633–7.
170. Jinzaki M, Ohkuma K, Tanimoto A, et al. Small solid renal lesions: usefulness of power Doppler US. *Radiology* 1998;**209**:543–50.
171. Koch J, Jensen AL, Wenck A, et al. Duplex Doppler measurements of renal blood flow in a dog with Addison's disease. *J Small Anim Pract* 1997;**38**:124–6.
172. Newell SM, Ellison GW, Graham JP, et al. Scintigraphic, sonographic, and histologic evaluation of renal autotransplantation in cats. *Am J Vet Res* 1999;**60**:775–9.
173. Halling KB, Graham JP, Newell SP, et al. Sonographic and scintigraphic evaluation of acute renal allograft rejection in cats. *Vet Radiol Ultrasound* 2003;**44**:707–13.
174. Pozniak MA, Dodd GD 3rd, Kelcz F. Ultrasonographic evaluation of renal transplantation. *Radiol Clin North Am* 1992;**30**:1053–66.
175. Brown ED, Chen MY, Wolfman NT, et al. Complications of renal transplantation: evaluation with US and radionuclide imaging. *Radiographics* 2000;**20**:607–22.
176. Baxter GM. Ultrasound of renal transplantation. *Clin Radiol* 2001;**56**:802–18.
177. Akbar SA, Jafri SZ, Amendola MA, et al. Complications of renal transplantation. *Radiographics* 2005;**25**:1335–56.
178. Friedewald SM, Molmenti EP, Friedewald JJ, et al. Vascular and nonvascular complications of renal transplants: sonographic evaluation and correlation with other imaging modalities, surgery, and pathology. *J Clin Ultrasound* 2005;**33**:127–39.
179. Schmiedt CW, Delaney FA, McAnulty JF. Ultrasonographic determination of resistive index and graft size for evaluating clinical feline renal allografts. *Vet Radiol Ultrasound* 2008;**49**:73–80.
180. Sandhu C, Patel U. Renal transplantation dysfunction: the role of interventional radiology. *Clin Radiol* 2002;**57**:772–83.
181. Datta R, Sandhu M, Saxena AK, et al. Role of duplex Doppler and power Doppler sonography in transplanted kidneys with acute renal parenchymal dysfunction. *Australas Radiol* 2005;**49**:15–20.
182. Chudek J, Kolonko A, Krol R, et al. The intrarenal vascular resistance parameters measured by duplex Doppler ultrasound shortly after kidney transplantation in patients with immediate, slow, and delayed graft function. *Transplant Proc* 2006;**38**:42–5.
183. Hricak H, Toledo-Pereyra LH, Eyler WR, et al. Evaluation of acute post-transplant renal failure by ultrasound. *Radiology* 1979;**133**:443–7.
184. Griffin JF, McNicholas MM. Morphological appearance of renal allografts in transplant failure. *J Clin Ultrasound* 1992;**20**:529–37.
185. Hilborn MD, Bude RO, Murphy KJ, et al. Renal transplant evaluation with power Doppler sonography. *Br J Radiol* 1997;**70**:39–42.
186. Sidhu MK, Gambhir S, Jeffrey RB Jr, et al. Power Doppler imaging of acute renal transplant rejection. *J Clin Ultrasound* 1999;**27**:171–5.
187. Baxter GM, Morley P, Dall B. Acute renal vein thrombosis in renal allografts: new Doppler ultrasonic findings. *Clin Radiol* 1991;**43**:125–7.
188. Dodd GD 3rd, Tublin ME, Shah A, et al. Imaging of vascular complications associated with renal transplants. *AJR Am J Roentgenol* 1991;**157**:449–59.
189. Grenier N, Douws C, Morel D, et al. Detection of vascular complications in renal allografts with color Doppler flow imaging. *Radiology* 1991;**178**:217–23.
190. Ojo AO, Hanson JA, Wolfe RA, et al. Dialysis modality and the risk of allograft thrombosis in adult renal transplant recipients. *Kidney Int* 1999;**55**:1952–60.
191. Silver TM, Campbell D, Wicks JD, et al. Peritransplant fluid collections. *Radiology* 1981;**138**:145–51.
192. Letourneau JG, Day DL, Ascher NL, et al. Imaging of renal transplants. *AJR Am J Roentgenol* 1988;**150**:833–8.
193. Genkins SM, Sanfilippo FP, Carroll BA. Duplex Doppler sonography of renal transplants: lack of sensitivity and specificity in establishing pathologic diagnosis [see comments]. *AJR Am J Roentgenol* 1989;**152**:535–9.
194. Kelcz F, Pozniak MA, Pirsch JD, et al. Pyramidal appearance and resistive index: insensitive and nonspecific sonographic indicators of renal transplant rejection [see comments]. *AJR Am J Roentgenol* 1990;**155**:531–5.
195. Perrella RR, Duerinckx AJ, Tessler FN, et al. Evaluation of renal transplant dysfunction by duplex Doppler sonography: a prospective study and review of the literature. *Am J Kidney Dis* 1990;**15**:544–50.
196. Berland LL, Lawson TL, Adams MB. Evaluation of canine renal transplants with pulsed Doppler duplex sonography. *J Surg Res* 1985;**39**:433–8.
197. Takahashi S, Narumi Y, Takahara S, et al. Acute renal allograft rejection in the canine: evaluation with serial duplex Doppler ultrasonography. *Transplant Proc* 1999;**31**:1731–4.
198. Leveille R. Ultrasonography of urinary bladder disorders. *Vet Clin North Am Small Anim Pract* 1998;**28**:799–821.
199. Douglass JP. Ultrasound corner: bladder wall mass effect caused by the intramural portion of the canine ureter. *Vet Radiol Ultrasound* 1993;**34**:107.
200. Finn-Bodner ST. The urinary bladder. In: Cartee RE, editor. *Practical veterinary ultrasound*. Philadelphia: Williams & Wilkins; 1995. p. 200–35.
201. Geisse AL, Lowry JE, Schaeffer DJ, et al. Sonographic evaluation of urinary bladder wall thickness in normal dogs. *Vet Radiol Ultrasound* 1997;**38**:132–7.
202. Dubbins PA, Kurtz AB, Darby J, et al. Ureteric jet effect: the echographic appearance of urine entering the bladder. A means of identifying the bladder trigone and assessing ureteral function. *Radiology* 1981;**140**:513–15.
203. Price CI, Adler RS, Rubin JM. Ultrasound detection of differences in density. Explanation of the ureteric jet phenomenon and implications for new ultrasound applications [published erratum appears in *Invest Radiol* 1990 May;25(5):621]. *Invest Radiol* 1989;**24**:876–83.
204. Baker SM, Middleton WD. Color Doppler sonography of ureteral jets in normal volunteers: importance of the relative specific gravity of urine in the ureter and bladder. *AJR Am J Roentgenol* 1992;**159**:773–5.
205. Hanbury DC, Coulden RA, Farman P, et al. Ultrasound cystography in the diagnosis of vesicoureteric reflux. *Br J Urol* 1990;**65**:250–3.

206. Berrocal T, Gaya F, Arjonilla A, et al. Vesicoureteral reflux: diagnosis and grading with echo-enhanced cysto-sonography versus voiding cystourethrography. *Radiology* 2001;**221**:359–65.

207. Allen WE, Webbon PM. Two cases of urinary incontinence in cats associated with acquired vagino-ureteral fistula. *J Small Anim Pract* 1980;**21**:367–71.

208. De Baerdemaecker GC. Post spaying vaginal discharge in a bitch caused by acquired vaginoureteral fistula. *Vet Rec* 1984;**115**:62.

209. Banks SE, Fleming IR, Browning TN. Urinary incontinence in a bitch caused by vaginoureteral fistulation. *Vet Rec* 1991;**128**:108.

210. Hayes HM. Breed associations of ectopic ureter: a study of 217 female cases. *J Small Anim Pract* 1984;**25**:501–4.

211. Grauer GF, Freeman LF, Nelson AW. Urinary incontinence associated with an ectopic ureter in a female cat. *J Am Vet Med Assoc* 1983;**182**:707–8.

212. Rutgers C, Chew DJ, Burt JK. Bilateral ectopic ureters in a female cat without urinary incontinence. *J Am Vet Med Assoc* 1984;**184**:1394–5.

213. Burbidge HM, Jones BR, Mora MT. Ectopic ureter in a male cat. *N Z Vet J* 1989;**37**:123–5.

214. Holt PE, Gibbs C. Congenital urinary incontinence in cats: a review of 19 cases. *Vet Rec* 1992;**130**:437–42.

215. Steffey MA, Brockman DJ. Congenital ectopic ureters in a continent male dog and cat. *J Am Vet Med Assoc* 2004;**224**:1607–10, 1605.

216. Oglesby PA, Carter A. Ultrasonographic diagnosis of unilateral ectopic ureter in a Labrador dog. *J S Afr Vet Assoc* 2003;**74**.84–6.

217. Cannizzo KL, McLoughlin MA, Mattoon JS, et al. Evaluation of transurethral cystoscopy and excretory urography for diagnosis of ectopic ureters in female dogs: 25 cases (1992-2000). *J Am Vet Med Assoc* 2003;**223**:475–81.

218. Samii VF, McLoughlin MA, Mattoon JS, et al. Digital fluoroscopic excretory urography, digital fluoroscopic urethrography, helical computed tomography, and cystoscopy in 24 dogs with suspected ureteral ectopia. *J Vet Intern Med* 2004;**18**:271–81.

219. Takiguchi M, Yasuda J, Ochiai K, et al. Ultrasonographic appearance of orthotopic ureterocele in a dog. *Vet Radiol Ultrasound* 1997;**38**:398–9.

220. Green TA, Arble JB, Chew DJ, et al. Diagnosis and management of ureteroceles in two female dogs. *J Am Anim Hosp Assoc* 2011;**47**:138–44.

221. McLoughlin MA, Hauptman JG, Spaulding K. Classification and management of canine ureteroceles: a case report and literature review. *J Am Anim Hosp Assoc* 1989;**25**:699–706.

222. Janssens LA, Peeters S. Comparisons between stress incontinence in women and sphincter mechanism incompetence in the female dog. *Vet Rec* 1997;**141**:620–5.

223. Atalan G, Holt PE, Barr FJ. Ultrasonographic assessment of bladder neck mobility in continent bitches and bitches with urinary incontinence attributable to urethral sphincter mechanism incompetence. *Am J Vet Res* 1998;**59**:673–9.

224. Dicuio M, Pomara G, Fabris FM, et al. Measurements of urinary bladder volume: comparison of five ultrasound calculation methods in volunteers. *Arch Ital Urol Androl* 2005;**77**:60–2.

225. Roehrborn CG, Peters PC. Can transabdominal ultrasound estimation of postvoiding residual (PVR) replace catheterization? *Urology* 1988;**31**:445–9.

226. Atalan G, Barr FJ, Holt PE. Assessment of urinary bladder volume in dogs by use of linear ultrasonographic measurements. *Am J Vet Res* 1998;**59**:10–15.

227. Atalan G, Barr FJ, Holt PE. Comparison of ultrasonographic and radiographic measurements of bladder dimensions and volume determinations. *Res Vet Sci* 1999;**66**:175–7.

228. Atalan G, Holt PE, Barr FJ. Effect of body position on ultrasonographic estimations of bladder volume. *J Small Anim Pract* 1999;**40**:177–9.

229. Atalan G, Holt PE, Barr FJ. Effect of body position on ultrasonographic estimations of bladder volume [published erratum appears in *J Small Anim Pract* 1999 May;40(5):215]. *J Small Anim Pract* 1999;**40**:177–9.

230. Atalan G, Barr FJ, Holt PE. Frequency of urination and ultrasonographic estimation of residual urine in normal and dysuric dogs. *Res Vet Sci* 1999;**67**:295–9.

231. Atalan G, Parkinson TJ, Barr FJ, et al. Urine volume estimations in dogs recovering from intervertebral disc prolapse surgery. *Berl Munch Tierarztl Wochenschr* 2002;**115**:303–5.

232. Lobetti RG, Goldin JP. Emphysematous cystitis and bladder trigone diverticulum in a dog. *J Small Anim Pract* 1998;**39**:144–7.

233. Adin CA, Chew DJ, Heng HG, et al. Bladder inversion and secondary hematuria in a 6-month-old domestic shorthair cat. *J Am Vet Med Assoc* 2011;**239**:370–3.

234. Voros K, Wladar S, Marsi A, et al. Ultrasonographic study of feline lower urinary tract diseases: 32 cases. *Acta Vet Hung* 1997;**45**:387–95.

235. Martinez I, Mattoon JS, Eaton KA, et al. Polypoid cystitis in 17 dogs (1978-2001). *J Vet Intern Med* 2003;**17**:499–509.

236. Takiguchi M, Inaba M. Diagnostic ultrasound of polypoid cystitis in dogs. *J Vet Med Sci* 2005;**67**:57–61.

237. Root CR, Scott RC. Emphysematous cystitis and other radiographic manifestations of diabetes mellitus in dogs and cats. *J Am Vet Med Assoc* 1971;**158**:721–8.

238. Sherding RG, Chew DJ. Nondiabetic emphysematous cystitis in two dogs. *J Am Vet Med Assoc* 1979;**174**:1105–9.

239. Middleton DJ, Lomas GR. Emphysematous cystitis due to *Clostridium perfringens* in a non-diabetic dog. *J Small Anim Pract* 1979;**20**.433–8.

240. Petite A, Busoni V, Heinen MP, et al. Radiographic and ultrasonographic findings of emphysematous cystitis in four nondiabetic female dogs. *Vet Radiol Ultrasound* 2006;**47**:90–3.

241. Boedec K, le Pastor ML, Lavoue R, et al. Pseudomembranous cystitis, an unusual condition associated with feline urine outflow obstruction: four cases. *J Feline Med Surg* 2011;**13**:588–93.

242. Johnston GR, Walter PA, Feeney DA. Radiographic and ultrasonographic features of uroliths and other urinary tract filling defects. *Vet Clin North Am Small Anim Pract* 1986;**16**:261–92.

243. Weichselbaum RC, Feeney DA, Jessen CR, et al. Urocystolith detection: comparison of survey, contrast radiographic and ultrasonographic techniques in an in vitro bladder phantom. *Vet Radiol Ultrasound* 1999;**40**:386–400.

244. Cherbinsky O, Westropp J, Tinga S, et al. Ultrasonographic features of grass awns in the urinary bladder. *Vet Radio Ultrasound* 2010;**51**:462–5.

245. Norris AM, Laing EJ, Valli VE, et al. Canine bladder and urethral tumors: a retrospective study of 115 cases (1980-1985). *J Vet Intern Med* 1992;**6**:145–53.

246. Crow SE. Urinary tract neoplasms in dogs and cats. *Comp Cont Educ* 1985;**7**:607–18.

247. Knapp DW, Glickman NW, DeNicola DB, et al. Naturally occurring canine transitional cell carcinoma of the urinary bladder. A relevant model of human invasive bladder cancer. *Urol Oncol* 2000;**5**:47–59.

248. Wilson HM, Chun R, Larson VS, et al. Clinical signs, treatments, and outcome in cats with transitional cell carcinoma of the urinary bladder: 20 cases (1990-2004). *J Am Vet Med Assoc* 2007;**231**:101–6.

249. Schwartz PD, Greene RW, Patnaik AK. Urinary bladder tumors in the cat. *J Am Anim Hosp Assoc* 1985;**21**:237–45.

250. Cerf DJ, Lundquist EC. Palliative ultrasound-guided endoscopic diode laser ablation of transitional cell carcinomas of the lower urinary tract in dogs. *J Am Vet Med Assoc* 2012;**240**:51–60.

251. Nyland TG, Wallack ST, Wisner ER. Needle-tract implantation following us-guided fine-needle aspiration biopsy of transitional cell carcinoma of the bladder, urethra, and prostate. *Vet Radiol Ultrasound* 2002;**43**:50–3.

252. Vignoli M, Rossi F, Chierici C, et al. Needle tract implantation after fine needle aspiration biopsy (FNAB) of transitional cell carcinoma of the urinary bladder and adenocarcinoma of the lung. *Schweiz Arch Tierheilkd* 2007;**149**:314–18.

253. Lamb CR, Trower ND, Gregory SP. Ultrasound-guided catheter biopsy of the lower urinary tract: technique and results in 12 dogs. *J Small Anim Pract* 1996;**37**:413–16.

254. Henry CJ. Management of transitional cell carcinoma. *Vet Clin North Am Small Anim Pract* 2003;**33**:597–613.

255. Owen LN. *TNM classification of tumours in domestic animals.* Geneva: World Health Organization; 1980. p. 34.

256. Vallancien G, Veillon B, Charton M, et al. Can transabdominal ultrasonography of the bladder replace cystoscopy in the followup of superficial bladder tumors? *J Urol* 1986;**136**:32–4.

257. Zhang J, Gerst S, Lefkowitz RA, et al. Imaging of bladder cancer. *Radiol Clin North Am* 2007;**45**:183–205.

258. Singer D, Itzchak Y, Fischelovitch Y. Ultrasonographic assessment of bladder tumors. II. Clinical staging. *J Urol* 1981;**126**:34–6.

259. Akdas A, Turkeri L, Ersev D, et al. Transurethral ultrasonography, fiberoptic cystoscopy and bladder washout cytology in the evaluation of bladder tumours. *Int Urol Nephrol* 1992;**24**:503–8.

260. Barentsz JO, Jager GJ, Witjes JA, et al. Primary staging of urinary bladder carcinoma: the role of MRI and a comparison with CT. *Eur Radiol* 1996;**6**:129–33.

261. Barentsz JO, Witjes JA, Ruijs JH. What is new in bladder cancer imaging. *Urol Clin North Am* 1997;**24**:583–602.

262. Reynolds D, Campbell BG. Delayed urethral obstruction after uterine torsion in a pregnant dog. *J Am Anim Hosp Assoc* 2011;**47**:e71–6.

263. Struble AL, Lawson GW, Ling GV. Urethral obstruction in a dog: an unusual presentation of T-cell lymphoma. *J Am Anim Hosp Assoc* 1997;**33**:423–6.

264. Mellanby RJ, Chantrey JC, Baines EA, et al. Urethral haemangiosarcoma in a boxer. *J Small Anim Pract* 2004;**45**:154–6.

265. Tarvin G, Patnaik A, Greene R. Primary urethral tumors in dogs. *J Am Vet Med Assoc* 1978;**172**:931–3.

CHAPTER 17
Prostate and Testes

John S. Mattoon • Thomas G. Nyland

Ultrasonographic study of the prostate and testes is a common diagnostic imaging procedure. Patients may present with clinical signs of lower urinary tract disease (hematuria), urethral discharge, systemic illness, gastrointestinal tract disorders (tenesmus), locomotor disease, and infertility.[1,2] Prostate enlargement or testicular abnormalities found during routine physical examination may warrant further work-up, even without corresponding clinical signs. Blood work, urinalysis, and abdominal and thoracic radiography are additional diagnostic procedures recommended when thorough investigation of the male canine reproductive tract is indicated.

Ultrasonographic evaluation of the prostate and testes allows assessment of anatomy, organ parenchyma, surrounding related structures such as lymph nodes, and distant organs such as the liver. Ultrasound imaging cannot reliably determine the histologic structure of disease processes, nor is it always capable of differentiating neoplastic from inflammatory conditions. Educated diagnoses can still be made, however, when all of the case data are reviewed. Ultrasound-guided aspiration of material for cytologic analysis and culture as well as tissue-core biopsy to obtain specimens for histopathologic examination can be performed easily and safely, often with minimal sedation. The role of ultrasonography in reproductive disease lies therefore in its ability to detect anatomic abnormalities, with the further capability of guiding interventional procedures to procure tissue samples for a more definitive diagnosis.

EXAMINATION TECHNIQUE

High-frequency transducers should be used whenever possible; 7.5- to 10-MHz units are typical. A 5-MHz or lower transducer may not provide sufficient resolution to detect small lesions or subtle parenchymal changes. Imaging the structures within the focal zone of the transducer is important for optimal resolution, regardless of the frequency used. Transabdominal (prepubic) examination is currently the standard in ultrasonography of small animals. Transrectal units are routinely used in reproductive studies of large animals. The advantage of transrectal scanning is enhanced image quality because of the lack of overlying anatomic structures and the ability to optimize the short focal zone. Disadvantages in small animal practice are inconvenience, discomfort of the patient, and necessity of sedation or anesthesia. Transrectal scanning is now the standard for evaluation of the human prostate gland, and its use in the dog has been reported.[3,4] Transrectal ultrasound scanning has been shown to be superior in detecting alterations in canine prostatic parenchymal echogenicity, caudal prostatic lesions, capsular abnormalities, and prostatic

urethral disease but failed to identify cranial lesions that were diagnosed by transabdominal imaging.[4] Transrectal imaging of the prostate may become more commonplace as specialized equipment becomes available to small animal veterinarians.

As a general rule, the ventral abdominal hair coat should be closely clipped. However, the caudoventral abdominal hair of many patients is sparse enough to allow adequate imaging without clipping. This is usually true of the scrotum as well. We avoid clipping the scrotum for most testicular examinations because of potential irritation and resultant self-traumatization. Acoustic gel or alcohol is mandatory to achieve the necessary transducer-patient contact.

The patient is generally placed in dorsal recumbency for a ventral transabdominal approach. Various scanning positions may be used and may be necessary to fully examine a particular structure. Localizing the prostate gland is usually simple. The transducer is placed on the caudoventral abdomen, to one side of the penis or prepuce, cranial to the pubis. Identification of the urinary bladder followed by caudal direction of the scan plane is necessary. Once it is identified, the prostate gland should be carefully scanned in both longitudinal and transverse planes. A dorsal (frontal) plane may be required for access to the prostate if it is within the pelvic inlet. Transrectal imaging is done with the patient in sternal, lateral, or dorsal recumbency. Sedation or general anesthesia is preferred to ensure the patient's comfort and to optimize scanning technique. The transducer must be well lubricated, and a probe sheath should be used. Image planes are transducer dependent (e.g., end-fire, radial 360 degrees, biplanar).

A distended urinary bladder may pull the prostate gland craniad for easier visualization. A small intravenous dose of a diuretic such as furosemide will usually cause the bladder to fill during the examination. The bladder may be filled with sterile saline through catheterization, although this will lead to nonspecular echo formation within the bladder from the presence of microbubbles. Tilting the examination table so that the hind end of the patient is elevated above the head also pulls the prostate gland craniad. Conversely, tilting the table so that the hind end is lower than the head is helpful in distending the trigone of the urinary bladder and the prostatic portion of the urethra, two areas that must be critically evaluated during prostate examination.

Testicular examination is a straightforward procedure. The testes should be scanned in transverse, longitudinal, and dorsal planes. A standoff pad often enhances the study, allowing better near-field structural visualization. Alternatively, one testis may be used as a standoff to image the opposite one. Linear-array transducers work especially well for testicular examinations because of excellent near-field resolution, although the entire testis may not fit within the field of view in larger patients.

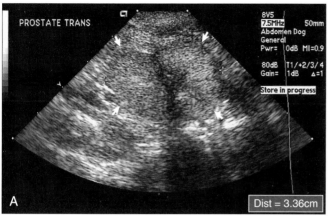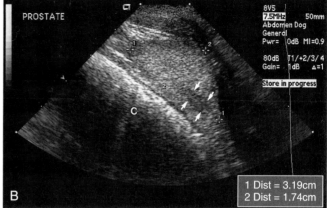

Figure 17-1 Normal prostate in an intact 3-year-old beagle; transverse (**A**) and sagittal (**B**) images. The prostatic parenchyma is echogenic, homogeneous, and finely textured. **A,** The prostate (*white arrows*) is a bilobed gland. The hypoechoic round structure near midline represents the urethra (*red arrows*). A faint hypoechoic peripheral rim can be seen in the ventral prostatic tissue. An acoustic shadow is created by the dorsal indentation and median raphe between the right and left lobes, seen as a hypoechoic, vertically oriented midline structure. The width of the gland is 3.36 cm, denoted by electronic cursors. **B,** The prostate is demarcated by electronic cursors and measures 3.19 cm in length, 1.74 cm in depth. A faint hypoechoic region (*arrows*) represents a portion of the urethra. The highly echogenic linear region dorsal to the prostate is the gas-filled colon (C).

NORMAL PROSTATE GLAND

The prostate gland is the lone accessory sex gland in the canine and is well developed. Pathologic conditions are fairly common in the dog although rarely reported in cats.[1,2,5-8]

The prostate gland surrounds the pelvic urethra, beginning at the level of the trigone of the urinary bladder. The urethra may be eccentrically located dorsally in the gland[9] or course through the center of it.[10] It is bounded cranially by the urinary bladder, ventrally by the floor of the pelvis and abdominal wall, and dorsally by the rectum, from which it is separated by two layers of folded peritoneum (rectogenital space).[9] These layers may be normally joined by fibrous connections.[11] In the transverse plane, it is semioval, flattened dorsally adjacent to the rectum. It is a bilobed structure, separated by a median septum and surrounded by a capsule composed of smooth muscle and fibrous connective tissue.[12] The capsule has septa extending into the parenchyma of the gland, forming lobules of prostatic parenchyma consisting of compound tubuloalveolar glands. The glands secrete serous fluid into the prostatic urethra. The paired ductus deferens course from each epididymis, enter the craniodorsal surface of the prostate gland, and course caudoventrally, entering the prostatic urethra at the colliculus seminalis. Blood supply to the prostate is through paired, dorsally located prostatic arteries, arising from the internal pudendal arteries. Branches off the prostatic arteries penetrate the capsule, become subcapsular, and course deep into the gland along the septa to supply glandular tissue. Venous drainage is provided by the prostatic and urethral veins into the internal iliac veins. Lymphatic drainage from the prostate gland is to the medial iliac and hypogastric lymph nodes.[9]

Ultrasonography of the normal and abnormal canine prostate has been reported.[2,3,10,13-17] It is apparent that the ultrasonographic appearance of the normal prostate varies with age, intact or neutered status, type and quality of the ultrasound equipment, and machine settings. The normal prostate in a young to middle-aged intact dog has a fairly homogeneous parenchymal pattern with a medium to fine texture. Echogenicity is variable, from hyperechoic to hypoechoic, although moderate echogenicity is most common. Prostatic lobules cannot be individually resolved. The bilobed shape of the prostate gland can generally be recognized on the transverse image plane (Figures 17-1, *A*, and 17-2, *B*; see also Figures 17-5, *A*; 17-6, *A*; 17-7 *A*; and 17-8, *A*). It should be smoothly marginated, and a thin hyperechoic rim representing the capsule may be identified. The prostatic urethra can often be imaged; it appears as a hypoechoic to anechoic round structure on midline, within the central, dorsal, or ventral portion of the gland. The prostate is round to oval on sagittal images (Figures 17-3; 17-4; 17-5, *B*; 17-6, *B*; 17-7, *B*; 17-8 *B*; and 17-9; see also Figures 17-1, *B*, and 17-2, *C*). The prostate may be in contact with the trigone of the urinary bladder or be separated from it by a small portion of pelvic urethra. The urethra can often be seen as a hypoechoic round or oval (transverse image) or linear (sagittal image) structure, especially with the use of high-frequency transducers (see Figures 17-1 and 17-2B; and 17-6, *B*; and 17-7 to 17-9). It may course obliquely within the prostate on a sagittal image. Rarely, the ductus deferens can be seen as hypoechoic linear echoes coursing obliquely through the dorsal portion of the gland. Visualization of a dilated urethra or ductus deferens warrants special attention to a potential abnormality. Dorsal to the prostate, the distal colon is often imaged as a hyperechoic linear or curvilinear structure, with acoustic shadowing secondary to colonic gas.

The ultrasound appearance of the canine prostate with histologic correlation has been reported.[18] In this study, prostate glands were harvested and studied in a water bath, an ideal setting. In transverse section, sexually mature prostatic parenchyma had an echogenic butterfly-shaped appearance extending laterally into both lobes, corresponding to collagenous fibers surrounding the ductal system. Dorsal and ventral to this were roughly triangular hypoechoic regions corresponding to glandular tissue. Glandular tissue was also located in the periphery of the prostate, creating a thin hypoechoic

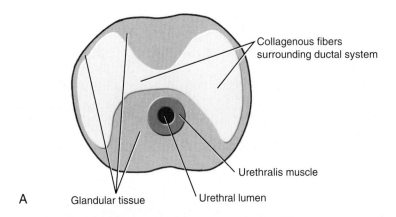

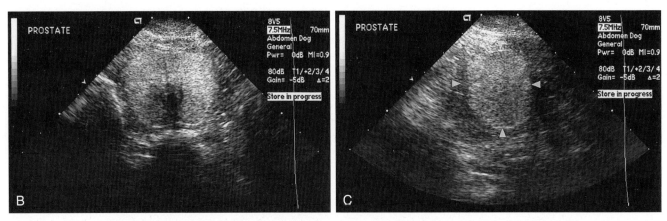

Figure 17-2 Normal prostate in a 10-month-old intact Samoyed, transverse illustration (**A**) and transverse (**B**) and sagittal (**C**) images. **A,** Illustration of a transverse section of the prostate corresponding to **B. B,** Echogenic butterfly-shaped parenchyma extending laterally into both lobes. Between the echogenic parenchyma dorsally and ventrally are hypoechoic regions representing glandular tissue. The prostatic capsule is easily seen along the ventral and dorsal surface but is not clearly defined laterally. **C,** The prostate (*arrowheads*) is nearly round in sagittal section, taken to the left of midline. The parenchyma is fairly homogeneous, finely textured, and echogenic.

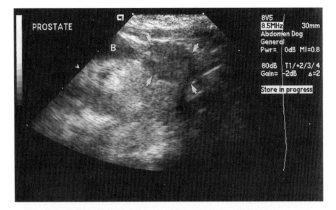

Figure 17-3 **Normal prostate in a 2-month-old intact mixed-breed dog, sagittal image.** The prostate is a small, relatively hypoechoic structure (*arrows*). The trigone of the urinary bladder (*B*) is noted. An 8.5-MHz Vector wide-view array transducer was used.

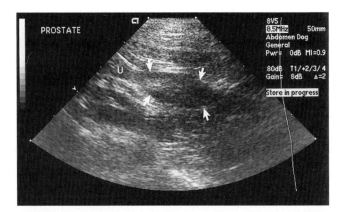

Figure 17-4 Normal prostate in a 9-year-old neutered cocker spaniel, sagittal image. The prostate (*arrows*) is hypoechoic, essentially isoechoic with the surrounding soft tissues. It is small and elongated. A thin hyperechoic capsule is visualized. The pelvic urethra (*U*) just cranial to the prostate is noted.

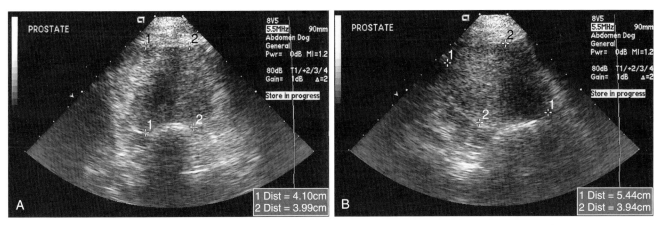

Figure 17-5 Prostate in a 6-year-old intact rottweiler, transverse (A) and sagittal (B) images. The prostate is considered normal for the age and intact status of this patient; it is probable that mild benign hyperplasia is present. A, The prostate has varying echogenicity but is homogeneous, has maintained a normal shape, and is judged to be normal size. The thin echogenic capsular margins are clearly defined ventrally and dorsally. Electronic cursors define height of the left and right prostate lobes. B, The prostate is homogeneous, hypoechoic cranially, and nearly anechoic caudally. It is smooth in shape, and thin echogenic capsular margins are seen. Electronic cursors define the craniocaudal (longitudinal) and ventrodorsal (depth) dimensions.

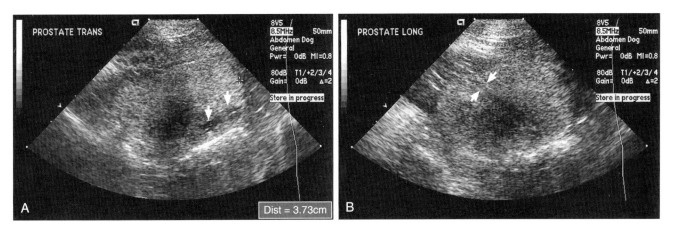

Figure 17-6 Prostate in an 11-year-old intact Shetland sheepdog, transverse (A) and sagittal (B) images. Mild benign prostatic hyperplasia is suspected, given the age and intact status of this patient. A, Normal internal architecture is maintained with hyperechoic and hypoechoic parenchyma. The prostate is smoothly margined. An irregular, nearly anechoic area is present within the left dorsal lobe (arrows), representing coalescing prostatic cysts. Electronic cursors define the width of the prostate (3.73 cm). B, The shape of the prostate on the sagittal image is similar to that on the transverse image, suggesting some enlargement. A portion of the cranial prostatic urethra (arrows) can be seen entering obliquely.

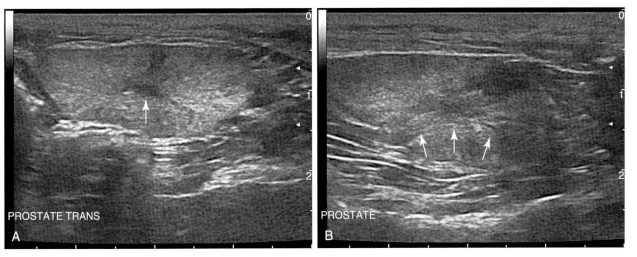

Figure 17-7 Normal prostate in a 1-year-old intact male Pekinese with gastrointestinal signs. A, Transverse image of the normal prostate gland. The urethra can be seen centrally as a hypoechoic structure (arrow). B, Sagittal image of the normal prostate gland, showing an arched urethra (arrows).

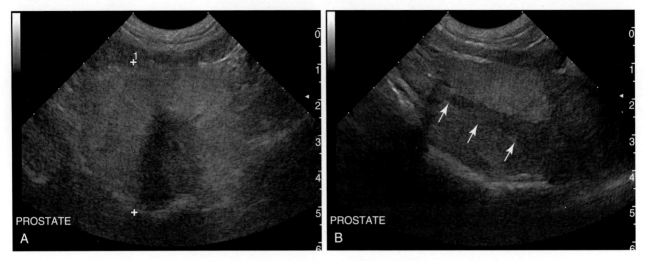

Figure 17-8 **Normal prostate in a 3-year-old male vizsla with a cutaneous mast cell tumor. A,** Transverse image of the prostate gland shows the normal bilobed nature of the gland. The right lobe is 4.20 cm in height (between electronic cursors). The hypoechoic central area represents the urethra and associated attenuation that is often seen in transverse view. **B,** Sagittal view showing the prostatic urethra (*arrows*) centrally in the gland.

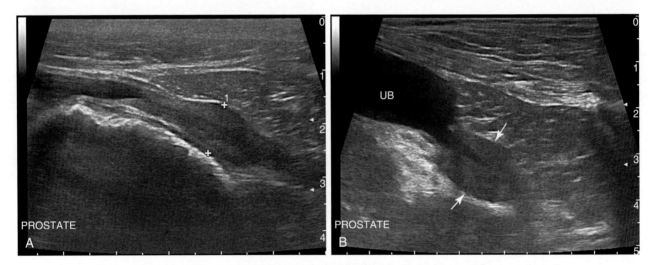

Figure 17-9 **Atrophied prostate gland in neutered male dogs. A,** Sagittal image of a normal small prostate gland in a 2-year-old English setter. The gland is less than 1 cm in height (0.95 cm, between electronic cursors). The hypoechoic urethra can be seen centrally within the gland. The trigone of the urinary bladder is to the left, the hyperechoic colonic wall is directly adjacent in the far field. **B,** Sagittal image of the normal small prostate gland (between arrows) in a neutered 10-year-old English springer spaniel. The urinary bladder (*UB*) is to the left and the prostatic urethra can be seen transitioning from the bladder centrally. This animal was neutered early in life.

rim around the circumference of the prostate. Glandular tissue was noted to be less apparent at the cranial-most extent of the prostate. On sagittal section, there was an oval central area of hyperechogenicity surrounded by hypoechoic tissue, corresponding to collagenous and glandular tissue, respectively. Sexually immature dogs showed diffusely hyperechoic prostate glands, reflecting lack of glandular development and a preponderance of collagen. When seen, the lumen of the prostatic urethra is hypoechoic. Periurethral tissue is hyperechoic because of collagenous tissue, except near the midpoint of the prostatic urethra, where it may be hypoechoic because the prostatic ducts enter the urethra at this level and relatively more glandular tissue is present. A hypoechoic ring surrounds the caudal-most portion of the prostatic urethra, corresponding to the urethralis muscle. In our experience, it is unusual to see this degree of anatomic detail in situ (see Figure 17-2, *B*).

The size and position of the normal canine prostate gland vary with age and with the intact or neutered status of the animal. In sexually immature or neutered dogs, the prostate is much smaller and often has a relatively hypoechoic and homogeneous appearance (see Figures 17-3 and 17-4). The prostate may be difficult to visualize in these patients. The prostate is reported to be within the abdominal cavity at birth until about 2 months of age, when it moves to the pelvic cavity, subsequent to breakdown of the urachal remnant. It enlarges at sexual maturity secondary to hormone influences, becoming progressively more intraabdominal in location.[19,20] The neutered canine has a small prostate gland that rapidly decreases in size after castration in normal dogs. It also decreases in size after hormone therapy and has been studied in this regard by ultrasonography.[21] The size of the normal canine prostate varies with body size and age and perhaps breed; the Scottish terrier has been reported to have a larger prostate than that of other breeds.[20]

Investigators have studied the size of the prostate grossly, radiographically, and with ultrasonography in intact and neutered dogs as well as in vitro.[2,3,13,17,20-28] Studies have shown a positive correlation between prostate size and parameters related to body size and age in intact dogs[24,26] but not in neutered dogs.[26] It has also been shown that there is good correlation between ultrasound-derived prostate measurements, radiographic measurements,[25] and actual prostate measurements.[23,25,26,28]

Determination of prostate size by length (L), depth (height) (D), and width (W) measurements is straightforward with use of electronic cursors. The basic equation used to determine prostate volume (V) is an ellipsoid model (V = $0.524 \times L \times W \times D$). Two investigations have refined prostate volume formulas from multiple regression analyses using ultrasound-derived values compared with actual volume determined by a water displacement method.[26,28] One study[28] using 12 intact adult dogs calculated prostate volume (V) from ultrasound-determined length, width, and depth measurements by the formula V = $[1/2.6 (L \times W \times D)] + 1.8$ (cm^3). In a study of 77 male dogs (17 neutered), prostate volume was determined by the formula $0.487 \times L \times W \times (DL + DT)/2 + 6.38$ (DL, depth on long-axis image; DT, depth on transverse image).[26] This group of dogs included histologically confirmed normal and abnormal prostates (atrophy, hyperplasia, prostatitis, and neoplasia).

Although determining the size and volume of the prostate has been refined, deciding when a particular patient has prostate enlargement is a more difficult question because of body size and age considerations. One investigation addressed this question by studying 100 clinically normal, intact, sexually mature dogs.[24] Multiple regression analyses established formulas for calculation of maximal predicted value of prostate length (L), width (W), height (Hsag, height on sagittal image; and Htr, height on transverse image), and volume (V) based on body weight (BW) in kilograms and age (A) in years:

$$L = (0.055 \times BW) + (0.143 \times A) + 3.31$$

$$W = (0.047 \times BW) + (0.089 \times A) + 3.45$$

$$Hsag = (0.046 \times BW) + (0.069 \times A) + 2.68$$

$$Htr = (0.044 \times BW) + (0.083 \times A) + 2.25$$

$$V = (0.867 \times BW) + (1.885 \times A) + 15.88$$

However, because live animals were studied, it is unknown how many of these prostate glands were normal histologically. Enlarged prostate glands in some of these subjects may have been due to benign prostatic hyperplasia, considered a normal occurrence as intact dogs age.

One study stated that the length (craniocaudal dimension) or depth (ventrodorsal dimension) of the canine prostate should not be larger than 70% of the distance between the sacral promontory and the pubis on a lateral radiograph.[22] Another author stated that the canine prostate should not be larger in diameter than one half to two thirds the width of the pelvic inlet based on a ventrodorsal radiograph.[29] A study compared transabdominal ultrasound measurement of the canine prostate with lateral radiographic assessment.[25] Good agreement of prostate length determination was noted, but significant differences in depth measurement existed.

What these various studies indicate is that the primary value of accurately determining the size of the canine prostate gland is in assessing the resolution or progression of disease. Although recent work in ultrasound determination of prostate size is promising, it is debatable whether ultrasound imaging can accurately assess what is normal or abnormal for a particular patient at that point in time. Prostate enlargement, especially mild enlargement, is still subjective, influenced by palpation and radiographic assessment as well as by ultrasound findings.

Doppler blood flow evaluation of the canine prostate gland has been described.[30] Maximal and minimal velocities and resistive indices were determined for prostatic, capsular, and parenchymal arteries. Prostatic arteries have a spectral waveform characteristic of high-impedance vessels with a sharp, narrow systolic peak and antegrade low diastolic flow. Capsular and parenchymal arteries have lower impedance and lower velocities. The resistive index of prostatic arteries and capsular arterial velocities were significantly lower in dogs sedated with acepromazine than in nonsedated subjects. In this same study, 5 of 16 dogs with normal ultrasound examination findings had chronic lymphocytic-lymphoplasmacytic prostatitis diagnosed on histopathologic evaluation. These dogs had prostatic blood flow characteristics indistinguishable from those of normal dogs. In the future, Doppler characteristics of the canine prostate may be helpful in distinguishing between different disease processes. Currently, Doppler analysis of the canine prostate is primarily used to assess vascularity and blood flow characteristics before biopsy procedures.

Recent studies have evaluated the use of contrast-enhanced color Doppler assessment of the prostate gland.[31-33] Russo and colleagues[31] showed that the prostatic artery could be seen along the dorsolateral surface of the gland, branching into small arteries toward the central prostatic urethra after tunneling through the capsule. Prostatic parenchyma enhanced by 15 seconds after injection of microbubble contrast agent, with homogeneous wash-in and wash-out observed. Bigliardi and co-workers[32] studied 10 normal dogs before and after ultrasound contrast administration. They classified noncontrast Doppler imaging as poorly depicting prostatic blood flow, whereas contrast-enhanced Doppler analysis allowed moderate (3 dogs) or good (7 dogs) blood flow to be observed. Vignoli and associates[33] studied contrast-enhanced ultrasound in normal dogs and in dogs with prostatic disease. They found no significant difference in contrast enhancement between normal prostate glands and benign prostatic disease (hyperplasia and prostatitis). Time to peak contrast intensity (TPI) was 33.6 ± 6.4 seconds with a peak perfusion intensity (PPI) of 14.8% for normal dogs. Interestingly, whereas the small number of malignant prostatic conditions differed from normal values, values higher and lower than normal were observed. They concluded that contrast-enhanced ultrasound may be useful in differentiating benign from malignant prostatic disease.

Radiography of the caudal abdomen is recommended in addition to ultrasound evaluation whenever disease of the prostate is suspected. It may detect mineralization or gas within the prostatic parenchyma; sublumbar lymph node enlargement; reactive bone response of the caudal lumbar vertebrae, pelvis, and femur; and displacement of the urinary bladder or colon. Contrast radiographic studies (cystography, urethrography) are also important adjuncts that can corroborate ultrasonographic findings as well as provide additional information, such as subtle urethral irregularities and prostatic reflux. The role of survey radiographs as well as of special radiographic studies should therefore not be ignored but thought of as complementary.

PATHOLOGY OF THE PROSTATE

Benign Prostatic Hyperplasia

Benign hyperplasia is an enlargement of the prostate gland in which glandular hyperplasia or squamous metaplasia, or both, result from hormone imbalance in intact male dogs.[34] It is a disease of older dogs, usually older than 4 years, and can be considered a variation of normal physiologic manifestations in both dog and man. Prostatic hyperplasia is often an incidental finding on physical examination, but significant enlargement can lead to signs affecting defecation or urination. In some cases, it may lead to clinical signs that are more commonly associated with prostatitis or neoplasia, such as bloody urethral discharge.[35]

The ultrasonographic appearance of benign prostatic hyperplasia may be subtle inhomogeneity of the parenchyma without obvious enlargement (see Figure 17-5). Often, but not always, the prostate is enlarged, in severe cases four times normal size.[34] The enlargement may be symmetric or asymmetric, smooth or nodular, distorting the margin of the gland (Figures 17-10 to 17-14). Diffuse enlargement may cause loss of the normal bilobed appearance of the prostate (see Figures 17-12, *A*, and 17-13, *A*). The margins of the gland should be seen and differentiated from the surrounding tissues. The echogenicity of the gland varies. It may be diffusely homogeneous and hypoechoic to hyperechoic, but some degree of inhomogeneity is noted in most cases. Parenchymal texture varies from smooth to coarse. Scattered hyperechoic foci, thought to be secondary to increased vascularity and

fibrosis, may be present. Mineralization is not typically seen with benign prostatic hyperplasia. Intraparenchymal cysts of varying size and number can be present; these probably represent dilated acini and ducts secondary to hyperplasia (see Figures 17-6 and 17-13, *A*). Pathologic changes resulting in a heterogeneous appearance can make the diagnosis of benign prostatic hypertrophy difficult; differential diagnosis includes inflammation, infection, and neoplasia. As a general consideration, the ultrasonographic changes are usually less severe with benign prostatic hyperplasia than with inflammatory or neoplastic conditions. Hyperplasia should not disrupt the capsule of the prostate gland, nor should there be evidence of sublumbar lymph node enlargement. It is fairly common to find multiple pathologic processes occurring simultaneously, underlining the need for biopsy and culture for a definitive diagnosis. Multiple biopsies of various portions of the gland are recommended. Diminishment of gland size after castration can be monitored with serial ultrasound examinations.

Infection and Inflammation

Bacterial prostatitis can be an acute or chronic condition. A multitude of microorganisms have been cultured. Ascending urinary tract infection or septicemia is a common cause, although descending urinary tract infections or extension from testicular or epididymal disease can occur. A recent report describes an outbreak of *Brucellosis canis* in which it was noted that the prostate gland was a common site of bacterial isolation.[36]

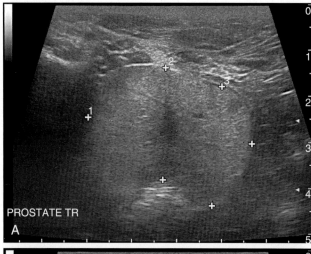

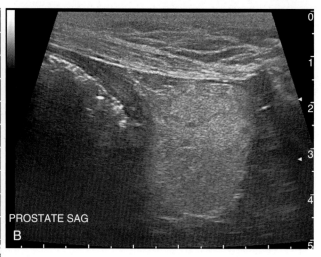

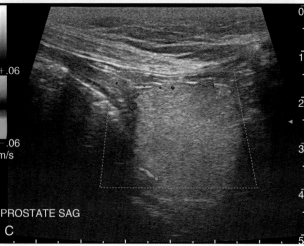

Figure 17-10 **Benign prostatic hyperplasia in a 9-year-old male Welsh Pembroke corgi. A,** Transverse image showing symmetric enlargement of the gland (between electronic cursors). The gland is solid, relatively hyperechoic, and has maintained its bilobed shape. Its margins are clearly demarcated from the surrounding tissues. The prostatic urethra is seen as a hypoechoic central structure. **B,** Sagittal image shows an echogenic, solid appearance of the gland, clearly demarcated from the surrounding tissues. **C,** Color Doppler image of the prostate gland shows peripheral blood flow.

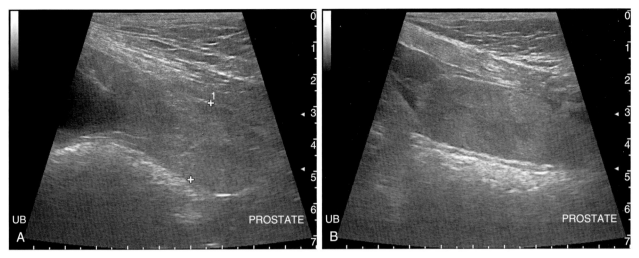

Figure 17-11 **Benign prostatic hyperplasia in a 9-year-old male Labrador retriever with a history of hematuria.** **A,** Sagittal image of the mildly enlarged prostate gland (2.46 cm, between electronic cursors), solid and homogeneous in appearance, with distinct margins. Note how the cranial portion of the gland encroaches on the urinary bladder. **B,** Sagittal image positioned further caudally shows the entire length of the enlarged prostate, over 6 cm long. Histology was diagnostic for prostatic hyperplasia complex with mild lymphoplasmacytic and histiocytic prostatitis.

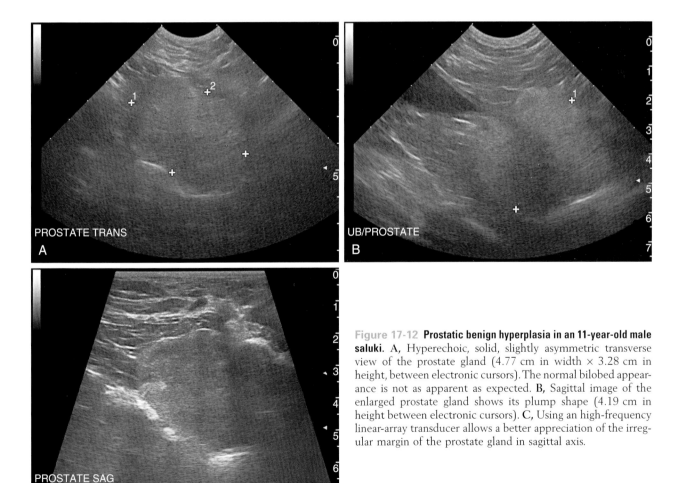

Figure 17-12 **Prostatic benign hyperplasia in an 11-year-old male saluki.** **A,** Hyperechoic, solid, slightly asymmetric transverse view of the prostate gland (4.77 cm in width × 3.28 cm in height, between electronic cursors). The normal bilobed appearance is not as apparent as expected. **B,** Sagittal image of the enlarged prostate gland shows its plump shape (4.19 cm in height between electronic cursors). **C,** Using an high-frequency linear-array transducer allows a better appreciation of the irregular margin of the prostate gland in sagittal axis.

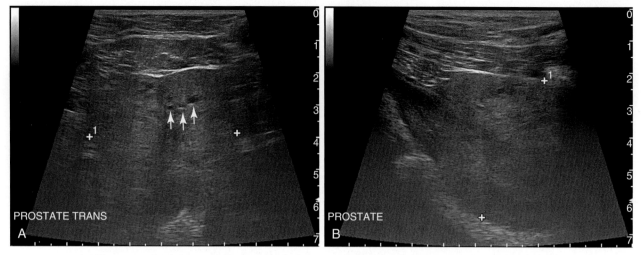

Figure 17-13 **Benign prostatic hyperplasia in an 8-year-old dog. A,** Transverse image shows some asymmetry to the gland (4.68 cm in width, between electronic cursors). There are several small anechoic cysts in the ventral portion of the left lobe (*arrows*). **B,** Sagittal image of the enlarged prostate gland (4.69 cm in height, between electronic cursors). The parenchyma is mildly heterogeneous.

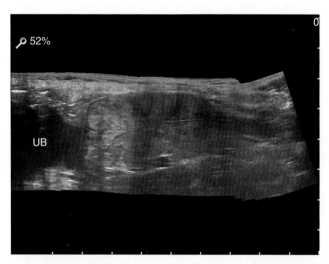

Figure 17-14 **Severe benign prostatic hyperplasia.** This extended field of view image allows excellent appreciation of the abnormal length, shape, margination, and altered internal echogenicity in this intact 9-year-old male Labrador retriever. *UB,* Urinary bladder.

Symmetric or asymmetric enlargement may be present, depending on whether the disease is focal, multifocal, or diffuse. The overall appearance of the parenchyma is usually a heterogeneous, mixed pattern of varying echogenicity (Figures 17-15 to 17-18). Focal or multifocal areas of poorly marginated hypoechogenicity or hyperechogenicity may be present. Variably sized cysts or cystlike structures may be present, including abscesses (Figures 17-19 and 17-20). We have observed abscess formation in which the entire gland filled with pus (Figure 17-21). Foci of intense echo formation may be secondary to fibrosis, gas, or mineralization (see Figure 17-18). The capsule of the gland is usually intact, and it is uncommon to detect anything more than mild lymphadenopathy with inflammation alone. Agut and co-workers[37] reported the formation of a uerthrorectal fistula secondary to

a prostatic abscess, attributed to urolithiasis. Diffuse inflammation may rarely appear homogeneous and may be either hyperechoic or hypoechoic. In this instance, the ultrasonographic appearance of bacterial prostatitis may be similar to that of benign hyperplasia. In a study of Doppler ultrasound characteristics of the canine prostate, 5 of 16 subjects had normal ultrasound examination findings, yet histologically confirmed lymphocytic-lymphoplasmacytic prostatitis was present.[30] This underscores that a definitive diagnosis must be made by aspiration for culture and sensitivity analyses and by biopsy.

Whereas bacterial prostatitis is common, fungal prostatitis is rarely seen but has been reported secondary to blastomycosis[1] and systemic candidiasis[38] in a dog. Granulomatous prostatitis has been described in humans.[39] Prostatomegaly was usually present, with hypoechoic foci of various sizes in all portions of the glands. One patient had a solitary peripheral hypoechoic lesion. These inflammatory lesions are similar to those described in prostatic neoplasia in humans.

Castration appears to be beneficial in the resolution of chronic bacterial prostatitis.[40] Serial ultrasound examinations may be useful in the assessment of prostatic parenchymal lesion resolution and size reduction after neutering. Conversely, if serial examinations do not show improvement, it is possible that an underlying neoplastic process is present.

Neoplasia
Prostatic neoplasia occurs in older, intact dogs of medium to large breeds and has been found to be more common in neutered males.[41-43] Adenocarcinomas and undifferentiated carcinomas are the most common histologic types,[34,44] whereas transitional cell carcinoma (urothelium and ductal rather than acinar epithelium neoplasia) is highest in neutered male dogs.[43] There may also be breed predisposition, suggesting genetic factors play a role in prostatic cancer.[43] Lymphoma of the prostate gland has been reported.[45-46]

Prostatic neoplasia can manifest a plethora of ultrasonographic appearances (Figures 17-22 to 17-26). Typically, the gland is enlarged, is irregular in shape, and has a heterogeneous echo texture. Hyperechoic foci may be dispersed throughout the parenchyma or be confined to focal areas.

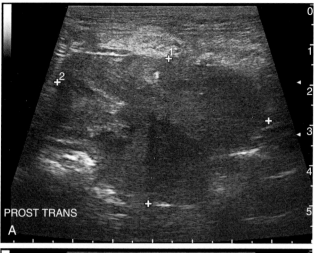

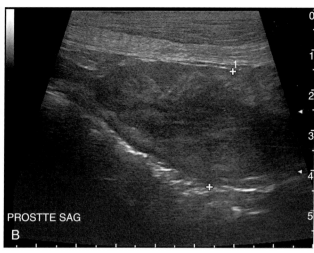

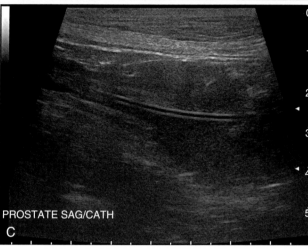

Figure 17-15 **Bacterial prostatitis in an 8-year-old male Siberian husky with difficulty urinating and overall poor health. A,** Transverse image showing irregular enlargement, heterogeneous parenchyma with diminished demarcation from the surrounding tissues (3.63 cm in height × 5.39 cm in width, between electronic cursors). **B,** Sagittal image of the enlarged, heterogeneous prostate gland (2.93 cm in height, between electronic cursors). **C,** Sagittal image showing placement of a urinary catheter. *Staphylococcus* was cultured from the prostate gland, multiple organs, and the blood.

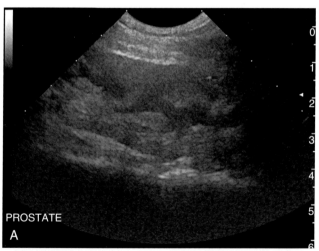

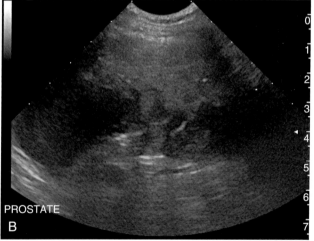

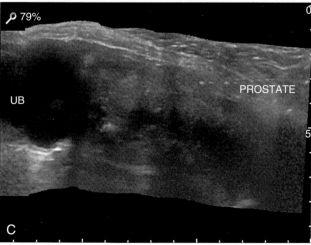

Figure 17-16 **Bacterial prostatitis in an 8-year-old male Labrador retriever. A,** Sagittal image shows an enlarged, irregular prostate gland with very heterogeneous parenchyma. A dilated, tortuous prostatic urethra is present. **B,** Sagittal image shows how the enlarged prostate gland is encroaching on the neck of the urinary bladder. **C,** Sagittal extended field of view image shows the extensive nature of the prostatic enlargement and the overall heterogeneity of the infected parenchyma. *UB,* Urinary bladder.

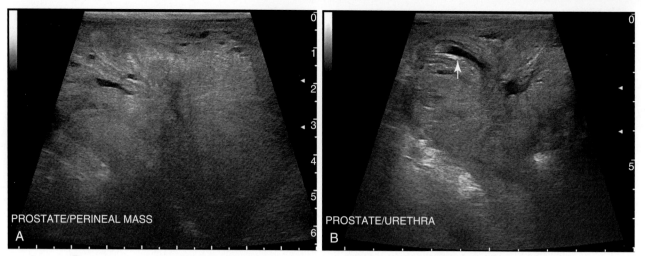

Figure 17-17 **Bacterial prostatitis in a 9-year-old male rottweiler with perineal swelling. A,** Transverse image of a very enlarged, misshapen prostate gland. The gland is fairly solid but several linear to small focal anechoic areas are present, representing dilated ducts and parenchymal cysts or abscesses. **B,** Sagittal image shows an oblique section through the prostatic urethra (*arrow*). Note the periprostatic tissues are indistinct.

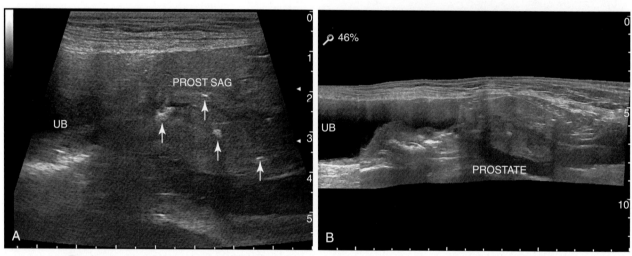

Figure 17-18 **Bacterial prostatitis with mineralization in a 10-year-old male golden retriever. A,** Sagittal image of the heterogeneous prostate gland with multifocal areas of mineralization (*arrows*). **B,** Extended sagittal field of view image. The histologic diagnosis was bacterial prostatitis with osseous metaplasia.

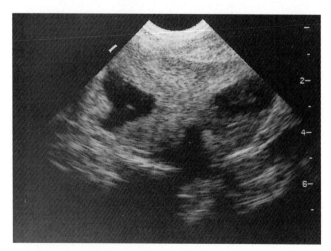

Figure 17-19 **Eight-year-old intact Old English sheepdog, transverse image.** The prostate is enlarged and misshapen. Within the parenchyma are irregularly shaped anechoic to hypoechoic areas that contained pus on aspiration.

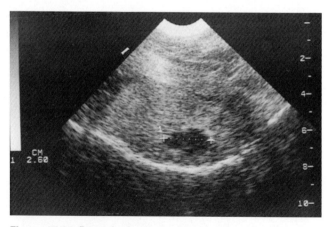

Figure 17-20 **Prostatic abscess in a 6-year-old intact Doberman pinscher, sagittal image.** A focal hypoechoic region (between electronic cursors, 2.6 cm) is present within a markedly enlarged prostate.

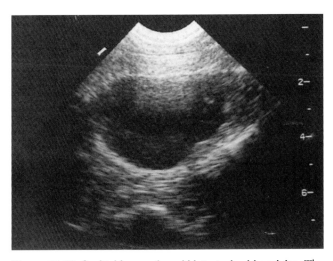

Figure 17-21 Sagittal image of an old intact mixed-breed dog. The margin of the prostate, containing hypoechoic material (pus), is well defined. Virtually the entire prostate gland was abscessed.

Hyperechoic foci with acoustic shadowing representing mineralization may be present. Bradbury and colleagues[47] found that prostatic mineralization in neutered dogs had a 100% positive predictive value for malignancy, whereas intact dogs without prostatic mineralization were unlikely to have prostatic neoplasia. Cavitary, cystlike lesions may be present and vary in size, shape, and number (Figure 17-27). True cystic lesions are probably less common than in benign prostatic hyperplasia and inflammatory disease. Rohleder and Jones[48] reported emphysematous prostatitis in a dog with prostatic carcinoma.

Distinguishing neoplasia from prostatitis can be difficult solely on the basis of ultrasonographic findings, and indeed, both may be present. As with prostatitis, the changes can be severe. However, several important criteria are strongly suggestive of neoplasia. As mentioned previously, mineralization in prostatic disease in neutered dogs is an ominous sign.[47] Extension of pathologic changes to the urethra or neck of the urinary bladder, regional lymph node enlargement, and disruption of the capsule with extension to the surrounding tissues are ominous signs indicating neoplasia. Figure 17-26 is

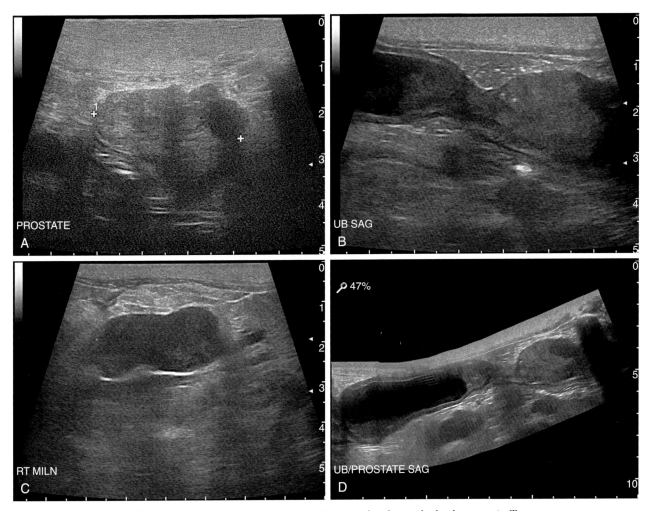

Figure 17-22 Prostatic neoplasia in a 6-year-old neutered male standard schnauzer. A, Transverse image shows asymmetry of the prostate gland and heterogeneity of the parenchyma (3.27 cm in width, between electronic cursors). **B,** Sagittal image shows extensive nature of the disease encroaching into the trigone of the urinary bladder, heterogeneous parenchyma, and multifocal mineralization. **C,** Enlarged metastatic medial iliac lymph node. **D,** Extended field of view image better depicts the extensive nature of the disease.

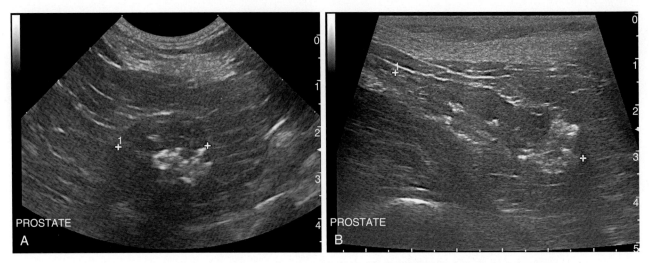

Figure 17-23 Prostatic neoplasia in an 11-year-old neutered mixed-breed dog. A, Transverse image shows an irregular, heterogeneous prostate gland with multifocal mineralization (1.97 cm in width, between electronic cursors). The gland, while small, is larger than expected for a neutered dog. **B,** Sagittal image showing extensive intraparenchymal mineralization and heterogeneity of the gland (4.51 cm in length, between electronic cursors).

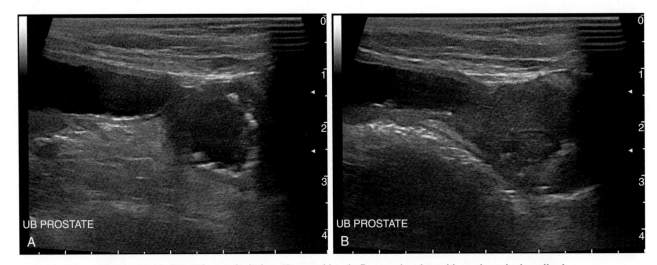

Figure 17-24 Prostatic neoplasia in a 15-year-old male Pomeranian dog with cystic and mineralized components. A, Sagittal image showing a large cystic component to one lobe of the gland, lined with mineralization. **B,** Sagittal image of the opposite lobe showing its solid nature, with several tiny mineralized foci evident. On both images the urinary bladder is seen to the left.

an example of hydroureter and hydronephrosis secondary to prostatic tumor invasion of the urinary bladder trigone. Prostatic neoplasms have a high rate of metastasis to regional lymph nodes (see Figure 17-22, C) and bony structures, lungs, and distant bony sites.[41,44,49,50] Shor and colleagues[51] reported an epithelioid hemangiosarcoma that mimicked metastatic prostatic neoplasia. Whereas the majority of prostatic neoplasms are malignant, a benign tumor occupying one lobe of the prostate has been reported.[52] Biopsy should be used to confirm the diagnosis.[53] We routinely sample multiple sites because more than one disease process may be occurring. However, it has been reported that seeding of neoplastic cells along the needle tract can occur, although rare.[54] In men, reports have suggested the benefit of random biopsies of the prostate in addition to sampling of the focal lesions.[55]

Cysts

Prostatic cysts have been described in the preceding accounts of hyperplasia, prostatitis, and neoplasia. They may be developmental or congenital; in the dog, they are classified into cysts associated with prostatic hypertrophy or squamous metaplasia, retention cysts, and paraprostatic cysts.[34] In our experience, prostatic cysts are often identified as an incidental finding in intact dogs. This has been documented by others as well.[24,56] Aspiration revealed that approximately half of the cysts found incidentally were infected, however.[56] True cysts are characterized by anechoic contents surrounded by a thin hyperechoic wall with distal acoustic enhancement (Figure 17-28, *B*). Prostatic cysts vary in size and number. A solitary cyst originating from the right prostate lobe became large enough to obstruct the ureters and cause hydronephrosis

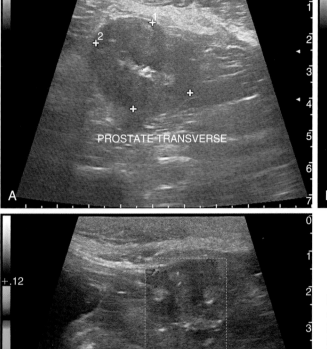

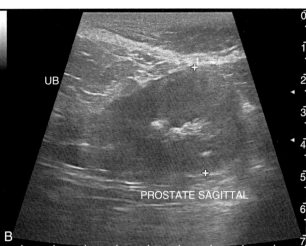

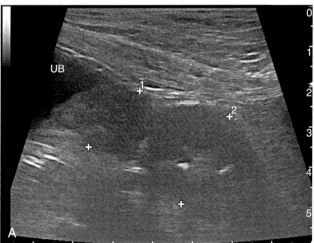

Figure 17-25 **Prostatic neoplasia in a 9-year-old neutered male chow chow.** **A,** Transverse image shows an irregular gland with heterogeneous, solid parenchyma and mineralization (2.75 cm in height × 3.34 cm in width, between electronic cursors). **B,** Sagittal image (3.30 cm in height, between electronic cursors). **C,** Sagittal color Doppler image.

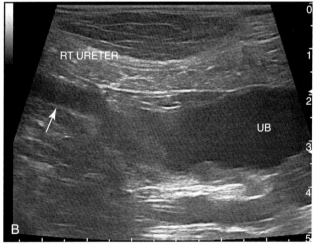

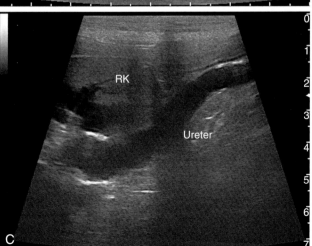

Figure 17-26 **Prostatic carcinoma with ureteral obstruction in an 11-year-old neutered male Labrador retriever.** **A,** Sagittal image of the neoplastic prostate gland (1.89 cm and 2.48 cm, between electronic cursors). It is overall hypoechoic and contains several foci of mineralization. *UB,* Urinary bladder. **B,** Sagittal image showing the enlarged right ureter (*RT URETER, arrow*) as it nears the urinary bladder (*UB*). **C,** Sagittal image of right hydronephrosis (*RK*) and hydroureter (*Ureter*) secondary to blockage by prostatic tumor extension into the trigone of the urinary bladder.

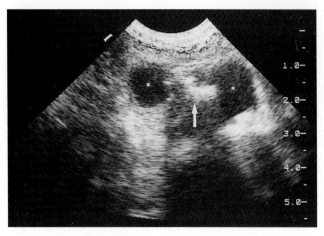

Figure 17-27 Prostatic adenocarcinoma in a neutered old mixed-breed dog, transverse image. Two large anechoic to hypoechoic cystlike structures are present (*asterisks*), irregular in shape. Strong acoustic enhancement is present. Multiple hyperechoic foci (*arrow*) are present within the central portion of the gland, with evidence of acoustic shadowing. Aspiration of the anechoic areas yielded nondiagnostic fluid; adenocarcinoma was the biopsy diagnosis.

(Figure 17-29). If cysts are very small and numerous, they can render the prostatic parenchyma diffusely hyperechoic.

A study in humans showed that prostatic cystic lesions were associated with benign prostatic hypertrophy, inflammation (abscesses), and anatomic variants (Müllerian duct remnants), ranging in size from 2 to 30 mm.[57] Cysts related to previous biopsy were also reported. Size of the cysts increased with the severity of benign prostatic hypertrophy. Abscesses contained inhomogeneous echogenic material, pathologically correlated with inflamed tissue, pus, and debris.

Paraprostatic Cysts
Paraprostatic cysts are not uncommon. They are thought to originate from embryological remnants of müllerian ducts or as extensions from a prostate lobe.[34] They may be attached to the prostate by a thin stalk, or broad fibrous adhesions may be present. Communication directly with the prostate gland and urethra can occur. The "double bladder" sign, in which there appear to be two urinary bladders present in addition to the prostate gland, may be seen radiographically. Indeed, these cysts can become large, dominating the caudal abdomen and sometimes extending into the pelvic canal. On occasion, paraprostatic cysts may be bilobed structures.

The radiologic and ultrasonographic appearances of paraprostatic cysts in dogs have been discussed.[58,59] The ultrasound evaluation of paraprostatic cysts typically reveals an anechoic, fluid-filled structure (see Figure 17-28, C). Wall thickness can vary. It may be thin, thick, smooth, or irregular, even within a particular patient. Size varies, but the cysts are usually large at the time of clinical presentation. The contents of the cyst may have focal echogenicities, perhaps demonstrating a swirling movement when agitated with transducer pressure (Figure 17-30). Sedimentation of the contents can occasionally be demonstrated, with hyperechoic echoes seen in the dependent portion of the cyst, capped by anechoic or hypoechoic fluid. These large cysts can become infected and be reflected in the clinical signs. Membranous, linear echoes may be present, and internal septa may divide the cyst into irregularly shaped compartments. Paraprostatic cysts can appear as predominantly solid structures, with complex, multilocular echo

formation. Infection by gas-forming bacteria can lead to hyperechoic foci within the cyst. Concurrent prostate disease may be present. Bilateral prostatic cysts have been reported in association with a Sertoli cell tumor of a retained testis.[60]

Difficulty can sometimes arise in differentiating the paraprostatic cyst from the urinary bladder, but careful study of the location of the prostate gland and trigone usually suffices to distinguish the two. Because centesis and antibiotic therapy alone are not curative, surgical intervention is usually recommended.

NORMAL TESTES

The testes should be imaged ultrasonographically whenever there is clinical evidence of urogenital tract disease or reproductive disorders. Testicular disease may be the source of the clinical signs, or concurrent disease processes may be present.

The paired testes are contained within the scrotum, separated from one another by the median septum. The testes are covered by connective tissue, the tunica albuginea, which gives off septa that radiate centrally to join the mediastinum testis, which is oriented in a sagittal plane. The septa divide the testicular parenchyma into lobules, composed of seminiferous tubules. The seminiferous tubules are composed of spermatogenic cells and Sertoli cells. The seminiferous tubules form a collecting system, straight tubules, which in turn form the rete testis, located within the mediastinum testis. Efferent ductules leave the testicle, joining the head of the epididymis. Interstitial (Leydig) cells are present within the connective tissue separating the tubules; these cells are responsible for testosterone production.[9]

The epididymis is composed of a head, body, and tail. The head lies in a cranial direction; the body is located along the lateral and dorsal aspect of the testicle and courses caudad. The tail of the epididymis is attached by the proper ligament of the testis caudally and continues craniad along the dorsal-medial surface as the ductus deferens in the spermatic cord, entering the abdomen through the inguinal canal to enter the prostate gland dorsally.[9] Figure 17-31 illustrates normal testes anatomy.

The canine testis is echogenic with a homogeneous, medium echo texture[61] (Figure 17-32). The parietal and visceral tunics form a thin hyperechoic peripheral echo. The mediastinum testis is seen as an echogenic central linear structure on the midsagittal plane and as a central focal echo on a midtransverse scan plane. Both testes can often be imaged in one scan plane. Imaging of each testicle in a transverse or dorsal section is helpful for direct comparison (see Figure 17-32, E).

The tail of the epididymis is generally less echoic than the testicular parenchyma and at times can appear nearly anechoic (see Figure 17-32, C and D). The tail also has a coarser echo texture than the testis. The head and body of the epididymis are nearly isoechoic with the testis (see Figure 17-32, B, and D to G). The head is cranially located, and from it the body can be followed caudally in both sagittal and transverse planes to the tail, which is reported to be the most consistently imaged portion of the canine epididymis.[61] The ductus deferens is difficult to follow because it becomes small. It is rarely seen entering the prostate gland in a normal state.

Color flow Doppler ultrasound examination of the testes has been reported in men[62]; Günzel-Apel and co-workers[63] and Gumbsch and colleagues[64] reported on the Doppler characteristics of dog testes over a decade ago. Arterial blood flow to the testis and spermatic cord is normally detected, but it is not seen in the epididymis. Venous blood flow is not normally detected anywhere in the scrotum. Doppler examination of

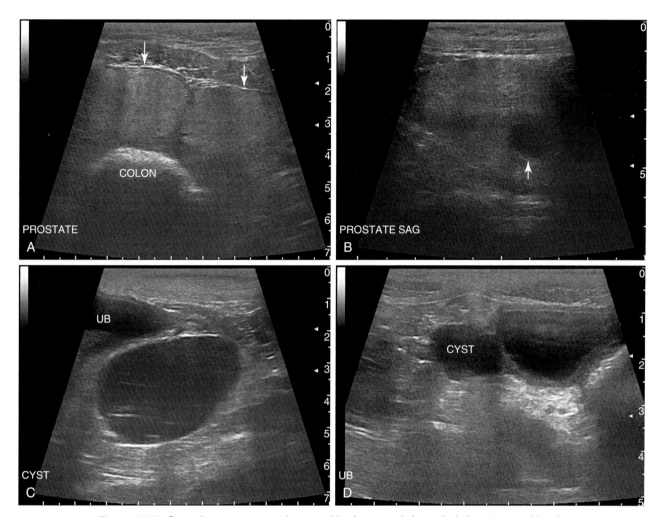

Figure 17-28 Prostatic cyst, paraprostatic cyst and benign prostatic hyperplasia in an 11-year-old male Belgian Malinois with a 2-month history of straining to defecate. A, Transverse image of an enlarged, very bilobed prostate gland (*arrows*). The parenchyma is very homogeneous and hyperechoic. **B,** Sagittal image shows the presence of a prostatic cyst (*arrow*). **C,** Sagittal image shows the presence of a large paraprostatic cyst with the urinary bladder (*UB*) in the near field. **D,** Transverse view shows both the paraprostatic cyst (*CYST*) and the urinary bladder.

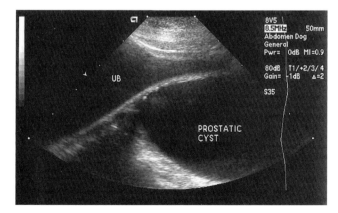

Figure 17-29 Large prostatic cyst in a middle-aged intact springer spaniel, sagittal image. A large anechoic prostatic cyst originated within the right prostate lobe. It extended along the pelvic urethra to the level of the trigone of the urinary bladder (*UB*), compressing the ureters and causing hydronephrosis. The left lobe of the gland was normal (not shown).

canine testes consistently detects the presence of an artery located dorsally between the testis and the epididymis (see Figure 17-32). Although duplex and color Doppler studies may not be able to detect the low blood flow of the testicular and epididymal parenchyma, power Doppler imaging does document blood flow (see Figure 17-32).

Two studies have evaluated ultrasound mensuration of dog testicles, comparing results with caliper measurements (orchidometer).[65,66] The both found ultrasound to be more reliable than orchidometry, using the formula L × W × H × 0.71 (L, length; W, width; H, height).

TESTICULAR PATHOLOGY

Ultrasonography of the testes and scrotum is performed in veterinary and human medicine. It is used to assess palpable and nonpalpable changes, to differentiate testicular from epididymal and scrotal disease, and to localize undescended testicles. As with disease of other organs, histologic diagnoses cannot be made on the basis of ultrasonographic appearance. Detection of a testicular abnormality warrants examination of abdominal organs for evidence of metastatic lesions or

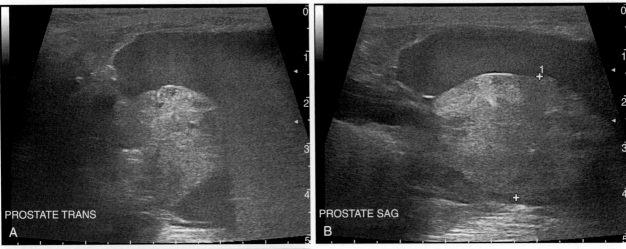

PROSTATE TRANS

A

PROSTATE SAG

B

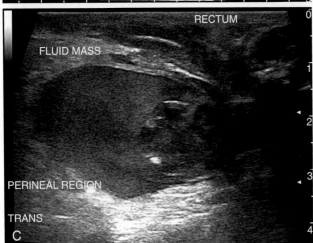

RECTUM

FLUID MASS

PERINEAL REGION

TRANS

C

Figure 17-30 **Paraprostatic cyst and benign prostatic hyperplasia is an 8-year-old male dachshund with a perineal hernia.** **A,** Transverse image of a highly hyperechoic prostate gland with several tiny cysts. A large, echogenic structure (paraprostatic cyst) is to the right of the prostate gland, which in real-time examination showed this to be fluid filled and contained by a thin wall. **B,** Sagittal image of the hyperechoic prostate gland (between electronic cursors) surrounded in the near field by swirling echogenic fluid contained within the paraprostatic cyst. The neck of the urinary bladder is present to the left of the image. **C,** Transverse image of the perineum showing the caudal extent of the paraprostatic cyst with a heterogeneous caudal extent of the prostate gland within it. The pathology diagnosis following surgical resection and biopsy was a large hemorrhagic paraprostatic cyst and benign prostatic hyperplasia.

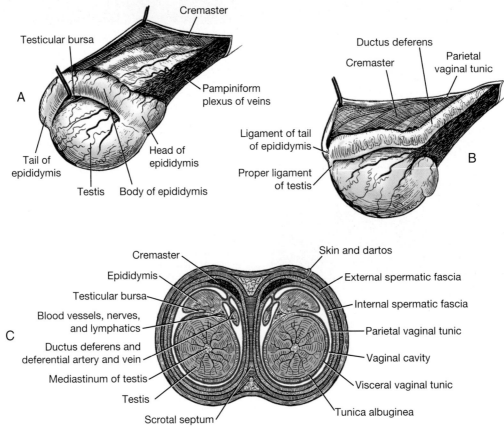

Figure 17-31 **Structures of testes and scrotum.** **A,** Right testis, lateral aspect. **B,** Left testis, medial aspect. **C,** Schematic cross section through scrotum and testes. (From Evans H. *Guide to the dissection of the dog,* 7th ed. St. Louis: Saunders; 2010.)

systemic disease. The testicles should be examined when prostate disease is present or suspected clinically.

Neoplasia

Three common types of testicular tumors are seen: interstitial cell, Sertoli cell, and seminomas. Interstitial cell tumors are composed of small nodules that may be singular or become confluent to form large nodular masses; they are poorly encapsulated and are yellowish, soft, and greasy on cut surface. They may be bilateral and associated with hormone abnormalities. Sertoli cell tumors often cause testicular enlargement and are associated with feminizing syndrome and bone marrow suppression due to high estrogen production. The opposite (normal) testicle will atrophy. One report describes the ultrasonographic diagnosis of nonpalpable Sertoli cell tumors in infertile dogs.[67] Seminomas are often large, solitary, unilateral lesions, with internal necrosis and hemorrhage. The cut surface is white to gray and may exude a milky fluid. Seminomas are not associated with hormone production. Mixed testicular tumors can occur as well.[34]

Several reports describe the ultrasonographic appearance of testicular neoplasia in dogs.[68-72] The ultrasonographic appearance of testicular neoplasms varies and is not specific for tumor type (Figures 17-33 to 17-36). Large lesions generally have a mixed or complex parenchymal pattern, which may be secondary to hemorrhage and necrosis. They may cause generalized testicular enlargement and obliteration of the mediastinum testis and epididymis ultrasonographically.[69] Focal and multifocal lesions occur and may be hypoechoic or hyperechoic. In one report, four of five interstitial cell tumors were focal hypoechoic lesions less than 3 cm in diameter.[9] The ultrasonographic appearance of cryptorchid neoplastic testes has also been described in the dog.[68-70] Sertoli cell tumors are the most common. They often become large when they are intraabdominal and have a mixed or complex echo texture. The small size of nonneoplastic retained testes makes them

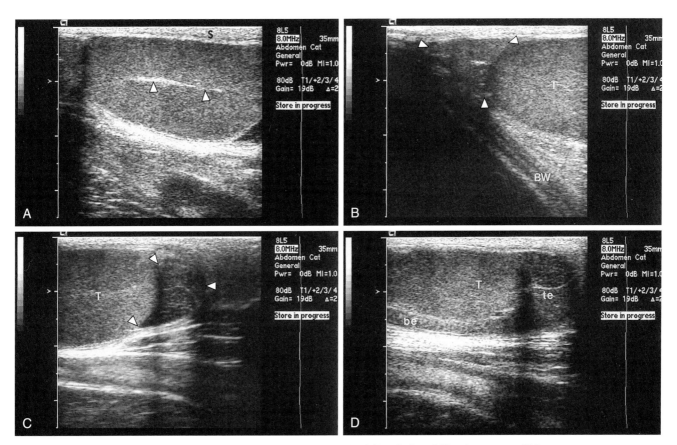

Figure 17-32 Normal testes in a 1-year-old dog, sagittal (A to D, F, and G) and transverse (E) images. **A,** The testis is an echogenic, homogeneous organ with a medium parenchymal echo texture. The mediastinum testis is an echogenic linear structure in the central portion of the testicle (*arrowheads*). The scrotal wall is a thin, striated structure in the near field (*S*). **B,** The cranial to mid portion of the testis is imaged to include the head of the epididymis. The head of the epididymis (*arrowheads*) is isoechoic with the testis (*T*), has a similar echo texture, and is roughly triangular. The ventral abdominal body wall (*BW*) is a multilayered, striated structure composed of muscle, fascia, and adipose layers. **C,** The mid to caudal portion of the testis (*T*) including the tail of the epididymis (*arrowheads*). The tail of the epididymis is generally less echogenic than the testis with a slightly coarser echo texture. Acoustic shadows are created by the junction between the testis and the tail of the epididymis and by the curved caudal margin of the epididymis. **D,** Rotating the transducer to image the dorsolateral surface of the testis (*T*) allows imaging of the body of the epididymis (*be*). The body of the epididymis is similar to the testis in echogenicity and echo texture and hyperechoic relative to the tail of the epididymis (*te*).   *Continued*

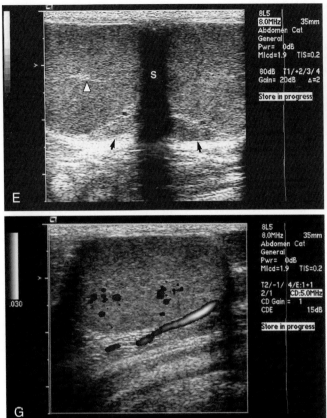

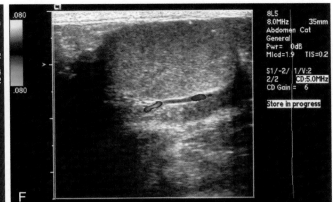

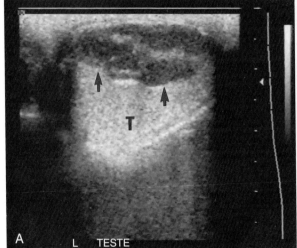

Figure 17-32, cont'd **E,** Transverse image of both testes. The mediastinum testis is a small echogenic focus centrally within the right testis. The scrotal septum has created a strong acoustic shadow (*S*) between the testes. The body of each epididymis (*arrows*) is seen as a flattened triangular structure dorsally (*arrowhead,* mediastinum testis). **F,** Color Doppler analysis shows an artery located between the testis and the body of the epididymis. The testicular parenchyma is devoid of large vessels; blood flow is too low to be detected by conventional color Doppler imaging. **G,** Power Doppler evaluation detects extremely low blood flow (without direction or velocity information), indicated by multiple small red patches within the testicular parenchyma.

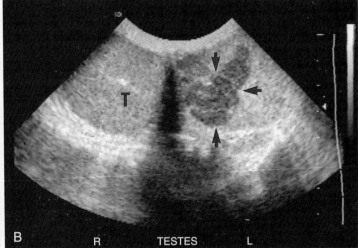

Figure 17-33 Interstitial cell tumor in the left testis of a 10-year-old mixed-breed dog, sagittal (**A**) and transverse (**B**) images. **A,** The tumor (*arrows*) is hypoechoic relative to the normal testicular parenchyma (*T*). Linear echogenic areas are noted within the tumor, which has a smooth, slightly lobular margin. **B,** The tumor (*arrows*) is hypoechoic, lobular, and roughly V shaped. The opposite right testicle (*T*) is normal.

difficult to identify in many instances (Figure 17-37). They may be located anywhere caudal to the kidneys to the inguinal canal. The key to identification is recognition of the presence of the centrally echogenic mediastinum testis; this helps differentiate it from an intraabdominal lymph node. Figures 17-38 and 17-39 are examples of retained testes.

Orchitis

Orchitis is often found concurrently with epididymitis in the canine. Retrograde infection through the ductus deferens from urinary bladder, prostate, or urethral infections is the most common route, although penetrating wounds can occur. Abscess formation is common.[34] The ultrasonographic

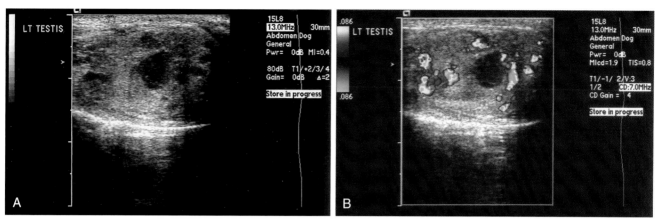

Figure 17-34 **Mixed testicular tumor (interstitial cell and seminoma) in a 15-year-old mixed-breed dog, sagittal images. A,** The majority of the testicular parenchyma has been replaced by hypoechoic to anechoic foci of various sizes and shapes. **B,** Color Doppler imaging indicates abnormal blood flow in all but the largest central hypoechoic foci.

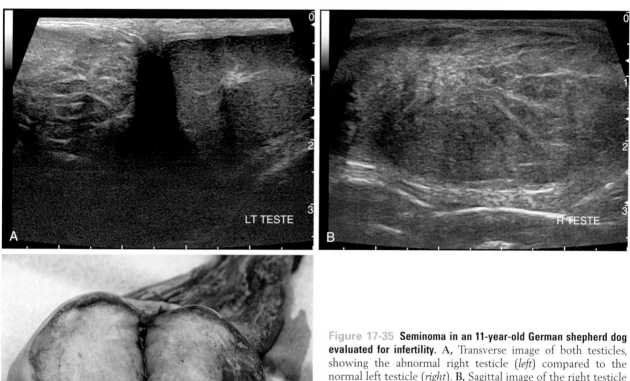

Figure 17-35 **Seminoma in an 11-year-old German shepherd dog evaluated for infertility. A,** Transverse image of both testicles, showing the abnormal right testicle (*left*) compared to the normal left testicle (*right*). **B,** Sagittal image of the right testicle shows complete obliteration of the normal parenchyma. The parenchyma is hyperechoic and there are multiple linear striations present. **C,** Gross specimen of the seminoma.

appearance of acute infectious testicular disease has been described as a diffuse, patchy, hypoechoic parenchymal pattern, usually with testicular and epididymal enlargement.[70] Orchitis as a result of Rocky Mountain spotted fever has been reported, where ultrasound was valuable in differentiating it from torsion and testicular neoplasia.[73]

Epididymitis can occur without testicular disease and vice versa (Figure 17-40). Infection may extend to include the ductus deferens. Abscesses, characterized by an irregular hyperechoic wall and anechoic to hypoechoic central contents, can occur. Chronic infection may reveal a hyperechoic or mixed echogenic parenchyma, and the testicle may be

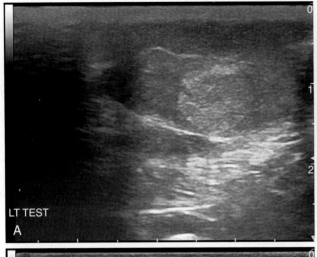

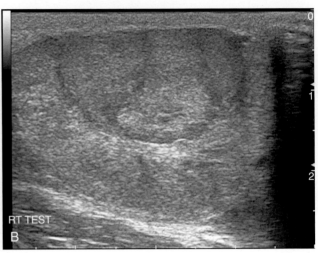

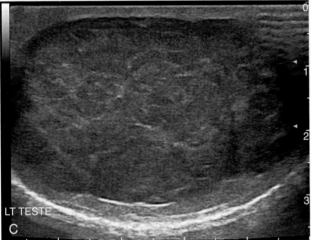

Figure 17-36 Testicular neoplasias. A, Sagittal image of a discrete hyperechoic testicular nodule in a 12-year-old male smooth fox terrier. **B,** Sagittal image of a very large testicular mass in a 10-year-old dog. **C,** Complex mass completely obliterating the normal testicular architecture in a 15-year-old Norwich terrier.

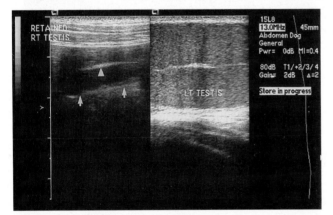

Figure 17-37 Retained (cryptorchid) and contralateral normal testes in a 1-year-old German shorthaired pointer, sagittal images. The right testis (*arrows*) was intraabdominal. It is hypoechoic and considerably smaller than the left testis. The linear echogenic right mediastinum testis (*arrowhead*) was an important sonographic landmark that allowed positive identification of the retained testis.

reduced in size. Orchitis can appear similar to neoplasia, although extratesticular fluid and epididymal enlargement may more commonly be associated with infection.[70] Color flow Doppler characteristics of epididymo-orchitis in men include focal or diffuse hypervascularity.[62]

Atrophy

In addition to small size, the parenchyma has been described as hypoechoic to isoechoic (normal)[70] (Figure 17-41). We have observed diffusely hyperechoic atrophied testicles as well. Atrophied testes may be a senile change and normally located in the scrotum, or they may be present with cryptorchidism or occur unilaterally as a result of a neoplasm in the opposite testicle.

Torsion

The ultrasonographic appearance of experimentally induced testicular torsion in the dog has been reported.[74-76] Testicular enlargement typically characterized by diffusely decreased parenchymal echogenicity, concurrent enlargement of the epididymis and spermatic cord, scrotal thickening, and loss of Doppler signal were consistently identified. These changes occurred rapidly, from 15 to 60 minutes after torsion. Ultrasound evaluation is used to diagnose testicular torsion and to differentiate it from acute orchitis or epididymitis in men. Doppler ultrasonography (including color flow) and nuclear scintigraphy are sensitive indicators of compromised testicular blood flow.[62] Figure 17-42 is an example of testicular torsion. Of interest is that the testicular parenchyma is much more echogenic than expected.

Infarction of a testicle caused by obliteration of vascular supply by an aggressive retroperitoneal hemangiosarcoma has been seen. The testicle was diffusely hypoechoic with areas of almost anechoic parenchyma. The mediastinum testis was still present (Figure 17-43).

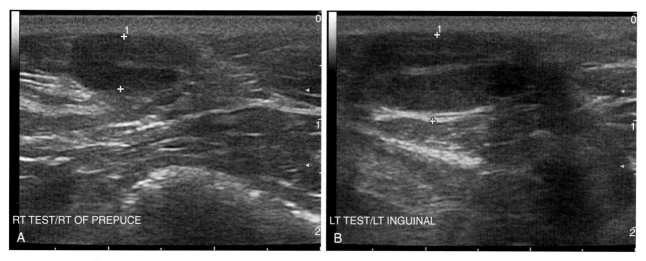

Figure 17-38 Bilateral retained testes in a 14-month-old male Pekinese. A, Sagittal image of the small retained right testis (0.49 cm, between electronic cursors), found along the prepuce. Note the presence of the mediastinum testis, seen centrally as a hyperechoic linear structure. **B,** Sagittal image of the left testis (0.80 cm, between electronic cursors) found at the left inguinal area. It is notably larger than the right testis, and the mediastinum testis is readily identified.

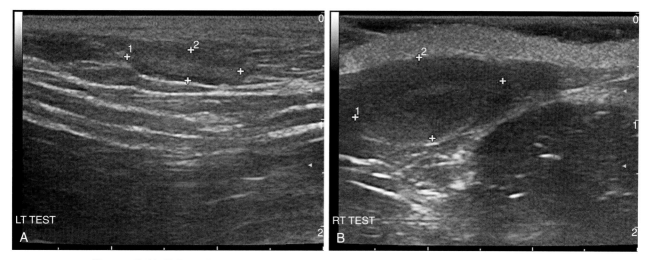

Figure 17-39 Unilateral cryptorchid in a 4-month-old silken windhound. A, Sagittal image of the retained left testicle located along the left inguinal region (1.08 × 0.29 cm, between electronic cursors). **B,** Sagittal image of the normal juvenile descended right testicle, measuring 1.45 × 0.76 cm, between electronic cursors.

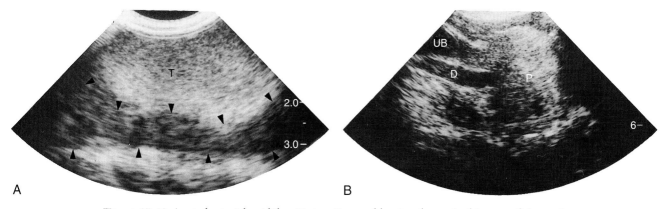

Figure 17-40 Acute bacterial epididymitis in a 7-year-old rottweiler; sagittal images of the testis (**A**) and prostate (**B**). **A,** A greatly enlarged body of the epididymis (*arrowheads*) is hypoechoic and has a coarse texture. Normal echoic testicular parenchyma (*T*) is present in the near field. **B,** A dilated ductus deferens (*D*) is seen as it enters the infected prostate gland (*P*). *UB,* Urinary bladder. A 7.5-MHz mechanical transducer was used with a standoff pad for **A,** and a 5-MHz mechanical transducer was used for **B.**

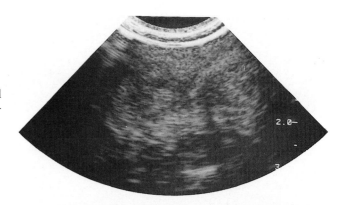

Figure 17-41 **Testicular atrophy, sagittal image.** The testicle is small with inhomogeneous parenchyma. A 7.5-MHz mechanical transducer was used with a standoff pad.

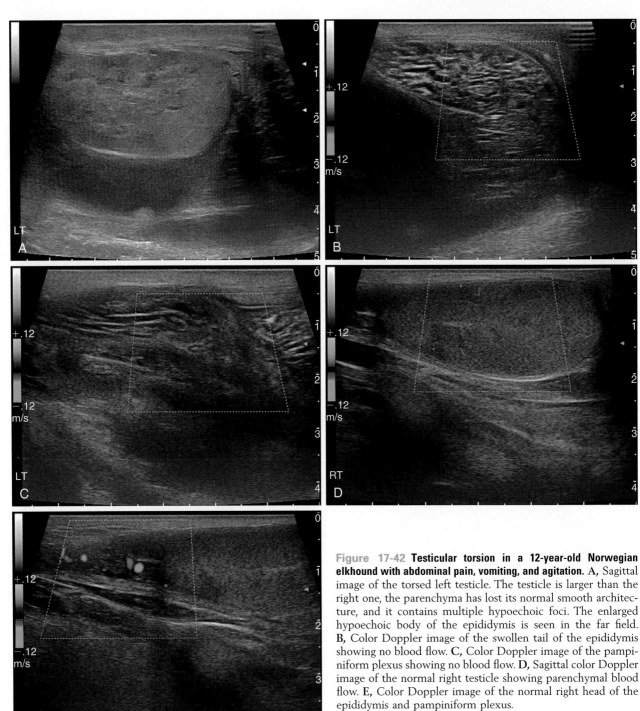

Figure 17-42 **Testicular torsion in a 12-year-old Norwegian elkhound with abdominal pain, vomiting, and agitation. A,** Sagittal image of the torsed left testicle. The testicle is larger than the right one, the parenchyma has lost its normal smooth architecture, and it contains multiple hypoechoic foci. The enlarged hypoechoic body of the epididymis is seen in the far field. **B,** Color Doppler image of the swollen tail of the epididymis showing no blood flow. **C,** Color Doppler image of the pampiniform plexus showing no blood flow. **D,** Sagittal color Doppler image of the normal right testicle showing parenchymal blood flow. **E,** Color Doppler image of the normal right head of the epididymis and pampiniform plexus.

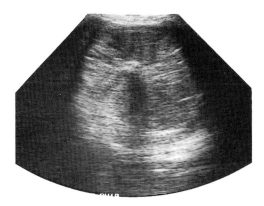

Figure 17-43 Testicular infarction, transverse image. The testis is diffusely inhomogeneous. The mediastinum testis is the hyperechoic structure in the center of the testicle with acoustic shadowing. (Courtesy Dr. Charles R. Pugh, Lafayette, Colorado.)

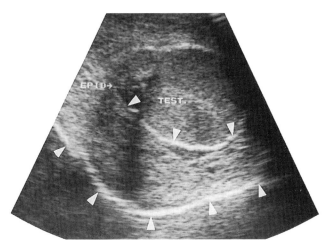

Figure 17-44 Scrotal edema in a 5-year-old Scottish deerhound, transverse sonogram. The scrotum (*arrowheads*) is markedly thickened and slightly hyperechoic compared with the normal testis (*TEST*). The head of the epididymis (*EPID*) is seen. (Courtesy Dr. Charles R. Pugh, Lafayette, Colorado.)

SCROTUM

Several reports of scrotal ultrasonography in the dog are available.[70,77] Evaluation of the scrotum is useful in assessing scrotal dermatitis, penetrating wounds, foreign bodies, edema, neoplasia, and hernias and in differentiating scrotal from testicular disease. Scrotal disease usually manifests as a thickened scrotum that is isoechoic to hyperechoic compared with the testes in cases of edema and vascular tumors (Figures 17-44 and 17-45). Herniation of small bowel into the scrotal sac may be detected by observing peristalsis.

A patient has presented with the observation of a unilateral small "testis" but with a history of castration 3 months earlier. A small, complex structure was identified within the scrotal sac compatible with a chronic, organized hematoma. Color Doppler and color Doppler energy evaluation confirmed the absence of blood flow (Figure 17-46).

REFERENCES

1. Krawiec DR, Heflin D. Study of prostatic disease in dogs. *J Am Vet Med Assoc* 1992;**200**:1119–22.

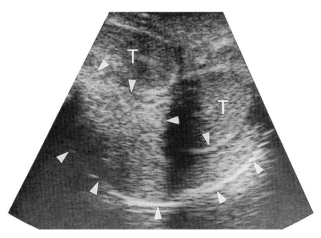

Figure 17-45 Varicose scrotal tumor in a 5-year-old bullmastiff, transverse sonogram. There is marked scrotal thickening (*arrowheads*), which is diffusely isoechoic to hyperechoic compared with the normal testes (*T*). (Courtesy Dr. Charles R. Pugh, Lafayette, Colorado.)

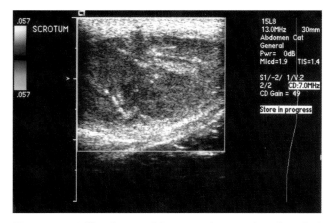

Figure 17-46 Chronic scrotal hematoma in a greyhound, sagittal image. A firm, small structure was palpated in the scrotum after uneventful castration 3 months previously. An inhomogeneous structure was present within the scrotum. It did not resemble testicular parenchyma, and color Doppler and power Doppler evaluation revealed absence of blood flow.

2. Smith J. Canine prostatic disease: a review of anatomy, pathology, diagnosis, and treatment. *Theriogenology* 2008;**70**(3):375–83.
3. Miyashita H, Watanabe H, Ohe H, et al. Transrectal ultrasonotomography of the canine prostate. *Prostate* 1984;**5**:453–7.
4. Zohil AM, Castellano C. Prepubic and transrectal ultrasonography of the canine prostate: a comparative study. *Vet Radiol Ultrasound* 1995;**36**:393–6.
5. Barsanti JA, Finco DR. Prostatic diseases. In: Ettinger SJ, Feldman EC, editors. *Textbook of Veterinary Internal Medicine*. 4th ed. Philadelphia: WB Saunders; 1995. p. 1662–85.
6. Hawe RS. What is your diagnosis? *J Am Vet Med Assoc* 1983;**182**:405–9.
7. Hubbard BS, Vulgamott JC, Liska WD. Prostatic adenocarcinoma in a cat. *J Am Vet Med Assoc* 1990;**197**:1493–4.

8. Pointer E, Murray L. Chronic prostatitis, cystitis, pyelonephritis, and balanoposthitis in a cat. *J Am Anim Hosp Assoc* 2011;**47**(4):2588–61.

9. Christensen GC. The urogenital apparatus. In: Evans HE, Christensen GF, editors. *Miller's anatomy of the dog*. 2nd ed. Philadelphia: WB Saunders; 1979. p. 544–601.

10. Feeney DA, Fletcher TF, Hardy RM. Abdomen and pelvis. In: Feeney DA, Fletcher TF, Hardy RM, editors. *Atlas of correlative imaging anatomy of the normal dog—ultrasound and computed tomography*. Philadelphia: WB Saunders; 1991. p. 219–333.

11. Gordon N. Surgical anatomy of the bladder, prostate gland and urethra in the male dog. *J Am Vet Med Assoc* 1960;**136**:215–21.

12. Bacha WJ, Wood LM. Male reproductive system. In: *Color atlas of veterinary histology*. Philadelphia: Lea & Febiger; 1990. p. 189–205.

13. Cartee RE, Rowles T. Transabdominal sonographic evaluation of the canine prostate. *Vet Radiol* 1983;**24**:156–64.

14. Foss RR, Wrigley RH, Park RD, et al. A new frontier—veterinary ultrasound: the prostate. Part 2. *Med Ultrasound* 1984;**8**:15–19.

15. Johnston GR, Feeney DA. Comparative organ imaging—lower urinary tract. *Vet Radiol* 1984;**25**:146–53.

16. Feeney DA, Johnston GR, Klausner JS. Two-dimensional gray-scale ultrasonography: applications in canine prostatic disease. *Vet Clin North Am Small Anim Pract* 1985;**15**:1159–76.

17. Feeney DA, Johnston GR, Klausner JS, et al. Canine prostatic disease—comparison of ultrasonographic appearance with morphologic and microbiologic findings: 30 cases (1981-1985). *J Am Vet Med Assoc* 1987;**190**:1027–34.

18. Cooney JC, Cartee RE, Gray BW, et al. Ultrasonography of the canine prostate with histologic correlation. *Theriogenology* 1992;**38**:877–95.

19. Gordon N. The position of the canine prostate gland. *Am J Vet Res* 1961;**22**:215–21.

20. O'Shea JD. Studies on the canine prostate gland. Factors influencing its size and weight. *J Comp Pathol* 1962;**72**:321–31.

21. Cartee RE, Rumph PF, Kenter DC, et al. Evaluation of drug-induced prostatic involution in dogs by transabdominal B-mode ultrasonography. *Am J Vet Res* 1990;**51**:1773–8.

22. Feeney DA, Johnston GR, Klausner JS, et al. Canine prostatic disease—comparison of radiographic appearance with morphologic and microbiologic findings: 30 cases (1981-1985). *J Am Vet Med Assoc* 1987;**190**:1027–34.

23. Suzuki K, Ito K, Okazaki H, et al. Estimation of canine prostatic volume: nomogram based on prostatic cubic volume. *Int Urol Nephrol* 1998;**30**:725–30.

24. Ruel Y, Barthez PY, Mailles A, et al. Ultrasonographic evaluation of the prostate in healthy intact dogs. *Vet Radiol Ultrasound* 1998;**39**:212–16.

25. Atalan G, Barr FJ, Holt PE. Comparison of ultrasonographic and radiographic measurements of canine prostate dimensions. *Vet Radiol Ultrasound* 1999;**40**:408–12.

26. Atalan G, Holt PE, Barr FJ, et al. Ultrasonographic estimation of prostatic size in canine cadavers. *Res Vet Sci* 1999;**67**:7–15.

27. Dorso L, Chanut F, Howroyd P, et al. Variability in weight and histological appearance of the prostate of beagle dogs used in toxicology studies. *Toxicol Pathol* 2008;**36**(7):917–25.

28. Kamolpatana K, Johnston GR, Johnston SD. Determination of canine prostatic volume using transabdominal ultrasonography. *Vet Radiol Ultrasound* 2000;**41**:73–7.

29. Lattimer JC. The prostate gland. In: Thrall DE, editor. *Textbook of veterinary diagnostic radiology*. 3rd ed. Philadelphia: WB Saunders; 1998. p. 499–511.

30. Newell SM, Neuwirth L, Ginn PE, et al. Doppler ultrasound of the prostate in normal dogs and in dogs with chronic lymphocytic-lymphoplasmacytic prostatitis. *Vet Radiol Ultrasound* 1998;**39**:332–6.

31. Russo M, Vignoli M, Catone G, et al. Prostatic perfusion in the dog using contrast-enhanced Doppler ultrasound. *Reprod Domest Anim* 2009;**44**(Suppl. 2):334–5.

32. Bigliardi E, Ferrari L. Contrast-enhanced ultrasound of the normal canine prostate gland. *Vet Radiol Ultrasound* 2011;**52**(1):107–10.

33. Vignoli M, Russo M, Catone G, et al. Assessment of vascular perfusion kinetics using contrast-enhanced ultrasound for the diagnosis of prostatic disease in dogs. *Reprod Domest Anim* 2011;**46**(2):209–13.

34. Ladds PW. The male genital system. In: Jubb KVF, Kennedy PC, Palmer N, editors. *Pathology of Domestic Animals*. 4th ed. Orlando, Fla: Academic Press; 1993. p. 471–529.

35. Kustritz MV, Merkel L. Theriogenology question of the month. Benign prostatic hypertrophy (BPH), prostatitis, and prostatic neoplasia. *J Am Vet Med Assoc* 1998;**213**:807–9.

36. Brennan SJ, Ngeleka M, Philibert HM, et al. Canine brucellosis in a Saskatchewan kennel. *Can Vet J* 2008;**49**(7):703–8.

37. Agut A, Lucas X, Castro A, et al. A urethrorectal fistula due to prostatic abscess associated with urolithiasis in a dog. *Reprod Domest Anim* 2006;**41**(3):247–50.

38. Kuwamura M, Ide M, Yamate J, et al. Systemic candidiasis in a dog, developing spondylitis. *J Vet Med Sci* 2006;**68**(10):1117–19.

39. Bude R, Bree RL, Adler RS, et al. Transrectal ultrasound appearance of granulomatous prostatitis. *J Ultrasound Med* 1990;**9**:677–80.

40. Cowan LA, Barsanti JA, Crowell W, et al. Effects of castration on chronic bacterial prostatitis in dogs. *J Am Vet Med Assoc* 1991;**199**:346–50.

41. Bell FW, Klausner JS, Hayden DW, et al. Clinical and pathologic features of prostatic adenocarcinoma in sexually intact and castrated dogs: 31 cases (1970-1987). *J Am Vet Med Assoc* 1991;**199**:1623–30.

42. Teske E, Naan EC, van Dijk EM, et al. Canine prostate carcinoma: epidemiological evidence of an increased risk in castrated dogs. *Mol Cell Endocrinol* 2002;**197**(1–2):251–5.

43. Bryan JN, Keeler MR, Henry CJ, et al. A population study of neutering status as a risk factor for canine prostate cancer. *Prostate* 2007;**67**(11):1174–81.

44. Nielsen SW, Kennedy PC. Tumors of the genital system. In: Moulton JE, editor. *Tumors in Domestic Animals*. 3rd ed. Berkeley: University of California Press; 1990. p. 479–517.

45. Winter MD, Locke JE, Penninck DG. Imaging diagnosis—urinary obstruction secondary to prostatic lymphoma in a young dog. *Vet Radiol Ultrasound* 2006;**47**(6):597–601.

46. Assin R, Baldi A, Citro G, et al. Prostate as sole unusual recurrence site of lymphoma in a dog. *In Vivo* 2008;**22**(6):755–7.

47. Bradbury CA, Westropp JL, Pollard RE. Relationship between prostatomegaly, prostatic mineralization, and cytologic diagnosis. *Vet Radiol Ultrasound* 2009;**50**(2):167–71.

48. Rohleder JJ, Jones JC. Emphysematous prostatitis and carcinoma in a dog. *J Am Anim Hosp Assoc* 2002;**38**(5):478–81.

49. Lee-Parritz DE, Lamb CR. Prostatic adenocarcinoma with osseous metastasis in a dog. *J Am Vet Med Assoc* 1988;**192**:1569–72.
50. LeBlanc CJ, Roberts CS, Bauer RW, et al. Firm rib mass aspirate from a dog. *Vet Clin Pathol* 2004;**33**(4):253–6.
51. Shor S, Helfand SC, Gorman E, et al. Diagnostic exercise: epithelioid hemangiosarcoma mimicking metastatic prostatic neoplasia in a dog. *Vet Pathol* 2009;**46**(3):548–52.
52. Gilson SD, Miller RT, Hardie EM, et al. Unusual prostatic mass in a dog. *J Am Vet Med Assoc* 1992;**200**:702–4.
53. Powe JR, Canfield PJ, Martin PA. Evaluation of the cytologic diagnosis of canine prostatic disorders. *Vet Clin Pathol* 2004;**33**(3):150–4.
54. Nyland TG, Wallack ST, Wisner ER. Needle-tract implantation following US-guided fine-needle aspiration biopsy of transitional cell carcinoma of the bladder, urethra, and prostate. *Vet Radiol Ultrasound* 2002;**43**(1):50–3.
55. Dyke CH, Toi A, Sweet JM. Value of random US-guided transrectal prostate biopsy. *Radiology* 1990;**176**:345–9.
56. Marquez GA, Nyland TG, Ling GV, et al. *Prevalence of canine prostatic cysts in adult large breed dogs. Proceedings of the Sixteenth Annual House Officer Seminar Day.* School of Veterinary Medicine, University of California Davis; 1994. p. 30.
57. Hamper UM, Epstein JI, Sheth S, et al. Cystic lesions of the prostate gland—a sonographic-pathologic correlation. *J Ultrasound Med* 1990;**9**:395–402.
58. Atiola MAO, Pennock PW. Cystic uterus masculinus in the dog. *Vet Radiol* 1986;**27**:8–14.
59. Stowater JL, Lamb CR. Ultrasonographic features of paraprostatic cysts in dogs. *Vet Radiol* 1989;**30**:232–9.
60. Spackman CJ, Roth L. Prostatic cyst and concurrent Sertoli cell tumor in a dog. *J Am Vet Med Assoc* 1988;**192**:1096–8.
61. Pugh CR, Konde LJ, Park RD. Testicular ultrasound in the normal dog. *Vet Radiol* 1990;**31**:195–9.
62. Horstman WG, Middleton WD, Melson GL, et al. Color Doppler US of the scrotum. *Radiographics* 1991;**11**:941–57.
63. Günzel-Apel AR, Möhrke C, Poulsen Nautrup C. Colour-coded and pulsed Doppler sonography of the canine testis, epididymis and prostate gland: physiological and pathological findings. *Reprod Domest Anim* 2001;**36**(5):236–40.
64. Gumbsch P, Gabler C, Holzmann A. Colour-coded duplex sonography of the testes of dogs. *Vet Rec* 2002;**151**(5):140–4.
65. Paltiel HJ, Diamond DA, Di Canzio J, et al. Testicular volume: comparison of orchidometer and US measurements in dogs. *Radiology* 2002;**222**(1):114–19.
66. Gouletsou PG, Galatos AD, Leontides LS. Comparison between ultrasonographic and caliper measurements of testicular volume in the dog. *Anim Reprod Sci* 2008;**108**(1–2):1–12.
67. England GCW. Ultrasonographic diagnosis of nonpalpable Sertoli cell tumours in infertile dogs. *J Small Anim Pract* 1995;**36**:476–89.
68. Eilts BE, Pechman RD, Hedlund CS, et al. Use of ultrasonography to diagnose Sertoli cell neoplasia and cryptorchidism in a dog. *J Am Vet Med Assoc* 1988;**192**:533–4.
69. Johnston GR, Feeney DA, Johnston SD, et al. Ultrasonographic features of testicular neoplasia in dogs: 16 cases (1980-1988). *J Am Vet Med Assoc* 1991;**198**:1779–84.
70. Pugh CR, Konde LJ. Sonographic evaluation of canine testicular and scrotal abnormalities: a review of 26 case histories. *Vet Radiol* 1991;**32**:243–50.
71. Archbald LF, Waldow D, Gelatt K. Interstitial cell tumor. *J Am Vet Med Assoc* 1997;**210**:1423–4.
72. Vascellari M, Carminato A, Camali G, et al. Malignant mesothelioma of the tunica vaginalis testis in a dog: histological and immunohistochemical characterization. *J Vet Diagn Invest* 2011;**23**(1):135–9.
73. Ober CP, Spaulding K, Breitschwerdt EB, et al. Orchitis in two dogs with Rocky Mountain spotted fever. *Vet Radiol Ultrasound* 2004;**45**(5):458–65.
74. Hricak H, Lue T, Filly RA, et al. Experimental study of the sonographic diagnosis of testicular torsion. *J Ultrasound Med* 1983;**2**:349–56.
75. Tarhan F, Erbay ME, Erdogan E, et al. Effects of unilateral testicular torsion on the blood flow of contralateral testis—an experimental study on dogs. *Scand J Urol Nephrol* 2000;**34**(4):229–32.
76. Pinto CR, Paccamonti DL, Partington B, et al. Theriogenology question of the month. Torsion of the spermatic cord. *J Am Vet Med Assoc* 2001;**219**(10):1343–5.
77. Mitchner KL, Toal RL, Held JP, et al. Use of ultrasound and nuclear imaging to diagnose scrotal hernia in a dog. *J Am Vet Med Assoc* 1990;**196**:1834–5.

CHAPTER 18
Ovaries and Uterus

John S. Mattoon • Thomas G. Nyland

Ultrasonography has been used extensively to diagnose pregnancy in the queen and bitch.[1] Pregnancy can be reliably diagnosed during the first trimester by ultrasound imaging, before palpation and well before radiography. Ultrasound evaluation may be used to predict parturition dates, to provide an estimate of fetal number, and to assess fetal stress. Evaluation of a number of reproductive disorders has also become common. In patients of unknown medical history, it can be used to establish intact versus ovariohysterectomized status.

EXAMINATION TECHNIQUE

High-frequency transducers (7.5 to 10 MHz or higher) are ideal for transabdominal evaluation of the normal ovaries and uterus in the dog and cat. A 5.0-MHz transducer is satisfactory for diagnosis of midterm to late-term pregnancy, pyometra, and ovarian tumors, but it may not provide adequate resolution for study of more subtle pathologic changes of the reproductive tract.

The patient is routinely placed in dorsal recumbency. However, many positions are possible for optimal scanning, including right or left lateral recumbency for scanning from the dependent or nondependent side, and scanning with the animal standing. Scanning the animal in a standing position seems to appease the occasional client who objects to positioning his or her animal on her back. Having the patient stand on the floor is advantageous for large or giant-breed dogs. Multiple positions and scanning planes may be needed to visualize the entire reproductive tract.

Owners of show animals may object to clipping of the ventral abdominal hair coat, which is standard protocol to obtain the best image. Wetting with alcohol or other agents before the acoustic gel is applied to an unclipped hair coat may improve image quality by reducing air between the transducer and skin. When a negative result is obtained under this less than ideal condition in early pregnancy, the ultrasound examination should be repeated several weeks later to confirm a false-negative diagnosis. Midterm and late-term pregnancies can usually be diagnosed without clipping the hair coat, as can pyometra and other conditions in which the reproductive tract is markedly enlarged.

The anatomic landmark for identifying each ovary is the caudal pole of the kidney. The adjacent area is scanned in sagittal and transverse planes to locate the ovary, which may contact the caudal pole of the kidney or be located up to several centimeters caudal. It is usually caudolateral to the kidney, although it may lie caudomedial, or ventral to the caudal pole of the kidney.[2] Although the sonographer is usually able to identify each ovary, nonvisualization of the ovaries in the dog and cat can occur and is due to their small size, the fact that they are often surrounded by adipose tissue, and interference by overlying bowel gas. This becomes important when assessing the intact versus spayed status of a patient. In addition, the ovaries are not as routinely scanned as other abdominal organs are because many animals examined for nonreproductive disease have undergone ovariohysterectomy.

A moderately full urinary bladder enhances visualization of the uterus. The bladder serves as an acoustic window by which to view the uterine body, located between the urinary bladder ventrally and the colon dorsally. Transverse images with the bladder in the near field, the colon in the far field, the uterine body in between is perhaps the easiest method to locate a small, anestrous uterus, seen as a hypoechoic round structure in cross section. Once identified, the transducer may be rotated into a sagittal scan plane to visualize the uterus in its long axis. The uterus is usually close to midline but may be displaced to the right or left by the bladder and be positioned laterally instead of ventrally to the bladder. The uterine horns are sometimes seen cranially as they branch from the uterine body, but they may be difficult to identify unless they are enlarged from pregnancy or disease.

Visualization of the pelvic inlet region can be difficult with an empty bladder, compounded by colonic gas and fecal artifacts. Diuretics such as furosemide may be administered in low doses to produce urinary bladder distention if needed.

NORMAL OVARY

The female reproductive tract consists of the ovaries, uterine tubes (oviducts), uterus, cervix, vagina, and vulva. The uterus and ovaries are well imaged with ultrasound; the vagina and vulva are usually better evaluated by direct visual inspection or by contrast radiography.

The ovaries are oval to round structures measuring approximately 1.5 cm in length, 0.7 cm in width, and 0.5 cm in thickness in a 25-pound dog on gross evaluation.[3] Ultrasound measurements of canine ovaries are similar, and although large dogs had slightly larger ovaries than small dogs, the mean difference was less than 0.2 cm.[2] Feline ovaries are smaller.[4] The ovary is made up of a cortex and a medulla, which are not distinguished sonographically. The cortex contains the follicles, which consist of an oocyte and granulosa cells. Stromal parenchymal tissue surrounds the follicles. During estrus, multiple follicles mature, become fluid filled, and may eventually rupture, releasing ova into the ovarian bursa followed by migration down the uterine tube. After ovulation, the follicular cavity fills with blood (corpus hemorrhagicum), which is resorbed, forming the corpus luteum. The corpus luteum

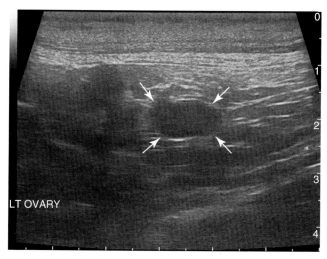

Figure 18-1 Inactive left ovary in a 10-year-old anestrous Labrador retriever. The ovary (*arrows*) is homogeneous, solid, and hypoechoic to the surrounding mesentery. It measures approximately 1 × 0.8 cm.

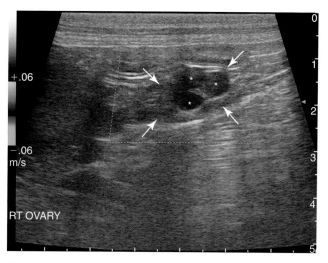

Figure 18-2 Multicystic ovary in a 2-year-old treeing walker coonhound in late proestrus. Three discrete follicular cysts (*asterisks*) are present within right ovary (*arrows*). There is mild acoustic and far-wall enhancement. The follicular cysts measured 5 to 6 mm. Color Doppler analysis showed no detectable blood flow at this relatively sensitive setting.

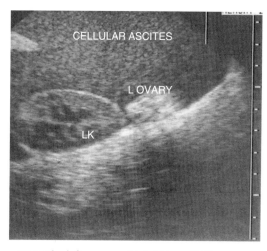

Figure 18-3 The left ovary and left kidney (*LK*) are seen in this sagittal plane, illustrating their close anatomic relationship. The hyperechoic left ovary contained multiple small cysts, not individually resolved but collectively creating a very echoic structure. Free abdominal fluid is present secondary to carcinomatosis. The fluid is echoic with swirling of the echoes observed in real time. Intraabdominal hemorrhage, peritonitis, and chylous effusions may look identical to this example.

remains throughout pregnancy (or throughout diestrus if pregnancy does not occur), producing progesterone; it then degenerates at parturition into a focal area of scar tissue, the corpus albicans.[3]

The sonographic appearance of the ovaries varies during the estrous cycle. During anestrus and early proestrus, they are small, usually oval to bean shaped, and have a homogeneous echogenicity similar to that of the renal cortex, sometimes with indistinct margins[2] (Figure 18-1). The cortex and medulla are not usually differentiated in dogs and cats, but a hyperechoic medulla surrounded by a hypoechoic cortex is often observed in women during endovaginal scanning.[5]

Follicular development begins in proestrus, reaching maturation during estrus when ovulation occurs. Ovulation occurs 24 to 48 hours after a peak in luteinizing hormone (LH) at the same time there is a rise in progesterone levels above baseline anestrous levels.[6] The anechoic fluid-filled follicles become hypoechoic solid corpora lutea, secreting high levels of progesterone.

Sonographic evaluation of canine follicular maturation and ovulation has been well studied.[2,7-11] Anechoic preovulatory follicular cysts may initially be identified at day 1 to day 7 of proestrus.[2,10] Multiple small anechoic follicles are seen, enlarging with time until ovulation occurs[2,10] (Figure 18-2), at which time 3 to 4 follicles are typically seen on each ovary.[10] Size ranges from nearly microscopic to greater than 1 cm as ovulation approaches.[2] More specifically, Hayer and colleagues[10] found follicular size increases from 3.7 ± 0.6 mm to 6.9 ± 0.7 mm between day −5 (pre LH surge) and LH surge (day 0), with further increases to 7.5 ± 0.7 mm until 2 days after the LH surge. Enlargement continues during corpus luteum development, reaching up to 8.1 ± 0.6 mm on the first day of diestrus. The presence of many small cysts may result in a diffusely hyperechoic ovary, without resolution of individual cysts (Figure 18-3). Larger follicular cysts are characterized by a thin wall, anechoic fluid center, distinct far wall, and distal acoustic enhancement (Figure 18-4). The exterior surface of the ovary may be irregular or lumpy. As the follicular cysts enlarge, the ovary also becomes larger, making it easier to identify.

In the dog, ovulation may be detected sonographically when there is a decrease in the number and size of follicles from one day to the next.[2] Although at least one large follicle remained in an ovary of most dogs (7 of 10), several dogs (3 of 10) had no evidence of follicles in either ovary on the day of ovulation. In another study, it was observed that the anechoic appearance of the ovary (follicles) changed dramatically to a mixed hypoechogenicity and hyperechogenicity between days 2 and 4 post LH peak (ovulation).[11] By day 6 post LH peak, the ovaries were hypoechoic because of the presence of corpora lutea. The ovaries change from oval to a more rounded shape and are frequently multilobular (see Figure 18-21, *Aa*). In another study, rapid disappearance of the anechoic follicle, corresponding to ovulation, was detected in only 2 of 15 bitches; in the remaining cases, follicular rupture was not detected. However, a gradual thickening of

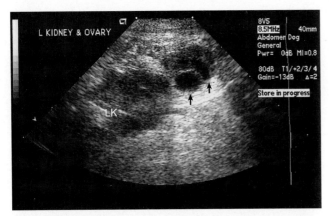

Figure 18-4 **Ovary in a 7-month-old Lhasa apso during early estrus, sagittal image.** Two discrete anechoic follicles (*arrows*) are present with acoustic enhancement. The ovary is almost round with a lumpy contour. Hypoechoic ovarian tissue is present in the near field. A portion of the left kidney (*LK*) is noted.

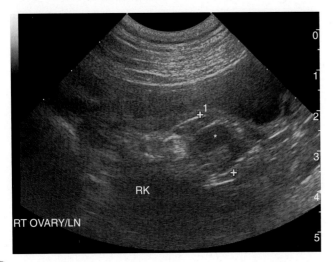

Figure 18-5 Solitary, hypoechoic corpus luteum (*asterisk*) within the ovary (between electronic cursors +, 1.66 cm) of a 4-year-old pregnant Labrador retriever in late second trimester. A wideband microconvex transducer operating in midzone was used. *RK*, Right kidney (not seen in this particular image).

the antral wall was observed beginning with the LH surge, progressing to obliteration of the anechoic region, characteristic of corpora lutea.[10] Thus anechoic cystic structures may still be recognized postovulation, indistinguishable from follicles, although number and size are reduced compared to preovulation. In most dogs, these anechoic structures gradually increase in size, followed by a decrease in size or an increase in echogenicity, or both. Multifocal, anechoic to hypoechoic areas as well as hyperechoic areas are present at the onset of diestrus, representing corpora lutea and perhaps corpora hemorrhagica[2] (Figure 18-5). A small amount of fluid surrounding one ovary was noted in 3 of 10 dogs several days after ovulation.[2] This may be similar to the pelvic ascites noted in women before impending ovulation.

It is probably safe to say that ultrasound detection of ovulation in the dog requires daily serial scanning to identify these changes in the appearance of the ovary. Correlation with more traditional screening procedures, such as vaginal cytology, progesterone levels, and LH peak, is also helpful. There is disagreement concerning whether sonographic evaluation can

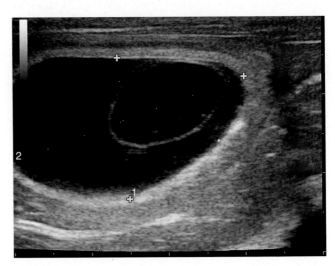

Figure 18-6 **Large follicular cyst in a young cat in estrus.** Though the ovary appears huge because of the magnification, it measures only 3.2 × 1.8 cm. The image was obtained with a wide bandwidth high-frequency linear-array transducer operating at 12 MHz.

reliably detect the precise time of canine ovulation because canine follicles do not collapse after ovulation.[8]

Doppler evaluation of dog ovaries during estrus has been reported.[12] It was shown that intraovarian perfusion gradually increased during proestrus. During the preovulatory phase, blood flow increased as the pulsatility and resistive indices decreased. Maximum perfusion was found during ovulation and the early luteal phase. Doppler analysis of ovarian blood flow during the estrus cycle is at least complimentary and could prove to be more definitive than anatomic B-mode findings for determination of ovulation.

Large ovarian follicles are seen in cats in estrus. Their relative size can be alarming, especially when examined with high resolution transducers (actual size may be in the 3 cm range) (Figure 18-6).

OVARIAN DISEASE

Cystic Ovarian Disease
Canine follicular and luteinizing cysts have been sonographically described.[13] The ultrasound appearance of cystic ovaries is that of true cystic lesions within the ovary, characterized by anechoic contents, thin walls, and acoustic enhancement (Figures 18-7 and 18-8). Ovarian cysts may be solitary or multiple, unilateral or bilateral. Cyst size varies from small (Figure 18-9) to large, and the overall size of the ovary is generally increased. Ultrasonography cannot reliably distinguish the various types of ovarian cysts, but solitary luteinizing cysts have a thicker wall than follicular cysts grossly, which potentially could help differentiate between luteinizing and follicular cysts sonographically.[14] Associated pathologic changes include pyometra, cystic endometrial hyperplasia, and hydrometra. Ultimately, interpretation of ultrasound findings is made with clinical signs, vaginal cytologic assessment, and hormone analysis.

Neoplasia
Three categories of ovarian neoplasms are recognized: surface epithelium tumors (adenoma and adenocarcinoma), sex cord–gonadal stromal tumors (granulosa cell tumor, thecoma, and luteoma), and germ cell tumors (dysgerminoma).[15] The

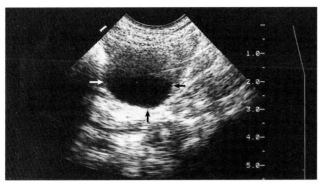

Figure 18-7 Unilateral cystic ovary (*arrows*), transverse image. This 1-year-old boxer had prolonged estrus lasting more than 2 months. She also had persistent vulval swelling, and multiple vaginal cytologic analyses were indicative of estrus. The ovary was markedly enlarged and was composed almost entirely of a large, solitary cyst, with strong acoustic enhancement. The uterus in this bitch was also enlarged. A 7.5-MHz mechanical transducer was used.

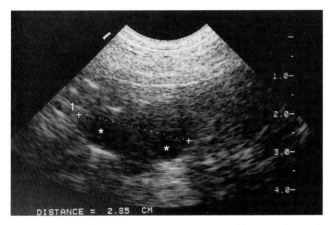

Figure 18-8 Polycystic ovary (+) in a 9-year-old rottweiler with depression and vomiting several weeks after her last breeding; sagittal image. The ovary is enlarged (2.85 cm between electronic cursors) and contains two large cysts (*asterisks*) with distal acoustic enhancement. The other ovary was similar in appearance. Pyometra was diagnosed sonographically and confirmed at surgery. A 7.5-MHz mechanical transducer was used.

ultrasonographic appearance of ovarian tumors has been reported for the dog.[13,16-18] Clinical signs associated with canine ovarian tumors include anorexia, weight loss, lethargy, abdominal distention, palpable abdominal mass, vulvovaginal discharge, abnormal estrous behavior, and polyuria-polydipsia.[17,18] Laboratory workup is often unremarkable.[17] Unilateral tumors are most common, but bilateral ovarian adenocarcinomas have been described.[16-18]

Ovarian tumors can be recognized ultrasonographically as a mass lesion in the location of one or both ovaries. If they become large enough, a midabdominal mass will be apparent. Tumors may be predominantly solid, solid with a cystic component (Figure 18-10), or primarily cystic and complex[17] (Figure 18-11). Margins may be smooth or irregular.[16,17] Concurrent findings may include pyometra or cystic endometrial hyperplasia, ascites, and carcinomatosis.[16,17] Although most ovarian neoplasms are readily identified, a diagnosis of an ovarian mass lesion is sometimes made by exclusion, that is, by ruling out splenic, renal, or lymph node masses. The remaining internal organs should be evaluated for evidence of metastatic disease.

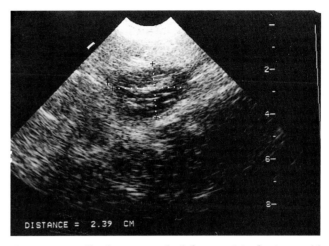

Figure 18-9 Follicular cysts in the left ovary (+) of a 6-year-old Labrador retriever with a history of epistaxis, vaginal bleeding, and pancytopenia; sagittal image. The ovary is enlarged, is misshapen, and has a heterogeneous parenchyma. On histologic examination, more than 50 cysts were present. A 5-MHz mechanical transducer was used.

Ovarian Stump Granuloma

We have infrequently identified complex mass lesions in the region of the ovary that have been diagnosed at surgery and at pathologic examination as granulomas associated with prior ovariohysterectomy. These may vary in size, shape, and echo texture. Complex lesions predominate. Occlusion of the adjacent ureter can be a secondary finding, leading to hydronephrosis.

NORMAL UTERUS

The uterus is composed of three layers: the mucosa, the muscularis, and the serosa. It is located between the urinary bladder ventrally and the descending colon dorsally. The size of the uterus varies, depending on the size of the animal, number of previous pregnancies, disease states, and whether the animal is pregnant. Nulliparous bitches weighing 25 pounds are reported to have uterine horns in the range of 10 to 14 cm in length and 0.5 to 1.0 cm in diameter.[3] The uterine body is slightly larger in diameter and is 1.4 to 3 cm long. The bifurcation of the uterine body is cranial to the pubis. The cervix is 1.5 to 2 cm in length and 0.8 cm in diameter.

A normal, small, nongravid uterus can usually be imaged (Figures 18-12 to 18-14). It is identified as a solid, homogeneous, relatively hypoechoic structure. The endometrium and myometrium cannot usually be differentiated. A thin hyperechoic border may be evident peripherally. The uterine lumen is generally not seen, although it might be visible as a bright echogenic central area, thought to represent a small amount of intraluminal mucus, or a hypoechoic to anechoic region if a small amount of fluid is present. Even when the nongravid uterine body is identified, it is challenging to identify and follow the uterine horns, which are small and become lost in small bowel echoes and mesenteric fat (see Figure 18-14, *B*). However, following each uterine horn cranially is one method of locating the ovaries. The uterus can be differentiated from small bowel by lack of peristalsis, lack of intraluminal gas, and absence of the layered appearance characteristic of small intestine.

The cervix is often seen in dogs and cats when good visualization of the uterine body is obtained. It is recognized as an oblique hyperechoic linear structure on a sagittal view. The

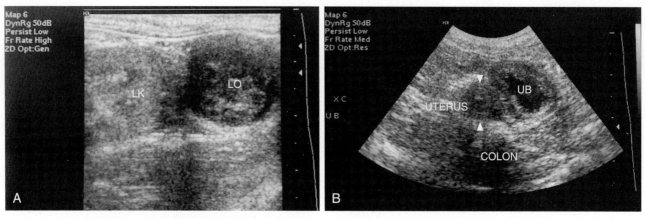

Figure 18-10 Ovarian cystadenoma in an older mixed-breed dog with mild, persistent vaginal discharge; sagittal image of the left ovary (**A**) and transverse image of the uterine body (**B**). **A,** The left ovary (*LO*) is round and heterogeneous. Small anechoic islands are scattered throughout the ovary, accounting for the distal acoustic enhancement. The adjacent, relatively hyperechoic caudal pole of the left kidney (*LK*) is noted. A 10-MHz linear-array transducer was used. **B,** The uterine body (*arrowheads*) is seen as a hypoechoic, relatively homogeneous structure abutting the trigone portion of the minimally distended urinary bladder (*UB*). Various portions of the uterine wall had small anechoic cysts, and a small amount of hypoechoic luminal fluid representing cystic endometrial hyperplasia was noted. Acoustic shadowing from the colon is noted dorsal to the uterus and bladder in the far field.

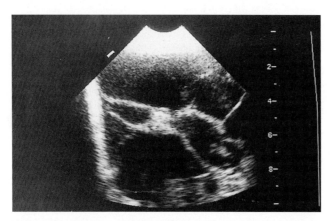

Figure 18-11 Large, complex ovarian tumor, primarily cystic in nature. Anechoic fluid-filled areas are separated by echogenic septa. A 5-MHz mechanical transducer was used.

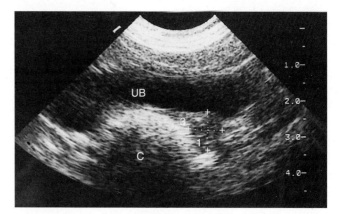

Figure 18-12 Transverse image of the uterine body (+) at the level of the urinary bladder in a 12-year-old anestrous golden retriever. The uterine body is hypoechoic and homogeneous. The distance between the electronic cursors is 9×9 mm. The compressed urinary bladder (*UB*) is an acoustic window. C, Colon. A 7.5-MHz mechanical transducer was used.

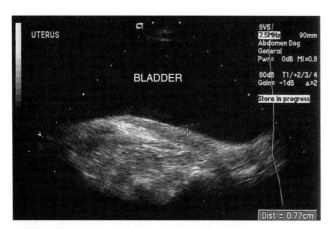

Figure 18-13 Sagittal image of the uterus in a 2-year-old anestrous Doberman pinscher. Uterine body diameter (+) is 7.7 mm. A markedly distended anechoic urinary bladder is in the near field.

proximal part of the vagina may also be identified. Instillation of saline into the vaginal vault through a Foley catheter and scanning by a transabdominal approach can facilitate imaging of this portion of the reproductive tract, although direct endoscopic evaluation is preferred.

UTERINE DISEASE

Pyometra

Canine cystic endometrial hyperplasia–pyometra complex is secondary to an abnormal response to repeated progesterone stimulation and uterine infection. Cystic endometrial hyperplasia (CEH) usually precedes pyometra in bitches older than 6 years, whereas younger bitches may develop pyometra without concurrent cystic endometrial hyperplasia. With cystic endometrial hyperplasia, endometrial thickening occurs

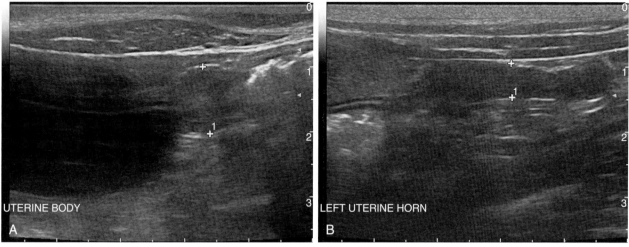

Figure 18-14 Uterine body (**A**) and left uterine horn (**B**) in an anestrous 2-year-old dog. **A,** The uterine body is seen as a solid, hypoechoic structure in transverse section between electronic cursors (1.04 cm). The anechoic, moderately distended urinary bladder is present to the left. **B,** The hypoechoic left uterine horn is seen in its long axis between electronic cursors (0.52 cm).

as endometrial glands increase in size and number in response to progesterone. Sterile luminal mucin fluid accumulation may occur, causing hydrometra or mucometra (the difference depends on degree of mucin hydration). Uterine infection leads to pyometra.[19]

Ultrasound imaging is the modality of choice to diagnose pyometra.[20] An ultrasound examination is usually performed to confirm a clinical diagnosis of pyometra, either from signs referable to an open pyometra or from systemic illness when the cervix is closed. Ultrasound evaluation has also been used to diagnose pyometra before the appearance of clinical signs.[21] The ultrasonographic findings include an enlarged uterus and uterine horns (Figure 18-15). The enlargement may be minimal or dramatic. The enlargement is usually symmetric, but segmental or focal changes can occur. The luminal contents are usually homogeneous and may be anechoic with strong distal enhancement; or they may be echogenic, in which case movement, characterized by slow, swirling patterns, is often noted. Intraluminal focal hyperechoic structures believed to represent resorption of fetuses and placental tissue have been reported.[21]

The uterine wall is variable in appearance, from smooth and thin to thick and irregular. Segmental variations in wall thickness can occur. The wall may be more echoic than the uterine contents or be relatively hypoechoic. Within the thickened endometrium are often islets of anechoic foci that represent dilated cystic glands, tortuous glandular ducts, and vascular structures. A thickened endometrium with cystic structures is diagnostic of cystic endometrial hyperplasia,[22] with or without pyometra (Figure 18-16). Arnold and co-workers[23] reported the ultrasound diagnosis of segmental CEH; pathology revealed serosal inclusion cysts. Evaluation of the ovaries may show the presence of cysts, hypoechoic solid foci representing corpora lutea, or complex mass lesions. Often, however, the ovaries are small, solid, and appear normal, if imaged at all.

Additional differential diagnoses for a fluid-filled uterus include hydrometra and mucometra. These two conditions are less common than pyometra. They may be suspected if the luminal contents are anechoic (hydrometra) or echogenic (mucometra) and the clinical signs of pyometra are lacking.[24] When massive uterine distention is identified, the uterine wall is usually thin, regardless of fluid type.

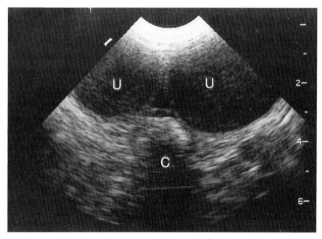

Figure 18-15 **Right and left uterine horns (U) in a mixed-breed dog with pyometra, transverse image.** The uterine horns are markedly enlarged and contain hypoechoic material that showed movement in real time. The uterine walls are thin. A small amount of anechoic fluid is noted between the two uterine horns. C, Colon. A 7.5-MHz mechanical transducer was used.

We do not usually advocate centesis of the uterine fluid, particularly if pyometra is suspected clinically. The potential for peritoneal contamination is high in cases where the uterine wall is thin. Most of these animals are scheduled for ovariohysterectomies. Although surgical removal of the reproductive tract is usually regarded as the therapy of choice, veterinarians encounter animals valuable for their breeding potential. Medical therapy consisting of prostaglandins and antibiotics may be a treatment alternative in select cases, prescribed after a diagnosis is made from the ultrasonographic findings and other pertinent clinical, biochemical, and cytologic findings. Response to therapy can be monitored with serial ultrasound examinations (Figure 18-17). Uterine diameter will decrease as luminal fluid diminishes, and the uterine wall will become progressively thinner. Rapid improvement has been observed, with a marked response seen in 1 week. Other cases take 3 to 4 weeks before the uterus returns to a normal or nearly normal appearance sonographically.

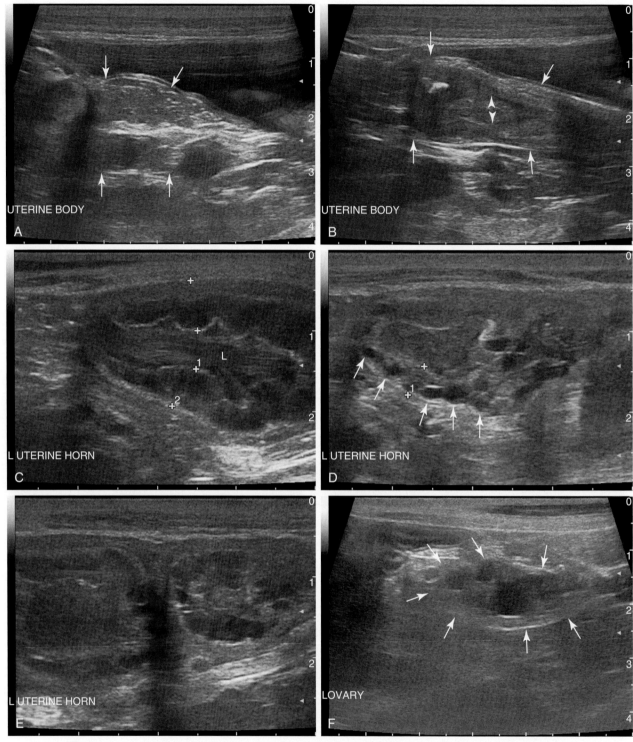

▶ **Figure 18-16 Cystic endometrial hyperplasia (CEH)-mucometra.** Uterus and ovaries (A to F) of a 4-year-old German shepherd dog presented following reproductive failure and abortion. **A,** Sagittal image of the uterine body (*arrows*) showing thickened walls. **B,** Sagittal image of a more proximal portion of the uterine body (*arrows*). A hyperechoic focus with shadowing is present within the uterine lumen, representing gas or perhaps mineralized fetal remnants. The lumen (*arrowheads*) also contains abnormal material. **C,** Sagittal view of the left uterine horn shows thickened walls (0.47 cm) and a horn diameter of 1.56 cm. The lumen (*L*) contains echogenic strands of material, shown to be sterile mucus. The hypoechoic endometrium can be differentiated from the more echogenic muscular layer in this example. **D,** Another sagittal section of the left uterine horn shows the presence of multiple small cysts (*arrows*) within the uterine wall (0.41 cm). **E,** Abnormal right and left uterine horns side-by-side in transverse axes. **F,** Enlarged left ovary (*arrows*) shows the presence of multiple anechoic cysts with an irregular contour.

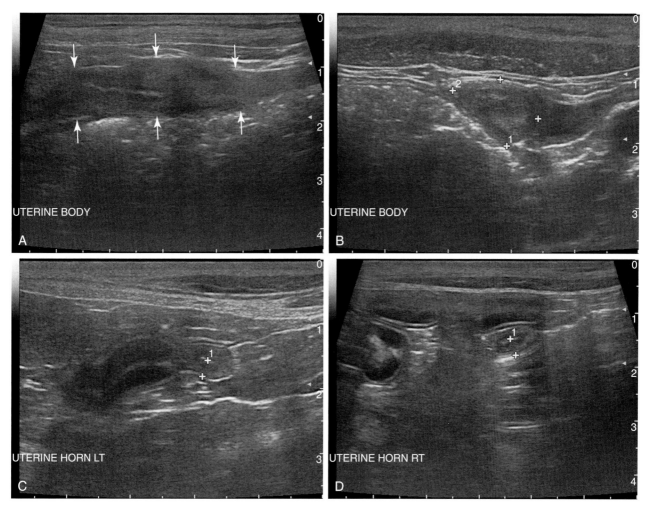

Figure 18-17 **Images from same dog used in Figure 18-16.** Fifty days later, following therapy, a normal reproductive tract (**A** to **D**) was found. **A,** Sagittal image of the normal uterine body (*arrows*). The colon is adjacent to the uterus in the far field. **B,** Transverse view of the normal uterine body (1.03 × 1.42 cm, between electronic cursors). **C,** The left uterine horn is now normal, showing dramatic reduction ins size (0.26 cm wall thickness). A segment of small intestine is seen to the left. **D,** Normal right uterine horn, the wall is 0.32 cm thick. Multiple loops of the small intestinal are present. This dog became pregnant about 6 weeks after these images were taken and had a healthy litter of puppies.

Uterine Stump Pyometra

Stump granuloma (stump pyometra) can be a challenge to diagnose without the aid of ultrasonography. Survey radiographs may show a soft tissue mass between the colon and the urinary bladder and focal loss of serosal detail. A vaginogram may provide the diagnosis if the cervix is open. Clinical signs may be referable to a persistent vaginitis or discharge, or it may be associated with dysuria secondary to scarring and adhesions of the uterine stump to the urinary bladder. The ultrasonographic appearance of stump pyometra varies. The uterine remnant will be located just cranial to the pubis, between the bladder and colon. A large, complex mass lesion is classically identified (Figure 18-18). Smaller lesions are more difficult to image, their uterine origin less certain. We have seen a case of a uterine stump hematoma that developed several days postovariohysterectomy (Figure 18-19).

Neoplasia

Although uterine neoplasms are rare in the dog and cat, adenomas, adenocarcinomas, leiomyomas, and leiomyosarcomas do occur. Multiple uterine leiomyomas associated with generalized nodular dermatofibrosis and renal cystadenocarcinomas in German shepherd dogs have been reported.[25] The sonographic appearance of a canine uterine leiomyoma has been reported as isoechoic to the surrounding uterine tissue, projecting into the uterine lumen.[13] This is similar in appearance to the condition in women, although it may become necrotic and develop a complex internal architecture or undergo cystic degeneration and have a significant cystic component.[26] This is the typical appearance of large hepatic, intestinal, and splenic leiomyosarcomas diagnosed sonographically in dogs. Stöcklin-Gautschi and co-workers[27] reported two cases of uterine adenomyosis, presenting as knobbly uterine enlargements with a diameter of 4 to 8 cm. One patient had chronic vaginal discharge. The second patient was in generally poor health with presenting symptoms of an acute abdomen; a uterine horn torsion was identified at surgery.

Sontas and co-workers[28] reported an interesting case of uterine stump leiomyoma, occurring 8 years following (incomplete) ovariohysterectomy. The patient developed tenesmus and was attracting male dogs and willing to mate. A large, caudal abdominal heterogeneous multicystic mass was identified with anechoic structures adjacent to the caudal pole of

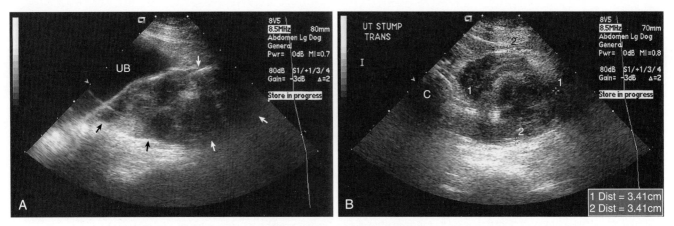

Figure 18-18 **Stump pyometra in a dog.** **A,** Sagittal image. The infected uterine remnant (*arrows*) is a heterogeneous mass dorsal to the urinary bladder (*UB*). **B,** Transverse image caudal to the urinary bladder. The uterine remnant (+) measures 3.4 × 3.4 cm. C, Colon.

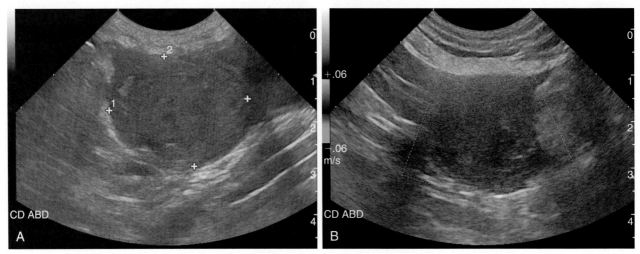

Figure 18-19 Uterine stump hematoma (**A** and **B**). This patient developed lethargy and an enlarging abdomen several days following ovariohysterectomy. **A,** A hypoechoic, homogeneous mass was found in the pelvic inlet, consistent with a uterine remnant. **B,** Color Doppler ultrasound showed lack of blood flow. Abdominal hemorrhage from the uterine stump was found at surgery.

each kidney. Ovarian remnants showed cysts and papillary cystic adenomas to be present.

PREGNANCY DIAGNOSIS AND FETAL DEVELOPMENT

Early diagnosis of pregnancy has become a common request of the veterinary ultrasonographer. Breeders of animals are often anxious to confirm pregnancy and determine the number of fetuses. Cases of unwanted or accidental matings and potential pregnancy may also require a definitive answer of pregnancy status. Early detection of pregnancy has classically been confirmed by careful palpation of an enlarged uterus and the presence of gestational sacs. A period of 21 to 35 days after breeding is the easiest and most accurate time for pregnancy detection. Earlier detection is difficult owing to the small size of the uterus. Beyond 35 days, the individual gestational sacs may become nonpalpable as a result of generalized uterine enlargement. Whereas radiography can demonstrate an enlarged uterus that is consistent with early pregnancy, fetal mineralization, which is the definitive radiographic finding of

pregnancy, does not occur until day 45 post LH surge in the bitch[29] and day 36 to day 45 of gestation in the queen.[30] Ultrasound imaging has been used to detect pregnancy as early as 10 days after breeding in the bitch[31] and 11 days after breeding in the cat.[32] A study using 55 bitches compared palpation, radiography, and ultrasonography in pregnancy detection and estimation of fetal number.[33] It was shown that radiography was 100% accurate in detection in the last trimester and 93% accurate in determining fetal number. Ultrasonography was 94% accurate and palpation was 88% accurate in detecting pregnancy.

There has been general acceptance that fetal number cannot be accurately judged with ultrasound evaluation.[31-35] It is our experience that absolute, accurate determination of fetal number is unreliable, especially at early pregnancy and late in gestation. Bondestam and colleagues[35] believed that day 28 to day 35 is the easiest time to predict fetal number, and this is our impression as well. The problem lies in the fact that only small portions of the reproductive tract can be imaged in a given scan plane. Fetuses may be counted more than once or not at all. In the clinical setting, we inform the client that estimation of fetal number is not completely accurate. If this information is essential, radiography is recommended late in gestation, after fetal mineralization has occurred.

Before the specifics of pregnancy diagnosis and fetal development are discussed, several important points regarding ovulation, conception, and definition of gestational age must be addressed. Ovulation in the bitch occurs 24 to 72 hours after a peak in blood LH.[6,36] Estrus begins a day or two before the LH surge and lasts 5 to 9 days.[6] During estrus, breeding may occur once or on multiple occasions. Canine sperm are hardy and may remain fertile for at least 4 to 6 days.[6,37] Therefore the exact time of conception (and thus gestational or fetal age) is unknown. This can complicate prediction of gestational age or number of days before parturition from sonogram images and measurements. As an example, the owner of a breeding bitch may know that servicing occurred on days 1, 3, and 5 of estrus. Suppose conception took place on the last breeding date (day 5). If, by convention, the middle date (day 3) is taken as the date of conception, it would be 2 days off if fertilization actually occurred on day 5. Taking into account long canine sperm fertility, actual conception could take place up to 7 days from the last breeding. The point is that actual gestational age may be less than an estimate based on breeding date. The clinical danger is that this underestimate of gestational age will lead to a false negative pregnancy diagnosis early in pregnancy. The cat is different from the bitch; queens are induced ovulators, so conception takes place rapidly after copulation.[38] However, many cat owners are unaware of when their queen was bred, so similar challenges to predicting gestational age or days before parturition exist.

Pregnancy detection ultrasonographically is similar in the dog and cat, although some variation in timing undoubtedly exists. The earliest detectable change (nonspecific) is visualization of an enlarging uterus (Figure 18-20). Uterine enlargement may be seen as early as 7 days after breeding in the bitch[31] and 4 days in the queen.[32] Although uterine enlargement is a sensitive indicator of a hormonally influenced uterus and may indicate pregnancy, it is not at all specific because a normally cycling bitch and queen will have identical hormonally induced uterine enlargement, regardless of pregnancy status.

The first sign confirming pregnancy is detection of a gestational sac (also referred to as blastocyst, chorionic cavity, and embryonic vesicle). The gestational sac is simply a maturing blastocyst, inside of which is the developing embryo. The gestational sac (blastocyst) is anechoic and only several millimeters in diameter, but it may be detected under the best of conditions (Figure 18-21, *Ab*). Day 17 post LH peak in the dog is the earliest that we have detected gestational sacs. It is possible to overlook such an early pregnancy when only one or two gestational sacs are present because of overlying bowel gas or other suboptimal conditions. Clinically, we prefer to have the client wait until day 30 after the last breeding date for ultrasonographic evaluation of pregnancy; gestational sacs with viable embryos can be identified with a high level of confidence by that time. Thirty days from the last breeding means that the pregnancy cannot be less than 23 to 25 days under any circumstance because that is about the maximum fertile life span of canine sperm. The rapid growth rate that can be appreciated during such a short period is astounding (Table 18-1).

TABLE 18-1

Time of Sonographic Recognition of Canine Fetal Structures

Fetal Structure	Days Post LH Surge	Days Before Parturition (65 ± 1) Based on LH Surge
Gestational sac	20	45
Embryo	23-25	40-42
Cardiac activity	23-25	40-42
Yolk sac, U shaped	25-28	37-40
Yolk sac, tubular	27-31	34-38
Fetal orientation (head and body)	28	37
Limb buds, fetal movement	35	30
Fetal skeleton	33-39	26-32
Stomach, urinary bladder	35-39	26-30
Lungs—hyperechoic vs. liver	38-42	23-27
Kidneys, eyes	39-47	18-26
Cardiac chambers	40	25
Intestines	57-63	2-8

LH, Luteinizing hormone.
Adapted from Yeager AE, Mohammed HO, Meyers-Wallen V, et al. Ultrasonographic appearance of the uterus, placenta, fetus, and fetal membranes throughout accurately timed pregnancy in beagles. *Am J Vet Res* 1992;53:342-1.

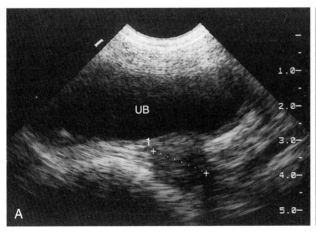
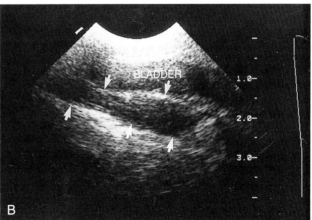

Figure 18-20 **Uterine enlargement in early pregnancy. A,** In this transverse image, the uterine body is mildly enlarged (1.6 cm between electronic cursors), hypoechoic, and solid. *UB,* Urinary bladder. **B,** Sagittal image of the uterus (*arrows*). This image was obtained after the patient expressed her urinary bladder. A 7.5-MHz mechanical transducer was used.

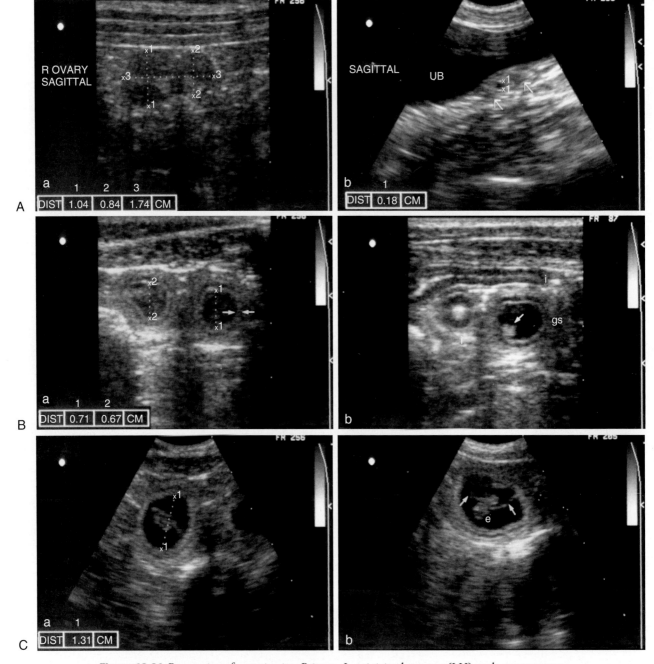

Figure 18-21 Progression of gestation in a Brittany. Luteinizing hormone (LH) peak, progesterone rise, and vaginal smear consisting entirely of cornified epithelial cells defined the onset of estrus April 13. Natural breedings April 14, April 16, and April 18. Whelping, 10 pups, occurred on June 15. A 10.0-MHz microconvex-array and 10.0-MHz and 7.5-MHz linear-array transducers were used. **A,** Day 17 post LH peak (April 30). **a,** Right ovary, sagittal image. The ovary is hypoechoic and multilobular, representing corpora lutea separated by slightly more echogenic stromal parenchymal tissue. The left ovary was similar in appearance. Electronic cursors define the margins of the ovary and indicate its size. **b,** Blastocyst, sagittal image. A tiny (1.8 mm) anechoic blastocyst (gestational sac) is identified between the electronic cursors (*x*). The section of uterus seen (*arrows*) is homogeneous, just dorsal to the neck of the urinary bladder (*UB*). **B,** Day 22 post LH peak (May 5). **a,** Two gestational sacs in the right and left uterine horns, transverse image. The gestational sacs are anechoic and surrounded by a thin, developing echogenic placenta (between arrows) that is surrounded by the uterine wall. Electronic cursors indicate the gestational sac sizes of 0.67 cm and 0.71 cm. Predicted gestational age is 24 days (± 3 days) [(6 × 0.67) + 20]. **b,** A single uterine horn and gestational sac, transverse image. The embryonic mass (*arrow*) is seen as an echogenic focus along the wall of the anechoic gestational sac (*gs*). Note the adjacent small intestine (*i*) seen in transverse section to the left and in sagittal section in the near field. Flickering cardiac activity could be seen during imaging. **C,** Day 25 post LH peak (May 8). **a,** The gestational sac is larger (1.31 cm), nearly doubling in size in 3 days. Flickering cardiac activity was observed within the centrally located embryo. Predicted gestational age is 27 days (±3 days) [(1.31 × 6) + 20]. **b,** The embryo (*e*) is an echogenic structure now positioned more centrally within the anechoic gestational sac. The linear echo is the yolk sac membrane (*arrows*).

Two excellent studies evaluated the ultrasonographic appearance of canine fetal development and determination of gestational age.[39,40] A gestational sac was consistently detected within the uterine horn on day 20 after LH surge in Beagles (18 days after ovulation).[40] At this time, gestational sacs are seen as 2-mm anechoic structures (primarily chorionic fluid) surrounded by a thin, hyperechoic wall (trophoblasts). The uterine tissue surrounding the gestational sac becomes focally thickened and is hyperechoic relative to adjacent uterine tissue. Reports vary as to the earliest detection of gestational sacs in the bitch, ranging from 10 to 20 days.[31,34,39,40] In the cat, gestational sacs may be seen as early as 11 days after breeding.[32] Much of the variation in the literature is due to differences in defining pregnancy timing and spatial resolution of ultrasound equipment. We define gestational or fetal age by days post LH surge, unless otherwise noted. By use of this criterion, gestational length in the bitch is 65 ± 1 days.

The embryo is first seen at day 23 to day 25 as an oblong echogenic structure several millimeters in length,[40] eccentrically located within the rapidly enlarging, spherical gestational sac (Figure 18-21, B). The gestational sac is encompassed by a thin, peripheral hyperechoic inner layer of the uterus, which is the developing placenta (see Figure 18-21, Ba). The gestational sac begins to change shape from spherical to oblong by day 28 (Figure 18-22). Distinct zonary placentation may be recognized by day 27 to day 30 as focal cylindrical thickening of the placenta, becoming evident by day 36. The embryo

moves away from the uterine wall, attached to it by the yolk sac membrane, on day 25 to day 28 (see Figures 18-21, C, and 18-22). The yolk sac membrane is imaged as an echogenic linear structure, initially U shaped, changing to a tubular structure by day 27 to day 31; it extends from pole to pole of the gestational sac with eventual infolding on itself by day 31 to day 35. The yolk sac membrane appears as two parallel echogenic lines on a sagittal section (see Figures 18-21, Cb, and 18-22), round in a transverse plane, separated by anechoic fluid. As it infolds, the lumen is obliterated and becomes hyperechoic. The allantoic membrane can be recognized as a thin, less echoic membrane surrounding the embryo and yolk sac on day 27 to day 31.[40]

Whereas the detection of a gestational sac is diagnostic of pregnancy, visualization of cardiac activity and, later, fetal movement indicates fetal viability. Cardiac activity in the dog is detected at the same time the embryo is recognized, day 23 to day 25 post LH surge,[40] which corresponds to day 23 to 29 according to the study by Verstegen and colleagues.[41] In cats, cardiac activity is seen 18 to 25 days postbreeding.[41] Cardiac activity is recognized as a small focus of rapidly fluttering echoes within the embryo. This occurs before recognizable gross anatomic features are seen. Cardiac rate in the fetus has been reported to be approximately twice the maternal rate.[42,43] In dogs, heart rates were 230.2 ± 15.4 beats per minute (bpm). Initially values were 214 ± 13.3 bpm with significant increases to 238.2 ± 16.1 bpm at day 40. A reduction was noted near

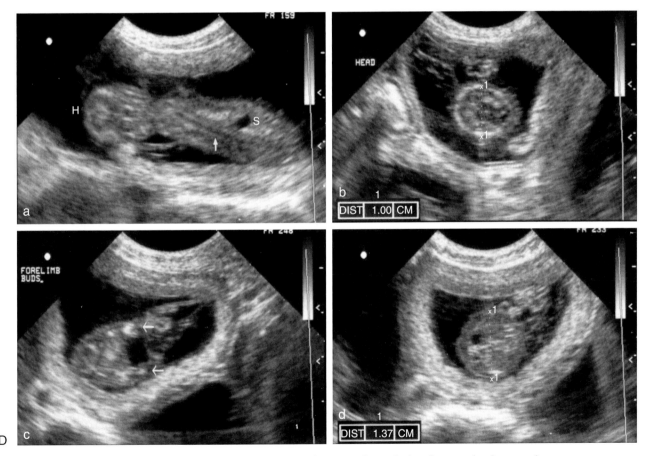

D

Figure 18-21, cont'd D, Day 37 post LH peak (May 20). Marked embryonic development has occurred. Fetal orientation can be determined, with identification of the head, neck, thorax, abdomen, and limb buds. a, Dorsal image, fetal head (H) to the left. The stomach (s) and spine and spinal cord (arrow) are seen, b, Head diameter is 1.00 cm. Predicted gestational age is 35 days (±3 days) [(15 × 1.0) + 20]. c, Transverse image, forelimb buds (arrows). d, Body diameter at the level of the stomach is 1.37 cm. Predicted gestational age is 38 days (±3 days) [(7 × 1.37) + 29].

Continued

parturition. In queens, heart rate was 228.2 ± 35.5 bpm. This study found that cardiac frequencies remained stable during pregnancy.[41]

Fetal development progresses rapidly from day 30, allowing recognition of organogenesis sonographically (Figure 18-23; see also Figure 18-21, *D* to *I*). Fetal orientation can be recognized with confidence, with the head and body seen by day 28. Within the head is an initial anechoic focus, followed by development during the next week of the echogenic bilobed choroid plexus, surrounded by an anechoic cerebral ventricle. Limb buds and fetal movement are recognized on about day 35.[40] The fetal skeleton can be identified on day 33

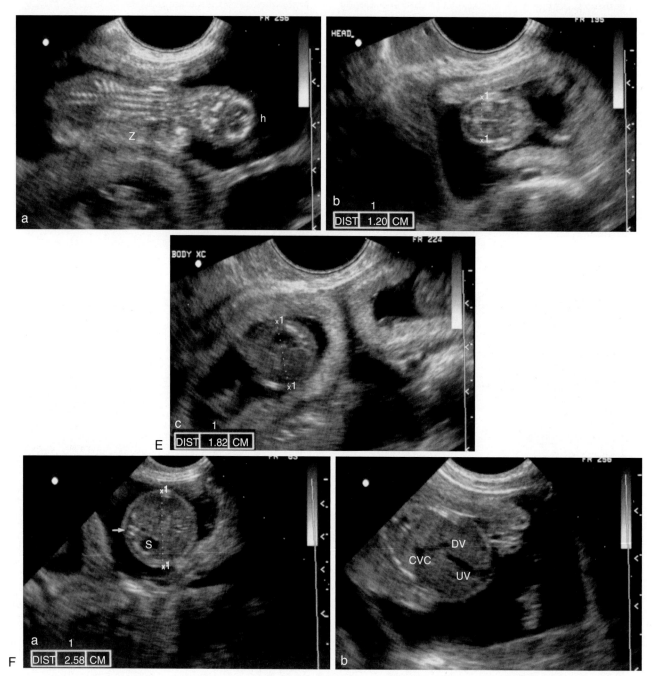

Figure 18-21, cont'd **E**, Day 40 post LH peak (May 23). Multiple anatomic features are recognized as fetal maturation continues. Fetal heart rate was 240 beats per minute; maternal rate was 102 beats per minute. **a**, Dorsal image. The head (*h*), spine, ribs, and zonary placenta (*z*) are clearly identified. **b**, Transverse image. The head diameter (*H*) is 1.20 cm. Predicted gestational age is 38 days (±3 days) [(15 × 1.20) + 20]. **c**, Transverse image. Body diameter at the level of the stomach is 1.82 cm. Predicted gestational age is 41 days (±3 days) [(7 × 1.82) + 29]. **F**, Day 44 post LH peak (May 27). **a**, Body diameter at the level of the liver and stomach (*s*) is 2.58 cm. A vertebra in transverse section (*arrow*) is noted as three tiny echogenic foci. Predicted gestational age is 47 days (±3 days) [(7 × 2.58) + 29]. **b**, The umbilical vein (*UV*), ductus venosus (*DV*), and caudal vena cava (*CVC*) are shown in this dorsal image.

to day 39 and is seen as hyperechoic structures with acoustic shadows.[39] The head is detected first, followed by rapid mineralization of the thoracic spine and ribs, then the cervical spine and appendicular skeleton. The urinary bladder and stomach are the first abdominal organs identified sonographically, by day 35 to day 39, and appear as anechoic focal areas.[40] Because the stomach and urinary bladder fill and empty for a time, various degrees of distention may be observed, and these may change during the course of the examination.

The lung has been shown to vary in echogenicity during development. The lung and liver are relatively isoechoic when they are initially seen, without clear definition between them. Orientation is made by location of the heart, stomach, and urinary bladder. The lungs become hyperechoic relative to the liver as the fetus develops by day 38 to day 42.[40] The kidneys and the eyes are seen by day 39 to day 47 (see Figure 18-21, *Ic*).[40] The kidneys are hypoechoic with prominent anechoic pelves.[40] With time, the renal cortex and medulla can be differentiated and the pelves become less dilated. The heart is hypoechoic to anechoic, with linear septate echoes representing the chamber walls and heart valves. The four chambers of the heart are seen by about day 40 (see Figure 18-21, *Ga*, *Hb*, and *Ia*). Several days later, the great cardiac vessels can be

imaged. The intestine is seen late, by day 57 to day 63 (see Figure 18-21, *Ha* and *Ib*).[40]

FETAL MEASUREMENTS AND ESTIMATION OF FETAL AGE

Ultrasonographic fetal mensuration of the dog was first reported in 1984[31] and followed by two excellent papers in the early 1990s.[39,40] Beck and colleagues[44] first reported fetal mensuration and prediction of parturition in cats in 1990. Four newer studies have investigated the role of ultrasound in predicting parturition dates in dogs.[45-48]

Chorionic cavity diameter (gestational sac diameter) was shown to be the most accurate predictor of gestational age between days 20 and 37 in the dog.[40] From days 38 to 60, fetal head diameter (known as biparietal diameter in human sonography) was the most accurate predictor of gestational age, but fetal crown-rump length and body diameter were also significant.[40] It was noted that fetal crown-rump length was difficult to measure after day 48 because of fetal flexion and fetal size, which exceeded the sector image field. The recent study by Beccaglia and co-workers[46] confirmed that

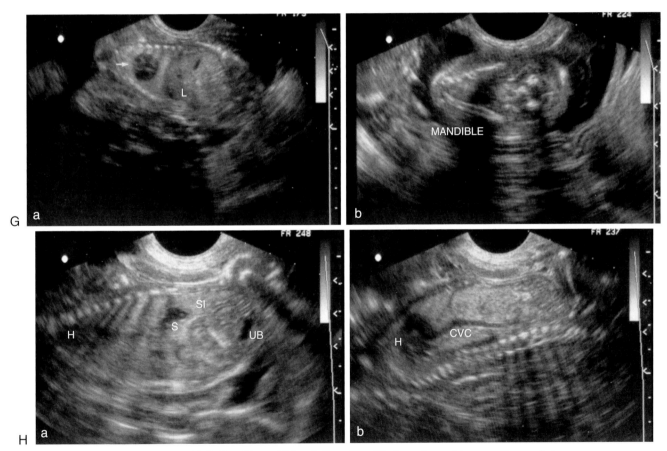

Figure 18-21, cont'd G, Day 51 post LH peak (June 3). **a,** The heart (*arrow*) is a round hypoechoic to anechoic structure surrounded by echogenic lung. The liver (*L*) is less echoic than lung. Echogenic foci with acoustic shadows represent vertebral bodies and sternebrae. Body diameter (not shown) was 3.63 cm. **b,** In this dorsal image of the skull, the V-shaped mandible is noted. **H,** Day 58 post LH peak (June 9). **a,** The heart (*H*), stomach (*S*), small intestine (*SI*), and urinary bladder (*UB*) are identified. The vertebrae are creating strong acoustic shadows, indicating mineralization. **b,** The heart (*H*), caudal vena cava (*CVC*), and vertebral bodies are present with strong acoustic shadowing. An anechoic curvilinear diaphragm separates the liver from the lung. The fetus is in dorsal recumbency. *Continued*

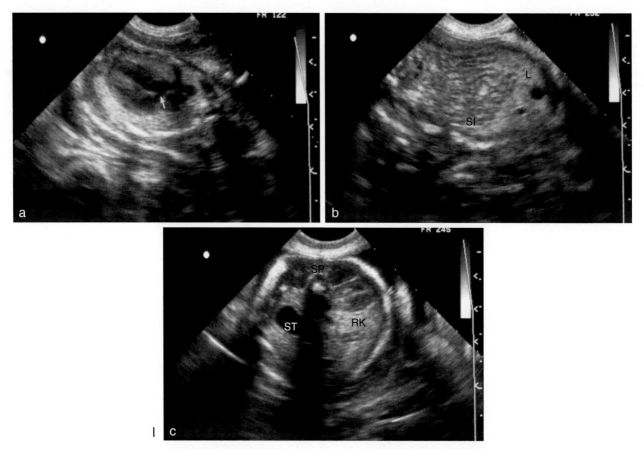

Figure 18-21, cont'd **I,** Day 61 post LH peak (June 13). **a,** Fetal cardiac anatomy is clearly seen. The foramen ovale (*arrow*) is noted. Echogenic lung surrounds the heart. **b,** Small intestines (*SI*) are seen. The echogenic, homogeneous liver (*L*) is to the right. The gallbladder is the round anechoic structure within the liver centrally. **c,** A transverse image through the cranial abdomen identifies the echogenic spine (*SP*), hypoechoic surrounding epaxial musculature, echogenic ribs, fluid-filled stomach (*ST*), and right kidney (*RK*). The body diameter was 4.51 cm.

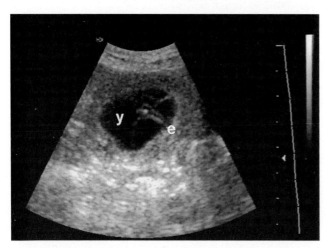

Figure 18-22 A 28-day canine embryo. The embryo (*e*) is an elongate echogenic structure. The gestational sac is slightly oblong. The developing placenta is seen as a thin echogenic layer internal to the homogeneous hypoechoic uterine wall. *y,* Yolk sac.

parturition predictions can be accurately made early in pregnancy by chorionic mensuration, and late in pregnancy using biparietal diameter.

Biparietal and body diameters of the cat fetus have been published.[44] Body diameter increased more rapidly than head diameter. Fetal morphology was recognized by 38 to 35 days before parturition, or 23 to 28 days after breeding. Using these values and known queening dates, a fetal maturation chart was generated. Accurate calculation of queening dates for cats with unknown breeding dates was demonstrated.

Subsequently, we used the work of these investigators[39,40,44] to develop easy-to-use formulas to predict gestational age and number of days until parturition in the dog and cat (Box 18-1). Gestational sac (chorionic cavity) diameter is measured until approximately day 40 in the dog (approximately 3 cm in diameter) (see Figure 18-21, *Ba* and *Ca*), after which head diameter and body diameter are easier to determine accurately. Crown-rump length is also useful in early to midgestation for predicting gestational age, but as mentioned earlier, it can be difficult to measure accurately because it matures much beyond 45 to 48 days (6 to 7 cm). Biparietal diameter and body diameter should be measured when the fetus is large enough for these structures to be identified. Head diameter is measured in the transverse plane (see Figure 18-21, *Db* and *Eb*). Maximal body diameter measurements are also obtained in a transverse plane at the level of the liver (see Figure 18-21, *Dd, Ec,* and *Fd*). Prediction of gestational age is believed to be most accurate in the early to midpart of gestation, when rapid growth of the fetus is taking place. Over the years we have found this simple formula to be acceptably accurate.

In human medicine, guidelines were established for obstetric ultrasound examination in 1985 through cooperative

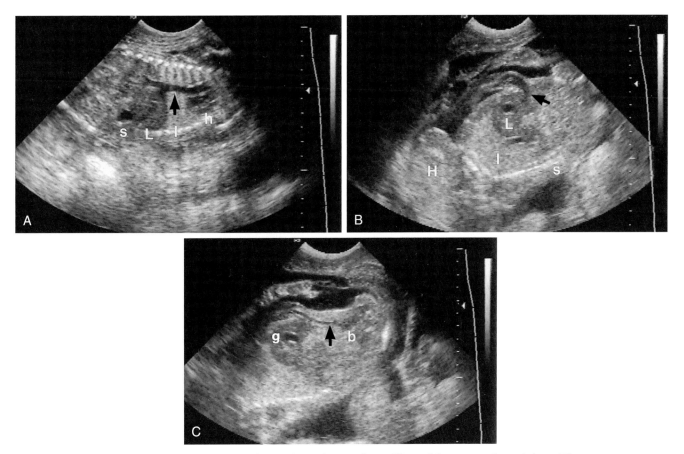

Figure 18-23 **Late feline gestation.** A, Sagittal image, heart (*h*), caudal vena cava (*arrow*), liver (*L*), and fluid-filled stomach (*s*) caudal to the liver. The lung parenchyma (*I*) is hyperechoic relative to the hypoechoic liver. Vertebrae and sternebrae are mineralized, seen as echogenic foci creating acoustic shadows. B, Sagittal image of a fetus in dorsal recumbency. The umbilical vein (*arrow*), umbilicus, and fetal membranes are seen. *H,* Head; *L,* liver; *I,* lung; *s,* spine. The lung is more echogenic than the liver. C, Same fetus as in B, this sagittal image shows the urachus (*arrow*) and an empty urinary bladder (*b*). The round, anechoic gallbladder (*g*) is surrounded by hypoechoic liver parenchyma.

efforts between the Ultrasound Commission of the American College of Radiology, Obstetricians, and the Section of Obstetrical and Gynecological Ultrasound of the American Institute of Ultrasound in Medicine.[49] Briefly, these guidelines discuss equipment, documentation, and first-, second-, and third-trimester criteria. Guidelines for the first trimester include documentation of the location of the gestational sac. The embryo's crown-rump length is recorded, and biparietal and other measurements may be made. The presence or absence of fetal life is noted, as is the number of fetuses. Also included is an examination of the uterus and associated structures. During the second and third trimesters, fetal life, fetal number, and fetal presentation are recorded. Heart rate is evaluated, as is the amount of amniotic fluid and the location of the placenta. Gestational age is determined by biparietal diameter and femur length, and growth is assessed by abdominal circumference and comparison with earlier measurements if previous examinations have been performed. Fetal anatomy is evaluated, including the umbilical cord insertion site and anterior abdominal wall, cerebral ventricles, heart, spine, stomach, urinary bladder, and kidneys.

Assessment of human fetal well-being on the basis of biophysical parameters has become routine with the advent of real-time ultrasonographic imaging of the fetus.[50] Some of these parameters are body and respiratory movements, fetal tone, fetal heart rate, umbilical blood flow, suckling, swallowing, amniotic fluid volume, and placental assessment.

POSTPARTUM UTERUS

Normal involution of the canine postpartum uterus is usually complete in 3 to 4 weeks. At this time, the uterine body will be only a centimeter or so in diameter and may be difficult to identify on a sonogram. Ultrasonographic evaluation of the canine postpartum uterus has been described in detail.[51,52] From 1 to 4 days postpartum, the uterus is enlarged and echogenic, containing fluid and remnants of fetal and maternal membranes (Figure 18-24). Sites of placentation are larger than the interplacental uterus (2.2 to 2.8 cm versus 1 to 1.5 cm in diameter in medium-sized bitches weighing 15 to 25 kg). The placentation sites are oval on longitudinal scans. The uterine wall is thick and irregular, and blood vessels can sometimes be imaged. The uterine wall becomes thinner later in the postpartum period (8 to 24 days), and luminal contents decrease and become more homogeneous as involution progresses. Distinguishing luminal contents from the adjacent uterine wall can be difficult, but luminal contents become hypoechoic in some cases and contrast nicely with the adjacent hyperechoic endometrium. The hyperechoic

BOX 18-1

Formulas to Predict Gestational Age and Days Before Parturition in the Dog and Cat*

GESTATIONAL AGE IN THE DOG (±3 DAYS)

Less Than 40 Days
GA = (6 × GSD) + 20
GA = (3 × CRL) + 27

More Than 40 Days
GA = (15 × HD) + 20
GA = (7 × BD) + 29
GA = (6 × HD) + (3 × BD) + 30

Days Before Parturition In The Dog
DBP = 65 − GA

GESTATIONAL AGE IN THE CAT (±2 DAYS)

Greater Than 40 Days
GA = 25 × HD + 3
GA = 11 × BD + 21

Days Before Parturition in the Cat
DBP = 61 − GA

*Gestational age (GA) is based on days post luteinizing hormone (LH) surge in the dog and days post breeding in the cat. Gestational sac diameter (GSD), crown-rump length (CRL), head diameter (HD), and body diameter (BD) measurements are in centimeters. Days before parturition (DBP) is based on 65 ± 1 days post LH surge in the dog and 61 days post breeding in the cat. Data modified and adapted from England et al.,[39] Yeager et al.,[40] and Beck et al.[44]

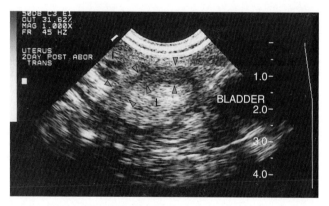

Figure 18-24 **Transverse image of a uterine horn 2 days after abortion.** The lumen (*L*) contains echogenic material, and the uterine wall is hypoechoic and irregular (*arrowheads*). The anechoic urinary bladder is to the right. *I*, Small intestine. A 7.5-MHz mechanical transducer was used.

endometrium is surrounded by relatively hypoechoic myometrium and is thicker at placentation sites compared with the interplacental endometrium. Some bitches had an additional hyperechoic ring of fat between the uterine serosa and myometrium. By day 24 postpartum, the diameter of the uterus at placentation sites was 1 to 1.4 cm, 0.6 to 0.9 cm in the interplacental zones.

Normal involution of the feline uterus was shown to occur by day 24 postpartum in a study of six cats.[53] Immediately after parturition, feline uterine diameter ranges from 6.5 to 30.5 mm. Uterine contents are isoechoic to the adjacent echogenic endometrium. By day 7, uterine diameter is 7.3 to 13.1 mm; at day 14, it is 4.3 to 7.8 mm. Uterine contents are of mixed echogenicity during this interval. Three distinct layers of the uterus are recognized during the first 14 days postpartum: a thick echogenic endometrium, a thin hypoechoic myometrium, and a thin echogenic serosal surface. By 24 days, uterine diameter is small (2.5 to 6.3 mm), and visualization of uterine wall layers is lost. Thickening of the uterine wall at zonary placentation sites was not identified in this group of cats, unlike in the dog.

Doppler ultrasonography has been used to study maternal and fetal blood flow during pregnancy. Three significant studies have been published, with similar results.[54-56]

In 1998, Nautrup[54] used color flow and pulsed wave Doppler ultrasonography for the first time to study the quality and quantity of the normal blood flow of maternal circulation and the development of fetal vascularization in six Beagles during normal gestation. They found pulsatility index, resistance index, and A:B ratio (systolic-to-diastolic ratio, S/D) decreased in nearly all vessels during gestation; only the fetal common carotid artery had constant pulsatility and resistance indices.

Di Salvo and co-workers[55] studied blood waveforms of the uteroplacental arteries, aorta, caudal vena cava, and umbilical cord of the fetuses in 16 pregnant bitches in 2006. Weekly measurements of peak systolic velocity (PSV), end-diastolic velocity (EDV), resistance index (RI), and pulsatility index (PI) were reported. Uteroplacental blood flow was biphasic, whereas the umbilical artery and aorta were initially systolic and became diastolic. The vena cava displayed a venous waveform. During gestation the EDV and PSV of fetal vessels increased while the PI and RI of all vessels examined decreased except for the PI of the aorta.

Recently, Miranda and Domingues[56] found that RI and PI of the uterine artery (UA) and umbilical artery (Uma) decreased significantly during pregnancy. For the UA, RI and PI were 0.95 ± 0.02 and 2.75 ± 0.41, respectively, on day −44; and they were 0.60 ± 0.01 and 0.99 ± 0.03 on day −4. For the Uma, RI and PI were 0.99 ± 0.01 and 2.42 ± 0.03 on day −31; and they were 0.62 ± 0.01 and 1.15 ± 0.02 on day −4. The complete disappearance of the early diastolic notch in the UA and the appearance of diastolic flow in the Uma occurred on days −16 ± 5 and −21 ± 1. The authors concluded that UA and Uma perfusion were important end points to assess fetal vitality in bitches.

ABNORMAL PREGNANCY

Ultrasonography is used to detect a variety of conditions that may occur during abnormal pregnancies.[57] These include fetal resorption, abortion, delayed embryonic development, fetal abnormalities, fetal death just before or during parturition, fetal stress, and a variety of other conditions.

England and Russo[58] reported on ultrasound characteristics of reproductive failure in bitches. Resorption of conceptuses occurred in 6 of 20 bitches. One or more conceptuses were resorbed in each bitch, with continuation of the remaining pregnancy to term. Impending resorption may be predicted by detecting a delay in the time of development of a specific embryologic feature or measuring a slow growth rate.

Small or underdeveloped conceptuses are best recognized by direct comparison with adjacent conceptuses. It is difficult to make an accurate determination on the basis of one measurement on any given day. Serial examinations allow documentation of normal gestational sac diameter growth, essentially linear at 1 mm/day from day 17 to day 30 post LH surge.[57]

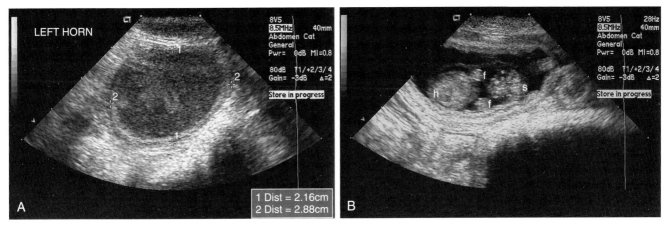

Figure 18-25 Fetal death and a healthy fetus in a 1-year-old Siamese cat bred 32 days ago, examined for vaginal bleeding and abortion. **A,** Transverse image of the left uterine horn. Focal dilation of the uterus is present. The lumen contains echogenic fluid and debris. This was thought to represent the site of prior fetal implantation and subsequent abortion. The remaining left uterine horn also contained echogenic fluid but was smaller in diameter. **B,** Transverse image of one of two viable fetuses identified, *f,* Forelimb buds; *h,* heart; *s,* skull.

If embryonic death occurs before 25 days after ovulation, complete resorption of the embryo results.[59] Resorption is recognized by a reduction in size of the embryo compared with adjacent conceptuses, a change in embryonic fluid from anechoic to hypoechoic, the presence of echogenic particles, and the absence of a heartbeat. The gestational sac collapses, and the adjacent uterine wall may be relatively hypoechoic. These changes occur rapidly, within hours to several days.[57]

Fetal death after about 35 days results in abortion, generally but not always affecting the entire litter[57] (Figure 18-25). Deceased fetuses rapidly lose a normal sonographic appearance and are expelled in a few days. The uterus will be similar in appearance to a postpartum uterus.

Recognition of fetal death at or near parturition is of extreme importance. Fetal death is recognized by a loss of cardiac activity. On assessment of near-term or term fetuses, cardiac activity should immediately be recognized. Fetal movements, such as swallowing, hiccoughs, and body and limb movements, should also be seen. Sonographic recognition of fetal structures rapidly diminishes after death. After a day or two, only mineralized skeletal structures may be recognized by characteristic hyperechogenicity and acoustic shadows. Intrauterine or intrafetal gas may also be identified.

Fetal stress is diagnosed by reduced fetal heart rate that is due to hypoxia. Normal fetal heart rate is approximately twice the maternal heart rate. An increased or decreased heart rate may indicate stress of the fetus and is used clinically in human medicine. Increased fetal heart rate in response to stress is a positive sign, indicating fetal vigor.

M-mode evaluation is an accurate method of determining fetal heart rate (Figure 18-26). With dystocia or prolonged parturition, some fetuses may have normal heart rates while littermates are bradycardic. It is not unusual in these cases that some degree of fetal mortality is present.

A recent paper describes a prolonged interval between parturition of normal puppies.[60] The last pup was born 37 hours after initiation of parturition, 34 hours after expulsion of the last fetus. Multiple doses of oxytocin were administered to overcome uterine inertia. Both radiography and ultrasound are commonly used to ascertain the presence or absence of a remaining fetus.

Ultrasound examination for fetal abnormalities is commonplace in human medicine but infrequently reported in

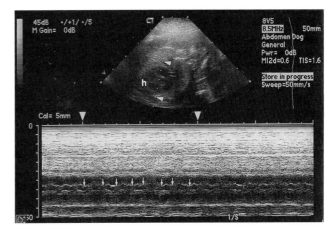

Figure 18-26 **Fetal heart rate.** *Top,* Transverse B-mode sector image of a fetal thorax with the M-mode cursor (*small arrowheads*) directed through the heart (*h*). *Bottom,* M-mode image. Fetal heart rate is determined by counting fetal heart contractions (*arrows at systole*). In this example, there are eight heartbeats during a 2-second interval (*large arrowheads*). Heart rate is 240 beats per minute.

small animal veterinary medicine.[13,61-63] The importance of recognizing fetal abnormalities in veterinary medicine is not as great as it is in human medicine, because it does not change overall management of the patient.

MAMMARY GLAND

The normal mammary gland at parturition is echogenic and homogeneous (Figure 18-27). Large vessels are seen entering the gland. With mastitis, the gland may become inhomogeneous and enlarged. Hyperechoic foci representing gas may be detected (Figure 18-28). Abscessation can occur.

Ultrasound evaluation of mammary neoplasia may help define the extent of the lesion, including body wall invasion (Figure 18-29), although ultrasound is an insensitive test, as Figure 18-30 illustrates. Regional lymph nodes should be evaluated for evidence of enlargement, which suggests metastasis.

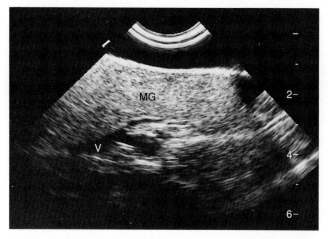

Figure 18-27 Sagittal image of a normal mammary gland (*MG*) at parturition. The gland is homogeneous and hyperechoic. Large vessels (*V*) are seen. A standoff pad and a 7.5-MHz mechanical transducer were used to obtain this image.

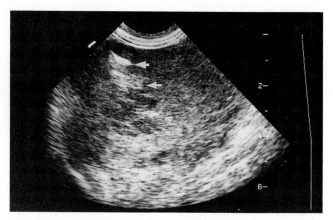

Figure 18-28 Mastitis. The mammary gland is enlarged and inhomogeneous. Discrete hyperechoic foci represent gas within the tissue (*arrows*). A 5-MHz mechanical transducer was used.

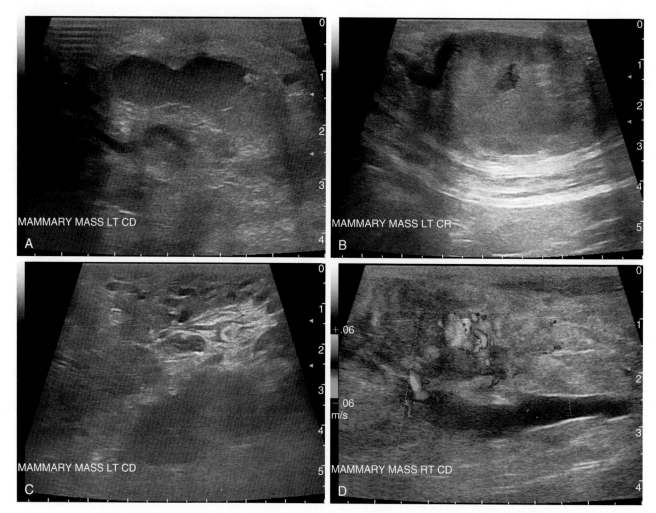

Figure 18-29 Extensive mammary gland tumors in an intact 10-year-old Labrador retriever mix (**A** to **D**). **A,** This portion of the mass has a large cavitary component. **B,** A very heterogeneous region of the mass. **C,** A predominantly solid area of the mass. **D,** Color Doppler image shows high vascularization of the mass. This was a complex, anaplastic adenocarcinoma with metastasis to the medial iliac lymph nodes and the lungs.

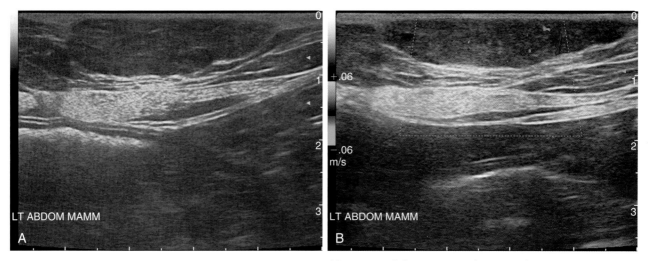

Figure 18-30 Mammary carcinoma in a 7-year-old intact English setter (**A** and **B**). **A,** A homogeneous, apparently well-circumscribed mass is present in the near field, arising from the mammary gland. **B,** Color Doppler evaluation shows moderate vascularization. The histologic diagnosis was an aggressive mammary carcinoma with extensive invasion of the vessels in and around the mass.

REFERENCES

1. Davidson AP, Baker TW. Reproductive ultrasound of the bitch and queen. *Top Companion Anim Med* 2009;**24**(2): 55–63.
2. Wallace SS, Mahaffey MB, Miller DM, et al. Ultrasonographic appearance of the ovaries of dogs during the follicular and luteal phases of the estrous cycle. *Am J Vet Res* 1992;**53**:209–15.
3. Christensen GC. The urogenital apparatus. In: Evans HE, Christensen GC, editors. *Miller's anatomy of the dog.* 2nd ed. Philadelphia: WB Saunders; 1979. p. 544–601.
4. Ellenport CR. Female genitalia. In: Getty R, editor. *The anatomy of the domestic animals.* 5th ed. Philadelphia: WB Saunders; 1975. p. 1584–9.
5. Neiman HL, Mendelson EB. Ultrasound evaluation of the ovary. In: Callen PW, editor. *Ultrasonography in obstetrics and gynecology.* 2nd ed. Philadelphia: WB Saunders; 1988. p. 423–46.
6. Feldman EC, Nelson RW. Ovarian cycle and vaginal cytology. In: *Canine and feline endocrinology and reproduction.* 2nd ed. Philadelphia: WB Saunders; 1996. p. 526–46.
7. Inaba T, Matsui N, Shimizu R, et al. Use of echography in bitches for detection of ovulation and pregnancy. *Vet Rec* 1984;**115**:276–7.
8. England GCW, Allen WE. Ultrasonography and histological appearance of the canine ovary. *Vet Rec* 1989;**125**: 555–6.
9. England GCW, Yeager AE. Ultrasonographic appearance of the ovary and uterus of the bitch during oestrus, ovulation and early pregnancy. *J Reprod Fertil Suppl* 1993;**47**: 107–17.
10. Hayer P, Günzel-Apel AR, Lüerssen D, et al. Ultrasonographic monitoring of follicular development, ovulation and the early luteal phase in the bitch. *J Reprod Fertil Suppl* 1993;**47**:93–100.
11. Silva LDM, Onclin K, Verstegen JP. Assessment of ovarian changes around ovulation in bitches by ultrasonography, laparoscopy and hormonal assays. *Vet Radiol Ultrasound* 1996;**37**:313–20.
12. Köster K, Poulsen Nautrup C, Günzel-Apel AR. A Doppler ultrasonographic study of cyclic changes of ovarian perfusion in the Beagle bitch. *Reproduction* 2001;**122**(3):453–61.
13. Poffenbarger EM, Feeney DA. Use of gray-scale ultrasonography in the diagnosis of reproductive disease in the bitch: 18 cases (1981-1984). *J Am Vet Med Assoc* 1986; **189**:90–5.
14. Dow C. Ovarian abnormalities in the bitch. *J Comp Pathol* 1960;**70**:59–70.
15. Nielsen SW, Kennedy PC. Tumors of the genital systems. In: Moulton JE, editor. *Tumors in domestic animals.* 3rd ed. Berkeley: University of California Press; 1990. p. 479–517.
16. Goodwin J-K, Hager D, Phillips L, et al. Bilateral ovarian adenocarcinoma in a dog: ultrasonographic-aided diagnosis. *Vet Radiol* 1990;**31**:265–7.
17. Diez-Bru N, Garcia-Real I, Martinez EM, et al. Ultrasonographic appearance of ovarian tumors in 10 dogs. *Vet Radiol Ultrasound* 1998;**39**:226–33.
18. Purswell BJ, Parker NA, Bailey TL, et al. Theriogenology question of the month. Persistent estrus caused by functional granulosa cell tumor of the left ovary. *J Am Vet Med Assoc* 1999;**215**:193–5.
19. Feldman EC, Nelson RW. Cystic endometrial hyperplasia/ pyometra complex. In: *Canine and feline endocrinology and reproduction.* 2nd ed. Philadelphia: WB Saunders; 1996. p. 605–18.
20. Bigliardi E, Parmigiani E, Cavirani S, et al. Ultrasonography and cystic hyperplasia-pyometra complex in the bitch. *Reprod Domest Anim* 2004;**39**(3):136–40.
21. Fayrer-Hosken RA, Mahaffey M, Miller-Liebl D, et al. Early diagnosis of canine pyometra using ultrasonography. *Vet Radiol* 1991;**32**:287–9.
22. Voges AK, Neuwirth L. Cystic uterine hyperplasia. *Vet Radiol Ultrasound* 1996;**37**:131–2.
23. Arnold S, Hubler M, Hauser B, et al. Uterine serosal inclusion cysts in a bitch. *J Small Anim Pract* 1996;**37**(5): 235–7.
24. van Haaften B, Taverne MAM. Sonographic diagnosis of a mucometra in a cat. *Vet Rec* 1989;**124**:346–7.
25. Lium B, Moe L. Hereditary multifocal renal cystadenocarcinomas and nodular dermatofibrosis in the German shepherd dog: macroscopic and histopathologic changes. *Vet Pathol* 1985;**22**:447–55.

26. Green WJ, Fendley SM, Wintzell EC, et al. Cystic degeneration of a large uterine leiomyoma. *Invest Radiol* 1989; **24**:626–9.

27. Stöcklin-Gautschi NM, Guscetti F, Reichler IM, et al. Identification of focal adenomyosis as a uterine lesion in two dogs. *J Small Anim Pract* 2001;**42**(8):413–16.

28. Sontas BH, Ozyogurtcu H, Turna O, et al. Uterine leiomyoma in a spayed poodle bitch: a case report. *Reprod Domest Anim* 2010;**45**(3):550–4.

29. Rendano VT. Radiographic evaluation of fetal development in the bitch and fetal death in the bitch and queen. In: Kirk RW, editor. *Current veterinary therapy*, vol. 8. Philadelphia: WB Saunders; 1983. p. 947–52.

30. Boyd JS. Radiographic identification of the various stages of pregnancy in the domestic cat. *J Small Anim Pract* 1971;**12**:501–6.

31. Cartee RE, Rowles T. Preliminary study of the ultrasonographic diagnosis of pregnancy and fetal development in the dog. *Am J Vet Res* 1984;**45**:1259–65.

32. Davidson AP, Nyland TG, Tsutsui T. Pregnancy diagnosis with ultrasound in the domestic cat. *Vet Radiol* 1986;**27**:109–14.

33. Toal RL, Walker MA, Henry GA. A comparison of real-time ultrasound, palpation and radiography in pregnancy detection and litter size determination in the bitch. *Vet Radiol* 1986;**17**:102–8.

34. Shille VM, Gontarek J. The use of ultrasonography for pregnancy diagnosis in the bitch. *J Am Vet Med Assoc* 1985;**187**:1021–5.

35. Bondestam S, Alitalo I, Karkkainen M. Real-time ultrasound pregnancy diagnosis in the bitch. *J Small Anim Pract* 1983;**24**:145–51.

36. Wildt DE, Chakraborty PK, Panko WB, et al. Relationship of reproductive behavior, serum luteinizing hormone and time of ovulation in the bitch. *Biol Reprod* 1978;**18**:561–70.

37. Holst PA, Phemister RD. Onset of diestrus in the Beagle bitch: definition and significance. *Am J Vet Res* 1974;**35**:401–6.

38. Feldman EC, Nelson RW. Feline reproduction. In: *Canine and feline endocrinology and reproduction*. 2nd ed. Philadelphia: WB Saunders; 1996. p. 741–68.

39. England GCW, Allen WE, Porter DJ. Studies on canine pregnancy using B-mode ultrasound: Development of the conceptus and determination of gestational age. *J Small Anim Pract* 1990;**31**:324–9.

40. Yeager AE, Mohammed HO, Meyers-Wallen V, et al. Ultrasonographic appearance of the uterus, placenta, fetus, and fetal membranes throughout accurately timed pregnancy in beagles. *Am J Vet Res* 1992;**53**:342–51.

41. Verstegen JP, Silva LD, Onclin K, et al. Echocardiographic study of heart rate in dog and cat fetuses in utero. *J Reprod Fertil Suppl* 1993;**47**:175–80.

42. Barr FJ. Pregnancy diagnosis and assessment of fetal viability in the dog: a review. *J Small Anim Pract* 1988;**29**:647–56.

43. Helper LC. Diagnosis of pregnancy in the bitch with an ultrasonic Doppler instrument. *J Am Vet Med Assoc* 1970;**156**:60–2.

44. Beck KA, Baldwin CJ, Bosu WTK. Ultrasound prediction of parturition in the queen. *Vet Radiol* 1990;**31**:32–5.

45. Luvoni GC, Beccaglia M. The prediction of parturition date in canine pregnancy. *Reprod Domest Anim* 2006; **41**(1):27–32.

46. Beccaglia M, Luvoni GC. Comparison of the accuracy of two ultrasonographic measurements in predicting the parturition date in the bitch. *J Small Anim Pract* 2006; **47**(11):670–3.

47. Kim Y, Travis AJ, Meyers-Wallen VN. Parturition prediction and timing of canine pregnancy. *Theriogenology* 2007;**68**(8):1177–82.

48. Lopate C. Estimation of gestational age and assessment of canine fetal maturation using radiology and ultrasonography: a review. *Theriogenology* 2008;**70**(3):397–402.

49. Leopold GR. Antepartum obstetrical ultrasound examination guidelines. *J Ultrasound Med* 1986;**5**:241–2. (ed).

50. Brar HS, Platt LD, DeVore GR. Assessment of fetal wellbeing: The biophysical profile. In: Callen PW, editor. *Ultrasonography in Obstetrics and Gynecology*. 2nd ed. Philadelphia: WB Saunders; 1988. p. 335–50.

51. Yeager AE, Concannon PW. Serial ultrasonographic appearance of postpartum uterine involution in beagle dogs. *Theriogenology* 1990;**34**:523–33.

52. Pharr JW, Post K. Ultrasonography and radiography of the canine postpartum uterus. *Vet Radiol Ultrasound* 1992; **33**:35–40.

53. Ferretti LM, Newel SM, Graham JP, et al. Radiographic and ultrasonographic evaluation of the normal feline postpartum uterus. *Vet Radiol Ultrasound* 2000;**41**:287–91.

54. Nautrup CP. Doppler ultrasonography of canine maternal and fetal arteries during normal gestation. *J Reprod Fertil* 1998;**112**(2):301–14.

55. Di Salvo P, Bocci F, Zelli R, et al. Doppler evaluation of maternal and fetal vessels during normal gestation in the bitch. *Res Vet Sci* 2006;**81**(3):382–8.

56. Miranda SA, Domingues SF. Conceptus ecobiometry and triplex Doppler ultrasonography of uterine and umbilical arteries for assessment of fetal viability in dogs. *Theriogenology* 2010;**74**(4):608–17.

57. England GCW. Ultrasonographic assessment of abnormal pregnancy. *Vet Clin North Am Small Anim Pract* 1998; **28**:849–68.

58. England GC, Russo M. Ultrasonographic characteristics of early pregnancy failure in bitches. *Theriogenology* 2006; **66**(6–7):1694–8.

59. Christensen GC. Reproduction and prenatal development. In: Evans HE, Christensen GC, editors. *Miller's Anatomy of the Dog*. 2nd ed. Philadelphia: WB Saunders; 1979. p. 13–77.

60. Romagnoli S, de Souza FF, Rota A, et al. Prolonged interval between parturition of normal live pups in a bitch. *J Small Anim Pract* 2004;**45**(5):249–53.

61. Allen WE, England GCW, White KB. Hydrops foetalis diagnosed by real time ultrasonography in a Bichon Frise bitch. *J Small Anim Pract* 1989;**30**:465.

62. Adams WH, Toal RL, Breider MA. Ultrasonographic findings in ethylene glycol (antifreeze) poisoning in a pregnant queen and 4 fetal kittens. *Vet Radiol* 1991; **32**:60–2.

63. Heng HG, Randall E, Williams K, et al. What is your diagnosis? Hydrops fetalis. *J Am Vet Med Assoc* 2011; **239**(1):51–2.

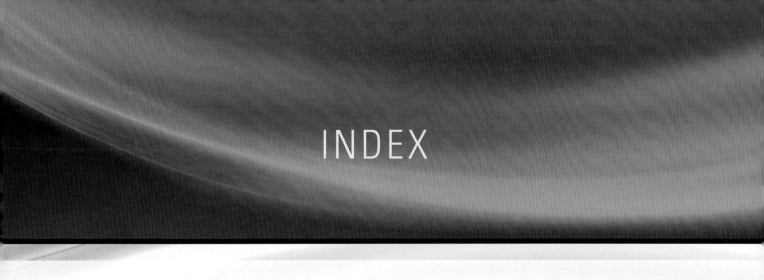

INDEX

Page numbers followed by "f" indicate figures, "t" indicate tables, and "b" indicate boxes.

Carcinomatosis, 506f
Cardiac arrhythmias, 305
Cardiac auscultation, 217
Cardiac catheterization, with angiography, 219
Cardiac chamber size
    assessment of, 267-279, 268t-272t, 267.e1t-267.e3t
    limitations and suggested approach to assessment of, 267-270
Cardiac cycle, 249-250, 251f
Cardiac diseases. *see also* Heart disease.
    transesophageal echocardiography for diagnosis of, 243
Cardiac image processing, advanced, 220b
Cardiac imaging, nomenclature and display of, 227-228
Cardiac masses, 312-314, 313f
Cardiac measurements, echocardiographic, 267-279, 268t-272t
Cardiac output, 242
Cardiac related neoplasms, in dogs, 312-314
Cardiac remodeling, in mitral regurgitation, 294-295
Cardiac shunts, contrast echocardiography for, 242, 242f
Cardiac studies
    Doppler, 244-248
    instrumentation for, 220-224, 221t
Cardiac tamponade, 312
Cardiac ultrasound (US), 217
Cardiomegaly, 267, 268t
Cardiomyopathy, 304-312
    arrhythmogenic right ventricular, 311-312
    dilated, 310-311, 310f
    in dogs, 305-307
    essential imaging characteristics of, 305
    etiologies of, 305-307
    hypertrophic, 305, 307-310, 308f
    other assessments for, 305
    practical considerations for, 304-307
    restrictive, 305, 311
    unclassified, 305
Cardiovascular diseases, echocardiography for, 217
Carotid artery(ies), 155-160
    arteriovenous malformations of, 159
    common, examination of, 191, 192f
    neoplasia of, 159-160
    stenosis of, 159
    thrombosis of, 159
Carotid bifurcation, 155, 159f
Carotid body tumors, 160
Castration, chronic bacterial prostatitis and, 616
Cataracts, 142-144, 143f-144f
Catheterization
    cardiac, with angiography, 219
    interventional, 243
Caudal cruciate ligaments, 525
Caudal vena cava
    abnormalities of, 382-383, 384f
    2D and CDI of, 236
    examination of, 101-103, 123f-126f, 125-126, 333-335, 334f-337f
    Doppler, 126, 127f, 338-339, 382-391
    fetal, 644f-649f
    heartworms within, 515f
    thrombosis of, 383, 513, 515f
    adrenal tumors and, 551-552, 551f
Cavitary lesions, aspiration of, 71-72
CDI. *see* Color Doppler imaging (CDI).
Cecum, abnormalities of, 493-496
Celiac artery, 126-127, 127f

Cellulitis
    neck, 182, 182f-184f
    retrobulbar, 146f
    skin, subcutaneous tissues and muscle, 517, 518f
Cervical lesions, chemical ablation of, 78
Cervical musculature, 180
Cervical region, fine needle aspiration and biopsy of, 60, 61f
Cervical tumors, ethanol ablation of, 78
Cervix
    examination of, 120-121
    normal appearance of, 637-638
Chemical ablation, 78
Chemodectomas, 312-314
Cholangitis/cholangiohepatitis complex, 373, 375f
Cholecystitis, 66, 66f, 373-376, 375f
    acute, 373
    chronic, 370f-371f, 376
    emphysematous, 373-376
    gangrenous, 376
    necrotizing, 376
Cholecystocentesis, 379
Cholecystography, percutaneous, 66
Cholecystostomy, percutaneous, 66
Choledocholithiasis, 380f
Cholelithiasis, 373
Chordae tendineae, 230
Chorionic cavity. *see* Gestational sac.
Choroid, 128
Choroidal excavation, 135
Chronic enteropathies, 492
Chronic hepatitis, 359
Chronic hypertrophic gastritis, 479
Chronic hypertrophic pyloric gastropathy (CHPG), 472, 475f
Chronic lymphocytic thyroiditis, 164
Chronic mitral endocarditis lesions, 293
Chronic pancreatitis, 451, 452f-454f
Ciliary body, 135
Cirrhosis, hepatic, 359
"Clean" acoustic shadowing, 190, 191f
Clots
    in bladder, 593
    in eye, 137
    in ureter, 576-577
Coil embolization, 388
Colic lymph nodes, 125. *see also* Lymph nodes.
Colon
    abnormalities of, 493-496
    evaluation of, 110f, 117-119, 119f
    normal ultrasound appearance of, 471-472, 473f
Color Doppler imaging (CDI), 259, 260f-261f
    advantage of, 259
    instrumentation for, 261-263
    interpretation and quantitation in, 263-264
    limitations and pitfalls of, 264, 264t-265t
    normal findings of, 263
Color Doppler ultrasonography, 36-39, 37f, 40f
    advantages and disadvantages of, 39t
    bar, 37-38, 38f
    gastrointestinal, 491-492
    hepatic, 357
    spectral Doppler *versus*, 36-37, 37f
Color flow mapping. *see* Color Doppler imaging (CDI).
Color M-mode echocardiography, 238-240, 262f, 266f
Color mapping, 259-261, 260f-261f

Color write priority, in Doppler ultrasonography, 43
Colorized gray-scale maps, 11, 15f
Comet-tail artifacts, 27-28, 204, 205f, 207f-208f, 212f
Common bile duct, 125, 334f
    obstruction of, 380-381, 380f, 383f
Common carotid artery, 155, 157f, 159f-162f. *see also* Carotid artery(ies).
Compartmental syndrome, 527-528
Complex masses, renal, 563-566
Computed tomography (CT)
    of adrenal glands, 541
    ultrasound-guided, 80-81, 81f
Concentric hypertrophy, 274
Concurrent pleural effusions, 312
Congenital heart disease, echocardiography in, 218. *see also* Echocardiography.
Congenital hypertrophic pyloric stenosis, 472, 474f
Congenital/idiopathic disorders, in dilated ureter and renal pelvis, 574
Congenital pancreatic cysts, 458f
Congenital peritoneopericardial diaphragmatic hernia (CPDH), 210
Congenital shunts, 314-317, 315f
    practical considerations for, 314
Congestion, splenic, 425, 425f
Congestive heart failure (CHF), 228
Consolidation, of lung, 204, 208f-210f, 212f
Constrictive pericardial disease, 312
Constrictive pericarditis, 241
Continuity relationship, 258, 258f
Continuous wave (CW) Doppler ultrasonography, 35
Continuous wave (CW) spectral waveforms, *versus* pulse wave Doppler spectral waveforms, 35, 36f
Continuous-wave Doppler (CWD) echocardiography, 255-264, 256f
    hemodynamic quantitation using, 255-259
    inherent limitations of, 255
    of mitral regurgitation, 297
Contrast agents
    bioeffects of, 87
    in echocardiography, 242
    for hepatic imaging, 357
    for ultrasound, 82-83, 83f, 87f
Contrast echocardiography, 242, 242f. *see also* Echocardiography.
Contrast-enhanced harmonic imaging, 86, 86f
    of metastatic hemangiosarcoma, 85-86, 86f
Contusions, muscles, 528
Core biopsy, 536. *see also* Biopsy.
Core examination, in echocardiography, 226-227
Corncobs, 474-475, 475f
Cornea, 141-142, 142f
Corneal technique, 130
Coronary artery disease, in dilated cardiomyopathy, 305
Corpora hemorrhagica, 635-636, 636f
Corpus cavernosum urethrae, 586
Corpus luteum, within ovary, 636f
Corrugated bowel pattern, 480, 481f
Corticomedullary rim sign, 572f
Coxofemoral joint
    aspiration of, 536
    examination of, 525, 526f
Cranial cruciate ligaments, 525
Cranial mesenteric artery, 126-127, 127f
Cranial vena cava, persistent left, 234, 235f